SAMUEL L. MOSCHELLA, M.D., F.A.C.P.

Chairman, Department of Allergy and Dermatology, The Lahey Clinic, Boston

DONALD M. PILLSBURY, M.D., D.Sc.(Hon.), F.A.C.P.

Professor of Dermatology and Chairman Emeritus of the Department of Dermatology, University of Pennsylvania School of Medicine, Philadelphia

HARRY J. HURLEY, Jr., M.D., D.Sc.(Med.), F.A.C.P.

Professor of Clinical Dermatology, University of Pennsylvania School of Medicine, Philadelphia

DERMATOLOGY

VOLUME I

W. B. Saunders Company

PHILADELPHIA · LONDON · TORONTO

W. B. Saunders Company: West Washington Square
Philadelphia, PA 19105

1 St. Anne's Road
Eastbourne, East Sussex BN21 3UN, England

1 Goldthorne Avenue
Toronto, Ontario M8Z 5T9, Canada

Library of Congress Cataloging in Publication Data

Moschella, Samuel L

Dermatology.

Includes index.

1. Dermatology.   I. Pillsbury, Donald Marion, 1902–
joint author.   II. Hurley, Harry J., joint author.
[DNLM: 1. Skin diseases. WR140 M895d]

RL71.P65 1975   616.5   73–88263

ISBN 0–7216–6565–9 (v. 1)

ISBN 0–7216–6566–7 (v. 2)

Dermatology   ISBN Vol I: 0-7216-6565-9
                                               ISBN Vol II: 0-7216-6566-7

Print No: 9   8   7   6   5   4   3

Dedicated to

Those who taught us

and to

Those who helped us

CONTRIBUTORS

A. BERNARD ACKERMAN, M.D.

Development, Morphology, and Physiology of Skin

Associate Professor, Departments of Dermatology and Pathology, New York University Hospital and Bellevue Hospital, New York, New York.

HARVEY BAKER, M.D., F.R.C.P.

Physiologic Reaction Patterns of Skin

Consultant Dermatologist, The London Hospital, London, England.

RICHARD D. BAUGHMAN, M.D.

Systemic Bacterial Infections

Assistant Clinical Professor of Dermatology, Dartmouth Medical School; Chairman, Section of Dermatology, Mary Hitchcock Memorial Hospital, Hanover, New Hampshire.

DONALD L. BAXTER, M.D.

Mycotic Infections

Captain, Medical Corps, United States Navy, Retired; Clinical Associate Professor of Medicine (Dermatology), Hahnemann Medical College and Hospital, Philadelphia; Staff Dermatologist, Riddle Memorial Hospital, Media, Pennsylvania.

HERMAN BEERMAN, M.D., D.Sc. (Med.), F.A.C.P.

Drug Eruptions

Professor Emeritus, Department of Dermatology, The University of Pennsylvania School of Medicine and Hospital of the University of Pennsylvania; Consultant in Dermatology, Graduate Hospital of the University of Pennsylvania and Pennsylvania Hospital, Philadelphia, and Veterans Administration Hospital, Coatesville; Honorary Consultant in Dermatology, Philadelphia General Hospital; Consultant to Laboratory, Children's Hospital; Consultant in Dermatopathology, United States Naval Hospital, Philadelphia, Pennsylvania.

GARY JULES BRAUNER, M.D.

Cutaneous Diseases in Black Races

Assistant Clinical Professor of Medicine, Albert Einstein College of Medicine of Yeshiva University; Assistant Attending Physician, Montefiore Hospital and Medical Center, Bronx, New York.

JOSEPH W. BURNETT, M.D

Viral and Rickettsial Infections

Associate Professor of Medicine in Dermatology, University of Maryland School of Medicine, Baltimore, Maryland.

ORLANDO CANIZARES, M.D.

Nontreponemal Venereal Infections

Professor of Clinical Dermatology, New York University School of Medicine; Attending Dermatologist, Bellevue Hospital and St. Vincent's Hospital (Chief), New York; Consultant, Dermatologist, Veterans Administration Hospital, Bronx, and United States Public Health Hospital, Staten Island, New York.

WILLIAM A. CARO, M.D.

Tumors of Skin

Associate Professor of Clinical Dermatology, Northwestern University Medical School; Associate Attending Physician, Northwestern Memorial Hospital; Attending Pathologist, Veterans Administration Research Hospital; Consulting Dermopathologist, Children's Memorial Hospital, Chicago, Illinois.

D. MARTIN CARTER, M.D., Ph.D.

Hereditary Cutaneous Disorders

Associate Professor of Dermatology and Howard Hughes Medical Investigator, Yale University School of Medicine; Attending Physician, Yale University School of Medicine, New Haven, Connecticut.

WILLIAM A. CRUTCHER, M.D.

Viral and Rickettsial Infections

Staff Dermatologist, Queen of the Valley Hospital, Napa, California.

HUGH M. CRUMAY, M.D.

Surgical Diathermy, Ultraviolet Light and Cryosurgical Therapy

Associate in Dermatology, The University of Pennsylvania School of Medicine, Philadelphia; Dermatologist Emeritus, Harrisburg General Hospital; Consulting Dermatologist, Holy Spirit Hospital and Harrisburg State Hospital and Rehabilitation Center, Harrisburg, Pennsylvania.

THOMAS B. FITZPATRICK, M.D.

Mechanisms of Pigmentation

Professor, Department of Dermatology, Harvard Medical School; Chief of Dermatology, Massachusetts General Hospital, Boston, Massachusetts.

RAUL FLEISCHMAJER, M.D.

Diseases of Corium and Subcutaneous Tissue

Professor of Medicine and Director, Division of Dermatology, Hahnemann Medical College and Hospital, Philadelphia, Pennsylvania.

JOHN L. FROMER, M.D.

Lymphomas

Chairman Emeritus, Department of Dermatology and Allergy, Lahey Clinic Foundation; Dermatologist, New England Deaconess Hospital and Massachusetts General Hospital, Boston, Massachusetts.

PHILLIP FROST, M.D.

Disorders of Cornification

Chairman, Department of Dermatology, Mount Sinai Medical Center, Miami Beach, Florida.

HERBERT GOLDSCHMIDT, M.D., F.A.C.P.

Dermatologic Radiation Therapy

Associate Clinical Professor of Dermatology, The University of Pennsylvania School of Medicine; Attending Dermatologist, Hospital of the University of Pennsylvania, Philadelphia, Pennsylvania.

PETER HACKER, M.D., F.R.C.P. (C)

Bacterial Infections

Assistant Professor of Medicine (Dermatology), McGill Medical School; Consulting Staff, Royal Victoria Hospital and Montreal Children's Hospital, Montreal, Quebec, Canada.

JOSEPH HONIGMAN, M.D.

Psychogenic and Neurogenic Skin Diseases

Commander, Medical Corps, United States Navy; Chief of Dermatology, United States Naval Hospital and Naval Regional Medical Center, Jacksonville, Florida.

HARRY J. HURLEY, M.D., D.Sc. (Med.)

Permeability of Skin, Papulosquamous Eruptions, Exfoliative Dermatitis, Diseases of Sweat Glands, Dermatologic Therapy

Professor of Clinical Dermatology, The University of Pennsylvania School of Medicine; Attending Dermatologist, Hospital of the University of Pennsylvania and Mercy Catholic Medical Center, Philadelphia, Pennsylvania.

BERNETT L. JOHNSON, Jr., M.D.

Histopathologic Reaction Patterns of Skin

Chairman, Department of Dermatology, United States Naval Hospital; Adjunct Assistant Professor of Dermatology, Temple University School of Medicine, Philadelphia, Pennsylvania; Special Lecturer, Dermatology, Howard University College of Medicine, Washington, D.C.

HARRY IRVING KATZ, M.D.

Anaphylactic Syndromes

Clinical Associate Professor of Dermatology, University of Minnesota, Minneapolis, School of Medicine; Assistant Director of Dermatology, Ramsay County Hospital, St. Paul; Active Staff (Dermatology), Mount Sinai Hospital and Unity Hospital, Minneapolis, Minnesota.

BERNARD A. KIRSHBAUM, M.D., M.S.

Drug Eruptions

Clinical Associate Professor of Medicine (Dermatology), Medical College of Pennsylvania; Dermatologist, St. Mary's Hospital and West Park Hospital, Philadelphia, Pennsylvania.

ALLAN L. LORINCZ, M.D.

Disturbances of Melanin Pigmentation

Professor of Dermatology, The University of Chicago, Pritzker School of Medicine; Head, Section of Dermatology, The University of Chicago Hospitals and Clinics, Chicago, Illinois.

EDMUND D. LOWNEY, M.D., Ph.D.

Contact Dermatitis

Professor of Medicine and Director of Division of Dermatology, Ohio State University College of Medicine, Columbus, Ohio.

HENRY C. MAGUIRE, Jr., M.D.

Diseases of Hair

Clinical Associate Professor of Medicine and Associate Professor of Microbiology, Hahnemann Medical College and Hospital; Visiting Scientist, Institute for Cancer Research, Philadelphia, Pennsylvania.

HOWARD I. MAIBACH, M.D.

Bacterial Infections

Professor of Dermatology, University of California, San Francisco, School of Medicine, San Francisco, California.

RICHARD R. MARPLES, B.M., M.Sc., M.R.C. (Path.)

Cutaneous Microbiology

Consultant Microbiologist, Cross Infection Reference Laboratory, Central Public Health Laboratory, London, England.

NANCY MATUS, M.D.

Diseases of Corium and Subcutaneous Tissue

Clinical Senior Instructor, Department of Medicine, Division of Dermatology, Hahnemann Medical College and Hospital, Philadelphia, Pennsylvania.

PHILIP L. McCARTHY, M.D.

Disorders of the Oral Cavity

Associate Clinical Professor, Oral Pathology, Tufts University School of Dental Medicine; Assistant Dermatologist, Massachusetts General Hospital, Boston; Chief of Dermatology, Carney Hospital, Boston, and Quincy City Hospital, Quincy; Visiting Dermatologist, Boston City Hospital, Boston; Consultant in Dermatology, Norfolk County Hospital, Braintree, and Milton Hospital, Milton, Massachusetts.

SAMUEL L. MOSCHELLA, M.D.

Hypersensitivity, Bullous Diseases, Reticuloendothelial Diseases, Diseases of Peripheral Vessels, Connective Tissue Disease, Diseases of Nutrition and Metabolism, Parasitology and Tropical Dermatology, Dermatologic Surgery, Rare and Controversial Diseases

Chairman, Department of Allergy and Dermatology, The Lahey Clinic Foundation; Clinical Instructor, Harvard Medical School, Boston, Massachusetts; Consultant, United States Naval Hospital, Philadelphia, Pennsylvania, and United States Public Health Service Hospitals, Boston, Massachusetts, and Carville, Louisiana.

LESLIE NICHOLAS, M.D.

Treponemal Infections

Professor of Medicine (Dermatology) and Attending Dermatologist, Hahnemann Medical College and Hospital, Philadelphia, Pennsylvania.

LAWRENCE A. NORTON, M.D.

Disorders of Nails

Instructor, Dermatology, Boston University School of Medicine; Attending Dermatologist, University Hospital, Boston, and Newton-Wellesley Hospital, Newton, Massachusetts.

EDWARD J. O'KEEFE, M.D.

Hereditary Cutaneous Disorders

Assistant Professor of Dermatology and Assistant Professor of Pharmacology and Experimental Therapeutics, The Johns Hopkins University School of Medicine; Assistant Physician, Johns Hopkins Hospital, Baltimore, Maryland.

JOHN M. O'LOUGHLIN, M.D.

Clinical Immunology

Senior Staff, Department of Allergy and Dermatology, Lahey Clinic Foundation, Boston, Massachusetts.

DONALD M. PILLSBURY, M.A., M.D., D.Sc. (Hon.)

Principles of Clinical Diagnosis, Eczema

Professor Emeritus, Department of Dermatology, The University of Pennsylvania School of Medicine; Dermatologist, Hospital of the University of Pennsylvania; Senior Consultant in Dermatology, Philadelphia General Hospital, Philadelphia; Consultant in Dermatology, Children's Hospital, Philadelphia, and Bryn Mawr Hospital, Bryn Mawr, Pennsylvania.

PETER E. POCHI, M.D.

Sebum

Associate Professor of Dermatology, Boston University School of Medicine; Associate Visiting Physician for Dermatology, University Hospital and Boston City Hospital, Boston, Massachusetts.

M. H. SAMITZ, M.D., M.Sc. (Med.)

Industrial Dermatoses

Professor of Dermatology, The University of Pennsylvania School of Medicine; Chief, Department of Dermatology, Graduate Hospital of the University of Pennsylvania; Associate Physician, Hospital of the University of Pennsylvania, Philadelphia, Pennsylvania.

ARTHUR J. SOBER, M.D.

Mechanisms of Pigmentation

Instructor, Department of Dermatology, Harvard Medical School; Assistant in Dermatology, Massachusetts General Hospital, Boston, Massachusetts.

LAWRENCE M. SOLOMON, M.D.

Atopic Dermatitis

Professor and Head, Department of Dermatology, University of Illinois College of Medicine; Associate Professor of Dermatology, The Abraham Lincoln School of Medicine, University of Illinois; Attending Physician, University of Illinois Hospitals, Chicago, Illinois.

E. LAURIE TOLMAN, M.D.

Acne

Senior Staff, Lahey Clinic Foundation; Clinical Instructor in Dermatology, Harvard Medical School, Boston, Massachusetts.

FREDERICK URBACH, M.D., F.A.C.P.

Reactions to Physical Agents

Professor and Chairman, Department of Dermatology, Temple University School of Medicine; Medical Director, The Skin and Cancer Hospital of Philadelphia; Dermatologist, Temple University Hospital; Consultant in Dermatology, St. Christopher's Hospital for Children, Philadelphia, Pennsylvania.

ISAAC WILLIS, M.D.

Photosensitivity

Assistant Professor of Medicine (Dermatology), Emory University School of Medicine; Chief of Dermatology, Veterans Administration Hospital; Staff Physician, Veterans Administration Hospital; Attending Physician, Grady Memorial Hospital, Crawford W. Long Memorial Hospital of Emory University, Henrietta Egleston Hospital for Children, Holy Family Hospital, Hughes Spalding Pavilion, Atlanta, Georgia.

PREFACE

There is nothing permanent except change.
HERACLITUS (513 B.C.)

This work is a successor to but not a revision of the Pillsbury-Shelley-Kligman DERMATOLOGY (1956).

These volumes are, like the earlier text, based on a clinical and laboratory approach to diseases affecting the skin, either primarily in this organ or as a manifestation of systemic disease. With the stimulus of significant advances in facilities for study of cutaneous disease and a widening world-wide scope of fundamental understanding of the basic factors involved in the normal physiology of the skin, and of the etiology of disease disturbances affecting it, a considerable expansion of previous morphologic approaches to skin diseases is now possible.

The main purpose of these volumes may be summarized as follows: To provide a detailed presentation in text and picture of those skin diseases that are encountered most frequently by generalists and specialists alike, and that may be recognized by distinctive primary and secondary lesions and patterns, distribution of lesions, and associated systemic signs and symptoms, without resort, at least initially, to endoscopic, radiologic, histopathologic, immunologic, or biochemical techniques. Few diseases of man present invariable courses and patterns, or do not simulate other diseases, and hence alternative diagnoses are outlined in some detail. It is hoped that assistance is provided in differentiating between the common and the uncommon, and outlining what further studies may be necessary to establish diagnosis more precisely.

To achieve these objectives this new DERMATOLOGY is intended to be complete in coverage. Not only are morphologic features of each skin disease emphasized in both text and illustration but the modalities of laboratory diagnosis are also stressed and for each chapter references are provided to enable the inquisitive reader to pursue each subject further. It is hoped that the citations to literature represent a kind of plateau of advance demonstrating the intellectual health of the discipline of dermatology. The format for each disease description includes a discussion of the responsible pathogenetic mechanisms, as they are understood, and of histopathologic features and available treatment. As for terminology, we have endeavored to focus on the preferred term for each disease, but with references to others of historical significance or to common usage of other terms. Unfortunately such designations have varying degrees of importance, and repeated attempts by international and national committees and study groups have resulted in failure to reach complete agreement.

All of medicine has become increasingly global. Though certain diseases may be concentrated in a particular climatological environment, or country, or ethnic group, or isolated area, individuals with these diseases are moving about the world in increasing frequency and numbers. The possibility of an "exotic" disease must be considered more often. American medicine has been guilty of diagnostic parochialism at times in the past, and we have tried to avoid this as much as possible. We have accordingly given special consideration to parasitologic and tropical medicine; indeed, scabies has been described in detail because of its current striking increased incidence.

All physicians, of whatever specialty persuasion, are at times bewildered in determining the clinical significance of the streams of data emanating from basic science laboratories. Much of this information, in the fields of histochemistry, immunology, immunofluorescence, electron microscopy, microbiology, and experimental pharmacology has achieved clinical importance in dermatology, though, unfortunately, often not in a form readily available to the practicing physician. Of the advances having significance, we have attempted to supply details and interpretation. There are others on the horizon which are mentioned only briefly.

Heritable diseases especially are under intense investigative study. They are currently better diagnosed through the use of advanced laboratory techniques, and, until therapeutic approaches keep pace with theoretical knowledge, the main function of the capable and interested physician must be to provide wise genetic counseling. Therefore, an emphasis on genetics is timely and necessary. Similarly, it is essential that specialists in dermatology be aware of and familiar with the cutaneous manifestations of systemic disorders; consequently, internal medicine is emphasized in the considerable space allocated to it throughout the text.

In view of the frequency of cutaneous manifestations of systemic infection, the sections concerned with viral and systemic bacterial diseases have been enlarged. Scarlet fever, the result of a bacterial infection, is described in the chapter on viral diseases because it is frequently considered in the differential diagnosis of viral enanthems.

The broadening responsibilities, interests, and abilities of dermatologists, especially in the surgical and physical areas of therapy, are reflected in generous coverage of these topics. Radiation therapy (conventional and electron beam therapy) is still today a useful tool in the treatment of cutaneous malignant disease. Ultraviolet therapy, as part of the effective Goeckerman regimen or of the more recent and exciting but not fully established photochemotherapy for psoriasis, is emphasized, and its inherent problems are reviewed. With the advent of not only local therapeutic medicines but also systemic drugs for skin diseases, it has also been thought necessary to provide some explanation, especially in a text with a clinical concentration, of the role of chemotherapy and its potential problems and hazards; therefore, systemic chemotherapy has been discussed not only in the chapter on Therapy but also in the final chapter on Rare and Controversial Diseases and Conditions.

Pursuit of these aims made apparent that assistance from other clinicians and investigators would be required, if a balanced and reasonably complete presentation of the rapidly expanding field of dermatologic diseases and their origins were to be presented. A multi-authored text has therefore resulted, with many chapters written by individual authorities in special fields, but with, it is hoped, a continuity of editorial style and presentation which will not jar the sensibilities of those who might peruse the volumes as a whole. Some duplication has been inevitable, principally in areas where repeated emphasis of important points has seemed advisable.

Our purpose, then, has been to put a complex medical subject within the perspective of practical clinical usefulness. We therefore owe an immense debt of gratitude to our contributing authors, who have been willing to distill for us the results of wise observation of extensive clinical experience. We owe a similar debt of gratitude to Doctors Shelley and Kligman, who were unable to participate in this new book but who graciously allowed us reuse of some of the material and several of the fine and unique photographs appearing in the original DERMATOLOGY.

Since no big work of this type is ever accomplished without the dedicated effort of behind-the-scenes help, we offer also a more than perfunctory word of appreciation to Penny Doran, Jane McWilliams, Ann Ryan, Margaret Scheiter, Ella Slingluff, and Pauline Zorolow, who spent many hours typing manuscript. An expression of appreciation would not be complete without a very special thank you and a warm extension of gratitude to our families who endured much and assisted greatly. Their support has been invaluable.

It is our belief that the material contained in these volumes demonstrates that dermatology is a rapidly expanding branch of medicine, in terms of the skin as a complex multipurpose body organ, as a significant reflector of systemic disease, and as a rewarding focus of study by physicians and scientists in many disciplines.

SAMUEL L. MOSCHELLA, M.D.
DONALD M. PILLSBURY, M.D.
HARRY J. HURLEY, M.D.

CONTENTS

CHAPTER
1

STRUCTURE AND FUNCTION OF THE SKIN

Section I

DEVELOPMENT, MORPHOLOGY, AND PHYSIOLOGY

A. Bernard Ackerman

In the English language, no other organ of the body is invoked more frequently or more flavorfully than the skin. This conspicuous usage in common parlance reflects the unique significance of the skin in the life of contemporary man: skin is synonymous with "life" in the phrase "to save my skin"; human sensibilities are measured by "thin-skinned" or "thick-skinned"; a shallow person is "skin-deep" and a miser is a "skin-flint"; a friendly greeting is "give me a little skin" and an unfriendly feeling is "skin him alive"; relief is expressed by "the skin of my teeth," unconcern by "no skin off my back," and annoyance by "getting under my skin"; a sylph is "skinny" and nude swimming is "skinny dipping."

To many students of medicine, the skin is merely the body's largest organ; to others, it is the most fascinating.

The author gratefully acknowledges the constructive criticism of this chapter by: Gary Cage, M.D.; Ervin Epstein, Jr., M.D.; Phillip Frost, M.D.; Edward Gomez, M.D., Ph.D.; Kenneth Halprin, M.D.; Ken Hashimoto, M.D.; Robert Hsia, Ph.D.; Douglas E. Kelly, Ph.D.; Albert Kligman, M.D., Ph.D.; William Montagna, Ph,D.; Leopold Montes, M.D.; George F. Odland, M.D.; Neal Penneys, M.D., Ph.D.; Herman Pinkus, M.D.; Peter Pochi, M.D.; Arkadi M. Rywlin, M.D.; Inga Silverberg, M.D.; Richard Winkelmann, M.D.; Fred Woessner, Ph.D.; and Nardo Zaias, M.D., residents in dermatology and pathology at the University of Miami School of Medicine.

THE DEVELOPMENT OF SKIN

All constituents of human skin are derived from either ectoderm or mesoderm. The epithelial structures (epidermis, pilosebaceous-apocrine unit, eccrine unit, and nails) are ectodermal derivatives. Nerves and melanocytes emanate from neuroectoderm and neural crest. Mesenchymal structures (collagen, reticulum, and elastic fibers; blood vessels, muscles, and fat) originate from mesoderm.

Initially, embryonal dermis consists of stellate mesenchymal cells suspended in an acid mucopolysaccharide matrix. At about six weeks, the first delicate reticular fibers appear; by 12 weeks, collagen bundles can be recognized, and by 24 weeks, elastic fibers are also present within this myxomatous matrix. The collagen fibers in the upper part of the dermis are arranged in thinner bundles than they are in the deeper part. As the fibrillar component steadily increases and the cellular content relatively declines, the dermis acquires features typical of connective tissue.

Blood vessels are formed within the dermis from mesenchymal cells. A vascular network begins to organize at about the twelfth week, but characteristic vascular patterns, with venous and arterial pathways and capillary loops into the dermal papillae, are not apparent until the final weeks of fetal development. Beneath the dermis, mesenchymal cells surrounding newly formed blood vessels differentiate into lipid-filled cells to form the subcutaneous fat. The brown fat cell of the fetus is more active metabolically than the white fat cell of the infant.

Cutaneous nerves originate from neural crest and are detectable in the embryonic dermis at about five weeks. In the succeeding weeks, an elaborate nerve network develops. Deeper nerve trunks send out ascending branches that terminate as slender fibrils in the papillary dermis, and Meissner's corpuscles appear at the tips of the papillae in acral areas, such as fingers. Pacini's corpuscles appear later, deep in the dermis and in subcutaneous fat.

The epidermis, which develops from the surface ectoderm, consists of one layer of undifferentiated cells in a three-week old embryo (Fig. 1–1). By four weeks, it has an inner germinative layer of cuboidal cells with dark, compact nuclei and an outer layer of slightly flatter cells covered by microvilli. At 10 weeks, a third intermediate single row of cells forms by multi-

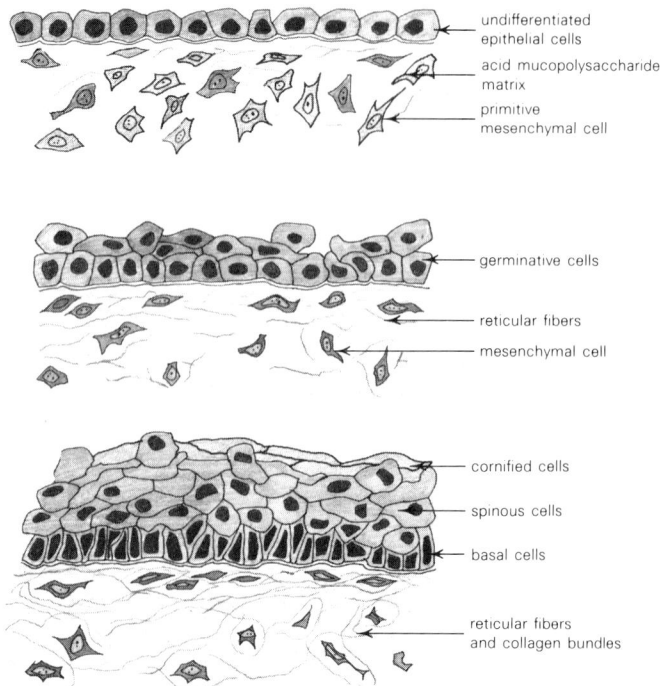

undifferentiated epithelial cells

acid mucopolysaccharide matrix

primitive mesenchymal cell

germinative cells

reticular fibers

mesenchymal cell

cornified cells

spinous cells

basal cells

reticular fibers and collagen bundles

Figure 1–1 Histogenesis of epidermis from a single layer of undifferentiated epithelial cells to a multilayered cornifying epithelium.

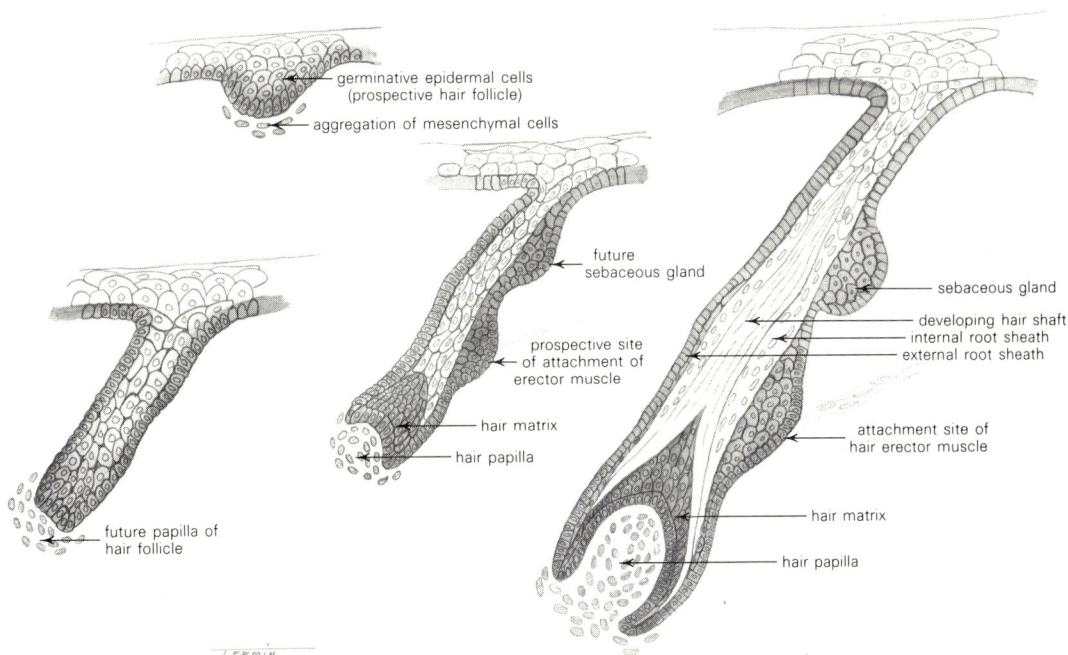

Figure 1–2 The pilar unit begins with the massing of primitive mesenchymal cells, the prospective hair papilla, beneath a focus of undifferentiated epidermal cells, the prospective hair follicle. The sebaceous gland and the attachment site of the hair erector muscle develop from hair follicle epithelium.

plication of germinative cells. At about this time, dendritic cells (melanocytes) derived from neural crest are first seen at the base of the epidermis. Between the fourteenth and sixteenth weeks, several layers of glycogen-rich, pale cells have been added to the intermediate zone. With the light microscope, these cells appear to be joined together by delicate bridges that resemble "spines." Granules (keratohyaline) become increasingly prominent in the upper part of the spinous zone. When, after the seventeenth week, the germinative cells become columnar and the surface cells lose their nuclei and begin to cornify, the fetal epidermis resembles the newborn epidermis. From inside outward, there are basal, spinous, granular, and cornified layers. The epidermis is a characteristic epithelium with contiguous cells and a minimum of extracellular material.

In the early stages of skin development, the interface between the epidermis and dermis is flat. At about 10 weeks, this boundary becomes wavy. The dermal papillae result from nipple-shaped insertions of connective tissue into hollows of the epidermal undersurface. The papillae contain terminal capillary loops and sensory nerve endings. A "basement membrane," contributed partly by the adjacent epidermal cells, develops at the junction between dermis and epidermis.

The first indication of impending hair follicle differentiation is seen at 10 weeks when nubbins of mesenchymal cells aggregate beneath discrete foci of closely crowded elongate germinative epidermal cells (Fig. 1–2). These rapidly dividing cells grow downward as solid, slanting columns that penetrate through the developing dermis into the subcutaneous fat. The germinative cells also proliferate upward as a cord piercing the epidermis to establish the funnel-shaped opening of the hair canal and to provide a wall for the hair shaft. Each descending column of epithelial cells advances, as if in pursuit of the knob of mesenchymal cells. The base of the epithelial column becomes bulbous as it finally catches and partially encloses the spade-shaped connective tissue that will serve as the hair papilla. Continuous with the papilla, in crescent-shaped array, are the germinative, or matrix, cells of the hair follicle. This hair unit of papilla and matrix cells is analogous to the unit formed by the papillary dermis and the basal cells.

The hair-matrix cells proliferate and maturate into several concentrically arranged cellular tubes of the hair follicle. From inside outward, they are the hair cortex, hair cuticle, inner root-sheath cuticle, Huxley's layer, Henle's layer, and outer root-sheath (trichilemmal sheath). The hair cortex (shaft), in the center of the follicle, is pushed upward by the stream of cornifying cells supplied by the matrix. By the thirteenth week, wisps of hair (lanugo) emerge from orifices on the eyebrow, upper lip, and chin. These hairs eventually cover the whole skin surface, except for the palms and soles.

As it slants downward into the dermis, the prospective hair follicle is bilaterally symmetrical. Near the sixteenth week, epithelial cells crowd together at three discrete loci on the side of the follicle that forms the widest angle with the epidermis. These three buds of epithelial cells expand outward into the mesenchyme. The lowest of these linearly arranged outgrowths forms the inferior attachment site, the bulge, of the hair erector muscle. This smooth muscle develops from elongate mesenchymal cells aligned from the bulge to the superior attachment site beneath the epidermis. As its cells become lipid laden, the middle bud develops into the lobulated sebaceous gland. The sebaceous gland connects to the central hair canal by a narrow duct. The uppermost outgrowth of the follicular epithelial cells forms the apocrine gland, which grows down into the subcutaneous fat as a solid cord of cells that, by 24 weeks, becomes coiled. A lumen, formed by a cleft between the cells, usually opens into the hair canal above. Less commonly, the lumen of the apocrine duct empties directly onto the skin surface. Apocrine glands are located primarily in the axillary and genital regions.

Initially, the epidermis that will become the future nail unit is indistinguishable from the surrounding surface epithelium (Fig. 1–3). At 10 weeks, a smooth, shiny quadrangular area, demarcated laterally and proximally by a continuous shallow groove, can be recognized on the distal dorsal surface of each digit. The epidermis in this circumscribed area consists of three layers: surface, intermediate, and germinative. At 11 weeks, the column of germinative and intermediate cells, the anlage of the nail matrix, grows proximally downward at a slant for a short distance into the dermis. The acute angle formed between and matrix and the surface epidermis becomes the proximal nail fold. Later, the distal boundary of the matrix will be represented by the lunula, a whitish half-moon–shaped area that extends beyond the proximal nail fold and is best seen in the thumbnail.

At 13 weeks, four layers can be recognized in the epidermis of the prospective nail area: basal, spinous, granular, and cornified. This area, now called the nail bed, loses its granular layer by the twentieth week. At 14 weeks, the proximal part of the nail bed acquires an additional cover of cornified cells, the nail plate or actual nail. The nail plate is produced by the matrix, without an intermediary granular layer. The cornified layer that extends from the undersurface of the proximal nail fold onto the surface of the newly formed nail plate is called the cuticle. Histochemical stains can distinguish cornified cells of the nail plate, with their abundant sulfhydryl groups, from those of the cuticle. The germinative cells of the epidermis, hair, and nail produce a similar end product: cornified cells composed mainly of the protein, keratin. Cells in skin that make keratin are called keratinocytes.

At 16 weeks, the nail plate has advanced from the matrix distally to cover one-half of the nail bed and completely covers it by 21 weeks, at which age the fetal nail resembles that of the adult.

Eccrine sweat glands develop first on palms and soles of 10-week-old embryos as focal massings of germinative cells at the bases of the epidermal ridges (Fig. 1–4). This apparently occurs without the formation of mesenchymal papillae. Slender cords of glycogen-filled epithelial cells project perpendicularly downward into the dermis and upward through the epidermis. The epithelial columns' outer layers of cells are continous with the germinative layer of the epidermis, whereas the columns' inner cores connect with the intermediate layer. When the epithelial downgrowths reach the subcutaneous fat, their deepest portions become coiled. At

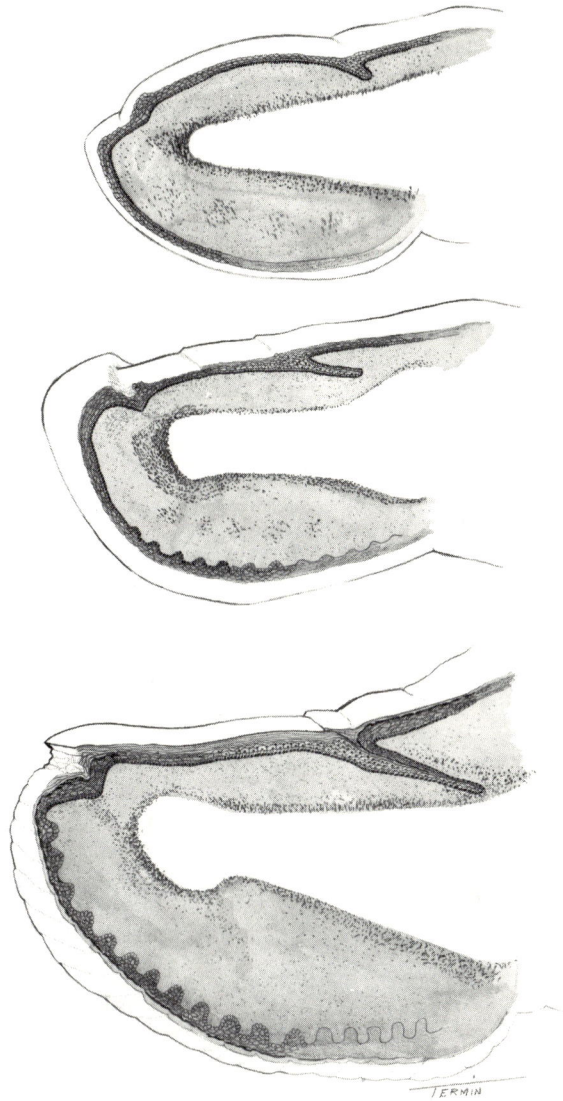

Figure 1–3   The nail unit evolves in a fashion similar to the hair follicle. Cornified cells of the nail plate, hair shaft, and epidermal cornified layer are the respective end products of germinative nail, hair, and epidermal cells.

about the thirtieth week, these cellular cords acquire lumens. From the base upward, the mature eccrine sweat unit consists of a coiled secretory gland, coiled intradermal duct, straight intradermal duct, and spiraled intradermal duct.

The mechanisms that govern the development of skin are fragmentarily understood; however, some insight into cutaneous differentiation has been gained from experimental studies. In the beginning of embryonic life, an unidentified diffusible mesenchymal substance appears to be responsible for the induction of epithelial differentiation. At this early stage, mesenchyme from different embryonic sources can alter presumptive epidermis so that it will fail to cornify and even become ciliated. Mesenchyme also induces the epidermal cells to produce adnexa: hairs, nails, and glands. These events require a continuous mesenchymal influence, but do not necessitate direct contact between mesenchyme and epithelium. Once epidermal development is sufficiently advanced, the epithelium becomes partially autonomous and, in addition, exerts an influence on mesenchymal behavior.

Stratification of the epidermal cells is dependent upon an intact basal lamina. This is witnessed in re-epithelialization of healing wounds. Epithelial cells from hair

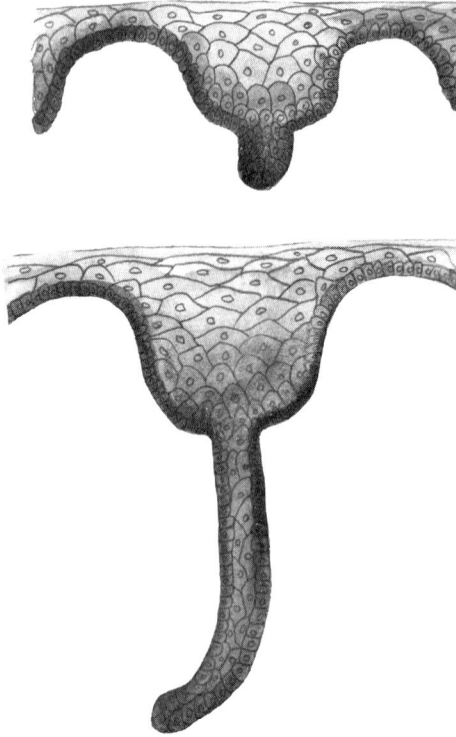

Figure 1–4   The eccrine sweat unit develops from undifferentiated cells at the nadir of the epidermal rete, in the absence of a connective tissue papilla.

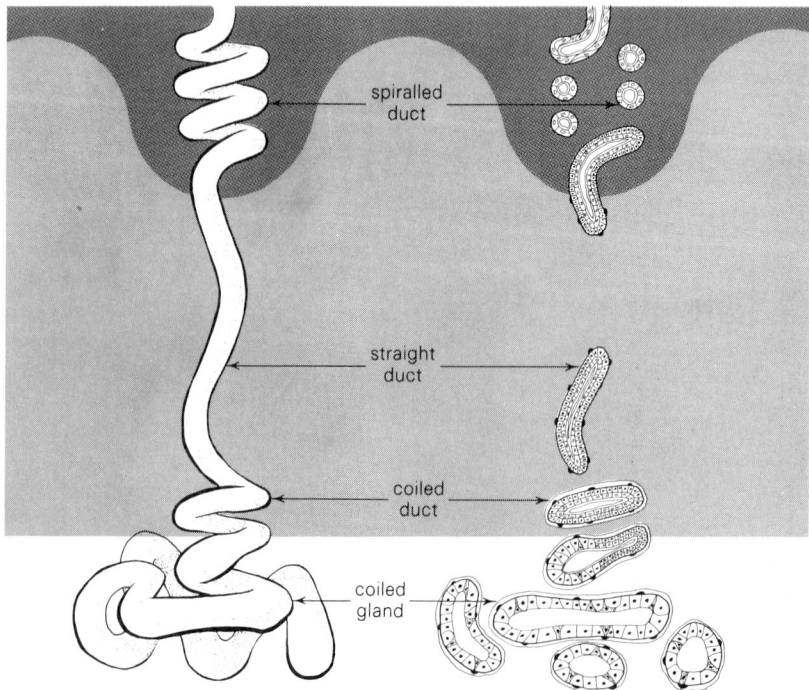

spiralled duct

straight duct

coiled duct

coiled gland

follicles and eccrine ducts, as well as from surrounding basal and spinous cells, migrate, in a single row, to cover the denuded epidermis. When the defect has been covered and the epithelial cells are firmly fixed to the basal lamina, stratification commences. These new germinative cells in contact with the basal lamina generate an epidermis, despite their adnexal and spinous-cell origins. The reconstitution of epidermis from keratinocytes of all ectodermally derived structures in skin demonstrates keratinocytic pluripotentiality.

The interdependence of epithelium and mesenchyme is particularly well illustrated in the development of the pilosebaceous-apocrine apparatus. This epithelial unit will not develop from epidermis in the absence of a mesenchymal papilla and, conversely, a papilla will not form in the absence of an epithelium. This reciprocal influence of adnexal epithelium upon its surrounding connective tissue, and vice versa, persists into adult life.

In conclusion, the development and maintenance of skin depends upon interactions between epithelium and mesenchyme, germinative cells and components of their basal lamina, and interactions of epithelial cells with one another. These interactions result in a heterogeneous but unified structure with marked regional differences in form, color, and consistence.

TOPOGRAPHY OF THE SKIN

The skin's terrain is intricate and varied. Regional differences in skin structure represent adaptations to particular functions or the vestiges of prehuman life. The reader should use his own skin as a demonstration model while perusing the following few paragraphs.

The skin of infants is traversed by a subtle maze of markings which develops during the third and fourth months of fetal life and which becomes increasingly prominent during childhood. The designs remain unchanged throughout life and are nearly indestructible. Swirled patterns typify palms and soles. Small, roughly diamond-shaped outlines crisscross the rest of the body surface and are particularly well seen in the skin over the volar aspects of the wrists and elbows, in the antecubital fossae, and between the knuckles (Fig. 1–5). The developmental conditions that determine the orientation of the surface ridges are unknown, but they are thought to result from the combined effect of: (1) epidermal rete–dermal papillae configuration (2) arrangement of underlying collagen bundles, and (3) muscle and fascial pull on the dermis. Just as the epidermal surface is marked by diverse figurations, so too the epidermal undersurface on different body regions is distinguished by varied contours (Fig. 1–6).

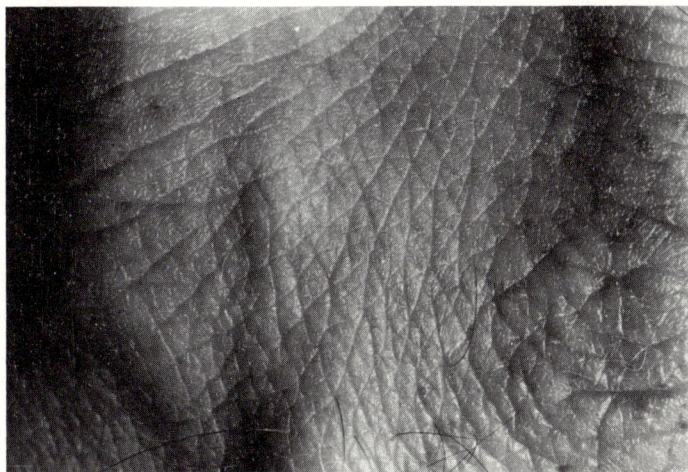

Figure 1–5 Diamond-shaped outlines crisscross most of the body surface, as in the skin between the knuckles.

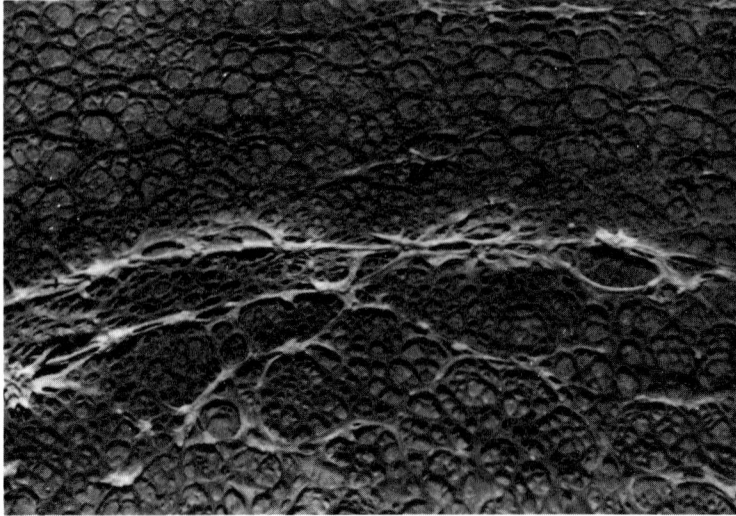

Figure 1–6 The variegate moldings of the epidermal undersurface at the junction of the female nipple and areola. (Courtesy of William Montagna, Ph.D.)

The etchings that cover the entire surface of the palms and soles, excluding flexion and other secondary creases, are collectively termed "dermatoglyphic patterns." Parallel ridges and furrows form whorls, loops, and arches on the fingertips in a pattern so highly individualistic that fingerprinting has been used as a reliable method of personal identification, even permitting the distinction between identical twins (Fig. 1–7). There are noticeable differences in dermatoglyphic patterns on the palms and fingers of the same individual. Statistically, the patterns of women contain fewer whorls and more arches than those of men. The study of dermatoglyphics has enabled early detection of genetic abnormalities, such as Down's syndrome, and of defects caused in utero by infectious agents, such as German measles virus. Histologically, palmar and plantar skin is characterized by a thick cornified layer, prominent retia and papillae, numerous nerve endings and eccrine sweat units, and the absence of hair follicles. The corrugated palmar surface, like the tread of a tire, is ideally suited for grasping and gripping. The tactile properties of the fingertips were utilized by Braille to compensate for eyesight.

The dense, luxurious pelage that covers the scalp is reflected microscopically in numerous deeply rooted hair follicles. In man, hair is largely ornamental compared to other mammals in whom hair serves primarily as a furry blanket to conserve heat. Although on casual observation man is an apparently naked animal, except for

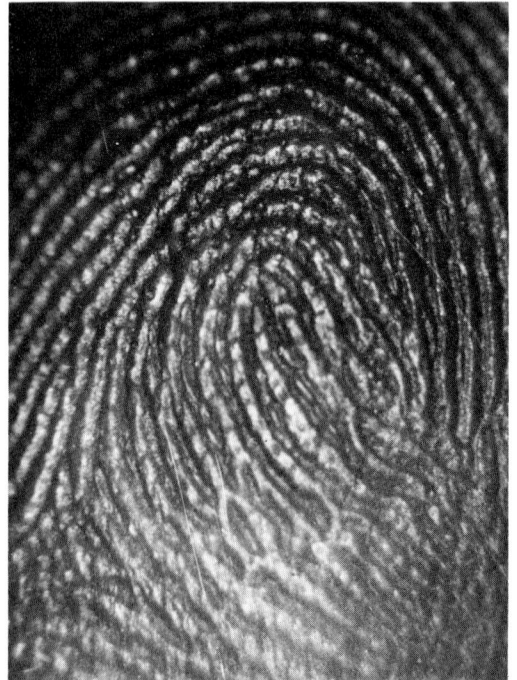

Figure 1–7 Dermatoglyphic pattern of the human thumb.

the scalp, pubis, and axillae, in actuality the entire body surface, excluding acral volar skin and mucocutaneous junctions, is dotted by hairs, many of them slim and diminutive. The follicular orifices from which these slender vellus hairs emerge are easily detected on the forearm. Vellus hairs on the face of women, such as those above the lip, are usually inconspicuous until menopause, when hormonal changes cause them to enlarge.

The taut skin of the back, composed of a thick dermis with broad collagen bundles, is well constructed to withstand the stress of man's upright posture. In contrast, the distensible skin of the eyelids, with its thin dermis, is aptly designed for the rapid movements necessary to protect the eye. In general, skin is elastic.

At the body openings, skin is continuous with mucous membrane. Mucocutaneous junctions occur at the eyelids, nares, vulva, prepuce, clitoris, and anus. Histologically, skin differs from mucous membrane by possessing an anucleate, fully cornified layer.

Other regions of the skin also have distinguishing features: the greasy middle third of the face, especially in adolescence, results from secretions of the numerous large sebaceous glands associated with small hair follicles having prominent follicular orifices (Fig. 1–8); the helix of the ear is covered by many tiny vellus hairs (Fig. 1–9), seen microscopically as closely set minute hair follicles in a dermis devoid of sweat glands; pigmented zones

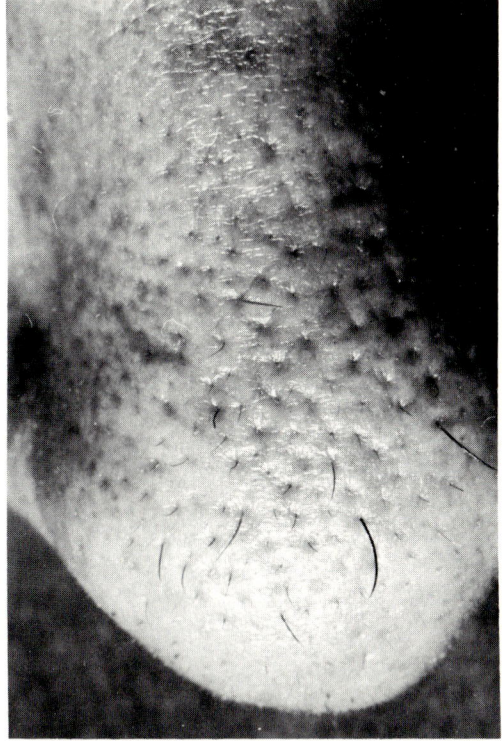

Figure 1–8 Orifices of hair follicles are particularly prominent on the nose.

like the areola contain increased amounts of epidermal melanin, whereas the Mongolian spot over the infant's sacrum is due to dermal melanocytes; the common occipital "port-wine stain" results from telangiectases; the hairy, sweaty axilla is an adnexal potpourri of hair follicles and

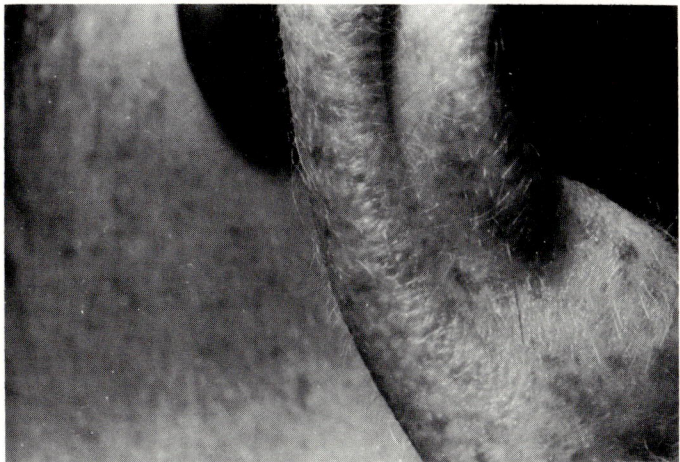

Figure 1–9 Vellus covers the pinna of the ear.

sebaceous glands and myriads of apocrine and eccrine glands; and erectile tissues, such as nipples, clitoris, and penis, are endowed with highly vascularized smooth muscles. The skin's vasculature also eloquently expresses intense emotions, betraying shame and anger (reddening) and fear (pallor). Telltale signs of anxiety are cold hands and sweaty palms (clammy palms).

THE DERMIS

The skin is composed of three anatomically distinct layers. From the surface inward, these are the epidermis, dermis, and subcutaneous fat. The epidermis has a thickness about equal to the paper of this page and is the thinnest layer, varying from 0.04 mm. on the eyelids to 1.6 mm. on the palms. It is a stratified squamous epithelium with a high metabolic rate. By contrast, the dermis is mostly composed of dense, relatively noncellular fibroelastic tissue in which are embedded the pilosebaceous-apocrine and eccrine units, blood vessels, and lymphatics, muscles, and nerves. The dermis is 15 to 40 times thicker than the epidermis, depending upon the locale, but its energy needs are low. The dermis rests on a thick pad of fat.

Embryologically, mesenchymal cells of the mesoderm give rise to the following dermal components:

1. Cells
   a. Fibrocytes (fibroblasts)
   b. Endothelial cells
2. Fibers
   a. Reticular
   b. Collagen
   c. Elastic
3. Ground substance
   a. Hyaluronic acid
   b. Chondroitin sulfate
   c. Dermatan sulfate

The fully formed dermis can be conveniently divided into two distinct compartments: (1) the thin zone immediately beneath the epidermal rete ridges (papillary dermis) and around adnexa (periadnexal dermis), and (2) the thick reticular dermis. The combined anatomic unit of papillary and periadnexal dermis is called the "adventitial dermis." It is charac-

terized by thin, haphazardly arranged collagen fibers; many reticular fibers; delicate branching elastic fibers; numerous elongate, plump, and stellate-shaped fibroblasts; abundant ground substance, and plentiful capillaries linked to superficial arterial and venous plexuses (Fig. 1–10). The papillary dermis and epidermis together form a morphologic and functional unit, whose intimacy is reflected in their joint alteration by common inflammatory diseases. A similar relationship exists between periadnexal connective tissue and its epithelia. The major component of the dermis (reticular dermis) extends from the base of the papillary dermis to the subcutaneous fat. It is composed of thick collagen bundles mostly arranged parallel to the skin surface in orthogonal wicker-work. A network of coarse, elastic fibers enmeshes the collagen bundles. Proportionally, there are fewer reticular fibers, fibroblasts, and blood vessels and less ground substance in the broad reticular dermis than in the narrow adventitial dermis. Occasionally, cells of the subcutaneous fat can be found within the dermis, and striated muscle is commonly seen in the dermis of facial skin. The fibrous trabeculae of the subcutaneous fat are comparable to the connective tissue of the adventitial dermis (Fig. 1–11).

The dermis varies in thickness in different regions, being thinnest on the eyelids and thickest on the back (Fig. 1–12). The total thickness of the papillary dermis increases when the skin is subjected to long-standing rubbing (lichen simplex chronicus), and the entire reticular dermis thickens in the disease scleredema. Individual collagen bundles become thinner in an atrophic scar and wider in a keloid. Like other tissues, the dermis decreases in thickness with advancing age.

The fibroblast is the master cell of the dermis. It produces all three types of fibers and the ground substance. As seen with the light microscope, the fibroblast has a spindle- or stellate-shaped nucleus and indistinct cytoplasm. The electron microscope discloses that the fibroblast cytoplasm contains numerous dilated cisternae lined by ribosomes, many mitochondria, and a well-defined Golgi apparatus. These are features of a metabolically active cell, and it is likely that the fibroblast contrib-

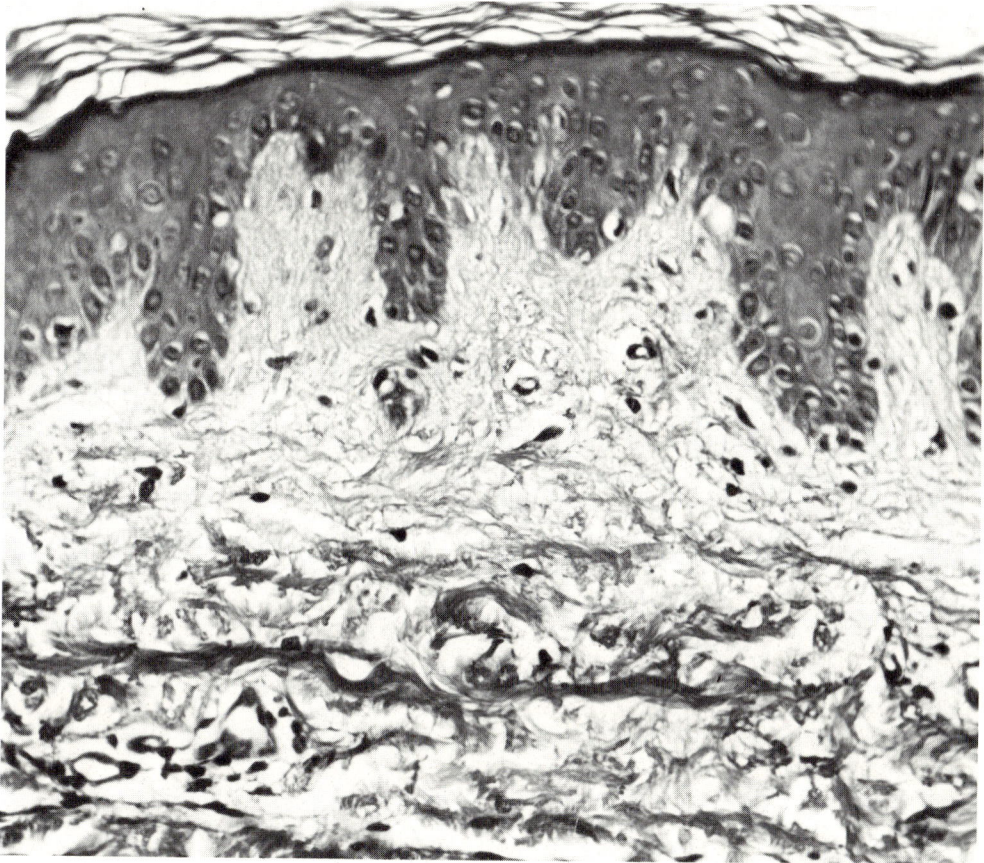

Figure 1–10 The superficial (papillary) dermis is composed of thin, haphazardly arranged collagen fibers in contrast to the deeper (reticular) dermis which is formed by thick collagen bundles. (× 374).

utes not only to connective-tissue synthesis, but to its catabolism as well.

Connective tissue fiber proteins are formed from relatively small, soluble monomeric units synthesized on ribosomes within the cell and conveyed to the outside where they are polymerized. Collagen, reticular and elastic fibers appear to be fashioned, in their final form, outside the fibroblast.

The initial stages of collagen synthesis proceed within the fibroblast cytoplasm. Amino acids are assembled into polypeptide chains of about 120,000 molecular weight. Lysine and proline are hydroxylated, and the disaccharide unit, glucosegalactose, is added to certain hydroxylysine residues. Three of the polypeptide chains then wind up into a triple helix, forming the tropocollagen molecule, a

long rodlike structure, 14 × 2800 Å, with a total molecular weight of 285,000. The ends of the chains are clipped off by a protease to give chains of 95,000 molecular weight each. Apparently, the discarded pieces had helped to align the three chains before the winding process. Soluble tropocollagen molecules are next transported from the fibroblast into the immediate surroundings where, in subsequent steps, collagen fibril formation takes place by the aggregation of tropocollagen molecules. Covalent links form between tropocollagen molecules; these links involve lysine and hydroxylysine residues in various combinations. These bonds hold the fiber together and give it tensile strength. Covalent links continue to develop with aging, causing rigidity and loss of resiliency.

papillary dermis

periadnexal dermis

reticular dermis

adventitial dermis
papillary
plus
periadnexal

fibrous trabeculae

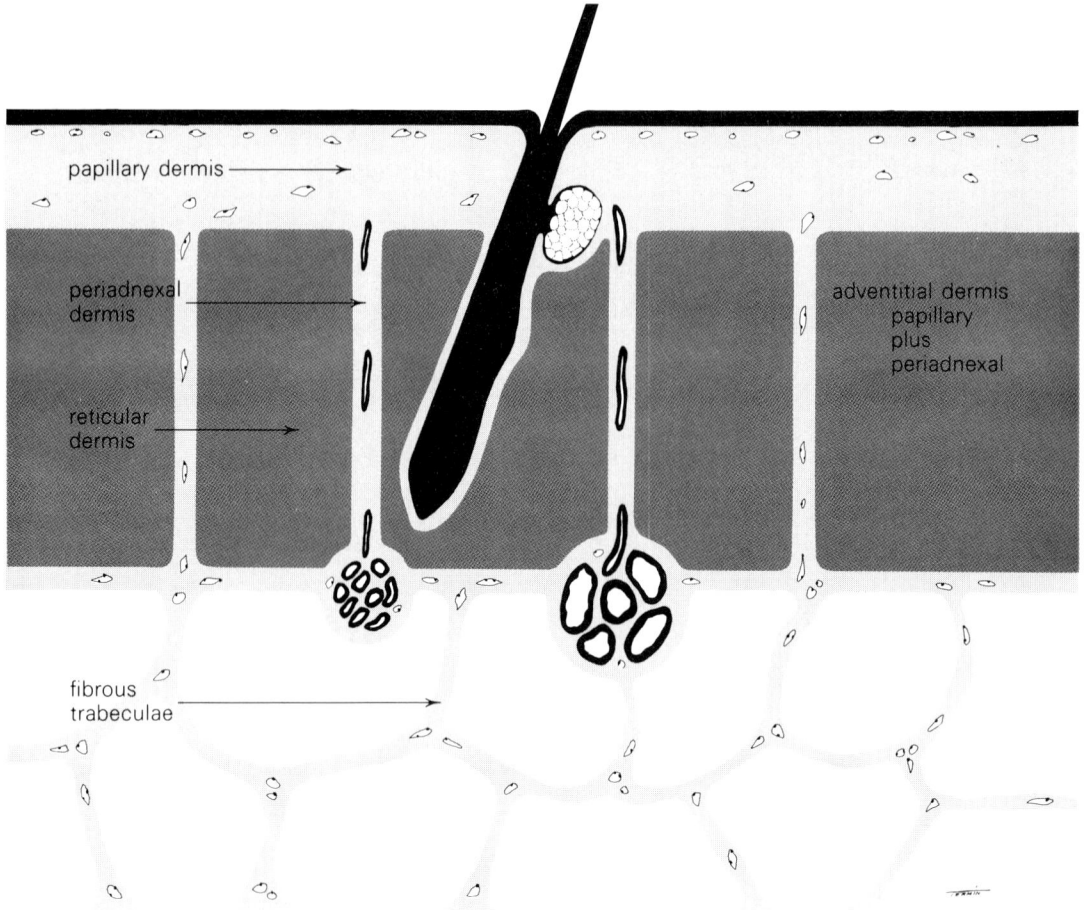

Figure 1–11   The connective tissue of the papillary and periadnexal dermis, which together are called the adventitial dermis, has a similar appearance and function. The fibrous trabeculae of the subcutaneous fat are analogues of the adventitial dermis.

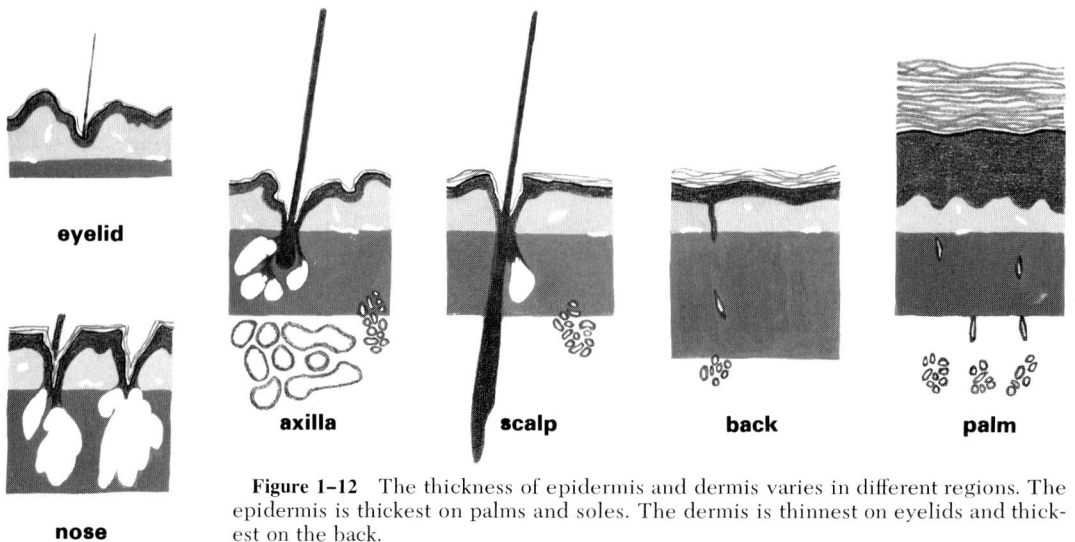

eyelid

nose

axilla

scalp

back

palm

Figure 1–12   The thickness of epidermis and dermis varies in different regions. The epidermis is thickest on palms and soles. The dermis is thinnest on eyelids and thickest on the back.

Mature collagen fibrils have a width of about 1000 Å and distinct cross-banding, 680 Å apart (Fig. 1–13). A distinctive chemical feature of collagen is its content of hydroxyproline and hydroxylysine, amino acids not commonly present in other proteins. Glycine comprises one-third of the amino acid residues in collagen. Proline plus hydroxyproline account for another one-quarter of the collagen residues. Tyrosine and tryptophane are present in minuscule amounts.

Reticular fibers are young, finely formed collagen fibers with a similar periodicity but narrower diameter than mature collagen. These fibers are not visible with hematoxylin-and-eosin stains, but are blackened by silver stain (argyrophilic). Reticular fibers are prominent within and beneath the epidermal basement membrane, where they intermingle with mature collagen fibers. In this zone, reticular fibers and finer filaments coursing in and through the basal lamina apparently help anchor the epidermis to the dermis. This narrow subepidermal zone of densely packed reticular fibers separates the elastic fibers of the papillary dermis from the epidermis. In the papillary dermis, elastic fibers are thin and mostly oriented perpendicular to the epidermis. In the reticular dermis, elastic fibers are thicker and seemingly arranged mostly parallel to the skin surface (Fig. 1–14).

Immature elastic fibers are aggregates of protein microfibrils grouped in a long cylinder along the surface of the fibroblast (Fig. 1–15). Later, a second protein, elastin, is synthesized and secreted by the cell into the preformed tube of microfibrils. Elastic fibers then consist of microfibrils of about 110 Å in diameter and elastin with a molecular weight of 40,000. The elastic subunits become cross-linked into a three-dimensional network by reactions involving three or four lysines that join to form the complex. Cross-linkage in elastin is provided by two lysine-derived amino

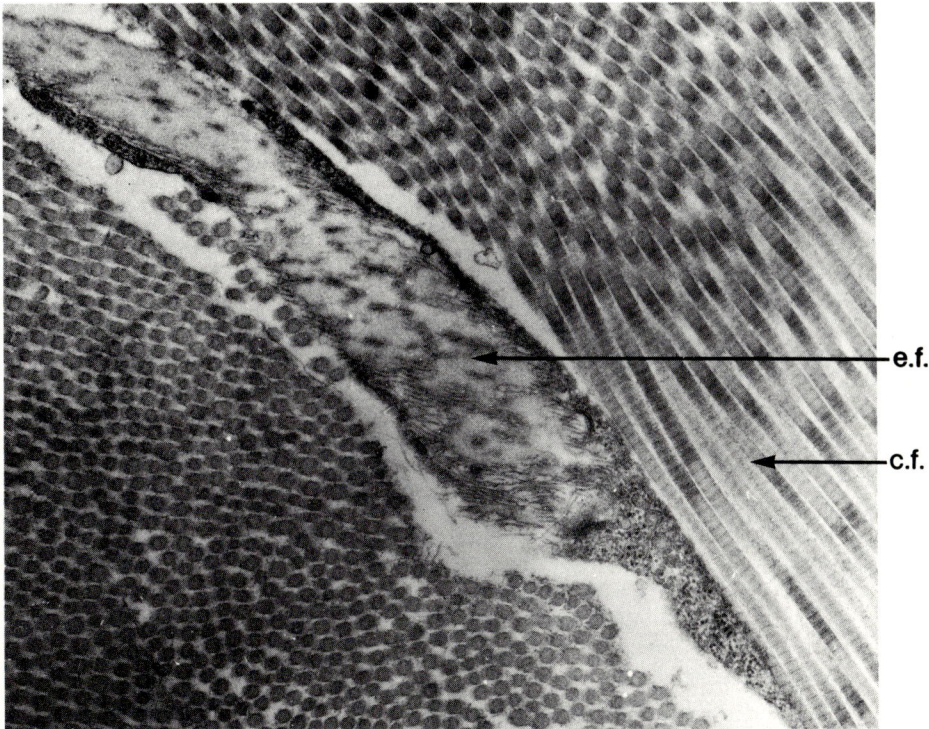

Figure 1–13 Longitudinally cut collagen fibrils have a width of about 1000 Å and a distinct cross-banding, 680 Å apart. An elastic fiber consists of non-collagenous fibrils embedded in homogeneous elastin. *e.f.*, elastic fiber; *c.f.*, collagen fibrils. (× 55,000.) (Courtesy of Richard Wood, Ph.D.)

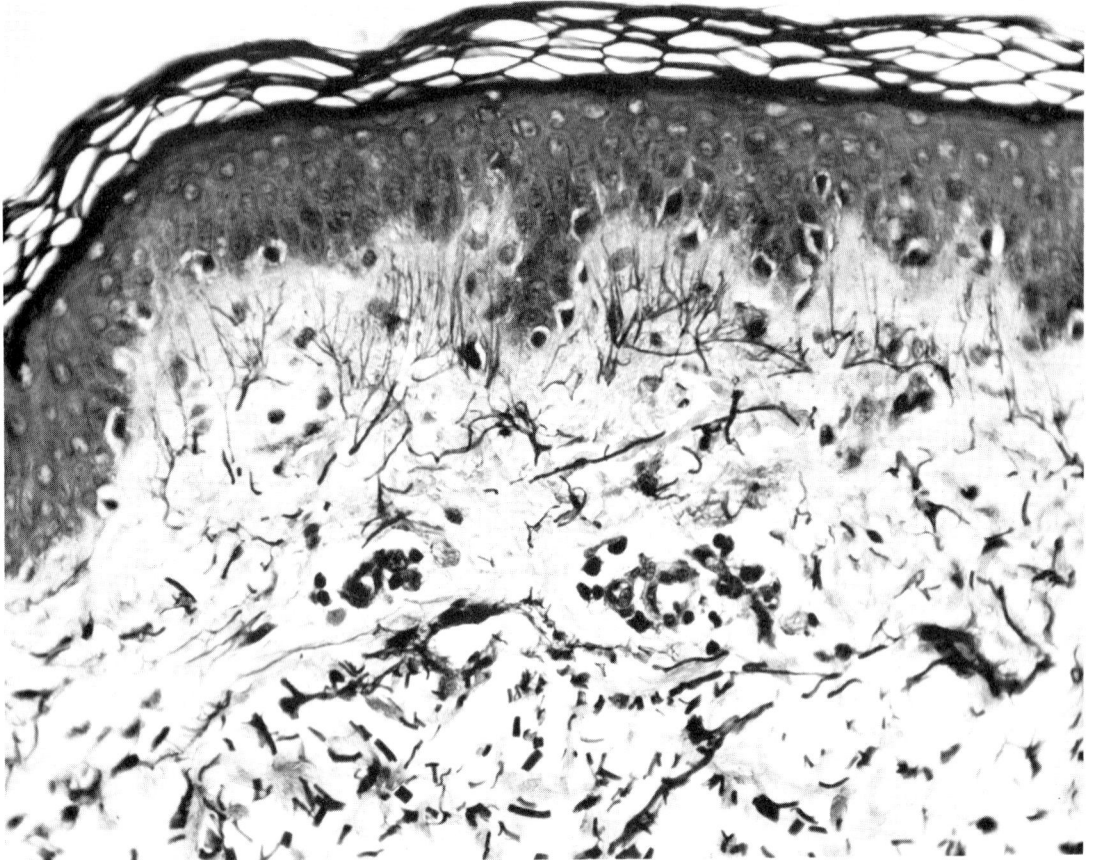

Figure 1–14   The thin elastic fibers in the papillary dermis appear to be mostly oriented perpendicular to the surface, whereas those in the reticular dermis are thicker and seemingly arranged mostly parallel to the skin surface. ($\times$ 462.)

acids, desmosine and isodesmosine, which are unique to this molecule.

Elastin differs chemically from collagen. It has one-third of its residue as glycine, but has more alanine and less hydroxyproline than collagen. Mature elastic fibers are refractile and exhibit autofluorescence. Whereas collagen comprises 90 per cent of the dry weight of the dermis, elastic tissue constitutes only 2 per cent. The two major fibers of the skin are closely associated with each other, elastic fibers being found only where there are collagen fibers. Collagen presumably provides the skin with tensile strength, whereas elastic fibers give the organ, and its larger blood vessels, elasticity. Diminution or absence of elastic fibers allows the skin to bulge in atrophic conditions such as stria and anetoderma. The abundance of elastic fibers is peculiar to human skin.

Fibroblasts also give rise to ground substance, the extracellular mucinous matrix of the dermis. In routine histologic sections, the ground substance is invisible, appearing as empty spaces between collagen bundles. Special stains, such as alcian blue and colloidal iron, reveal ground substance in normal skin, especially in the adventitial dermis. The ground substance accounts for only a minuscule fraction of the dermal weight, but for a substantial portion of the volume. Acid mucopolysaccharides, particularly hyaluronic acid, chondroitin sulfate, and dermatan sulfate, are the major elements of the ground substance. Chemically, acid mucopolysaccharides are long molecules with protein cores to which are attached many long side-chains composed of repeating disaccharide units. Other components of the ground substance are neutral mucopolysaccharides, proteins, and electrolytes. The ground substance, most abundant in the adventitial dermis, is concentrated in the papillae of anagen hair follicles and around eccrine sweat glands. Ground substance has a great capacity to bind water.

In certain pathologic states, the amount of acid mucopolysaccharides in the dermis increases. This deposition varies from the widespread myxedema to the localized focal mucinosis.

In addition to fibroblasts, there are other important "wandering" cells in the dermis. Scattered among the fibers are histiocytes, distinguished from fibroblasts not always by histologic appearance but by function. These are the scavengers of the dermis which engulf hemosiderin, melanin, lipid, and debris (Fig. 1–16). Histiocytes arise in the bone marrow as monocytes.

Mast cells, primarily located around blood vessels, can be recognized in hematoxylin and eosin–stained tissue sections by their darkly basophilic ovoid nuclei and granular amphophilic cytoplasm. The water soluble mast cell granules are revealed to be coarse and metachromatic when exposed to special stains of alcohol-fixed tissue. These granules contain the acid-mucopolysaccharide anticoagulant, heparin, and the vasoactive amine, histamine. Some believe that mast cells participate in the regulation of vascular permeability. During inflammatory processes, mast cells lose their granules, presumably releasing histamine. Mast cells are particularly numerous in association with neural tissue, such as neurofibroma, and are the dominant cell in the skin lesions of urticaria pigmentosa.

Vascular structures of skin are derived from primitive mesenchymal cells. An endothelial cell lining is common to all

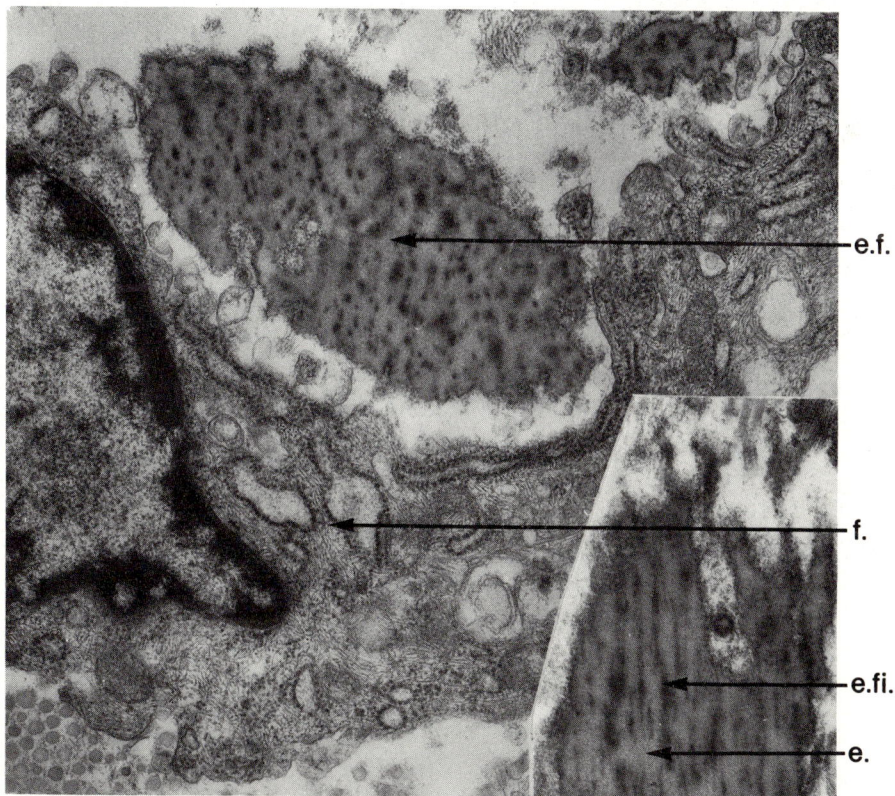

Figure 1–15 An elastic fiber is formed in the vicinity of a fibroblast that has a well-developed rough surfaced endoplasmic reticulum. In the insert, an elastic fiber is seen to consist of fibrils and homogeneous elastin. *e.f.*, elastic fiber; *f.*, fibroblast; *e.fi.*, elastic fibrils; *e.*, elastin. (× 22,500; insert × 41,750.) (Courtesy of Ken Hashimoto, M.D.)

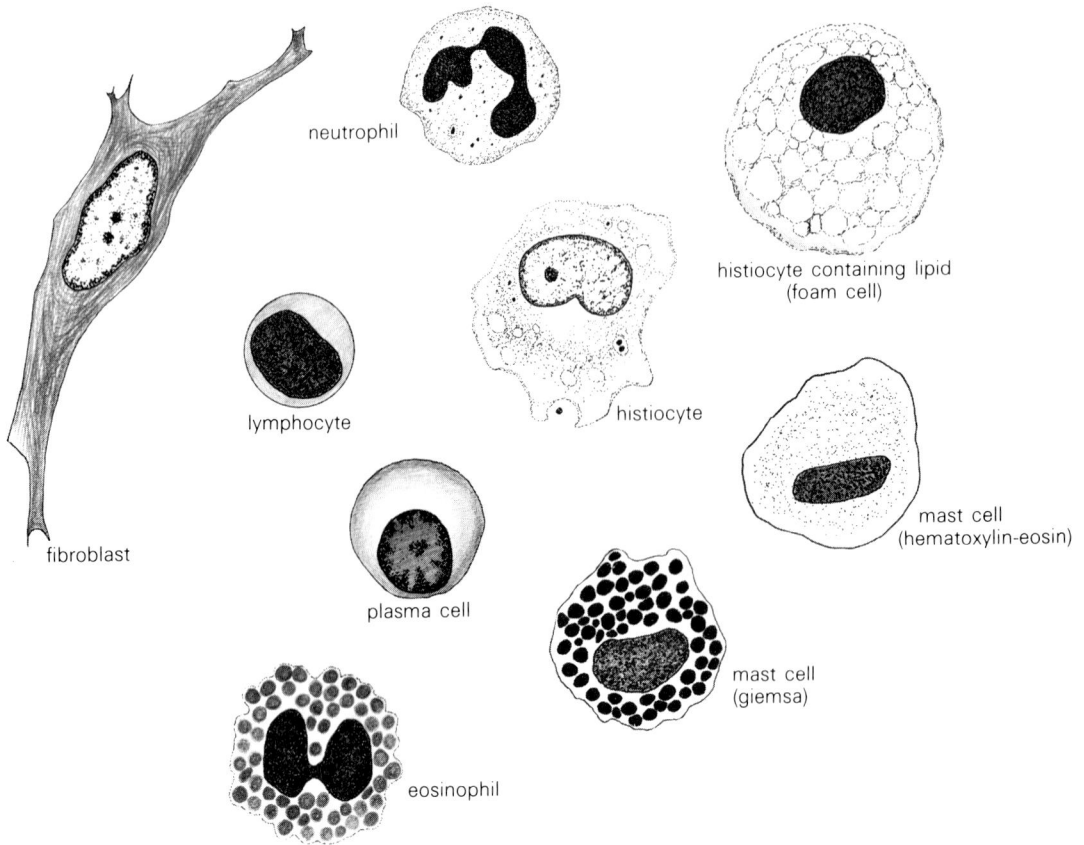

Figure 1–16   Comparative cytology of cells found in normal and inflamed skin.

parts of the vascular system. In the smallest cutaneous capillaries, a single endothelial cell may encircle the entire circumference of the vessel. In larger capillaries, a single layer of two to three flat endothelial cells, whose serrated edges interdigitate with each other, curve around the lumen. Capillary endothelial cells are ensheathed by thin collagen or reticular fibers. Arterioles have an intima of endothelial cells, a medium containing smooth muscle cells, and an adventitia composed of collagen and elastic fibers. An internal elastic membrane is present beneath the endothelium of larger arterioles. Arteries that supply the skin are located in the subcutaneous fat and they have both an internal and an external elastic membrane. Venules, veins of small caliber, consist only of endothelium surrounded by a thin zone of collagen fibers. In progressively larger venules, smooth muscle and elastic fibers appear. Pericytes lie just outside the endothelial cells of the microcirculation.

It is through the capillaries and venules that oxygen, water, nutrients, and hormones are distributed from the blood to the tissues and carbon dioxide and other products of skin metabolism are collected for transmission to the excretory organs. The endothelium of capillaries and venules functions as a porous membrane, permeable to water and crystalloids, but relatively impermeable to large molecules. Venules are more permeable than capillaries to intravenously injected dyes, as well as to histamine, serotonin, and other substances that increase vascular permeability. Venules are also of primary importance in changes associated with inflammation.

The architecture of the dermal vasculature is a three-dimensional network of two plexuses that parallel the skin surface. One plexus is in the lower part of the reticular dermis (deep plexus), the other courses beneath the papillary dermis (superficial plexus). Perpendicularly oriented communicating blood vessels connect the deep and superficial plexuses. The deeper blood vessels have larger diameters. From the subpapillary plexus, arcades of capillaries loop upward into the papillae. Similar vessels infuse the periadnexal dermis, The rich blood supply of the adventitial dermis constitutes a microcirculation, in contrast to the relatively straight, large conduits of the two parallel plexuses and their communicating vessels (Fig. 1–17).

Arteriovenous anastomoses are present in skin, especially in the digits. These segments, interposed between arteriole and venule, are surrounded by aggregates of uniform, ovoid, smooth-muscle cells that serve as sphincters. Each of these shunts, known as a "glomus," enables blood to by-

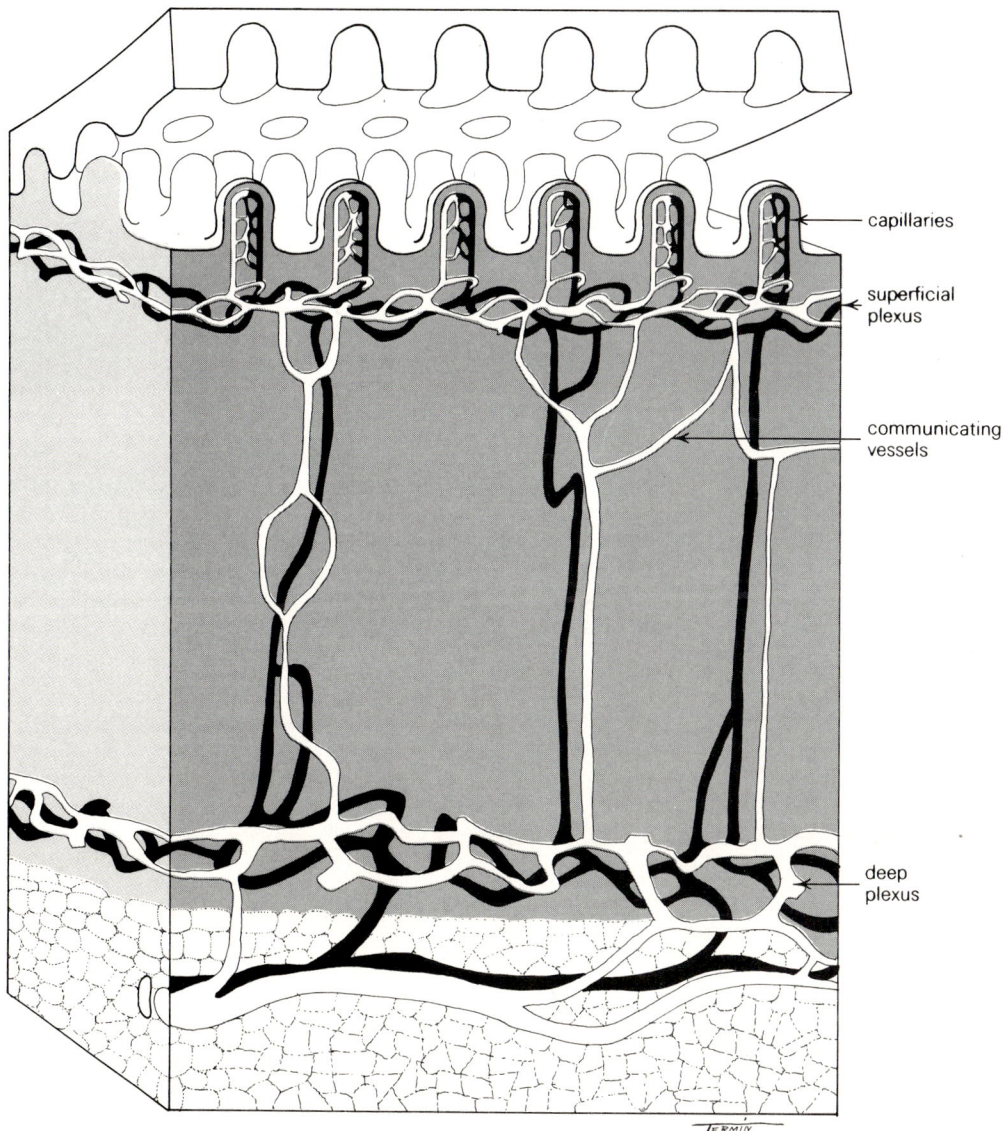

Figure 1–17 The dermal vasculature consists of a three-dimensional network of two plexuses that parallel the skin surface: one in the lower reticular dermis (deep plexus), the other beneath the papillary dermis (superficial plexus). Perpendicularly oriented communicating blood vessels connect the deep and superficial plexuses. The rich capillary supply of the adventitial dermis constitutes a microcirculation, in contrast to the relatively straight, large conduits of the two parallel plexuses and their communicating vessels.

pass the capillaries; this accelerates blood flow through the acral skin. Both the glomera and arterioles are under the control of the sympathetic nervous system. Arterioles also respond to a variety of pharmacologic agents; for example, epinephrine, Pitressin, and angiotensin cause vasoconstriction, whereas histamine, ethanol, and acetylcholine lead to vasodilation.

Thermoregulation is the cardinal function of the cutaneous vasculature. Blood vessels in the skin maintain the body at a constant temperature by buffering the effect of wide variations in the environmental and internal temperatures. Blood flow through the dermis varies in response to changes in the core temperature of the body and the temperature of the external environment. The control of dermal blood flow is partly directed from the hypothalamus and is mediated by the sympathetic nervous system.

Another function of the dermal blood vessels is to provide nutrition for the skin. The plentiful capillaries of the adventitial dermis supply epithelial structures whose oxidative requirements are greater than those of connective tissue. The total volume of blood that circulates through the dermis is requisite for thermoregulation but is considerably greater than necessary simply to nurture the skin.

Dermal blood vessels also play an important role in inflammation. The microcirculatory unit of the papillary dermis participates in skin diseases characterized by erythema. These include all the common inflammatory eruptions whose red color is imparted by blood. The entire dermal vasculature presumably reacts, albeit to a lesser degree, in these inflammatory disorders.

Skin also harbors an elaborate network of lymphatics that parallels the major vascular plexuses but is independent of them. Like capillaries, the walls of lymphatics are constructed of a single-layered endothelium, but unlike capillaries the lymphatics have no pericytes. Larger lymphatics can sometimes be distinguished from capillaries by the presence of valves. One terminus of a lymphatic tube ends blindly, the other empties into a vein. Lymphatics filter and transport a large portion of the capillary transudate, called "lymph" once it has entered the lymphatics, and return it to the venous system.

SUBCUTANEOUS FAT

Beneath the dermis, the connective tissue forms fat. Subcutaneous fat, like the dermis, is derived from mesenchyme, and mesenchymal cells give rise to lipocytes (fat cells), as well as to fibrocytes. Lipocytes manufacture so much fat in their cytoplasm that it presses and flattens the nucleus against the periphery of the cell. Electron microscopy of lipocytes demonstrates that their cytoplasm is replete with mitochondria. Human fat consists largely of triglycerides.

Strands of collagen divide the population of fat cells into lobules. These fibrous elements, known as trabeculae, house the major vascular networks, lymphatics and nerves, and are analogous to the adventitial dermis (Fig. 1–18). Lipomas, benign tumors of normal-appearing fat cells, are recognized histologically by the absence of a normal trabeculate framework. The coiled secretory tubules of eccrine and apocrine glands, as well as the bulbs of scalp hair follicles, may be found in the subcutis.

The subcutaneous fat varies in thickness from one part of the body to another, being especially broad in the waist of the middle-aged and practically nonexistent on the eyelid. There are also regional differences between the sexes in deposition of fat, most notable in the rounded contours of the female torso. Besides this aesthetic role, the subcutaneous fat functions as a heat insulator, shock absorber, and a caloric-reserve depot.

NERVES

The skin is a major sense organ, serving as a receptor for a barrage of stimuli and a perceptor of man's environment. The sensations of touch, pressure, temperature, pain, and itch are received by millions of microscopic dermal nerve endings (Fig. 1–19). They are most numerous on hair-

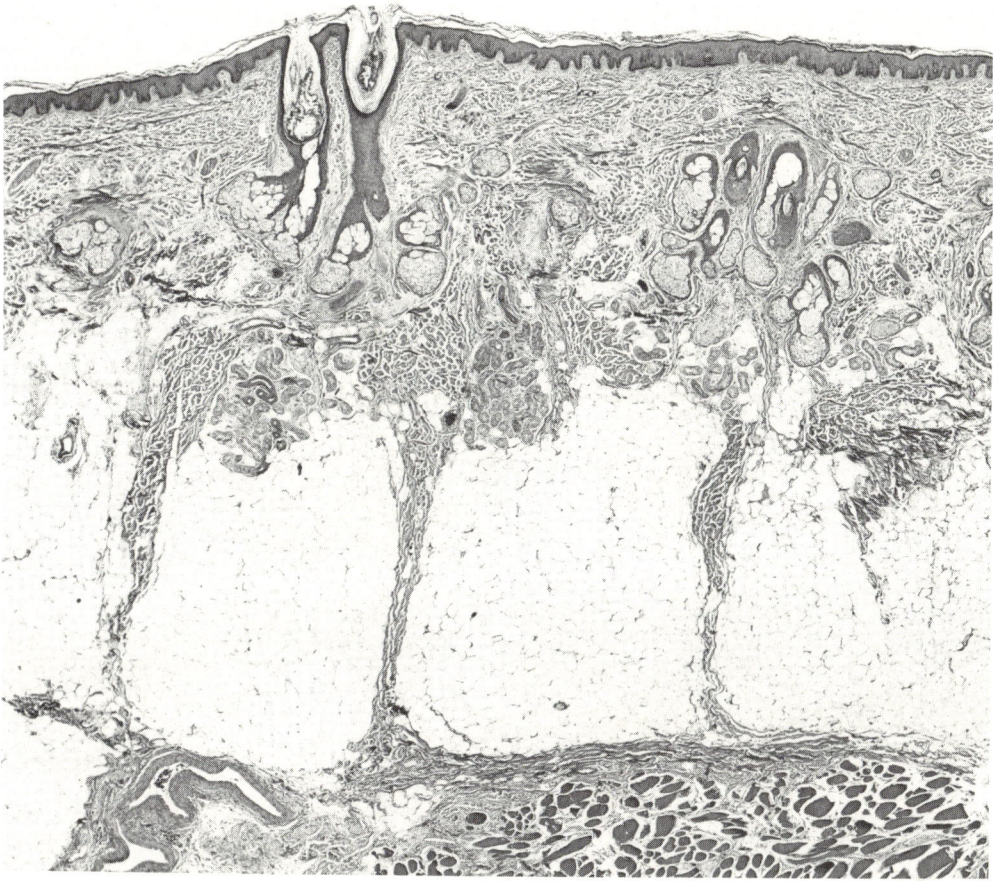

Figure 1–18 Strands of collagen divide the subcutaneous fat cells into lobules. These fibrous trabeculae house the major vascular networks, lymphatics, and nerves. (× 25.)

less parts (palms, soles, fingers) and mucocutaneous areas, especially the lips, glans penis, and clitoris, the erogenous zones. These tiny end organs terminate principally in the papillary dermis and around hair follicles. They are both free and encapsulated, myelinated and unmyelinated, and most are visualized with difficulty using the hematoxylin-and-eosin stain. Fine nerve endings require special staining with silver, methylene blue, or cholinesterase methods.

The sensations of temperature, pain, and itch are gathered by tiny unmyelinated nerves that end in the papillary dermis and surround the hair follicles. Stimuli received by these nerve endings are transmitted to the central nervous system by relatively slow conducting fibers.

Of all the sensations mediated by skin

receptors, itch is of greatest consequence to the patients of dermatologists. Itching is most simply defined as the desire to scratch and is conceived to be a type of mild pain. Although sensations of itch and pain are transmitted by the same fibers, the nerve impulse frequency in itching is appreciably lower than in pain. By scratching, especially furiously, the pruritic patient substitutes pain for itch, replacing the slower, maddening impulses with faster, more tolerable ones.

The sensations of touch and pressure are recorded by the specialized corpuscles of Meissner and Pacini. Anatomically, one can recognize Meissner's corpuscles in the papillary dermis on palms and soles as encapsulated nerve endings consisting of a cylindrical connective-tissue unit within which ramify myelinated and unmyelin-

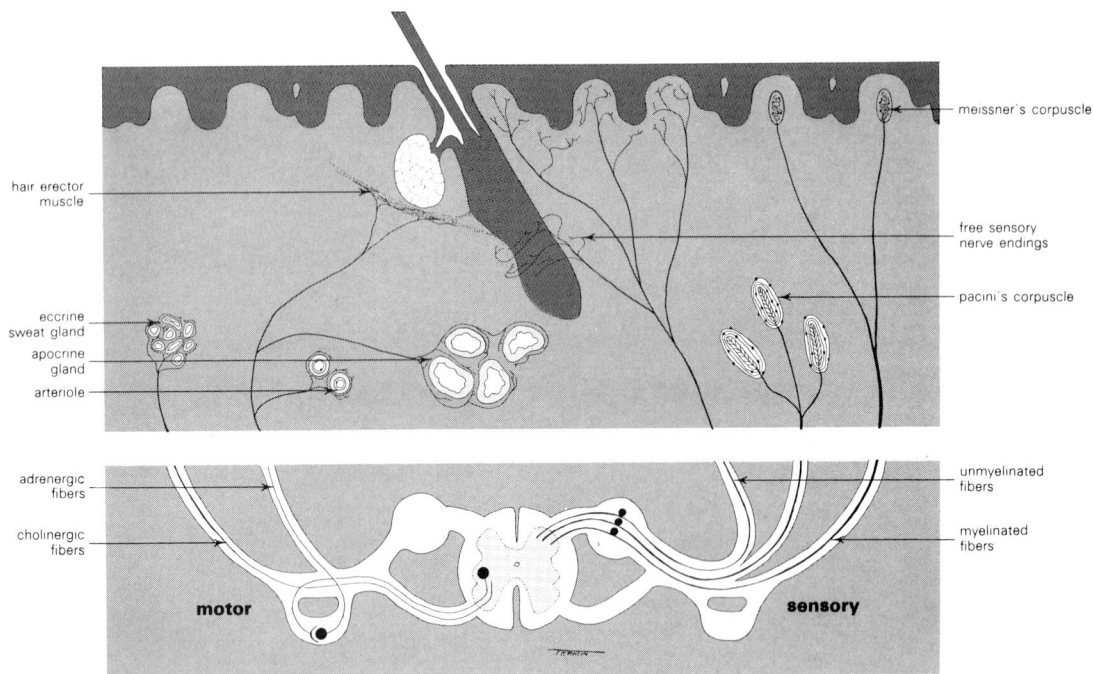

hair erector
muscle

eccrine
sweat gland

apocrine
gland

arteriole

adrenergic
fibers

cholinergic
fibers

motor

meissner's corpuscle

free sensory
nerve endings

pacini's corpuscle

unmyelinated
fibers

myelinated
fibers

sensory

Figure 1–19 Sensations of touch, pressure, temperature, pain, and itch are recorded by unmyelinated cutaneous nerve endings that transmit the impulses to the central nervous system via the dorsal root ganglia. All motor fibers in skin are supplied by the autonomic nervous system. Those that activate the arterioles, glomus body, hair erector muscle, and apocrine glands are adrenergic. Those that stimulate the eccrine sweat glands are cholinergic.

ated nerve fibers. Pacini's corpuscles are found particularly on weight-bearing surfaces. They are large encapsulated end organs composed of thin lamellae of fibrous tissue arranged in concentric fashion around the myelinated and unmyelinated nerve filaments. The impulses originating at these mechanoreceptors pass into myelinated fibers and are swiftly transmitted to the central nervous system.

All the cutaneous nerves, except those of the head, arise from the spinal cord. Peripheral sensory impulses return to the central nervous system via the dorsal root ganglia, where the cutaneous dendrites join their parent nerve cells and pass their signals on to the spinal cord.

The autonomic nervous system supplies the only motor fibers to the skin. The postganglionic fibers of the sympathetic nervous system conduct impulses that activate smooth-muscle cells in arteriole walls, the glomus body, and the myoepithelial cells of the apocrine gland. The fibers are adrenergic. Their stimulation of arteriolar

muscles produces vasoconstriction. Similar adrenergic nerves supply the hair erector muscles, which, upon contraction, pull the hair follicle into an upright position producing "goose flesh."

Cholinergic fibers form a rich bundle of terminal rami around the secretory portion of the eccrine gland and are instrumental in initiating production of sweat.

The sebaceous glands are mostly free of autonomic innervation and depend on endocrine stimuli for function.

THE EPIDERMIS

The epidermis is composed mostly of keratinocytes. The cells differentiate in the direction of the external environment to produce a cornified surface membrane. The process of differentiation whereby germinative keratinocytes move outward to become fully cornified cells takes approximately 14 days, and an additional 14 days are spent in transit through the cornified layer. The time required for a keratinocyte to traverse the entire epidermis is 28 days. The rate of epidermopoiesis varies slightly from one body site to another. Epidermal cells are constantly being shed from the body surface and continually being renewed in the germinative zone. Cell birth is in equilibrium with cell death.

The replacement of epidermal cells (mitosis) normally occurs at the bottom layer of the epidermis and, in very thick epidermis, in the second cell layer as well. In the basal layer, 3 to 5 per cent of the cells are synthesizing DNA at any given time. The daughter cells from each division may either remain in the basal layer or migrate upward and differentiate; about 50 per cent remain and 50 per cent move up. In pathologic processes such as psoriasis, or when the cornified layer is stripped with adhesive tape, a burst of mitosis occurs in the basal zone, causing replacement of the entire epidermal population in 24 to 72 hours. A similar phenomenon accounts for the scaling following sunburn.

During their upward migration toward maturation, keratinocytes undergo characteristic changes. One can recognize basal, spinous, granular, and cornified layers. These strata reflect stages in the conversion of a germinative keratinocyte to the end product of epidermal differentiation, the cornified keratinocyte. The four layers are not independent of one another but are interrelated and continuous phases in the life histories of epidermal cells. During the process of cornification, viable germinative keratinocytes are transformed by a series of biochemical events into dead keratinocytes (Fig. 1–20).

Three biologically separate species of keratinocytes live together in association within the epidermis (Fig. 1–21). Epidermal keratinocytes predominate, but adnexal keratinocytes course through the epidermis en route to the skin surface: intra-epidermal hair-follicle (acrotrichial) keratinocytes and intra-epidermal sweat-duct (acrosyringial) keratinocytes.

The single row of cuboidal-columnar–shaped basal keratinocytes contains relatively large round-oval nuclei and slightly more basophilic cytoplasm than the keratinocytes above it (Fig. 1–22). The polygonal-shaped cells of the suprabasal spinous layer assume a gradually more flattened configuration as they approach the surface. The spinous keratinocytes are named for the delicate "spines" (desmosomes) that are seen, with light microscopy, to cross the narrow intercellular spaces. Toward the surface, there are flattened diamond-shaped cells filled with coarse, irregularly shaped, darkly basophilic granules (keratohyaline granules). The outermost layer of the epidermis is formed by flat, anucleate, eosinophilic staining, cornified cells. In this manner, the vertically oriented, columnar basal cells are transformed into horizontally

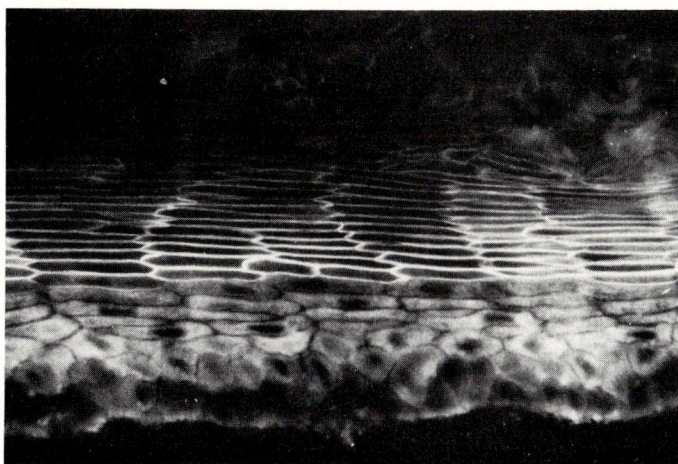

Figure 1–20 Cells in the cornified layer are arranged in vertical columns, resembling stacked pie plates. Cryostat section of guinea pig skin treated with 0.1 N sodium hydroxide. (Courtesy of Enno Christophers, M.D.)

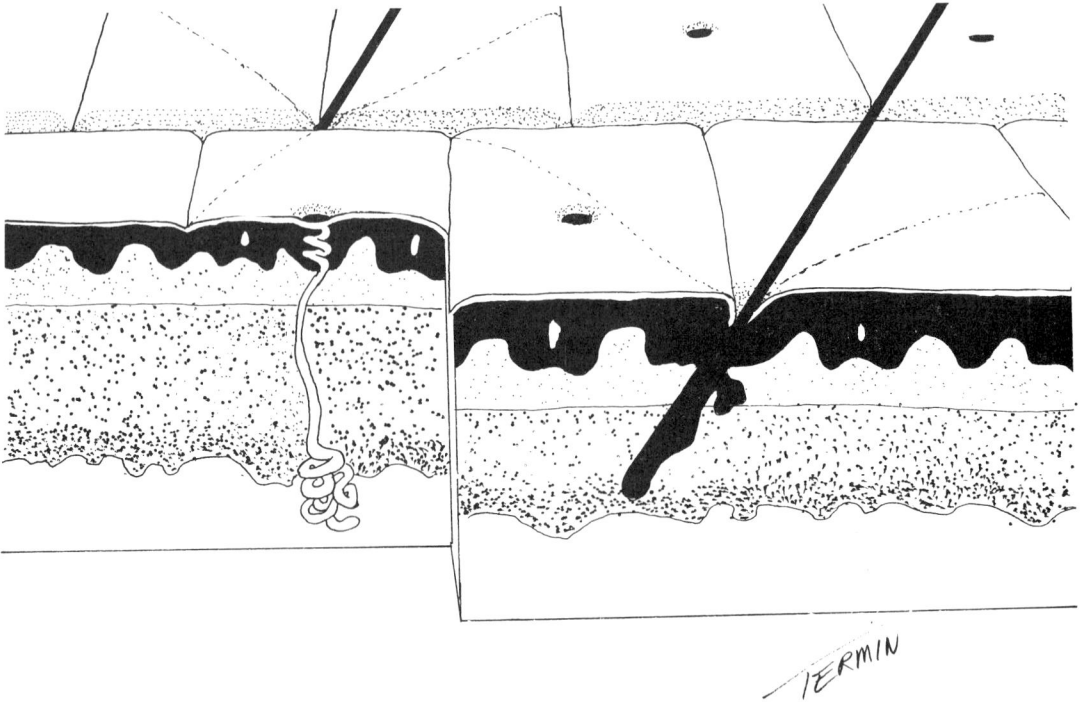

Figure 1–21 Adnexal keratinocytes pass through the epidermis en route to the skin surface. Intra-epidermal hair follicle keratinocytes and intra-epidermal sweat duct keratinocytes live together in intimate association with the dominant epidermal keratinocytes.

aligned, thin, cornified cells. Each pancake-shaped cornified cell covers the area occupied by about 25 basal cells.

With the electron microscope, one can obtain a more detailed view of the keratinocytic structural alterations during ascent. The basal-cell cytoplasm is packed with ribosomes which impart basophilia to hematoxylin and eosin–stained sections and indicate that the cell synthesizes protein. Present in basal-cell cytoplasm is a fundamental structure of all keratinocytes, the tonofibril, composed of a bundle of threads, 40 to 50 Å in width, called "tonofilaments." The basal-cell nucleus is large, with a prominent chromatin network and one or more nucleoli. Each cell is enclosed by a well-defined, highly convoluted cell membrane (Fig. 1–23). As the offspring of basal keratinocytes journey upward, the number of tonofibrils progressively increases, tonofilaments thicken to 70 Å, and the number of ribosomes decreases (Fig. 1–24). The tonofibrils are responsible for the eosinophilia of cornified cells stained with hema-

toxylin and eosin. At the top of the spinous layer, granules with a highly ordered lamellar internal structure appear near Golgi complexes and then scatter throughout the cytoplasm. Next, dense osmiophilic bodies that lack internal structure appear in what becomes the granular layer (Fig. 1–25). As the osmiophilic bodies and tonofibrils accumulate, the nucleus and most of the intracellular organelles disappear. The lamellar granules move to the region of the plasma membrane and are discharged into the intercellular space, presumably acting as a cementing substance for adherence of cornified cells. Concurrently, the thickness of the cell membranes in the cornified layer doubles, presumably owing to deposits upon them (Fig. 1–26).

The filamentous protein complex formed during epidermal differentiation results from the linking together of amino acid units into polypeptide chains. The basic molecule is hundreds of times longer than it is wide. The molecular chains are arranged side by side, with their long axis parallel and with numerous

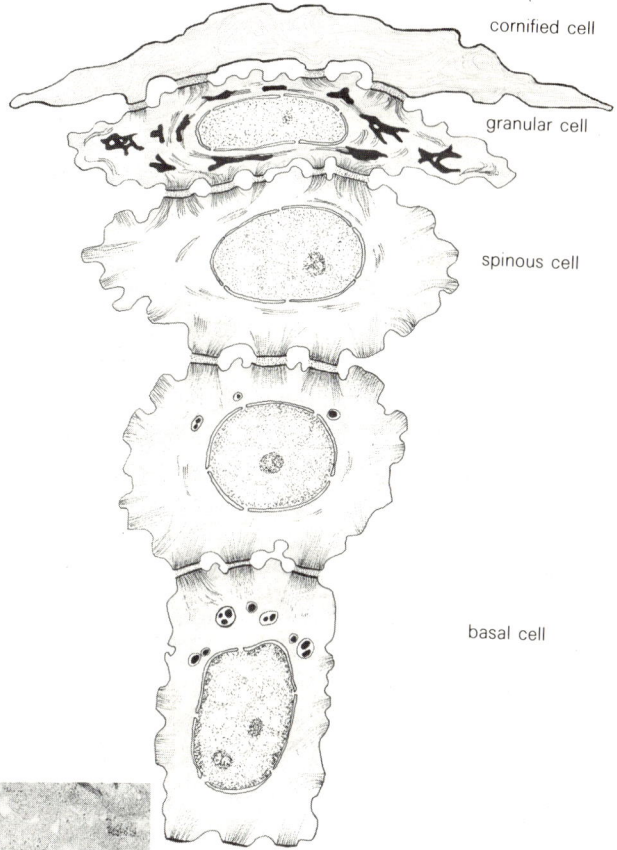

cornified cell

granular cell

spinous cell

basal cell

Figure 1–22 The basal, spinous, granular, and cornified layers reflect stages in the conversion of a germinative keratinocyte to the end product of epidermal differentiation, the cornified keratinocyte. The vertically oriented, columnar basal cells are transformed into horizontally aligned, thin cornified cells.

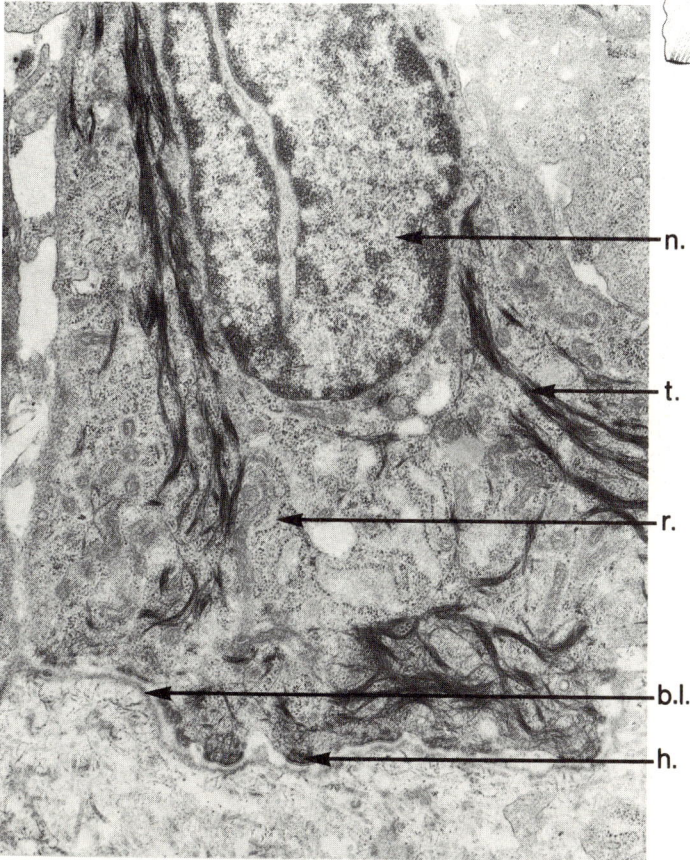

n.

t.

r.

b.l.

h.

Figure 1–23 Basal cell cytoplasm contains abundant mitochondria and ribosomes and relatively few tonofibrils, the fundamental structure of all keratinocytes. A basal cell is situated upon the basal lamina and is connected to it by a number of hemidesmosomes. *n.*, nucleus; *t.*, tonofibrils; *r.*, ribosomes; *b.l.*, basal lamina; *h.*, hemidesmosome. × 25,000. (Courtesy of Ken Hashimoto, M.D.)

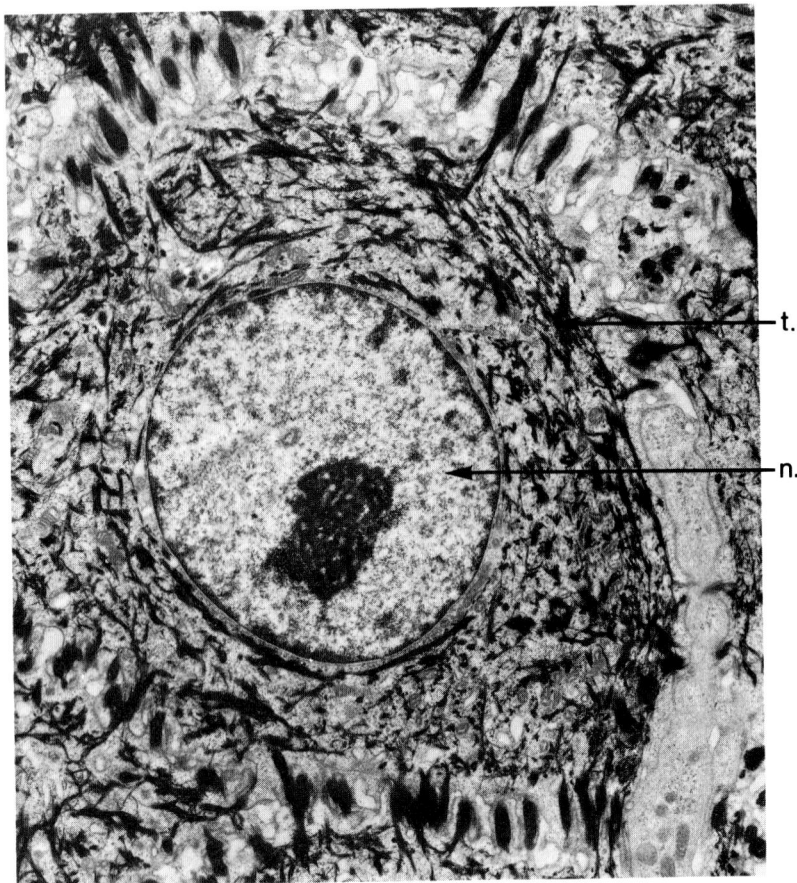

Figure 1–24 Spinous cell cytoplasm is almost entirely occupied by tonofibrils, except for a small number of mitochondria and scattered free ribosomes. The tonofibrils surround the nucleus and radiate toward the periphery, particularly converging upon desmosomes. *t.*, tonofibrils; *n.*, nucleus. (× 9,500.) (Courtesy of Ken Hashimoto, M.D.)

cross-linkages between them. The most important cross-linkages are the covalent disulfide bonds that stabilize the structure. Other cross-linkages that tend to keep the fibers in place are the weaker hydrogen and ionic bonds. The nonfilamentous matrix is sulfur-rich. In addition to the production of proteins during epidermal differentiation, lipids are also synthesized. Some fatty substances in the lipid film on the skin's surface arise from the epidermis, but most come from sebaceous glands.

In summary, epidermal cornified cells bear little resemblance to their progenitor basal cells. Nucleus and organelles are absent. The cell is filled with closely packed tonofibrils encased in a protein matrix. During differentiation, among other changes, keratinocytes: (1) change shape (flatten), (2) lose organelles, (3)

form fibrous proteins, (4) become dehydrated, and (5) thicken their cell membrane.

This same type of tough fibrous protein that constitutes the cornified cells of skin also forms the major component of claws and armor of reptiles, feathers and beaks of birds, and hooves, horns, hair, and nails of mammals. This protein, keratin, possesses enormously versatile properties. The principle differences among these various cornified end products of keratinocytic differentiation appear to be: (1) the mode of packing of the tonofibrils and (2) the amount and constitution of the sulfur-rich matrix in which they are embedded. By electron microscopic examination, the tonofibrils themselves seem to possess a remarkably uniform structure.

Epidermal cells are joined to one an-

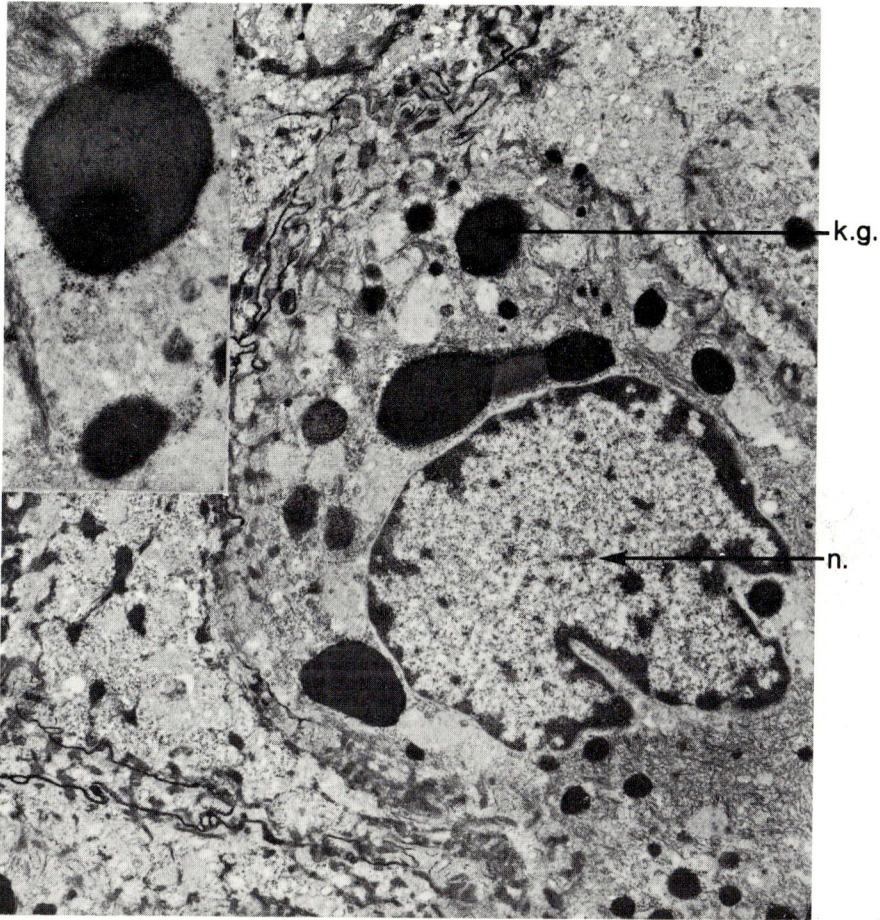

Figure 1–25   Granular cell cytoplasm contains keratohyaline granules, as well as tonofibrils and a few ribosomes. Smaller keratohyline granules represent immature forms, whereas larger ones often result from fusion of granules. *k.g.*, keratohyaline granule; *n.*, nucleus. (× 11,500; insert × 20,000.) (Courtesy of Ken Hashimoto, M.D.)

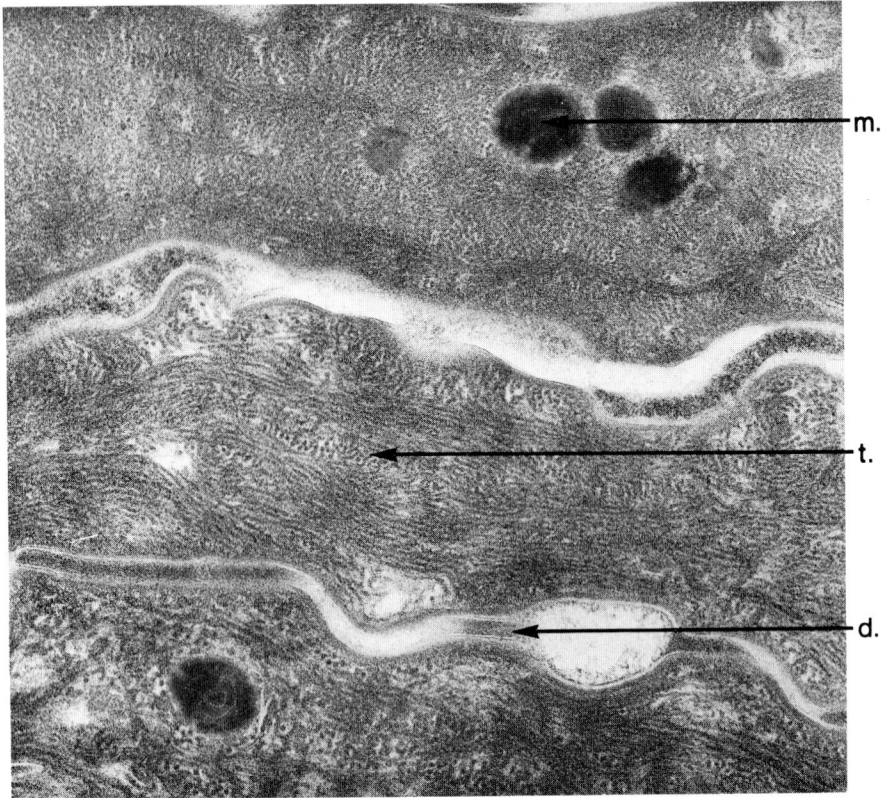

Figure 1-26 Cornified cells are still attached by vestigial desmosomes. The cornified cell is a package of tonofibrils that are encased in a protein matrix. The nucleus and cytoplasmic organelles have been lost during maturation. Pigment organelles, melanosomes, are contained within keratinocytes at all levels of the epidermis, including the cornified layer. *m.,* melanosome; *t.,* tonofibrils; *d.,* desmosome. (× 75,000.) (Courtesy of Ken Hashimoto, M.D.)

other by specialized intercellular attachment devices called desmosomes, characteristic of all epithelia (Fig. 1–27). These specializations along the plasma membrane are formed by multilayered electron-dense materials that occur on both sides of adjacent cell membranes. Tonofibrils sweep across the interior of the cell, where some loop and attach to the plasma membrane at the desmosome. Desmosomes provide firm mechanical attachment between adjacent cells, but they are thought to break and reform during the process of keratinocytic migration and maturation. Cleavage between desmosomes in the cornified layer results in desquamation.

Immediately beneath the basal layer, a thin zone of neutral mucopolysaccharide, the basement membrane, can be demonstrated with the light microscope, especially by the periodic acid-Schiff (PAS) stain

(Fig. 1–28). The basement membrane is usually not evident with hematoxylin and eosin stain. With the electron microscope, individual components of the basement membrane can be visualized: a basal lamina parallels the lower border of the basal-cell plasma membrane, from which it is separated by a thin electron-lucent intermembranous space (lamina lucida). Beneath the basal lamina are fibers of the papillary dermis. Hemidesmosomes attach the basal-cell plasma membrane to the basal lamina (Fig. 1–29).

The cornified layer, situated at the interface between man and his environment, serves as a shield without which life is not possible. This thin, flexible, transparent covering of cornified cells functions as:

1. *The body's major barrier,* possessing the vital properties of:
    a. Relative impermeability to water and electrolytes that prevents de-

hydration by loss of internal fluids and limits penetration by external fluids and gases.

b. Resistance against damaging corrosives.

c. Physical toughness that mutes the injurious effects of external trauma, such as mechanical injury.

d. High electrical impedance that restricts passage of electrical current.

e. Relatively dry surface that retards proliferation of microorganisms.

2. *A rate-limiting membrane* for passage of water and other molecules between the "wet" internal environment of the body and the "dry" external environment.

3. *A reservoir* for topical medications.

All of the cell strata of the cornified layer, 15 to 40 depending on the site, contribute to its barrier function. Although this layer is an effective barrier against the penetration of most substances, it is a perfect barrier to only a few. The ability of molecules, such as the oleoresin of poison ivy, to diffuse through the cornified layer enables development of allergic contact dermatitis.

There are three pathways by which external substances can be transported through the skin: (1) through adnexal orifices (pilosebaceous and sweat), (2) via intercellular spaces between the cornified cells, and (3) directly through the cornified cells.

Although the adnexal orifices account for only a fraction of the skin's total surface area, they are important to the transport of certain classes of molecules. During the first stage of transepidermal transport, before diffusion reaches a steady state, the adnexal orifices are the principal pathway

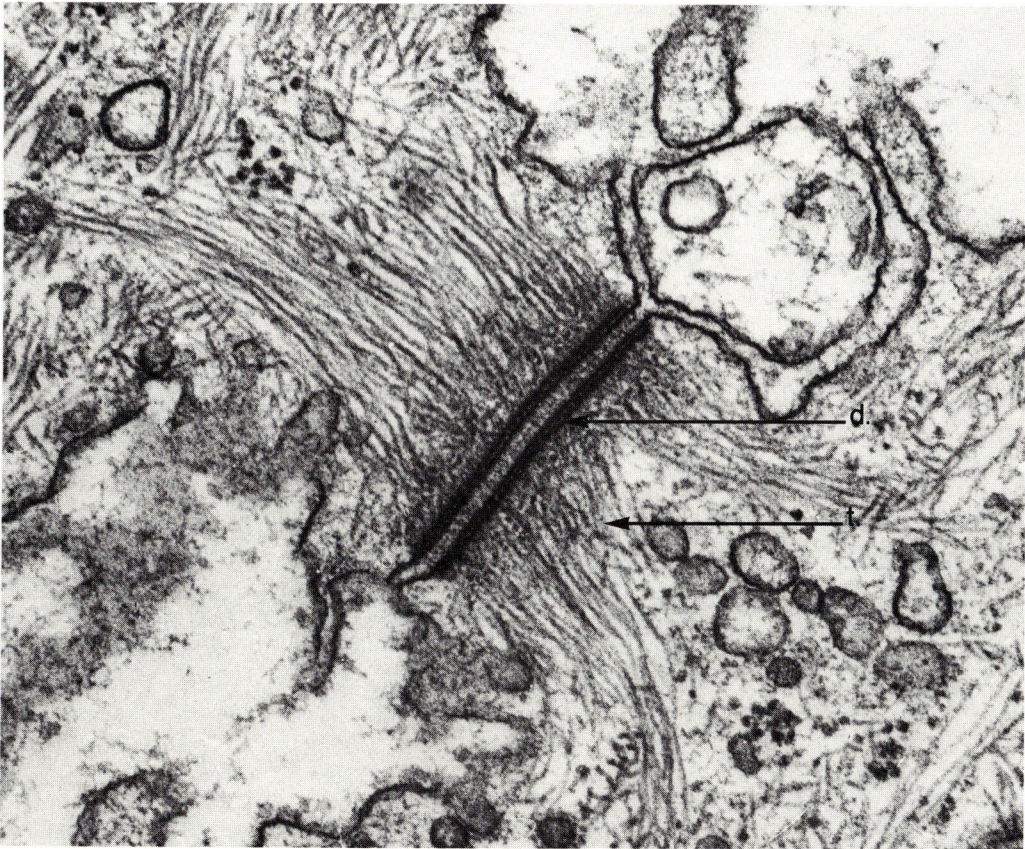

Figure 1–27 Looping of tonofibrils at the desmosomes between adjacent keratinocytes. *d.,* desmosome; *t.,* tonofilaments. (× 132,300.) (Courtesy of Douglas E. Kelly, Ph.D.)

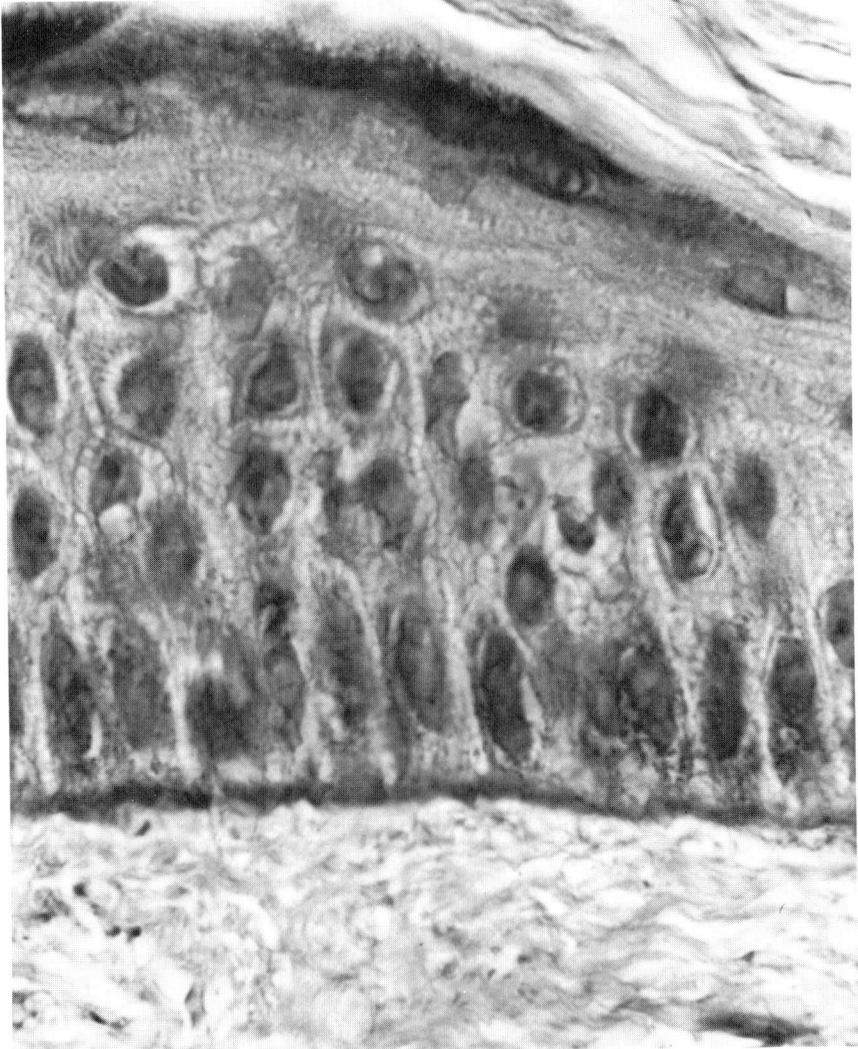

Figure 1–28   With the light microscope, the basement membrane is seen to be a band of PAS-positive neutral-mucopolysaccharide located immediately beneath the epidermal basal cell layer.

for penetration. The adnexal shortcut to percutaneous absorption is taken by molecules with very low permeability coefficients, and by large molecules.

Very little passage occurs via the intercellular route, except for water and low molecular weight, polar alcohols.

Most molecules move into the skin directly through the cell membranes and through the cells of the cornified layer. Experimentally, the isolated cornified layer is almost as impermeable as the whole skin. Once a substance has penetrated the cornified layer, it encounters very little further resistance en route to blood vessels and lymphatics in the papillary dermis. The relatively impermeable membrane formed by the cornified layer can be traversed more readily by: (1) increasing skin hydration, (2) increasing skin temperature, and (3) exposing it to lipid solvents. The cornified layer can imbibe up to several times its weight in water and, as hydration increases, so too does the transport of molecules through it.

The current mode of augmenting penetration of topical medications is to occlude the skin surface with plastic membranes. This method works by hydrating the cornified cells with trapped water of perspiration and insensible water loss and by increasing the skin's temperature. It has been shown that the cornified layer also acts as a reservoir for topically applied corticosteroids, releasing these over a period of days after a single application.

Several factors affect the absorption of substances through human skin including (1) the anatomic site which varies in thickness of the cornified layer and the number of adnexal orifices, (2) the local cutaneous circulation, (3) the properties of the vehicle, and (4) the properties of the penetrating molecule, such as its size, shape and lipid/water solubility characteristics.

Unique permeability properties of the cornified layer underlie its essential function in the maintenance of the body's water content and electrolyte concentration. When the cornified layer is altered, water loss and percutaneous absorption are increased; if the injury to the cornified layer is severe and widespread, death may result from dehydration or toxicity.

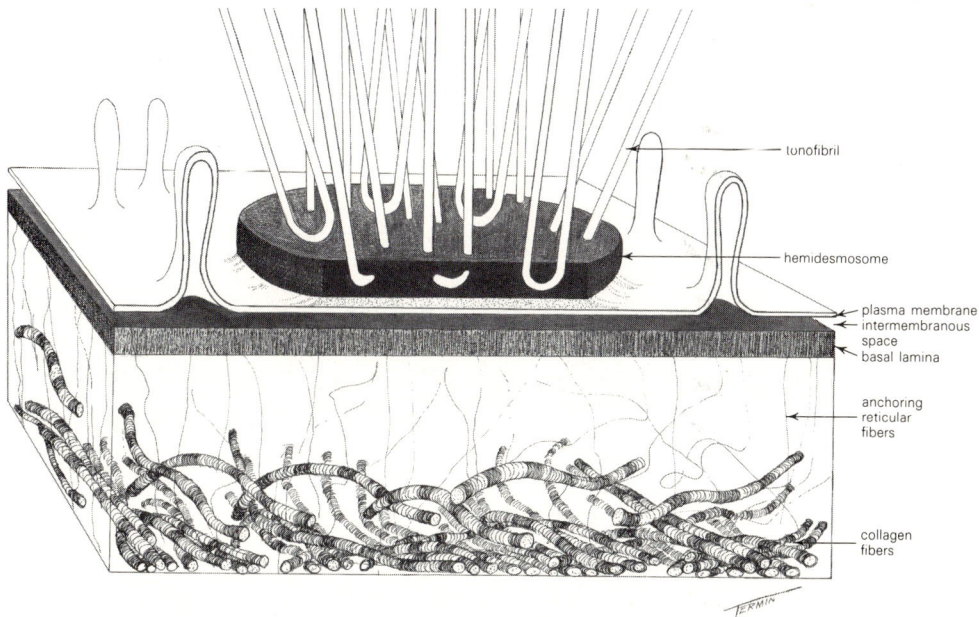

Figure 1–29 When studied with the electron microscope, the basement membrane is resolvable into several components. A basal lamina parallels the lower border of the basal cell plasma membrane, from which it is separated by a thin electron lucent intermembranous space (lamina lucida). Beneath the basal lamina are fibers of the papillary dermis. Hemidesmosomes attach the basal cell plasma membrane to the basal lamina. (After Douglas E. Kelly, Ph.D.)

THE MELANOCYTE

Melanocytes are dendritic cells that synthesize and secrete melanin pigment. Presumably, they are derived from the neural crest and migrate to the epidermis, mucous membrane epithelia, dermis, hair follicles, leptomeninges, uveal tract, retina, and other tissues (Fig. 1–30). In the skin, melanocytes are situated at the dermo-epidermal junction, except for those that remain behind in the dermis. Dermal melanocytes are seen in blue sacral patches (Mongolian spots) and other blue nevi.

On the skin, melanocytes are present in all body sites, but their distribution varies. For example, they are more abundant on the cheek than on the trunk, and the ratio of melanocytes to keratinocytes in the basal layer varies from 1:4 to 1:10 depending on the region. With advancing age, the ratio shifts further in favor of the keratinocytes. The relative number of melanocytes is the same for both sexes and for all races. Differences in coloration among the races result, not from differences in the number of melanocytes, but from their activity as gauged by the rate and amount of melanin produced; melanocytes of dark races make more melanin. The intensity of skin coloration is further determined by the total number, size, and intracellular distribution of melanin granules within epidermal keratinocytes.

With the light microscope, epidermal melanocytes appear as "clear cells" in and immediately beneath the basal cell layer (Fig. 1–31). The clear space is an artifact of fixation due to the collapse of the melanocytic cytoplasm around the nucleus. The melanocyte nucleus is smaller and more deeply basophilic than that of the

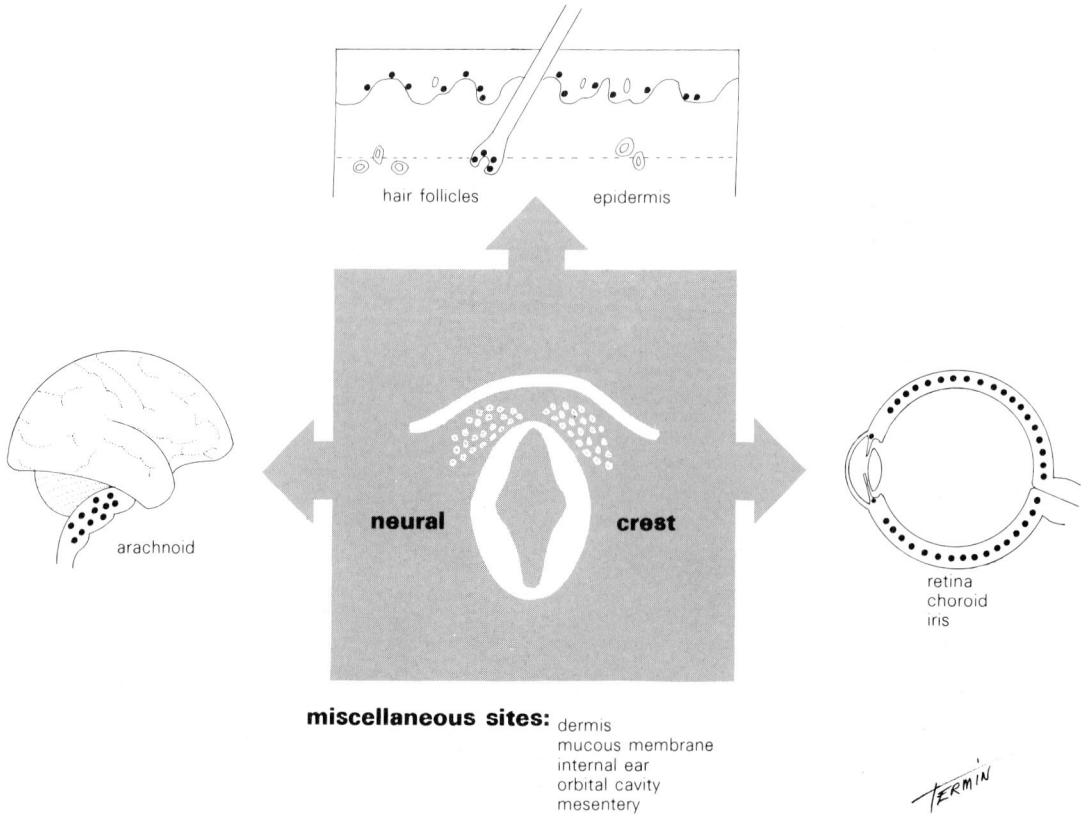

Figure 1–30   Melanocytes are presumably derived from the neural crest and migrate to the epidermis, mucous membrane epithelia, dermis, hair follicles, leptomeninges, uveal tract, retina, and other tissues. Black dots represent melanocytes.

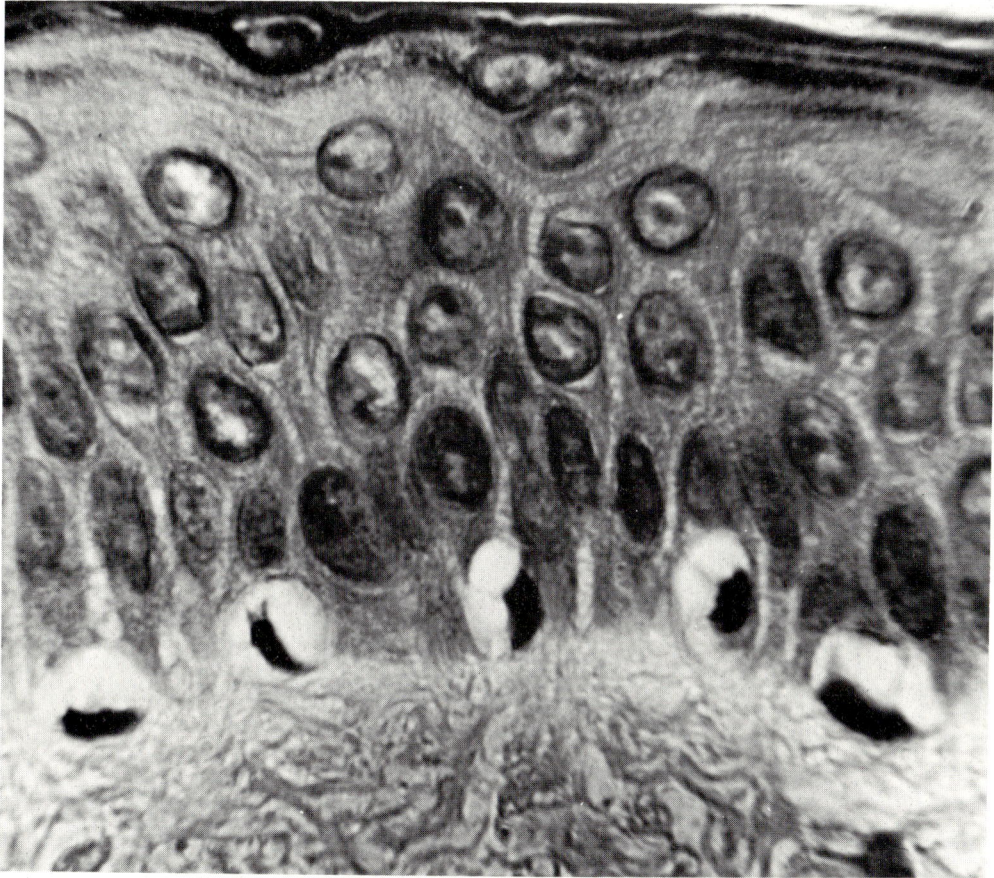

Figure 1–31 With the light microscope, epidermal melanocytes appear as "clear cells" in and immediately beneath the basal cell layer. This clear space is an artifact of fixation due to collapse of the melanocyte cytoplasm around the nucleus. The melanocyte nucleus is smaller and more deeply basophilic than that of the contiguous keratinocytes. (× 1350.)

keratinocytes. Although all levels of the epidermis, including the cornified layer, contain melanin pigment, the basal layer is the most heavily pigmented. Melanocytes can be better seen by staining with silver salts, which combine with the melanin pigment to form a black deposit. Melanin granules are concentrated in umbrella-like array above each nucleus on the side toward the skin surface. Melanocyte dendrites extend in all directions, laterally along the basal layer, downward toward the dermis, and upward between the keratinocytes in the spinous layer (Figs. 1–32 and 1–33).

Seen under the electron microscope, the melanocyte appears to be a protein-synthesizing cell with large mitochondria, rough endoplasmic reticulum containing many ribosomes, prominent Golgi apparatus, and no tonofibrils or desmosomes. Inside the cytoplasm of melanocytes are special organelles called "melanosomes" (Fig. 1–34). These are spherical or ellipsoid membrane-bounded particles (Fig. 1–35) with a highly organized internal structure composed of longitudinally oriented concentric lamellae with a characteristic periodicity (Fig. 1–36).

Melanosomes are the site of melanin formation. This process unfolds as follows:

1. Tyrosinase, a copper-containing enzyme, is synthesized in ribosomes.

2. Tyrosinase is transferred to the region of the Golgi apparatus by way of rough endoplastic reticulum.

3. Tyrosinase is assembled into units surrounded by a smooth-surfaced mem-

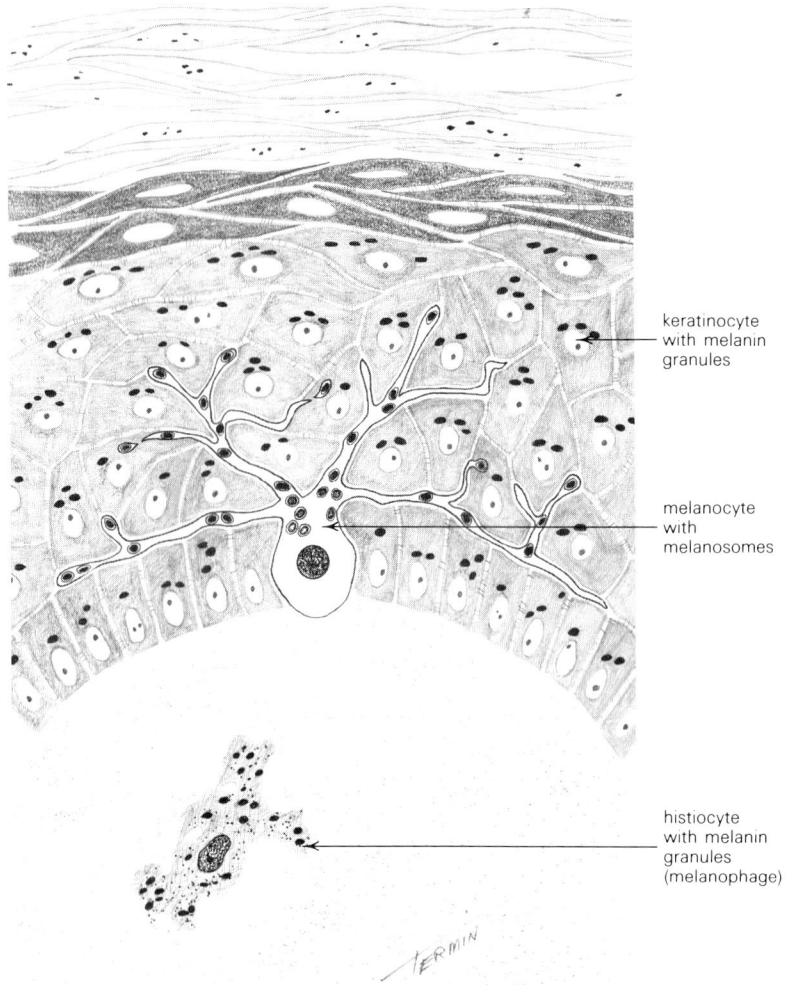

keratinocyte
with melanin
granules

melanocyte
with
melanosomes

histiocyte
with melanin
granules
(melanophage)

Figure 1–32   Melanocyte dendrites extend in all directions, especially laterally along the basal cell layer and upward between the keratinocytes in the spinous layer. Once melanin is formed, it is transferred from melanocytes into keratinocytes by apocopation.

brane, forming a vesicle called a "melanosome." This vesicle contains protein filaments that have a distinct periodicity of 100 Å.

4. Melanin particles are gradually deposited on the inner membranes, partly obscuring the internal structure of the melanosomes.

5. Melanin deposits eventually fill the entire melanosome, which then becomes a dense melanin granule.

The biochemical concomitants of these morphologic events are still being elucidated. Melanogenesis occurs entirely within the melanosome and involves the conversion of the colorless amino acid tyrosine into the brown-black polymer, melanin, which binds to a protein to form melanoprotein. During the initial step of the reaction, the enzyme tyrosinase, in the presence of oxygen, catalyzes the hydroxylation of tyrosine to form dihydroxyphenylalanine (DOPA). Tyrosinase then oxidizes DOPA to form DOPA-quinone. The remainder of the reaction proceeds in the absence of tyrosinase and ends with the formation of melanoprotein. In the process, the enzymatically active melanosomes are transferred into inert melanin granules.

Melanin is a complex polymer containing many quinone groups, with an extremely high molecular weight; it is insoluble in most solvents and resistant to most chemical treatments. The general absorption spectrum of melanin, in the range of 200 to 2400 nm., covers the entire range of ultraviolet and visible light. Once melanin is formed, it is transferred from melanocytes into keratinocytes by apocopation. The keratinocytes actively engulf the melanin-filled tips of melanocytic dendrites, resulting in the discharge of melanin granules into both epidermal and hair keratinocytes. Thus, melanin-making cells (melanocytes) and melanin-taking cells (keratinocytes) constitute a biologic unit. The interdependence and interaction of melanocytes and keratinocytes are witnessed in a variety of pathologic processes ranging from blockage of melanosome transfer in certain keratinocytic hyperplasias and neoplasias to excessive transfer of melanosomes in postinflammatory hyperpigmentation. Once transferred to the keratinocyte, the fully melanized melanosomes are partially degraded by

lysosomal enzymes or desquamated with the cornified cells. Exposure to ultraviolet light expedites the delivery of melanosomes to keratinocytes. During the tanning of skin by ultraviolet light, more melanosomes are manufactured and available for discharge into newly formed keratinocytes.

The principal function of melanin is to screen the skin from the sun's harmful ultraviolet rays by absorbing their radiant energy. Melanosomes both scatter and absorb the ultraviolet light. The damaging effects of sunlight on unpigmented skin are evident in albinism. In this condition, melanocytes are present, but their melanosomes lack the enzyme tryrosinase requisite for melanin production. Solar keratosis and all forms of skin cancer develop in albinos who are exposed to the sun's rays.

There are three major controls of melanin production: (1) genetic, (2) environmental, and (3) hormonal. The prime examples of genetic influence are differences in skin coloration among the races. Diseases resulting in altered pigmentation,

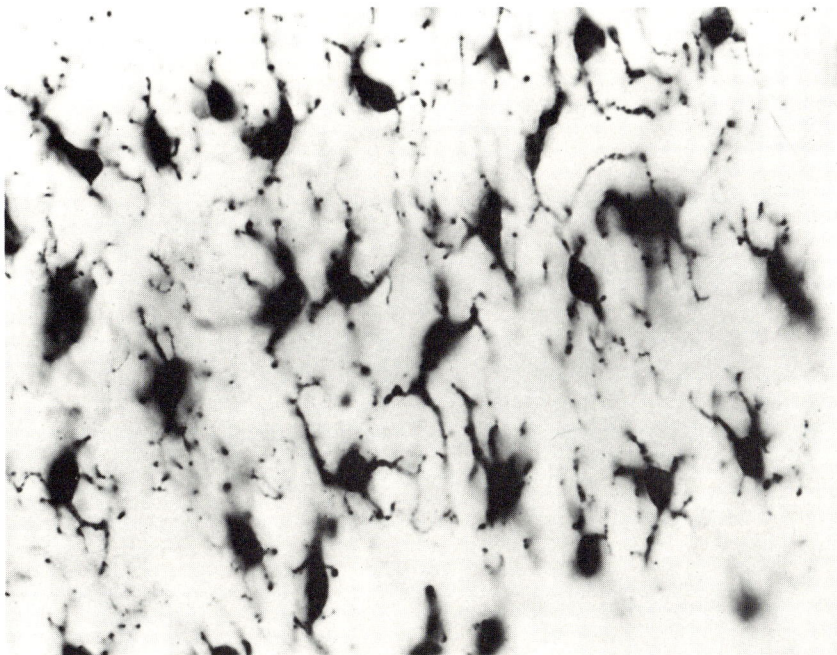

Figure 1–33 Melanocyte dendrites are particularly well demonstrated in this split-skin preparation from a Rhesus monkey that has been irradiated for 28 days with ultraviolet light and stained with DOPA. (Courtesy of William Montagna, Ph.D.)

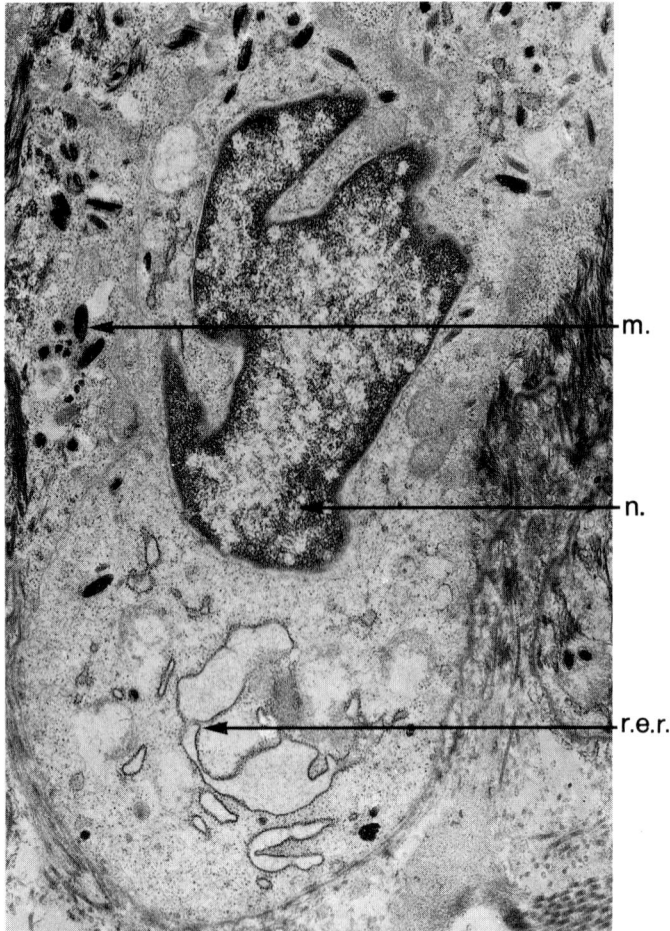

Figure 1–34 A melanocyte is distinguished by the presence of melanosomes and the absence of tonofibrils. *m.,* melanosome; *n.,* nucleus; *r.e.r.,* rough endoplasmic reticulum. (× 17,000.) (Courtesy of Ken Hashimoto, M.D.)

such as albinism and phenylketonuria, are also transmitted genetically.

Examples of environmental influences on skin and appendageal pigmentation, in addition to ultraviolet light, are: (1) depigmenting effects of chemical compounds, such as the various hydroquinones, (2) the conversion of dark hair to blond with hydrogen peroxide by the oxidation of melanin to a colorless compound, and (3) altered pigmentation that often follows inflammatory reaction in the skin.

Overproduction of the pituitary peptides, melanocyte stimulating hormone (MSH) and adrenocorticotropic hormone (ACTH), is responsible for the hyperpigmentation of Addison's disease and adrenogenital syndrome, whereas their absence in panhypopituitarism causes generalized hypopigmentation. In pregnancy, darkening of the nipples and patchy facial hyperpigmentation (melasma) result from the combined effects of MSH, estrogen, and possibly progesterone. Another illustration of the role of sex hormones in promoting pigmentation is found in eunuchs, who tan poorly when exposed to ultraviolet light, unless they are given androgens.

Melatonin, a hormone synthesized in the pineal gland, lightens the skin of adult frogs by aggregating melanin granules around the nuclei. MSH and adrenalin reverse this process, causing dispersion of the granules within the cytoplasm and darkening of the frog's skin. There is scant evidence for these reactions in man.

In addition to melanocytes, other

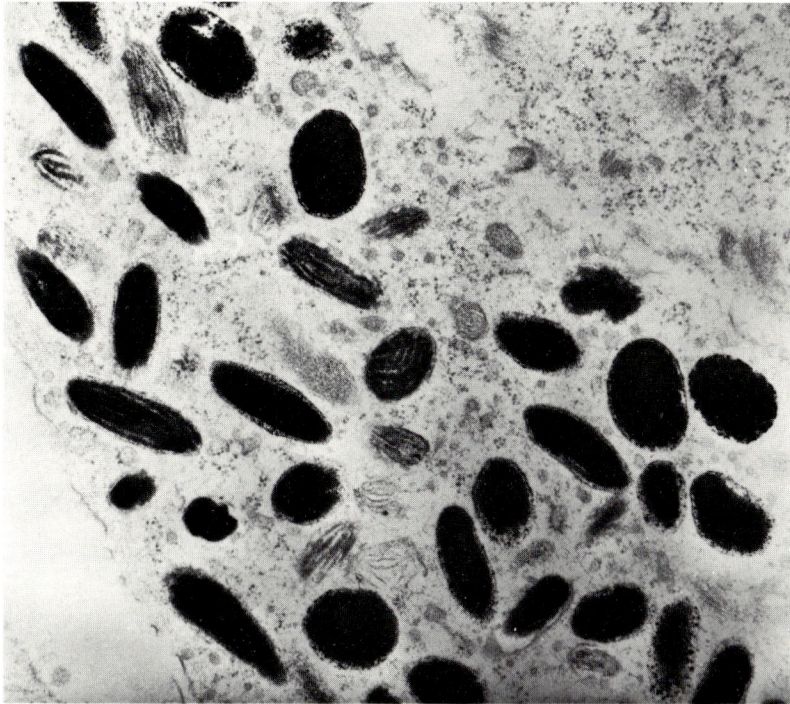

Figure 1–35 Melanosomes, spherical and ellipsoidal membrane-bounded particles, at various stages of development. (Courtesy of Alvin Zelickson, M.D.)

dendritic clear cells are found within the normal epidermis as early as the fourteenth week of fetal life. These cells, called Langerhans' cells, are often referred to as "high-level dendritic cells" because

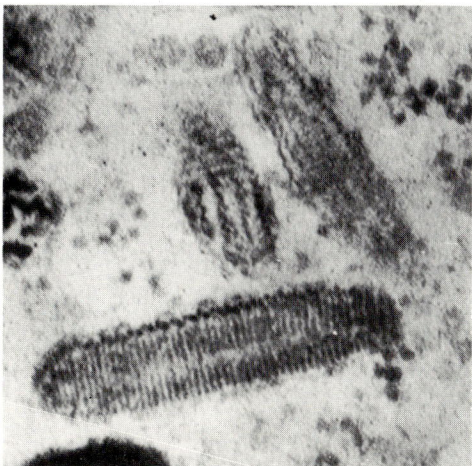

Figure 1–36 Melanosomes have a highly organized internal structure composed of longitudinally oriented concentric lamellae with a characteristic periodicity. (× 92,900.) (Courtesy of Alvin Zelickson, M.D.)

they usually reside in the upper part of the epidermis. Unlike melanocytes, Langerhans' cells do not possess tyrosinase (as evidenced by their negative staining reaction with DOPA), do not increase in number after stimulation by ultraviolet light, are relatively constant in number from one region of the body to another, are stained by gold chloride, and increase in number in vitiligo, a condition characterized by the virtual absence of melanocytes.

Electron microscopy is reliable for distinguishing Langerhans' cells from melanocytes. Langerhans' cells have a convoluted notched nucleus and contain characteristic granules with a "tennis-racquet" configuration resulting from vesicular dilatation at one end of the organelle (Fig. 1–37). Langerhans' cells, like other non-melanin-making cells, such as keratinocytes and histiocytes, may also possess melanin granules. These granules are contributed solely by melanocytes, the only cells known to be capable of melanin synthesis. The function of Langerhans' cells is unknown.

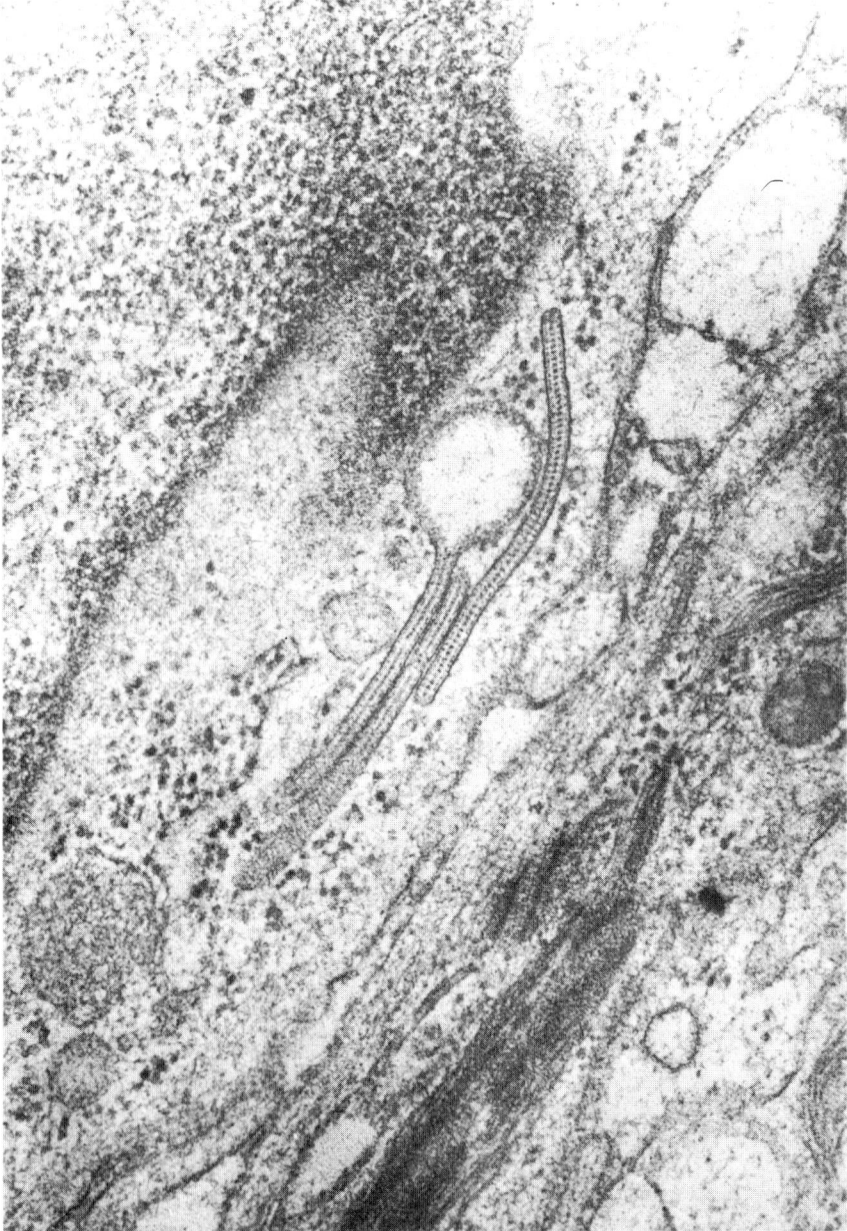

Figure 1–37   Langerhans' granules have a tennis-racquet configuration resulting from vesicular dilatation at one end of the organelle. (× 82,600.) (Courtesy of Alvin Zelickson, M.D.)

THE HAIR FOLLICLE

Man is, at the same time, a naked and a hairy animal. Only the palms, soles, and a few other areas do not contain hair. Over most of the body surface the hairs are vestigial. Even the apparently hairless baby is covered with inconspicuous hairs.

The protective value of hair, so important in furry animals against heat loss in the cold and against sunburn in the tropics, is insignificant in man.

The fetus is covered by wisps of lightly pigmented hairs, called "lanugo." Similar fine hairs in the adult are termed "vellus." Even when an individual seems bald, vellus hairs are actually present. In the adult, the coarse pigmented hairs, named "terminal hairs," are best developed on the scalp, beard, and pubic and axillary regions. A single scalp follicle initially produces a lanugo hair, later a terminal hair, and finally, with baldness, a vellus hair.

Hair is different, morphologically and biologically, on different parts of the body. Hairs vary in structure, length, rate of growth, and responses to various stimuli. For instance, sex hormones do not directly govern the development of eyelashes and eyebrows, yet body, axillary, pubic, and facial hairs are directly dependent upon hormonal stimulation for their adult characteristics. These latter hairs are part of the ensemble composing the secondary sexual characteristics. They wax and wane with the physiologic flow of sex hormones, becoming prominent at puberty and regressing with senescence.

The same hormone may simultaneously influence the growth of hairs in different regions in opposite ways. This is illustrated by the administration of testosterone to eunuchs. Ordinarily, male castrates do not become bald, yet they have no significant pelage over the rest of the body other than the scalp. When androgens are given, this situation is reversed: they begin losing their scalp hair in typical male-baldness patterns and acquire hair elsewhere on the body, characteristic of normal men.

Morphologic and quantitative differences in hair exist among the races. Caucasoids are hairiest and Mongoloids least hairy, with Negroids in between. Morphologically, hairs can be divided into four major categories: straight, wavy, helical, and spiral. Mongoloid hairs are straight, because the hair follicle is oriented at right angles to the skin surface. Negroid hairs are spiral owing to curvature of the hair follicle with the concavity facing the skin surface. Caucasoid hairs include all of the major classes. Physically and chemically, there are no significant differences in hair properties among the races.

The hair follicle and its hair are fundamentally one structure, derived from undifferentiated cells of the fetal epidermis. In longitudinal sections, the hair structure can be divided anatomically into three segments: (1) infundibular, the upper, funnel-shaped invagination that extends from the pilar orifice above to the entrance of the sebaceous duct below, (2) isthmus, the short midsection of the follicle bounded superiorly by the sebaceous duct and inferiorly by the insertion of the hair erector muscle, and (3) inferior, extending from the muscle insertion to the base of the follicle (Fig. 1–38).

The expanded lower terminus of the follicle is the hair bulb, which encloses an ovoid-shaped vascular, connective-tissue papilla. The round, uniform-appearing matrix cells of the bulb have a relationship to the hair papilla similar to that of the basal cells of the epidermis to the papillary dermis. Through a narrow outlet at the distal end of the bulb, the papilla emerges to

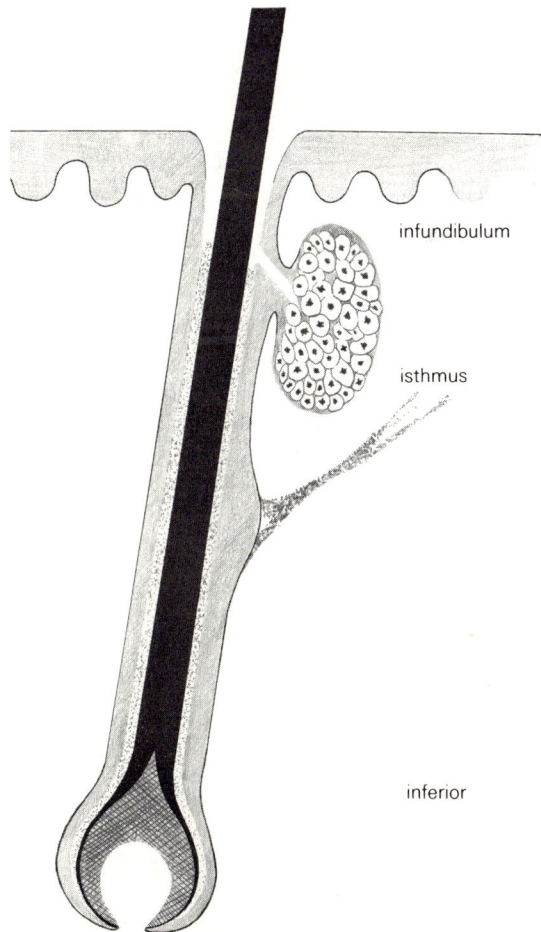

Figure 1–38 The three I's of pilar anatomy: infundibular, isthmus, and inferior.

become continuous with the connective-tissue sheath that envelops the entire follicle (periadnexal dermis). Concentric circular and longitudinal layers of collagen fibers, with their associated fibroblasts, comprise the outermost fibrous sheath. A "glassy" PAS-positive basement membrane, composed of reticular fibers and neutral mucopolysaccharides, separates the fibrous sheath from the follicular epi-

thelium of the outer root sheath. A thin rim of outer root sheath epithelial cells encloses the hair bulb (Fig. 1–39). Most of the mitotic activity occurs within the matrix cells in the bottom half of the bulb. Melanocytes are situated mostly in the upper half of the bulb (Fig. 1–40) and, to a lesser extent, in the outer root sheath.

Unlike epidermal germinative cells, which produce only one population (spin-

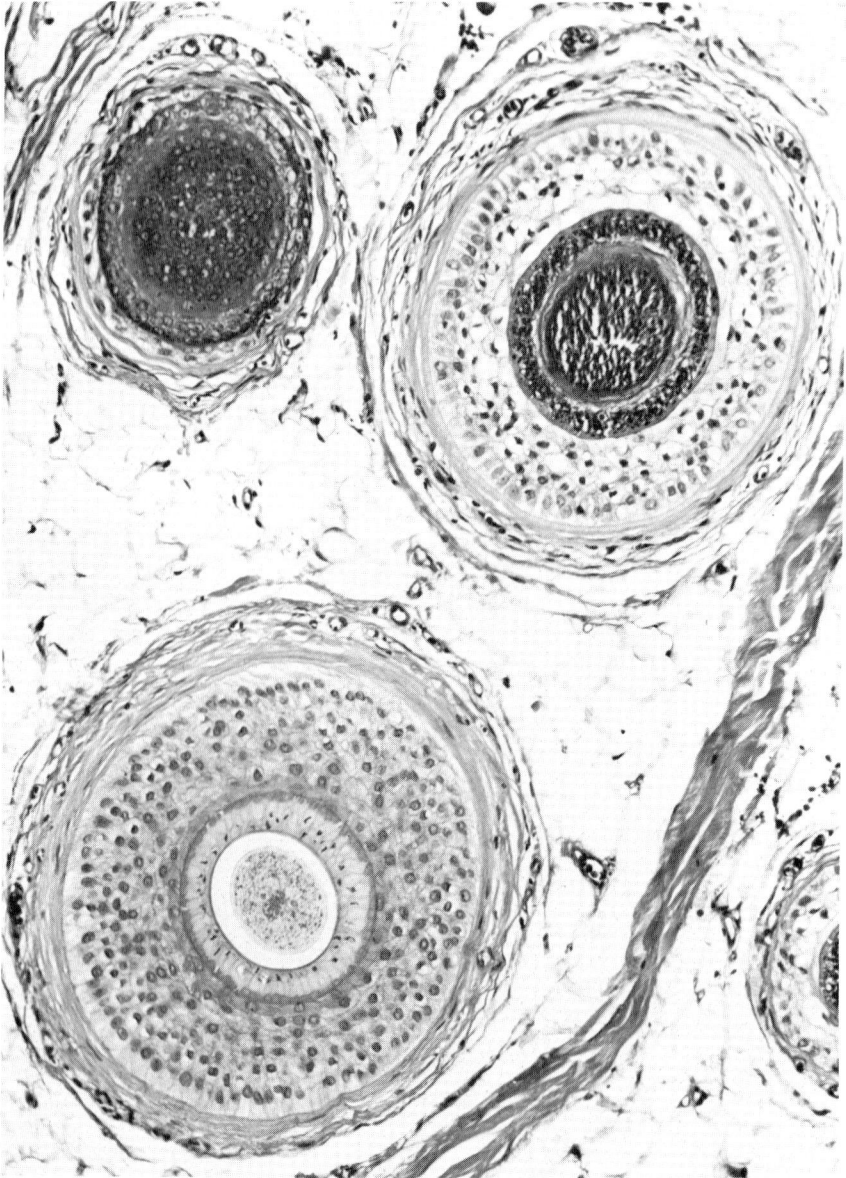

Figure 1–39 Cross-sections through different levels of the inferior segment of the hair follicle. ($\times$ 176.)

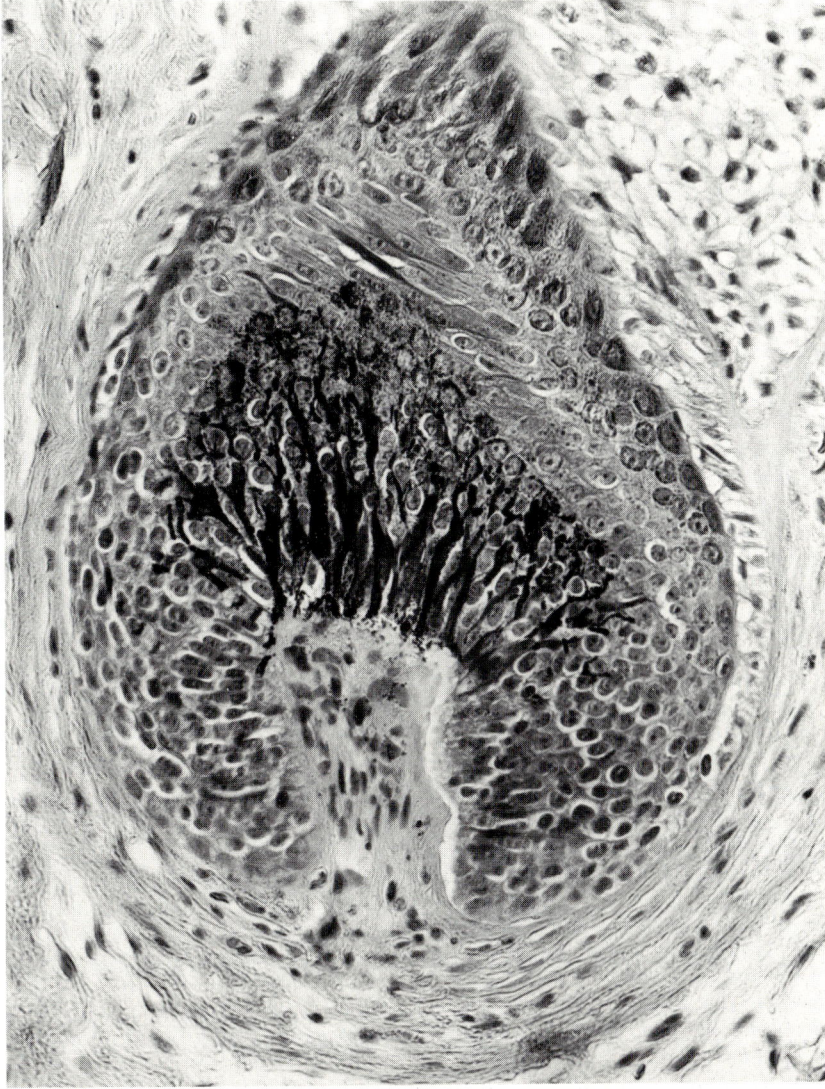

Figure 1–40   Dendritic melanocytes are situated in the upper half of the hair bulb. (× 352.)

ous cells), the cells of the hair matrix differentiate along six separate lines. These changes are first detected near the base of the bulb. Here the plump matrix cells give rise to elongate cells that form the three concentric layers of the inner root sheath and the three concentric layers of the hair itself (Figs. 1–41 and 1–42). From the outside inward, these are (1) Henle's layer, the first to cornify and only one cell thick, (2) Huxley's layer, characterized by brightly eosinophilic-staining trichohyaline granules and two cells thick, (3) cuticle of the inner root sheath, (4) cuticle of the hair, (5) hair cortex, and (6) hair medulla. Enveloping this central core of matrix is the pale-staining, relatively broad, outer root sheath composed of glycogen-filled cells. The mechanism whereby a similar-appearing population of hair matrix cells produces six morphologically different end products in concentric arrangement is unknown. It has been proposed that cells at equal distance from the base of the egg-shaped papilla undergo the same type of differentiation.

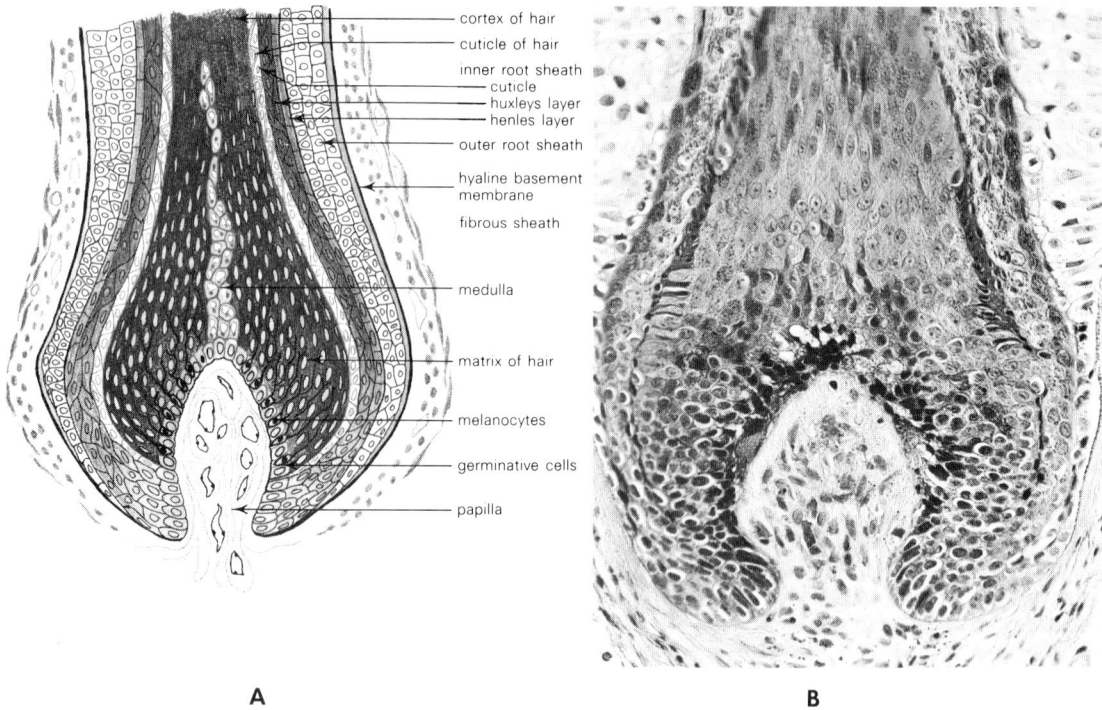

A   B

Figure 1-41   The cells of the hair matrix differentiate along six separate lines. From outside inward, as shown in *A*, these are Henle's layer, the first to cornify and only one cell thick; Huxley's layer, characterized by brightly eosinophilic-staining trichohyaline granules and two cells thick; cuticle of the inner root sheath; cuticle of the hair; hair cortex; and hair medulla. Surrounding the central core of matrix products is the pale staining, relatively broad, outer root sheath. Through a narrow outlet at the distal end of the bulb, the papilla emerges to become continuous with the connective tissue sheath that envelops the entire follicle. *B*, Photomicrograph of hair matrix. (× 374.)

All hair follicles are associated with some sensory nerves, suggesting that hairs also participate in the cutaneous sensory system (Fig. 1–43).

The matrix cells are a pool of undifferentiated cells with intense activity. The mitotic rate of the active hair matrix is greater than that of any other normal tissue, with the possible exception of bone marrow, being completely replaced every 12 to 24 hours. The matrix products, inner root sheath and hair, move outward, gliding over the passive, relatively stationary, outer root sheath. In contrast, the cuticle of the inner root sheath interdigitates with the cuticle of the hair so that the hair and inner root sheath ascend together at the same pace.

An anatomic change occurs at the isthmus. It is delimited below by the insertion of the hair erector muscle to which it is tied by elastic tissue (Fig. 1–44). The entire follicle beneath the isthmus, the inferior segment, can be considered "temporary" because it disappears during the involutional stage of the hair cycle and reforms again during the growth phase. The upper segments, isthmus and infundibulum, are "permanent." At the isthmus, the cells of the inner root sheath disintegrate, and the outer root sheath, no longer in contact with an inner root sheath, begins to cornify (Fig. 1–45).

Another anatomic boundary of the hair follicle is marked by the entry of the sebaceous duct into the follicular wall. This point forms the upper limit of the isthmus and the lower pole of the infundibulum. The infundibulum passes through the epidermis (acrotrichium) and opens onto the skin surface. Infundibular epithelium is morphologically identical to

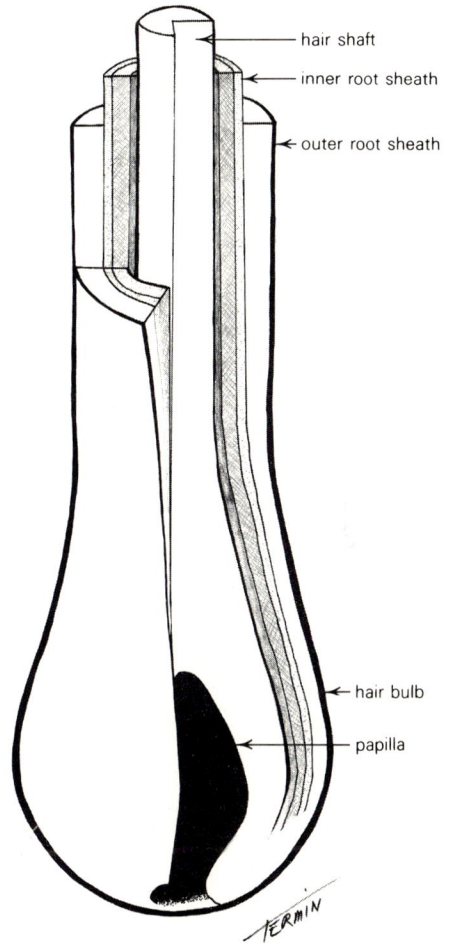

Figure 1–42   The inferior segment of the hair follicle.

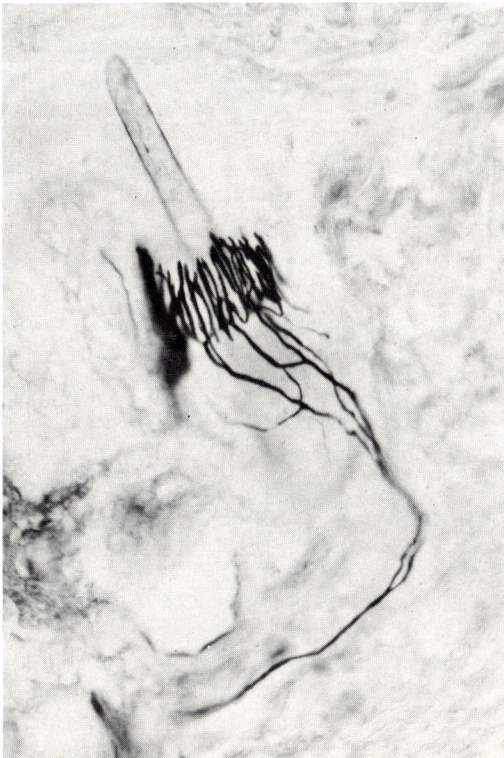

Figure 1–43   End organ of vellus hair follicle demonstrated by silver impregnation after cholinesterase. (Courtesy of William Montagna, Ph.D.)

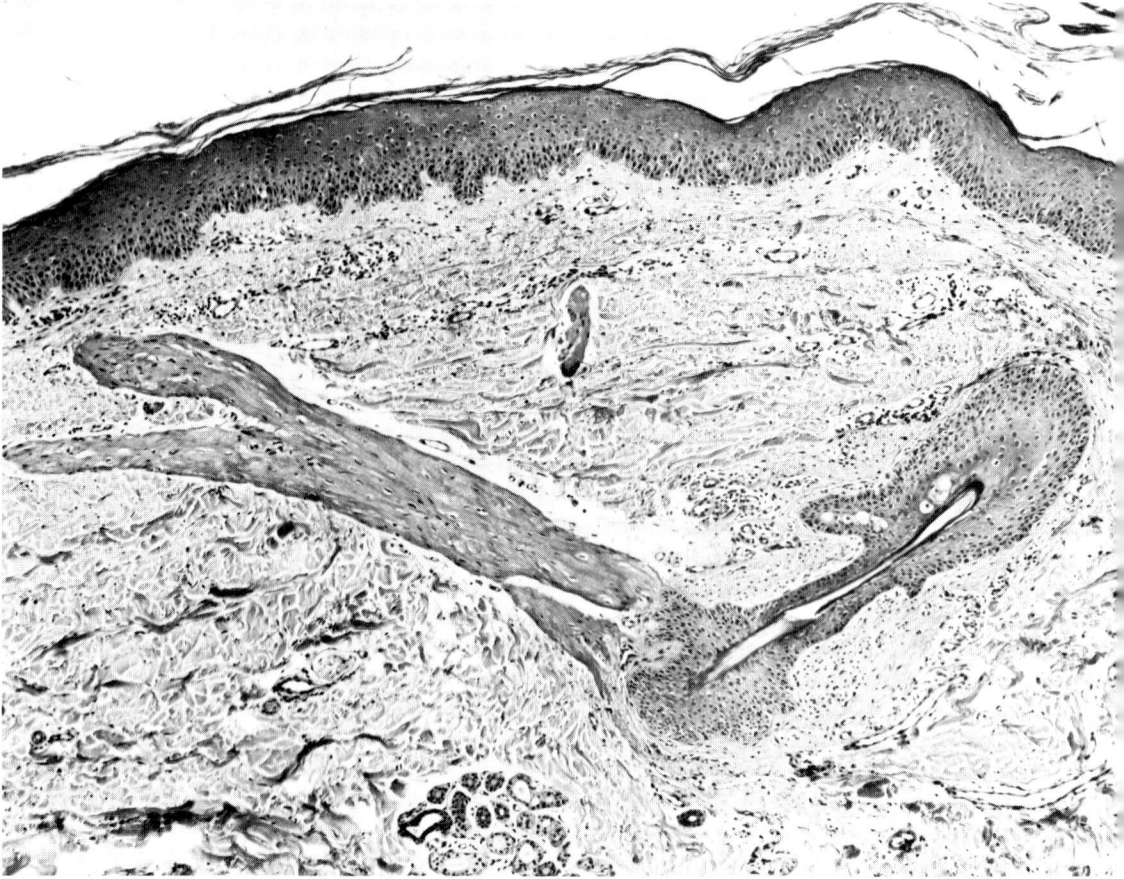

Figure 1–44   The hair erector muscle dwarfs this telogen hair, to which it is attached at "the bulge." In telogen, the entire follicle beneath the insertion of the hair erector muscle (inferior segment) disappears. (× 81.)

that of the epidermis with which it is continuous, even to the presence of keratohyaline granules and a basket-woven pattern to the cornified layer. However, infundibular keratinocytes are biologically different from epidermal keratinocytes, a phenomenon well illustrated in solar keratosis, a condition in which proliferation of atypical epidermal keratinocytes by-passes the normal-appearing keratinocytes of intra-epidermal adnexa.

The hair shaft is a dead cornified structure that extends from the follicle above the surface of the skin. It has three components: an outer cuticle, a cortex, and an inner medulla. The medulla in human hair is mostly discontinuous and sometimes absent. Fetal hairs have no medulla. Medullary cells are loosely arranged, in contrast to the fusiform, tightly packed keratinocytes of the cortex. Cortex cells are aligned with their long axis parallel to the length of the hair. The exterior cuticular squames overlap each other to form an imbricated capsule around the cortex (Fig. 1–46). The color of hair depends primarily upon the amount and distribution of melanin within it. In blond hair the bulbar melanocytes produce fewer melanosomes or incompletely melanized melanosomes resulting in a poorly pigmented hair shaft. Gray hair is a consequence of the relative absence of melanosomes in the hair shaft secondary to a diminished number of melanocytes in the hair bulb. The melanin in red hair is chemically distinct from that of black hair and the melanosomes are spherical rather

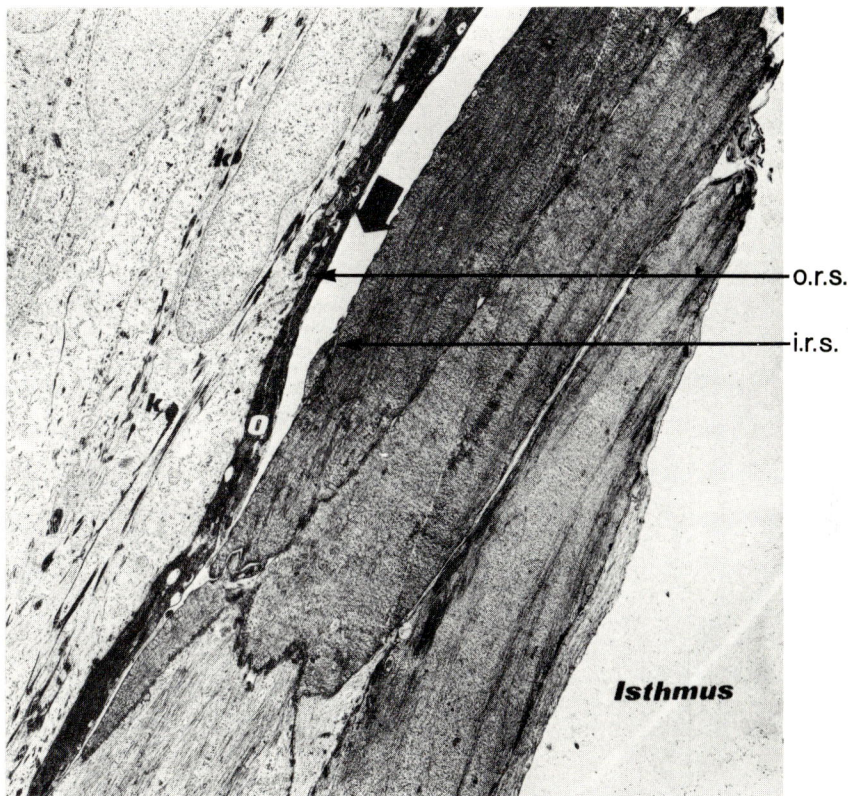

Figure 1–45 At the isthmus, the inner root sheath detaches from the outer root sheath. *o.r.s.*, outer root sheath; *i.r.s.*, inner root sheath. Hair of human embryo. (× 10,000.) (Courtesy of Ken Hashimoto, M.D.)

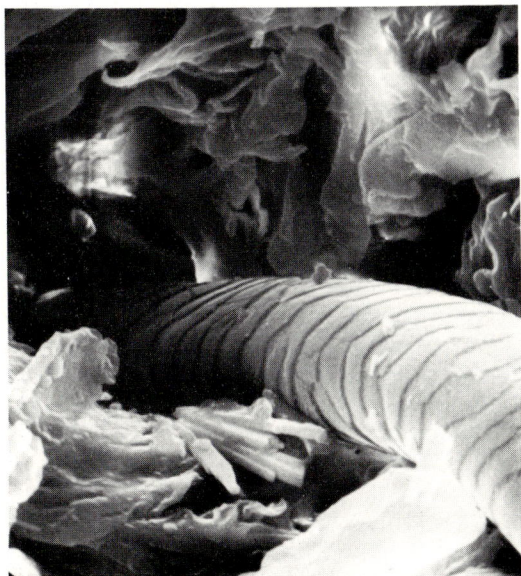

Figure 1–46 With the scanning electron microscope, the exterior cuticular squames of the hair shaft can be seen to overlap and form an imbricated capsule around the cortex. (Courtesy of Christopher Papa, M.D.)

than ellipsoidal. One hypothesis suggests that red color in hair results from iron-containing pigment. Melanocytes are absent in the snow-white hair of the aged.

The growth of hair is cyclical. The three phases in the life cycle of a hair are (1) growing (anagen), (2) involuting (catagen) and (3) resting (telogen) (Fig. 1–47).

At the end of the active growth phase, a remarkable series of involutional changes occurs in the hair bulb. Catagen is heralded by loss of metachromasia of the hair papilla, and the glycogen-filled outer root sheath retracts into a cornifying epithelial sac around the bulbous lower end of the hair shaft (club hair). Melanocytes of the hair bulb become inactive, and the cessation of melanin synthesis causes the expanded end of the club hair to turn white. A thin cord of epithelial cells, probably contributed by the matrix below and the outer root sheath above, replaces the entire inferior segment of the follicle. This epithelial column connects the

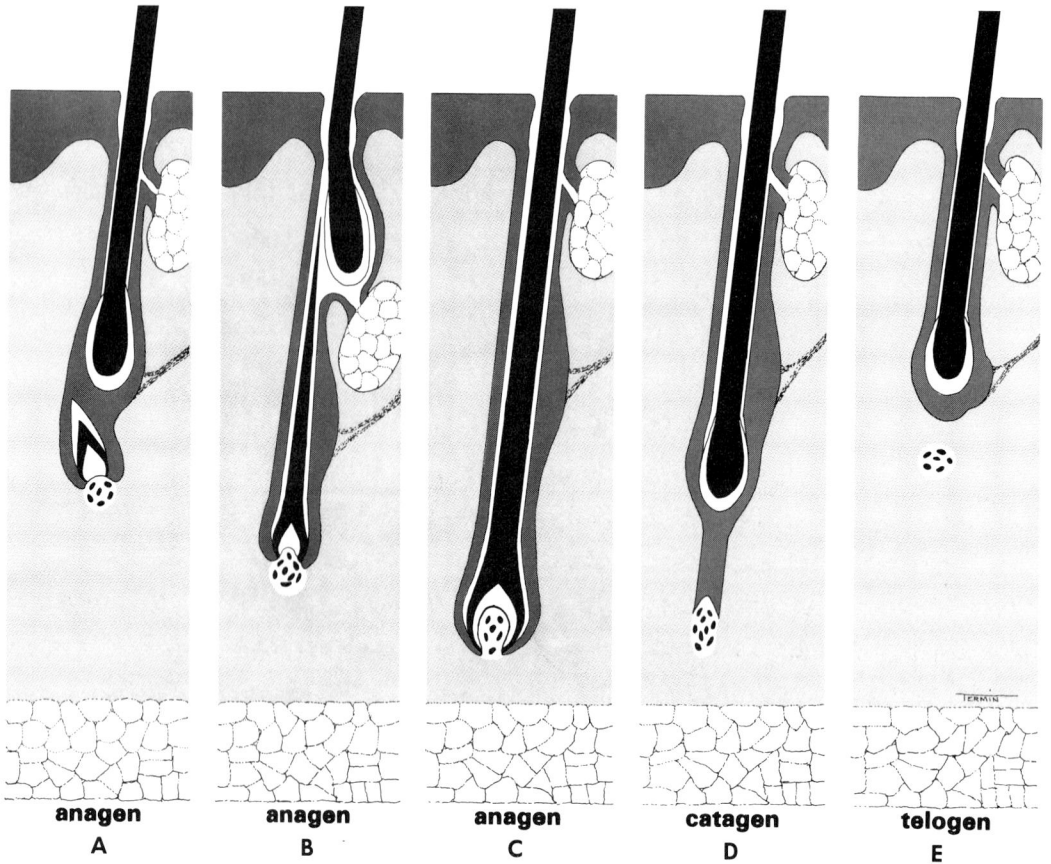

Figure 1–47   Phases in the life cycle of a hair. *A*, Anagen begins with a renewal of the intimate relationship between the papilla and the undifferentiated cells that partially enclose it. *B*, As anagen proceeds, matrix cells generate a new hair that pushes upward toward the surface and in the process dislodges the old club hair. *C*, Mature anagen hair follicle consists of infundibular, isthmus, and inferior segments. *D*, During catagen, the entire inferior segment of the follicle shrivels upward as a thin cord of epithelial cells and is followed upward by the papilla. *E*, During telogen, the club hair rests in its cornified sac at the level of the hair erector muscle.

papilla to the cornifying epithelial sac that encloses the club hair. The epithelial stalk is surrounded by an enormously thickened and corrugated "glassy" basement membrane. Eventually, the club hair ascends to the level of insertion of the pilary muscle.

During telogen, the club hair rests within its cornified sac, and the subjacent attached column of epithelial cells shrinks upward. As this strand shortens, it is followed upward by the liberated papilla that migrates behind in close proximity. Left in the wake of this shortened epithelial column is a streamer of fibrous connective tissue (Fig. 1–48). The epithelial column comes to rest as a ball of undifferentiated cells on the undersurface of the club hair

epithelial sac. During telogen, the hair melanocytes cease synthesizing melanin and then return to function with the advent of anagen.

The anagen phase of the cycle begins with a renewal of the intimate relationship between the papilla and the undifferentiated cells that partially enclose it. A new hair matrix is formed, and papilla and matrix descend together along the preformed fibrous-sheath pathway. Another epithelial column then develops in the reverse direction, and at the lower end, a new bulb forms. Its dedifferentiated matrix cells generate a new inner root sheath and hair. These events recapitulate the formation of the original hair from undifferentiated cells in the fetal epidermis. The new hair formed by the matrix pushes upward toward the surface, dislodging the old resting hair in the process. For a time there may be two hairs in a single follicle, the new hair and the old club hair. The root of the anagen hair is deeply pigmented and surrounded by a translucent sheath, whereas the bulbous tip of the telogen hair is unpigmented (Fig. 1–49). A graphic demonstration of these differences can be obtained by simply plucking hairs from your own scalp and eyebrows and comparing the roots.

Human hair follicles operate independently of one another, adjacent follicles being in different phases of the hair cycle. Human hairs are normally lost randomly and inconspicuously, unlike some animal hairs which are shed over territories at one

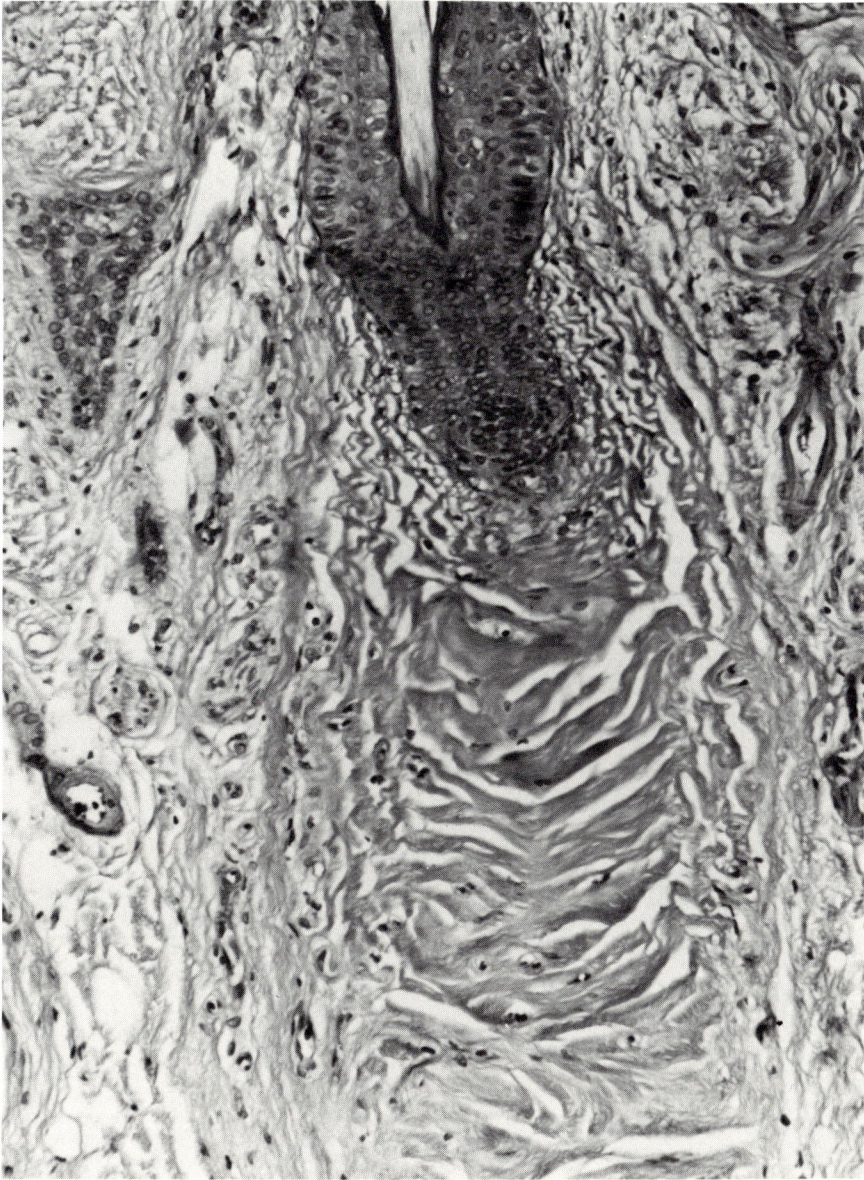

Figure 1–48   In telogen, a fibrous connective tissue streamer is left in the wake of the inferior segment of the hair follicle as it migrates upward. (× 241.)

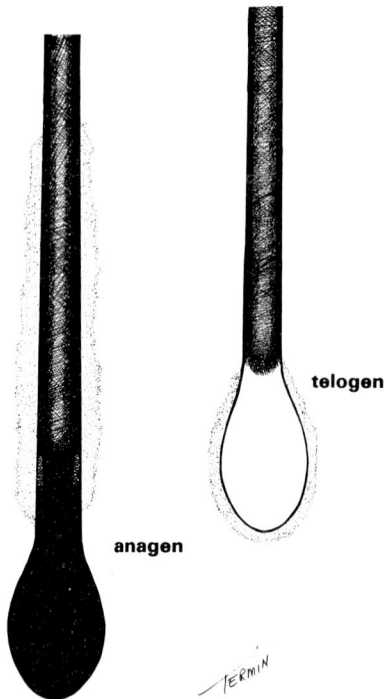

Figure 1–49 The root of the anagen hair is pigmented and is surrounded by a translucent sheath, whereas the bulbous tip of the telogen hair is unpigmented.

time (synchronous shedding) and then are sprouted as a crop anew.

The time interval between the growing, involuting, and resting phases is an important characteristic of the hair cycle. The hairs in different regions of the body spend different proportions of their time in anagen, resulting in the typical variation in the length of hair. Scalp hair grows from 3 to 10 years, involutes during about three weeks, and rests for approximately three months. In healthy young adults, less than 10 per cent of all scalp hairs are resting at a given time. The growing period of scalp hairs is much longer than that of hairs elsewhere on the body. As a rule, the growing phase of hairs on the extremities, trunk, and eyebrows does not exceed six months, and the duration of the resting phase is roughly the same. There is a relationship between the final length attained by a hair and the duration of its growing period. The longest hairs on the scalp grow for the longest time. Hair production is a continuous process in

each of the approximately 100,000 anagen follicles on the average scalp. The protein-synthesizing capacity of the hair matrix is enormous when one considers that scalp hair is practically pure protein and grows at a rate of about 0.35 mm. daily, resulting in the daily manufacture of approximately 100 feet of hair. Many factors, such as nutrition, hormones, temperature, and light, control the growth of hair.

Understanding the hair cycle has useful application in medical practice. Growing scalp hairs may enter the resting phase prematurely under stressful circumstances, such as parturition or systemic disease. Resting hairs are more easily lost from the follicle because they are anchored less securely. These resting hairs may be depilated during combing and washing, giving rise to a sudden hair loss that simulates partial baldness. When the inciting cause has passed or been remedied, new hairs will be generated during the next growing phase of the cycle. Thus, the alarmed patient can be assured that the hair loss is only temporary.

In contrast, "male pattern" baldness is permanent. This type of scalp baldness is somewhat related to the action of androgenic hormones in a genetically predisposed individual. Aristotle, who had a bald pate, proudly observed that eunuchs were never bald. Paradoxically, androgens are also responsible for the excessive body and facial hairiness known as hirsutism.

Knowledge of the hair cycle assists management of dermatophytic infections of hair. The causative fungi do not attack hairs that are in the resting phase, and a hair entering this phase spontaneously becomes free of infection. Thus dermatophytosis involving the eyelashes and eyebrows, in contrast to the scalp, never lasts more than a few months because of the relatively short period of hair growth in these locations.

The susceptibility of hair follicles to depilation by x-ray, antimetabolites, systemic disease, and other factors that interrupt hair growth is related to the length of the growth cycle; hairs that grow for years and then rest briefly are the most vulnerable. Beard hair will not be depilated by a dose of x-rays sufficient to cause scalp depilation. The scalp is most markedly affected in hair loss resulting from systemic administration of anti-metabolites and in alopecia associated with systemic disease.

An array of curious abnormalities of the hair shaft results from still undefined disturbances of the hair matrix. Beaded, ringed, twisted, "bamboo," and "bayonette" hairs are evidences of interferences, some of them doubtlessly genetic, with the hair matrix.

Hair screens the nasal passages from irritants, the scalp from the sun's rays, and the eyes from the sunlight and droplets of sweat. It mutes friction in intertriginous regions and aids in tactile perception. The major adaptive value of hair is ornamental, a means of sexual attraction.

THE APOCRINE UNIT

On the human body, the coiled, tubular aprocrine glands are found in the axillae, areolae, mons pubis, labia minora, prepuce, scrotum, the periumbilical and circumanal areas, the external ear canal (ceruminous glands), and on the eyelids (Moll's glands). Apocrine glands may also be found in the face and scalp and in the epithelial hamartomas, such as nevus sebaceus and syringocystadenoma papilliferum. Apocrine glands make a secretion the function of which is unknown.

In other mammals, such as dogs, monkeys, and apes, apocrine glands are distributed over the entire skin surface where they are believed to serve as protective or sexual scent organs. Concomitant with the diminution in hair cover in man, there has been a decrease in the number of apocrine glands. During the fifth month of gestation, the human fetus has anlagen of apocrine glands over the entire skin surface. These later regress so that by term, apocrine glands are confined to the aforementioned sites. These glands remain small until early puberty when they enlarge and begin to secrete.

Histologically, the apocrine gland consists of two portions: (1) a coiled secretory gland situated in the lower part of the dermis or in the subcutaneous tissue and (2) a straight excretory duct that empties into the infundibular part of the hair follicle just above the entrance of the sebaceous duct (Fig. 1–50). Occasionally, apocrine ducts open directly onto the epidermis. In cross-section, the apocrine secretory coil has a diameter several times wider than that of the eccrine coil (Fig. 1–51). These differences are best appreciated in the axilla, where apocrine glands are intermingled with eccrine glands.

The lumen of the secretory coil is lined by one layer of cells ranging in shape from cuboidal to columnar, with round nuclei located near the bases and abundant, pale-staining eosinophilic cytoplasm (Fig. 1–52). The convex apical borders of the secretory cells may project into the lumen at various heights, depending on their stage in the secretory cycle. These secretory cells are surrounded by one layer of myoepithelial cells, a PAS-positive basement membrane, and a network of elastic and reticular fibers.

The excretory duct is composed of two layers of cuboidal cells with an inner periluminal cuticle and no myoepithelial component. At its distal end, the apocrine duct merges with the epithelium of the infundibulum.

With the electron microscope, the apocrine secretory cells are seen to contain organellar components typical of secretory epithelia: many ribosomes, rough endoplasmic reticulum, mitochondria, lysosomes, and a prominent Golgi apparatus. The microvesicles present at the free border are further indications of an active secretory cell (Fig. 1–53). Histochemical stains show that secretory cells of apocrine glands also contain lipid, iron, lipofuscin and PAS-positive, diastase-resistant granules. The type of secretion seen in apocrine glands was dubbed "apocrine" ("apo" meaning "off") because of the appearance, under the light microscope, of "pinching off" (decapitation secretion) of apical cytoplasm into the lumen. The exact mode of apocrine secretion is still unresolved.

There are two separate aspects to the production of apocrine sweat: (1) secretion and (2) excretion. Secretion by the apocrine gland is a continuous process, but excretion is episodic. Excretion occurs when the reservoir of apocrine secretion is propelled upward by peristaltic waves, presumably provided by the myoepithelial

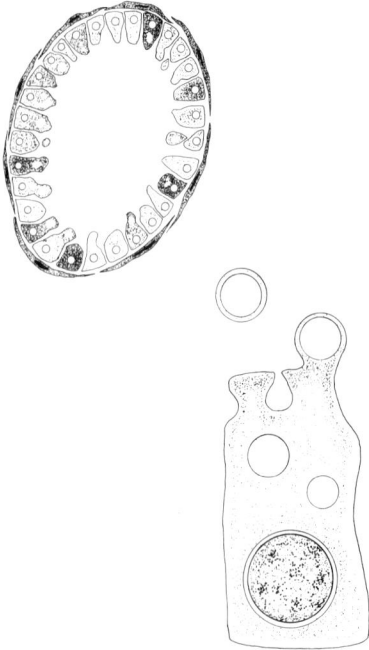

Figure 1–50 The apocrine gland consists of two portions: (1) a coiled secretory gland situated in the lower part of the dermis or in the subcutaneous fat and (2) a straight excretory duct that empties into the infundibular part of the hair follicle.

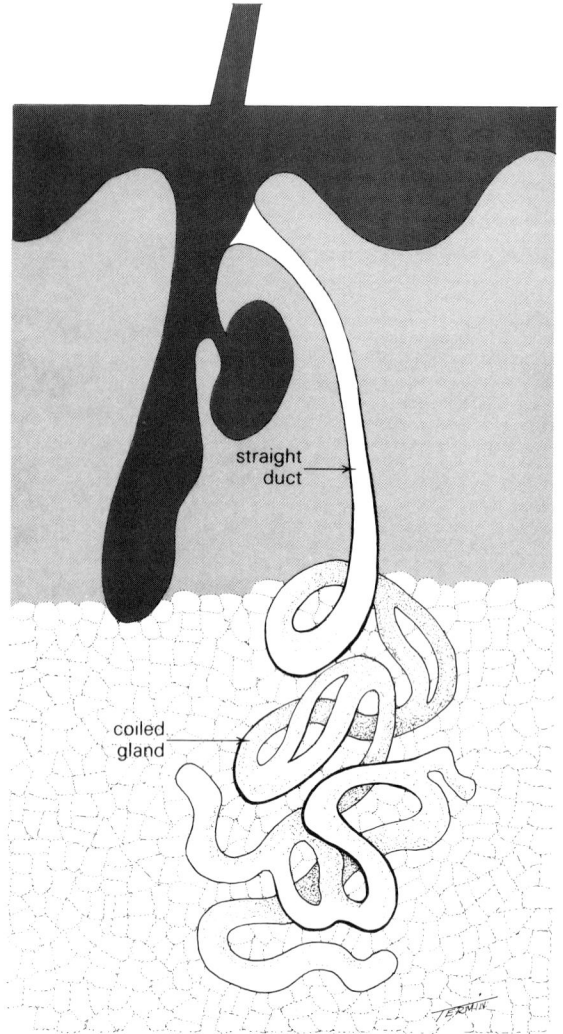

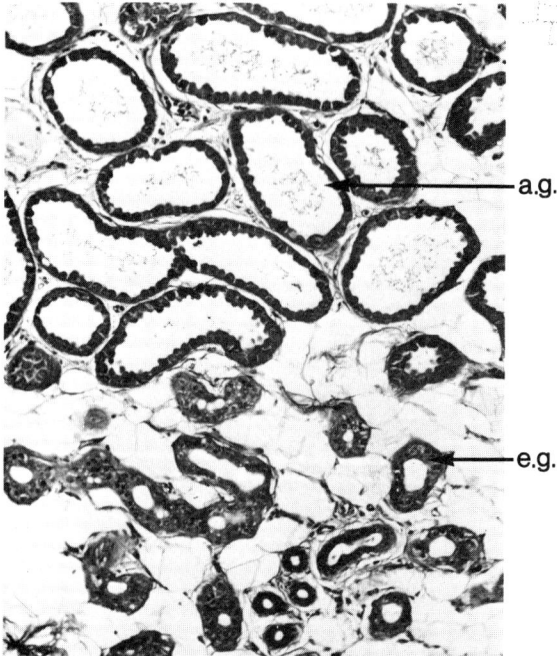

Figure 1–51 In cross-section, the apocrine secretory coil has a diameter several times wider than that of the eccrine coil. ($\times$ 176.)

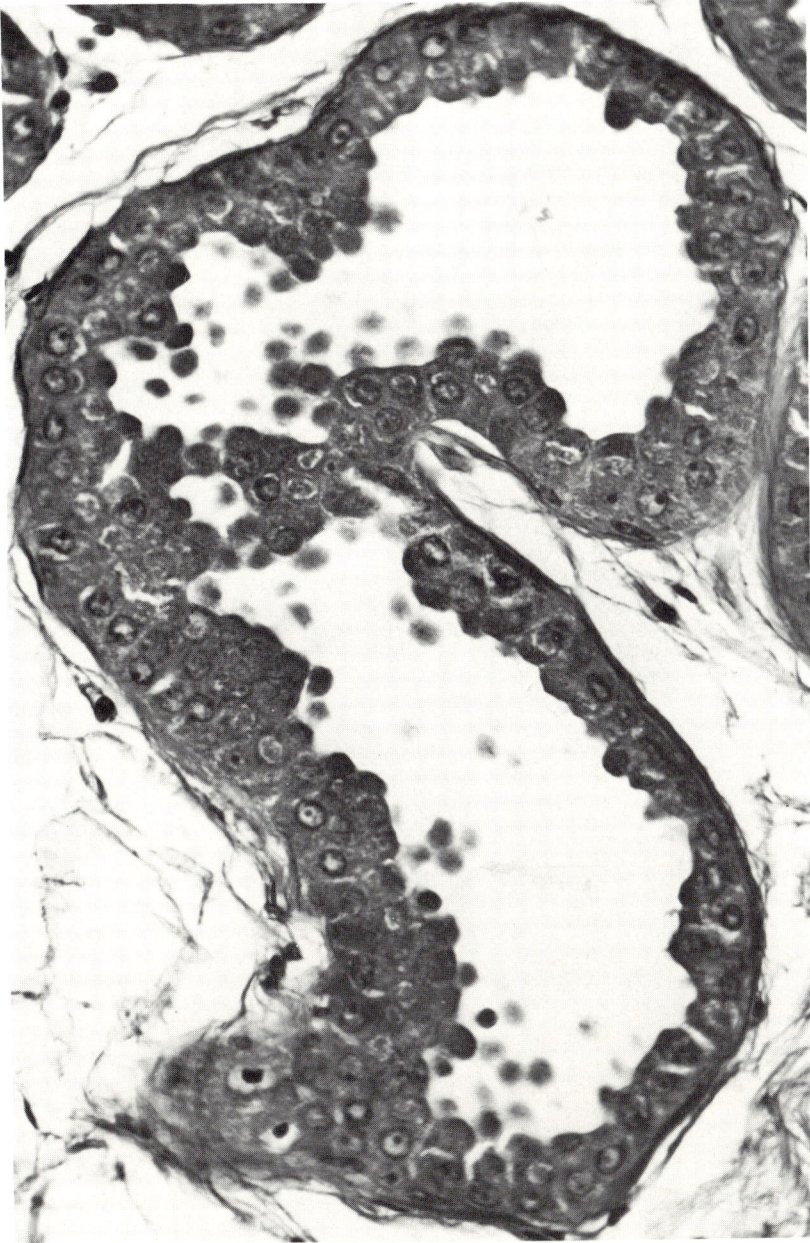

Figure 1–52 The lumen of the apocrine secretory coil is lined by one layer of cells ranging from cuboidal to columnar, with round nuclei near the bases and abundant pale-staining eosinophilic cytoplasm. The convex apical borders project into the lumen at various heights, giving the impression of "decapitation secretion." (× 479.)

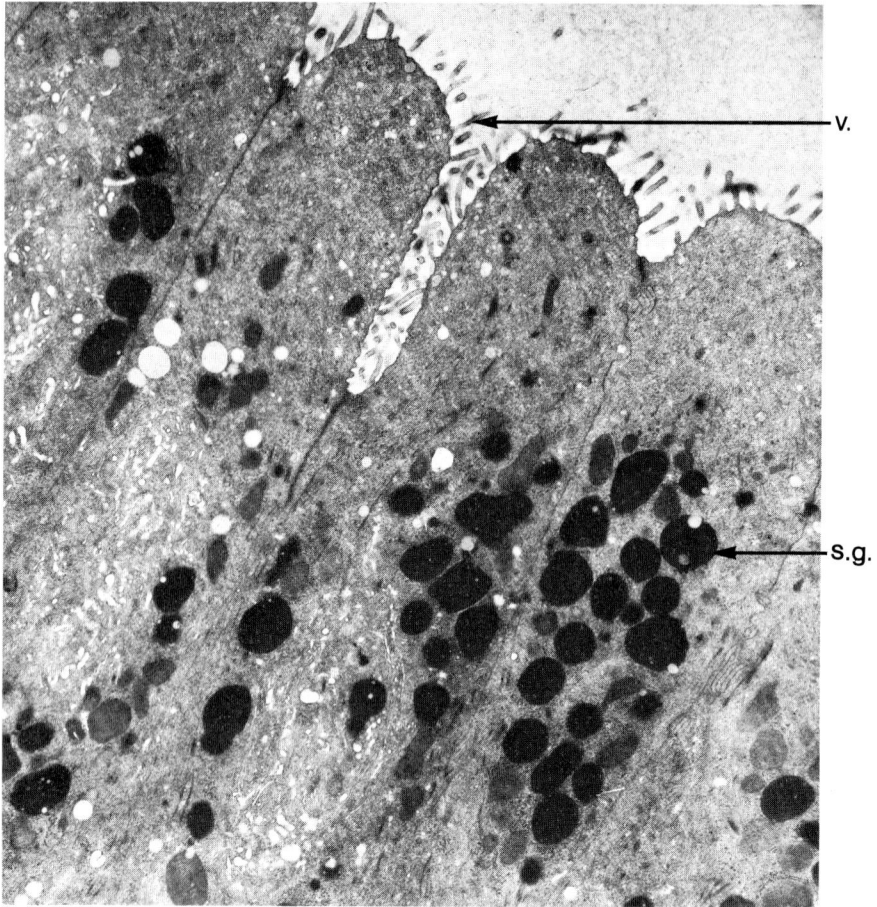

Figure 1–53   Columnar apocrine secretory cells contain many dense secretory granules, ribosomes, rough endoplasmic reticulum, mitochondria, lysosomes, and a well-developed Golgi apparatus. Villi at the free border of the lumen are also indications of an active secretory cell. *v.*, villi; *s.g.*, secretory granules. (×7,500.) (Courtesy of Ken Hashimoto, M.D.)

cell sheath. The myoepithelium is innervated by adrenergic nerve fibers. Myoepithelial contraction, and resultant apocrine excretion, are induced by pharmacologic agents (Pitocin and epinephrine) and by emotional stresses (fear and anger) that cause adrenergic sympathetic discharge.

The quantity of apocrine secretion is quite small, even in the axilla where the apocrine glands are most numerous. After an apocrine gland is emptied, a refractory period ensues, during which the duct refills with glandular secretion. Apocrine secretion has a milky color, contains protein and carbohydrates, may fluoresce, and quickly dries as a varnish-like cap over the follicular orifice. Within the duct, apocrine secretion is sterile and odorless. The ac-

tion of bacteria on apocrine secretion that has reached the skin surface causes the skin to become malodorous (body odor). Many underarm deodorants, as advertised, contain antibacterial ingredients that eliminate the offending microorganisms. There is no known function of the apocrine gland in humans.

THE SEBACEOUS GLAND

Sebaceous glands, specialized for lipid synthesis, arise embryologically as an epithelial bud from the outer root sheath at a point marking the junction of the future infundibulum and isthmus. Sebaceous glands are distributed over the entire body surface, except for the palms, soles, and dorsa of the feet. They are most populous and most productive on the face and scalp. Because of its mode of development, almost every sebaceous gland is joined to a hair follicle. As a rule, sebaceous gland size varies inversely as the diameter of the follicle with which it is associated, exceptions being the large glands adjoining sturdy follicles of the beard and scalp and the tiny glands attached to the vellus follicles. Some follicles containing puny hairs become an insignificant appendage of the sebaceous gland. The "sebaceous follicles" are found on the face (excluding the beard) and on the upper part of the back and chest. In some locales, sebaceous glands are not associated with hairs: buccal mucosa and vermillion border of the lip (Fordyce's spots), female areola (Montgomery's tubercles), prepuce (Tyson's glands), and the eyelids (Meibomian glands).

The several lobules that comprise a sebaceous gland are enveloped by a thin, highly vascular, fibrous tissue capsule (periadnexal dermis) (Fig. 1–54). No motor nerves appear to be affiliated with the gland. The peripheral germinative cells are somewhat flattened or cuboidal with a large nucleus and homogeneous basophilic cytoplasm. Germinative cells of the sebaceous gland correspond to the basal cells of the epidermis. During differentiation, lipid droplets accumulate, eventually filling the cytoplasm of the cell. The more centrally located cells have a characteristic vacuolated cytoplasm and a scalloped nucleus, owing to compression by lipid globules (Fig. 1–55). The continuous proliferation of undifferentiated peripheral cells gradually displaces the more differentiated vacuolated cells toward the center of the acinus. Finally, the boundaries of these bloated cells become indistinct, the cells disintegrate, and the mass of lipid and cellular debris (sebum) is discharged into the sebaceous duct, a short narrow common excretory duct connecting several sebaceous lobules with the wider follicular infundibulum. The sebace-

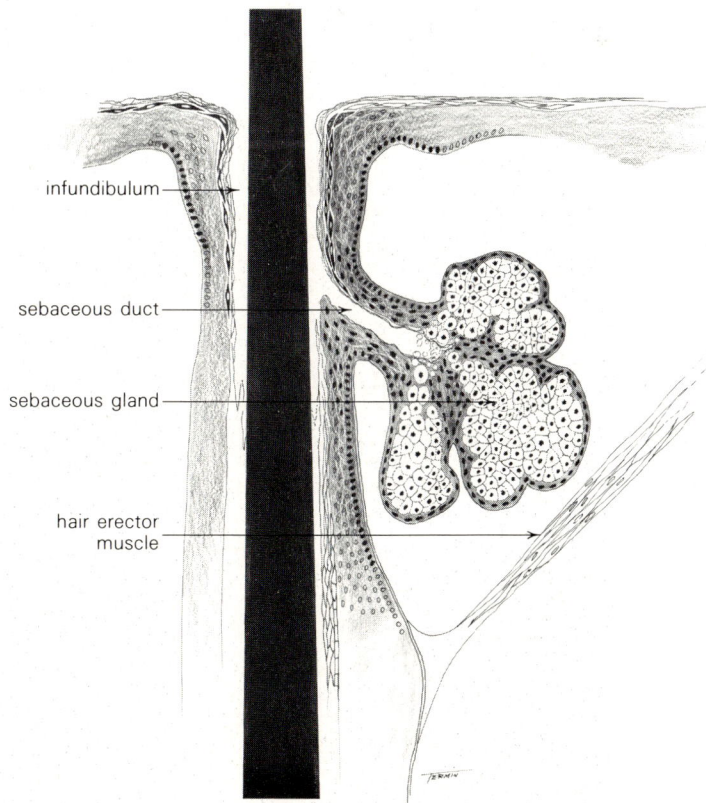

Figure 1–54 Almost every sebaceous gland is joined to a hair follicle. The peripheral germinative cells of the sebaceous gland correspond to the basal cells of the epidermis. During differentiation, lipid droplets accumulate, eventually filling the cytoplasm of the cell. Finally, the boundaries of these bloated cells become indistinct, the cells disintegrate and the mass of lipid and cellular debris (sebum) is discharged into the sebaceous duct, a short, narrow, common excretory duct connecting several sebaceous lobules with the wider follicular infundibulum.

infundibulum

sebaceous duct

sebaceous gland

hair erector muscle

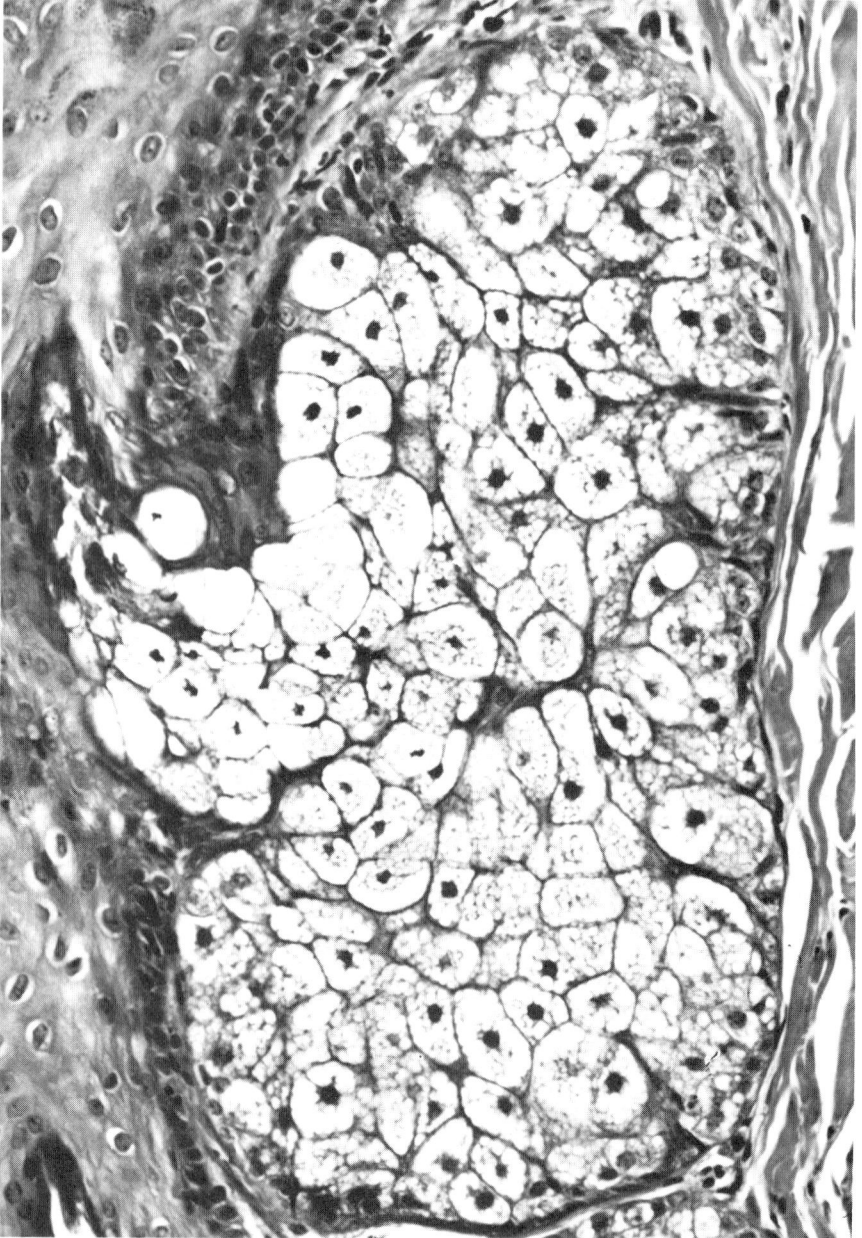

Figure 1–55 Sebaceous gland nuclei nearest to the peripheral germinative layer are round, but appear scalloped as they differentiate owing to compression by lipid droplets. (× 306.)

ous duct is lined by cornifying squamous epithelium. A mite, *Demodex folliculorum*, is so commonly present in the infundibulum and sebaceous duct that it is usually regarded as a normal inhabitant of facial pilosebaceous units (Fig. 1–56).

The sebaceous gland is a holocrine gland because in the process of secretion the entire cell is cast off, in a manner analogous to the production of desquamating cornified cells by the epidermis. Furthermore, the name "sebum" given to the secretory products of the sebaceous gland can be likened to the term "keratin": both represent the composite end product of their specific tissue differentiation.

Histochemical and ultrastructural findings during sebaceous gland differentiation clarify observations with the light microscope (Fig. 1–57). The undifferentiated peripheral cells are glycogen-laden and contain tonofilaments, rough and smooth endoplasmic reticulum, and many mitochondria. As differentiation proceeds, glycogen disappears, tonofibrils are displaced, and the cell cytoplasm fills with lipid vacuoles whose formation may be related to the numerous mitochondria,

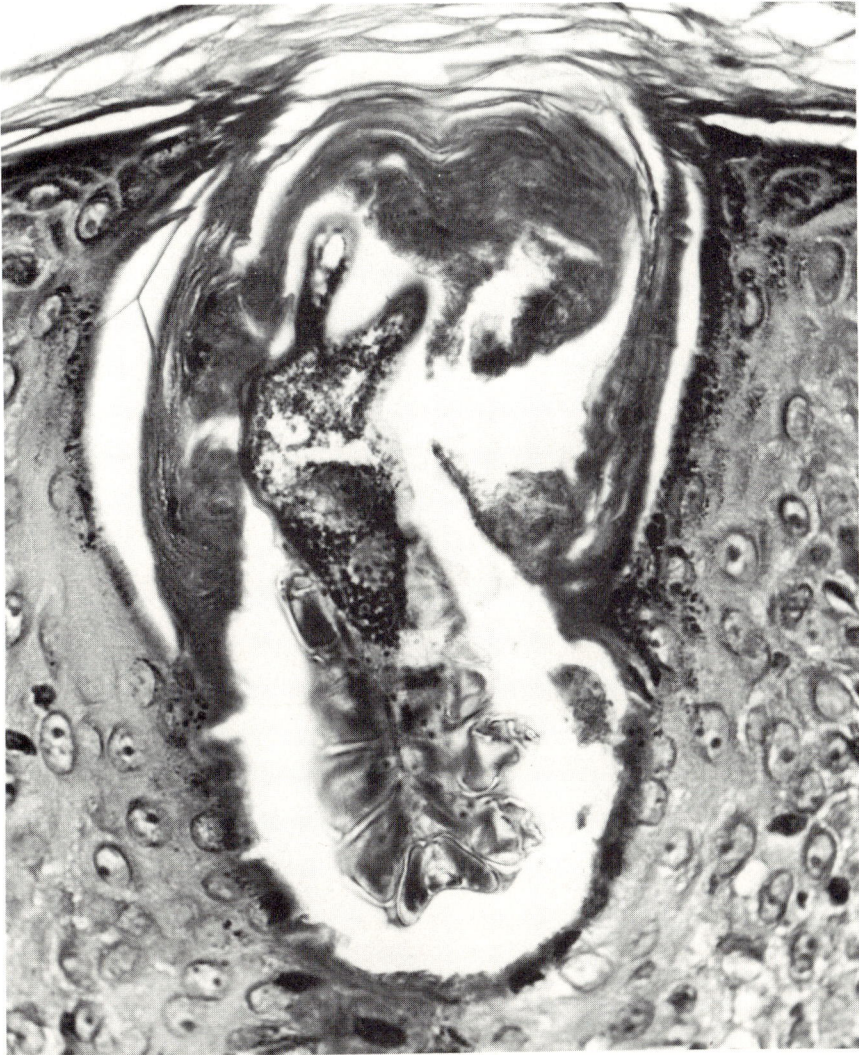

Figure 1–56   The mite, *Demodex folliculorum*, is so commonly present in the infundibulum of facial pilosebaceous units that it is regarded as a normal inhabitant. (× 670.)

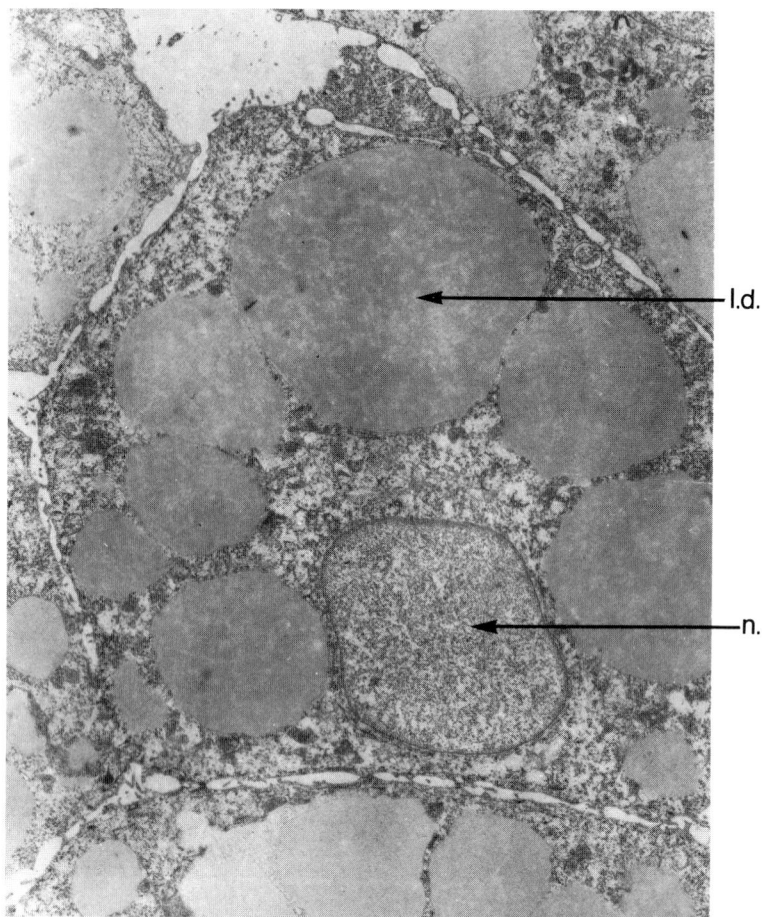

Figure 1–57 As differentiation proceeds, the sebaceous gland cell is filled with lipid. *l.d.*, lipid droplets; *n.*, nucleus. (× 14,500.) (Courtesy of Ken Hashimoto, M.D.)

smooth endoplasmic reticulum, and large Golgi apparatus. Eventually, the cell membrane disorganizes; the cell fragments and the cellular components, including nuclear remnants, disperse.

THE ECCRINE SWEAT UNIT

Eccrine sweat units derive from the surface epidermis, independent of hair follicles, and descend through the dermis, coming to rest near the junction of the dermis and subcutaneous fat. Eccrine sweat units are present everywhere on human skin except the mucocutaneous junctions and the ears. They are most highly concentrated on the palms, soles, and forehead, and in the axilla, and are least numerous on the arms and legs. It has been estimated that 3,000,000 eccrine sweat units are present at birth. Since no additional sweat glands are formed during life, the density is greatest in infant skin. Wide distribution of highly developed eccrine sweat units is unique to man. The eccrine sweat gland makes a hypotonic solution (sweat) that flows to the skin surface for evaporative cooling in times of heat stress. It is the eccrine rather than apocrine gland that is the true sweat gland in man. Eccrine sweat glands have been found only on the bodies of higher primates and horses.

The sweat pores, or openings of the sweat ducts on the skin surface, are not visible with the naked eye. With a hand lens, tiny pits can be seen on the summit of the ridges on the palms and soles. These regularly arranged pits represent the orifices of the eccrine sweat ducts. Minute droplets of sweat can be detected in some of these depressions. Elsewhere on the body, sweat can be observed to emerge from the pores only after special preparation of the skin surface, such as with starch and iodine.

Each eccrine sweat unit is a simple hollow tube bounded distally by an opening onto the skin surface and proximally by a cul-de-sac (Fig. 1–58). Both ends of the tube are wound and connected by a straight duct. The proximal portion coils in irregular fashion, like a ball of yarn, whereas the distal portion spirals through the epidermis. The eccrine unit can be divided into:

1. Coiled secretory gland.
2. Coiled dermal duct.
3. Straight dermal duct.
4. Spiraled intra-epidermal duct.

The intradermal portions of the eccrine unit are enclosed in a richly vascular connective-tissue sheath (periadnexal dermis) that is separated from the tubal epithelium by a PAS-positive basement membrane.

The coiled secretory gland is composed of two layers of cells (Fig. 1–59):

1. A thin outer row of spindle cells (myoepithelium).
2. An inner row of pyramidal, cuboidal epithelial cells (secretory epithelium). The single row of secretory cells that lines the lumen of the gland consists of two types of cells, distinguished by their staining characteristics:

    a. Small mucopolysaccharide-containing dark cells that are crowded toward the lumen.

    b. Large glycogen-containing pale cells peripherally.

The secretory gland is abundantly innervated by unmyelinated nerve fibers. The response of these fibers is mediated primarily by acetylcholine and inhibited

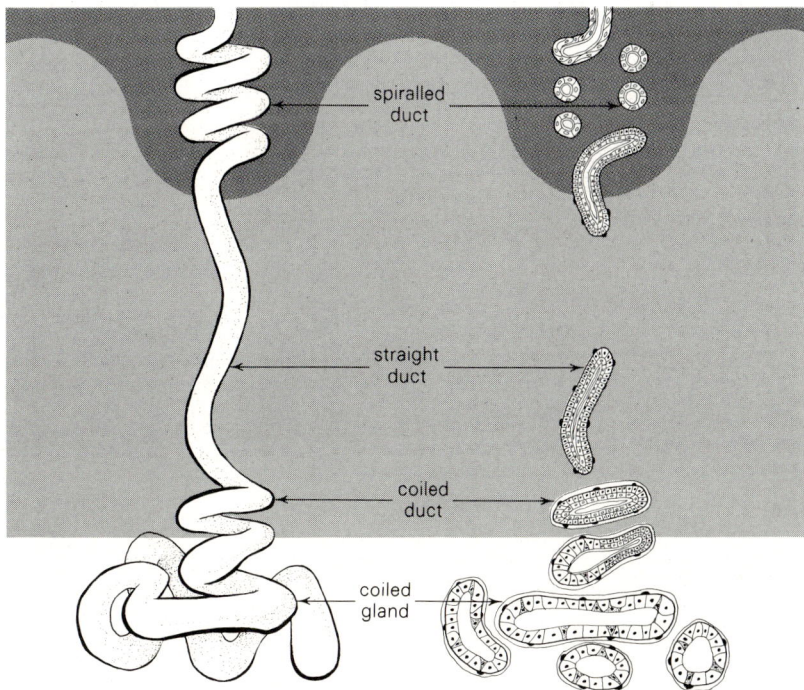

Figure 1–58 The eccrine sweat unit is a simple hollow tube bounded distally by an opening onto the skin surface and proximally by a cul-de-sac. Both ends of the tube are wound and connected by a straight duct. The proximal portion coils in irregular fashion, whereas the distal portion spirals through the epidermis.

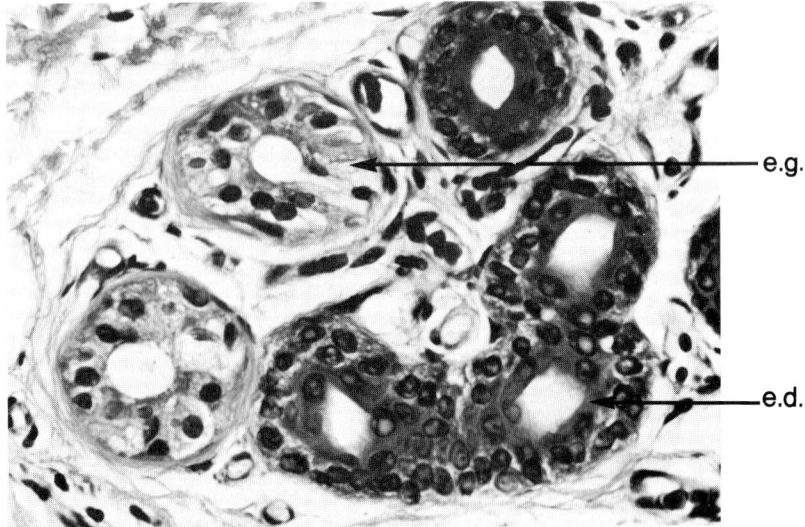

Figure 1–59   The secretory portion of the eccrine sweat gland is surrounded by a basement membrane and consists of two layers of cells: (1) a thin outer row of myoepithelial cells and (2) an inner row of cuboidal epithelial secretory cells. The ductal portion is lined by two layers of smaller cuboidal epithelial cells with a luminal edge rimmed by a homogeneous eosinophilic cuticle. (× 740.)

by atropine. Actually, the eccrine sweat glands respond to both parasympathomimetic and sympathomimetic drugs, being more sensitive to parasympathomimetic ones.

The secretory epithelium is easily differentiated from the ductal epithelium. The eccrine dermal duct is lined by two layers of small, darkly basophilic-staining, cuboidal epithelial cells. The luminal edge of these ductal cells is rimmed by a homogeneous eosinophilic cuticle. The duct narrows as it ascends from the coiled portion through the straight segment until the epidermis is reached. Here the duct again becomes coiled and widens as it spirals upward through the epidermis to open onto the skin surface. The intra-epidermal keratinocytes of the eccrine duct differ morphologically and biologically from their neighboring epidermal keratinocytes, to which they are linked by desmosomes. Keratohyaline granules are present within the eccrine duct cells and melanin granules are absent at almost all levels of the duct's twist through the epidermis. The intra-epidermal sweat duct keratinocytes cornify independently, reflected in the corkscrew pattern preserved within the cornified layer, which is best demon-strated on the palms and soles (Fig. 1–60). A cuticle lines the luminal border of the intra-epidermal duct, just as it does that of the dermal duct.

The process of making sweat begins in the pale cells of the secretory gland in which there are abundant mitochondria and glycogen particles (Fig. 1–61). Active sweating is accompanied by dramatic changes, indicative of intense metabolic activity, in these pale cells. Within minutes after the onset of sweating, glycogen is consumed and the number of other organelles is diminished. It is surmised that during this time anaerobic glycolysis depletes the pale cell cytoplasm, resulting in formation of lactate and hydrogen ions. These ions move in conduits, intercellular canaliculi, lined by microvilli, which connect the pale cells with one another. In the canaliculi, hydrogen ions are removed by reaction with bicarbonate, and the lactate-containing solution flows from the canaliculi into the secretory lumen.

The precise role of the dark cells is unknown. Cytoplasm of the dark cells contains abundant nucleic acids and vacuoles, but few mitochondria and no glycogen. During the process of active sweating, the numerous cytoplasmic vacuoles decrease in number and size. It has been suggested that the dark cells permit reabsorption of sodium, potassium, and chloride from the secretory lumen, but act as an impermeable membrane to lactate. The secretion formed in the lumen of the secretory coil by the combined efforts of pale and dark cells is isotonic, or slightly hypertonic, compared with plasma.

The secretion is altered during its passage through the dermal duct, where sodium is actively reabsorbed, followed passively by chloride and very little water. The ductal membrane is relatively impermeable to water compared to the membrane of the secretory coil. In summary, a solution is formed in the secretory coil that is isotonic or slightly hypertonic and contains large amounts of lactate and minute amounts of bicarbonate. As it passes through the dermal duct, this solution is altered by active reabsorption of sodium and passive absorption of chloride, and perhaps small amounts of water. As it

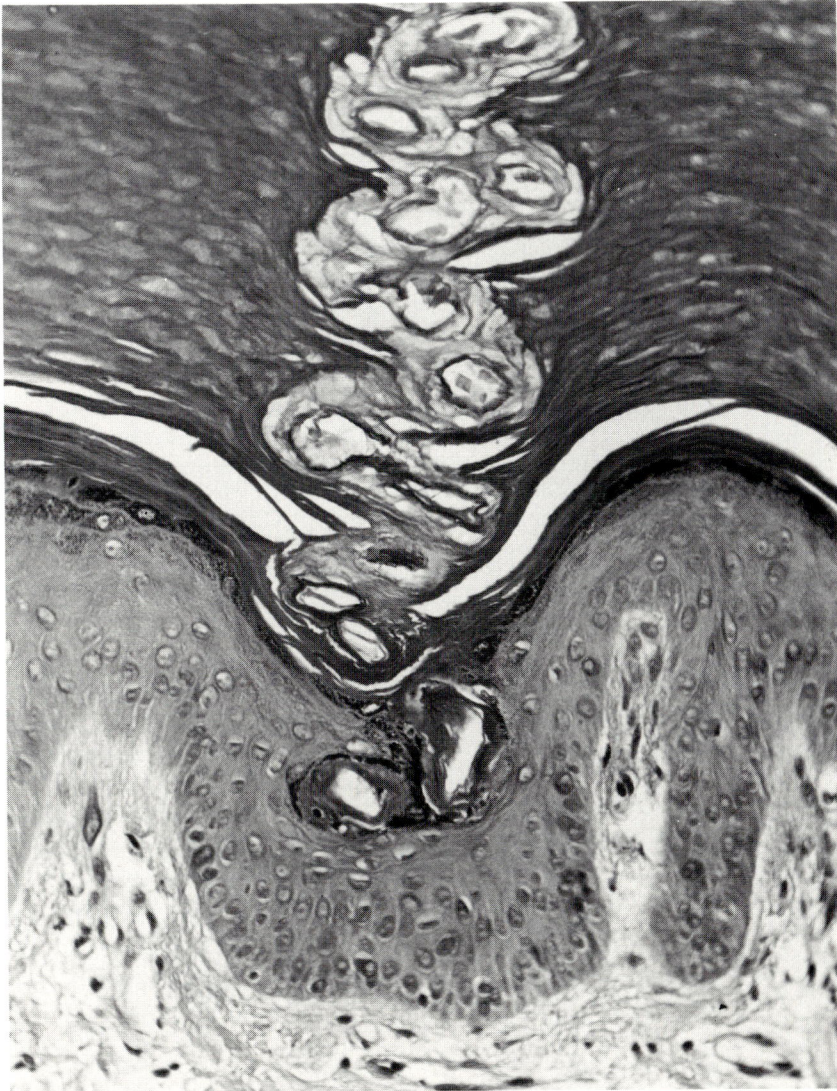

Figure 1–60 The intra-epidermal keratinocytes of the eccrine duct differ morphologically and biologically from their neighboring epidermal keratinocytes. That intra-epidermal sweat duct keratinocytes cornify independently is reflected in the corkscrew pattern preserved within the cornified layer, best demonstrated on the palms and soles. (× 352.)

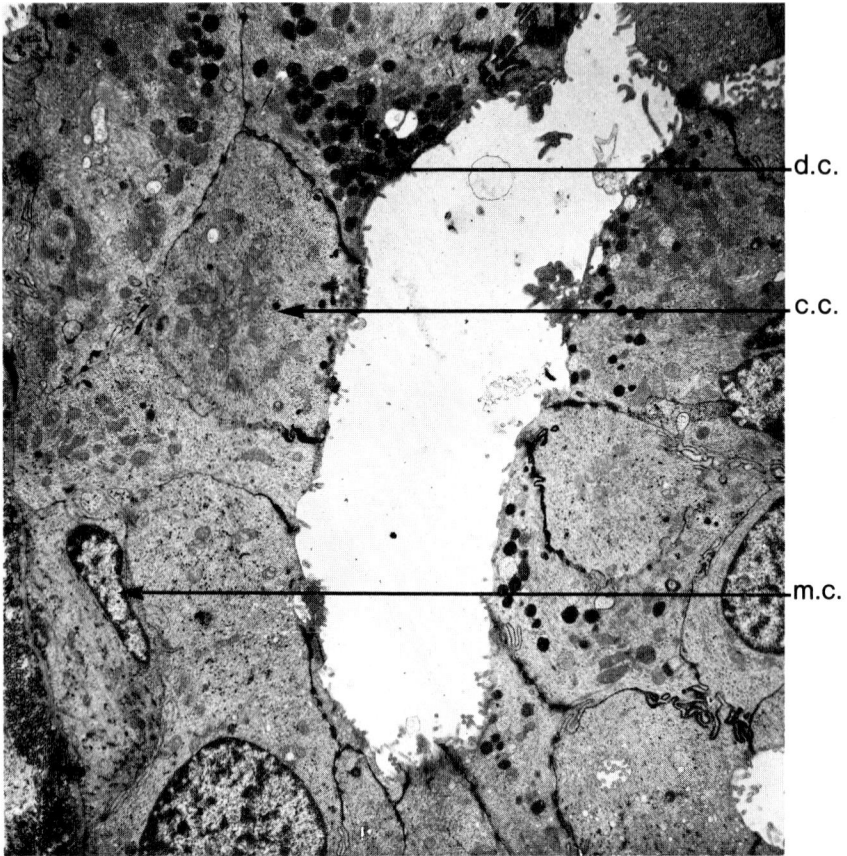

Figure 1–61   The single row of secretory cells that lines the lumen of the eccrine sweat gland consists of two types of cells: (1) clear cells containing abundant glycogen and mitochondria and (2) dark cells having dense granules. The luminal border of these secretory cells bears numerous villi. Myoepithelial cells surround the secretory cells. *d.c.*, dark cell; *c.c.*, clear cell; *m.c.*, myoepithelial cell. (Courtesy of Ken Hashimoto, M.D.)

emerges onto the skin surface, sweat is hypotonic.

The concentration of all substances in sweat has been shown to vary with the sweat rate. The concentrations of sodium and chloride increase with increased sweat rate, whereas those of potassium, lactate, and urea decline with increased sweat rate. The maximum capacity of the duct to reabsorb sodium is only one-fourth the capacity of the secretory coil to secrete sodium; therefore, large amounts of sodium will be lost at high sweat rates.

All eccrine sweat glands do not function all of the time. Some glands are more active than others, each discharging sweat in bursts. Eccrine glands respond promptly to heat stress, delivering the sweat to the skin surface shortly after its secretion,

unlike apocrine glands whose secretion is temporarily stored within the duct. The first response to elevated skin temperature is an increase in the number of eccrine glands that are activated. With increasing thermal stress, there is an increase in the amount of sweat produced by any given gland. The total amount of sweat manufactured by a single gland is small, yet, in aggregate, the quantity of sweat produced by an adult human is astounding—2 to 3 liters an hour by individuals exposed to extreme climatic stress. Each liter of evaporated sweat removes 540 calories of heat from the body.

Eccrine sweat is a colorless, odorless, hypotonic solution composed of water, 99 per cent by weight, and the remainder solutes, which in decreasing order are:

sodium, chloride, potassium, urea, protein, lipids, amino acids, calcium, phosphorus, and iron. All of the electrolytes present in plasma are found, to a lesser extent, in eccrine sweat. The specific gravity of sweat is approximately 1.005. Its pH is generally between 4.5 and 5.5, but as sweating progresses, the pH may increase to 7.0.

Man is a warm-blooded animal, his internal body temperature remaining constant despite enormous changes in the temperature of his external environment. This feature of having a thermoregulatory system that sets a constant internal environment has enabled man to escape the rigid climatic limitations placed upon cold-blooded organisms. Unlike more furry mammals, man cannot rely upon hair for protection against cold. An arctic fox, clothed in its winter fur, rests comfortably at a temperature of −50° C. without increasing its resting rate of metabolism. Man, if unclothed, begins to shiver and raise his metabolic rate when air temperature falls to 28° C. How does the body achieve thermal homeostasis? In large part the skin is responsible. As the natural interface between the body and the external environment, the skin plays a passive role in all heat exchange, but, in addition, the skin has a specialized part to play as an active organ regulating heat exchange. The eccrine sweat units and the cutaneous blood vessels evolved as cardinal structures to serve this function. The eccrine sweat glands flood the skin surface with water for cooling and the blood vessels dilate or constrict for dissipation or conservation of body heat. The capacity of the eccrine gland to make sweat for dissipation of excessive body heat is greatest in the human.

The prime stimulus for the eccrine sweat gland is heat. The control center of the sweat gland is the hypothalamus, which is responsible for thermoregulatory functions and is, in effect, a neural thermostat. It integrates the effect of thermosensory impulses arising in the skin with that of the blood temperature. The usual and most important general sudomotor stimulus is an increase in the body temperature (0.5° C.) which excites a hypothalamic discharge over cholinergic fibers of the sympathetic nervous system, causing immedi-

ate action of sweat glands over the entire body.

Exercise causes almost immediate generalized sweating. With continuation of exercise, increases in temperature of the blood perfusing the hypothalamic centers contribute to the sweating response.

Acclimatization to heat involves a readjustment of sweating mechanisms so that smaller elevations in body and skin temperature are required to produce a given sweat rate. The results of this sweating adaptation are dramatic: environmental conditions that result in collapse within one hour of the first day of exposure become tolerable for several hours after several days of exposure. Once acclimatization has been achieved, aldosterone secreted by the adrenal gland acts upon the duct to increase sodium reabsorption. Aldosterone diminishes sodium depletion during intense thermal stress. Although the decrease in sodium concentration in acclimatization is related to aldosterone activity, the increased sweat rate after acclimatization is probably not mediated by aldosterone. Thus, the process of acclimatization involves both a decrease in the sodium concentration of sweat and an increase in the sweat rate at smaller elevations of temperature. There is no significant effect of aldosterone in the unacclimatized person, even during intense exercise.

Regional heating of the skin can cause increases in the sweat rate over the heated region. This peripheral effect has been attributed to direct thermal action on the eccrine sweat apparatus.

Despite the fact that heat is the prime activator, eccrine sweat glands respond to other physiologic stimuli. All of these operate through the nervous system and usually produce localized sweat responses. An example in many individuals is facial sweating that results from the eating of spicy food, called "gustatory sweating." Sweating stimulated by emotional stresses such as pain, fear, or anger is a common experience and is usually localized to a few areas, the commonest sites being the palms, soles, axillae, and forehead. Extreme emotional stresses may result in a generalized sweating response. The palms and soles respond poorly to thermal stimulation, but their dramatic response to psychogenic stimuli forms one basis for the lie-detector test. This paradoxical sweating response of the palms is picturesquely illustrated in the contrast between the sweat-drenched ditchdigger who spits onto his palms in order to moisten them and the public speaker with stage fright whose skin and mouth are parched, but who continually has to dry his perspiration-soaked palms.

REFERENCES

Billingham, R. E., and Silvers, W. K.: Studies on the conservation of epidermal specificities of skin and certain mucosas in adult mammals. J. Exp. Med. *125*:429, 1967.

Cage, G. W., and Dobson, R. L.: Sodium secretion and reabsorption in the human eccrine sweat gland. J. Clin. Invest. *44*:1270, 1965.

Fitzpatrick, T. B., Miyamoto, M., and Ishikawa, K.: The evalution of concepts of melanin biology. Arch. Dermatol. *96*:305, 1967.

Gross, J.: Collagen. Sci. Am. *204*:121, 1961.

Hurley, H. J., and Shelley, W. B.: The Human Apocrine Gland in Health and Disease. Springfield, Illinois, Charles C Thomas, 1960.

Loewi, G.: The acid mucopolysaccharides of human skin. Biochim. Biophys. Acta 52:435, 1961.

Lynne, A. G., and Short, B. F.: The Biology of Skin and Hair Growth. Sydney, Angus and Robertson, 1965.

McLoughlin, C. B.: Mesenchymal influences on epithelial differentiation. Symp. Soc. Exp. Biol. *17*:359, 1963.

Mercer, E. H.: Keratin and Keratinization. New York, Pergamon Press, 1961.

Montagna, W.: The Structure and Function of Skin. New York, Academic Press, 1962.

Montagna, W., and Ellis, R. A.: Biology of Hair Growth. New York, Academic Press, 1958.

Montagna, W., and Lobitz, W. C.: The Epidermis. New York, Academic Press, 1964.

Montagna, W., Ellis, R. A., and Silver, A. F.: Advances in Biology of Skin. Vol. 4: The Sebaceous Glands. New York, Pergamon Press, 1963.

Odland, G.: The Skin. University of Washington School of Medicine, 1971.

Pinkus, H., and Mehregan, A. H.: A Guide to Dermatohistopathology. New York, Appleton-Century-Crofts, 1969.

Rich, A., and Crick, H. F. C.: The molecular structure of collagen. J. Mol. Biol. 3:483, 1961.

Scheuplein, R. J.: Mechanism of percutaneous absorption. I. Routes of penetration and influence of solubility. J. Invest. Dermatol. 45:334, 1965.

Scheuplein, R. J.: Mechanism of percutaneous absorption. II. Role of transient diffusion in determining relative importance of various routes of skin penetration. J. Invest. Dermatol. 48:79, 1966.

Weinstein, G. D., and Van Scott, E. J.: Autoradiographic analysis of turnover times of normal and psoriatic epidermis. J. Invest. Dermatol. 45:257, 1965.

Wessels, W. K.: Differentiation of epidermis and epidermal derivatives. N. Engl. J. Med. 277:21, 1967.

Zelickson, A. S.: Ultrastructure of Normal and Abnormal Skin. Philadelphia, Lea and Febiger, 1967.

Section II

SEBUM: ITS NATURE AND PHYSIOPATHOLOGIC RESPONSES

Peter E. Pochi

NATURE AND COMPOSITION OF SEBUM

The skin surface lipid film is a complex mixture of triglycerides, mono- and diglycerides, fatty acids, wax esters, squalene, sterols, sterol esters, and diol esters (Downing and Strauss, 1974). It derives from two principal sources: sebum, the secretory product of the sebaceous glands, and the lipid of keratinization. The composition of the lipids from these two sources differs, but since most of the surface lipid is of sebaceous gland origin, its relative composition varies little, even over a rather wide range of values for sebaceous gland secretion. Quantitatively, the major constituents of sebum are the glycerides (mostly triglycerides), wax esters, squalene, and fatty acids. Qualitatively, the wax esters and squalene appear to be derived solely from the sebaceous glands, and, accordingly, are markers for sebum. Studies of isolated sebaceous glands and of regional variations in surface lipid composition reveal that free fatty acids are not present in the freshly secreted sebum but are formed from intrafollicular glyceride lipolysis, presumably as the result of bacterial lipase action. These free fatty acids have inflammation-evoking properties and thus are of putative importance in acne. Only the fatty acids from glycerides appear to be involved, since the wax ester concentration is not altered with antibiotic treatment in contrast to the triglyceride fraction.

The nature of the fatty acids in sebum has been the subject of considerable investigation. They have chain lengths varying from C_3 to C_{32}, with quantitative predominance of acids (in triglycerides) from C_{14} to C_{18}. They consist of saturated and unsaturated acids, straight and branched chain, with a significantly higher percent of odd-numbered acids than are found in other tissue lipids. The unsaturated acids, both even and odd-chain lengths, include compounds having their double bonds in either the 6,7 or 8,9 positions, rather than in the more usual 9,10 configuration.

CONTROL OF SEBACEOUS GLAND SECRETION

The sebaceous glands develop in the fourth month of fetal life and at birth are moderately well developed. After birth the glands involute and remain quite small throughout childhood. Glandular redevelopment begins to take place between the ages of 8 and 10 as an early manifestation of puberty (Pochi and Strauss, 1974). Sebaceous maturation continues into adolescence, then remains essentially unchanged until later years, decreasing after the menopause in women and after the seventh decade in men.

The development of the sebaceous gland and the stimulation of sebum synthesis depend principally upon hormonal factors, with the prime direct stimulating effect being an androgenic one (Pochi and Strauss, 1974). Thus, the sebaceous gland is an androgen target organ. The administration of androgenic compounds to individuals with inadequately stimulated glands, such as children, eunuchs, or postmenopausal women, leads to an increase in sebum secretion. Estrogens can oppose this stimulating effect, but only in large gonadotropin-inhibiting doses. The effect of estrogen, then, appears to result from a suppression of androgens primarily at sites of androgen synthesis rather than at the level of the sebaceous gland. Progesterone in physiologic amounts has no effect on sebaceous gland secretion in man, and there is no significant fluctuation of sebum levels in the menstrual cycle. Since adrenocortical suppression with exogenous glucocorticoid can decrease sebum levels in women but not in men, adrenal androgens, in addition to gonadal androgen, are a source of sebaceous stimulation in women. The role of the pituitary on the sebaceous gland appears to be principally an indirect one through its release of tropic hormones (Shuster and Thody, 1974). Proof is lacking concerning the presence of a specific sebotropic hormone, but there is evidence from animal studies that melanocyte-stimulating hormone (MSH), growth hormone, or prolactin have functional activity in this regard. Their possible role in man, however, remains to be clarified.

The sebaceous glands are not innervated, and thus denervation or neuronal excitation exert minimal effects (Kligman and Shelley, 1958; Shuster and Thody, 1974). Moreover, the glands are essentially unresponsive to the administration of physiologic chemomediators of neurotransmission, such as norepinephrine and acetylcholine (Kligman and Shelley, 1958; Shuster and Thody, 1974).

Little is known of non-endocrine factors affecting sebaceous gland secretion. The effect of changes in sebum viscosity and skin temperature appears to be related more to the delivery of sebum once formed rather than to an influence on sebum synthesis per se (Shuster and Thody, 1974).

FUNCTIONS OF SEBUM

The physiologic significance of sebum in man remains an enigma. Its role in animals is that of coating the hair to protect it against wetting and of providing heat insulation. Also, sebaceous secretions in animals may be odoriferous possibly serving as sexual attractants or territorial markings. In man these functions are inoperable or irrelevant, but other roles have variously been ascribed to human sebum, namely (1) barrier protection, (2) regulation of percutaneous absorption, (3) emulsification, (4) antimicrobial activity, and (5) a vitamin D precursor. However, there is no proof that any of these are operative in man, and there is much evidence to suggest that none of them are (Kligman, 1963).

SEBUM ALTERATIONS IN DERMATOLOGIC DISEASE

From the result of various studies, sebaceous gland secretion in acne has been found to be greater than normal (Pochi and Strauss, 1974; Shuster and Thody, 1974). The differences cited are based on statistical comparisons of the average values of groups of acne patients versus normal controls. However, it is important to realize that sebum levels of given individuals in the two groups overlap, such that an acne patient may produce less sebum than a normal individual. This observation does not diminish the importance of sebum in the pathogenesis of acne, since severer cases of acne tend to show greater sebaceous secretion than do milder cases. On the basis of current knowledge, the principal pathologic role of sebum is its capability of evoking inflammation. It may have an added role of inducing faulty follicular epithelial keratinization leading to the formation of comedones.

Disorders in which sebum production is allegedly decreased include those with manifestations of dry skin, such as atopic dermatitis, asteatosis, xerosis, ichthyosis, and so forth. However, there are no convincing reports that sebum is reduced in any of these disorders. Noteworthy in this regard is the observation that dryness or oiliness of the skin may be related less to decreased or increased oil secretion and more to surface moisture content (Kligman and Shelley, 1958).

The composition of sebum in acne has also been studied by various investigators, but no consistent patterns of alterations have been seen, except possibly for an increase in the relative amount of squalene (Strauss et al., 1974). The free fatty acids, the component of the surface lipid having greatest potential significance in the pathogenesis of acne, have been reported variously to be normal, increased, or decreased in amount.

SEBACEOUS GLAND SECRETION IN SYSTEMIC DISEASE

Hormonal Disorders

Since sebaceous gland secretion is an androgen-dependent function, disorders of androgen excess in women (for example, adrenal hyperplasia, ovarian tumors, polycystic ovarian disease) or of androgen insufficiency in both sexes (for example, primary or secondary hypogonadism, adrenal insufficiency) are associated with increased or decreased sebum production levels, respectively (Burton et al., 1972; Pochi and Strauss, 1974; Shuster and Thody, 1974; Strauss and Pochi, 1968). Sebum secretion has also been reported to be excessive in patients with acromegaly (Shuster and Thody, 1974). Because the range of sebaceous gland activity is so variable from person to person whether normal or abnormal, an individual patient with any of these endocrine disorders may have a sebum level which is altered from his pre-diseased norm but which actually lies within the established range of normal values. Usually only by comparison of pathologic and normal groups do differences become apparent.

No changes in the composition of sebum have been observed or reported to date in patients with hormonal disturbances, except in instances in which sebaceous secretion is so low (for example, in panhypopituitarism) that the relative contribution of epidermal lipid becomes evident. With very high rates of sebum secretion, on the other hand, the proportion of individual components of the lipid surface film remains unchanged.

Breast Cancer

Postmenopausal women with breast cancer have statistically higher rates of sebum secretion than normal (Krant et al., 1968). There is considerable overlap, however, with normal values, so that the sebum level has limited diagnostic importance. However, since sebum levels are much lower on average in postmenopausal women, it is conceivable that prospective study of sebum production in individuals with a high risk for developing breast cancer may have prognostic value. The reason for excess sebaceous gland activity in this group of patients is unknown, but it is not likely an androgenic effect, since women with breast cancer are not virilized and have normal levels of circulating androgens.

Parkinson's Disease

Patients with parkinsonism, particularly of the post-encephalitic type, tend to show heightened levels of sebaceous gland activity (Pochi et al., 1962). However, as in the case of patients with endocrine disorders, much variation can occur, such that it is not possible to characterize an individual patient as having Parkinson's disease by the quantity of sebum produced. Treatment with the anti-parkinsonian drug L-dopa effects a lowering of sebum in many cases (Shuster and Thody, 1974), but there is no correlation between the degree of suppression and neurologic improvement (Kohn et al., 1973). The cause of the seborrhea in this disease has not been established, but it has been suggested that excess MSH elaboration is responsible (Shuster et al., 1973).

Starvation

Sebum secretion levels decrease under conditions of total or near total caloric deprivation (Downing and Strauss, 1974). This reduction is accompanied by a change in the composition of sebum in which there is a decrease in the synthesis of triglycerides and wax esters but no apparent inhibitory influence on the synthesis of squalene. This is the only instance yet uncovered in which a selective inhibition of sebum synthesis is known to occur. These effects on sebum production and composition are totally reversible on re-alimentation.

REFERENCES

Burton, J. L., Johnson, C., Libman, L., et al.: Skin virilism in women with hirsutism. J. Endocrinol. 53:349, 1972.

Downing, D. T., and Strauss, J. S.: Synthesis and composition of surface lipids of human skin. J. Invest. Dermatol. 62:228, 1974.

Kligman, A. M.: The uses of sebum? *In* Montagna, W., Ellis, R. A., and Silver, A. F., (eds.): Advances in Biology of Skin. Vol. 4. Oxford, Pergamon Press, 1963, pp. 110–124.

Kligman, A. M., and Shelley, W. B.: An investigation of the biology of the human sebaceous gland. J. Invest. Dermatol. 30:99, 1958.

Kohn, S. R., Pochi, P. E., Strauss, J. S., et al.: Sebaceous gland secretion in Parkinson's disease during L-dopa treatment. J. Invest. Dermatol. 60:134, 1973.

Krant, M. J., Brandrup, C. S., Greene, R. S. et al.: Sebaceous gland activity in breast cancer. Nature 217:463, 1968.

Pochi, P. E., and Strauss, J. S.: Endocrinologic control of the development and activity of the human sebaceous gland. J. Invest. Dermatol. 62:191, 1974.

Pochi, P. E., Strauss, J. S., and Mescon, H.: Sebum production and fractional 17-ketosteroid excretion in parkinsonism. J. Invest. Dermatol. 38:45, 1962.

Shuster, S., and Thody, A. J.: The control and measurement of sebum secretion. J. Invest. Dermatol. 62:172, 1974.

Shuster, S., Thody, A. J., Goolamali, S. K., et al.: Melanocyte-stimulating hormone and parkinsonism. Lancet 1:463, 1973.

Strauss, J. S., and Pochi, P. E.: The hormonal control of human sebaceous glands: Observations in certain endocrine disorders. *In* Astwood, E. B., and Cassidy, C. E., (eds.): Clinical Endocrinology II. New York, Grune & Stratton, 1968, pp. 798–808.

Strauss, J. S., Pochi, P. E., and Downing, D. T.: Acne: perspectives. J. Invest. Dermatol. 62:321, 1974.

Section III

PERMEABILITY OF THE SKIN

Harry J. Hurley

Misconceptions concerning the permeability of human skin abound in the minds of the laity and many medical personnel. Skin is neither an impregnable, impermeable envelope nor a fragile, freely permeable membrane. It is a durable, selectively permeable (more impermeable than permeable) cover, showing regional variations in absorptive capacity. It owes its durability to the dermis, but its chemical impermeability resides in the epidermis and almost exclusively in its dead outer layer, the stratum corneum. The cutaneous permeability of man cannot be equated with that of any other species although, in this property at least, the skin of the pig and guinea pig comes closest to that of man.

Skin should be viewed both as a membrane limiting water loss from the body and as a protective sheath regulating the penetration of water and other chemicals into the system. In the latter role, skin is both a barrier to the absorption of most substances and a system of routes or pathways permitting the selective entry of others. Physicians are concerned with both of these reciprocal aspects of cutaneous permeability since absorbed chemicals can produce cutaneous damage and systemic toxicity and the effective treatment of dermatologic disease requires topical application of medicaments. At the present state of medical knowledge, percutaneous treatment of systemic illness is neither possible nor desirable.

Present day concepts governing the permeability of skin have been derived from both clinical and investigative observations. Recent basic research has modified our appreciation of the significance of the stratum corneum as a barrier and of the roles of the sweat ducts and pilosebaceous units in absorption. However, the most important recent advance in topical dermatologic therapy (that is, the use of vapor-impermeable plastic films to enhance the absorption and thera-peutic effect of applied medications) resulted from a clinical application of an old observation (Garb, 1960; Rothman, 1954; Sulzberger and Witten, 1961). It should be stressed that the mechanisms involved in this therapeutic approach have not been fully clarified.

The most comprehensive recent reviews of cutaneous permeability are those of Wallberg (1973), Grasso and Lansdown (1972), Scheuplein (1972), Scheuplein and Blank (1971), and Tregear (1966). Kligman's evaluation (1964) of the stratum corneum is enlightening, as are the reports of McKenzie and Stoughton (1962) and Stoughton (1965) on the absorption of topical corticosteroids and the accelerant effects on absorption of dimethylsulfoxide and related compounds.

MEASUREMENT TECHNIQUES

A variety of in vivo and in vitro techniques have been developed to measure percutaneous absorption. Although the efficacy of the "barrier" may be determined by the water diffusion method or by electrical conductivity studies, these tests are not routinely performed in assessment of percutaneous absorption. The most useful in vivo method of measuring percutaneous absorption is the determination, employing chemical or radioisotopic tracer techniques, of the rate of disappearance of substances applied topically. Less sensitive are measurements of urinary, fecal, or respiratory excretion or deposition in internal organs and methods which are based on observation of pharmacologic, immunologic, or biochemical effects. Some of the latter have selected application, however, as in the vasoconstrictor assay of corticosteroid efficacy. Autoradiographic analysis permits the microscopic localization of applied compounds but has limitations as a quantitative tool. Absorption in vitro can be quantitated by measuring the passage of a substance across skin which has been mounted in a chamber. As in the in vivo methods, chemical or radioisotopic methods are used to measured concentration.

BARRIERS TO ABSORPTION

For many years it was taught that the principal barrier opposing percutaneous absorption was in the lower reaches of the stratum corneum in the region just above the stratum granulosum. It is a dense keratinous zone of compactly arranged layers of stratum corneum and has been called the stratum conjunctum. On electron microscopy, this "layer" presents a homogeneous lamellar appearance (Odland, 1973), and Szakall (1958) claims to have isolated it as a tough elastic membrane composed of interwoven fibrils. As part of this concept, the more loosely bound superficial portion of the stratum corneum, which was presumably more porous, was contrastingly named the stratum disjunctum. In objecting to division of the stratum corneum into disjunctum and conjunctum layers, Kligman (1964) envisioned the stratum corneum as a barrier gradient of increasing resistance from above to below. In this view, increased cohesiveness of the lower layers accounted for their increased resistance to penetration.

Subsequent studies have emphasized that the *entire* stratum corneum, not just its lower portion, is a uniformly good diffusion barrier and presents the major resistance to absorption (Scheuplein, 1972). The high DC and AC resistance of the skin resides in the entire bulk of the stratum corneum, not in any special zone or layer. Isotopic tracers applied to the skin appear in highest amount in the outer horny layers, decreasing proportionately toward the deeper levels. The conclusion that the entire stratum corneum is the principal permeability barrier is inescapable. Consonant with this is the finding that the overall thickness of the stratum corneum is also a factor influencing absorption. For most substances, the palms

and soles, with a stratum corneum of 600 microns in width, are less permeable than are other skin regions whose stratum corneum measures only 10 to 15 microns.

The surface lipid film limits water loss from the skin as well as the penetration of water and water-soluble substances into the skin but it is not a major factor slowing absorption. The presence of an additional barrier at the dermo-epidermal junction has also been postulated (Vickers, 1966) but apparently it is of negligible influence since most studies indicate rather free passage once the stratum corneum is traversed.

Much of the data on localization of the cutaneous barrier has been obtained with the adhesive stripping method (Vickers, 1966; Wolff, 1939). Although it has definite limitations and produces histologically demonstrable damage to the granular layer, this technique has broad application in permeability studies and has provided some of the most meaningful observations on the site of the cutaneous barrier. It may also be employed to facilitate penetration of applied materials.

ROUTES OF PERCUTANEOUS ABSORPTION

Discussion of the available routes by which substances may pass across the skin must include an analysis of anatomic features as well as of physical and chemical forces which influence absorption. Three possible pathways may be defined anatomically: (1) through the stratum corneum, (2) through the hair follicles, or (3) through the sweat ducts. The older literature stresses the importance of the hair follicles and sebaceous glands as an absorptive route but more recent studies indicate that the principal pathway lies across the stratum corneum. The hair follicles and sweat glands are now felt to play a minor, secondary role. Only during an early, brief period of perhaps five minutes immediately after the application of the test substance is absorption through the appendages greater than that through the stratum corneum. Transappendageal absorption occurs by diffusion and involves water and water-soluble substances primarily. After this initial phase, however, most of the percutaneous absorption takes place across the stratum corneum, which has a much greater surface area than do the hair follicles and sweat ducts.

A concentration gradient is probably the sole driving force behind the percutaneous absorption across the stratum corneum. Moreover, transcorneal movement is apparently directly through the cell walls of the compacted corneum and not via intercellular routes. Hydration of the stratum corneum increases its permeability, possibly by expanding pores or channels which fill readily with water. These channels may not be true pores but may simply represent protein filaments which act as pathways for polar compounds. Resistance along the polar pathway is offered by "bound" water present in fully hydrated stratum corneum, according to Scheuplein (1967). The lipids of the stratum corneum provide a route for nonpolar molecules. Lipid-soluble substances, however, which do not damage the stratum corneum, are also absorbed to a lesser extent through the pilosebaceous apparatus.

OTHER FACTORS INFLUENCING PERCUTANEOUS ABSORPTION

Increased skin temperature, like increased water content of the skin, clearly results in an increase in absorption through the skin. Changes in the pH of the applied solution influence absorption indirectly by altering the ionization of the compound. Ionization decreases the passage of chemicals through the stratum corneum. The rate of passage of ionized electrolytes is approximately equivalent to that of water, which traverses the stratum corneum with difficulty. Lipids and lipid-soluble substances pass through the skin comparatively easily, while organic compounds possessing hydrophilic groups do so less readily. Small molecules showing both water and lipid solubility are apparently the most easily absorbed. Compounds in the gaseous state, with the strange but fortunate exception of carbon monoxide, are readily absorbed through the skin. Their passage increases substan-

tially with increased skin temperature and with hydration of the stratum corneum.

Vehicles affect the absorption of incorporated compounds. The controlling factors include the nature and absorption characteristics of the vehicle, the degree of partition between the vehicle and the stratum corneum, and the concentration of the compound in the vehicle. The latter factor is especially important for aqueous solutions of electrolytes. The greater the partition coefficient between the vehicle and the stratum corneum the more independent will be the rates of absorption of the vehicle and incorporated compound. The problem is quite complicated, however, and the absorption of a compound from various vehicles is not completely predictable. Some vehicles injure the stratum corneum and increase absorption. The ease of release of the compound from its vehicle is another factor which must be recognized. Moreover, it is well to take into consideration also the degree to which vehicles duplicate physiologic changes which affect cutaneous permeability (Baker, 1969). For example, the application of an ointment to the skin surface may lead to relative occlusion so that the normal evaporation of water is impeded. Increased hydration of the stratum corneum results and, as emphasized earlier, penetration is enhanced. It is probably fair to state that only by careful experimentation using the given compound and the base intended for its incorporation can an accurate assessment of its absorption be made.

CLINICAL CORRELATION

Skin damaged by disease or chemicals, especially solvents, denaturants, and strong surfactants, is substantially more permeable than is intact skin. This change reflects the effect these agents have on the chemical or physical-chemical state of the stratum corneum, especially its lower levels. Hyperemic skin, which has long been known to show increased absorption, is usually associated with an abnormal epidermis which alters the absorptive capacity. Increased blood flow alone has not yet been critically evaluated as a factor influencing absorption because of the difficulty in separating epidermal alteration and hyperemia. Diseases, such as toxic epidermal necrolysis, bullous erythema multiforme, pemphigus, and burns, which produce complete denudation of the epidermis or of the entire stratum corneum, understandably also dramatically increase permeability. In addition, disorders of keratinization, such as psoriasis, in which the barrier is imperfectly formed, show increased percutaneous absorption. Mucous membranes are much more permeable, in the range of 10 to 50 times greater, than is skin, probably principally because of the absence of a stratum corneum, although the factors of increased temperature and hydration of mucosal surfaces are important also.

The organic solvents, dimethylsulfoxide (DMSO) and to a lesser extent dimethylacetamide and dimethylformamide, have been shown to increase significantly the penetration of many substances while not producing any visible damage to the skin. Chemical changes, in the form of extracted lipoprotein, do occur, however (Allenby et al., 1969), and morphologic alterations have been described under electron microscopy (Montes et al., 1967). The anticipated broad clinical application of DMSO as a carrier or accelerant of percutaneous absorption, which would enhance the efficacy of topical corticosteroids, local anesthetics, cytotoxic agents, and antibiotics, has not yet materialized.

The effective use of occlusive dressings, made possible in the 1960s by the development and availability of vapor-impermeable plastic films such as polyvinylidine and polyethylene, has added an extra dimension to topical dermatologic therapy. Limited application of the technique to small areas such as the hands or feet is possible with the use of plastic gloves or boots. Body suits or bags may be worn for treatment of wide areas of the skin surface. A special development simplifying the occlusive approach has been the incorporation of medications into adhesives applied to polyethylene tape which sticks to the diseased area. Surprising and previously unachievable beneficial effects have been seen with occlusive topical therapy but it is not without its hazards. Used on exudative surfaces, the prospect of complicating infection is greatly enhanced and the increased absorption the technique provides can produce undesirable local and even systemic effects of the applied compound.

The existence of a reservoir or depot in the stratum corneum which results in prolongation of the effect of topically applied materials seems well established, especially for corticosteroids (Vickers, 1972). This depot effect requires an occlusive method of application, however, and an essentially normal stratum corneum. Psoriatic skin, for example, does not exhibit the reservoir phenomenon. In contrast, in dermatoses with a stratum corneum which is relatively normal, such as in localized neurodermatitis and ichthyosis, the reservoir may be of therapeutic significance. One must conclude that the presence or absence of a clinically important reservoir in the stratum corneum must be determined for each disorder as well as for each medicament.

Over the last 20 years, topical dermatologic therapy has shown dramatic changes, reflecting pharmacologic and physiologic advances. The future should see continued progress in topical therapy, and much of it will result from the further study and application of the principles which govern cutaneous permeability.

REFERENCES

Allenby, A. C., Creasey, N. H., Edginton, J. A. G., et al.: Mechanism of action of accelerants on Skin Penetration. Br. J. Dermatol. *81* (Suppl. 4):47–55, 1969.

Baker, H.: Experimental studies on the influence of vehicles on percutaneous absorption. J. Soc. Cosmet. Chem. *20*:239–252, 1969.

Garb, J.: Nevus verricosus unilateris cured with Podophyllin ointment. Arch. Dermatol. *81*:606–609, 1960.

Grasso, P., and Lansdown, A. B. G.: Methods of measuring and factors affecting percutaneous absorption. J. Soc. Cosmet. Chem. *23*:481–521, 1972.

Kligman, A. M.: The Biology of the Stratum Corneum. *In* Montagna, W., and Lobitz, W. C., (eds.): Epidermis. New York, Academic Press, 1964.

McKenzie, A. W.: Percutaneous absorption of steroids. Arch. Dermatol. *86*:614, 1962.

McKenzie, A. W., and Stoughton, R. B.: Method for comparing percutaneous absorption of steroids. Arch. Dermatol. *86*:608–610, 1962.

Montes, L. F., Day, J. L., Wand, C. J., et al.: Ultrastructural changes in the horny layer following local application of dimethyl sulfoxide. J. Invest. Dermatol. *48*:184–196, 1967.

Odland, G.: Quoted by Malkinson and Rothman in Percutaneous Absorption, pp. 90–156. *In* J. Jadassohn's Handbuch Der Haut Und Geschlechtskrankheiten. Normale und Pathologische Physiologie Der Haut. I. Edited by A. Marchionini and H. W. Spier. Berlin, Springer-Verlag, 1963.

Rothman, S.: Physiology and Biochemistry of the Skin. Chicago, University of Chicago Press, 1954.

Scheuplein, R. J.: Mechanism of percutaneous absorption. II. Transient diffusion and the relative importance of various routes of skin penetration. J. Invest. Dermatol. *48*:79–88, 1967.

Scheuplein, R. J.: Properties of skin as a membrane. *In* Montagna, W., Van Scott, E. J., and Stoughton, R. B. (eds.): Advances in Biology of the Skin. Vol. XII. New York, Appleton-Century-Crofts, 1972.

Scheuplein, R. J., and Blank, I. H.: Permeability of the skin. Physiol. Rev. *51*:702–735, 1971.

Stoughton, R. B.: Dimethylsulfoxide (DMSO) induction of a steroid reservoir in human skin. Arch. Dermatol. *91*:657–660, 1965.

Sulzberger, M. B., and Witten, V. H.: Thin pliable plastic film in topical dermatologic therapy. Arch. Dermatol. *84*:1027–1028, 1961.

Szakall, A.: Experimentelle Daten zur Klärung der Funktion der Wasserbarriere in der Epiderms des Lebenden Menschen. Berufs-dermatosen *6*:171–191, 1958.

Tregear, R. T.: Physical Functions of the Skin. London, Academic Press, 1966.

Vickers, C. F. H.: *In* MacKenna, R. M. B., (ed.): Modern Trends in Dermatology. Vol. 3. London, Butterworth and Co. Ltd., 1966.

Vickers, C. F. H.: Stratum corneum reservoir for drugs. *In* Montagna, W., Van Scott, E. J., and Stoughton, R. B. (eds.): Advances in Biology of the Skin. Vol. XII. New York, Appleton-Century-Crofts, 1972.

Wallberg, J. E.: Percutaneous absorption. Curr. Probl. Dermatol. *5*:1, 1973.

Wolff, S.: Die Innere Struktur der Zellen des Stratum Desquamans der Menschlichen Epidermis. Z. Mikr. Anat. Forsch. *46*:170–202, 1939.

CHAPTER

2

BASIC PHYSIOLOGIC
AND HISTOPATHOLOGIC
REACTION PATTERNS

Section I

BASIC PHYSIOLOGIC REACTIONS
Harvey Baker

The purposes of this chapter are to describe briefly the changes at the cellular and tissue levels which accompany disease of the skin, to relate these changes to the spectrum of syndromes seen by the physician, and to describe briefly the patterns of pathophysiologic response seen in the skin.

The skin, like any other organ, is subject to a variety of pathologic processes which stem from its exposure to influences mediated by the vascular or nervous systems. In addition, it is peculiar in that it is exposed to a variety of external environmental insults, both physical and chemical.

The skin's main function is to act as a two-way barrier, preventing loss of body constituents and entry of noxious or unwanted molecules or irradiation from the environment. If pathologic changes of any sort lead to breakdown of this barrier function, secondary cutaneous, subcutaneous, or systemic reactions may follow.

Before the use of electron microscopy, it was convenient to recognize three basic tissue responses. These were: (1) functional impairment in the absence of morphologic change, (2) inflammatory and degenerative responses to cellular injury, and (3) neoplastic cellular proliferation, benign or malignant.

Such a division, however convenient, is

69

no longer tenable. Virtually every functional disorder is accompanied by morphologic changes, whether at the macroscopic, light microscopic, or electron microscopic level. The distinction between structure and function, therefore, no longer has meaning, and every pathologic change has to be viewed simultaneously in anatomical, physiological, biochemical, and biophysical terms. A process which starts in one type of cell (for instance, the keratinocytes) may rapidly implicate others. Nevertheless, for purposes of analysis, the skin presents a number of units (see Table 2-1) which can be conveniently looked at individually and which may and do undergo pathologic reactions.

The behavior of each of these cell lines needs to be considered individually and as a tissue component, but before embarking on this it is necessary to analyze the morphologic changes, visual or tactile, perceived by the clinician.

The clinician initially detects changes in either color or mass. Changes in mass are in turn due to increase or decrease of cells, extracellular deposits, or fluid. The particular shape of such alteration in mass may be important. Two or more of these fundamental changes may coexist. The causes of each of these are multiple and are listed in Table 2-2.

Change of color may be due to vascular or melanocytic changes or to the optical sequelae of increasing or decreasing mass. Examples of clinical situations in which color changes are so produced are given in Table 2-2. The causes of change of mass are equally complex; only fluid accumulation is a relatively simple process.

REACTION PATTERNS OF INDIVIDUAL CELL LINES

The pathologic alterations of each cell or unit may be further correlated with specific clinical entities.

The Keratinocyte

Of the three epidermal cell lines, the keratinocyte is by far the most numerous. Its sole function is to elaborate the stratum corneum which is the major component of the cutaneous barrier. The twin processes of keratinocyte maturation (cornification) and intracellular keratin formation (keratinization) depend upon a dynamic equilibrium between basal cellular division, migration, maturation, and shedding (Bullough, 1972). Thus:

$$\begin{matrix} \text{Rate of cellular} \\ \text{production by} \\ \text{division} \end{matrix} = \begin{matrix} \text{Rate of incorp-} \\ \text{oration of cells} \\ \text{into stratum} \\ \text{corneum} \end{matrix} = \begin{matrix} \text{Rate of shedding} \\ \text{of cells from} \\ \text{epidermal sur-} \\ \text{face} \end{matrix}$$

If production exceeds shedding, increased epidermal volume must follow, producing hypertrophy. According to the type of disorder, such epidermal hypertrophy can chiefly affect the living (Malpighian) epidermis, so-called acanthosis, or it can affect the stratum corneum, producing hyperkeratosis (if the corneal cells are mature, have lost their nuclei, and are firmly adherent) or parakeratosis (if the cells are less mature). If, on the other hand, cell loss by shedding predominates over the new cell production in the basal layer, epidermal atrophy must follow.

Table 2–1 FUNCTIONAL UNITS OF THE SKIN

	Cells	*Appendages*	*Systems*
Epidermis	Keratinocyte Melanocyte Langerhans' cells	Hair follicle Sebaceous gland Apocrine gland Eccrine gland	Vascular Neural Myeloid Reticuloendothelial (lymphoid)
Dermis	Fibroblast Histiocyte Mast cell Lymphocyte Plasma cell		

Table 2–2 COLOR AND MASS CHANGES OF CELL LINES

Change Perceived	*Pathology*	*Cause*
Change of Color (vascular)	Vasoconstriction	Cold
	Vasodilatation	Inflammation
	Telangiectasia	Rosacea
	Proliferation of capillaries	Angioma
	Disappearance of capillaries	Atrophie blanche
	Extravasation of red cells	Purpura
Change of Color (pigment)	Increased melanin in epidermis	Negro skin
	Increased melanin in dermis	Resolving lichen planus
	Reduced epidermal melanin	Vitiligo
	Presence of other pigments	Hemosiderosis
Change of Mass	Leukocytic immigration *into* epidermis	Pustular psoriasis
	Lymphoid immigration *into* epidermis	Mycosis fungoides
	Melanocyte immigration *into* epidermis	Malignant melanoma
	Increased keratinocyte mass	Psoriasis, lichen simplex
	Decreased keratinocyte mass	Lichen sclerosis
	Increased collagen mass	Scleroderma
	Decreased collagen mass	Exposed senile skin
Fluid Accumulation	Subcorneal blister	Impetigo
	Intra-epidermal blister	Pemphigus
	Subepidermal blister	Pemphigoid
	Intra-epidermal edema	Eczema
	Dermal edema	Urticaria
Altered Exfoliation	Accelerated epidermopoiesis	Psoriasis
	Maturation defects	Ichthyosis
	Retarded epidermopoiesis	Methotrexate erosions

Nevertheless, it is clear that an equilibrium state of the epidermal volume could be maintained at widely different levels of cell production, maturation, and shedding, provided these are in balance. Factors not yet understood must thus control epidermal turnover time (Marks, 1972). The dynamic state of the epidermis can be completely characterized by its rate of new cell production (mitotic rate) and turnover time.

The integrity of the epidermis depends upon its blood supply, conveyed ultimately by the capillaries of the dermal papillae. Reduction in the number of these capillaries, their obstruction by sluggish flow or extravasation of red cells, or the shunting of flow through the subpapillary venous plexus may all lead to epidermal atrophy.

Within the epidermis, cell dynamics around the intracorneal portions of sweat ducts and hair follicles are important and may cause obstruction (comedones, keratinous plugs), contributing to a variety of sebum and sweat retention disorders.

The keratinocyte mass of the epidermis gives a characteristic response to injury which is clinically dermatitis. Varying degrees of damage produce changes varying from erythema (due to secondary dermal vasodilation) to bullous formation. The appearance of vesicular loci of free fluid within the epidermis surrounded by intercellular and intracellular edema (spongiosis) is characteristic, whether the injury be chemical, thermal, radiant, or mechanical.

In other circumstances keratinocyte damage is specifically localized. Viruses may invade the cellular cytoplasm (vaccinia, variola) or the nuclear DNA (zoster, wart virus). Desmosomal complexes may become abnormal, leading to reduced intercellular adhesion and giving the acantholysis of pemphigus (Braun-Falco, 1969).

Maturation of the epidermis can be disordered in other ways. Individual cell keratinization may be genetically determined, as in Darier's disease, or due to carcinogenic stimuli, such as long-term sun exposure (actinic dyskeratosis) or inorganic arsenic administration. Such changes may progress to intra-epidermal carcinoma (Bowen's disease). Keratinization is also disordered in the ichthyoses which are a group of separate, inherited ectodermal defects (see Chapter 21). Localized, often unilateral, epidermal defects may be congenital (epidermal nevus or ichthyosis hystrix). Lastly, basal and squamous cell epitheliomata occur (Newbold, 1972).

The Melanocyte

Disorders of pigmentation are discussed in detail in Chapter 22. Melanocytes synthesize melanin within specific organelles, the melanosomes. These are injected, via the melanocytes' dendritic processes, into surrounding keratinocytes. For a variety of reasons, melanin production may be excessive or defective, leading to hyperpigmentation or hypopigmentation. Melanocytes may also actually disappear, as in the center of lesions of vitiligo (Duchon et al., 1968).

Localized hypopigmentation may be genetically determined, as in piebaldism, or result from drugs such as chloroquine taken internally or from chemicals applied externally (for example, hydroquinones). It may be postinflammatory or related to adjacent nevi (for example, halo nevus).

A similar range of factors determines localized hyperpigmentation. The cafe-au-lait macules of neurofibromatosis and polyostotic fibrous dysplasia are genetically determined. Pituitary melanocyte stimulating hormone determines chloasma (for example, in pregnancy or during oral contraceptive therapy).

Proliferation of abnormal melanocytes (nevus cells) at the epidermal-dermal junction in childhood and adolescence is responsible for the type of macular moles known as junctional nevi. These usually evolve into dermal moles. Neoplastic junctional proliferation of melanocytes later in life is the first feature of malignant melanoma.

THE EPIDERMAL APPENDAGES

Hair Follicle

Appreciation of the cyclic nature of hair growth (see Chapter 25) has in the last two decades led to a greatly increased understanding of pathologic responses of the follicle. Each hair follicle in the body has a constitutionally determined cyclic pattern of hair production (anagen) and rest (telogen). Catagen is a third brief phase of transition from growth to rest. The relative duration dose of the two main phases determine the natural length to which uncut hair will grow. On the normal scalp, anagen lasts two to five years; telogen approximately three months. By contrast, anagen is far shorter and telogen much longer in the eyebows or eyelashes (Montagna and Van Scott, 1958).

Against this constitutional pattern of follicular behavior, environmental factors such as age, circulating hormone levels, local inflammation, or ischemia influence the follicle. Nevertheless, the basic pathologic patterns of follicular disturbance can now be classified on a rational basis. The causes of alopecia are described in detail in Chapter 25 but illustrative patterns will be mentioned here. The follicle may be primarily affected during anagen without the cycle being disturbed. Thus, invasion of hair shafts by a dermatophyte may lead to breaking off of hairs. Antimitotic drugs, such as methotrexate or cyclophosphamide, directly inhibit new hair formation. This may distort the hair shaft or lead to its complete rupture (anagen alopecia). Clearly, follicles in telogen cannot be influenced by such drugs in the same way.

Hormonal, emotional, toxic, and other unknown factors may abruptly and prematurely terminate anagen, precipitating an apparently normal telogen phase. Such factors, acting simultaneously on a large number of follicles, have the effect of synchronizing their growth cycles. This results in a clinically apparent loss of large numbers of telogen hairs when the synchronized follicles go into anagen again approximately three months later. The hormonal events of childbirth and the toxemia of severe infection act in this way so that postpartum or postinfective alopecia characteristically occurs 10 to 14 weeks after the events which caused it (Kligman, 1961).

In male-patterned balding, a genetic prejudgment, exerting its influence only at a certain age and in certain areas (for example, the temples), in the presence of adequate circulating androgen, results in slow follicular involution with progressively shorter anagen phases, producing shorter and thinner hairs.

Inflammation of whatever cause in or around the follicle may produce loss of hair. Bacterial or fungal folliculitis does so. If the inflammation is transient, full follicular recovery can be expected. If it is chronic, as in lupus vulgaris or leprosy, or discoid lupus erythematosus, or if the inflammation is sufficiently severe although transient, as in lichen planus or opthalmic (trigeminal) zoster, alopecia may be permanent, associated with gross follicular destruction.

Sebaceous Gland

The sebaceous glands open into the upper pilar follicle. They remain dormant and inactive until stimulated by androgens at puberty. These lead to increase in size and activity of the glands and the excretion of sebum onto the hair and skin surface. The size and potential for activity of the glands is again constitutionally determined, being most marked on the scalp, face, and upper central trunk.

Hypofunction of sebaceous glands is not associated with any recognized pathologic state; specifically, it is not an important factor in dryness of the skin. Hyperfunction results in seborrhea. This may be recognized as greasiness of the skin or may go unnoticed. It may or may not be associated with acne vulgaris. The triglycerides in sebum may be broken down to free fatty acids by lipolytic, commensal bacteria, leading to inflammation of the follicular wall. Obstruction at the follicular pore, preventing the free flow of sebum onto the skin surface, may also be a factor in acne but the inflammation is known to be secondary to sebaceous rupture and release of acid sebum into the surrounding dermis. The physical signs of acne, namely, comedones, inflammatory papules, pustules, cysts, abscesses, and scarring, are explicable in terms of these basic pathologic reactions. Scarring may eventually destroy the glands and follicle completely, as may x-irradiation in high dosage (Strauss and Kligman, 1958).

Benign overgrowth of the sebaceous glands is common (for example, in nevus sebeceus of Jadassohn). Benign or malignant epidermal tumors may show varying degrees of sebaceous differentiation.

Apocrine Sweat Gland
(Hurley and Shelley, 1960)

The gland may rarely produce colored sweat secretion (localized chromidrosis) in the presence of bacteria. Again, the follicular orifice may be closed, leading to apocrine sweat retention. This may be asymptomatic or may result in rupture of the duct or the tubules (Fox-Fordyce disease). This is usually associated with intense itching, usually in the axillae.

Infection of the apocrine system is seen in hidradenitis suppurativa, associated with ductal obstruction and secondary granulomatous changes and sinus formation. The cause of this disease is unknown.

The apocrine glands may show heterotopic localization in the buccal mucosa and on the scalp, face, and trunk. Rarely, benign growths may be found which seem to originate from various components of the gland (for example, syringocystadenomas). Extramammary Paget's disease is a malignant intra-epidermal carcinoma originating from apocrine ductal cells. It may be seen, for instance, perianally.

Eccrine Sweat Gland

Rapid progress has been made in the understanding of eccrine sweat gland function in the last two decades. The glands constitute the principal organ of thermoregulation and may show abnormally increased or decreased function.

In the absence of thermal stress, excessive sweating is usually emotionally determined and is a common problem in adolescents and young adults in certain well-defined sites, namely, the palms, axillae, and face. Such hyperhidrosis tends to spontaneous improvement over a few years. Localized asymmetrical hyperhidrosis (for example, in one leg) may occasionally be the presenting manifestation of vascular disorders such as Buerger's disease. Granulosis rubra nasi is an uncommon condition of inflammation and hyperhidrosis confined to the nose, usually in young women.

Reduction in sweating, or hypohidrosis,

may be due to failure of the sweat coil to secrete, excessive tubular reabsorption of sweat, or, most commonly, to obstruction of the sweat duct within the epidermis. Transient failure to secrete may be due to anticholinergic drugs, taken systemically or applied topically, or to inflammatory damage to sweat coils by adjacent dermal disease (for example, a reticulocytic infiltrate). Increased tubular reabsorption does not have an established pathology but may be the means by which certain topical antiperspirants exert their effect. Obstruction of the sweat duct is common. Under hot conditions, poral closure is one of the factors contributing to the group of syndromes known as miliaria. Many disorders of epidermal maturation, such as psoriasis or ichthyosis, may cause obstruction within the intracorneal duct, leading to hypohidrosis. In addition, overhydration of the horny layer with consequent swelling temporarily blocks sweat ducts. Sweat gland necrosis may be produced by local pressure (for example, in patients with barbiturate poisoning). Chronic ingestion of the antimalarial, Atabrine, may also lead to long-standing anhidrosis.

Rarely, various tumors can arise from the cells constituting the sweat apparatus.

VASCULAR SYSTEM

The integrity of the skin is entirely dependent on its blood supply. Specifically, the epidermis depends on an adequate circulation through the papillary capillaries. The impact of vascular disorders on the skin depends entirely on the size and type of vessels involved. The clinical manifestations are of two sorts, the symptoms and signs caused by the disease itself (for example, the tender swellings of superficial thrombophlebitis) and the secondary local circulatory and nutritional consequences.

Gross, acute, or subacute arterial deprivation (for example, due to arterial thrombosis or embolism) produces full-thickness necrosis, that is, gangrene of skin. Ischemia may lead to focal necrosis which initially manifests itself as areas of erythematous swelling which rapidly become purpuric, then necrotic and pustular and which heal as a varioliform scar. Such a pathologic sequence is seen in allergic vasculitis (leukocytoclastic angiitis) and pityriasis lichenoides et varioliformis acuta. Obstruction due to inflammation and thrombosis of smaller arterioles may be insufficient to induce complete necrosis, but varying combinations of erythema, papules, nodules (for example, in nodular vasculitis), purpura, and blisters may follow, as in erythema multiforme or mild cold-induced perniosis (chilblains). If the ischemia is confined to the papillary capillaries because they are by-passed or blocked by sludged cells, only the immediately overlying epidermis will suffer. A combination of punctate purpura and overlying ischemic scaling of the epidermis is characteristic of capillaritis, as in, for example, the hypersensitivity reaction to carbromal. Interference with papillary capillary flow may also be due to chronic venous insufficiency in the lower limbs. It may lead to extensive white atrophy of the epidermis of the lower legs and ankles. The necrotic pustules of Behçet's syndrome are due to small vein thrombosis, inducing local ischemia. Thrombophlebitis of larger superficial veins is seen in Buerger's disease, after trauma, local infection, or intravenous cannulation and (as thrombophlebitis migrans) in association with internal carcinomata, especially of the stomach and pancreas.

Functional vascular disorders, due, for instance, to temporary vasoconstriction or vasodilatation, may produce distinctive clinical pictures. Raynaud's phenomenon of the hands is one such pattern. Livedo reticularis in the legs due to cold is another. Both of these patterns may be associated with organic vascular disease. Examples are systemic sclerosis with Raynaud's phenomenon (so-called acrosclerosis) and cutaneous polyarteritis nodosa underlying chronic livedo. Chronic minor functional abnormalities are also seen in the skin as telangiectasis (for example, in systemic sclerosis), spider nevi (in pregnancy and advanced cirrhosis), or venous stars.

Alterations in growth of the vascular system are common and may be genetically or congenitally determined, or be acquired later in life. The capillary hemangioma (port-wine stain) is present at birth and is permanent. The cavernous hemangioma (for example, strawberry nevus) in which larger and deeper capillary proliferation is seen, usually appears shortly after birth and, after a brief phase of growth for several months, slowly and spontaneously involutes. Other less common types of cavernous hemangioma may appear later or may be permanent. The common cherry angioma appears quite late in life and is harmless. Similar angiomata are seen, mostly about the tongue and face, in hereditary hemorrhagic telangectasia (Osler's disease).

Capillary proliferation may be intermixed with inflammatory changes, as in granulation tissue and the common granuloma telangiectaticum. Other benign overgrowths include glomus tumors. Malignant tumors occasionally develop. Malignant angio-endothelioma is rare. It may develop on a lymphedematous arm after radical mastectomy. Kaposi's hemorrhagic sarcoma characteristically appears at multiple sites in the lower limbs in elderly people.

In addition to the range of organic vascular reactions described, reversible functional changes may be provoked by drugs, toxins, and so forth. Toxic erythema of many different patterns may be induced by infections (for example, scarlet fever), drugs (for example, ampicillin, atropine, meprobamate), or endogenous metabolites, as in the flushing of the carcinoid syndrome or mastocytosis.

Purpura, in addition to being part of the picture of vasculitis, venous insufficiency, or drug-induced capillaritis, may be due to ascorbic acid deficiency (scurvy) or dysproteinemias such as macroglobulinemia or cryoglobulinemia.

DERMAL CELLULAR RESPONSES

Fibrocyte

This cell is responsible for laying down normal collagen and elastin in the dermis. Increased activity is its usual response to injury and is seen in granulation tissue as a temporary phenomenon. Unrestrained hyperactivity leads to hypertrophic scars and keloids. Chronic localized hyperplasia is common in middle life and leads to the simple dermal fibroma. Fibrosarcomata,

including dermatofibrosarcoma protuberans, is rare.

The collagen-elastin matrix of the dermis may be defective or damaged for genetic reasons, as in pseudo-xanthoma elasticum or the Ehlers-Danlos syndrome. Its bulk is reduced by aging, by the catabolic effects of prolonged systemic or local steroid therapy, and by actinic exposure. It may be the seat of mucinous degeneration in lichen myxedematosus or pretibial myxedema and of amyloid deposition. Various factors may induce necrobiosis of dermal collagen, known (as in necrobiosis lipoidica of diabetes) or unknown (as in granuloma annulare). Other rare abnormalities are elastosis perforans and perforating collagenosis.

Histiocyte (Macrophage)

Histiocytes phagocytose particulate matter, including melanin emanating from inflammatory processes at junctional level, lipids, hemosiderin following purpura, foreign pigments (as in tattoos), bacteria, fungi, and protozoa. Fusion of several cells leads to the formation of multinucleate foreign body giant cells. In certain xanthomata, multinucleated histiocytes filled with lipid droplets appear (Touton giant cells). In granulomata, histiocytes can become modified to epithelioid cells which form Langhans' giant cells. The latter are phagocytic and distinctive of the lesions of syphilis, tuberculosis, leprosy, sarcoidosis, and the deep mycoses.

Abnormal proliferation, involving skin, bones, liver, and spleen is seen in reticulohistiocystosis, histiocytosis X, and certain sarcomata. Examples of benign histiocytic proliferations are histiocytoma (localized, generalized, or eruptive) and xanthogranuloma of young children.

Mast Cells

These mesodermal cells are usually found in small numbers in the superficial dermis. Their granules are known to contain histamine and heparin. Discharge of the former under a variety of stimuli leads to a local urticarial reaction. The only disease in which hyperplasia of mast cells is recognized is mastocytosis (urticaria pigmentosa).

Lipocyte

The control of the fat organ is little understood. It is part of the metabolic pool and can be increased or reduced according to need. Fat may be injured by cold or ischemia (for example, due to vasculitis). Panniculitis is generally caused by vascular inflammation within the subcutaneous fat, but metabolic factors, such as circulating pancreatic enzymes (for example, in carcinoma of the pancreas), may be responsible. If the insult is severe enough, fat necrosis or liquefaction can occur. Benign tumors (lipoma) are common. They may be single or multiple. The latter may be painful and genetically determined. Liposarcoma is rare.

Myeloid-Lymphoid Cells

One final group of cells of mesodermal origin enters into cutaneous pathology, although the cells are not normally resident in the skin: the myeloid and lymphoid series of cells, very closely related to the reticular cells of the skin (fibrocyte, histiocyte, and mastocyte). The myeloid or blood leukocytes play major roles in the skin's reaction to injury. In bacterial infection, the polymorphonuclear leukocyte is predominant because of its ability to ingest bacteria (microphage). In atopic dermatitis and dermatitis herpetiformis, eosinophilic leukocytes are prominent. Basophils cannot be easily distinguished from the mastocytes. In malignant tumors of the myeloid system, an infiltrate of the immature and mature cells alike, may occasionally be found in the skin (leukemia cutis).

The lymphoid cells (lymphocytes) are found in large numbers in a very wide range of acute and chronic inflammatory changes. These cells are so common as to be considered by some as a normal constituent of skin. The most striking collections of lymphocytes are seen in the granulomas (so named because of histologic resemblance to granulation or scar tissue). Lichen planus and discoid lupus erythematosus are two other skin diseases in which the lymphoid infiltration is striking. Benign lymphocytic aggregates may be provoked by sunlight (actinic lymphocytoma) or insect bites. Malignant changes in the lymphoid system (lymphoma) may

be associated with massive cutaneous infiltrates of immature and mature cells.

Potentially malignant proliferation of the reticuloendothelial elements of the skin may lead to chronic and puzzling clinical reaction patterns lasting for years before frank tumors are clinically and histologically evident. Such patterns include generalized pruritus, acquired ichthyosis, generalized exfoliative dermatitis, poikiloderma, and curious psoriasiform and eczematoid lesions. When the reticulosis has frankly declared itself, tumors which may ulcerate are seen. These often have a characteristic bizarre configuration with curious serpiginous and horse-shoe shaped infiltrated plaques (late mycosis fungoides).

The plasma cell is infrequently present in the skin. It is seen in some infections involving the skin, such as syphilis and rhinoscleroma, and in malignancies such as mycosis fungoides and plasmacytoma. Some inflammatory processess of the mucous membranes, such as balanitis plasma cellularis (Zoon's disease) and lichen planus of the oral mucosa, have an unusual plasma-cell response.

INTERRELATION OF THE SKIN AND ITS ENVIRONMENT

Having considered cutaneous pathologic processes in terms of individual tissues, let us now look at how the whole skin is related to its internal and external environments. The relationships may be expressed as follows:

1. Systemic disturbance → Skin
2. External environmental disturbance → Skin
3. Skin → Systemic disturbance.

THE EFFECT OF SYSTEMIC DISTURBANCES ON THE SKIN

Microorganisms, toxins derived from such organisms, drugs, immune complexes, humoral and cell-bound antibodies, or malignant cells may reach the skin, usually via the blood stream. In addition, the skin may be affected by both excesses and deficiencies of hormones or vitamins reaching it. As a result of such mechanisms and others not yet understood, the skin is an important "marker" of systemic disease; many examples are described elsewhere in this book.

THE EFFECTS OF THE ENVIRONMENT ON THE SKIN

External effects may be immediate or cause long-term changes. The relevant factor can be physical or chemical and the impact may be primarily epidermal or dermal.

Physical factors include friction (leading to epidermal callus formation), heat (for example, erythema ab igne if chronic or the acute changes of a burn), and x-irradiation from industrial or medical sources. However sunlight is the most important and its effects may be due to quite separate components of the spectrum. Thus, short wave ultraviolet light (about 300 nm.) is responsible for normal sunburn and tanning. In certain subjects, for reasons unknown, it may also provoke a variety of pathologic responses. Long-term ultraviolet light exposure has direct dermal effects, leading to actinic elastosis and loss of collagen, and epidermal effects, that is, dyskeratosis and stimulation of epidermal carcinomata. Longer wave ultraviolet light (about 360 nm.) is important in certain photoallergic responses to drugs (either taken internally or applied topically). Skin containing abnormal amounts of porphyrins is activated by 400 nm. light. Waves of visible light longer than 400 nm. may provoke urticaria. The photodermatoses are fully described in Chapter 6.

Chemical agents reaching the skin surface may produce a variety of pathologic responses such as blistering, acantholysis (due to cantharidin, for example), or urticaria due to nettle stings or insect bites; however, dermatitis is the most common response. This may be provoked by primary irritants or by an allergic reaction resulting from the contact with allergens or haptens, to which the skin harbors sensitized lymphocytes. The subject of contact dermatitis is an enormous one and is of increasing industrial and socioeconomic importance.

Last, the skin may be subject to a variety of ectoparasitic infestations by mites (scabies), lice, causing pediculosis, and others.

THE SYSTEMIC EFFECTS OF CUTANEOUS DISEASE
(Shuster and Marks, 1970)

Generalized inflammation of the skin, especially if prolonged, may have profound effects on the whole body, particularly on thermoregulation, the circulation, the metabolism of water, protein and folates, and the gastrointestinal tract.

Thermoregulation

In the presence of generalized exfoliative eczema or psoriasis, the cutaneous component of heat regulation may break down. Obstruction of sweat ducts within the stratum corneum leads to hypohidrosis or complete anhidrosis and potentially to hyperthermia. At the same time, the vastly increased blood flow through the skin is responsible for a rise in skin temperature and increased surface heat loss by conduction and radiation. In addition, transepidermal water diffusion is greatly increased because of the impaired barrier function of an abnormal stratum corneum, and its evaporation takes heat from the body surface. These losses cannot be limited in a cool environment and hypothermia may follow. The patient is thus poikilothermic, tending towards the temperature of his environment.

Generally, excessive heat loss is predominant, and increased metabolic activity compensates for heat losses and eventually leads to tissue breakdown and loss of weight. The basal metabolic rate may be greatly increased but thyroid function remains essentially normal.

Hemodynamic Effects

The greatly increased blood flow through the skin augments the demands on the heart and circulation. Cardiac output (in the normal person) is likely to be at the high end of the normal range or above it and the usual signs of a hyperdynamic circulation, such as those seen in thyrotoxicosis and widespread Paget's disease of bone, or with a large arteriovenous aneurysm, are found. If preexisting heart disease limits cardiac response, failure may ensue. Diversion of blood flow may also be a feature of this situation and this could be a factor in causing disturbances in other organs. Occasionally, the onset of erythroderma may precipitate gangrene in an ischemic limb whose arterial supply was previously critical.

Metabolism

Although sweating is reduced, trans-epidermal water diffusion may be increased from the normal 100 to 150 ml. daily to 1.0 to 2.0 liters. This may lead to oliguria and increased thirst. The accelerated epidermopoiesis leading to scaling is responsible for protein loss which may reach 10.0 gm. per day or greater. Protein catabolism, hypoalbuminemia, and edema may follow. Increased utilization of available folates is the main cause of low serum folate levels. Minor abnormalities of iron and calcium metabolism are also present. The gynecomastia, loss of libido, and testicular atrophy found in some men with chronic exfoliative dermatitis appear to be due to increased levels of circulating estrogens, reflected in their increased urinary excretion; the source of these estrogens is uncertain.

Gastrointestinal Effects

The gastrointestinal effects of universal skin disease remain controversial but it has been claimed that an enteropathy may be produced and is characterized by abnormalities of jejunal mucosa and evidence of malabsorption. The enteropathy is reversible if the skin disease can be controlled.

REFERENCES

Braun-Falco, O.: The Pathology of Blister Formation. *In* Kopf, A. W., and Andrade, R.: Year Book of Dermatology. Chicago, Year Book Medical Publishers, Inc., 1969.

Bullough, W. S.: The control of epidermal growth. Br. J. Dermatol. 87:187, 1972.

Duchon, J., Fitzpatrick, T. B., and Seiji, M.: Melanin. *In* Kopf, A. W., and Andrade, R.: Year Book of Dermatology. Chicago, Year Book Medical Publishers, Inc., 1968.

Hurley, H. J., Jr., and Shelley, W. B.: The Human Apocrine Sweat Gland in Health and Disease. Springfield, Illinois, Charles C Thomas, 1960. (No. 376 American Lecture Series).

Kligman, A. M.: Pathologic dynamics of human hair loss. Arch. Dermatol. 83:175, 1961.

Marks, R.: The role of chalones in epidermal homeostasis. Br. J. Dermatol. 86:543, 1972.

Montagna, W., and Van Scott, E. J.: The Anatomy of the Hair Follicle. *In* Montagna, W., and Ellis, R. A.: Biology of Hair Growth. New York, Academic Press, 1958.

Newbold, P. C. H.: Precancer and the skin. Br. J. Dermatol. 86:417, 1972.

Pinkus, H.: The direction of growth of human epidermis. Br. J. Dermatol. 83:556, 1970.

Prunieras, M.: The Langerhans' cell. J. Invest. Dermatol. 52:1, 1969.

Shuster, S., and Marks, J.: Systemic Effects of Skin Disease. London, Heinemann Ltd., 1970.

Strauss, J. S., and Kligman, A. M.: Pathologic patterns of the sebaceous gland. J. Invest. Dermatol. 30:51, 1958.

Section II

BASIC HISTOPATHOLOGIC REACTION PATTERNS

Capt. Bernett L. Johnson MC USN

INTRODUCTION

Histopathology of the skin has significantly advanced over the past several years owing to the refined use of the electron microscope, histochemistry, enzyme histochemistry, and immunofluorescent studies.

The electron microscope has provided a more detailed look at the cell and subcellular particles. Histochemistry and enzyme histochemistry have identified the locations of enzyme systems within epidermal and adnexal structures and aid in a more precise definition and classification of adnexal tumors and metabolic diseases. Immunofluorescent techniques have made possible the identification and classification of the bullous diseases, lupus erythematosus, and others (Burnham et al., 1963). However, with all the advances and new techniques, 95 per cent of the diagnosis are established on the basis of correlating the clinical data with the histologic features observed in the light microscope with hematoxylin and eosin-stained sections. Thus, it is important that the students of dermatology and the practitioners be familiar with the basic changes and group concepts of dermal pathology.

Just as the clinician recognizes erythema, edema, scaling, exudation, papules, nodules, and tumors, the dermal pathologist has patterns, cellular response, and combinations that, together with the clinical information, lead to a diagnosis. Before one delves into these histologic details, the important aspects of obtaining an adequate specimen and submitting clinical data will be discussed.

SELECTION OF THE SPECIMEN

As with other aids to diagnosis, the biopsy can be diagnostic, confirmatory, helpful, or inconclusive, depending on the disease, selection of the specimen, adequacy of the specimen, and handling of the specimen after the biopsy. The impression should never be given that once a biopsy is obtained the answer will be magically forthcoming. The clinician's careful consideration and thoughtful preparation in obtaining the specimen are just as important as the interpretation of the section.

The following guidelines will ensure the most accurate interpretation possible:

A. Obtain a typical virginal, unadulterated lesion whenever possible. Avoid lesions with secondary changes and those affected by prior therapy.

B. Obtain a lesion early in the evolution of the disease.

C. Obtain an adequate specimen in all dimensions, including a margin of normal skin whenever possible as well as subcutaneous tissue (Fig. 2-1).

D. Place the specimen in the proper fixative (usually neutral buffered formalin) immediately after the biopsy.

E. Place each biopsy specimen in a separate container properly labeled.

F. Submit with each specimen a complete, concise, clinical description of the disease, including onset, duration, type of lesion biopsied, site of the biopsy (specifically), and the age, sex, and color of the individual biopsied. These points may seem elementary, but their importance cannot be stressed enough.

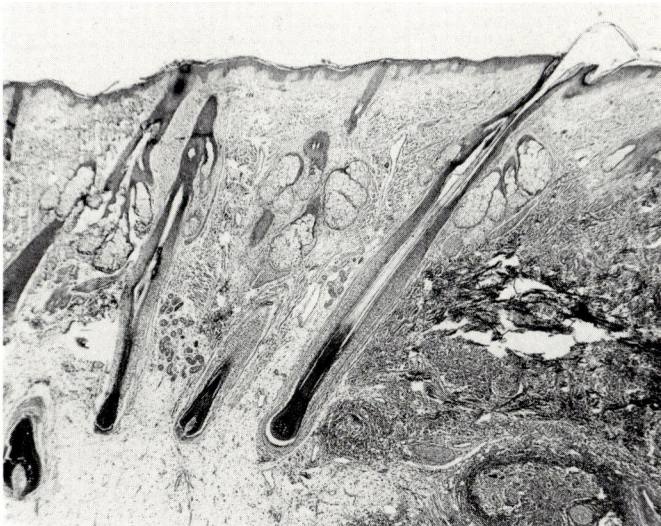

Figure 2–1   Normal skin. (Armed Forces Institute of Pathology, AFIP, photograph.) (× 40.)

HISTOCHEMISTRY

Histochemical techniques over the past several years have evolved from primarily a research tool to an important adjunct in the interpretation of histologic material (Johnson, 1972).

The use of histochemical and enzyme histochemical methods enables the pathol-

TABLE 2–3 HISTOCHEMICAL TECHNIQUES

Histochemical Technique	Reaction for:	Visual Representation	Remarks
		Organic Material	
Prussian Blue Reaction	Iron	Blue to blue-black granules	Differentiate hemosiderin from melanin; reaction positive in vascular lesions and following hemorrhage
Von Kossa	Calcium	Black	Identification of calcium tissue
		Acid Mucosaccharides°	
Colloidal Iron	Ground substance and muco-saccharides with acid groups in the tissue	Blue to blue green	Dermal mucinosis and conditions with increased ground substance
Colloidal Iron Technique with hyaluronidase digestion	Hyaluronic acid	No color	Sulfated acid mucopolysaccharides will still produce a blue-green color (mast cells, blood vessel walls, nerves, anagen hair papilla, etc.)
Periodic acid-Schiff (PAS)	Most mucosaccharides except hyaluronic acid will react. Fungi will react.	Red to red purple	
Periodic acid-Schiff (PAS) with diastase digestion	Glycogen	None	Glycogen will be digested by the diastase and will not stain. Those substances still staining will be mast cells, luminal cells, and secretory granules of apocrine glands, indicating the presence of acid mucosaccharides
Aldehyde-fuchsin: pH (1.7)	Epithelial mucins (breast, colon, respiratory tract) sulfated mucopolysaccharides, elastic tissue	Purple to purple brown	Hyaluronic acid (ground substance will not stain)
Aldehye-fuchsin: pH (1.0)	Strongly sulfated acid muco-polysaccharide	Purple to purple brown	Epithelial mucins will not stain. Mast cell granules, cartilage, and interfibrillar material of blood vessels will stain
		Tissue Elements	
Hematoxylin and eosin	Routine	Nuclei — blue Collagen — red Muscles — red Nerves — red	
Fontana-Masson	Melanin	Melanin granules — black to black green	
Masson's trichome	Muscle-collagen	Nuclei — black Muscle — red to red purple Nerves — red to red purple Collagen — green to blue green	
Oil red-O (formalin-fixed tissue not imbedded in paraffin)	Lipids	Lipids — red	
Gomori's aldehyde-fuchsin	Elastic tissue	Elastic fibers — purple	
Fite or Fite-Faraco	Acid-fast bacilli	Acid-fast bacilli — red	Leprosy, tuberculosis
Giemsa	Mast cell granules, Leishmania, histoplasmosis	Nuclei — blue Mast cell granules — purple to blue Organisms — blue to purple	
Immunofluorescence	Immunoglobulins Elastic tissue	Yellow-green fluorescence	Used in diagnosis of pemphigus, pemphigoid, vasculitis, lupus erythematosus, and the identification of elastic tissue
Alkaline phosphatase (Non-specific)	Endothelial cells of blood vessels	Blue to blue black	Shows blood vessels and their patterning very strikingly

°From Johnson and Helwig, 1963.

ogist to locate, in the tissues, inorganic substances, such as iron and calcium; infectious organisms, such as bacteria and fungi; and polysaccharides, such as glycogen in the group of simple polysaccharides and hyaluronic acid in the group of acid mucosaccharides (Johnson and Helwig, 1963; McKusick, et al., 1965).

Tissue elements such as collagen and elastic tissue can be made to stand out more distinctly with the use of histochemical techniques.

Enzyme histochemistry has enabled the pathologist to determine action sites of various enzymes within the components of the skin, such as alkaline phosphatase in blood vessels and phosphoralase in eccrine sweat structures. Representative types of histochemical procedures are summarized in Tables 2-3 and 2-4.

ELECTRON MICROSCOPY

The electron microscope, with newer refined techniques and improved sectioning and staining, has unfolded for the histopathologist a new world beyond the boundaries of the cell wall and its previous limiting membrane as viewed with the light microscope. Those things once viewed with awe at 2000 Å with the light microscope have vanished over the horizon with 6 to 8 Å resolution available and with no apparent end in sight (Zelickson, 1967).

Technical advances are made; the invisible becomes visible; new structures are identified; theories proposed. How do these advances relate to the student of dermatology, to the practitioner, to those who do not have these tools available?

The relationship is apparent when one correlates all the information obtained from the electron microscope with what is known from previous information from other sources.

The process of keratinization can be more accurately described. The basement membrane, which is elusive with the light microscope, is now well defined by the electron microscope. The distinct changes in many of the bullous diseases have been described with the specific localization of the basic process, as in epidermolysis bullosa and pemphigus.

The melanocyte and the process of melanin production defined, the Langerhans' cell defined, the indeterminant cell defined—once these were all lumped into one category as melanocyte and old melanocytes. Tissue components have been clearly identified and mechanisms of production delineated as in collagen, amyloid, and ground substance. Viral particles and inclusions have been defined and localized and their structure described; thus, viral diseases have been more clearly illustrated. The papovavirus, that of molluscum contagiosum, and the zoster-varicella group have been well studied.

Thus, the advances afforded by the electron microscope give a better basic understanding of the skin, its components, and its reaction in disease, enabling the student, practitioner, and researcher to have a firm grasp, a solid foundation, and a clear insight into the specialty of dermatology.

POLARISCOPIC EXAMINATIONS

Polariscopic examination of tissue is a simple, rapidly performed procedure

TABLE 2–4 REPRESENTATIVE HISTOCHEMICAL DIAGNOSTIC PROCEDURE

	Colloidal Iron		PAS		Aldehyde-Fuchsin	
Tumor	Without Digestion	With Hyaluronidase Digestion	Without Digestion	With Diastase Digestion	pH 1.7	pH 1.0
Extra mammary Paget's disease	4+	4+	4+	4+	4+	–
Bowen's disease	–	–	4+	–	–	–

°From Johnson and Helwig, 1963.

which is important in histopathology in assessing the presence or absence of doubly refractile material in the tissue. This procedure is done by placing two polarizing disks in the light path between the source and the viewer. One disk is placed over the light source, the other in the eye piece or over the specimen. When either disk is rotated, the path of light is interrupted. When a substance in the tissue is doubly refractile, the light is bent to the observer and the substances are viewed as bright white objects.

Lipids containing cholesterol esters can be visualized; collagen will be visible as orange-like rippling fibers; silica will be visualized; amyloid stained with Congo red can be visualized, with polarized light appearing green to red as the polarizing disk is rotated.

The polariscopic examination can be an invaluable aid in establishing the nature of many granulomatous reactions if they are caused by any of the above substances.

HISTOLOGY

Skin diseases reflect alterations in the structure and function of the skin, and just as the changes are observed by the clinician as lesions, color, or tumors, similar alterations in structure and function will be noted by the dermal histopathologist.

Essentially, three large group changes occur.

1. Inflammation—characterized by vascular dilatation, increased cellular infiltrate in the dermis and epidermis, edema fluid in the dermis and epidermis, and if severe enough, ulceration, necrosis, and tissue death.

2. Proliferation—an increase in the number of cells or elements present in the skin. If it is the epidermis, acanthosis results; if basal cells proliferate, a basal cell carcinoma results. Proliferative changes may be benign or malignant.

3. Alteration of function—function can be altered by inflammation and cellular proliferation. In conditions such as vitiligo, melasma, and freckles, there is an alteration of function without apparent external or internal cause, inflammation or proliferation.

EPIDERMAL REACTION PATTERNS

Inflammatory (Eczema-Dermatitis)

The hallmark of the inflammatory epidermal changes is spongiosis (Fig. 2-2), defined as edema between epidermal cells. If the spongiosis is marked or severe, intra-epidermal vesicles and bullae will be produced (Fig. 2–2 B). Accompanying the edema are inflammatory cells that migrate into the epidermis (exocytosis) from the underlying dermal papillary blood vessels. Early in the disease process one finds only spongiosis and minimal exocytosis of lymphocytes; later, larger intra-epidermal vesicles and a mixture of inflammatory cells will be present. The usual early cell is the lymphocyte, except in the case of primary irritant contact dermatitis, where the *early* exocytotic cell is the polymorphonuclear leukocyte.

The intense reaction in this group of diseases occurs in the epidermis; the dermal reaction is nonspecific. Although one should keep in mind that the source of the edema fluid and exocytotic cells is the papillary dermal vessels, on close inspection one may find disruptions of the basal cells and the basement membrane zone overlying the dermal papillae. The conditions that are included in this group are:

1. Acute allergic contact dermatitis.
2. Acute primary irritant contact dermatitis.
3. Seborrheic dermatitis.
4. Atopic dermatitis (active).
5. Nummular eczema (active).
6. Dyshidrosis.
7. Patch test reactions.
8. Stasis dermatitis (acute).
9. Pityriasis rosea.

Acanthotic (Psoriasiform)

This group of conditions could also be classified as subacute or chronic dermatitis. Here the hallmarks are increased thickness of the epidermis (acanthosis), imperfect keratinization with retained nuclei in the stratum corneum (parakeratosis), and exocytosis of inflammatory cells with the formation of microabscesses (Pinkus and Mehregan, 1969).

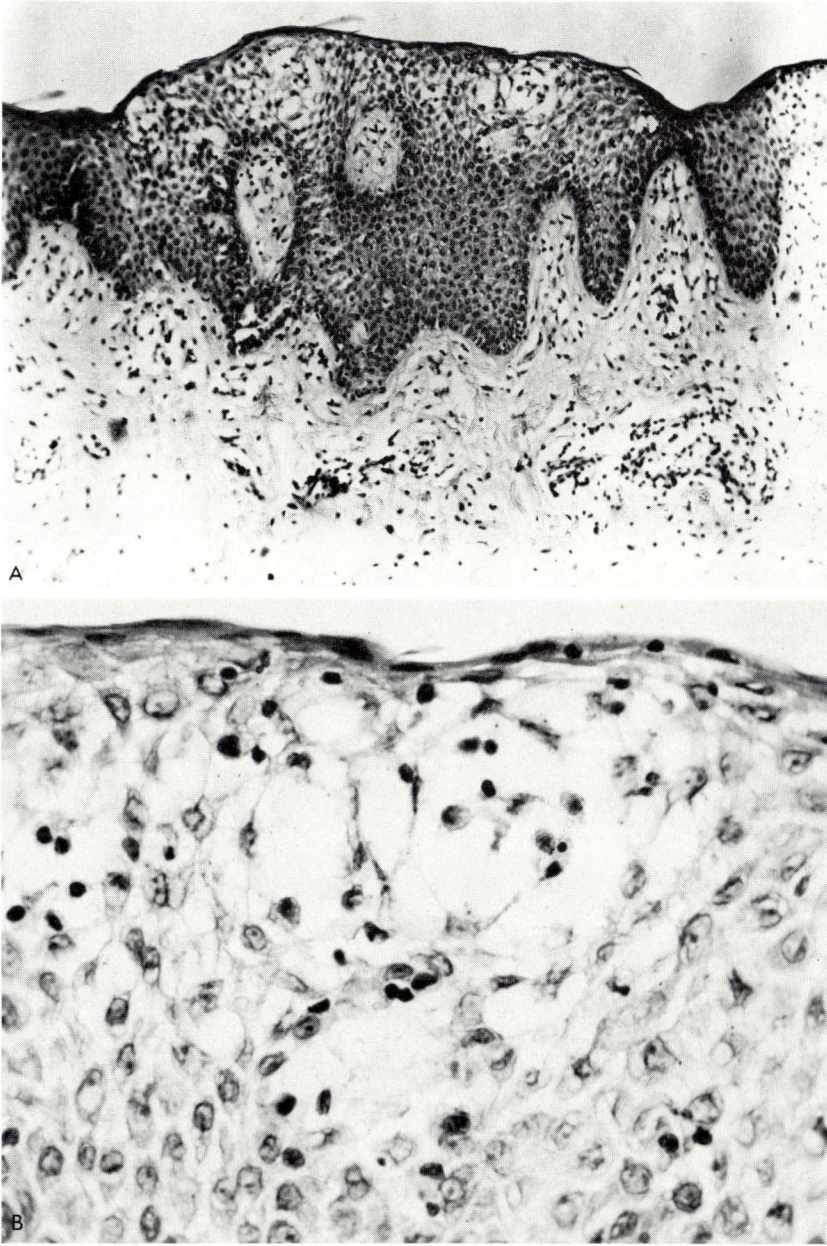

Figure 2-2 Spongiosis. (AFIP photograph.) ($A \times 125$; $B \times 610$)

Those conditions which show a regular, even acanthosis, parakeratosis, and minimal to absent spongiosis are psoriasis, seborrheic dermatitis chronic, atopic dermatitis chronic, lichen simplex chronicus, and nummular eczema. Of this group, psoriasis shows little spongiosis of the stratum malpighii whereas in seborrheic dermatitis, spongiosis may be marked (Fig. 2–3 *A* and *B*). In addition to acanthosis and parakeratosis, exocytosis is a constant feature, and its intensity and extent account for many variations seen within the group (Gordon and Johnson, 1967).

In nummular eczema, atopic dermatitis, and lichen simplex chronicus (Fig. 2-4) the primary exocytotic cell is the monocyte, and small microabscesses may be

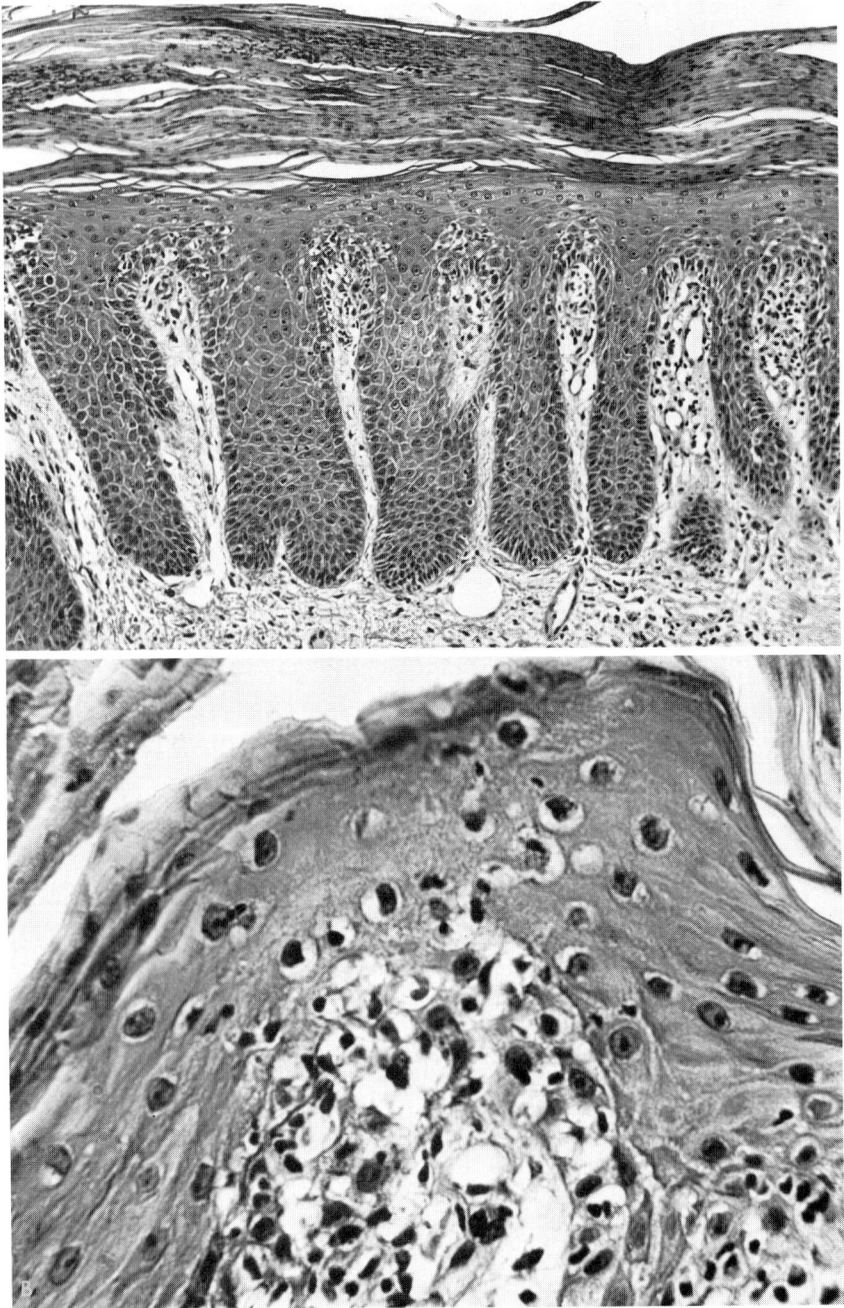

Figure 2–3   Psoriasis. Parakeratotic scale, acanthosis, and papillomatosis. Exocytosis at the supra papillary plate. (Courtesy of Waine C. Johnson, M.D.) (Reprinted from Archives of Dermatology, 95:402–407, 1967.) (*A* × 415; *B* × 500.)

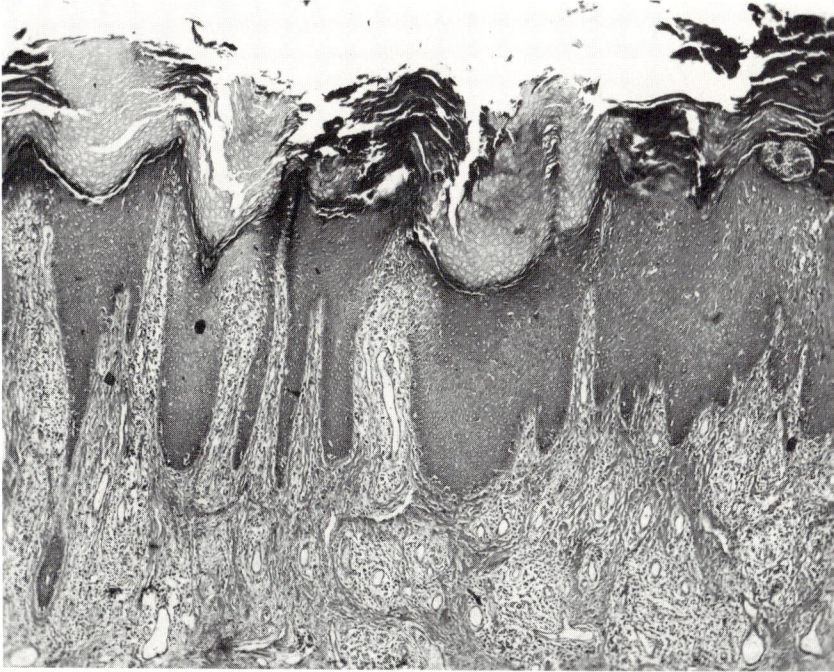

Figure 2–4 Neurodermatitis. Chronic dermatitis, hyperkeratosis, acanthosis, papillomatosis, and a chronic mononuclear inflammatory cellular infiltrate in the dermis. (AFIP photograph.) (× 35.)

seen in the epidermis. These can mimic those seen in mycosis fungoides (Graham and Mandrea, 1964).

Psoriasis and seborrheic dermatitis have the polymorphonuclear leukocyte as the primary exocytotic cell. This process is better developed in psoriasis than it is in seborrheic dermatitis. In psoriasis there are collections of polymorphonuclear leukocytes forming microabscesses (Munro microabscesses) in the superficial layers of the epidermis usually just below the zone of parakeratosis. In seborrheic dermatitis these are less well developed and smaller.

Dermal papillary vessel dilatation, with a perivascular round cell infiltrate, disruption in the overlying basement membrane with a focal edema, and exocytosis of polymorphonuclear cells in the epidermis, has been referred to as the squirting papilla by Pinkus and Mehregan in their text of histopathology, and is an explanation for the changes seen in psoriasis and seborrhea (Fig. 2-3*B*).

The epidermal response to the edema and exocytosis is epidermal proliferation and parakeratosis (imperfect cell keratinization with retention of nuclei in the stratum corneum). Parakeratosis is the usual finding in the inflammatory eczematous dermatosis, although normal keratinization (orthokeratosis) can occur. In severely inflamed processes with rapid epidermal turnover, hypokeratosis is noted.

The variants in this group, pustular psoriasis, acrodermatitis continua, impetigo herpetiformis, and keratoderma blennorrhagica, show the same even acanthosis and parakeratosis but the intensity of the leukocyte response is marked with the production of macroabscesses. In these diseases a diagnostic finding is the spongioform pustules of Kogoj, which represent collections of polymorphonuclear leukocytes within living epidermal cells.

The dermal participation is minimal in psoriasis, seborrheic dermatitis, nummular eczema, atopic dermatitis, and lichen simplex chronicus. There is usually papillomatosis (upward projection of the dermal papilla) with a mild perivascular chronic inflammatory cell infiltrate. In psoriasis, the papillary vessels are dilated and elongated, and have been described as rigid. The inflammatory infiltrate in Reiter's disease, impetigo herpetiformis, and acrodermatitis continua can be characterized by mononuclear cell infiltration about the superficial blood vessels, varying in intensity.

Lichenoid

The lichenoid dermatoses are those that resemble lichen planus histologically, and characteristically have bandlike or multiple nodular infiltrates in the papillary dermis that encroach upon and destroy the basal cells. The representative of this group is lichen planus (Fig. 2–5 *A* and *B*).

Lichen Planus

The typical histologic features of lichen planus are hyperkeratosis, hypergranulosis, and liquefaction degeneration of the basal cell zone, an infiltrate in the papillary dermis that invades the epidermis, producing edema of basal cells (liquefaction degeneration) as well as causing a ragged appearance of the rete that resembles the teeth of a saw (saw toothing).

Because of the loss of the continuity at the basal cell, basement membrane zone, pigment will be found in the upper dermis in dermal macrophages. Apparently because of the injury in this area, acidophilic oval-to-round bodies can be found. They probably result from cellular injury and a collection of protein or cell products on these cells; in many instances these same structures will fluoresce with the immunofluorescent technique. These bodies (Civatte bodies) are not unique to lichen planus but can be found in several diseases in which there are basal layer degeneration and exocytosis (lupus erythematosus, lichen nitidus, and actinic keratosis) (Hiroaki, 1969).

The infiltrate in the dermis is composed mainly of lymphocytes, although histiocytes and, rarely, plasma cells are present. The infiltrate is usually confined to the papillary dermis and if it extends deeply, a lichen planus-like drug eruption should be considered. Vascular dilatation and proliferation can be noted in the inflammatory infiltrate.

Lichen planus may be atrophic, having similar changes except for a thin epidermis; it may be hypertrophic with acanthosis, or bullous, showing epidermal-dermal separation.

Lichenoid Drug Eruption (Lichen Planus–like Drug Eruption)

Lichenoid drug eruption can closely resemble lichen planus. The features of this process are hyperkeratosis, spotted parakeratosis, hypergranulosis, saw toothing of the rete, exocytosis, and liquefaction degeneration.

In the upper corium is a high-hugging infiltrate that can be bandlike or focal, composed of lymphocytes, histiocytes, plasma cells, eosinophils, and rare giant cells. In addition to the superficial location, the infiltrate usually extends deeply into the mid- and lower corium about the blood vessels.

The differential features are spotted parakeratosis, a more distinctly polymorphous infiltrate with a variable number of eosinophils, and the extension of the infiltrate into the deeper corium and its location about the blood vessels.

Lichen Nitidus

Lichen nitidus and the early lichen planus papule may be indistinguishable histologically. The lesions of lichen nitidus remain the same size and retain their identity, while those of lichen planus develop into larger lesions and often plaques.

In lichen nitidus, there is a distinctly focal area of involvement usually confined to one papilla or an area between two rete ridges. There are parakeratosis, epidermal atrophy, and liquefaction degeneration. The infiltrate is distinctly granulomatous and composed of lymphocytes, histiocytes, epitheliod cells, and multinucleated giant cells. Melanophages with melanin pigment can also be found in the inflammatory infiltrate and are similar to those seen in lichen planus and lupus erythematosus.

Other conditions that may show a lichenoid configuration are lichenoid actinic keratosis, lichen sclerosis et atrophicus, lichen striatus, mycosis fungoides, and poikiloderma. These will be discussed later.

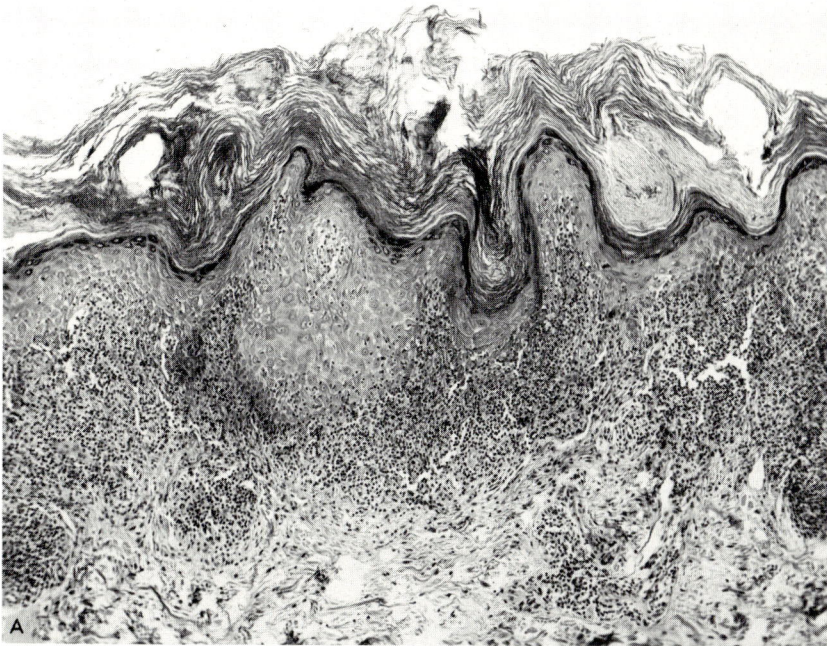

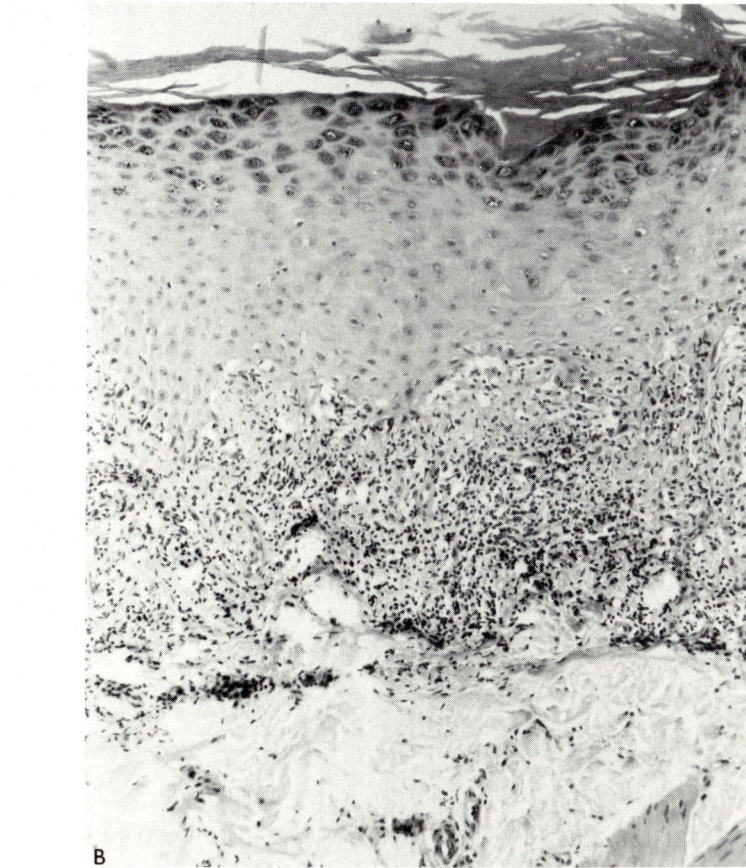

Figure 2–5 Lichen planus. Hyperkeratosis, hypergranulosis, basal cell layer liquefaction and obliteration. A bandlike lymphocytic cellular infiltrate at the dermo-epidermal junction. (*A*, AFIP photograph; × 80. *B*, Courtesy of T. R. Moore, Naval Hospital, Philadelphia, Pa.; × 450.)

Melanocytic Changes

Changes in color are very apparent to the clinician. A stark white patch on hyperpigmented skin is very noticeable. These changes are not as acute to the pathologist, especially when only the af-

fected area is biopsied; thus, it is important to obtain adjacent normal skin for more accurate interpretation. Basically two changes are noted histologically—hyperpigmentation, either epidermal or dermal, or hypopigmentation.

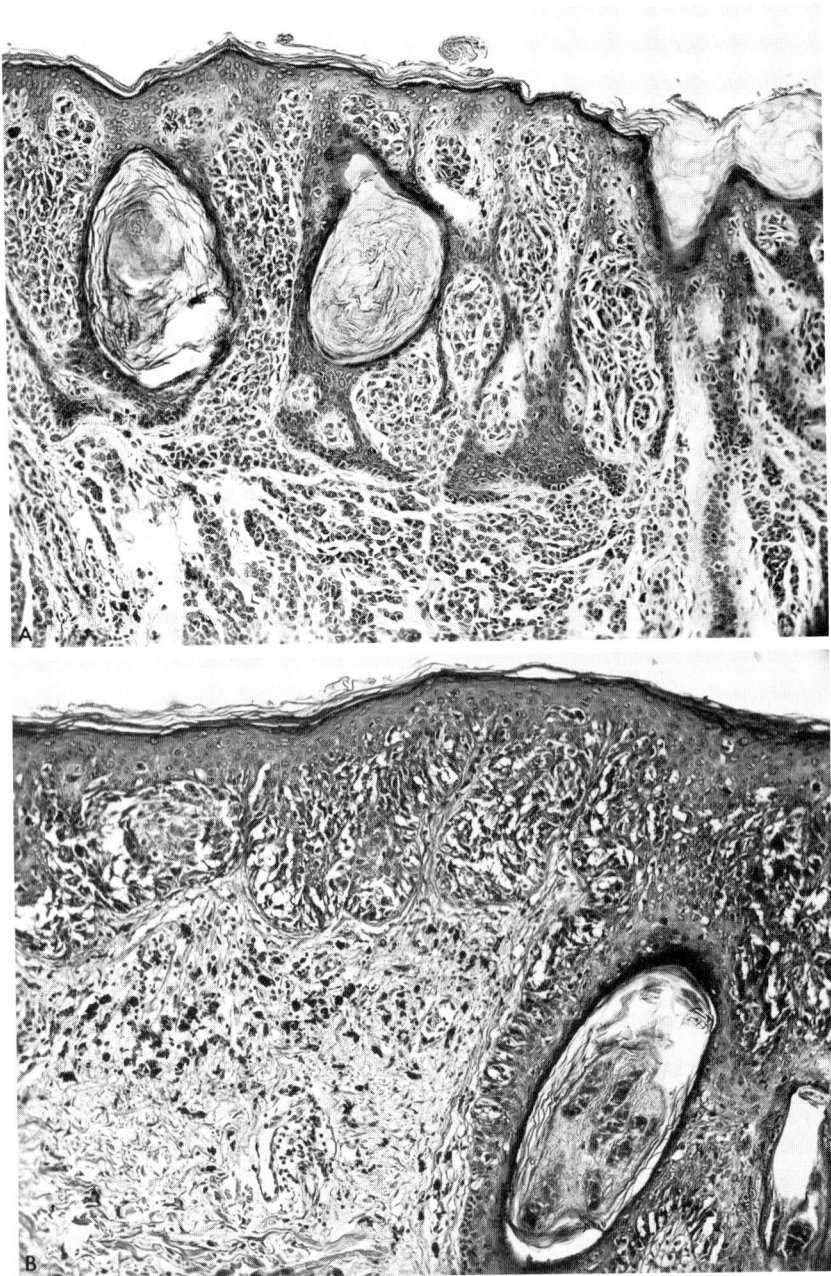

Figure 2–6 Nevi. *A*, Compound nevus. The main component of nevus cells is in the dermis. *B*, Compound nevus. The main component of nevus cells appears in the dermal-epidermal junction. (AFIP photographs.) (× 150.)

(Figure 2–6 continued on opposite page.)

Hyperpigmentation

Hyperpigmentation is an increase in pigmentation in the basal cell layer or pigment in dermal macrophages in the papillary or middermis. The increased pigmentation in the basal layer is a reflection of increased function of the melanocytes, as in freckles, or an increased function and number, as in café-au-lait spots.

On hematoxylin and eosin-stained sections increases or decreases in pigmentation of the epidermis will not be apparent unless there is a specimen of normally pigmented skin for comparison or unless dermal melanophages are present.

Conditions in which one can see increased basal layer pigmentation are freckles, café-au-lait spots, lentigines, nevi, hemochromatosis, chloasma, suntanning, and chronic inflammation (Johnson and Charneco, 1970). Dermal pigmentation (melanocytic) follows most acute inflammatory processes and is also seen in dermal nevi, blue nevi, and mongolian spots.

Hypopigmentation

Hypopigmentation is the loss of function of the melanocyte or absence of the melanocyte due to injury or disease. Again, comparison with the normal is essential for correct interpretation of a hypopigmented disorder.

On hematoxylin and eosin-stained sections there will be an absence of epidermal and/or dermal melanin. There may also be an absence or decrease in the number of "clear" cells in the basal layer.

Clear cells in the basal layer usually indicate melanocytes, although with more recent studies it has been shown that these clear cells may represent Langerhans' cells, which are increased in number in vitiligo, or indeterminant cells. Conditions that represent loss of epidermal melanin are vitiligo, postinflammatory hypopigmentation from various causes, and albinism.

Clinical pigment lightening is not always related to hypomelanization and may reflect vascular supply, scarring, and increased thickness of the granular cell layer. These conditions can be differentiated from hypomelanization on the basis of the histology.

Tumors (New Growths of Melanocytic Cells)

One of the most common skin tumors, the nevus, is a tumor of melanocytic cells. Nevi represent collections of nevus cells or melanocytic cells at varying locations in the skin; the name of the nevus is determined from this location.

NEVI (Fig. 2–6). The most common

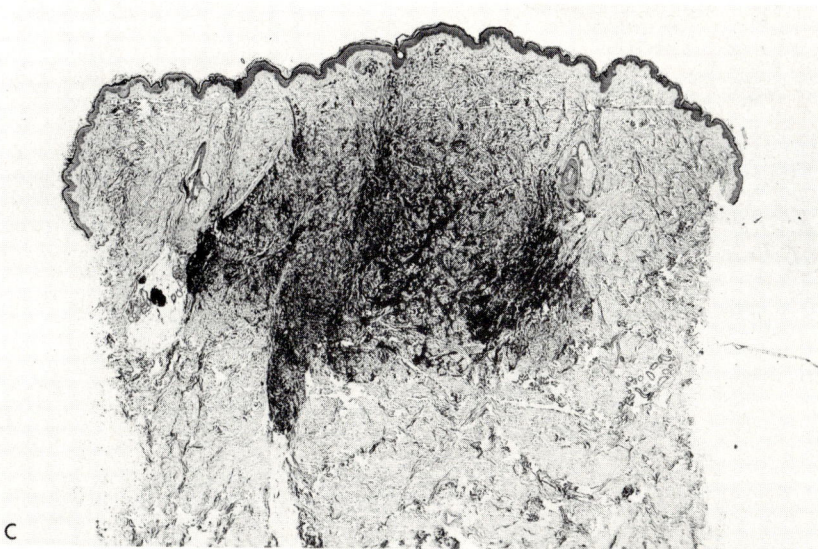

Figure 2–6 *Continued.*   *C*, Blue nevus. Spindled-shaped pigmented cells in the dermis. (AFIP photograph.) (× 16.)

skin tumor is divided histologically into three types:

Junctional – nests and thèques of nevus cells at the dermal-epidermal junction and in the basal layer of the epidermis.

Dermal – nests and thèques of nevus cells in the dermis. These may extend from the papillary dermis to the subcutis.

Compound – a combination of junctional and dermal. Melanin pigmentation is variable in these nevi, with the junctional and compound nevus possessing the most.

BLUE NEVI. This name is derived from the clinical blue color and not the histologic appearance. This type of nevus is usually located in the mid- to lower dermis and is composed of spindle-shaped cells that resemble fibrocytes because of their bipolar arrangement. Melanin pigment is present.

CELLULAR BLUE NEVI. These nevi are also located deep in the dermis and, in addition to the spindle cell component, have a cellular component with the cells arranged into tubes, chords, and fasicles.

MELANOMA. This tumor is a malignant melanocytic tumor. It is usually pigmented, although nonpigmented forms do occur. There are atypical abnormal and proliferating melanocytes. The usual orderly arrangement of the cells into nest and thèques is lacking. The respect for the stroma is lost as evidenced by streaming of these cells into the deeper tissues as well as by invasion of the epidermis. There is also a loss of the normal maturation of these cells from the papillary dermis to the lower dermis. Normally, the nevus cells become smaller, more compact, and have less cytoplasm as they are observed from the basal layer to the subcutis.

BULLOUS DISEASES

Bullous diseases are classified histologically into two broad groups according to the site of separation – either intra-epidermal or subepidermal. Intra-epidermal bullae or vesicles may result from marked spongiosis (Fig. 2-7), as seen in the inflammatory dermatoses (dermatitis-eczema group), or the bullae may be filled with polymorphonuclear leukocytes and are represented by pustules, as is noted in

subcorneal pustular dermatosis and pustular psoriasis. Superficial acantholytic bullae are seen in pemphigus foliaceus and pemphigus erythematosus. Suprabasalar acantholytic bullae occur in pemphigus vulgaris, pemphigus vegetans, Hailey and Hailey disease, Darier's disease, and often in actinic keratosis.

Intra-epidermal bullae are produced by viral infections, by a process of reticular degeneration, acantholysis and some spongiosis. This type of bulla will be seen in herpes simplex and zoster, variola and vaccinia.

Subepidermal bullae, before more refined histochemical, immunofluorescent and electron microscopic techniques, were all lumped into one group. We now can separate the subepidermal bullous diseases into three groups depending on whether the separation is through the basal cells, above the basement membrane, or below the membrane. Some conditions in which the separation is within the basal cells include epidermolysis bullosa simplex, toxic epidermal necrolysis, and second degree burns. Noting early lesions is imperative for making the diag-

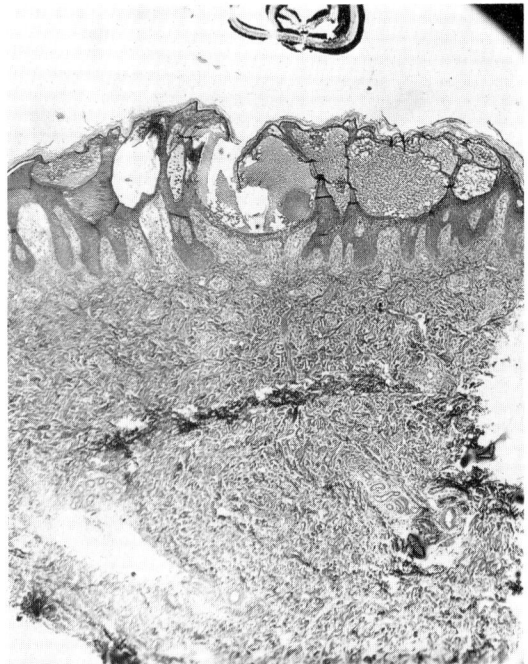

Figure 2-7 Intra-epidermal bullae (spongiotic). Contact dermatitis. (AFIP photograph.) (× 16.)

nosis since the disrupted basal cells rapidly degenerate. Thus in late lesions only a subepidermal bulla will be noted and none of the early changes of the basal cell edema and separation will be seen.

The second division of the subepidermal group are those bullous diseases occurring above the basement membrane as viewed with the light microscope when routine histochemical stains which show the basement membrane are used. An example of this type of stain is the periodic acid-Schiff (PAS), which stains the basement membrane red-purple, or the Snook's silver stain, which stains the basement membrane black; other fibers in the dermis and melanin will also stain black. If one correlates the findings of the light microscope and the electron microscope, the separation actually occurs in the intermembrane space (Pearson and Spargo, 1961). The intermembrane space has been defined as a space of low electrodensity measuring 300Å to 600Å in width and located between the plasma membrane of the basal cells and the basement membrane at the upper limits of the papillary dermis, this dermal portion being produced in all probability by the dermis.

It should be remembered that on routine sections with the special stains previously mentioned, the bulla will be above the basement membrane. Those bullous diseases in this group are dermatitis herpetiformis, bullous pemphigoid, and epidermolysis bullosa hereditaris letalis (Pearson, 1962).

The third division of the subepidermal bullous group are those subepidermal bullae occurring below the basement membrane. The separation occurs in the papillary dermis just below the basement membrane. Thus, with special stains, the basement membrane will be seen lining the roof of the bulla. The bullous diseases occurring in this group are epidermolysis bullosa dystrophica, erythema multiforme, porphyria cutanea tarda, and congenital erythropoietic porphyria.

Dermatoses that have liquefaction degeneration will also produce subepidermal bullae, although they are not classified in the group of bullous diseases. The bullae are produced in this group because of destruction of the basement membrane. Some examples of the disease in this group

that may become bullae on the basis of liquefaction degeneration are lichen planus, lupus erythematosus, lichen sclerosis et atrophicus, and lichenoid and bullous drug eruptions.

Pemphigus Vulgaris (Fig. 2–8)

The bullae develop in this disease by the process of acantholysis whereby the cohesion between epidermal cells is lost and they separate from one another and float free in the bullous spaces. This begins just above the basal cell layer (suprabasalar) and extends to one or two cell layers above, leaving a fairly thick roof. This suprabasalar separation extends into the follicular epithelium. The acantholytic epidermal cells show degenerative changes and are swollen with peripheral cytoplasmic condensation; dyskeratotic cells are not noted. Dermal papillae protrude into the bullous cavity and are lined by a single row of basal cells (villi).

In early lesions the reaction in the dermis is minimal. Slight inflammation and eosinophils may be present. Older lesions show considerable inflammation with a mixture of cells.

Recent immunologic, histochemical and electron microscopic studies (Hashimoto and Lever, 1970) show that the cause of the acantholysis in pemphigus is due to a defect in the intercellular cement substance or to an antigen-antibody reaction that causes a defect in the intercellular cement substance, leading to splitting of the desmosomes with complete separation of the epidermal cells.

Immunofluorescent studies have shown that immunoglobulin G (IgG) is bound to the intercellular cement substance. This can be demonstrated directly on a fresh lesion or indirectly by using the patient's serum and any normal tissue and fluorescence-labeled IgG.

In *pemphigus foliaceus* and *erythematosus,* acantholysis occurs in the superficial layers of the epidermis, usually in the granular cell layers. Distinct bullae are not usually noted. Rarely, isolated suprabasalar separations are noted. Older lesions show acanthosis, papillomatosis, and dyskeratosis in the granular cell layer. The

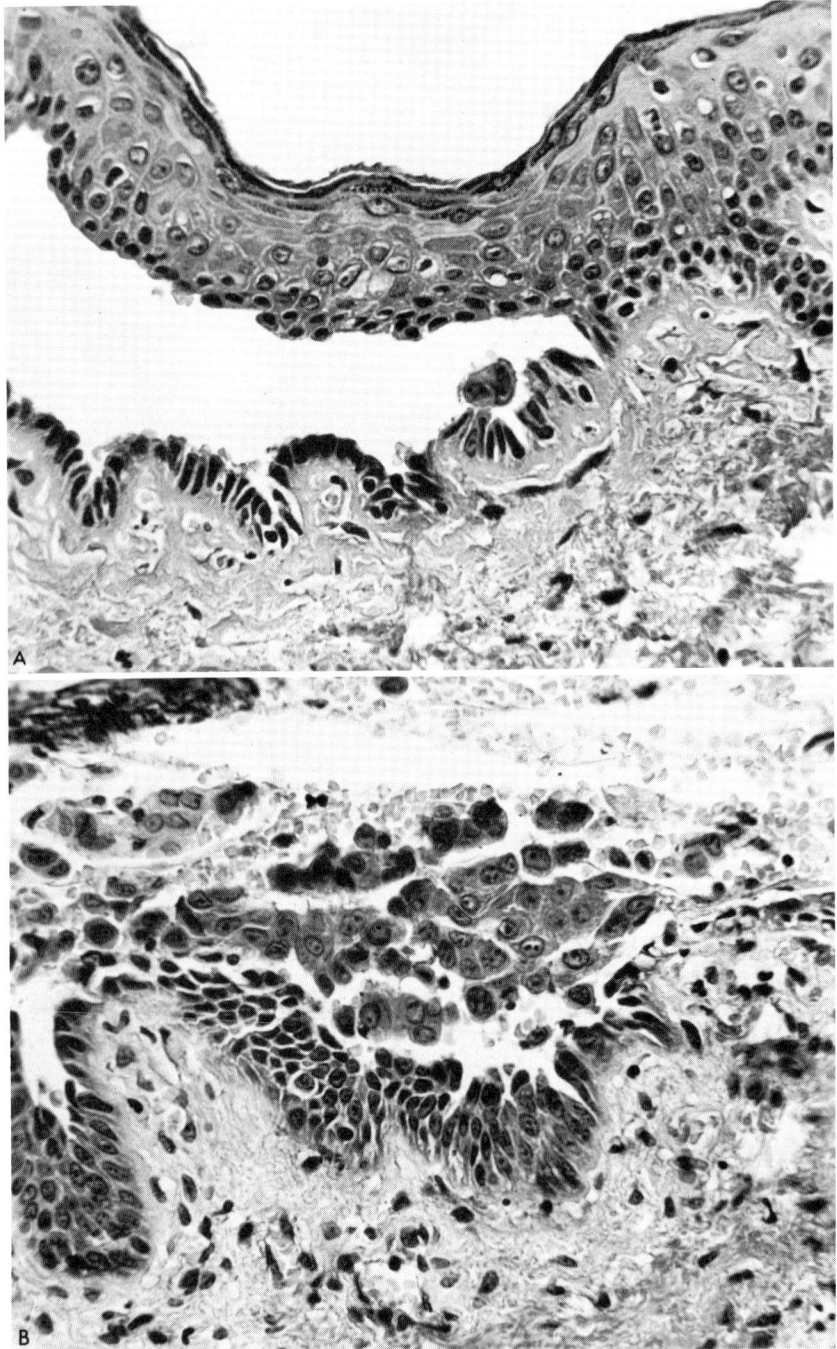

Figure 2-8 Intra-epidermal bullae (acantholytic). A, Pemphigus vulgaris. B, Acantholytic cells pemphigus. (AFIP photographs.) (× 395.)

dermis shows minimal inflammation (Lever, 1965, 1967).

Benign familial pemphigus (Hailey and Hailey disease) shows suprabasalar acantholysis with more extensive acantholysis of the overlying epidermal cells, producing a picture resembling "grapes suspended in jello." Dyskeratotic cells can be noted in this condition.

Darier's disease also has suprabasalar acantholysis with small areas of separation called lacunae, less extensive acantholysis of the upper epidermal cells, and extensive production of dyskeratotic cells called corps ronds and grains. There are distinct hyperkeratosis and follicular hyperkeratosis. The dermal reaction is minimal to moderate.

Dermatitis Herpetiformis

The early change is edema of the dermal papillae with collections of neutrophils, eosinophils, and lymphocytes. Subsequent to this there is separation of the epidermis just over the dermal papillae to form a multilocular bulla; as the process continues, a distinct unilocular bulla is produced. The dermal response consists of an inflammatory reaction about the papillary blood vessels that is composed mainly of lymphocytes with varying numbers of eosinophils and neutrophils. The PAS and Snooks stain will show the basement membrane on the floor of the bulla (MacVicar and Graham, 1965; MacVicar et al., 1963).

Bullous Pemphigoid

Early changes are edema of the dermal papilla without significant inflammation, as was noted in dermatitis herpetiformis. Because of the edema, the epidermis is separated from the dermis with a resultant subepidermal bulla. Epidermal regeneration occurs rather promptly (within one to two days); therefore, an early lesion is essential for accurate diagnosis. The dermal reaction is initially minimal with a few inflammatory cells consisting of lymphocytes and eosinophils. Older lesions or those with erythema may show a marked inflammatory response with some vasculitis.

Porphyria Cutanea Tarda

The striking feature of this process is a large subepidermal bulla with a minimal to absent inflammatory response in the dermis and naked papillae projecting into the bulla cavity (festooning). Electron microscopic studies have shown that the separation occurs in the papillary dermis just below the basement membrane.

Epidermolysis Bullosa Simplex (Fig. 2–9)

The early change here occurs in the basal cells with vacuolization and degeneration, with the production of an early intra-epidermal bulla, but with subsequent basal cell degeneration the bulla appears subepidermal. The dermal reaction is minimal to absent.

Epidermolysis Bullosa Dystrophica

Early lesions also show a subepidermal bulla with some festooning. The inflammatory response in the dermis is absent or minimal. Electron microscopic studies show that there is significant degeneration of the papillary dermal collagen; this is most severe in the recessive type.

Viral Bullous Diseases

The mechanism of bulla production in this group of diseases is reticular and ballooning degeneration. Because of the parasitization of the epidermal cells by the viruses, there is swelling and rounding of the epidermal cells (ballooning); as this proceeds, the cells rupture but leave remnants of intact cell walls to produce a net-like appearance (reticulation). As this process continues, a large intra-epidermal bulla is produced. Early lesions will show this change most characteristically. In older lesions, these changes will be noted at the margins of the bulla. In herpes simplex, zoster, and varicella, a unilocular bulla is usually produced. A multilocular bulla is usually produced in variola and vaccinia. Multinucleated viral giant cells can be found in herpes simplex, zoster, and varicella and are helpful in distinguishing this group from other such diseases. The inflammatory response is usually moderate to marked with significant

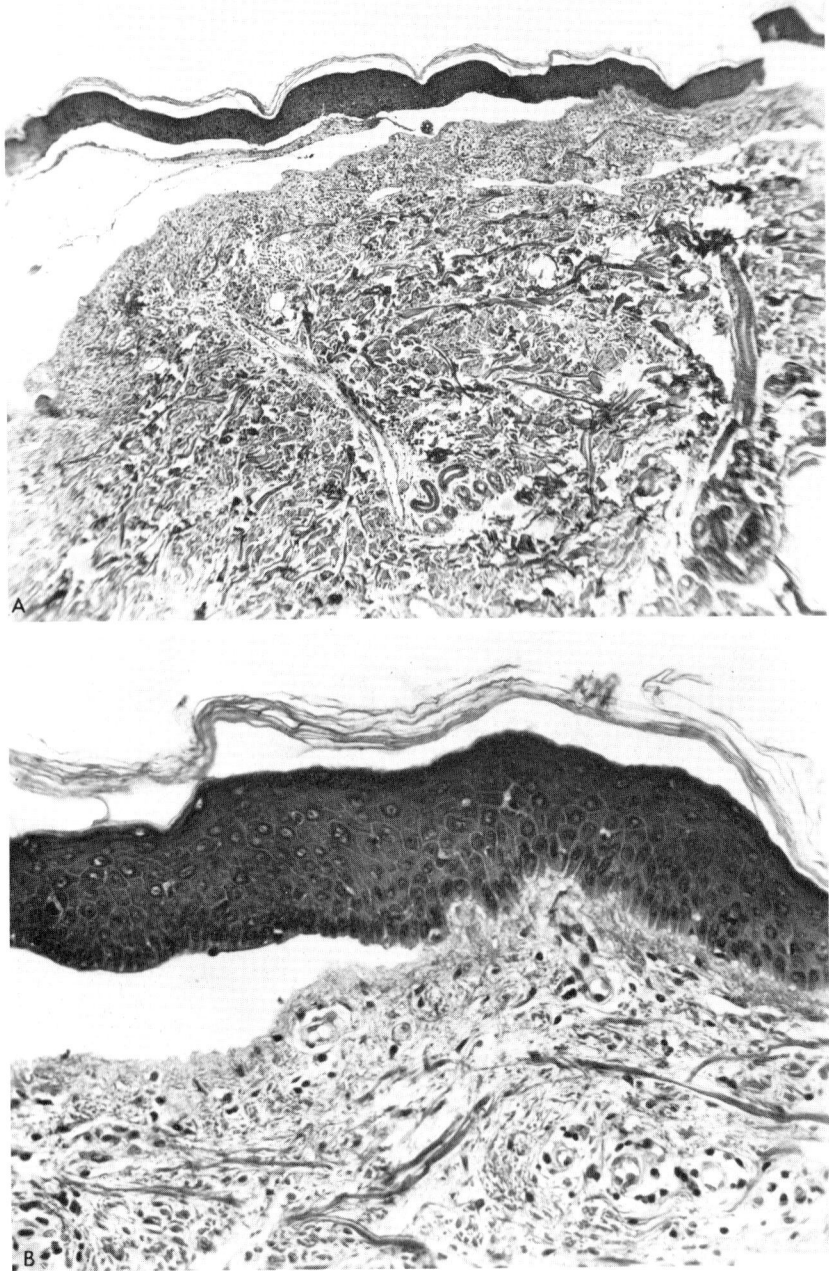

Figure 2–9 Subepidermal bulla. Epidermolysis bullosa. (AFIP photographs.) ($A \times 48$; $B \times 395$.)

exocytosis, the lymphocyte being the predominant cell.

VASCULAR REACTIONS

All dermatologic conditions will show histologically some vascular reaction, from simple ectasia to complete vessel occlusion. Although diseases are divided into groups that represent predominant epidermal involvement (dermatitis-eczema group) or connective tissue involvement, one should not overlook the fact that the dermal vessels play an active role in these processes through the release of cells, antibodies, or the mediators of the disease process.

Even though dermal vessels play some role in histologic patterns, certain groups of processes have been separated because the vascular reaction patterns are the most prominent feature, other changes being secondary.

The vascular reactions considered in this group are urticaria, dermal contact sensitivity, papular urticaria, allergic or leukocytoclastic angiitis, and periarteritis nodosa.

Urticaria

Urticaria represents the minimal end of the spectrum, showing histologically only dermal edema, vascular dilatation, mild endothelial swelling, and a banal perivascular infiltrate that consists of lymphocytes and a few eosinophils.

Erythema Multiforme

This process has been classified as a bullous disease in some texts and a vascular reaction in others. It probably is best classified as a vascular reaction, since the vessels may show a picture ranging from a mild perivascular infiltration to leukocytoclasis.

Histologically, erythema multiforme shows a mild perivascular infiltrate of lymphocytes in the dermis, mainly with a few eosinophils. As the clinical severity progresses, the histologic picture also progresses to that of a severe angiitis with leukocytoclasis, endothelial swelling, and vessel wall thickening. The epidermal reaction in the milder form is minimal and consists of spongiosis and exocytosis. In the severe reactions, bullae may occur on the basis of severe edema or liquefaction degeneration or both. Hemorrhage may occur in severe lesions.

Papular Urticaria (Lichen Urticatus)

This process is characterized by a more intense vascular reaction than that seen in urticaria. The dermal vessels are swollen and are surrounded by an inflammatory infiltrate consisting of lymphocytes, mainly with an admixture of eosinophils, plasma cells, and histiocytes.

The epidermis can show spongiosis, spongiotic vessels, and exocytosis.

Contact Dermatitis (Dermal Hypersensitivity Type)

This type of reaction is most often due to nickel sensitivity or neomycin. It can mimic atopic dermatitis clinically. Histologically, the epidermal changes are minimal acanthosis and occasional foci of parakeratosis. The major changes occur in the dermis about the upper and middermal blood vessels. These vessels are surrounded by a cellular infiltrate composed of lymphocytes, plasma cells, and few eosinophils and histiocytes.

Allergic Angiitis (Fig. 2–10)

The hallmarks of allergic angiitis are the following: vessel changes of the dermal blood vessels, endothelial swelling, thickening of the vessel wall, and a distinctive surrounding cellular infiltrate composed of lymphocytes, histiocytes, eosinophils and neutrophils. In many instances the predominant cell is the neutrophil, with few lymphocytes or eosinophils. These neutrophils may invade the vessel wall, and in some instances necrosis and occlusion of the vessel occur. Nuclear fragmentation (karyorrhexis) or so-called nuclear dusting is a distinctive feature of allergic angiitis.

Another feature of allergic angiitis is the presence of an eosinophilic homogeneous material (fibrinoid) about the blood vessels. This material is thought to be the result of altered connective tissue or the presence of an abnormal protein that has precipitated in this area because of the reaction. Hemorrhage (purpura) is a variable feature depending on the condition in which it occurs; it is a significant feature in Schoenlein-Henoch disease and is rare or absent in erythema elevatum diutinum.

These changes are usually confined to the smaller vessels of the dermis. When systemic changes are present and larger vessels involved, conditions such as periarteritis nodosa and allergic granulomatosis are considered. The vessel changes are essentially similar except for increasing vessel necrosis and a more granulomatous infiltrate about the blood vessels.

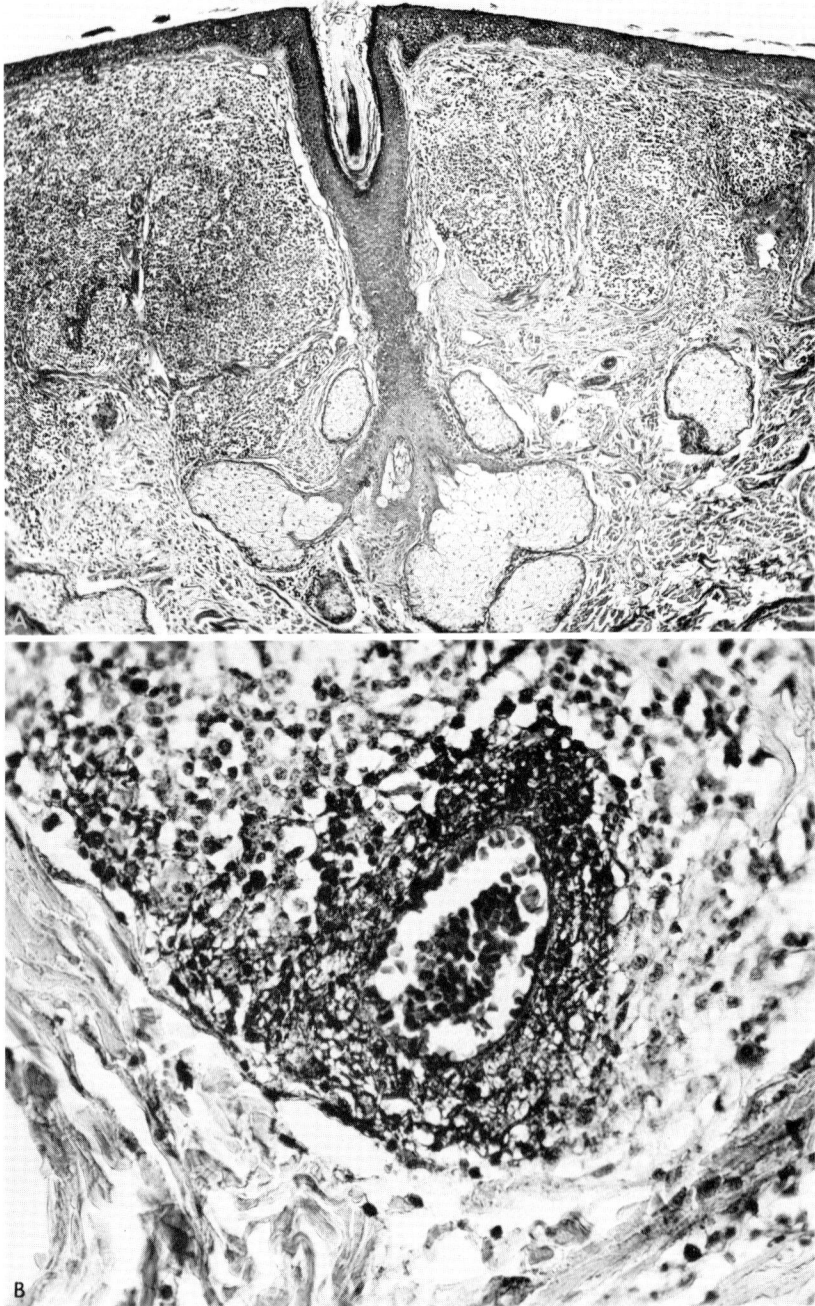

Figure 2-10 Allergic angiitis. *A*, Granuloma faciale. Granulomatosus infiltrate in the dermis, sparing the epidermis by a thin band of normal collagen (Grenz zone). (AFIP photograph.) ($\times$ 50.) *B*, Vessel involvement in allergic angiitis. Invasion of vessel wall by inflammatory cells. (AFIP photograph.) ($\times$ 35.)

Those processes considered to be a part of the spectrum of allergic angiitis are anaphylactoid purpura, Schoenlein-Henoch purpura, erythema elevatum diutinum, periarteritis nodosa, granuloma faciale, Gougerot's nodular dermal allergide, Ruiter's allergic arteriolitis, and Zeek's hypersensitivity angiitis.

CONNECTIVE TISSUE DISORDERS

Alterations in the dermal connective tissue (collagen and elastin) are presented in many forms; in the inflammatory dermatoses, edema and increased cellularity are noted, in bacterial and fungal diseases destruction and necrosis can be found. Other changes that are found are homogenization, sclerosis and proliferation of collagen, increased ground substance, foreign material, altered metabolic products, and atrophy. Connective tissue disorders can be grouped into those involving:

1. Collagen—dermatomyositis, lupus erythematosus, morphea-scleroderma, lichen sclerosis et atrophicus (balanitis xerotica obliterans, kraurosis vulvae).
2. Ground substance—dermal mucinosis and scleroderma.
3. Elastin—solar elastosis, pseudoxanthoma elasticum, elastosis perforans, cutis laxa, cutis hyperelastica (Ehlers-Danlos syndrome).
4. Proliferations of existing structures—dermatofibroma, neurofibroma, leiomyoma and keloid.

Dermatomyositis

The histologic features of this condition are not diagnostic but most often resemble lupus erythematosus. The significant feature in early skin lesions is dermal edema which can sometimes mimic a mucinosis. A dermal cellular infiltrate that is perivascular may extend throughout the dermis and is composed of lymphocytes. Occasionally, plasma cells and eosinophils may be seen.

The affected muscles show the most significant change, with inflammation, fragmentation of the muscle bundles, and proliferation of the sarcolemma nuclei. The end stage is fibrosis.

Morphea-Scleroderma

The histologic definition of these conditions is not always very distinctive, although early in the disease process an adequate deep biopsy will be of great value.

Early in the process, epidermal changes are insignificant. There are dermal edema and mild inflammation, but at the dermal subcutaneous junction there is a prominent inflammatory response involving the lower dermis and the subcutaneous tissue. Progression of the disease process leads to reduction of the inflammation in the area and replacement of the subcutis with new and altered collagen. The remainder of the dermis shows sclerosis; collagen bundles become thick and coarse. Appendages are lost, with sweat glands and arrector muscles of the hair remaining, usually appearing normal. The epidermal response is variable, usually appearing normal (Fig. 2–11).

Lichen Sclerosis et Atrophicus

Characteristically, there are hyperkeratosis, follicular plugging, epidermal atrophy with loss of distinct rete ridges, and basal layer liquefaction. A subepidermal zone of dermal edema is prominent and an inflammatory cell infiltrate is present below the zone of edema. Vascular ectasia may be present. Older lesions will show less edema and inflammation, some thickening of the collagen bundles, and atrophy of pilosebaceous structures. Sclerosis in this process is not as prominent as in morphea or scleroderma (Fig. 2–12).

Lupus Erythematosus

Although this process is grouped with the connective tissue disorders, the epidermal changes are very prominent and are important in establishing the diagnosis histologically. One could group this process with the lichenoid reactions, since the histology may closely resemble lichen planus. The essential epidermal features are: hyperkeratosis, hypergranulosis, follicular plugging, epidermal atrophy, and focal areas of liquefaction degeneration of the basal cell layer. The dermal features are: periappendageal and perivascular

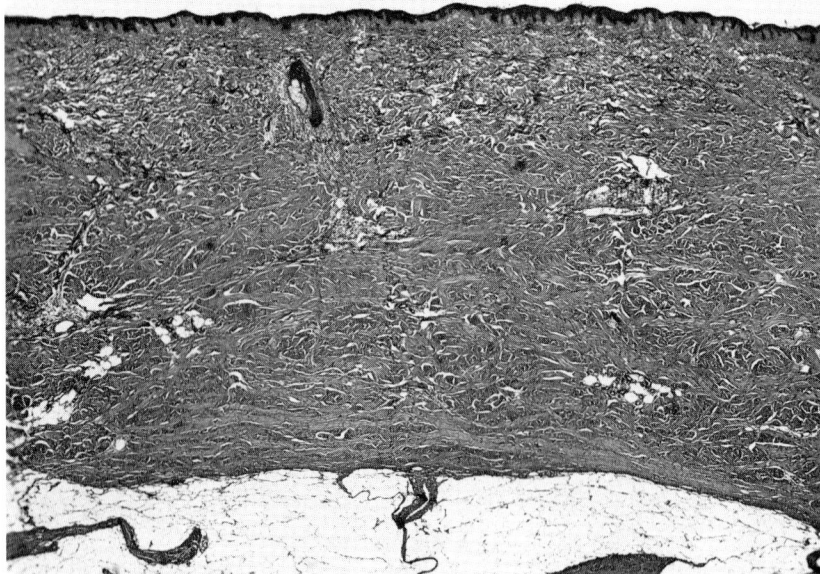

Figure 2-11 Morphea. Dermal sclerosis, loss of cellularity of collagen fat replacement by collagen. (AFIP photograph.) (× 17.)

round cell infiltration with invasion and subsequent atrophy of the pilary complexes. This infiltrate is almost purely lymphocytic. Pigment in dermal macrophages, ectatic dermal papillary blood vessels, and a variable amount of hyaluronic acid (edema) occur in the dermis. Although this is variable, it is almost always present (Fig. 2–13) (Johnson and Graham, 1965).

In some specimens a distinct eosinophilic (red) band is noted which corresponds to the basement membrane. On direct immunofluorescence this is the area that will fluoresce (Percy and Smyth, 1969). Eosinophilic globular bodies (Civatte bodies) may be noted at the dermal-epidermal junction or in the upper dermis. These bodies also fluoresce with the immunofluorescent technique.

Scleredema

In scleredema, one is immediately struck by the thickness and paleness of the dermis. The other structures, including the epidermis, appear normal. The thickness of the dermis is due to increased ground

substance and increased collagen. Some sclerosis of the collagen may occur but this is not a significant feature.

Dermal Mucinoses (Myxedema, generalized and localized; Lichen Myxedematosis; Cutaneous Focal Mucinosis; Cutaneous Myxoid Cyst; and the Genetic Mucinoses)

These conditions are presented as one group since they all have an essentially similar histologic picture. The epidermal changes are variable and are usually normal for the area biopsied or thinned if the accumulation of ground substance is great.

In the dermis, there is an accumulation of mucin which occurs between the collagen bundles, and fragmentation and splintering of the collagen occurs. This material appears stringy and basophilic (light blue) on hematoxylin and eosin-stained tissue. In focal cutaneous mucinosis the cutaneous myxoid cyst, the amount of mucin is large and a definite tumefaction results, producing large spaces in the dermis containing this bluish material.

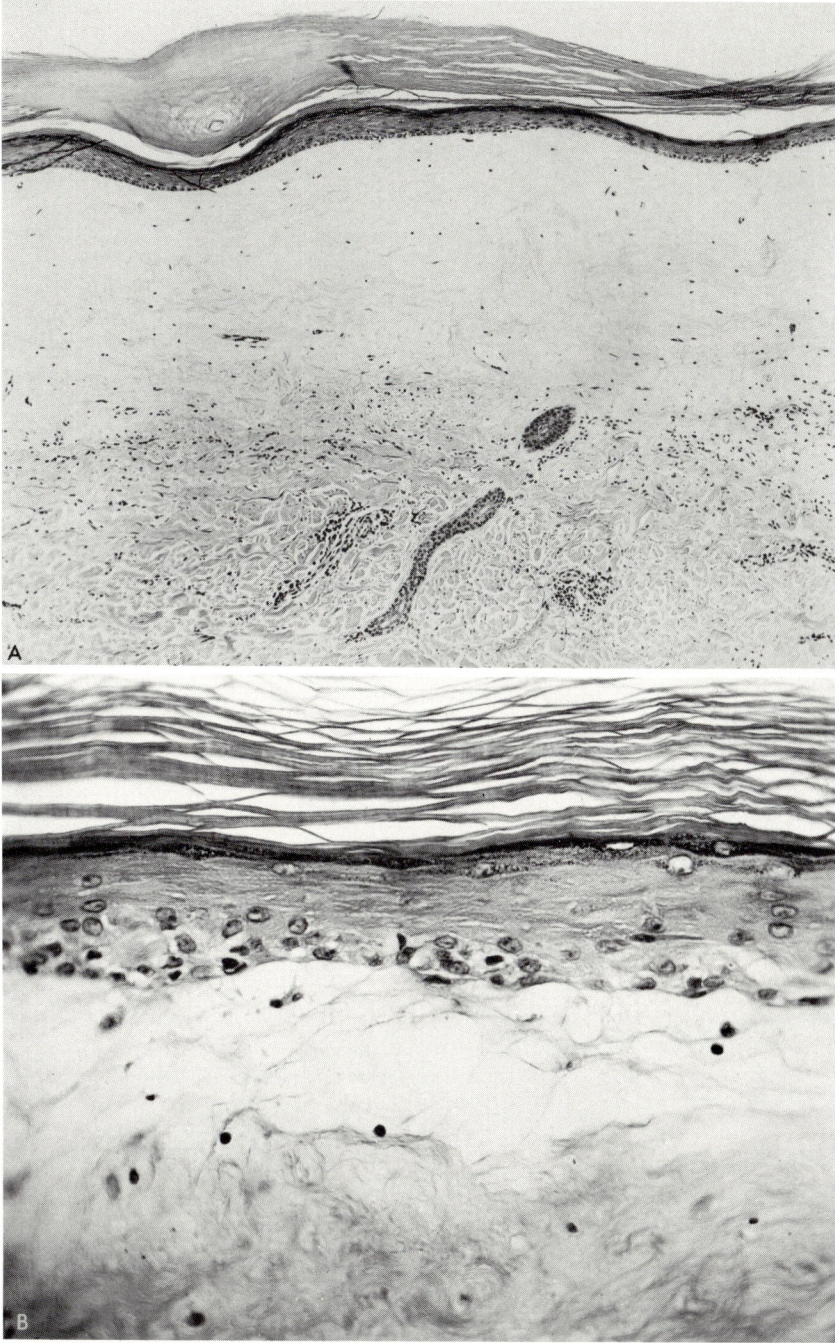

Figure 2-12   Lichen sclerosis et atrophicus. *A*, Hyperkeratosis, epidermal atrophy, and dermal homogenization. (Courtesy of Waine C. Johnson, M. D.) *B*, High-power view showing dermal-epidermal junction. (AFIP photograph.) (× 300.)

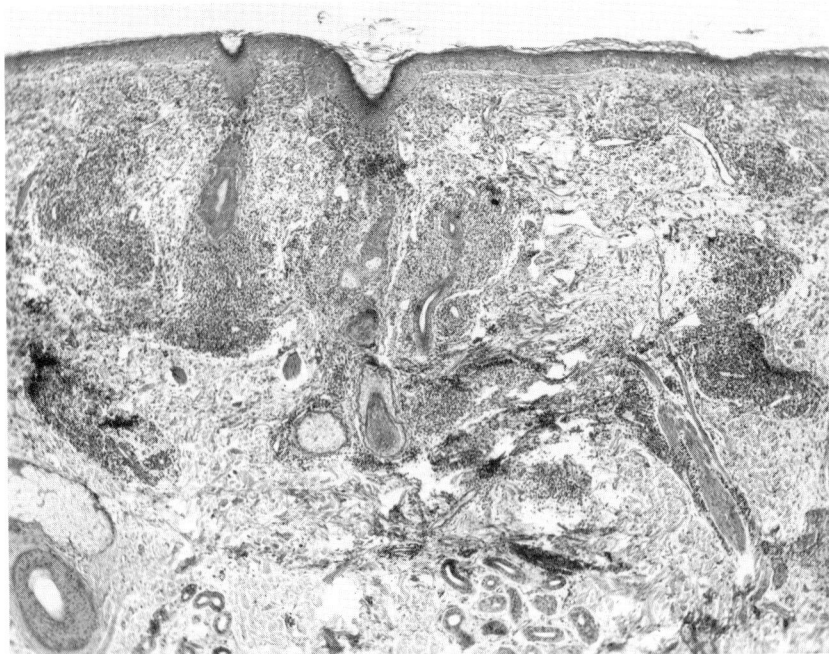

Figure 2–13 Lupus erythematosus. Hyperkeratosis, epidermal atrophy, follicular plugging, and a dermal lymphocytic adnexal infiltrate. (AFIP photograph.) (× 35.)

The other essential feature of this condition is the proliferation of stellate and spindle-shaped fibrocytes. The dermal mucin is mainly hyaluronic acid and can be identified by Hale's colloidal iron stain. When these mucinous changes occur and are limited to the pilosebaceous apparatus, the condition is called follicular mucinosis or alopecia mucinosa.

The finding of mucin is not limited to these conditions; it can be found in inflammatory dermatoses, tumors, and nevi.

Solar Elastosis

This represents the most common change seen in elastic tissue. This change does not occur to a significant degree in persons with prominent pigmentation of the epidermis.

The epidermis is usually normal or thinned. Just below the epidermis is a thin zone of normal or uninvolved collagen. In this upper and mid-corium is seen an amorphous homogeneous basophilic staining material in which there are coarse, thick, broken, granular basophilic fibers.

These usually occur together but may occur alone. It is probable that this condition not only represents altered elastic tissue but also altered collagen (Fig. 2–14).

Pseudoxanthoma Elasticum

A classic histologic picture that is diagnostic on routine stains occurs in the mid- and lower corium and consists of clumped, granular, fragmented, and basophilic-staining elastic fibers. Often they stain very dark blue purple with hematoxylin and eosin and appear granular owing to the collection of calcium on the altered elastic fibers. The epidermis is normal or thinned and there is usually a normal zone of collagen just below the epidermis.

Special stains for elastic tissue, including the aldehyde-fuchsin, Movat, and Weigert-Van Gieson, will demonstrate the fibers even more strikingly.

Elastosis Perforans Serpiginosa

This process shows another striking and diagnostic histologic picture. Histologically, there are focal areas of acanthosis that may be follicular or parafollicular. These acanthotic areas correspond to the clinical papules and are covered with ortho- and parakeratotic material. Within these areas of acanthosis are canals or channels that extend into the dermis. These channels are filled with parakeratotic cells at the margins and, centrally, basophilic granular debris which consists of degenerated and necrotic epithelial cells, inflammatory cells, and refractile eosinophilic fibers. At the surface of these canals (in the keratotic material just described) and at the base in the dermis, are a similar basophilic material, thick refractile eosinophilic fibers, and an inflammatory infiltrate. The infiltrate consists of histiocytes, fibroblasts, and occasionally multinucleated giant cells.

Special stains and electron microscopic studies have shown the refractile eosinophilic fibers to be elastic tissue. Conditions that may resemble elastosis perforans serpiginosa histologically are perforating folliculitis, reactive perforating collagenosis, and Kyrle's disease. These conditions do not demonstrate the altered elastic tissue in the epidermis and dermis as does elastosis perforans.

Cutis Laxa and Cutis Hyperelastica (Ehlers-Danlos syndrome)

These two conditions do not present diagnostic histologic features on routine stains and there is still doubt as to whether the alteration is purely with the elastic tissue or a combination of elastic and collagen alteration.

Sometimes in cutis hyperelastica an increased number of elastic fibers may be noted; this is not consistent, however. Frequently in cutis laxa the elastic fibers are granular, and they are fragmented when viewed under high power.

Dermatofibroma (Histiocytoma, Sclerosing Hemangioma, Nodular Subepidermal Fibrosis)

The name given to this lesion depends on the predominant type of process noted in the dermis. The essential features are hyperkeratosis and usually acanthosis, with basal cell proliferation. In the dermis, extending from just below the epidermis to the mid- or lower dermis, is a fibrocellular proliferation composed of histiocytes, fibroblasts, and a variable number of small blood vessels. the collagen is fi-

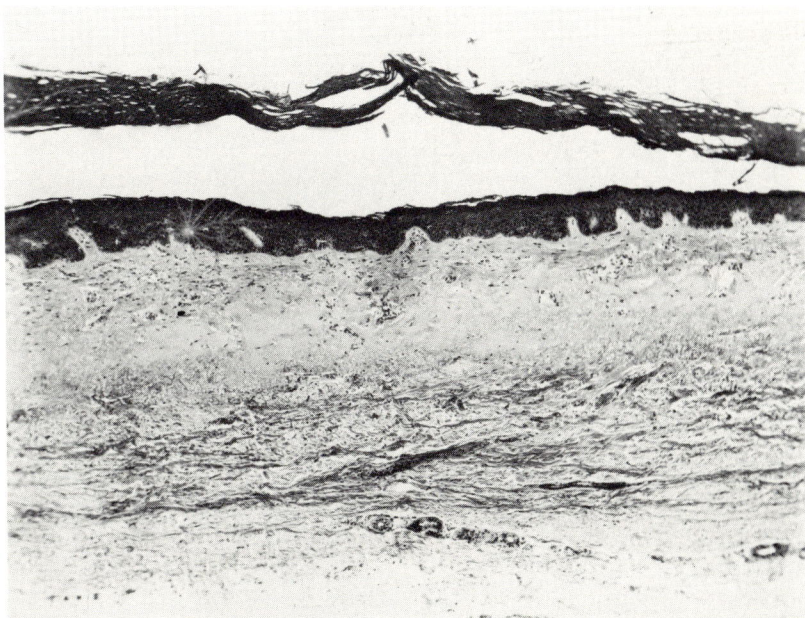

Figure 2–14 Solar elastosis. Homogeneous material in the middermis. Normal band of collagen just below the epidermis. (AFIP photograph.) (× 48.)

brotic, and there is anastomosing and intertwining of the collagen bundles. This mass extends into the corium at the lateral margins in fingerlike projections which surround normal islands of collagen (trapped collagen). Brown granular pigment may be present with the tumor and it can be melanin or hemosiderin. Lipids can also be found in this tumor, but on paraffin-blocked sections the lipid material will be removed and only clefts will be noted, often called cholesterol clefts (Fig. 2-15).

Neurofibroma

Neurofibroma is a dermal process that results from the proliferation of nerve sheath cells and fibers. The epidermis is thinned, with loss of distinct rete ridges. This dermal mass is well circumscribed but not encapsulated and may extend into the subcutaneous fat. It is composed of thin wavy fibers lying in loosely textured strands. These fibers stain pale blue on hematoxylin and eosin-stained sections.

The characteristic nuclei are narrow, bi-pointed, and serpentine. Many mast cells may also be noted in and about this tumor.

Leiomyoma

This tumor consists of a poorly defined proliferation of smooth muscle fibers that interlace and merge into the surrounding collagen. There is a zone (grenz) of unaffected collagen just below the epidermis that separates the epidermis from the tumor. The nuclei are long and thin and tend to have blunt ends, thus resembling a club. Special stains, such as the Movat penta-chrome or Masson trichrome, will aid in distinguishing muscle from collagen. In the trichrome stain, muscle will stain red and collagen, blue-green.

Keloid

The epidermis may be normal, acanthotic, or atrophied. In the corium one sees distinct sclerotic hyalinized eosinophilic bands of collagen, intertwined and intermingled with fibroblasts and some fibrous connective tissue. The fibrous portion of the lesion is more prominent at the periphery and staining is more basophilic. Extensive lesions may reach into the subcutis.

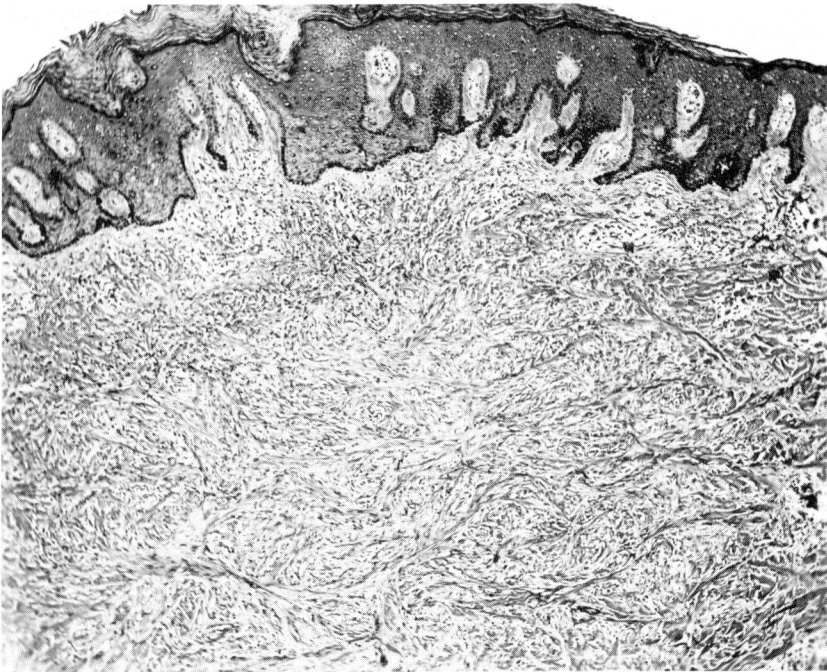

Figure 2-15 Dermatofibroma. Hyperkeratosis, acanthosis, a fibrocellular proliferation in the dermis. More normal appearing collagen at the margins of the cellular proliferate. (AFIP photograph.) ($\times$ 50.)

SUBCUTANEOUS REACTION PATTERNS

The separations of the subcutaneous inflammations and granulomatous processes are certainly less distinct than those of the epidermal or dermal reactions. The many clinical and histologic varieties, such as nodular vasculitis, Weber-Christian disease, erythema induratum, chronic relapsing micronodular hypodermatitis, Darier-Roussy hypodermal sarcoid, migrating epidermal panniculitis, and subcutaneous lipogranulomatosis, have common histologic features with certain variations that occur, depending on the time of biopsy, during the clinical course of the disease (Pierini et al., 1968).

Histologically, it is often difficult to place each of these processes into distinct, compact, well-defined, diagnostic packages. Thus, one should be familiar with the essential changes that occur. These are:

1. Inflammation, acute and granulomatous
2. Necrosis
3. Vasculitis (angiitis)
4. Fibrosis

The inflammatory process begins perivascularly in the septa, rarely in the lobules, and spreads to the fat lobules and even to the lower dermis. The cell types noted are lymphocytes, neutrophils, histiocytes, plasma cells, and eosinophils. If neutrophils predominate, and there is fragmentation, angiitis on an allergic basis is considered, with more emphasis toward nodular vasculitis or periarteritis nodosa, but certainly it is not highly specific.

As inflammation and angiitis progress, vascular endothelial proliferation, vessel wall thickening, invasion of the vessel by inflammatory cells, fibrinoid accumulations about the vessels, necrosis, fat liquefaction, and tissue death occur. With the liberation of fat from the cell, a foreign body reaction can occur and a granulomatous infiltrate will predominate with many histiocytes (lipophages) and foreign body giant cells. As the process resolves, fibrosis occurs with contraction and loss of some of the subcutaneous space.

Variations of this picture can be seen in any of these diseases. A unifying concept of these subcutaneous inflammations is more easily understood by separating them into entities which are based on both the histologic and the clinical course (Fig. 2–16).

GRANULOMATOUS REACTIONS

Granulomatous reactions represent a heterogeneous pattern of tissue reactions in response to varied stimuli.

There is no simple, precise way to define a granuloma histologically. It is defined on the basis of what is observed.

A granuloma or granulomatous inflammation may be defined as a circumscribed tissue reaction, subacute to chronic, located about one or more foci. The components of this reaction are: vascular changes dilatation of existing vessels or new vessel growth, or degenerative changes to the point of occlusion; connective tissue changes, including proliferation of fibrocytes and histiocytes, increased fibrous tissue with new fiber formation, or necrosis of the connective tissue; and cellular infiltration, with the characteristic cells being the giant cells (Langerhans,' foreign body, and Touton) epithelioid cells, lymphocytes, polymorphonuclear leukocytes, plasma cells, and fibrocytes.

This reaction is seen in response to many things; thus, the granulomatous reactions can be subdivided on the basis of the cause.

Infectious Granulomas

a. Treponemal diseases—syphilis, yaws, pinta, bejel.

b. Viral disease—lymphogranuloma venereum.

c. Bacterial diseases—leprosy, tuberculosis (Fig. 2–17), atypical mycobacterial infections, granuloma inguinale, rhinoscleroma.

d. Deep mycoses—histoplasmosis, blastomycosis, coccidioidomycosis, cryptococcosis, sporotrichosis, maduromycosis.

3. Superficial mycoses—T. rubrum, T. mentagrophytes, T. schoenleini.

f. Parasitic infections—amebiasis, onchocerciasis, leishmaniasis.

In the group of infectious granulomas, a specific diagnosis can be made if the organism can be identified in the tissue.

In leprosy and the mycotic infections, this is not too difficult owing to special stains, such as acid-fast and PAS, respectively.

The venereal diseases and tuberculosis

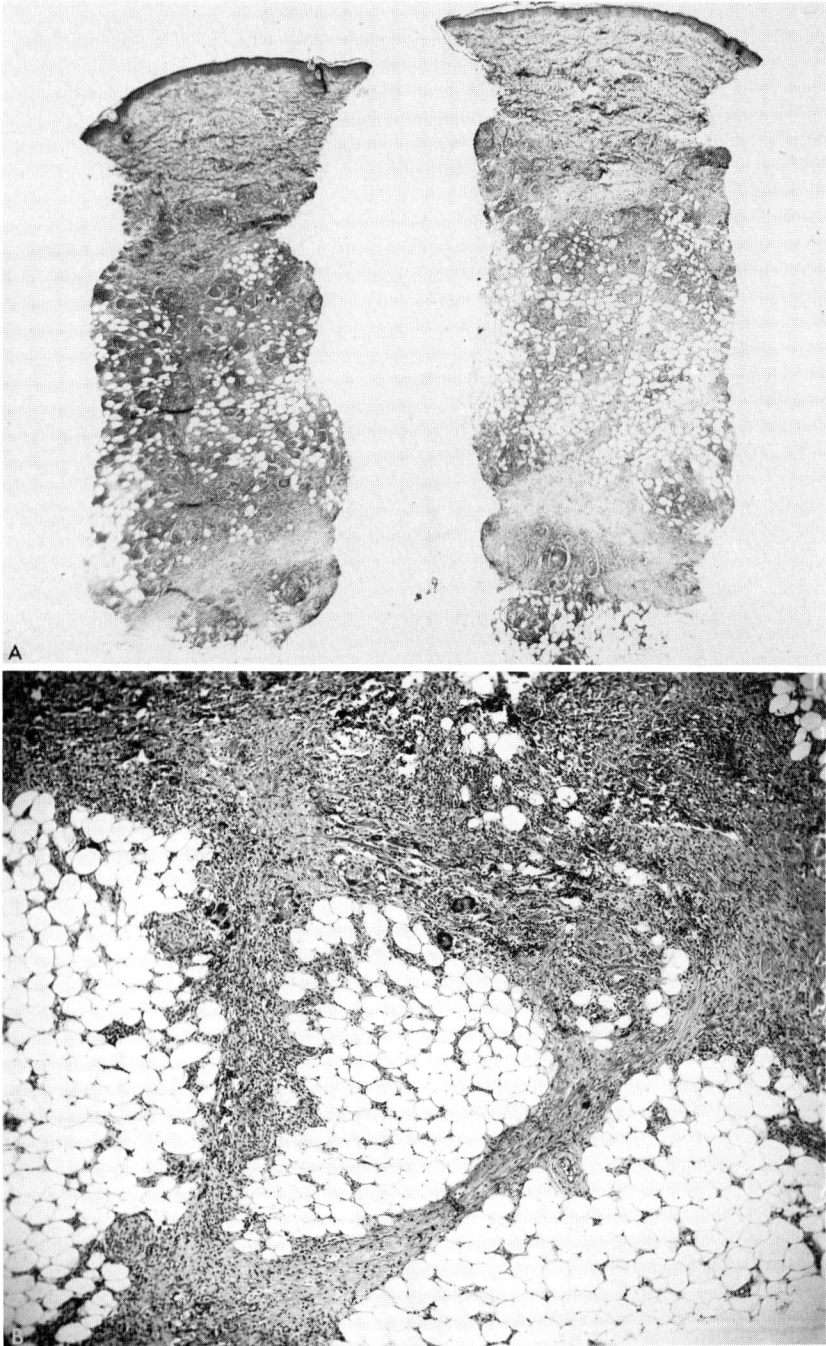

Figure 2-16 Erythema nodosum. *A*, Low-power view showing lower dermal and subcutaneous tissue inflammation. (Courtesy of Waine C. Johnson, M. D.) (× 4.) *B*, Panniculitis, mainly septal, granulomatous inflammation with giant cells and necrosis in the dermis. (AFIP photograph.) (× 48.)

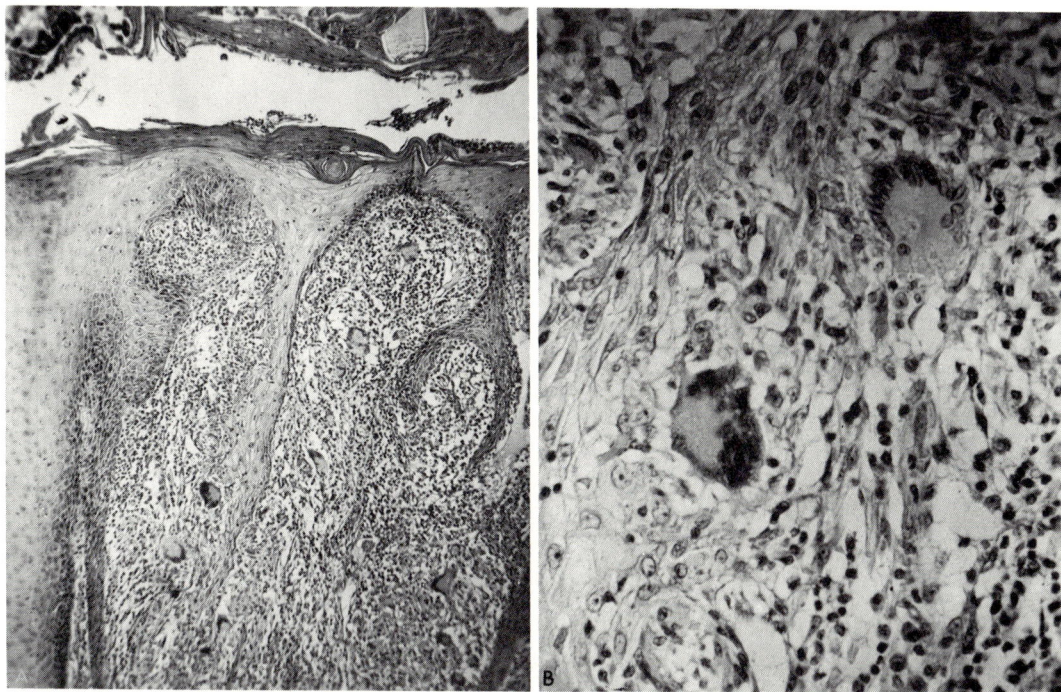

Figure 2-17 Infectious granuloma (tuberculosis). *A*, Parakeratosis, acanthosis, granulomatous inflammation with lymphocytes, epithelial cells, and giant cells. (AFIP photograph.) (× 75.) *B*, High-power view. (AFIP photograph.) (× 400.)

present a more difficult problem for tissue identification of the causative organism. Whenever possible, cultural studies should be performed for specific confirmation; these can easily be done at the time of biopsy by the tissue imprint method or by mincing a portion of the biopsy specimen for culture.

Sarcoidosis

Sarcoidosis is a granulomatous reaction of doubtful causes. This condition shows more cellular response with epithelioid cells being the predominant cells (Fig. 2-18).

Foreign Body Granulomas (Fig. 2-19)

a. Paraffin
b. Zirconium
c. Keratin (ruptured cysts)
d. Beryllium
e. Tattoo dyes
f. Silicon
g. Other material not usually found in tissue.

Palisading Granulomas

The classic histologic feature of this group of granulomatous processes is necrobiosis of the collagen with a palisading arrangement of epithelioid cells and histiocytes about the areas of necrobiosis. The collagen here appears washed out, with loss of fibrillation and cellularity but with remnants of cells and cell nuclei still present. There may also be an associated increased amount of mucin or ground substance present in these areas.

The granulomas in this group are (Fig. 2-20):

1. Granuloma annulare
2. Necrobiosis lipoidica
3. Rheumatoid nodules
4. Rheumatic nodules
5. Pseudorheumatoid nodules

Nonspecific Granulomas

1. Bromoderma
2. Lichen nitidus
3. Granuloma faciale

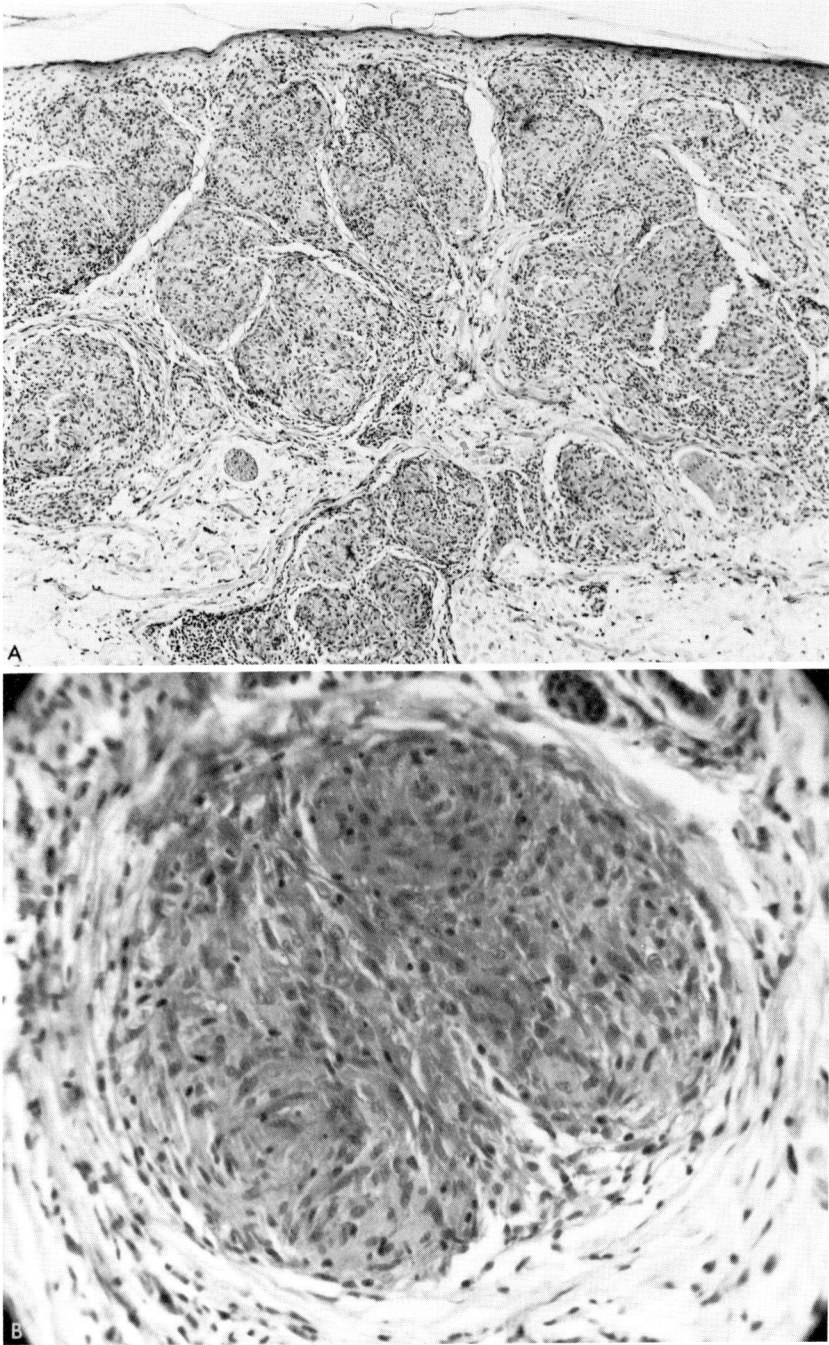

Figure 2–18 Sarcoidosis. *A,* Epithelioid cell granulomas in the dermis. Minimal inflammatory cellular response. (Courtesy of Waine C. Johnson, M.D.) (× 150.) *B,* Sarcoidal granuloma. (AFIP photograph.) (× 500.)

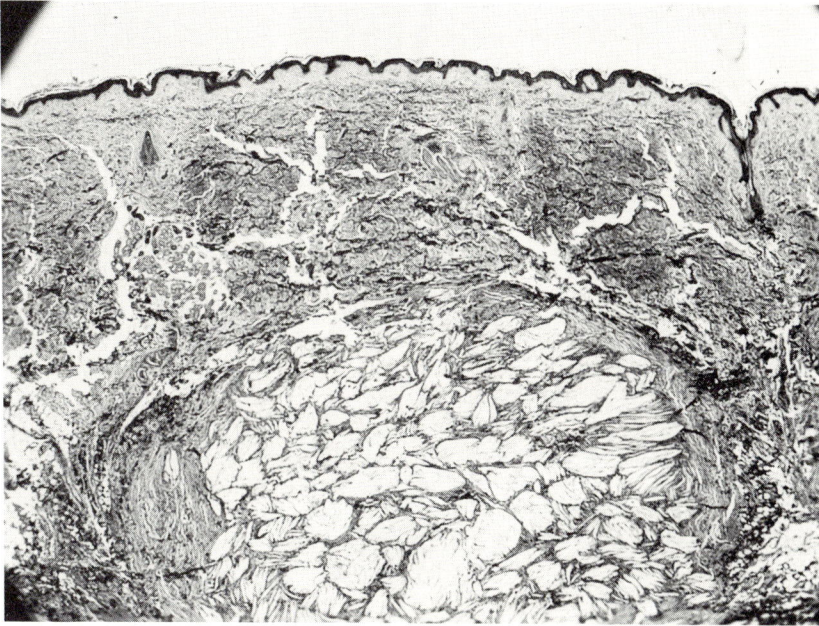

Figure 2-19 Foreign body granuloma. Granuloma due to paraffin, in mid- and lower dermis. Minimal inflammatory response. (AFIP photograph.) (× 18.)

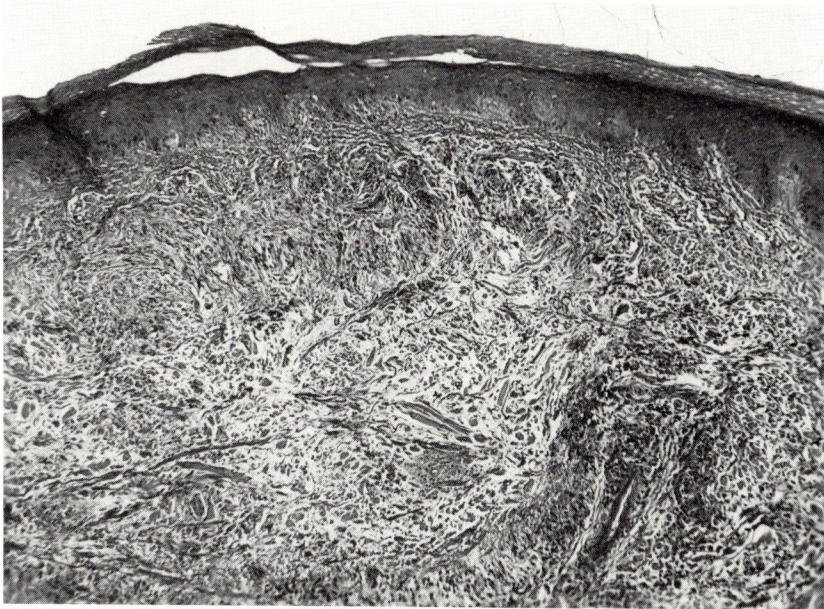

Figure 2-20 Palisading granuloma (granuloma annulare). Focal area of necrobiosis in the middermis with epithelial cells surrounding this area. (AFIP photograph.) (× 68.)

BACTERIAL DISEASES

Bacterial diseases of the skin are not frequently biopsied, although they occur rather commonly. The most commonly seen are bacterial folliculitis and impetigo.

Folliculitis

Superficial folliculitis consists of a pustule beneath the stratum corneum and a dense, inflammatory infiltrate about the upper portion of the follicles with invasion of the follicular epithelium. The infiltrate is composed of neutrophils and lymphocytes (Fig. 2–21).

Deep folliculitis (furuncle) is a more severe reaction with abscess formation in the follicular epithelium composed of neutrophils; the reaction in the dermis is more intense, with perivascular accumulations of lymphocytes. As this progresses, there will be complete destruction of the pilary complex.

Impetigo Contagiosa

This process can also be classified as a subcorneal pustular dermatosis, especially in young children and babies. A subcorneal pustule is noted, along with exocytosis of neutrophils and spotty areas of liquefaction degeneration. In the dermis is a variable perivascular cellular infiltrate of lymphocytes and neutrophils. Acantholysis can occur in this condition, and the histologic picture may mimic pemphigus foliaceus.

Impetigo herpetiformis and subcorneal pustular dermatosis have histologic findings very similar to impetigo contagiosa and must be differentiated from this condition.

CUTANEOUS MALIGNANCIES

Malignant tumors of the skin have distinct histologic features and present the most common lesion biopsied. Those considered are basal cell carcinoma, Bowen's disease, and squamous cell carcinoma. Actinic keratosis is also considered in this group, although it is usually thought of as a premalignant new growth.

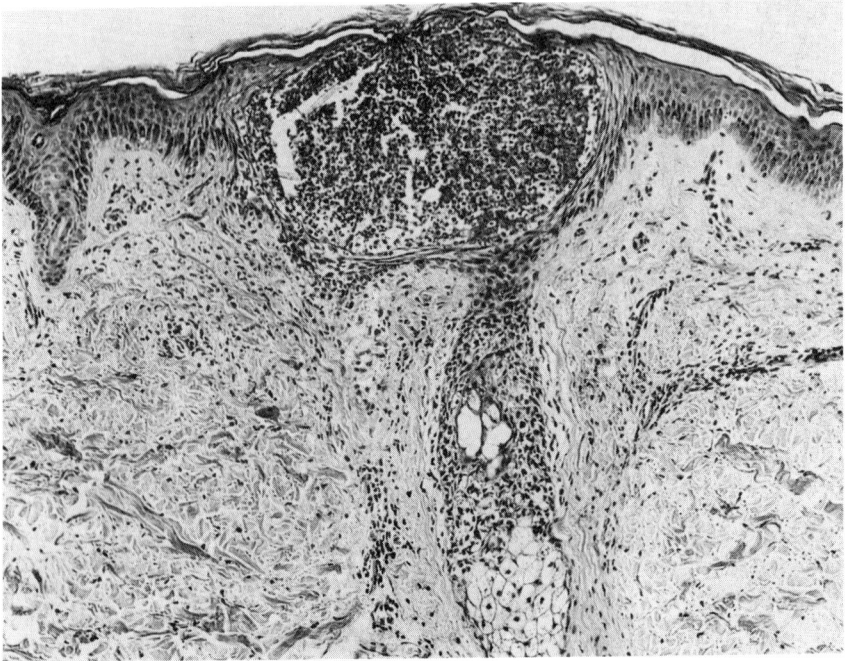

Figure 2–21 Folliculitis. Intra-epidermal pustule within and expanding the follicle at its intra-epidermal portion. (Courtesy of Waine C. Johnson, M.D.) (× 150.)

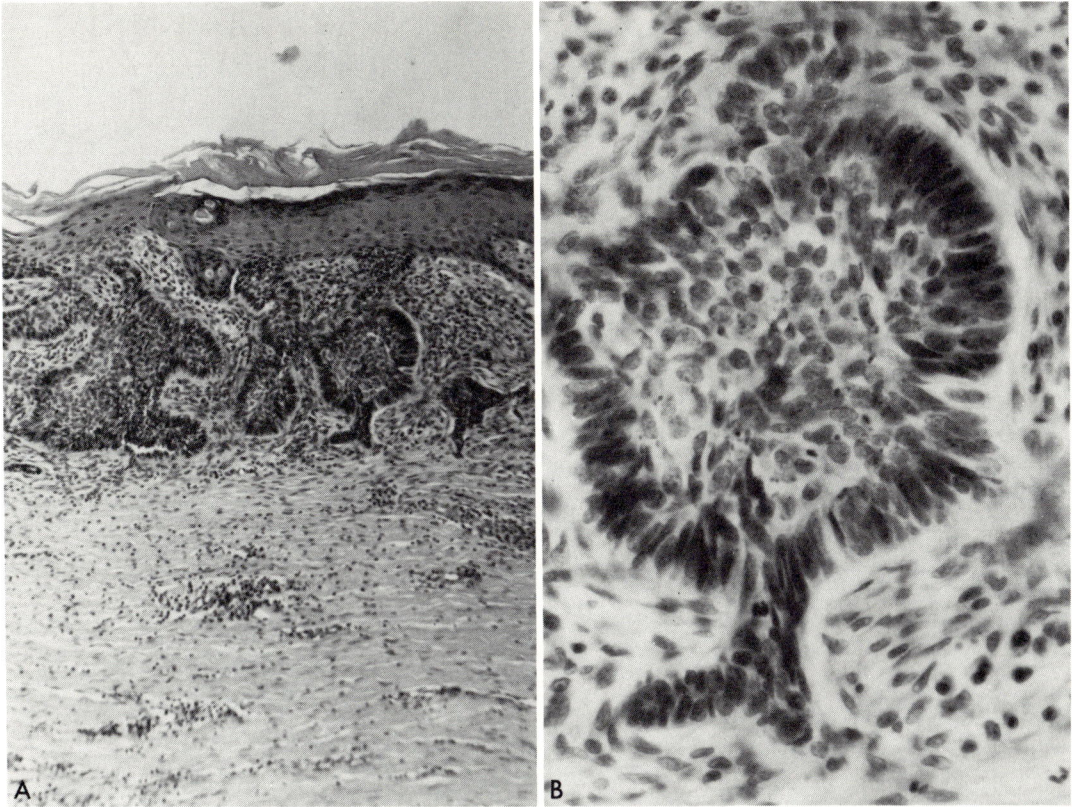

Figure 2-22   Basal cell carcinoma. *A*, New growths of proliferating basal cells from the epidermis. *B*, Island of tumor in the dermis, showing peripheral palisading. (Courtesy of E. Moore and D. Smith, Naval Hospital, Philadelphia, Pa.) (*A* × 80; *B* × 200.)

Basal Cell Carcinoma

This tumor arises from the epidermis at the basal layer or from the follicular epithelium. It is characterized by downgrowths or buds from the basal layer of follicles which produce islands, strands, or nodules of atypical basal cells in the dermis. These tumor islands show a picket fence–like arrangement of the cells at the periphery (peripheral palisading).

The stroma also participates in this reaction with an increase in ground substance and new fiber formation.

On processed tissue, spaces may be noted between the tumor lobules and the connective tissue (retraction spaces). These result from loss of ground substance and shrinkage of the connective tissue. This is a rather common finding in this tumor. Various patterns may be noted in basal cell carcinoma — adenoid, superficial (multiple epidermal buds), cystic, sclerotic (dense fibrous reaction in the dermis), and keratotic. In all these patterns, however, there are proliferations of atypical basal cells. Mitotic figures are present but do not overpower the observer (Fig. 2–22).

Bowen's Disease

This process can be best described as a proliferating epidermis without direction. There is a loss of the normal progression of epidermal cells from the basal layer to the stratum corneum. Large, atypical, dyskeratotic cells are seen throughout the epidermis; abnormal mitotic figures are abundant. Large pale cells loaded with glycogen, as demonstrated by the PAS technique, are noted. All these changes are confined to the epidermis. Other epidermal changes are acanthosis and parakeratosis. Normal areas of epidermis may be found between abnormal areas. The

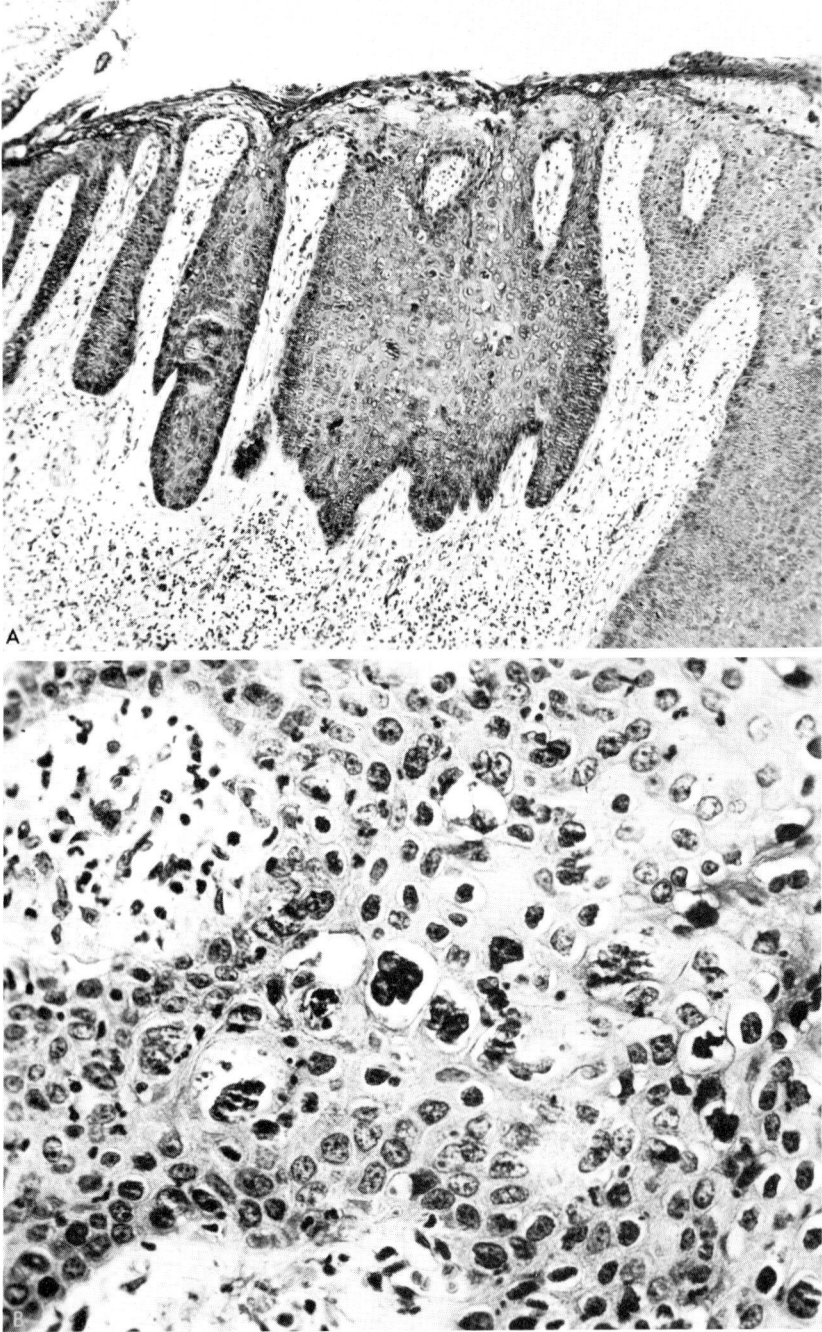

Figure 2-23 Bowen's disease. Abnormal intra-epidermal proliferation with atypical and dyskeratotic cells. (AFIP photographs.) (A × 80; B × 300.)

dermal reaction is variable, with inflammatory cells found focally and about blood vessels. When this reaction invades the dermis, it is termed invasive Bowen's disease or squamous cell carcinoma (Fig. 2–23) (Graham and Helwig, 1961).

Squamous Cell Carcinoma

This tumor may arise *de novo* or in an actinic keratosis. Prognostically this is important, since those that arise in actinic keratosis metastasize at a very low frequency and simple destruction and removal are usually curative.

Squamous cell carcinomas are proliferations of atypical and keratinizing epidermal cells into the adjacent dermis. These cells are larger and stain eosinophilic (pink) on hematoxylin and eosin sections. Mitotic figures are common, as are dyskeratotic cells. Keratinization commonly occurs in the form of so-called horn pearls which are concentric layers of squamous cells increasingly keratinized toward the center of the structure. The invading cells may be in sheets, buds, or islands, projecting into the dermis. The dermal response to this intrusion is an inflammatory cellular reaction composed of lymphocytes mainly, and histiocytes. The inflammatory response appears to be most intense in the least anaplastic varieties.

Acantholysis can occur in this tumor, and keratinization does not always take place.

Actinic Keratosis

This lesion has been described as squamous cell carcinoma grade ½ by Lever (1967). This description is borne out by the histologic findings. The distinctive findings are hyperkeratosis and focal areas of parakeratosis. The epidermis is usually atrophic and may show focal areas of acanthosis. Within the epidermis, atypical cells are noted; these are usually confined to the basal cell layer. These changes in the basal cells form the distinctive histologic feature of this lesion. The basal cells are larger, appearing more squamous in size and staining characteristics. These atypical basal cells proliferate and bud into the dermis, and in many instances clefts or separations, as well as acantholy-sis, occur between the basal cell layer and the remainder of the epidermis. Although the atypia is essentially confined to the basal cell layer, changes which resemble Bowen's disease may occur throughout the epidermis.

A distinctive phenomenon occurs in this lesion. In the areas where there is adnexal epithelium, the more normal appearing cells of the adnexae proliferate over and cover the dysplastic epithelium. At the junction of these two, a distinct and sharp division occurs in an arciform arrangement. This has been referred to as the umbrella concept by Pinkus, and is helpful in diagnosing an actinic keratosis (Pinkus, 1958).

In the dermis there is solar elastosis, a distinct and pronounced chronic inflammatory infiltrate composed mainly of lymphocytes. The infiltrate in some instances is distinctly lichenoid and the lesion may closely resemble lichen planus.

The presence of hyperkeratosis, parakeratosis, cellular atypia, especially basal cell budding, and the distinctive changes between the adnexal epithelium and the dysplastic epithelium make the actinic keratosis a distinctive lesion (Fig. 2–24).

Appendages

The appendages, hair, and eccrine and apocrine sweat glands produce tumors and hamartomatous growths. Clinically most of these are indistinct as nondescript tumors. Histologically they show distinct features. A detailed description of all these entities is beyond the scope of this presentation but they will be listed for the sake of completeness. (Helwig, 1963; Johnson and Helwig, 1963).

Tumors of follicular origin:
1. Trichoepithelioma
2. Basal cell carcinoma
3. Trichofolliculoma
4. Inverted follicular keratosis
5. Pilomatrixoma
6. Tricholemmoma

Tumors of eccrine origin:
1. Eccrine poroma
2. Eccrine acrospiroma
3. Cylindroma
4. Spiradenoma
5. Syringoma

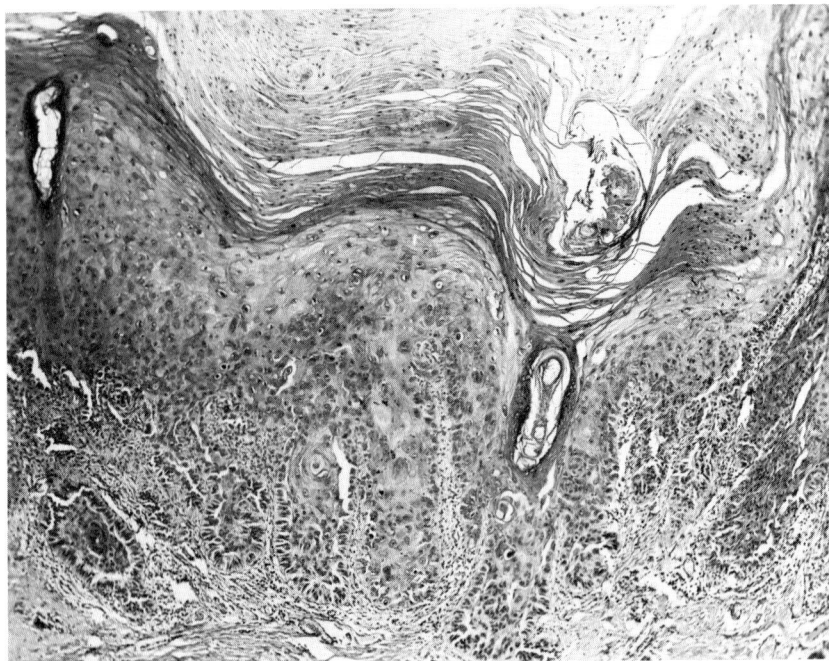

Figure 2-24   Actinic keratosis. Hyper- and parakeratosis, atypical and dyskeratotic cells primarily at the basal cell zone and one to two cell layers above. (AFIP photograph.) (× 50.)

6. Chondroid syringoma
7. Eccrine cystadenoma

Tumors of apocrine origin:
1. Syringocystadenoma papilliferum
2. Hidradenoma papilliferum
3. Apocrine cyst

The histologic descriptions are in no way intended to be a comprehensive review of dermal pathology; their purpose is to acquaint the student of dermatology with some of the concepts, patterns, and groups into which skin diseases are classified histologically.

REFERENCES

Burnham, T. K., Neblett, T. R., and Fine, G.: The application of the fluorescent antibody technique to the investigation of lupus erythematosus and various dermatoses. J. Invest. Dermatol. *41*:451, 1963.

Gordon, M., and Johnson, W. C.: Histopathology and histochemistry of psoriasis. Arch. Dermatol. *95*: 402, 1967.

Graham, J. H., and Helwig, E. B.: Bowen's disease and its relationship to systemic cancer. Arch. Dermatol. *83*:738, 1961.

Graham, J. H., and Mandrea, E.: Lichen simplex

chronicus: A clinicopathologic study. Am. J. Pathol. *44*:36a, 1964.

Hashimoto, K., and Lever, W. F.: An ultrastructural study of cell functions in pemphigus vulgaris. Arch. Dermatol. *101*:287, 1970.

Helwig, E. B.: Tumor seminar. Tex. Med. 59:652, 1963.

Hiroaki, U.: Hyaline bodies in subepidermal papillae. Arch. Dermatol. *100*:610, 1969.

Johnson, B. L., and Charneco, D. R.: Café-au-lait spot in neurofibromatosis and in normal individuals. Arch. Dermatol. *102*:442, 1970.

Johnson, B. L., Jr., and Helwig, E. B.: Eccrine acrospiroma: A clinicopathologic study. Cancer 23:641, 1969.

Johnson, W. C.: Histochemistry of the Skin. *In* Helwig, E. B., (ed.): Pathologic Physiology and Anatomy of the Skin. Baltimore, Williams and Wilkins Company, 1972.

Johnson, W. C., and Graham, J. H.: Cutaneous ground substance changes in lupus erythematosus. Lab. Invest. *14*(5):580, 1965.

Johnson, W. C., and Helwig, E. B.: Histochemistry of the acid mucopolysaccharides of skin in normal and certain pathologic conditions. Am. J. Clin. Pathol. *40*:123, 1963.

Lever, W. F.: Pemphigus and Pemphigoid. Springfield, Illinois, Charles C Thomas, 1965.

Lever, W. F.: Histopathology of the Skin. 4th ed. Philadelphia, J. B. Lippincott Company, 1967.

MacVicar, D. N., and Graham, J. H.: Pathodynamics of subepidermal bullous dermatoses: Basement membrane studies. Am. J. Pathol. *46*:372, 1965.

MacVicar, D. N., Graham, J. H., and Burgoon, C. F.,

Jr.: Dermatitis herpetiformis, erythema multiforme and bullous pemphigoid: A comparative histopathological and histochemical study. J. Invest. Dermatol. *41*:289, 1963.

McKusick, V. A., Kaplan, D., Wise, D., et al.: The genetic mucopolysaccharidoses. Medicine *44*:445, 1965.

Pearson, R. W.: Studies on the pathogenesis of epidermolysis bullosa. J. Invest. Dermatol. *39*:551, 1962.

Pearson, R. W., and Spargo, B. S.: Electron microscopic studies of dermo-epidermal separation in human skin. J. Invest. Dermatol. *36*:213, 1961.

Percy, J. S., and Smyth, C. J.: Immunofluorescent skin test in systemic lupus erythematosus. J.A.M.A. *208*:485, 1969.

Pierini, L. E., Abulafia, J., and Weinfeld, S.: Idiopathic lipogranulomatosous hypodermatitis. Arch. Dermatol. *98*:290, 1968.

Pinkus, H.: Keratosis senilis. Am. J. Clin. Pathol. *29*:193, 1958.

Pinkus, H., and Mehregan, A. J.: A Guide to Histopathology. New York, Appleton-Century-Crofts, Meredith Corporation, 1969.

Zelickson, A. S.: Ultrastructure of Normal and Abnormal Skin. Philadelphia, Lea and Febiger, 1967.

PRINCIPLES OF
CLINICAL DIAGNOSIS

Donald M. Pillsbury

THE MEDICAL HISTORY IN DERMATOLOGIC PATIENTS

The medical history in a patient with a disease affecting the skin obviously should be obtained with the same care that is exercised in a patient with any general medical or surgical illness. However, it frequently is not. Skin lesions are often too quickly assessed as trivial and unimportant. As a result, the history and physical examination may be totally inadequate, the precise extent of the skin lesions undetermined, and their possible general medical importance unsuspected.

The "chief complaint" of a patient with a skin condition is frequently expressed in such colloquial terms or may be so misleading as not to be worth recording verbatim. It is useful to delay putting it down until at least the preliminary history and examination have been completed. The symptomatic attributes of a dermatologic complaint may at times be helpful; for example, absence of itching eliminates atopic dermatitis as a diagnostic possibility, but symptoms such as pain, burning, and itching vary so greatly among different patients with the same disease as to make these symptoms sometimes misleading. It is useful to include in the chief complaint some indication as to (a) the type of skin lesions and whether they are localized or diffuse, (b) whether the dermatosis is acute or chronic, and (c) if chronic, whether or not the course has been characterized by remissions and exacerbations. Among the first questions to be asked, *without fail,* is whether or not any topical treatment of the lesion has been carried out.

It is unfortunately true that, because skin lesions are by their nature superficial and frequently of limited extent, superficiality in examination is regarded as adequate. It is also frequently a penalty of dispensary or office practice that initial examinations are hurried because of the press of patients and the distractions of many interruptions. A remarkable diagnostic acumen may be evident when a specialist with long experience with skin diseases merely inspects the presenting lesions, but this is an occupational trap for the unwary, and it may sometimes lead to serious diagnostic errors from the general medical standpoint. Diseases, like criminals, are sometimes trapped by sudden flashes of intuitive diagnostic genius, but this is a hazardous substitute for painstaking collection of the essential medical evidence.

Certain important questions must be answered during the initial contact with the patient, and this may be done quite rapidly if necessary. The more important and pressing of these are as follows:

1. What is the general character of the eruption, and is it more extensive than the patient indicates? If so, what is its distribution? Does this have any characteristic pattern?

2. Essential questions in regard to the history include information as to the duration of the eruption, whether or not it is recurrent, and *whether or not the patient feels ill generally*. It is important to determine promptly whether or not the patient is taking any medicine regularly, or whether topical medicaments have recently been applied to the skin.

3. In the course of this abbreviated initial questioning, it is of importance for the physician to sense whether or not the patient regards his skin disease as of great moment. Until recent years, a high proportion of dermatologic patients labored under a fear that the condition of the skin might be an evidence of syphilis. This type of apprehension has largely disappeared, but it has been replaced in many patients by an overwhelming fear of cancer. This may be present in patients with dermatoses which have no possible relation to any neoplastic process. Under such circumstances, immediate reassurance of the patient, even if he has not expressed a fear of tumor, is often very gratefully received and increases patient-physician rapport.

4. The initial survey of the patient may indicate quite clearly to the physician that further study or consultation will be necessary. It is probably best with most patients to indicate the need for this casually and by degrees, rather than to proceed with the examination with an air of omniscience

and then, suddenly and with no previous conditioning, to confront the patient with advice as to the performance of a variety of procedures.

5. Since skin lesions are common, are ordinarily visible to the patient, and cause patients to seek medical advice promptly as a rule, they may serve as a very effective means of directing the patient into proper channels of preventive medicine. Not infrequently, a few words of advice as to the value of preventive health examinations will be most gratefully received, especially by patients in the fifth decade or more. We have observed many patients in whom a wart or small keratosis, for instance, led directly to medical surveys which revealed significant early systemic disease.

To summarize, the objectives of a complete medical history in a patient with a disease affecting the skin are precisely the same as those of any other medical history; namely, to trace the development of the disease as accurately as possible; to determine those elements in the patient's past history which may be related to the disease in question and those which are not; to establish the relation of the patient and his disease to his heredity, personal and occupational environment, psychic and emotional status, and previous medical attention; and to establish a physician-patient rapport by an attitude of kindly interest and a willingness to listen. Patients frequently express ideas concerning the causes and progress of their disease which the physician may instinctively feel to be quite erroneous; nevertheless, information of much importance is sometimes contained in what may appear to be irrelevant statements by the patient.

Family History

In addition to inquiry concerning familial tendencies to diabetes, cardiovascular disease and tumors, questioning concerning the familial incidence of allergic diseases is of great importance in a wide variety of skin conditions. It is not sufficient simply to ask the question "Is there any allergy in your family?" Hives, eczema, hay fever, and asthma should be specifically mentioned. Other common familial trends in relation to skin diseases include ichthyosis of moderate to marked degree, acne, baldness, rosacea, and psoriasis. Uncommonly, certain other specific congenital malformations may be noted as hereditary traits.

Age

As with many other diseases, certain groups of skin conditions are seen much more frequently in various age groups. Nevertheless, *great caution should be exerted not to allow age to become too much of a determining factor in arriving at a diagnosis.* This is particularly true in the case of tumors. Cancer of the skin shows an increased incidence with age, but failure to consider the possibility of malignant tumor in children or in young adults has sometimes led to irretrievable error. The following common examples of age incidence in various dermatoses may be cited. Acne reaches its height in adolescence, and rosacea in early to late middle age, but these conditions are by no means entirely confined to these age groups. Atrophy and keratoses are characteristic of age and senility, but they may be seen in children with xeroderma pigmentosum. Atopic dermatitis frequently has an age periodicity and is fortunately not frequent after late adolescence; nevertheless, it may sometimes persist in severe or restricted forms. The common types of ringworm of the scalp are seen entirely in children, but an adult form is endemic in the southwestern and western United States. Age of the patient in the consideration of various diagnostic possibilities serves some usefulness, but its importance in the particular patient and disease in question should be interpreted with much care.

Race

Again, this may have some influence in the general consideration leading to diagnosis, but it is rarely a crucial determining factor. In the melting pot of America and in many parts of Europe and Asia, pure racial strains are uncommon. While pemphigus occurs more frequently in Jews than in non-Jews, the racial influence is not strong enough to have serious consideration in such a diagnosis. Kaposi's sarcoma is seen more frequently in patients whose personal or familial environment was originally in southeastern Europe, but again this is only a matter of interest and not a determining factor. Psoriasis is seen infrequently in pureblooded Negroes, but a majority of Negroes outside Africa are not pure-blooded. This list could be considerably extended, but there is no point in doing so here. Too great emphasis upon race in respect to diagnosis may lead to error.

Race may, however, be of considerable importance in the prognosis. Just as tuberculosis has had an extremely serious prognosis in American Indians, so does coccidioidomycosis frequently produce death in Negroes. Negroes may develop more bizarre and exuberant cutaneous reactions in the skin than do whites; for example, bizarre marked skin lesions of secondary syphilis or profuse annular lesions in sarcoid. Negro skin appears to be more prone to lichenification, especially with follicular involvement, when rubbed. Orientals have a greater tendency toward atopic dermatitis or lichen simplex chronicus as well as atypical clinical patterns of these conditions.

Geographic Origin

Some diseases can be acquired only under climatic and other conditions which render the diseases contagious and endemic in certain areas. An individual can almost never, for instance, acquire leprosy if he has not lived for extended periods in an environment other than the temperate parts of Europe or North America. Certain of the treponemal diseases, such as yaws, pinta, and bejel, are seen only in tropical environments; indeed, bejel is encountered only in the eastern Mediterranean area. Rhus contact dermatitis does not occur in England because the plant does not grow there.

While the strong geographic tendencies of certain diseases are useful in extending differential diagnostic considerations, they may also lead to error. If a patient states that he has spent some time in the tropics, too great emphasis may be placed upon the esoteric and the bizarre, with neglect of the common diseases. An individual who spends some time in a tropical climate, but who is not a native, is much more likely to have some very aggravated form of common disease, such as a bacterial or fungal infection of the skin, than he is to have a disease which is peculiarly and uniquely tropical. Moreoever, in respect to other diseases which are presumed to have a particular geographic point of origin, it must be kept in mind that the endemic foci of disease are constantly expanding and contracting, for reasons which may not be immediately apparent. Coccidioidomycosis is common in the San Joaquin Valley of California, but there are other areas in the United States and Mexico in which it is found, depending, apparently, upon certain conditions of prolonged heat and the type of soil. Rocky Mountain spotted fever is by no means confined to the area in which it was originally described, but has also been reported in the New England and Middle Atlantic areas. Certain endothrix infections of the scalp are far more common in Mexico and the southwestern United States, but patients with this disease have been observed in many far-removed areas of the United States and have escaped proper diagnosis for years because of mistaken ideas regarding the strict geographic origin of the infection.

Season

Certain diseases have seasonal peaks; at times the reasons for this may be apparent, but not infrequently they remain a mystery. Contact dermatitis from plants will obviously be seen far more frequently during seasons when plants are growing. Contact dermatitis from ragweed pollen will invariably be seen during the ragweed season when the disease first starts; however, with repeated recurrences of the disease, the seasonal onset may become less and less apparent. Photosensitization reactions will obviously be at their peak during the summer season, but in some patients they may persist for so long thereafter as to obscure this etiologic factor considerably. In patients with chronic recurrent skin disorders, the history of *climatic and other factors at the time of onset* is of great importance but may require prolonged questioning to elicit in proper perspective and detail.

Many diseases, including dermatitis and superficial fungal infections, become much worse during seasons of high environmental temperature. Miliaria is caused entirely by this factor. This item in the history is obviously worth noting. Certain common diseases, such as acne, show variable responses in relation to season. While acne is ordinarily improved by exposure of the skin to sun, it may sometimes become very much worse if the sunny climate is one of great heat and humidity. Papular urticaria in children has a marked seasonal incidence during the summer, which is explainable on the basis that a high proportion of cases are the result of insect bites. Sunlight may aggravate rosacea, and cases of benign familial pemphigus are made worse by the heat and sweat of summer.

The patient with congenital ichthyosis or a dry old skin is often worse during the winter because of the low humidity of artificially heated houses and exposure of the skin to the grateful pleasure of long hot baths. Recognition of this seasonal incidence may be useful in both diagnosis and treatment. Psoriasis and atopic dermatitis are ordinarily much improved during the summer months, though not invariably so. A common disease such as pityriasis rosea shows increased incidence in the spring and fall, for reasons which are a complete mystery. Erythema multiforme of the recurrent type may occur principally during the spring, through factors which are likewise quite unknown.

Personal, Environmental, and Occupational Factors

The skin is subjected to a wider variety of stimuli than any other organ of the body. Through a number of finely adjusted physiologic mechanisms, some of them still not well understood, the skin performs a vital service in preserving the life of the animal contained in it. It does this with a surprising capacity to maintain its own integrity and functions. Few organs of the body possess a comparable ability to repair structure and regroup forces while under the continuous and unremitting pressure of assault of many types.

There are few diseases of the skin in which environmental factors require no consideration. They manifest themselves in the calloused hands of the workman, the whealing of the skin in a patient with dermographism, the characteristic patch of pigmented thickened skin on the neck which marks the violin player, the characteristic keratosis and skin cancers which may mark the sailor long home from the sea, the bullous reactions to trauma occurring in patients with epidermolysis bullosa, fungal infections of the feet as a penalty for wearing shoes, and dermatitic reactions to innumerable sensitizing and irritant occupational contactants. This list of environmental excitants of cutaneous disease could be extended to include hundreds of examples. In view of the wide variety of physical, chemical, and microbiologic mechanisms of attack to which the skin is constantly subjected, it is apparent that such factors must receive consideration in almost every patient with a disease affecting the skin. Certain of these are most common and of prime importance, as follows:

PREVIOUS TOPICAL TREATMENT. This is often of crucial importance, both in the interpretation of the dermatosis under consideration and the selection of treatment. Until 1930 to 1935, the number of strongly sensitizing chemical compounds in use for the topical treatment of skin diseases was reasonably limited. Since that time, however, a very large number have become available and are frequently used. New therapeutic agents are undergoing constant trial, and the ultimate sensitizing capacity of these may not be exactly determined for several years.

Questioning of the patient as to local treatment which has been used must be routine. In many patients with dermatitis, it will be found that the objective changes are in large part due to the treatment which has been employed rather than to the primary disease. It will be found of value to list all the preparations, proprietary or otherwise, which have been used. It should be kept in mind that the patient may regard many common topical medicaments simply as cosmetics or "home remedies" incapable of causing difficulty.

The topical corticosteroids are prescribed very frequently and indiscriminately for inflammatory conditions. As a result of such treatment, ringworm (tinea) infections of the skin are masked so that their clinical appearance and patterns of presentation are altered and more difficult to recognize. Other conditions may also be aggravated, such as candidal (monilial) infections of skin, rosacea, and perioral dermatitis.

INTERNAL MEDICATION. There are few dermatologic syndromes which reactions to drugs may not simulate. In inflammatory and urticarial eruptions of the skin, in particular, it is essential that the patient be questioned regarding all internal medication. In this connection, it must be kept in mind that many individuals are so in the habit of taking tonics, vitamins, sedatives, cathartics, and so forth, that they hardly regard these as medicines. With some patients, the questioning in regard to these must be very detailed and may require repetition to elicit the essential information.

Corticosteroid therapy is now administered so frequently for such a wide variety of conditions that it is generally advisable to ask the patient specifically about this. It is also increasingly necessary to ask about other specific antibacterial agents, because information regarding reactions to these may be highly instructive. Vaginal monilial infections may be precipitated or aggravated by the use of antibiotics such as tetracycline or the anovulatory pill used for the treatment of acne vulgaris.

PHYSICAL THERAPY. Patients with chronic dermatoses may be subjected to various types of physical therapy. Of these, x-ray therapy is of great importance since its effects are cumulative and, in excess, potentially harmful. The number of treatments and sites of exposure should be recorded. In patients who have received considerable amounts of irradiation, it will frequently be advisable to complete the record by writing to the physician who administered it.

PEDIATRIC DERMATOLOGIC DIAGNOSIS

Diseases of the skin in newborn infants and young children often present patterns which diverge from those of the same diseases in adults. There are certain increased vulnerabilities to bacterial, viral, physicochemical, and allergic insults in the baby and child. A few cutaneous diseases are peculiar to children. Some of the anatomic and physiologic reasons for these differences are apparent, but others are entirely unknown or can only be conjectured. It seems worthwhile, therefore, to attempt to summarize, though perforce broadly, some of the main variations in diagnostic characteristics and clinical course of skin diseases in the infant and child.

The skin of the infant is characterized by certain features, as follows:

1. A greatly increased susceptibility to *superficial bacterial infections*, particularly by micrococci. This is seen in the extent and severity with which impetigo may occur in the newborn, and may be demonstrated experimentally in very young laboratory animals.

2. The skin and mucous membranes of the infant are sometimes peculiarly susceptible to *primary infection* with the virus of *herpes simplex*, with the production of an extensive local reaction and serious systemic symptoms. In general, no great susceptibility to other viral infections of the skin is apparent.

3. The cohesion at the dermo-epidermal junction in infants is apparently less firm than in adults, and certain diseases which rarely or never produce *bullous reactions* in the adult may do so in the child. The outstanding example of this is congenital syphilis, now fortunately rare, in which an overwhelming spirochetemia may induce bullous lesions of the skin, whereas this almost never occurs in the adult. Impetigo tends to be bullous in infants and children. It is possible that extreme bullous reactions noted occasionally in erythema multiforme and drug reactions in children may in part be related to this anatomic peculiarity.

4. Inflammatory contact dermatitis in infants is more likely to be due to a *primary irritant effect* than to sensitization. True eczematous sensitivity to external contactants is not present in the newborn infant. The infant also has not yet been stimulated to the formation of specific antibodies for the production of atopic reactions.

5. The most critical of all skin diseases affecting the newborn are those which are *nevoid* or *developmental*. These include moles and angiomas of all types, which may not become fully apparent for weeks or even years after birth. Ectodermal dysplasias of various types, neurocutaneous syndromes, and various other uncommon congenital abnormalities may offer immediate or potential difficulty.

6. *Eczema*, the largest group of skin diseases encountered in the infant and young child, offers many uncertainties in classification and prognosis. The patterns of lesions and of distribution may be entirely different from those seen in the older child or adult, as in atopic dermatitis. There are also many curious types of dermatitis which even the most experienced pediatrician or dermatologist must be content to call "rashes" and remain otherwise baffled.

The diseases in the following rather random grouping have been selected for mention because they are almost unique in children, because they offer a serious medical threat if they do occur in infancy or childhood, or because they occasionally begin in childhood and tend to persist through adult life, with the production of significant disability.

Bacterial Infections

The very great susceptibility of the skin of the newborn infant to micrococcal infections was frighteningly demonstrated in epidemics in nurseries prior to the availability of adequate antibacterial drugs. These widespread superficial infections, which were sometimes fatal, were variously called impetigo, "pemphigus" neonatorum, or Ritter's disease. Epidemics sometimes recurred even in nurseries from which the babies had all been removed and the interior and furniture scrubbed and painted. It seems probable that, in many such instances, a nurse or doctor who was disseminating a pathogenic strain of staphylococci or streptococci from the nose and throat or from the skin might have been too readily excluded as a source of infection. Such epidemics are ordinarily controllable by (a) immediate isolation and adequate treatment of the affected newborn, (b) the use of an antibacterial detergent in place of soap on the rest of the infants, and (c) relentless precautions to prevent contamination from the bodies of the professional and other attendants, insofar as possible. In older children, impetigo tends to be bullous and extensive but does not carry the grave systemic risk which it presents to infants. However, acute or chronic bacterial infections of the skin of children are almost certainly the bacterial source of glomerulonephritis at times. Attention is called to the not infrequent association of toxic epidermal necrolysis with phagetype 71 staphylococcal infection.

ECTHYMA (ulcerative impetigo) is common in children. It is particularly prone to occur on the lower legs as a result of repeated minor traumas which occur in this area. An alternate term for the disease in children is "traumatic infected ulcer." Once pathogenic micrococci have become established in large numbers on the skin of a child, any disturbance in the integrity of the skin, whether by injury, insect bites, or dermatitis, is prone to result in a superficial infected ulcer. Ordinarily such ulcers carry no implication of serious systemic disease. Furunculosis is probably not as common in children, unless they are immunologically compromised or have defective polymorphonucleocytes, as in adults but is occasionally encountered in very persistent and recurrent form. No truly satisfactory explanation for recurrent furunculosis is available, but its occurrence in localized areas would suggest that pathogenic bacteria have become established there and, for reasons which are poorly understood, repeatedly establish themselves in the pilosebaceous unit of the skin. Erysipelas has become something of a rarity in adults and children alike. The complication of noma, a frightening gangrenous and infected ulceration of the skin in children, seems almost extinct, probably because of early recognition and better available methods, such as systemic antibiotics, of treating early ulcerative pyogenic infections of the skin and subcutaneous tissues.

Eczema

The term "eczema" has persisted in the designation of chronic dermatitis affections in childhood much more than it has in those of adults, possibly because such eruptions often defy accurate classification in infants and young children, and it is necessary for the physician, in some confusion, to use a not too specific diagnostic term understandable to the laity. Almost any chronic dermatitis process in infants and very young children must be considered to be *atopic dermatitis* until proved otherwise. A majority of eczematous processes on the face in infants will eventually prove to be this disease. If the child comes from strongly atopic stock, the probability of this being the case is greatly increased, and it is worthwhile to examine the family history carefully in this regard.

Certain other eczematous syndromes in the infant or young child have fairly clearcut patterns and offer a good prognosis. One of these is *seborrheic dermatitis*, which in its simplest form is seen as ordinary cradle cap. This may be accompanied by rather marked localized erythema of the cheeks, sometimes with a yellowish seborrheic scaling and often some evidence of low-grade bacterial infection. In the chubby infant, intertrigo is a frequent accompaniment of seborrheic dermatitis, and every fold of the body may be affected. The prognosis in such infants is ordinarily good, and properly selected local treatment, along with a diet which will prevent overweight, may be effective.

Primary irritant dermatitis is common in infants and young children. A substance such as orange juice, or even an excess of saliva, may frequently irritate the infant's skin but not that of older children or adults. Even bland soaps may sometimes prove irritating, particularly in atopic children. Extremes of heat or cold or exposure to wind or wintry weather may produce quite surprising reactions of erythema and resultant dermatitis. Prolonged pressure on a toilet seat, or rubbing of the skin from crawling on a carpet may induce reactions which are representative of the early irritability of the skin of the infant and child, without the intervention of any specific sensitization mechanisms.

Two complications of eczema are probably more apparent in the infantile phase of life than at any other time; that is, uncontrolled excoriation and subacute or acute bacterial infection. If the infant experiences sensations of itching, he promptly responds, asleep or awake, with scratching by any means available—prolonged rubbing with hand or foot or rubbing of the affected area against the sheet or the side of the crib. Autoerotic mechanisms are often concerned in this response.

While some areas of eczema in infants and children never show any evidence of bacterial infection, others do, particularly in infants who are seborrheic or fat. It also seems probable that blockage of sweat ducts, with resultant sweat retention, itching, and miliaria, plays a significant role in infantile eczema which is frequently not appreciated. In infants who are solicitously kept in a too warm, semitropical environment, this mechanism may be predominant because of the continued stimulation of the eccrine sweat glands.

Diaper rashes are, of course, a characteristic disease of infantile life. A popular theory of their causation is that the surface pH of the skin has been raised by ammoniac decomposition of urine, with resultant inflammation, though there is no convincing experimental proof of this mechanism. Simple maceration undoubtedly plays a role; the stratum corneum becomes waterlogged, and various bacteria and yeasts can more easily gain a foothold in such fertile terrain. Another sequence of events follows with absolute certainty, namely, varying degrees of sweat retention. It has been shown experimentally that many types of superficial injury to the skin, including the application of a wet compress for 24 to 48 hours, will produce blockage of many sweat ducts. The diapered incontinent infant, no matter how careful and solicitous his nursing care, spends a good many hours each day with a urinary or fecal compress in the diaper region. There is, moreover, usually a fairly continuous stimulus to sweating, through the subtropical environment in which many infants are kept. It is clinically certain that many diaper eruptions have their onset with lesions which are entirely characteristic of miliaria, sometimes of pustular type.

Circumscribed neurodermatitis is commonly seen in adults but is almost never observed in children. The reason for this is not clearly understood, but possibly other forms of traumatic habit tics related to the skin are more characteristic of childhood. The nails frequently are a source of attention, in the form of nail biting. Less frequently, but still not uncommonly, the young child pulls or breaks the hair, producing varying degrees of alopecia (trichotillomania). Sucking and biting of a thumb or finger is, of course, a common childhood pastime which frequently produces characteristic calloused and hyperkeratotic areas, especially as the child becomes dentulous.

Various conditions which on initial inspection seem to be forms of dermatitis may offer grave systemic risks to the infant. Congenital ichthyosiform dermatitis is an example; Leiner's disease, in which one of the signs is an apparent severe and extensive seborrheic dermatitis, is another.

Although the clinical evidences of various types of eczema may be severe in children, there is rarely any permanent evidence of the previous involvement when the condition finally clears. Mothers are frequently justifiably concerned about the possibility of scarring, but this almost never occurs. Various degrees of hyperpigmentation, thickening, and occasional partial depigmentation may persist for a time, but these ordinarily disappear completely. The skin of the infant has a remarkable capacity for self-restoration.

A considerable number of *systemic infections* of childhood may produce overt manifestations in the skin. Possibly the largest representative of this group is *toxic erythema*, in which a variety of inflammatory lesions of the skin may occur, usually with fever, but ordinarily with no specific ascertainable cause. Reactions to *drugs* and various types of infections may be responsible. Another very large group is, of course, the *exanthemata*, chiefly viral in origin. True *scarlet fever* or severe scarlatiniform eruptions are not commonly seen in childhood at the present time, probably because of better means of controlling streptococcal infections at their onset. Various spirochetal infections are seen in childhood. Congenital syphilis is becoming almost a rarity in populations where adequate maternal care is available, and represents an inexcusable medical error because the means for prevention are so adequate. Yaws has almost been treated out of existence in certain areas, particularly Central America, and presumably bejel is still being encountered in the eastern Mediterranean basin. Tuberculosis of the skin, which was previously seen most commonly in the form of scrofulo-derma, lupus vulgaris, primary inoculation tuberculosis, and various types of tuberculids, is becoming rare indeed. There is no more striking example of the contribution of veterinary medicine than the decrease in tuberculous adenitis and resultant scrofuloderma; this has been brought about by the elimination of milk from tuberculous cows. Leprosy is, unfortunately, still very common among children in many areas of the world.

Fungal Infections

Fungal infections are, in general, not common in infants and young children. The ordinary adult types of tinea pedis and tinea cruris are strikingly uncommon in children of all ages. Typical ringed lesions of the glabrous skin due to ring-worm infection are seen, but ordinarily lesions of this type are more likely to be due to some other cause. *Tinea capitis* is common, though in urban centers of the United States it appears to have dropped somewhat in incidence since a peak reached in the five years following World War II. The incidence of endothrix infections, very common in Mexico and affecting children and adults alike, is not known precisely, but it appears to be increasing.

Oral thrush is the classic example of candidiasis of the buccal mucous membranes in infants. We have been impressed with the rapid disappearance of thrush as a common clinical entity in pediatric dermatology during the past decade. Cases are found among patients who are being treated with prolonged courses of antibiotics, who are on the anovulatory "pill," or who are immunosuppressed by their disease or treatment or a combination of both.

A common mucocutaneous disturbance in children, perlèche, has been attributed to Candida, but probably falsely. This disease is characterized by inflammation and fissuring at the angles of the mouth. It is ordinarily worse during winter months, and the zone of inflammation may sometimes extend out over the cheeks or involve the entire perioral region. It is extremely doubtful that the Candida recoverable from such lesions are of more than incidental importance. Vitamin deficiencies have been implicated, particularly deficiencies of the B complex, but we have never encountered a child in whom this could be proved. Dental malocclusion and unusual folds at the angles of the mouth are common findings in older patients. The condition may be due in part also to a habit tic of constantly licking the affected area, and residual deposits of food, fruit juices, and tooth paste may be contributory.

Deep Fungal Infections are not common among children, at least insofar as evidence of involvement of the skin is concerned. It is probable that a high proportion of children living in areas in which coccidioidomycosis is endemic become infected, but the initial infection may be asymptomatic or evidenced by a mild febrile illness, sometimes with *erythema nodosum*, from which the child recovers rapidly and has no further sequelae. In such a child, a strongly positive coccidioidin test will result. Histoplasmosis is common in children in some areas of the midwestern and southern United States, on the basis of surveys by means of the histoplasmin test and chest x-rays.

Certain of the more or less common papulosquamous eruptions of adults are seen with varying frequency in children. *Psoriasis* is probably uncommon in children below the age of three or four, but its onset is not uncommon in children older than this. Occasionally a child may present persistent patches of what appears to be seborrheic dermatitis, which may then develop into frank psoriasis in adult life. Bizarre low-grade inflammatory lesions, particularly about the hands or feet in children, may also eventuate in psoriasis at times. *Pityriasis rosea* is by no means uncommon in children; it is usually diagnosed as a ringworm infection.

Reactions to Actinic Trauma

Diseases which are representative of reactions to acute or chronic *actinic trauma* are common in childhood and deserve the most careful evaluation. The only type of skin which is physiologically fitted for unlimited exposure to sunlight is that of the dark full-blooded Negro. All other types of skin present varying degrees of tolerance, which reaches its lowest limits in blond or rufous (red-headed) persons. Children with obvious signs of intolerance to sunlight, such as very ready susceptibility to sunburn, excessive freckling, or areas (such as the bridge of the nose) which remain pink and scaling on continued exposure to sunlight, must be taught to adapt themselves to this circumstance early in life. These are the individuals from whom the vast majority of actinic (senile) keratoses and squamous cell skin cancers will be harvested later in life. Intolerance to sunlight may be particularly evident on the lips, sometimes in children who, because of individual lip conformation or malocclusion, present more of the mucous surface of the lower lip to the action of sunlight. This may be a forerunner of leukoplakia and squamous cell cancer, possibly fully as important as smoking. Such children can, without too much frustration or limitation of activity, learn the habit of avoiding undue prolonged exposure to sunlight or take the simple means of partial protection when play or sport makes such exposure necessary.

Certain other reactions to sunlight are more acute but less common. *Hydroa aestivale* is an example of this, vesicles and bullae appearing at the sites of greatest exposure to sunlight, such as on the bridge of the nose and on the malar prominences after exposure during the summer months. Although this entity is unquestionable, it is rare in our experience. Such children are ordinarily perfectly well, and elaborate studies of the liver function or of porphyrin metabolism are unavailing. The lesions fortunately do not often produce severe scarring, and the disorder tends to clear up at puberty. A somewhat similar disease in respect to incidence on exposure to sunlight is pellagra, a B vitamin deficiency disease, in which characteristic, sharply marginated, inflammatory plaques occur as an evidence of photosensitivity. This disease, formerly common in the southern United States and occasionally seen in chronic alcoholics on deficient diets, has all but disappeared. *Herpes simplex* is commonly precipitated by exposure to sunlight, most frequently on the lips, though other exposed sites may be involved.

A rare condition characterized by intolerance to sunlight and seen in young children is *xeroderma pigmentosum*. In this malignant inherited disease, the aging of the skin, which ordinarily requires prolonged exposure to sunlight for many years, is compressed into a very short period. Indeed, it would sometimes appear that even a short succession of moderate exposures may be sufficient to stimulate the skin through an irreversible cycle of aging, keratosis, and skin cancer. Reported cases have rarely survived longer than early adult life, but if the disease is recognized in its earliest phases, complete avoidance of exposure to direct sunlight might be lifesaving.

Discoid mucocutaneous lupus erythematosus is rare in children. *Systemic lupus erythematosus* is also very uncommon, other collagen diseases appearing more likely to affect children; for example, dermatomyositis and diffuse scleroderma. *Polymorphous light eruptions* of the type seen with some frequency in adults are not common in children, though they should be considered in eruptions which are in areas exposed to sunlight.

Viral Infections

The manifestations of *viral infections* of the skin in infants and children are numerous and varied. The systemic viral infections, varicella, variola, rubeola, and rubella, need only be mentioned. In children, infection with the virus of varicella will occasionally produce *herpes zoster,* but this ordinarily follows a surprisingly mild and almost painless course. *Herpes simplex* is, of course, very common in children. Activation of the infection is produced by a wide variety of agents, including fever, exposure to sunlight, and, possibly, foods or drugs. In girls, the onset of menstruation may induce recurrent herpes simplex. In infants, the primary infection with herpes simplex may be productive of severe systemic reaction and extensive mucocutaneous lesions. Herpes simplex may be associated with recurrent erythema multiforme.

Infants and adults with various types of chronic dermatitis, particularly atopic dermatitis, may experience a widespread *varicelliform eruption* as a result of infection with the virus of either herpes simplex or vaccinia. Great care should be exercised not to vaccinate a child who has a chronic dermatitis of any significance. Under ordinary circumstances, the risk of this child's developing eczema vaccinatum (Kaposi's varicelliform eruption) is considerably greater than the risk of smallpox when the disease is not endemic. Also, an adult with an active cold sore may be a source of danger to a child with eczema.

Warts of all types are common childhood complaints. Their only distinctive feature in the child is the greater readiness with which they may respond to suggestion therapy. It is possible that *flat warts* (verruca plana juvenilis) are somewhat more common in children, though this type is by no means infrequent in adults.

Another disease which is presumably of viral origin is *cat-scratch disease.* Inoculation occurs through a superficial abrasion of the skin, frequently a cat scratch, with, occasionally, a significant local reaction and often a persistent regional adenitis. The presence of a positive skin reaction to cat-scratch antigen is highly suggestive of the diagnosis, if the presenting clinical characteristics are appropriate.

A viral infection which is common in children is *molluscum contagiosum.* Among young adults, this disease, as well as that of herpes progenitalis and infestations with scabies and pediculosis pubis, is being seen more frequently because of their current living habits and change in sexual attitudes. The early lesion of molluscum contagiosum is highly characteristic, consisting of a small white to yellow nodule on the surface of the skin, ordinarily measuring 2 to 5 mm. in diameter. Occasionally, such lesions may be very large, "giant" mollusca. The lesions sometimes become inflamed and may at first glance appear to be small furuncles, though the differential diagnosis is easy to make. Solitary lesions in older people have been misdiagnosed as basal cell epitheliomas. Treatment is simple; all that needs to be done is to extrude the lesion. This virus infection is highly auto-inoculable, but we have never observed instances of its apparent spread to other children in a family, though this undoubtedly must occur at times.

Vascular Reactions

Evanescent urticaria of the type commonly seen in adults is not common in children in our experience, though this is at variance with statements to be found in many textbooks. It is perfectly true that urticarial lesions are frequently a component of eruptions seen in the child, but there is ordinarily an admixture of erythema or bulla formation, or purpura. Perhaps this is a reflection of the generally more fragile and immature structure of the blood vessels and cutis of the skins of very young children, and a lessened capacity to contain mild vascular reactions in the form of a simple localized tissue edema. Angioedema (giant urticaria) is occasionally observed in children, more commonly in the older age group, but it is not as commonly encountered as it is in adults. Acute reactions to drugs or foods are common causes of urticarial eruptions.

Purpura of almost all types is fairly common in children, with the allergic nonthrombocytopenic variety most frequent. Another vascular reaction pattern which is commonly related to sensitivity to microbiologic agents, *erythema nodosum,* is occasionally encountered in children and justifies most searching study to determine the cause. The chronic progressive systemic vascular reaction pattern known as *periarteritis nodosa* occurs rarely in children.

Functional vascular patterns, such as congenital erythema of the palms, or reactions to cold, such as *pernio* and *Raynaud's disease,* are by no means unknown in children. Repeated pernio may set a pattern of vascular response to alternate heat and cold which may make residence in temperate zone areas increasingly uncomfortable and disabling. This is rather strikingly seen in the female population of the British Isles, where variations in temperature, both within and without dwelling places, produce a very high incidence of changing vascular patterns listed under the pernio (erythrocyanosis) group. In such persons, the incidence of *nodular vasculitis* of the lower legs or its ulcerative analogue *erythema induratum* (nontuberculous type) may be much increased in later life.

Acrodynia is a curious and uncommon

pediatric disease in which erythema of the palms and soles is a sign. The erythema is so marked in some patients as to have led to the designation of "pink disease." There is associated extreme irritability, and the child appears sick, listless, and thoroughly miserable. Absorption of mercury, often from topical medication, is the etiologic factor.

Urticaria pigmentosa is characteristically a childhood disease, though a rather uncommon one. It consists of more or less pigmented macules and nodules which, upon irritation by stroking, are capable of producing marked urtication through the release of histamine and heparin from the numerous mast cells. The passage of fluid through the capillaries may be abrupt and voluminous enough to lead to bulla formation. The disease is relatively harmless, however, and the outlook for disappearance of the lesions in adult life is good.

Papular urticaria, a common disease among children in temperate parts of the world, has little relation to true urticaria. It is becoming increasingly clear that the disease is induced by the bites of fleas, bedbugs, and other insects, following which a persistent scratch dermatitis results. The synonym *lichen urticatus* is perhaps a better designation for the disease.

Diseases of Keratinization

A very large number of cutaneous diseases in children are associated with inherited or induced abnormalities of keratinization. Mention has been made above of ichthyosis, ichthyosiform erythroderma, and congenital ectodermal defects. To these may be added abnormalities of hair and nail growth, again either inherited or induced by trauma, inflammation, or infection.

Palmar and plantar keratosis is a not uncommon inherited abnormality. It is frequently associated with ichthyosis (for example, lamellar ichthyosis). In very marked forms of the disease, the palmar surfaces may show extreme hyperkeratinization, with complete obliteration of the normal skin markings. Such plaques may become fissured, the splits extending well down into the underlying viable tissues. Although such patients do not ordinarily sweat profusely, increase in emo-

tional sweating may cause a severe malodor. A geographically unique form of the disease is mal de Melada, so called because it is found on an island in the Adriatic Sea and is apparently related to the consanguinity of the parents of many of the children on the island.

Another characteristic disturbance of keratinization is seen in the various forms of *keratosis pilaris*. This is a regular accompaniment of ichthyosis during cold weather and is then rather diffuse over the extensor surfaces of the extremities, the back and buttocks, and sometimes the face. It also occurs in a form which is more circumscribed, which would appear to be a true nevoid abnormality, and which is little influenced by varying seasonal environments. This form is sometimes associated with abnormalities of hair growth, for example, *monilethrix*. The condition has no significance other than the cosmetic appearance but is sometimes very annoying in this regard.

Alopecia areata is a fairly common disturbance of hair growth in childhood. It may be confined to a few small patches or may be total. There is no disturbance of general health. Alopecia areata appearing before puberty has a much more serious prognosis than that appearing in adult life, in terms both of probable early regrowth of hair and of recurrence of the disease in the future.

Keratosis follicularis (Darier's disease) is a rare type of keratotic affection seen in children. This disorder is more frequently noted in the scalp and on the neck, presternal, and interscapular areas, but the distribution may be extensive at times. The pathologic picture is entirely characteristic. Clear evidence of a hereditary influence is sometimes apparent. In some patients with the disease, evidence of vitamin A deficiency either through inadequate intake or disturbance of liver function has been reported. This has, however, proved to be a most disappointing theory of the origin of the disease, and the administration of vitamin A either by mouth or by injection has usually proved ineffective in this author's experience. The disease is much worse during the warm summer months.

Another group of diseases in part at least dependent upon abnormalities of keratinization is composed of those which are more or less related to the pilosebaceous unit. *Milia*, which are simply superficial keratinized cysts, are quite common in infants, though they are ordinarily sloughed off within a few months. Comedones and even small acneiform lesions may also be seen in infants. In some children, typical comedones heralding the onset of acne may appear long before puberty, and they have been observed not infrequently in children of eight or nine. A measure of the general ineffectiveness of the treatment of acne is seen in the fact that in many such patients, there are no satisfactory means of warding off the eventual development of full-fledged acne. The application of retinoic acid, 0.1 per cent "Retin-A," may be helpful in reducing the number of comedones.

Disturbances of keratinization resulting in *sweat duct obstruction* are exceedingly frequent in childhood. Mention has been made of the participation of this phenomenon in the syndrome of diaper dermatitis. Any chronic eczematous process, of which atopic dermatitis and seborrheic dermatitis are the best examples, will induce obstruction of a large number of sweat ducts. In a cool environment and in the absence of "emotional" sweating, this duct obstruction offers no difficulty.

Bullous Dermatoses

Diseases characterized by the formation of *bullae* are fairly common in childhood. Mention has previously been made of the "rupturability" of the skin of infants and young children, particularly in regard to the cohesion between the epidermis and dermis. Stimuli which in adults may lead only to local tissue edema may, in children, result in the collection of free fluid; that is, a vesicle or bulla.

Erythema multiforme is particularly prone to be of bullous character in a child. "Simple" erythema multiforme of the recurrent, often seasonal, type, in which the lesions are urticarial, ringed, and sometimes purpuric, is uncommon in young childhood. Severe bullous erythema multiforme of the *Stevens-Johnson* type is by no means rare and is often alarming in the rapidity of its onset and the severity of the local manifestations. It is nearly always febrile. The chief sites of bullous involvement are around various body orifices and the eyes, though lesions of mixed bullous, urticarial, and purpuric character may be noted extensively elsewhere. Drug sensitivity may occasionally be an etiologic factor, but in most cases the cause remains unknown.

Another characteristically bullous and often highly mutilating dermatosis of children is *epidermolysis bullosa*. In this condition, because of a curious inherited reaction pattern of the skin to trauma, bullae and severe dystrophic changes may occur at the sites of greatest trauma to the skin, namely, on pressure points of the feet, the fingers and knuckles, elbows, knees, buttocks, and sometimes elsewhere.

Disorders of Pigmentation

While the formation of melanin proceeds normally in utero, the melanocytes commonly do not reach full activity until after birth. This is sometimes strikingly seen in newborn Negro infants, in whom the skin may be rather light, later becoming much darker. Macular pigmented moles are frequently invisible or hardly evident at birth and then become more and more prominent. It is not possible by examination of a newborn infant to assess the final extent or number of any of the nevoid growths affecting the skin. New pigmented moles may appear with the passage of time, and some of them do not become evident until puberty or even until a physiologic change such as pregnancy.

Moles and melanoma present an important pediatric problem which is dealt with in Chapter 28. There is one strong reassuring fact concerning moles in childhood, however; namely, that malignant melanoma is exceedingly rare among children, and no great concern as to this possibility need be felt until puberty is reached. Certain types of moles may, on excision, be diagnosed histologically as "juvenile melanoma," but this is a benign tumor.

Large congenital nevi and giant hairy nevus (bathing-trunk nevus) of children are considered premalignant lesions and prophylactic excision is recommended.

Mongolian blue spots, which represent

melanin deposited in the corium rather than in the epidermis, are found on the lower back and elsewhere in all Mongolian infants. They are common in Negro infants and sometimes occur in whites. They ordinarily disappear before late childhood is reached and are harmless. An analogous process pathologically is the *blue nevus*, which is also essentially harmless, but which may at times be very suggestive of melanoma.

A striking though uncommon disorder of pigmentation is seen in *acanthosis nigricans*. In this condition, which is localized principally to the axillae and anogenital region, dark pigmentation occurs along with varying degrees of a rather velvety thickening of the skin surface. When the disease occurs in childhood (juvenile type) it is of no apparent general medical significance; in adult life, on the other hand, the pigmentary and acanthotic changes may be evidence of internal malignant disease.

Various grades of *depigmentation* are common in childhood. This may be seen in the form of a *macular depigmented nevus*. Or the apparent lighter color may be due to *nevus anemicus;* in this condition the contrast between the nevus and the surrounding normal skin may be heightened by the application of ice. True *vitiligo* is not rare. In many children, particularly Negroes, various inflammatory eruptions of the skin may be followed by partial depigmentation, which is impermanent. This may occur in seborrheic dermatitis, particularly about the hair line. Scaling patches on the face, somewhat misnamed *achromia parasitica*, may be accompanied by hypopigmentation. Sometimes, on the other hand, the amount of melanin deposition is increased.

Freckling is a common phenomenon in childhood and waxes and wanes to some extent depending upon the recentness of exposure to sunlight. It is to be distinguished from *lentigines,* which are pigment depositions which do not wax and wane. Freckling is exceedingly marked in the rare condition of xeroderma pigmentosum. A similar type of pigmentation, though not in areas exposed to sunlight, was formerly noted in patients who received oral or systemic arsenicals for a long time.

Yellowish discoloration of the skin is common in infants, especially wellnourished ones. The layer of sebum over the skin may be quite yellow, or various areas of skin may be definitely orangeyellow in color. The condition is due to xantholipids and, as indicated by the diagnostic term *carotinemia*, is related to the vitamin A precursor, carotin. The pigment is harmless and is evidence of adequate, perhaps more than adequate, intake of orange juice, carrots, and the like.

Yellowish tumors and plaques are sometimes noted, and these should be considered in the light of a possible xanthoma, familial hyperlipemia, and cardiovascular disease. A description of the various types of xanthoma is found in Chapter 27.

Juvenile xanthogranuloma (nevoxanthoendothelioma) is another yellowish tumor of the skin, though an uncommon one. The lesions appear shortly after birth or no later than early childhood, in the form of one or more yellowish to brownish slightly raised nodules, usually on the face. Recognition of it is important, because the pathologic picture may be mistaken for sarcoma, but the disease is eventually selflimited and undergoes spontaneous involution. The old term is a complete misnomer; the condition is not a nevus, not a xanthoma, and not an endothelioma.

Tumors

While malignant tumors of the skin are uncommon in childhood, the possibility of them can by no means be completely discounted. It is important that the evaluation of any tumorous growth of the skin in a child be made on the clinical and *pathologic* findings, without regard to age. The principal tumors are, of course, nevoid growths, either vascular or pigmentary, and these rarely give rise to concern as to the possibility of invasive and metastatic malignancy in childhood. Certain other benign tumors are commonly encountered. Keloids are a common finding after injury and may be of importance by reason of marked cosmetic disfigurement, itching, or tenderness of the lesion. They are well known to occur more frequently in Negroes. Hypertrophic scars which will eventually disappear may easily be confused with keloids, which do not disappear and which tend to become larger. In any event, the tendency of the skin of any child to undergo hypertrophic scarring or keloid formation should be duly noted, particularly in respect to the undertaking of any elective surgical procedure in the future.

Another common tumor, occurring almost entirely in Negroes, is *dermatosis papulosa nigra*. These lesions are pathologically indistinguishable from seborrheic keratoses but often begin to appear on the face in Negroes during childhood.

Squamous cell carcinoma in childhood is rare. It has been observed in scars of burns and of lupus vulgaris and following excessive irradiation. Mention has been made of its multiple occurrence in xeroderma pigmentosum. *Basal cell epithelioma* is uncommon in children but by no means unknown. The nodules of neurofibromatosis may become evident during childhood, but their full development does not ordinarily occur until adult life. The nevoid tumor of the face, *adenoma sebaceum*, though rare, is of the greatest importance in the evaluation of some neurologic syndromes. The diagnosis may easily be made clinically by finding the "ash-leaf" hypomelanotic macule or performing a biopsy of nevoid skin papules or plaques.

Parasitic Infestations

The effects of bites of various arthropods on the skin of children are numerous and varied. The bites of mosquitoes, flies of various types, chiggers, fleas, and bedbugs may be the source of very fretful episodes in infants and young children. The effects are sometimes greater than in adults because excoriation by a child is likely to be completely uncontrolled, and the skin is more vulnerable to secondary bacterial infection. Mention has been made of a specific syndrome, *lichen urticatus*, which appears in most instances to be due initially to the bites of fleas. The local reaction following insect bites in children varies enormously from a very evanescent wheal to a large and even purpuric or bullous lesion. The duration of the itching varies greatly as well, as it does in adults. With some types of bites, for example, chiggers, the itching may persist for months.

Because of frequent close skin-to-skin contacts with infested adults, scabies is a disease frequently encountered in children if the infestation is endemic in the community. However, scabies has now reached epidemic proportions in certain countries such as Mexico and is not infrequent among young adults in the United States. In infants, there is a striking variation of the distribution of the lesions from that encountered in adults in that the infant's face is often the site of scabetic burrows and secondary lesions, while this is almost never the case in adults. Bullous impetigo is more commonly encountered as a complication of scabies in infants and young children.

Pediculosis of all types is seen less frequently than it was in 1940 but is being more frequently seen among young adults. A striking feature of pediculosis in children is that pediculosis capitis rarely affects Negroes, in part because of the shortness of hair of many of them, but also possibly because of some specific racial factor. Pediculosis pubis does not occur prior to the pubertal growth of hair in the anogenital region. Pediculosis of the eyelashes is more common in children than in adults and may be acquired by nursing infants.

Creeping eruption is a common and often very resistant infestation encountered particularly in the mid-coastal and southern United States. It results from the burrowing of the larva of cat or dog hookworm and is acquired by lying on wet sandy soil which has been contaminated by feline or canine feces. The disease may affect adults, but the exposure in children is likely to be much greater. The larva burrows in the upper portions of the skin and forms concentric and irregular inflammatory outlines which are very striking.

GERIATRIC DERMATOLOGIC DIAGNOSIS

The aging skin presents certain problems in diagnosis which are encountered more frequently than in the child or young adult. As with all other organs of the body, aging of the skin proceeds at a varying rate. It is possible that the skin shows greater local or general variations in this regard than does any other organ system of the body. In spite of this variability, it is possible to outline broadly the dermatoses which will be encountered most frequently in senile skin and to indicate some of the anatomic and physiologic reasons for the incidence of certain diseases, though there are many etiologic factors which are still poorly understood.

The principal anatomic and physiologic characteristics of aging of the skin are as follows:

1. The *stratum corneum* of senile skin reflects abnormalities of keratinization which are of much clinical significance. In general, the horny layer of the older person is thinner, though some areas show hyperplasia in the form of marked keratotic thickening. Visible scaling of the skin is usually more marked in an elderly person than in a young individual. This would seem to be due in part to decreased sebaceous secretion and, possibly, to qualitative or quantitative changes in the lipids within the stratum corneum. The water content of the stratum corneum is probably lower in the older person; this may well be related to changes in the surface lipids and to a resultant decrease in its water holding capacity. All of this results in greater susceptibility to dryness, chapping, and fissuring.

2. Aging skin is characterized by *thinning of the epidermis*, with flattening of the epidermal extensions between the papillae of the corium. In some areas, however, evidences of epidermal hyperplasia may be marked.

3. All of the *skin appendages* show evidences of decreased function in old age. The hair follicles are fewer and less prominent, and the number of "club" or resting hairs may be increased. The hairs of the eyebrows, nasal orifices, and ears frequently become coarser and attain greater length in older men. The sebaceous glands become smaller and less active, though sebaceous adenomas and comedones are frequently encountered in certain areas in older individuals. The apocrine gland undergoes atrophy at the menopause. The eccrine gland also participates in this gradual reduction of function, though again at a variable rate.

4. The *nails* age rather strikingly in many people. The manufacture of hard keratin becomes more slovenly, with resultant brittleness, ridging, flaking, and distortion. This often occurs in the absence of any local changes or obvious systemic disease.

5. The *corium* decreases in thickness, with loss of elastic and collagen fibers. The elastic fibers also become increasingly amorphous, and the collagen fibers are thin. The condition termed "senile elastosis," at one time presumed to be due to an increase in the elastic fibers, has now been shown to be a misnomer; a change in the collagen fibers is responsible. There are undoubtedly other changes in the corium which are less well delineated. All of these result in a corium which is structurally less firm. Loss of elasticity may be demonstrated very easily in an aged person: the stretched skin does not regain its former conformation rapidly. The skin appears grossly thinner and underlying blood vessels may become rather prominently visualized. Yellowing occurs for various reasons. The wrinkling so characteristic of aging is related to the thinness of the skin, its loss of elasticity, and the lessened firmness of support from the cutis and subcutaneous tissues. In many ways, the anatomic behavior of senile skin as compared to young skin is much like the contrast between an old, well-worn quilt and a sheet of newly manufactured sponge rubber padding.

6. The decrease in *subcutaneous fat* varies greatly with age, but it is commonly encountered. As a result of the decreased subcutaneous padding, the already thin and more vulnerable senile skin has inadequate cushioning to assist it in withstanding external physical trauma. In areas subjected to repeated trauma, this may result in disturbances of cutaneous integrity and slowness of healing.

7. It has been shown experimentally that the *percutaneous absorption* of materials coming in contact with the skin is significantly reduced in old age. This may be due in part to the atrophic changes of the pilosebaceous unit through which such substances are chiefly absorbed. It is a clinical fact that severe sensitization reactions to contactants are less commonly encountered in the older patient. In addition to lowered absorption, there may be a decreased immunologic response.

8. Disorders of *pigmentation* are characteristic of senile skin. The capacity of the melanocytes to lay down melanin granules in an orderly even fashion, particularly in response to various stimuli, seems disturbed. Freckles and "liver spots" are prominent. In many areas, considerable depigmentation may be noted, sometimes due to gross visible atrophy of the skin. In response to processes in which there is hyperplasia of the epidermis (that is, seborrheic keratoses, senile keratoses, and basal cell epitheliomas), excessive amounts of pigment may be formed. Lentigines may become melanomatous in old age, sometimes without the rapid course and metastasizing capacity of true malignant melanoma. In addition to disturbances of melanin deposition, pigmentation due to accumulations of hemosiderin following repeated deposition of red cells in the cutis may become marked, especially on the lower legs. Changes in color due to disturbed vascular states may be striking; in general, the vascular reactions of the aged skin tend to be slowed down and less responsive to external stimuli.

The following selection of diseases is necessarily somewhat arbitrary, but it includes most of the diseases of the skin which will be encountered most frequently among older patients.

Tumors

All types of tumors, benign and malignant, with the exception only of those of nevoid origin, occur with far greater frequency in the aging skin. These are discussed at some length in Chapter 28. It must be re-emphasized, however, that because a particular tumor is most common in the older skin *it will not necessarily be rare* in younger persons. In the congenital dysfunction of the skin known as xeroderma pigmentosum, the skin of a child of three may, in terms of keratoses, disturbance of pigmentation, and tumor formation, be entirely comparable to the skin of a person of 90. It must also be kept in mind that actinic irradiation from sunlight accelerates the aging process enormously and that the gross morphologic differences between the exposed and unexposed skin of a patient of 50 may be striking indeed. The term "senile" keratoses is

more frequently than not a misnomer, though they inevitably occur if a person lives long enough. They are more properly termed "actinic" keratoses. Middle-aged patients with such lesions on the skin often object to the designation "senile," and are appreciative of a more accurate qualifying adjective for their keratotic skin lesions.

The most common skin tumors of older patients are undoubtedly seborrheic keratoses, which may sometimes be seen in profusion in persons of 30 but which are almost always demonstrable in patients of over 70. Basal and prickle cell epitheliomas are the next most common group, the former being seen in areas with the greatest number of sebaceous glands. Though malignant melanoma begins somewhat less frequently in the aged, it is by no means a respecter of any age group, except for its rarity prior to puberty. Many of the tumors of the skin of older patients can be differentiated as benign or malignant on the basis of inspection, but some of them cannot; the use of biopsy examination in any tumor suggestive of a malignant lesion is essential.

Vascular dilatations and tumors are exceedingly common in the aging skin but are rarely of more than cosmetic significance. Telangiectatic vessels, especially in the flush areas and on the lower legs, are found in almost every patient over 60. "Cherry" angiomas of varying size are common on the trunk, especially in men. "Spider" angiomas may be present in association with hepatic disease, but such lesions are so common in healthy individuals as to make the lesion, of and by itself, of uncertain significance in this regard. Small cavernous hemangiomas of the "strawberry" type seen in infants are virtually unknown in adults. Extensive port-wine stains ordinarily persist unchanged throughout life. Extensive cavernous hemangiomas may persist into old age unless adequate treatment has been undertaken fairly early in life or spontaneous cicatrization has taken place.

Dermatitis

Some of the more common forms of dermatitis encountered in infancy and young adult life are uncommon or greatly altered in pattern in the aged. Mention has been made previously of the decreased frequency of severe contact dermatitis in the aged, though it is by no means rare. This author has the distinct clinical impression that when it occurs, it is more likely to pursue a more protracted course in elderly patients than in young adults.

One of the most surprising of all dermatologic phenomena in the older patient is the development of evidence that the skin has become sensitized to a contactant to which there has been intermittent exposure throughout life without any previous reaction. This is not uncommonly seen in sensitivity to poison ivy, which may first become manifest in the seventh or eighth decade of life. Such reactions are occasionally rather marked, because the patient, with a feeling of complete security, has exposed himself to massive quantities of the antigen. Contact dermatitis is often a source of much difficulty in the interpretation of industrial dermatologic diseases in older workers, because it may be due to an occupational contactant to which the patient has been exposed for from one to several decades without previous difficulty.

Ordinary seborrheic dermatitis sometimes becomes less marked in aged people who have had the condition intermittently for a lifetime. On the other hand, in an occasional patient, an intractable generalized exfoliative dermatitis may have its origin from a lifelong mild to moderate seborrheic dermatitis.

Dermatitis related to peripheral vascular disturbances is common in aged persons; *stasis dermatitis* is the leading example. *Nummular dermatitis* is more common in persons of middle adult life to old age and is sometimes exceedingly difficult to control, though the outlook is for eventual involution if the therapeutic management is adequate and competent. This dermatitis occasionally occurs in a person with an atopic history; it may follow a primary irritant or sensitization reaction to some contactant, for example, nickel; or it may arise as a complication of stasis dermatitis.

Atopic dermatitis in the classic distribution seen in young adults is practically unknown in old age. It may, nevertheless, remain as an extremely persistent dermatitis of varying pattern, sometimes localized to the hands, but occasionally generalized.

Localized neurodermatitis is common in the aging patient. Probably the single most common form of localized neurodermatitis in adult and older patients is itching of the perianal and vulvar regions. The psychic roots of such itching may be deep indeed, and relief of the condition in the aged patient by either medicinal means or psychotherapy is often impossible. More extensive forms of neurodermatitis are encountered, including a widespread unusual eruption known as *chronic discoid and lichenoid dermatosis* or an extensive very thick papular lichenification, sometimes of extensive areas on the arms and legs.

The senile skin is extraordinarily subject to "itchiness," with or without any evidence of inflammatory reaction. The dry, slightly chapped skin may become very pruritic following tactile and other stimuli which would ordinarily go unnoticed. A draft of air on undressing, a wisp of scratchy material on the skin, or a mildly stressful situation may induce a paroxysm of itching. This sometimes has a peculiar burning quality which is highly uncomfortable.

By far the most serious and medically important dermatitis encountered in the aged person is that in which dry erythematous moderately scaling plaques, or even generalized exfoliative dermatitis, develop for no apparent reason. Such a process may be the prodrome of mycosis fungoides or some other member of the lymphoma group, but it may be impossible to establish such a diagnosis with accuracy except by following the evolution of the disease for prolonged periods, sometimes for many years. In some older patients, extensive or generalized exfoliative dermatitis may have had its genesis in seborrheic dermatitis or psoriasis. There are also forms of generalized erythema and scaling, with or without thickening of the skin, which have been characterized by a variety of terms but of which almost nothing is known etiologically. In such patients, it is often impossible to detect any systemic abnormality in the early phases of the disease. The dermatitis may be completely disabling by reason of uninterrupted severe itching, marked exfoliation, and decreased capacity for adaptation to environmental temperature changes and to the systemic sequelae of significant prolonged protein losses through the loss of keratin. In such patients, the most careful and meticulous study from all standpoints is indicated as early as possible in the disease. In some older patients, the only method of treatment which will keep the process under control is the administration of corticosteroid therapy, often in amounts which may present very real physiologic hazards.

Urticaria and other forms of angioedema are not as commonly encountered in older patients as in young adults, though there is no accurate statistical information on this point. Urticaria may tend to be more of the "fixed" type, merging into the group of persistent and/or gyrate erythemas, in which lesions resembling urticaria clinically persist for long periods, often with gradual progression of the lesion and the formation of striking circinate outlines. *Erythema multiforme* of the bullous variety is probably not common in old age. When it does occur, the possibility of an associated visceral malignancy must be considered. In any bullous eruption, the possibility of a reaction to *drugs* or of *pemphigus* must be considered promptly. Since a severe bullous eruption with involvement of mucous membrane can severely affect nutrition and is easily complicated by septicemia in the aged, it should be dealt with vigorously.

In some processes which appear superficially to be dermatitic in older persons, the possibility of some underlying malignant disease must sometimes be considered. One of the best examples of this is Paget's disease of the areolar area in women, in which underlying tumor may be demonstrable. Superficial epitheliomatosis, or irritated basal cell epitheliomas, may, unless examined carefully and critically, be passed off as dermatitic. Leukemia and other forms of hematologic malignancy may be associated with a wide variety of nondescript skin changes, dermatitic and otherwise.

Rosacea

Though rosacea is primarily a disease of middle age, its most marked late effects may not be attained for many years. A striking feature is the gradual thickening of the skin which occurs, sometimes producing marked bulbous deformities of the nose, with thickening elsewhere on the face. Acneiform pustules may continue unabated, and the unusual complication of rosacea keratitis may not be seen until the disease has been present for many years.

Pigmentary Changes

Pigmentary changes are common in old age, and have been mentioned briefly previously. Vitiligo does not ordinarily arise in persons past 60 but may reach significant levels of cosmetic disfigurement and intolerance to sunlight at this time. The localized variations in pigmentation and depigmentation in the senile skin are often striking and sometimes difficult to assess accurately.

Keratoses

Various keratotic diseases frequently reach full flower in old age. Previously mild xerosis almost always becomes more pronounced. The congenital abnormality of keratosis of the palms and soles may become drier, thicker, and more fissured. Calluses and corns achieve greater clinical significance, particularly if they become ulcerated through trauma or overuse of keratolytic topical remedies. They may be especially troublesome in patients with diabetes or peripheral vascular disease or both. Keratotic lesions of the external ears, of varying types and often painful, are increasingly common with age. In some persons, increased keratinization of plaques of psoriasis on the palms and soles becomes evident, or keratotic plaques may occur after the menopause.

Bacterial Infections

Acute bacterial infections, at least of the superficial impetiginous type, do not occur with great frequency in the aged. When they do, there is a greater tendency for them to produce bullae with striking superficial erosions. Evidences of chronic superficial disturbances of the bacterial flora are common, especially in intertriginous areas. Recurrent cellulitis, with permanent resultant lymphedema, may reach its height in old age. Ulcerative processes of all types are common in the aged skin, and it is a safe rule to assume that an ulcer of the skin in an older person may *not* be due primarily to bacterial invasion but to some underlying local or systemic factor. These include, particularly, diseases of the peripheral vascular system, tumors, factitial lesions, diabetes, or some hematologic disorder. It is particularly important not to subject the older patient with an ulcerative process of the skin to a succession of trials of topical or systemic antibacterial therapy without careful consideration of all possible contributory factors.

Factitial Eruptions

Factitial eruptions in patients of upper middle age and old age are fairly common and extremely varied. They reflect many things, including tension regarding the physical and financial uncertainties of approaching old age, "skin fixation," preoccupation with fancied or real decrease in general physical attractiveness, the despairing prospect of loneliness, the need for attention and the fear of not obtaining it, and delusions of parasitophobia. The means of injuring the skin vary from simple scratching of a small area to deep excoriation or the application of escharotic chemicals. It is obvious that under such circumstances disturbances in the psychic background may vary greatly in depth and seriousness.

Atrophy and Scarring

Atrophy and scarring conditions of the skin offer much diagnostic difficulty at times, and differentiation of them may be of considerable importance in respect to malignancies of the skin. Included particularly are *kraurosis* (especially of the genitalia), *leukoplakia,* and the characteristic scarring condition known as *lichen sclerosus et atrophicus.* For unknown reasons, long-standing scars may sometimes begin to burn and itch in older people.

Viral Infections

Viral infections which commonly affect the skin of older persons are somewhat smaller in number than those seen in young adults or children. The common exanthemata will obviously be seen rather rarely, because immunity has usually long since been conferred by a previous infection. *Herpes zoster* is the most important viral dermatologic disease in the aged. The likelihood of severe neuralgic pain is almost directly proportional to the age of the patient, and this pain may be completely intractable. The individual lesions are, moreover, much more likely to produce severe local destructive changes. It should be kept in mind that the older person exposed to chickenpox may develop herpes zoster; numerous instances of this succession of events are on record. Among patients of upper middle age to old age, increasing consideration must be given to the possibility that herpes zoster may be an expression of malignant disease, particularly of the hematologic system. This association seems to occur much more frequently than can be explained by the laws of chance.

Metabolic Diseases

Finally, the dermatologic expressions of "degenerative" or metabolic diseases will obviously be found more frequently in aging patients. It is often extremely difficult to relate particular skin changes directly to the systemic disease. The most common groups concerned are xanthoma, systemic cardiovascular disease, and diabetes. These associations are discussed in some detail in Chapter 27.

DERMATOLOGIC DIAGNOSIS IN TROPICAL AREAS* ("TROPICAL DERMATOLOGY")

The diagnosis of a dermatologic lesion or syndrome is often greatly influenced, or even prejudiced, if the patient is seen in a tropical area, if he has ever been in one, or if his immediate forebears came from one. Consideration of a possible "tropical" origin of medical disease is both helpful and restrictive; it may widen the diagnostic

---

*Simons, R. D. G. Ph. (ed.): Handbook of Tropical Dermatology. Vols. 1 and 2. New York and Amsterdam, Elsevier Press, Inc., 1952, 1953.

considerations sufficiently to include a disease which might otherwise have been missed; or it may blind the physician, in his preoccupation with things rare and esoteric, to consideration of the commonplace and usual.

The scope of tropical medicine (and dermatology) cannot be defined precisely. Prevalence of a disease between the Tropics of Cancer and Capricorn does not mark it as tropical; there are few diseases which are not found in this area. It is not accurate to restrict the designation of "tropical" to those diseases which are most abundant in an ordinarily hot and humid climate. Considerable extremes of climate, from steaming coastal areas to frigid plains and mountains, are found in tropical countries. Some areas in the temperate zones regularly or occasionally offer prolonged periods of moist or dry extreme heat. New Orleans, Houston, Washington, and Philadelphia in the U.S.A. are sometimes subjected to periods of coastal humid heat which markedly increase the incidence of "tropical" rashes among the "natives."

The status of tropical medicine is further complicated by several other factors. The terminology is enormously complicated; the same disease may be designated by many synonyms, depending upon varying concepts of the etiology of the disease, the particular race affected, or the country (or even village) in which the disease is observed. Some tropical diseases have never been studied with the benefit of modern technical methods. On the side of solid knowledge of the greatest value, the work of a number' of students of diseases particularly endemic in tropical areas is available. Through long and intimate personal experience, and with extraordinary clinical acumen and an ability to overcome the limitations of working under less than favorable conditions, these workers have contributed descriptions and concepts of disease which are unsurpassed.

The general principles and chief diagnostic considerations relating to dermatologic patients seen in tropical areas may be summarized briefly. In the following sections, no attempt at any detailed description of individual dermatoses is made; these will be found in the appropriate clinical chapters.

In general, the diagnostic possibilities will vary depending on the color of the patient's skin and on whether he is native or non-native. The white non-native will be more likely to suffer from miliaria, other sweat retention syndromes, and exacerbation of preexistent mild dermatologic disease, particularly chronic dermatitis, acne, and bacterial or mycotic infections. The native on the other hand, has developed a physiologic tolerance to his environment, but he has been long exposed to many endemic diseases and gradually falls prey to one or more of them.

Bacterial Infections

All types of bacterial infection of the skin, subcutaneous tissue, and even underlying tendons, bones, and joints are far more common in hot humid areas than in more temperate climates. Some of the reasons for this are quite apparent. Moisture of the skin surface greatly facilitates the establishment of pathogenic bacteria among the resident flora of the skin. Maceration of the surface offers a further inducement. Dermatitis, miliaria, and insect bites present a fertile soil and innumerable portals of entry for infection. Among the less privileged members of the native population, dietary deficiencies may further lessen resistance to bacteria.

Such infections occur most commonly in the following types:

Primary Superficial Micrococcic Infections of normal or abnormal skin. "Tropical" impetigo, acute and chronic secondary bacterial infection of all types of dermatitis, fungal infections, and many other dermatoses.

Pustular Miliaria.

Ulcerative Bacterial Infections of All Types. These occur in fascinating variety and severity, and a great number of diagnostic terms have been applied to them, with much consequent confusion. The differentiation of the various types clinically is not always possible and is probably somewhat futile if bacteriologic facilities and modern antibacterial drugs are available. The "classic" types are:

Tropical Ulcer. This is predominantly a disease of the hot, steaming jungle and coastal areas. It almost always follows some type of superficial injury, is frequently phagedenic, and has a moist sloughing base, undermining edges, and surrounding edema. In its more severe forms it is primarily a disease of the native population.

Desert Sore. This type of ulceration is seen most frequently in dry, hot areas. There is little to distinguish it from the "traumatic infected ulcer" of the lower legs which is seen not infrequently in children in temperate zones. It is essentially a persistent and recurrent multiple ecthymatous ulceration.

Diphtheria Cutis. This is the most common fatal dermatologic disease of nonnatives in the tropics. It was encountered frequently among troops in tropical areas (and on the European continent) during World War II. It occurred as a complication of all types of superficial inflammatory diseases of the skin, including eczematous dermatitis and "tropical ulcer."

Various Other Phagedenic and Gangrenous Infections. These are encountered almost entirely among the native populations. Their counterparts in terms of extraordinary severity and destructiveness (noma) are rarely encountered in medical practice in temperate zones.

Mucocutaneous Ulcers. Chancroid, early and late ulcerative mucocutaneous syphilis, granuloma, venereum, yaws, and bejel are other causes of mucocutaneous ulcers in the tropics. These diseases are variously unknown or increasingly uncommon in medical practice in most countries in temperate zones. Leprosy is, of course, a common cause of mucocutaneous ulcers among many native populaces through either direct bacterial invasion or the consequences of the superficial peripheral neuropathy.

Other Nonbacterial Ulcerative Diseases. Certain other ulcerative diseases of nonbacterial origin may require differentiation, and these will all be encountered almost exclusively among native populations. *Cutaneous leishmaniasis* (principally in countries bordering the Mediterranean) and *American leishmaniasis* (wholly in South America and principally in Brazil) produce characteristic ulceration. The *Leishmania* causing both types is indistinguishable, but differentiation has been maintained on clinical grounds which,

however, may not be completely valid. *Amebiasis cutis* is encountered but is rare.

Elephantiasis Nostras (elephantiasis due to recurrent streptococcal cellulitis) is encountered more frequently in tropical areas than in temperate. It may be confused with elephantiasis due to filariasis and, indeed, may sometimes be a complication of the latter disease. Progressive unexplained chronic lymphedema has been described in endemic areas; for example, Addis Ababa, Ethiopia.

Hidradenitis Suppurativa (recurrent infection associated with apocrine gland sweat retention—axillary and anogenital regions).

Sweat Retention Syndromes

In tropical areas with a moist humid climate, this is probably the most common and annoying single dermatologic entity. Its incidence is extremely high among nonacclimated whites, particularly if the change to a hot climate has been abrupt. All varieties are seen, but inflammatory types are particularly common, and pustular miliaria may give rise to suddenly developing and extensive bullous impetigo ("monkey pox"). Deep miliaria (*miliaria profunda*) may interfere with heat radiation so markedly as to produce fever and tropical asthenia. In the hot, moist tropics miliaria is a common source of apparent exacerbation of all types of superficial inflammatory diseases in which some sweat duct blockage has inevitably occurred. Though acclimatization ordinarily occurs eventually in patients with miliaria, the disease may persist in some persons so markedly as to make continued residence in a hot environment impossible.

The Mycoses

Superficial mycotic infections of the glabrous skin are encountered with great frequency in tropical and subtropical climates. While the incidence of infection is probably no higher than in temperate zones, the severity and resultant disability are much greater. As is the case with many "tropical" diseases, the diagnostic terms which have been used are numerous and often romantic; for example, mango toe, dhobie itch, Singapore foot, Hongkong foot, foot tetter, and so forth. Such superficial infections may also assume bizarre and extensive forms which are rarely encountered in temperate zones, as in extensive *T. rubrum* infections, tinea imbricata, or tinea nigra.

Deep mycotic infections, on the other hand, are not encountered with great frequency in the tropics.

Contact Dermatitis

The incidence of epidermal sensitivity reactions to plants is high, because of the lush vegetation in many areas and because of the greater exposure of the skin incident to tropical dress. Plants of the genus *Anacardiaceae*, of which Rhus is a species, have a world-wide distribution and are closely related immunochemically. The sumac used in the manufacture of Japanese lacquer, the black sap from the cashew nut commonly used for marking laundry, and the mango plant will produce contact dermatitis in a person who is sensitive to American poison ivy. Many other plants and trees are, of course, capable of sensitizing the human skin. In addition, certain plants or extracts therefrom—for example, wild parsnip and oil of bergamot—are capable of inducing a local photosensitization of the skin, and such reactions may be very marked in the tropics.

Contact dermatitis from topical medication is an exceedingly important consideration in the treatment of skin diseases in the tropics. Irritation or sensitization from treatment may induce a series of changes which are more severe and persistent than in patients treated in cool climates. Such reactions invariably produce some degree of sweat retention in the area affected and also increase the vulnerability of the site to secondary bacterial infection. Both of these factors assume increased significance in a continuously warm environment.

A further consideration is the fact that greasy topical medicaments are often unpleasant and uncomfortable when used by a warm, perspiring patient. They are particularly so when applied to intertriginous areas such as the interdigital spaces of the toes, the anogenital region, and under the breasts. Drying shake lotions and

paints are generally more acceptable and effective. If an emollient effect is desired, emulsions or pastes which are not too greasy are preferable to all-grease preparations such as petrolatum or lanolin. Increased ventilation and drying of the skin are essential to a return of the skin to normality in many dermatoses, and it is often preferable to allow intervals when the skin can "breathe" and not keep it occluded continuously with local medication.

Disorders of Pigmentation

Certain sources of changes in pigmentation encountered in the tropics are rarely seen in temperate countries; for example, pinta and yaws (both spirochetal infections) and leprosy. In addition, constant exposure to sunlight may accentuate the contrast of either hyperpigmented or depigmented areas with the surrounding normal skin. Thus, the partial depigmentation of the upper trunk associated with tinea versicolor may be very marked if the surrounding skin is deeply tanned. Partial depigmentation sometimes results from various types of dermatitis—for example, atopic and seborrheic—and the pigmentary patterns with these diseases may be striking. Similar contrasts are seen in any process which produces atrophy and scarring and, contrariwise, in various inflammatory diseases which result in hyperpigmentation.

Drug Eruptions

The tropical dermatologic hazards involved in the administration of drugs are, of course, entirely similar to those of temperate areas. In the tropics, however, because of the endemicity of some diseases, prolonged suppressive prophylaxis may be necessary. There are almost no drugs which are incapable of producing some type of reaction in occasional patients. If any drug is taken over long periods of time and if, moreover, it accumulates in body tissues, the possibility of toxic pharmacologic, cumulative, or allergic effects is increased. This occurred with Atabrine (Mepacrine) suppressive therapy for malaria during World War II. While the risk involved in such prophylaxis was fully justified because troops could not have been maintained in some malarial areas without it, much disability and some deaths resulted. The incidence of dermatologic reactions was considerable, and many thousands of troops became completely disabled thereby. In addition, hepatic and hematologic reactions of mortal severity occurred.

Arthropods

The problems of medical entomology in the tropics are indeed great, and the methods of fending off the varied hordes of insects bent upon paying their respects to the human skin are improving though still inadequate. The most important considerations relate, of course, to those insects which are known vectors of disease—the mosquito, the body louse, flies of many kinds, and ticks. In addition to these, many varieties of insects are capable of inducing irritative and allergic reactions of various types. These vary from the passing wheal of the mosquito bite to the bullous reaction which may be seen not infrequently in some sensitized persons following the bites of various insects. Itching papules may persist for weeks, as after chigger bites, or chronic nodular granulomas may sometimes result from imbedded bits of chitin. Scratch dermatitis is a common sequel, and insect bites are frequently the starting point of bacterial infection.

Tumors

Accurate statistics on the comparative incidence of skin cancer in the tropics are not available. The predominant factor in whites is excessive exposure to sunlight, but white races living in the tropics are ordinarily more circumspect in regard to overexposure to sunlight than those in temperate climates. Basal cell epitheliomas among Negroes are extremely rare. Isolated causes of cancer, such as betel nut chewing, exist. The presentation of melanoma on the feet is characteristic of the African Negro. An endemic belt of Kaposi's disease occurs south of the Sahara and is almost exclusive in the indigenous Negro, affects children as well, and manifests itself clinically differently in them.

Factors of Race and Custom

Some common diseases are much more frequently encountered in certain races. Localized neurodermatitis (lichen simplex chronicus) is more common among the Chinese than any other race. Negroes are more susceptible to keloids and to annular, exuberant cutaneous lesions of systemic diseases than are non-Negroes. This is distinctly a racial tendency, however, and has no relation to tropical residence. Factitial cutaneous manifestations of racial and religious superstition and of psychosexual fetishes are extraordinarily varied and interesting in the tropics. Tattooing of the face, abdomen, and genitalia in varied patterns is common. Factitial injury, followed by keloids, may produce manifestations which are bizarre in the extreme. These customs are a source of wonder and amazement to the occidental observer and are ordinarily regarded as evidences of a primitive culture and civilization. An objective appraisal in comparison with the cosmetic and psychosexual customs of "civilized" races, however, may lead to the conclusion that, while modern cosmetic customs lack some of the overt factitial practices of the primitives, much has been added through many subtle and curious variations.

CLINICAL EXAMINATION AND REGIONAL DIAGNOSIS

Inspection of the skin and mucous membrane is the simplest of all the procedures of physical examination. Adequate exposure, proper illumination, good vision, and systematic thoroughness are the essential requirements. Nevertheless, this inspection is often carried out very incompletely, and important lesions may be overlooked. Certain sites, such as folds in the skin, the scalp, the palms and soles, and the anogenital region, are often not examined. Poor positioning of the patient and bad illumination may make an adequate examination impossible.

Lighting

Many gross diagnostic errors have resulted solely from illumination which is insufficient to permit thorough inspection. In obsolescent hospital wards and clinic quarters, the available natural or artificial illumination is rarely satisfactory. A flashlight or, for that matter, almost any small bulb source of illumination is completely unsatisfactory. The physician places himself at a serious disadvantage if he makes a dermatologic examination with light sources which are deficient in candle power, glaring, or productive of distorted shadows.

Natural daylight without sun glare is the best source of illumination for general inspection of the skin. An ordinary stand lamp with at least a 60 watt bulb is also very satisfactory. In offices or clinics, a wall bracket source of illumination which permits positioning of the bulb is extremely convenient; it is a necessity if large numbers of examinations are being done. Fluorescent lighting furnishes a brilliant source of illumination, but there may be considerable color distortion and some flickering to which the examiner may have difficulty becoming accustomed. Certain special surgical type lamps are often extremely useful and produce superb shadowless, nonglaring lighting of the skin. The routine use of a hand lens or of a head loop is essential to the adequate interpretation of many small lesions of the skin, especially tumors.

Technique of Examination

A definite sequence of examination of various parts of the skin and mucous membranes will lead to efficiency and saving of time. The order of examination indicated in the following sections has proved convenient for inspection of both the skin and mucous membranes as part of a general physical examination and for the more searching and detailed inspection which may be indicated in a disease which is principally cutaneous.

REGIONAL DIAGNOSIS

Consideration of dermatologic diagnostic possibilities on a regional basis is a useful device, *though it has serious limitations.* Certain dermatoses have such a regular distribution pattern that involve-

ment of a particular area of the body by a particular type of lesion immediately excites a conditioned reflex in the mind of the experienced physician. The following lists may be regarded only as incomplete guides, useful principally in the diagnosis of common and fairly obvious dermatoses. To use a geographic metaphor, they are signs which point more or less accurately to large areas and well populated centers, but cannot include obscure but sometimes important diagnostic hamlets and byways.

Hands

The skin of the hands is subjected to a wider variety of trauma than any other portion of the body. Physical influences of various types are at work, from the mechanical trauma of the laborer and the overexposure to sunlight of the gardener to the effects of ionizing radiation in the radiologist. The vasomotor system of the hands is labile and variably responsive to changes in environmental temperature and to psychosomatic influences. The types of bacterial, mycologic, and viral infection to which the hands are subjected are numerous. Some general infections, such as syphilis and smallpox, may show a rather characteristic distribution on the palms.

Dermatitis and Eczema

CONTACT DERMATITIS. Reactions to irritants and sensitizers are common on the hands, especially in workers in industry, housewives, surgeons, and nurses. Such reactions may start under rings or in the interdigital spaces, possibly because of less thorough rinsing of those particular areas after contact. The palms are far less frequently involved with this type of reaction than are the backs of the hands, not primarily because of the thickness of the keratinous layer, but because of the absence of hair follicles which serve as channels to transmit the irritants to living cells.

ICHTHYOSIS is common in mild to moderate degree on the hands.

"ID" REACTIONS AND DYSHIDROSIFORM ERUPTIONS. This is a very large and rather poorly defined group—a reaction pattern, not a single disease. Various causes include excessive sweating, reactions to drugs, foods, and fungi, emotional stimuli, and factors which are as yet unknown. Coincident reactions on the hands and feet are exceedingly common.

ATOPIC DERMATITIS may occur on the hands in association with other areas, except in late adult phases of the disease, when only the hands may be involved.

NUMMULAR DERMATITIS AND VARIANTS.

Microbiologic Infections

PYOGENIC INFECTIONS. These are common on the hands and may be acute, subacute, or extremely chronic. Acute pyogenic infections of the hands are usually secondary to some underlying dermatosis or to injury. In the more chronic types, bacterial infection and/or candidal infections occur. Aside from streptococcal and staphylococcal infections, certain uncommon though extremely important infections may be noted on the hands: tuberculosis, atypical mycobacteria infection (*Mycobacterium balnei, M. buruli, M. ulcerans*), anthrax, tularemia, erysipeloid, erysipelas (acute or recurrent), and diphtheria cutis.

CHANCRE OR "PRIMARY INOCULATION" SYNDROMES. These are less common but significant diseases of bacterial, fungal, and viral origin in which the portal of entry of infection is often on the hands. A "chancre" reaction occurs at the site of inoculation with, ordinarily, lymphangitis or lymphadenitis, or both. "Primary inoculation" tuberculosis, atypical mycobacteriae, tularemia, syphilis, sporotrichosis, blastomycosis, cat-scratch disease, milker's nodules, orf, and accidental cowpox vaccination are examples. Ulcerative tumors with regional metastasis may simulate such infections.

Scabies

Itching papules in the interdigital spaces are strongly indicative of scabies. The palms are also involved, especially in children.

Expressions of Systemic Disease

ERYTHEMA MULTIFORME. Lesions of this syndrome commonly appear on hands.

DISEASES ASSOCIATED WITH PHOTOSENSITIZATION. Discoid and disseminated lupus erythematosus, pellagra, polymorphous photosensitivity reactions, hydroa aestivale, and erythropoietic porphyria.

DIFFUSE SCLERODERMA, RAYNAUD'S DISEASE, EMBOLIC PHENOMENA, PURPURA, DIGITAL GANGRENE OR NECROSIS SECONDARY TO INTRAVASCULAR COAGULOPATHY OR VASCULITIDES OF SO-CALLED COLLAGEN DISEASES, RHEUMATOID NODULES, AND GOUTY TOPHI.

Superficial Fungal Infections

In temperate climates, fungal infections are not a common cause of inflammatory eruptions of the hands, and the diagnosis is too frequently made without justification.

Warts

The hands are by far the most common site of this virus infection. It is particularly important to examine carefully for *all* lesions and to remember that early treatment of paronychial warts is essential if they are to be cured at all.

Systemic Infections

SYPHILIS. Inflammatory papules appearing on the palms must be considered as a possible evidence of syphilis until proved otherwise. It is a highly suggestive cutaneous sign. It may sometimes be confused with psoriasis, lichen planus, and drug eruptions. Viral infections such as hand-foot-mouth disease (Coxsackie A16, A5, and A10), smallpox, and dengue have predilection for hands. Rocky Mountain spotted fever exhibits early palmar and plantar eruption.

Tumors

NEVI AND MELANOMAS.

SENILE KERATOSES.

CANCER. Squamous cell cancer is more common on hands, and basal cell is less frequent. Keratoacanthoma may be misdiagnosed as a wart.

Fig. 3–1   Fig. 3–2

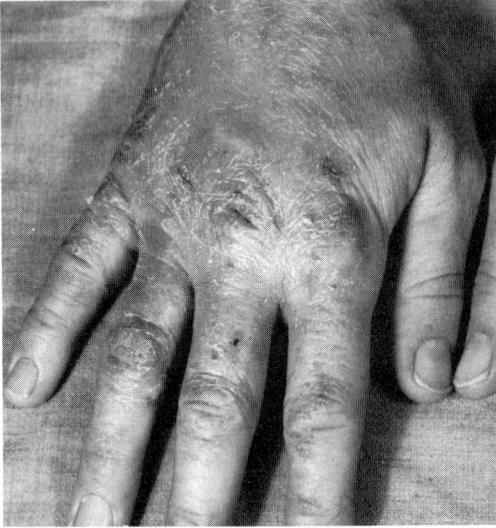
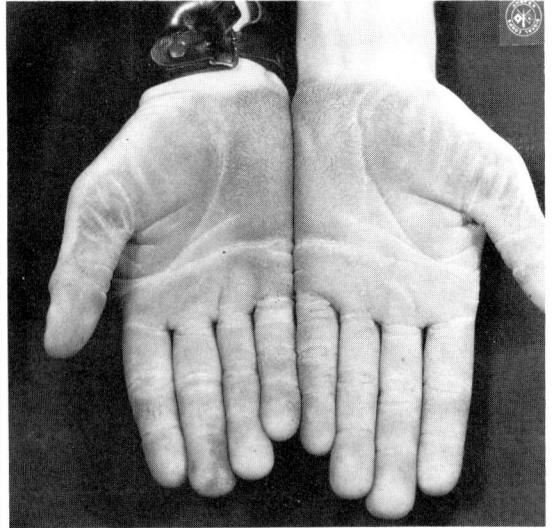

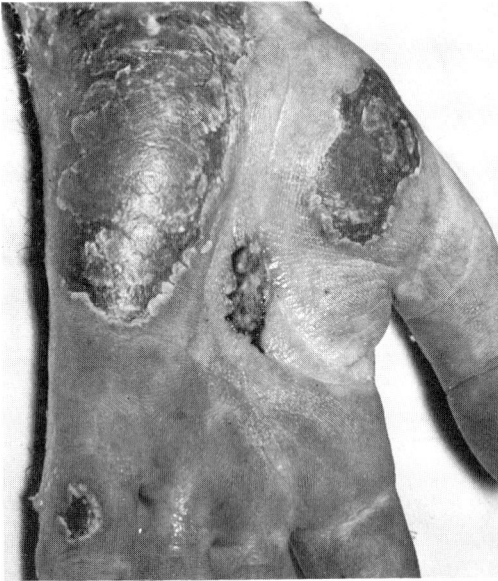
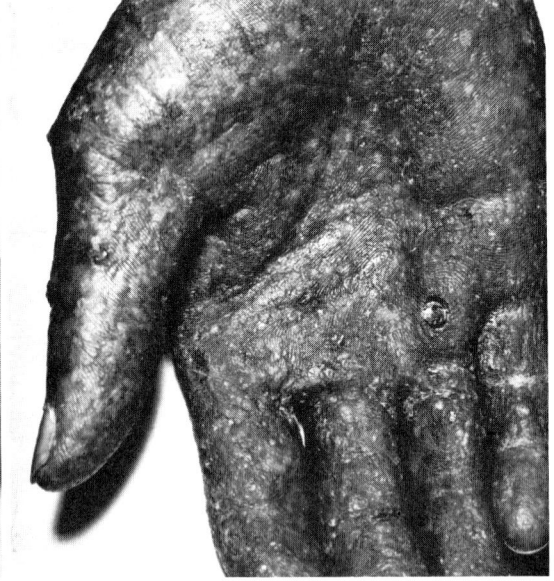

Figure 3–3   **Figure 3–4**

Figure 3–1   Subsiding phase of recurrent contact dermatitis. Note scaling and small fissures.

Figure 3–2   Congenital keratosis of the palms. The soles are almost always involved as well. Mild degrees of this condition occur.

Figure 3–3   Skin lesions of systemic lupus erythematosus. The precipitation of such lesions may be associated with moderate physical or actinic trauma.

Figure 3–4   Hyperpigmentation and multiple keratoses of the skin of a Negro. The patient was exposed to a tree spray containing arsenic, without any precautions, for several years.

Granuloma Annulare

This is a highly characteristic, uncommon annular dermatosis in which the hands are usually involved.

Diseases of Nails

A complex terminology with the common prefix *onycho-* has been applied to varying disturbances of nail growth. Some of these terms are meaningless and confusing and will not be referred to here. It is useful to describe nail changes rather exactly, however, in respect to presence or absence of inflammatory changes in the surrounding soft tissues, the degree of distortion of growth, loosening of the nail bed, the amount and character of scale and debris, and the appearance of the under-

Fig. 3–5

Figure 3–6

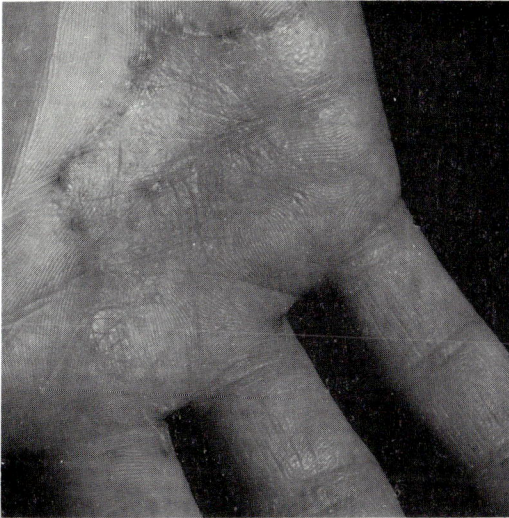
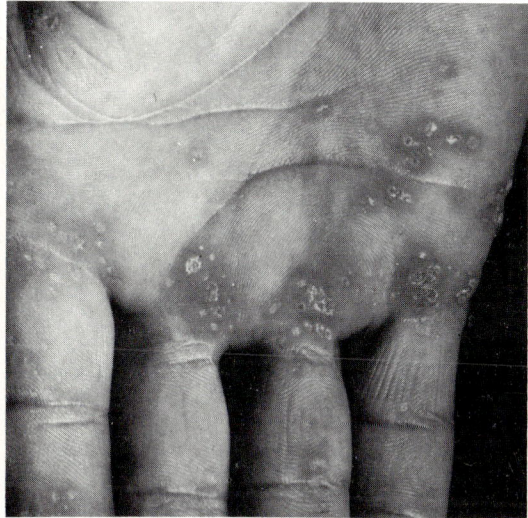

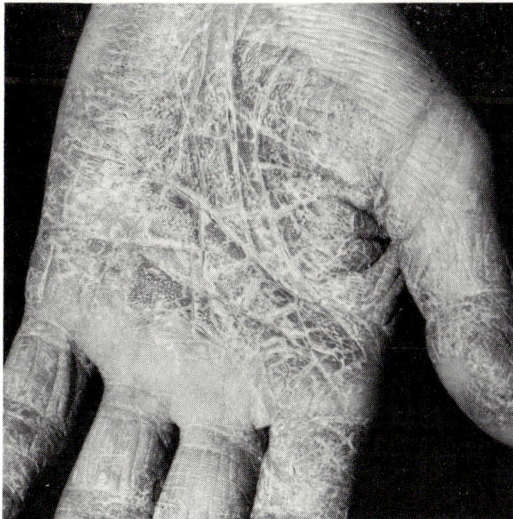
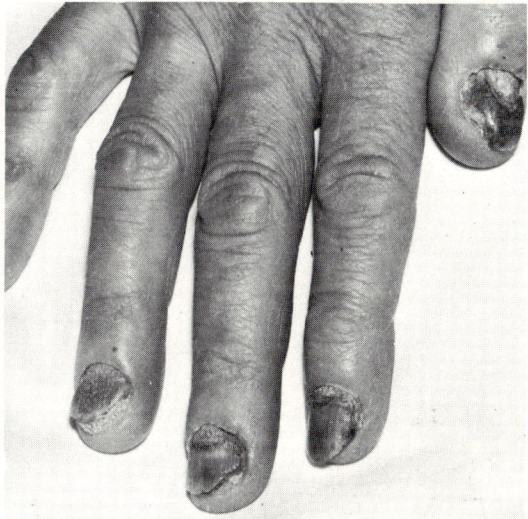

Fig. 3–7

Figure 3–8

Figure 3–5   Circinate ringworm infection of the palm (*T. rubrum*).

Figure 3–6   Warts of the palm, with aggregations of lesions in mosaic pattern in areas of greatest trauma.

Figure 3–7   Psoariasis of the palm. The diagnosis may depend upon the finding of psoriasis elsewhere on the skin surface.

Figure 3–8   Psoriasis of nails. This condition is frequently misdiagnosed as a fungal infection.

Fig. 3–9

Fig. 3–10

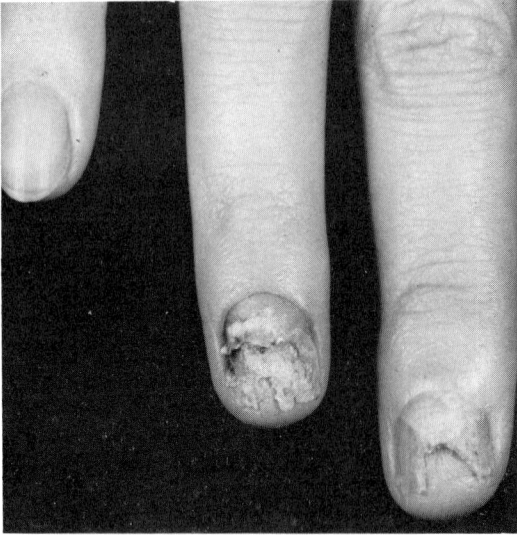

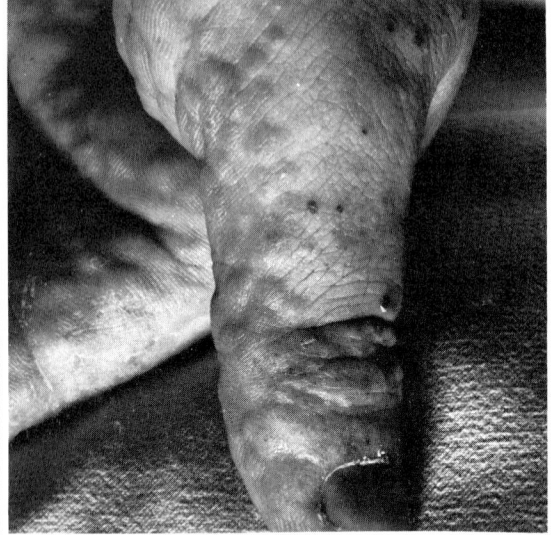

Fig. 3–11

Fig. 3–12

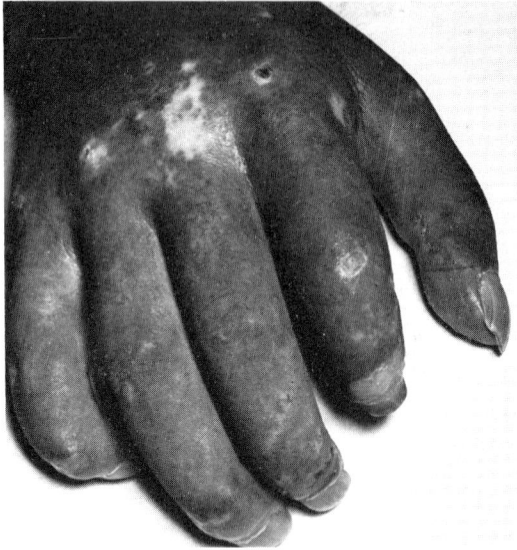

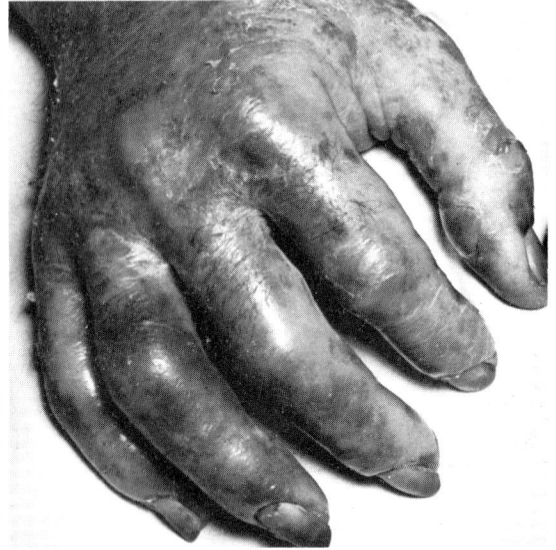

Figure 3–9 Fungal infection of fingernails due to *T. rubrum*. Note that the nail of the little finger is normal.

Figure 3–10 Marked pompholyx of hand. This is a type of dermatitic reaction peculiar to the hands and feet. The vesicles are not due to sweat retention.

Figure 3–11 Diffuse scleroderma of the hand. Atrophy and hardening, greatly decreased mobility, pigmentary changes, and beginning ulceration.

Figure 3–12 Subsiding severe dermatophytid eruption of the hand.

lying vascular bed. Pitting of the nail surface may be a highly suggestive feature, as in psoriasis. It is of especial value to note whether the fingernails and toenails are all involved to greater or less degree, or whether some are completely normal. Alopecia areata can be associated with the so-called plaid-nail change. Dystrophic

changes may occur with pterygium formation such as are seen in lichen planus.

Along broad lines, changes in the nails may usually be classified fairly promptly as follows:

1. Local changes (a) in or near the matrix which forms the nail, namely, paronychial dermatitis, trauma, any disturb-

ance of the posterior nail fold; or (b) involvement of the matrix itself (nevi) or of the nail bed.

2. Changes related to more extensive dermatoses, such as *psoriasis*, lichen planus, and alopecia areata.

3. Changes associated with general diseases; for example, congenital abnormalities, localized or generalized vascular disease, systemic infections, and neurologic disorders.

Wrists and Arms

The forearms and wrists are frequently the site of dermatoses which also involve

Fig. 3–13

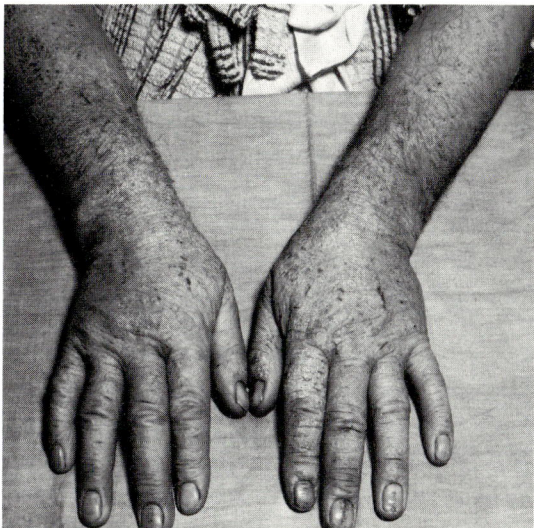

Fig. 3–14

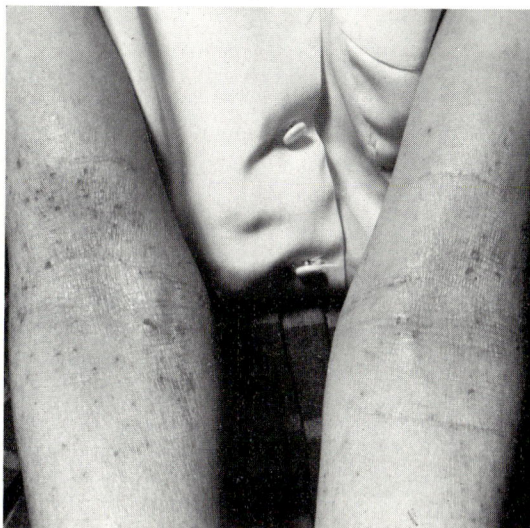

Fig. 3–15

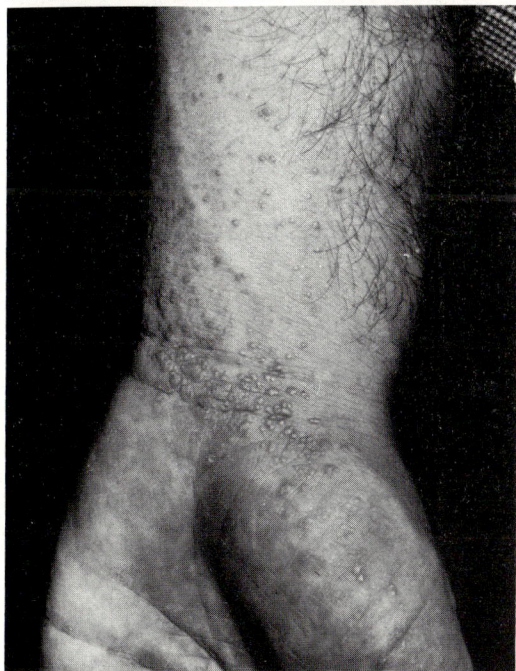

Fig. 3–16

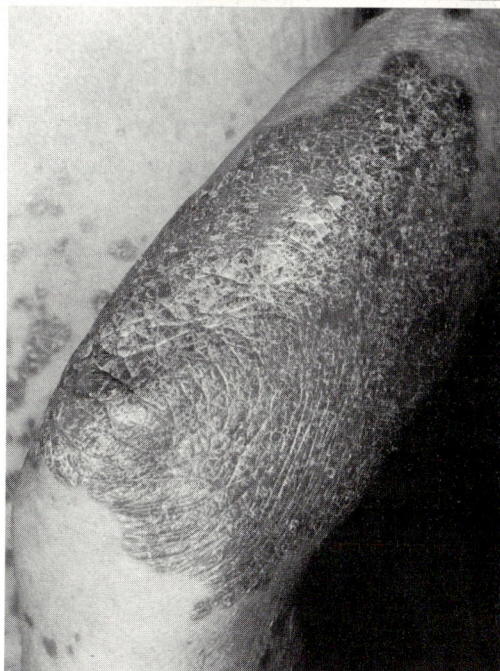

Figure 3–13 Chronic eczematoid dermatitis.
Figure 3–14 Atopic dermatitis.
Figure 3–15 Characteristic papular lesions of lichen planus in a location which is frequently involved in this disease.
Figure 3–16 Large plaque of subacute psoriasis about the elbow.

the hands. The upper arms are more often the site of lesions appearing coincidentally on the trunk. Certain common dermatoses characteristically may involve the arms; for example, scabies on the flexor surface of the wrists and on the elbows, atopic dermatitis in the antecubital fossa, psoriasis on the elbows, and lichen planus on the

Fig. 3–17

Fig. 3–18

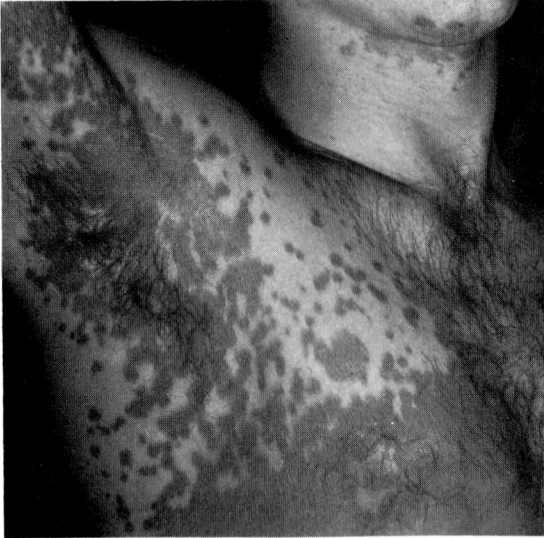 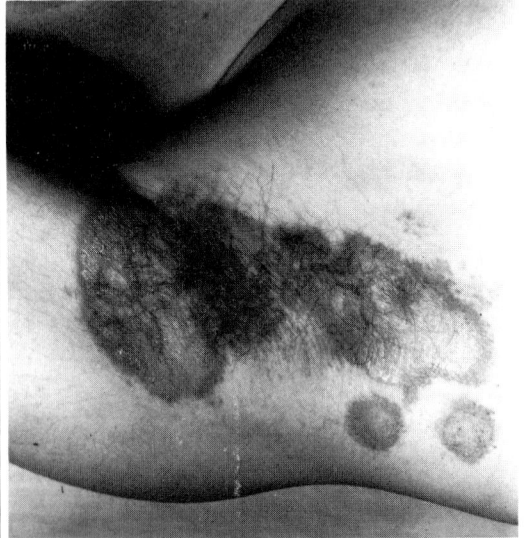

Figure 3–19

Fig. 3–20

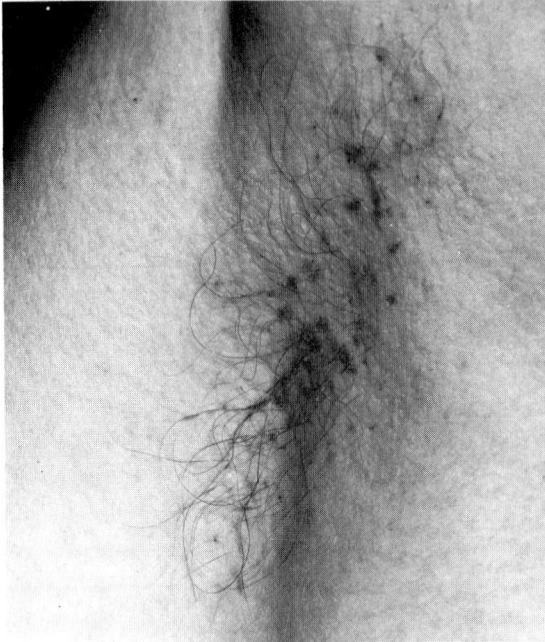 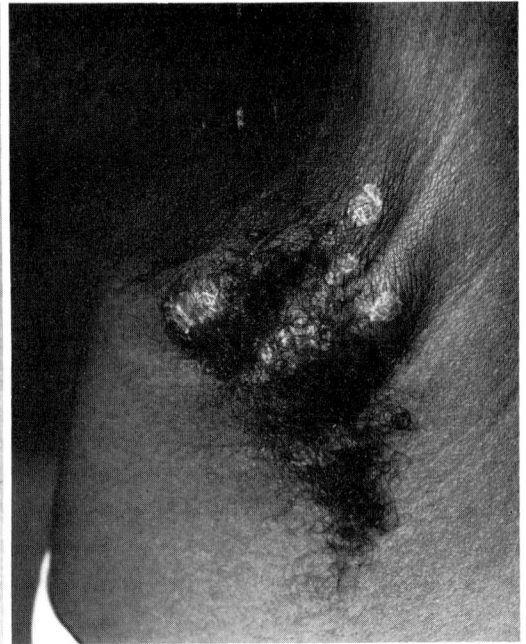

Figure 3–17 Acute active disseminating psoriasis. The lesions are principally in a "seborrheic" distribution.

Figure 3–18 Circinate lesions of superficial ringworm infection of the axilla. Psoriasis or seborrheic dermatitis may closely simulate this appearance. Fungi were present in abundance in the scaling border.

Figure 3–19 Pediculosis of the axillary hairs.

Figure 3–20 Suppurative nodules (hidradenitis suppurativa) resulting from apocrine gland infection in the axilla.

flexor surface of the wrists. The forearms are a very common site of contact dermatitis, and the extensor surfaces, particularly of the upper arms, are involved in nummular dermatitis. The arms frequently show scaling and keratosis pilaris in patients with moderate to marked degrees of ichthyosis.

Axillae

The axillae are frequently involved in a rather wide variety of skin lesions. This may be explained in part by consideration of the special structures present and the various types of trauma to which the axillae are subjected, as follows:

1. The presence of hair and of sebaceous, eccrine, and apocrine glands.

2. An unusual degree of mechanical and physical trauma, from rubbing of clothing, shaving, moisture, and, frequently, poor hygiene. The surface pH of the skin of the axilla is ordinarily rather alkaline, but the degree to which this contributes to the disease thereof has not been definitely established, though it has been the subject of much clinical speculation.

3. Constant exposure to a considerable variety of potential sensitizers, including particularly dress materials, perspiration shields, deodorants, and antiperspirants. For these and other reasons as yet undetermined, the axillae may be involved in the following types of dermatoses rather commonly:

CONTACT DERMATITIS. (The hairy area is ordinarily not involved.)

SEBORRHEIC DERMATITIS.

PSORIASIS.

SCABIES, particularly of the axillary folds. *Pediculosis* occasionally.

SUPERFICIAL BACTERIAL INFECTIONS, intertrigo and folliculitis, and particularly the recurrent and very troublesome infection known as hidradenitis suppurativa. Apparently because of the peculiar characteristics of the region, bacterial infection or pemphigus may induce a vegetative response.

ACANTHOSIS NIGRICANS, an important though uncommon disorder, is a dark hypertrophic change which in adults may be associated with visceral malignancy. Hyperpigmentation may occur in Addison's disease or from oral or topical use of drugs such as busulfan and topical psoralen.

FOX-FORDYCE DISEASE, a rare, ex-

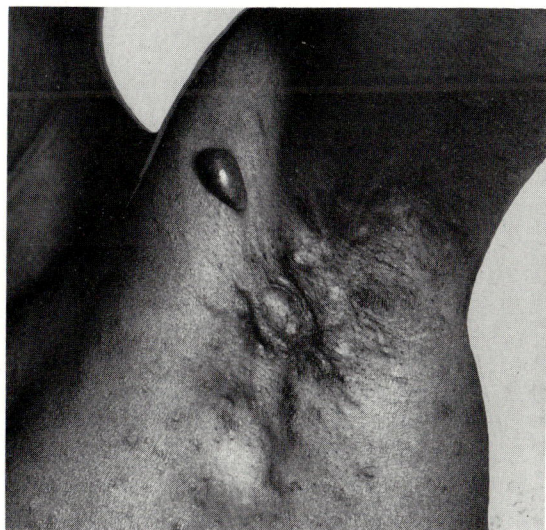

Fig. 3–21

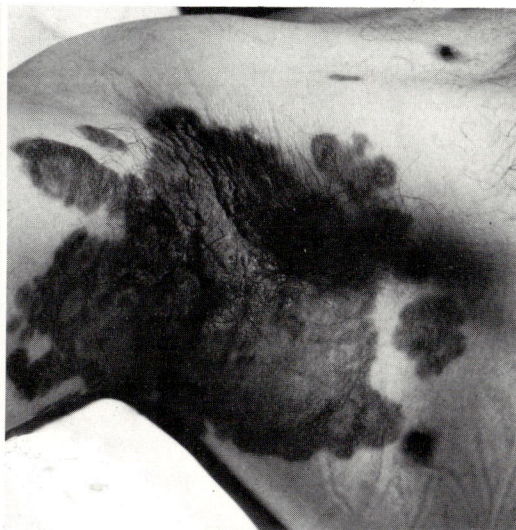

Fig. 3–22

Figure 3–21 Scarring incident to long-standing hidradenitis suppurativa, with keloid formation. Excision and plastic repair of the affected skin are sometimes necessary to prevent recurrences of this disease.

Figure 3–22 Hyperpigmented and hypertrophic lesions of pemphigus in the axilla. Bullae had been present; the disease was controlled and cured by corticosteroid therapy.

tremely pruritic involvement of the apocrine glands.

TRICHOMYCOSIS AXILLARIS, an unimportant common bacterial growth on hairs.

ERYTHRASMA, an unimportant superficial fungal infection.

MONILIASIS.

Face

The anatomic and physiologic peculiarities of the face and the wide variety of environmental stimuli to which it is subjected are the source of many skin lesions. The profusion of sebaceous glands is associated with seborrheic dermatitis, acne, various types of retention cysts, and acute and chronic infections. The stiff hairs in the bearded region, which are routinely subjected to the trauma of shaving, furnish another anatomic foothold for disease, folliculitis. Vasomotor responses in the face are frequently labile and very marked, and are greatly influenced by psychosomatic and dietary factors, leading to a variety of diseases having their basis in flushing of the skin. The face receives a greater total amount of sunlight during the lifetimes of many individuals than does any other portion of the body. This results in a variety of photosensitization reactions, pellagra, discoid lupus erythematosus, and the skin lesions of acute disseminate lupus erythematosus. Chronic reactions to sunlight include disorders of pigmentation and senile keratoses. The face is a favorite site for skin cancer and organoid tumors (sebaceous nevi, trichoepithelioma, syringoma, adenoma sebaceum). The sources of contact dermatitis are extremely varied, including cosmetics, materials transferred from the hands to the face, and airborne sensitizers such as ragweed pollen, sawdust, chemical vapors and insecticides. Superficial infections of the skin of the face are common, by reason of constant minor scratches and excoriations of the face and constant bacterial contamination, either through transfer by the hands or from bacteria in the nasopharynx. The face is also the chief site of the most common of viral infections affecting the skin, herpes simplex.

The diseases most commonly affecting the face may be listed in part as follows:

Diseases Associated with Obstruction or Stasis of Sebaceous Gland

MILIUM, a superficial keratinous cyst.

ACNE is a disease characterized by development of horny obstructive plugs at the follicular orifices. It is so common in adolescence as to represent a "physiologic" change rather than a disease. Inflammation may or may not be present.

INCLUSION CYSTS are common on the face and scalp (wens), extremely common about the ears.

FOLLICULAR INFLAMMATION is common on the face, either as part of a dermatitis or due to acute or chronic infection.

Dermatitis

Few persons escape some type of dermatitis on the face during their lifetimes.

CONTACT DERMATITIS. The cardinal features are erythema, vesiculation (either gross or microscopic), swelling, and itching. A feature highly suggestive of a contact dermatitis of the face is the fact that the involvement approaches but does not extend into the scalp. The dermatitis may be diffuse, with edema severe enough to close the eyes, as in a very marked reaction to poison ivy, or it may remain very localized, as in reactions to fingernail polish. The eyelids and sides of the neck are favorite sites for localized contact dermatitis such as nailpolish dermatitis. The number of compounds which have been reported to produce dermatitis of the face is enormous. A suggestion as to the source is sometimes obtained from the localization of the dermatitis, as in reactions to a hatband on the forehead or to a toothpaste or mouth wash about the mouth. Regardless of the type of dermatitis seen on the face, the possibility of some external contactant as a primary or secondary etiologic factor *should always be strongly considered.*

SEBORRHEIC DERMATITIS is commonly localized to the eyebrows, lid margins, and sides of the nose. It often occurs coincidentally with acne and rosacea.

INFANTILE ECZEMA. The face is almost invariably one of the sites involved in eczema of newborns and infants.

ATOPIC DERMATITIS. The face is one of the chief sites of involvement in the late childhood and adult phases of this chronic dermatitis.

LOCALIZED NEURODERMATITIS, EXCOR-
IATIONS.   Fingering and scratching of the
face is a common habit tic. Mild reactions
to repeated rubbing and excoriation are
therefore common. Severe, sharply marginated, circumscribed neurodermatitis is
not as common on the face as in other
areas, though it may occur, sometimes on
the eyelids. The results of excoriation,
which may be severe, are frequently seen
in patients who have or have had acne,
who are overconcerned about their appearance, or who suffer from parasitophobia.

Acute and Chronic
Reactions to Sunlight

ACUTE REACTIONS.   The phenomena
associated with sunburn are a part of
everyone's experience, with the exception
only of very dark-skinned Negroes. It is an
undesirable reaction; if repeated frequently through the years, it will inevitably leave its mark. Children with blond
or rufous (redhead) skins should be taught
early to avoid overexposure. The freckled,
redheaded urchin of childhood will almost
inevitably become an excrescence-laden
man if he does not mend his actinic habits.
SUBACUTE REACTIONS.   In many persons, exposure to sunlight in small amounts
produces either sunburn of unexpected
degree or localized lesions of varying
types. These patterns of reaction vary
greatly and fall into the following general
groups:
Polymorphous Light Eruptions. Urticarial, dermatitic, and erythema multiforme–like patches which may persist for
weeks after the exposure to sunlight. The
relation of these to photosensitivity is frequently overlooked.
Chronic Discoid Lupus Erythematosus.
The lesions of this disease of the skin and
mucous membranes almost always involve
the face. The disease may become activated and persist for many months after a
single overexposure to sunlight.
*Acute Disseminate Lupus Erythemato-
sus.* Exposure to sunlight is a common
"trigger" mechanism in producing exacerbations of this generalized disease of
collagen tissue and of the arterial system.
PHOTOSENSITIVITY ASSOCIATED WITH
NUTRITIONAL DEFICIENCIES. Pellagra.

RARITIES OF CHILDHOOD.   Xeroderma
pigmentosum, erythropoietic protoporphyria, and hydroa aestivale.
CHEMICALLY INDUCED PHOTOSENSI-
TIVITY.   Sulfonamides, and related compounds, chlorpromazine, tars, oil of bergamot, and many others.
CHRONIC EFFECTS OF SUNLIGHT.   The
effects of long-continued excessive exposure to sunlight are essentially an accele-
ration of the aging of the skin, with development of areas of pigmentation, diffuse or local atrophy, keratoses, and epitheliomata. Comparison of the exposed
and unexposed skin at the collar line of
sailors and farmers furnishes convincing
demonstration of the effects of sunlight
and weather; in the exposed area, the skin
of a person of 50 may be like that of a man
of 70, while a centimeter away it may be
indistinguishable from that of a young
adult. The final effects of aging and of exposure to sunlight may resemble late
changes produced by ionizing irradiation,
and it should be kept in mind that these
two types of physical trauma are additive.
Periorbital changes of solar elastosis,
comedones, and follicular cysts may be
seen in the aged and have been described
as the Favre-Racouchot syndrome.

Diseases Associated with Vasomotor
Instability

Individuals vary greatly in the vascular
responses of the skin, and nowhere more
than in the flush areas of the face. The
main disease associated with this is the
following:
ROSACEA.   An exaggeration of the vasodilatation normally seen in the flush area,
namely, the forehead, malar prominences,
nose, and chin. There may be associated
pustules (*acne rosacea*) or sometimes
thickening of the skin, especially of the
nose (*rhinophyma*). An important potential
ophthalmologic complication is *rosaceal
keratitis.*

Viral Infections

The face is a common site of involvement of a number of viral infections, including herpes simplex, warts, and (less
common) molluscum contagiosum. It is
also a frequent site of involvement in
certain systemic viral infections, including

Fig. 3–23

Fig. 3–24

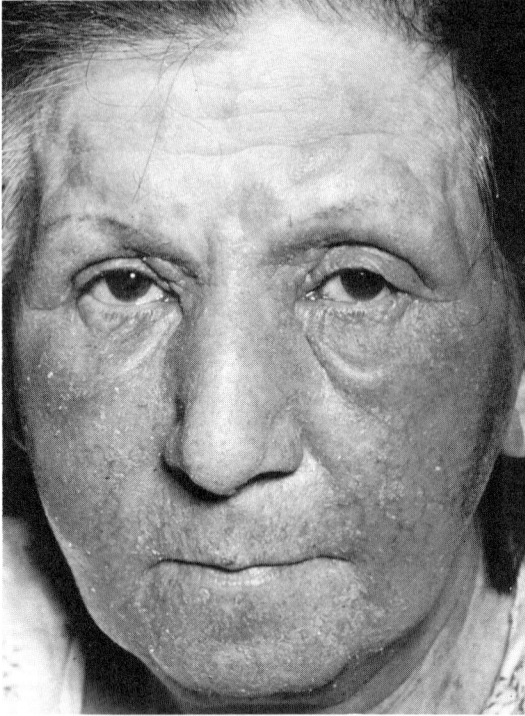
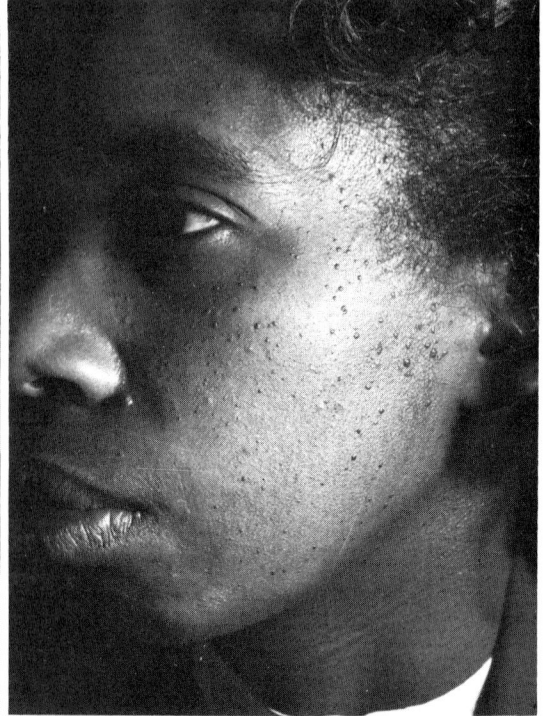

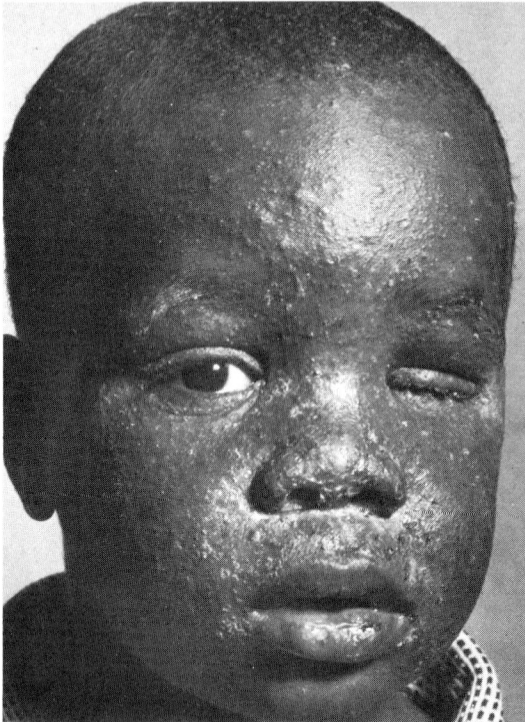
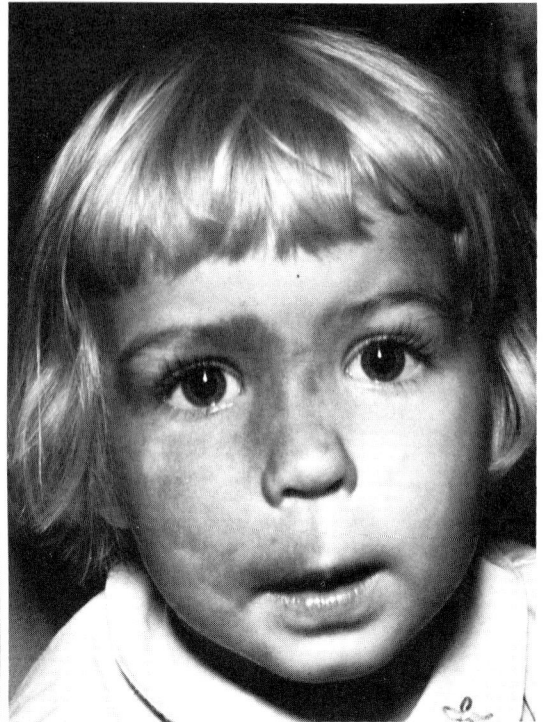

Fig. 3–25

Fig. 3–26

Figure 3–23   Reaction due to sensitivity to ointment containing benzocaine.

Figure 3–24   Dermatosis papulosa nigra, a very common lesion of the face in Negroes. The lesions are histologically indistinguishable from seborrheic keratoses.

Figure 3–25   Diffuse impetiginous dermatitis following acute nasopharyngitis.

Figure 3–26   Nevus flammeus (portwine stain) of face. There is no safe and satisfactory treatment for this condition, but the lesion is easily obscured by appropriate cosmetic creams.

zoster, varicella, vaccinia and variola, rubella, and rubeola.

Tumors

The face is more commonly the site of involvement by various tumors arising in the skin than any other area.

Miscellaneous

The face may also be involved rather characteristically in a wide variety of less common but important diseases. These include, for example, *leprosy, sarcoid, early* and *late syphilis, tuberculosis* of various types, *drug reactions*, including particularly reactions to iodides and bromides, and *erythema multiforme*. Chronic unusual responses to bacteria, or deep fungal infections such as *actinomycosis cryptococcosis*, and *blastomycosis*, may involve the face. The differentiation of these diseases sometimes offers great difficulty. They may escape diagnosis for much too long if not suspected early in the study of the patient.

Ears

The principal anatomic sites of cutaneous disease are (1) the ear canal, a blind pouch lined with skin (the only such area in the body); and (2) the pinna. The peculiar factors contributing to disease are (1) exposure to sunlight, cold, and trauma; (2) a multitude of specialized ceruminous glands; (3) relatively poor hygiene, including accumulation of dirt, bacteria, and wax; (4) a rather marked tendency to blockage of sebaceous glands in the area, with formation of cysts; (5) easy accessibility for scratching and transfer of irritant materials; and (6) secondary involvement by infectious drainage from middle ear disease. The ear is also frequently involved in cutaneous diseases of more generalized distribution, especially seborrheic dermatitis and psoriasis. The skin of the area is not frequently invaded by pathogenic fungi, and the commonly made diagnosis of otomycosis is rarely susceptible of proof.

The following are the chief diagnostic considerations in diseases of the external ears:

Dermatitis, Acute and Chronic (Otitis externa)

Localized Neurodermatitis (scratch dermatitis) is frequently seen in the external auditory canal. The habit of scratching the orifice of the canal, either with the finger or with various instruments such as hair pins, paper clips, and so forth is a very common one.

Seborrheic Dermatitis. In a patient with seborrheic dermatitis of any severity, the external ears are almost invariably involved. Scaling is seen particularly in the external auditory canal and in folds of the ears. Bacterial infection is a frequent complication.

Dermatitis from Irritants or Contactants. Spectacle frames which rest on the posterior external ear are a frequent source of dermatitis. The metal of spectacle frames is often somewhat abrasive, especially if the curve of the frame has been adjusted frequently. Sensitivity to nickel in the alloys of spectacles is common. About the ear, *chronic secondary infection* occurs very rapidly if the integrity of the skin is constantly disturbed. Another frequent source of dermatitis is medication, including ointments, lotions, and ear drops.

Recurrent Furunculosis

This is exceedingly painful and resistant in the external auditory canal.

Miscellaneous Chronic Diseases

In patients with discoid lupus erythematosus, the external ear is frequently involved. Vascular changes are common and the evidences of *pernio* (chilblains) may be marked. *Tumors* are quite common, including those ordinarily seen on the skin of the face elsewhere, and a troublesome painful type of nodule known as *nodular chondrodermatitis. Sebaceous cysts* are very frequent in the area, particularly near the lobule. The *tophi of gout* often occur on the ear. The ears are the usual presenting site of involvement of relapsing polychondritis. The Chiclero

Fig. 3-27

Fig. 3-28

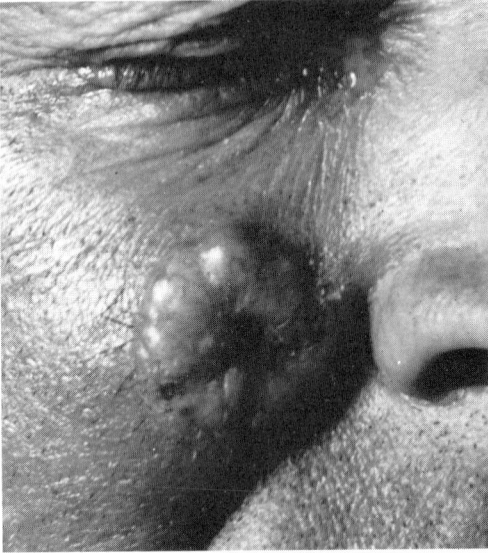

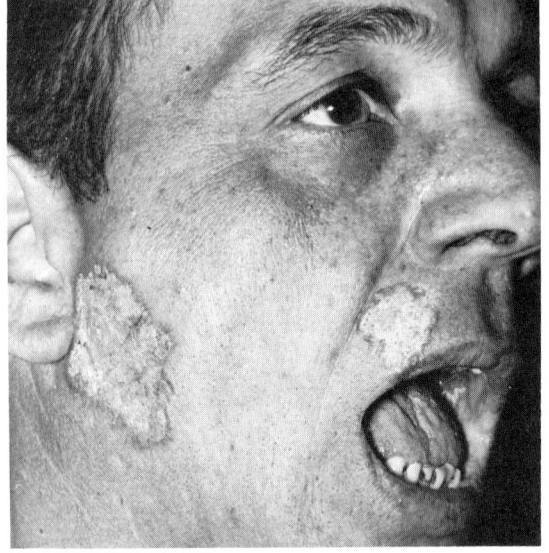

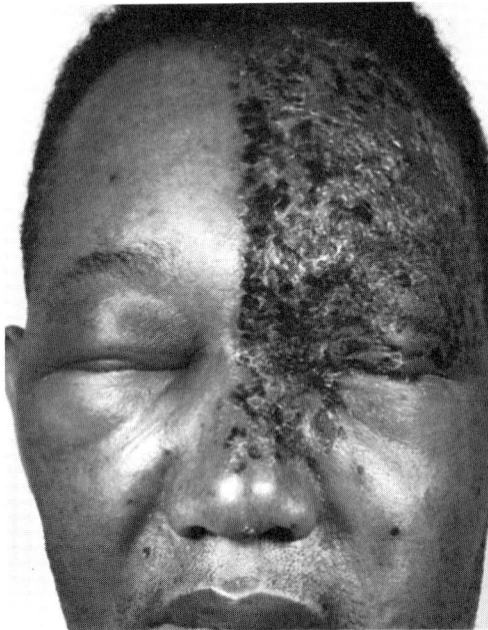

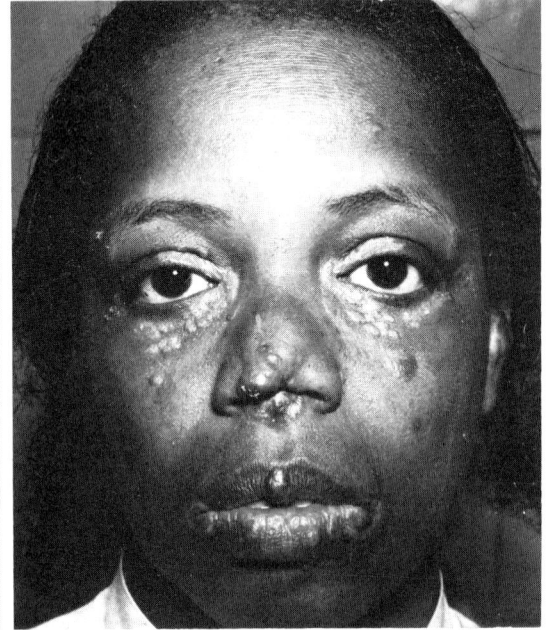

Fig. 3-29

Fig. 3-30

Figure 3-27   Characteristic basal cell epithelioma of cheek. "Pearly" border, telangiectasia, and central ulceration.

Figure 3-28   Discoid lupus erythematosus. Note patch on buccal surface of left cheek.

Figure 3-29   Herpes zoster of first branch of left trigeminal nerve. The ocular complications of zoster in this area may be extremely serious.

Figure 3-30   Sarcoidosis of skin. Diagnosis is dependent upon general medical study and biopsy of the skin lesion or other involved organ.

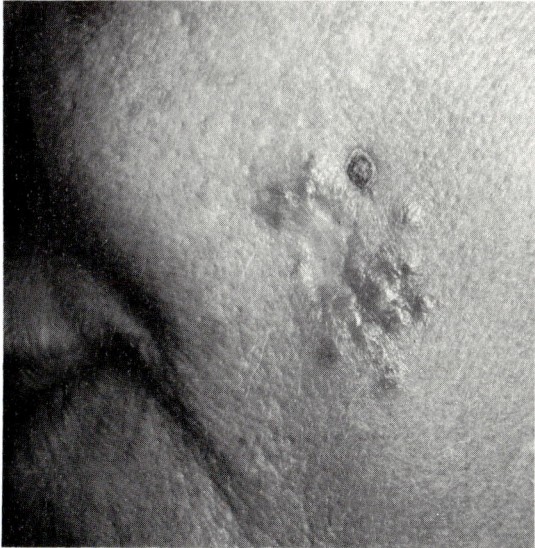 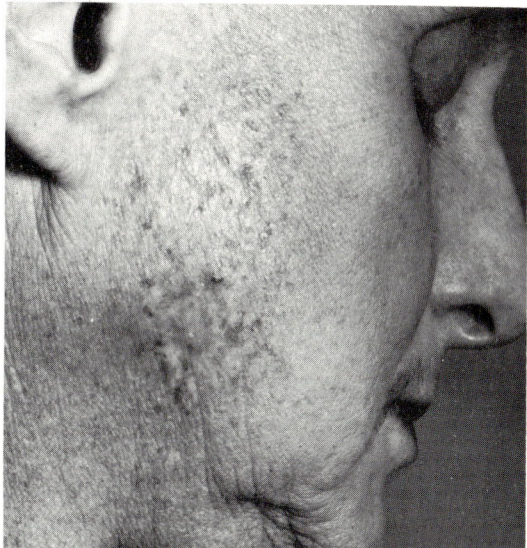

Fig. 3–31   Fig. 3–32

Figure 3–31   Nodules of lupus vulgaris. Diagnosis readily made by punch biopsy.
Figure 3–32   Moderate late x-ray atrophy of cheeks in patient to whom treatment for acne had been given some 25 years previously.

ulcer is a type of American leishmaniasis which is characterized by a chronic granulomatous ulcer of the ear.

Scalp

The scalp possesses certain anatomic and physiologic peculiarities which have a marked influence upon the diseases occurring in the area. These are (1) a loose tissue sliding over an aponeurosis, (2) cosmetic value often leading to mistreatment to satisfy personal eccentricities, (3) numerous hair follicles and sebaceous glands. Certain chronic diseases affecting the scalp, or tumors arising thereon, may exist for considerable time before they are noted.

Among the chief diagnostic possibilities in diseases affecting the scalp are the following:

Dermatitis

SEBORRHEIC DERMATITIS. The scales are frequently yellow and are cast off slowly because of adherence to and protection by the hair shafts. In mild form it is an exceedingly common, almost physio-logic, process. In infants it is known as "cradle cap."

LOCALIZED NEURODERMATITIS. Scratching of the scalp is a common habit tic which furnishes a convenient means of releasing tension. The most common site of involvement in this disease is usually in the occipital region in women, frequently over the area of the so-called physiologic birthmark (nevus flammeus). Small areas may become hypertrophic from scratching.

CONTACT DERMATITIS. A striking feature of the scalp is its relative immunity to dermatitis from external contactants. In a severe reaction to some airborne contactant, such as an insecticide, the scalp may hardly be involved at all. In reactions to hair tonics, the involvement is ordinarily in portions of the skin adjacent to the scalp. The reasons for this comparative immunity are not clear. In some instances, such as repeated scratching of the scalp by a patient with sensitivity to the fingernail polish on her fingers, a contact dermatitis may be induced.

PSORIASIS involves the scalp more regularly than any other portion of the body. The lesions are quite distinctive, having a rather heavy, thick white scale, and occur in sharply marginated patches

Fig. 3–33

Fig. 3–34

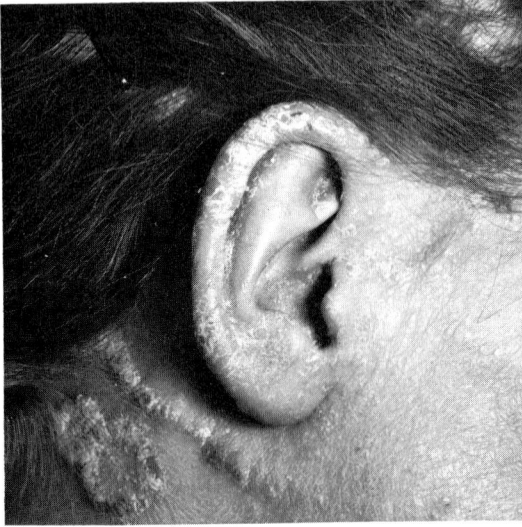
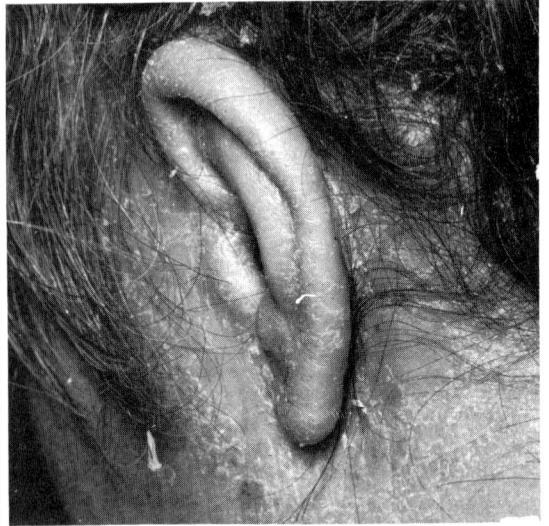

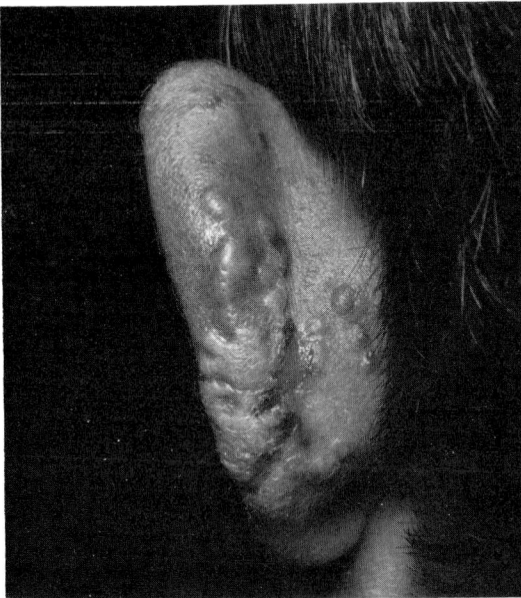
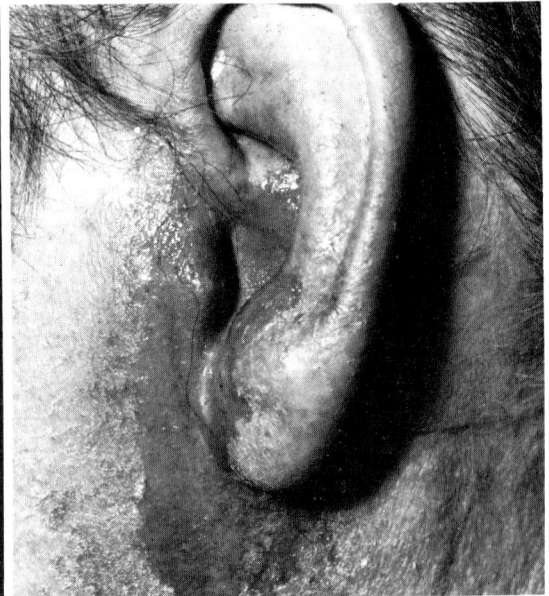

Fig. 3–35

Fig. 3–36

Figure 3–33 Characteristic lesions of psoriasis involving the ear and neck. Note linear and circinate lesions. The scalp of the patient was diffusely involved.

Figure 3–34 Seborrheic dermatitis, subsiding from an acute flare-up accompanied by secondary bacterial infection.

Figure 3–35 Recurrent herpes simplex involving the ear. This localization is not common, but the lesions of the disease are typical regardless of the site of involvement.

Figure 3–36 Infectious eczematoid dermatitis associated with draining middle ear disease. Cure is impossible until the middle ear infection has been controlled.

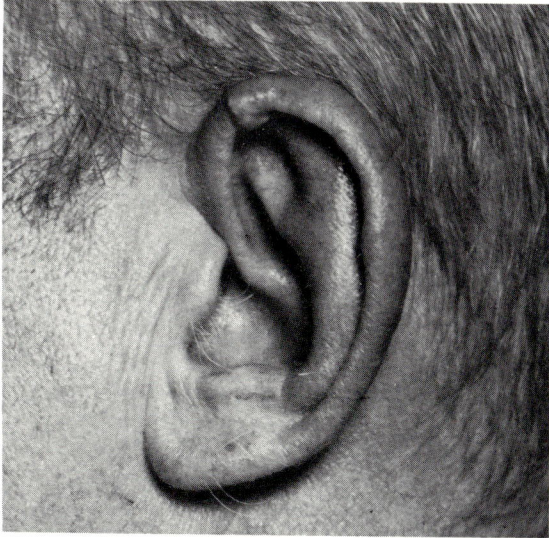
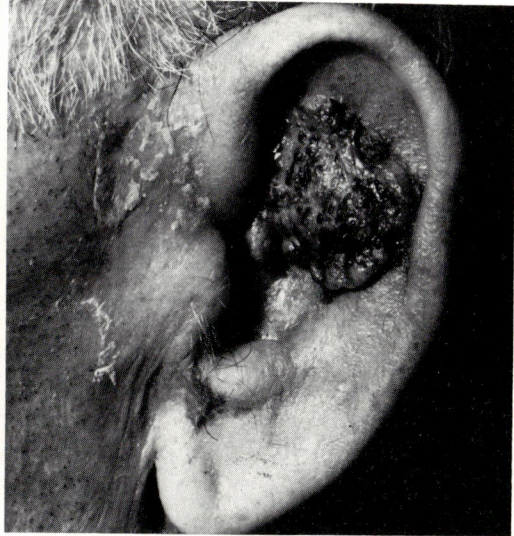

Fig. 3–37   **Fig. 3–38**

Figure 3–37   Nodular chondrodermatitis of ear. This lesion is often painful. Histologic differentiation from squamous cell epithelioma is mandatory.
Figure 3–38   Advanced squamous cell carcinoma of the external ear.

as a rule. This is a distinguishing point from seborrheic dermatitis, which is more diffuse. The two conditions may exist coincidentally or even alternately.

Superficial Infections

FUNGAL.   Tinea capitis was an extremely common disease in children prior to the availability of griseofulvin. The cardinal signs are broken-off hairs and partial alopecia. It frequently escapes detection for some time after the onset. A rather severe localized inflammatory reaction may occur (kerion), and this is frequently mistaken for a bacterial infection.

BACTERIAL.   Impetigo does not occur frequently on the normal scalp. However, it may be severe and extensive on the scalp which has been the site of dermatitis, infestation, or injury, and may be difficult to treat by topical medication because of the thick, matted, infectious debris, which is retained by the hair. Various types of folliculitis are common in the scalp, though not as much so as in the bearded region. Infection may play a small or predominant role in folliculitis, and the involvement may be superficial and minor or deep and persistent. Deep dissecting cellulitis of the scalp sometimes occurs and may be difficult to recognize promptly.

VIRAL.   Common warts may involve the scalp, sometimes recurrently for years. The scalp is not infrequently involved in herpes zoster. Other viral infections are not common in the scalp.

Tumors

The tumors occurring in the scalp are similar to those occurring on the rest of the head. An important practical difference, however, is that *tumors may be present in the scalp for a long time before being recognized*. A melanoma may be far past the point of any possibility of cure when it is first noted, and even a slowly invasive nonmetastasizing tumor such as basal cell epithelioma may become surprisingly extensive and may even involve underlying bone before it arouses the patient's suspicion. Barbers and hairdressers frequently perform a most helpful preventive medical function by calling the patient's attention to such lesions.

Alopecia

Loss of hair is by far the most common chief complaint related to the scalp. It is

Fig. 3–39

Fig. 3–40

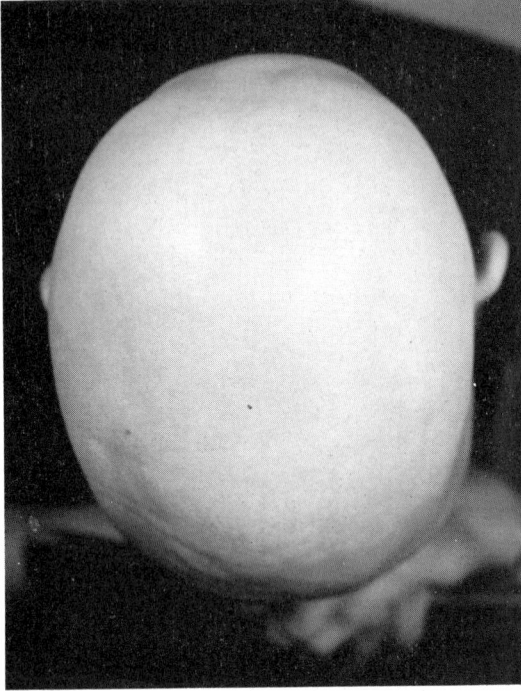
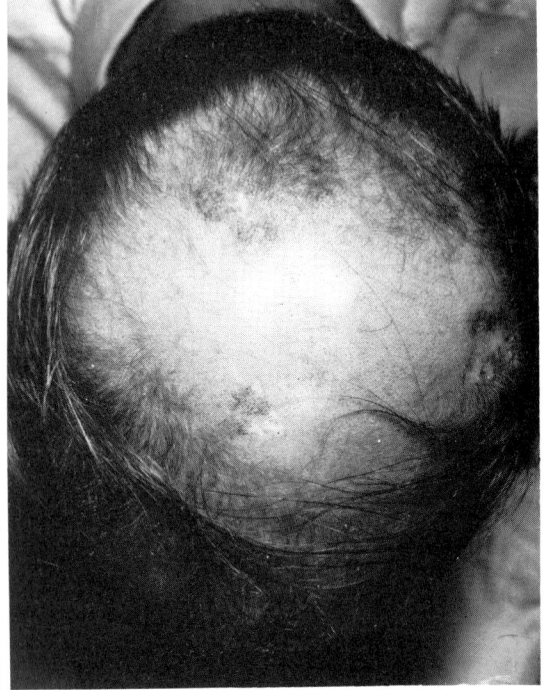

Fig. 3–41

Fig. 3–42

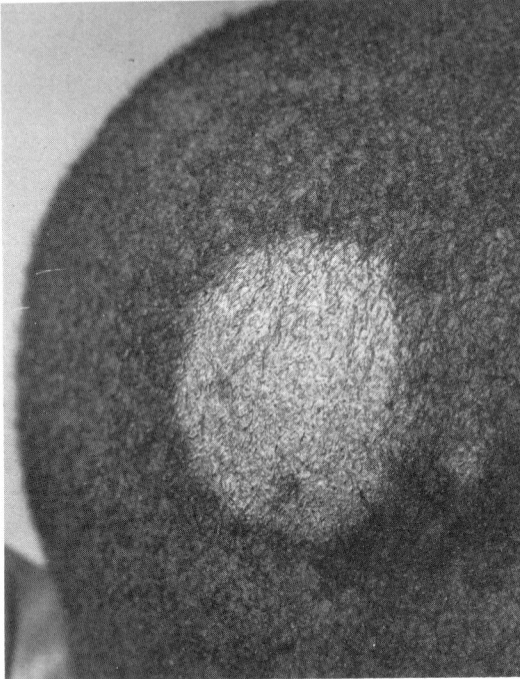
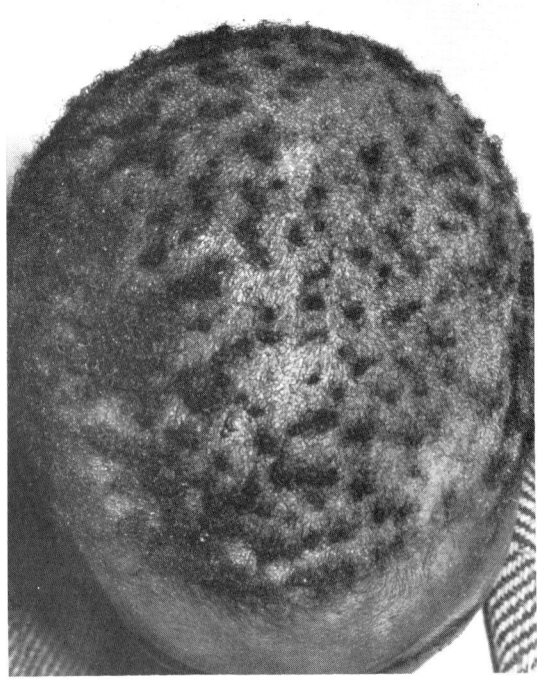

Figure 3–39   Alopecia totalis of the scalp. When this condition begins in childhood, the outlook for permanent regrowth of hair is exceedingly poor.

Figure 3–40   Typical patches of discoid lupus erythematosus at the margins of an area of idiopathic male baldness.

Figure 3–41   Localized tinea capitis due to *M. audouini.*

Figure 3–42   Diffuse tinea capitis due to *M. audouini.*

produced by a wide variety of etiologic agents. It is convenience to consider alopecia under two classifications.

1. That in which there is no scarring and in which the outlook for regrowth of hair in some diseases is excellent.

2. Alopecia with scarring, in which destruction of hair follicles has occurred.

ALOPECIA WITHOUT SCARRING (non-cicatricial):

Idiopathic Male Baldness

Alopecia Areata

Acute Systemic Infections; for example, scarlet fever, bacteremia with high fever, early syphilis, leprosy.

Fig. 3–43

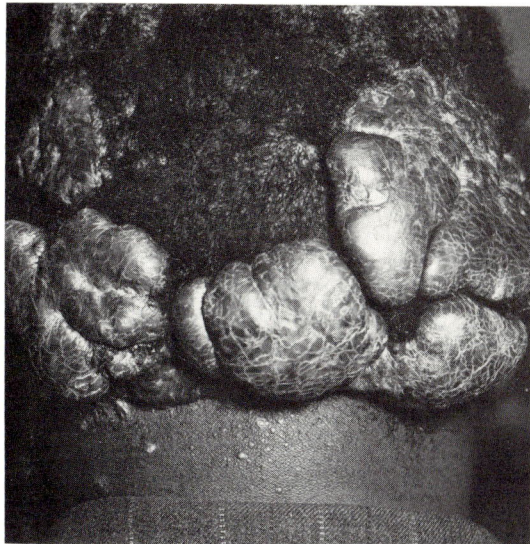

Fig. 3–44

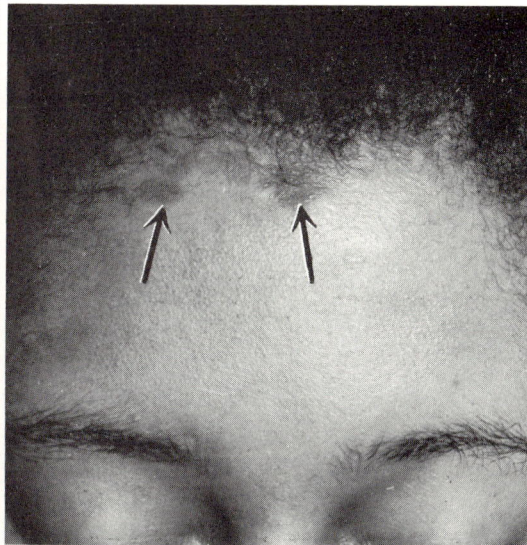

Fig. 3–45

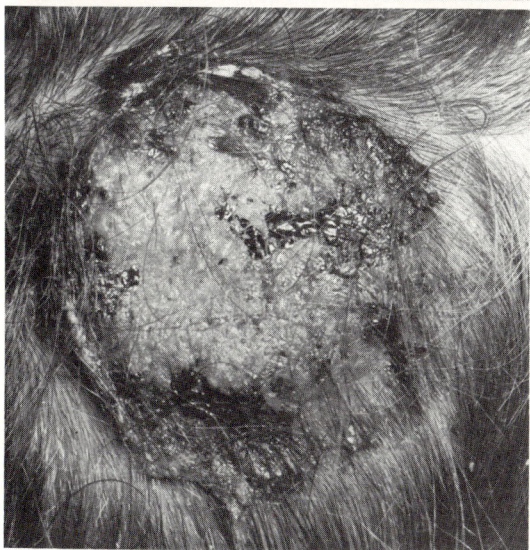

Fig. 3–46

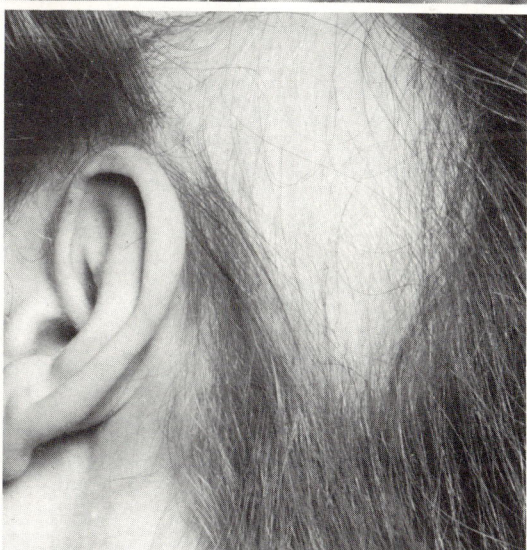

Figure 3–43 Extreme keloid formation following multiple follicular infections of the scalp.

Figure 3–44 Lesions of late secondary syphilis at scalp margin. Such lesions are often not prominent and may easily be missed.

Figure 3–45 Inflammatory kerion occurring in the evolution of tinea capitis. Spontaneous cure of the infection results, and permanent alopecia at the site is rare.

Figure 3–46 Typical alopecia areata in an adult. Some regrowth of hair has occurred in this patient. Many of the new hairs are depigmented.

Acute Disseminate Lupus Erythematosus (usually nonscarring).

Reaction to Toxic Drugs (thallium, arsenic, gold, and cytotoxic agents or antimetabolites).

Factitial. Rubbing of scalp by infants with eczema (very common).

Generalized Exfoliative Dermatitis.

Pulling of Hair (trichotillomania).

ALOPECIA WITH SCARRING (cicatricial):

Physical Trauma. Injuries, burns, ionizing irradiation.

Fungal Infections with Very Marked Inflammatory Changes. Deep fungal infections. (Ordinary tinea capitis rarely produces permanent alopecia.)

Local Bacterial Infections. Boils, carbuncles (rare if initial lesion is adequately treated). Acne (in severe cases at margin of scalp).

Acne varioliformis (rare disease). Deep perifolliculitis.

Systemic Infections with Local Destructive Changes. Late syphilis, tuberculoid leprosy, tuberculosis of various types, herpes zoster, variola and varicella.

Nevi and Cysts.

Lupus Erythematosus.

Circumscribed Scleroderma.

Diffuse Scleroderma.

Pseudopelade (rare).

Trunk

The skin area from the neck to the suprapubic region represents such a large portion of the body surface that it is impractical to attempt a complete listing of the diseases affecting it. Some conditions appear commonly in this area, and others are less common to extremely rare. From the etiologic standpoint, the occurrence of some diseases on the trunk may be explained quite reasonably; the reasons for the factors leading to a predominant distribution of others to the trunk are unknown. Diseases related to exposure to sunlight vary on the trunk, depending upon the habits of the patient. With increasing popularity of exposure to the sun and even bolder mores in respect to the area exposed, freckling, senile keratoses, and tumors of the trunk are being seen with increasing frequency. The profusion of sebaceous glands leads to acne, especially over the shoulders and upper portion of the trunk; and blockage of sweat ducts leads to miliaria, in which the trunk is the most commonly involved site. In obese persons, especially women, the intertriginous skin under the breasts and elsewhere affords a moist macerated surface on which bacterial and yeast infections and seborrheic dermatitis flourish. Seborrheic keratoses are common on the trunk. The umbilicus is a not infrequent site of low-grade infection, seborrheic dermatitis, and psoriasis.

Papulosquamous Eruptions

A commonly encountered differential diagnostic problem in lesions of the trunk is the sorting out of lesions which are papular and are characterized by varying degrees of scaling—the "papulosquamous" eruptions. On the basis of relative frequency and/or general medical importance, these may be listed as follows:

PITYRIASIS ROSEA. A very common disease, easily diagnosed on the basis of the morphology and distribution of the lesions.

SEBORRHEIC DERMATITIS. Ordinarily most marked in the presternal and interscapular region, but may be more extensive, with localization in intertriginous folds. In warm climates it is frequently coincident with miliaria.

PSORIASIS.

LICHEN PLANUS. The trunk is involved only in generalized phases of this disease, as a rule. The individual lesions are highly characteristic and easily recognized.

EARLY SYPHILIS. From 1945 to 1950 syphilis was a leading contender for consideration among the causes of papulosquamous eruptions of the trunk. It is again occurring more frequently.

DISCOID LUPUS ERYTHEMATOSUS. Principally on portions of the trunk exposed to sunlight.

SUPERFICIAL EPITHELIOMAS AND BOWEN'S DISEASE (INTRA-EPIDERMAL EPITHELIOMA). Not infrequently confused with psoriasis at onset.

PARAPSORIASIS. Rare.

TINEA VERSICOLOR. Scaling macules, varying in color. Very common; of cosmetic importance only.

NUMMULAR DERMATITIS. Patchy. Lesions principally on shoulders and back.

TINEA CORPORIS. Also follicular "ids" secondary to kerion.

Fig. 3–47

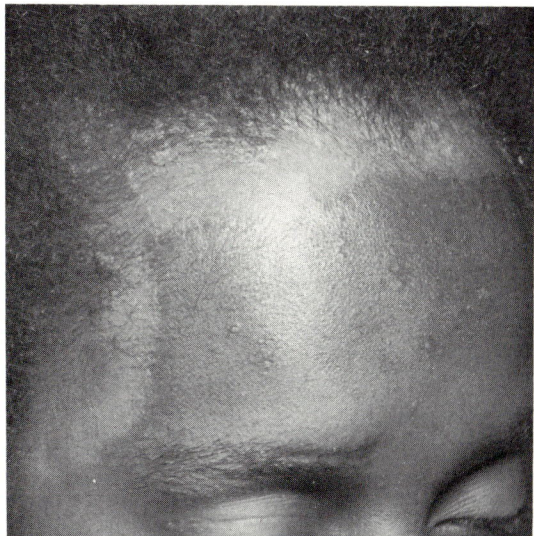

Fig. 3–48

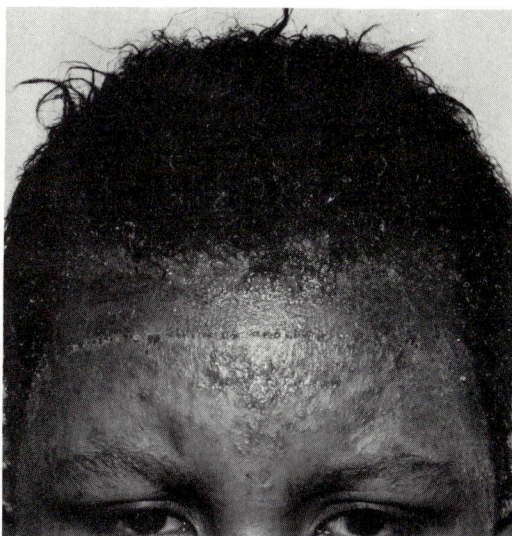

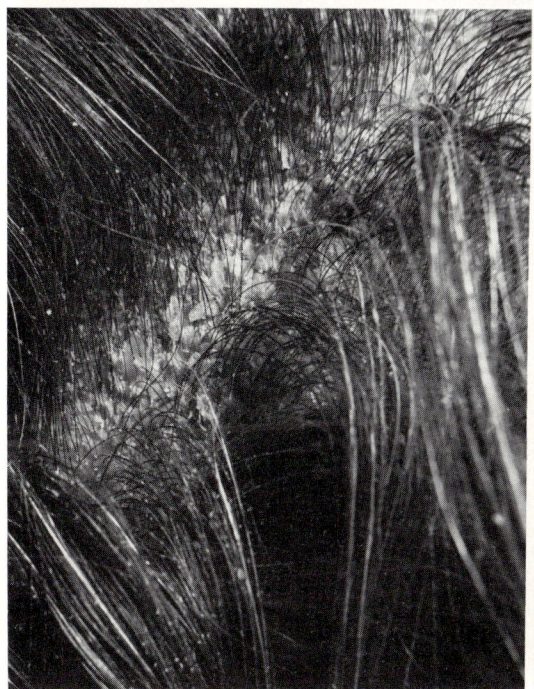

Fig. 3–49

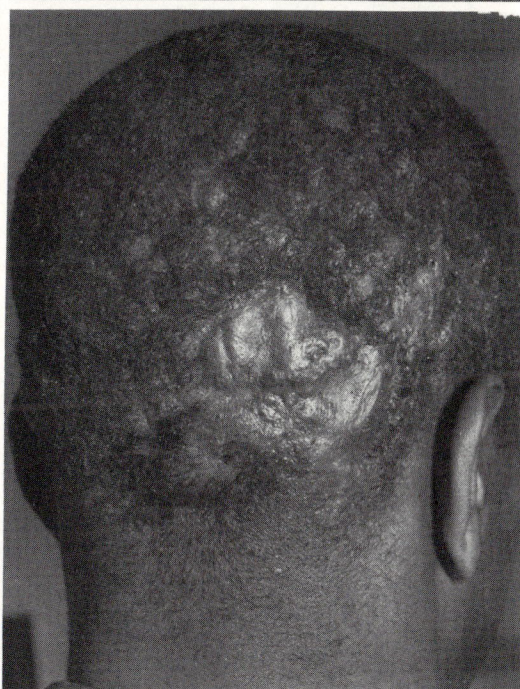

Fig. 3–50

Figure 3–47   Partial hypopigmentation at margins of scalp in patient with seborrheic dermatitis. The pigmentary response may sometimes be increased rather than decreased.

Figure 3–48   Contact dermatitis from hair dye. The reaction on the skin at the hair line is more severe than in the scalp itself.

Figure 3–49   Marked scaling of the scalp in chronic seborrheic dermatitis.

Figure 3–50   Deep chronic folliculitis of scalp. This disease is frequently very resistant to treatment, and keloid formation may follow (see Fig. 3–43).

Fig. 3–51

Fig. 3–52

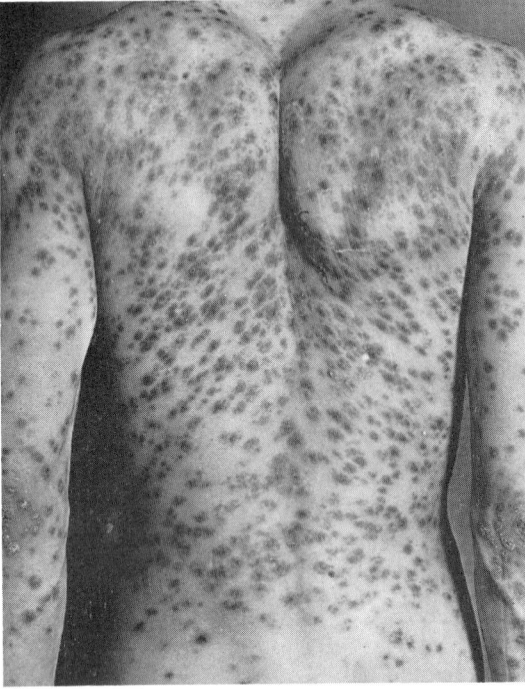

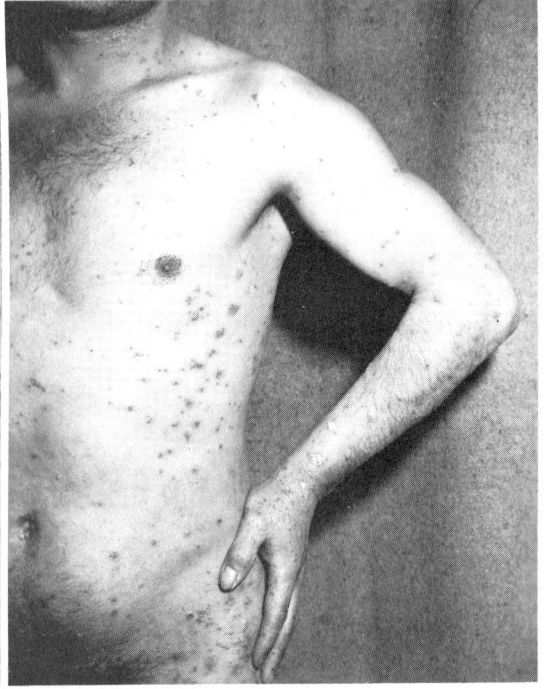

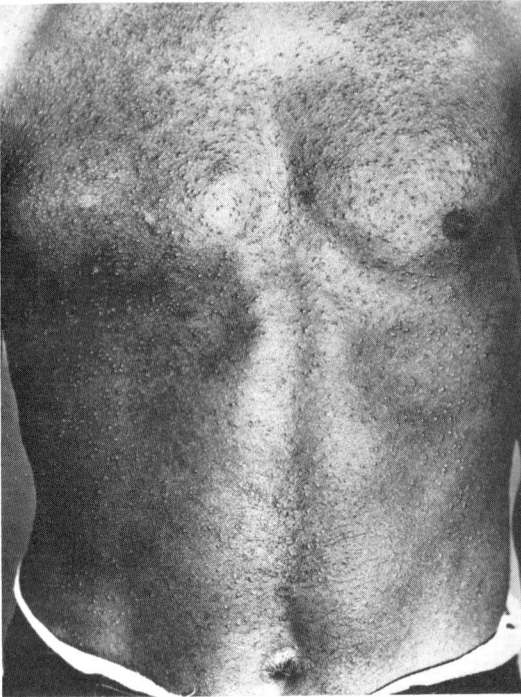

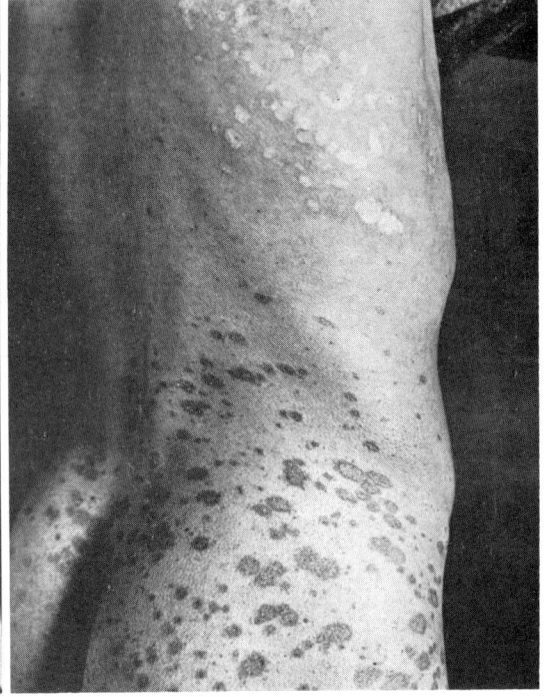

Fig. 3–53

Fig. 3–54

Figure 3–51 Extensive papular lesions occurring in early syphilis.
Figure 3–52 Extensive lesions of scabies.
Figure 3–53 Extensive severe miliaria (sweat retention).
Figure 3–54 Extensive pityriasis rosea.

Infestations

The trunk is commonly involved in scabies, with a predilection for the axillary folds, the breasts in women, and the belt line. Pediculosis corporis, with diffuse marked itching of the trunk and characteristic marks of deep excoriation, is rarely seen among populations whose hygiene is

Fig. 3–55

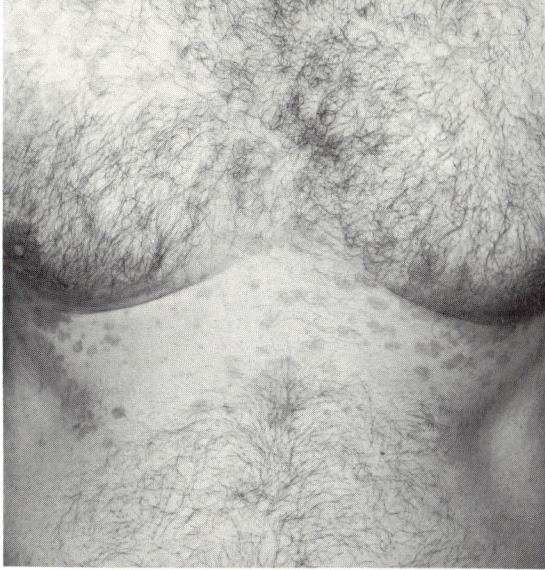

Fig. 3–56

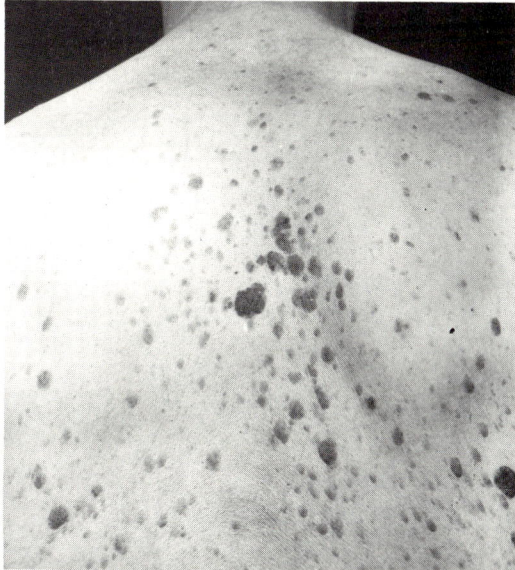

Fig. 3–57

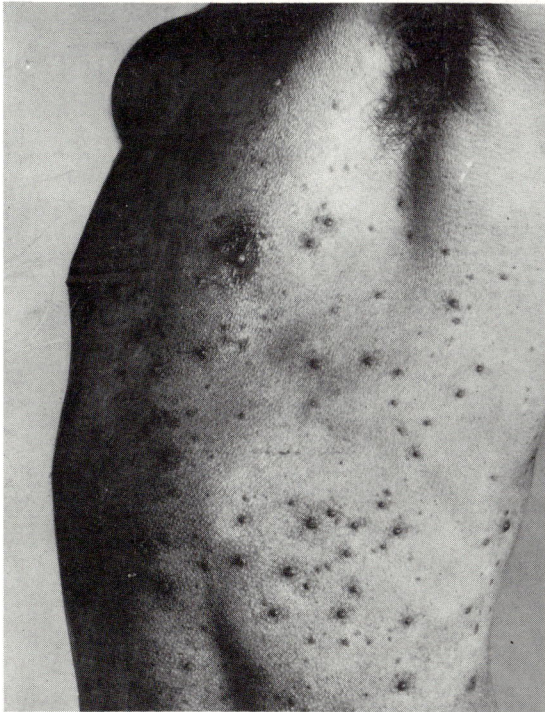

Fig. 3–58

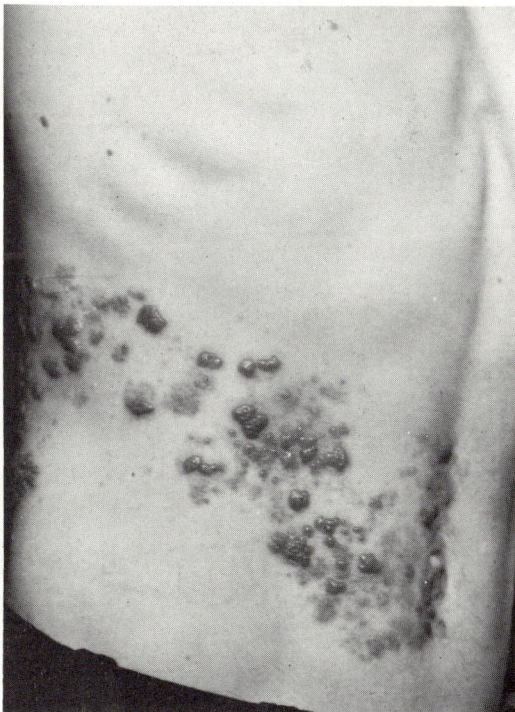

Figure 3–55 Pigmented slightly scaling lesions of tinea versicolor.
Figure 3–56 Multiple seborrheic keratoses. They are not "pre-malignant."
Figure 3–57 Characteristic lesions of varicella.
Figure 3–58 Grouped inflammatory unilateral lesions of herpes zoster.

even moderately good. Pediculosis pubis may produce some itching of the abdomen, and in hairy males the parasite may be found over the entire trunk.

Drug Eruptions

Numerous and varied.

Urticaria

Systemic Infections

Anogenital Region

This is a common site of involvement by a large number of dermatoses. Some dis-

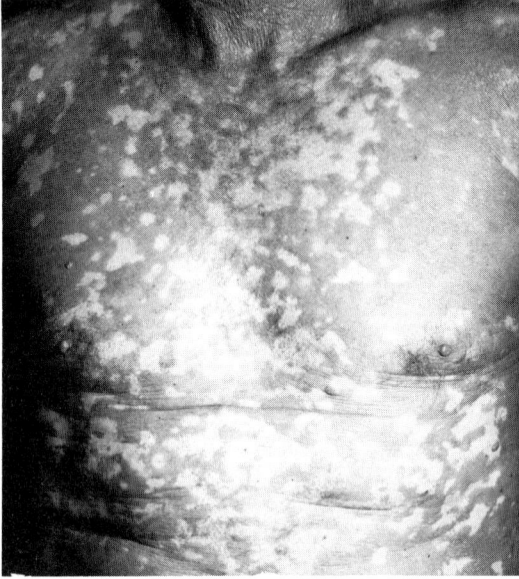

Fig. 3–59

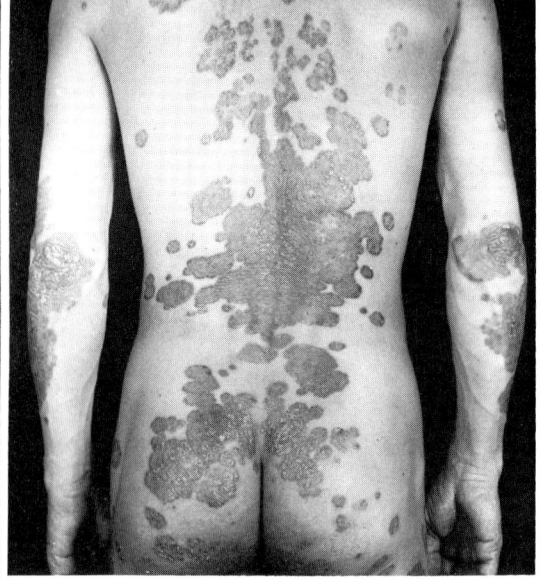

Fig. 3–60

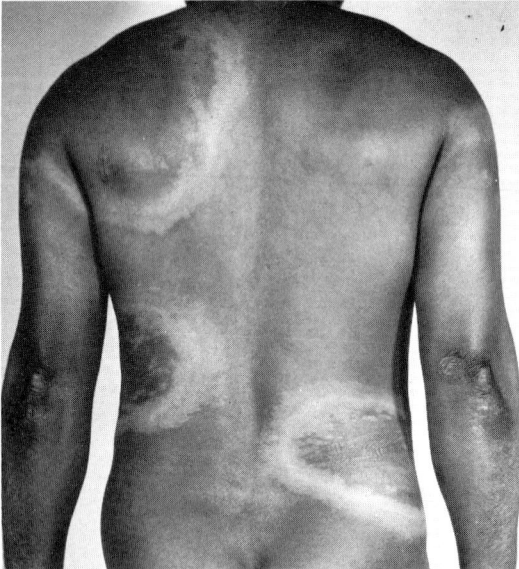

Fig. 3–61

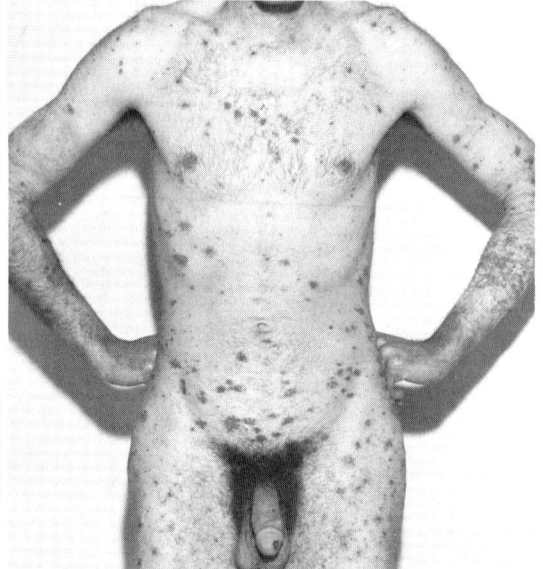

Fig. 3–62

Figure 3–59 Patchy progressive vitiligo of trunk.
Figure 3–60 Characteristic sharply outlined patches of psoriasis.
Figure 3–61 Anesthetic patches in a patient with tuberculoid leprosy (Major type).
Figure 3–62 Extensive patchy eczematid reaction occurring in patient who had developed contact dermatitis from topical antibiotic applied to the left forearm.

eases are much more liable to be extremely chronic in the region, because they may not be noted promptly after their onset and because many types of local medication are not as well tolerated as on some other parts of the skin surface and produce irritation. The anatomic characteristics which contribute to disease are the number of intertriginous folds, which make hygiene difficult and which interfere with the drying and aeration of the skin surface; the presence of a large number of specialized glands, including eccrine sweat glands, sebaceous glands, apocrine glands (as in the axillae), and smegma glands; and constant trauma from rubbing of the skin surface in walking, and rubbing from clothing, sanitary pads, and trusses. In the perianal region, there is regular irritation from fecal contamination and the results of inadequate or overadequate hygiene. Fissures develop easily at the mucocutaneous junction of the anal orifice and in the gluteal cleft and crural folds. The bacterial population is ordinarily very high. Nerve endings are abundant and alert; itching from minor irritation or inflammation tends to be extreme. The psychoerotic implications of itching, of oversolicitous hygienic and cosmetic attention to the region, and of preoccupation with minor abnormalities are marked. The region is subjected to potential irritation and sensitization by many cosmetic and medical preparations, much as are the axillae, with the addition of special hazards incident to "feminine hygiene" and contraception. In females, the region is occasionally subject to irritation and potential infection from discharge. A further source of trauma is the as yet poorly understood reactions in the anogenital region following the administration of broad-spectrum antibiotics. The region, unlike any other portion of the body, is, among civilized races, never the recipient of the benefits of adequate exposure to light and air.

Among the most common dermatoses affecting the anogenital region are the following:

Anal and/or Vulvar Pruritus

A symptom-complex, sometimes an extreme and very chronic one, resulting from a wide variety of factors.

"Intertrigo," Seborrheic Dermatitis, and Candidiasis

A sometimes indistinguishable group of conditions ordinarily arising initially in folds in the region, especially the gluteal cleft and crural areas.

Psoriasis

May be coincident with one of the preceeding conditions. It is frequently intractable in the anogenital region; symptoms are more marked than in psoriasis elsewhere on the body.

Venereal Diseases

Early syphilis, chancroid, lymphopathia venereum, and granuloma inguinale.

Viral Infections

Herpes simplex (progenitalis), fairly common and often misdiagnosed. Warts, usually large and exuberant.

Parasitic Infestations

Common site of involvement of scabies in male. Pediculosis pubis occasionally.

Bacterial Infections

Acute superficial bacterial infections of the anogenital region are not frequent, possibly because the region is thoroughly accustomed to a high bacterial count and to a widely varying transient flora. Folliculitis and boils are sometimes seen. Because of the presence of apocrine glands, hidradenitis suppurativa is seen in this region as well as in the axillae, though not commonly. Pustular miliaria may begin in the anogenital region as in the axillae. Dermatitis vegetans and diffuse granulomatous response to low-grade infection may occur.

Contact Dermatitis

Exceedingly common in this area. About the anus, the contact dermatitis may be followed by persistent localized neurodermatitis. If the scrotum is involved, the dermatitis may be surprisingly chronic.

Fig. 3–63

Fig. 3–64

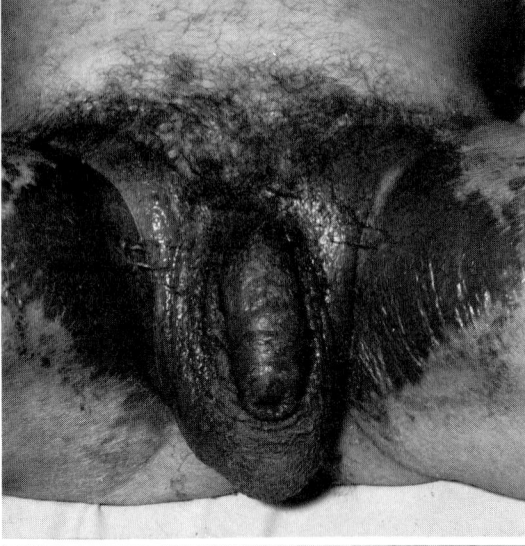 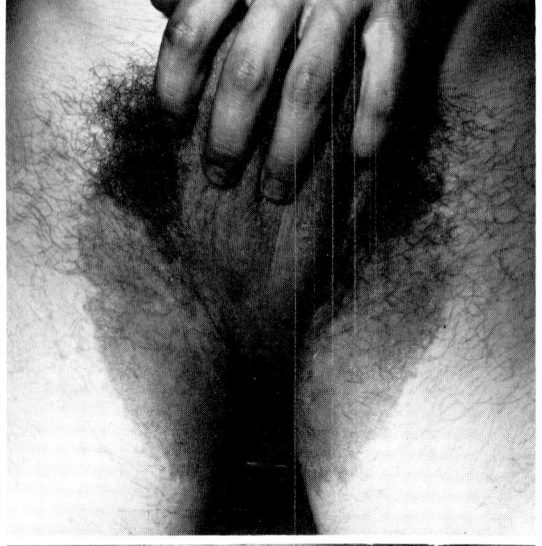

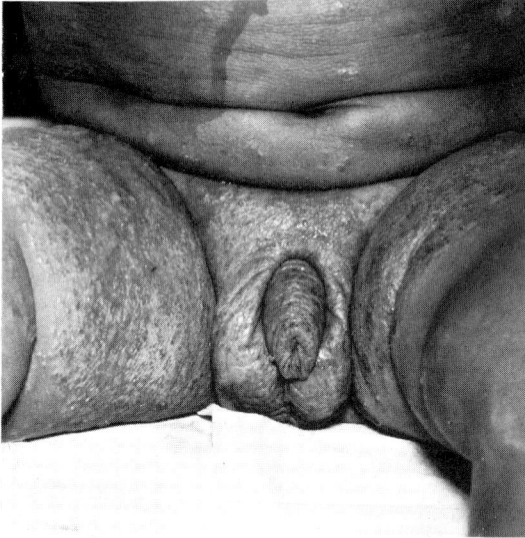 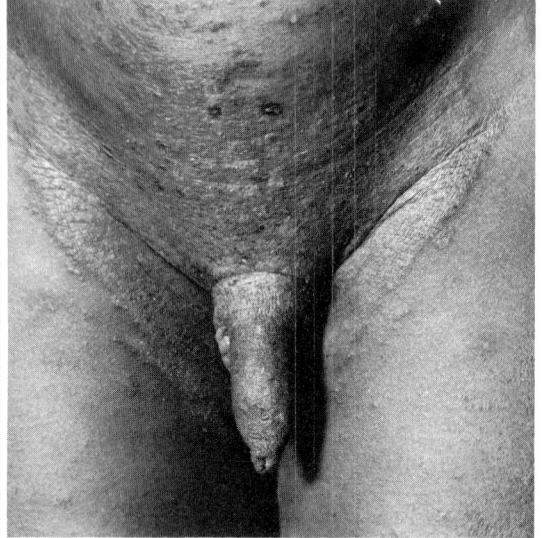

Fig. 3–65

Fig. 3–66

Figure 3–63   Severe inflammatory reaction to overtreatment. The anogenital region is particularly susceptible to such reaction.
Figure 3–64   Typical tinea cruris involving the upper inner thighs and scrotum.
Figure 3–65   Acute dermatitis confined to diaper region.
Figure 3–66   Lesions of lower abdomen and genitalia in patient with atopic dermatitis.

The most common source is local medication, but the region may be the site of poison ivy dermatitis by transfer of the contactant by the hands.

Bullous Eruptions

Fairly common and due to a variety of causes: drugs (phenolphthalein), the several types of erythema multiforme, pemphigus.

Lichen Planus

Commonly seen on the male genitalia, particularly the glans, and on the mucous surface of the vulva. May be confused with the following group:

Various lesions associated with *atrophy. Lichen sclerosus et atrophicus.* Localized scleroderma, *erythroplasia* (premalignant). *Leukoplakia* (premalignant).

Tinea Cruris

Common in males on upper inner thighs. Superficial ringworm infections are uncommon about the anus.

Fig. 3–67

Fig. 3–68

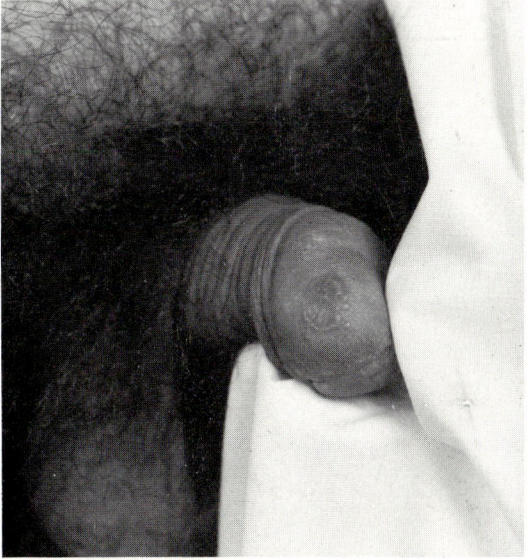
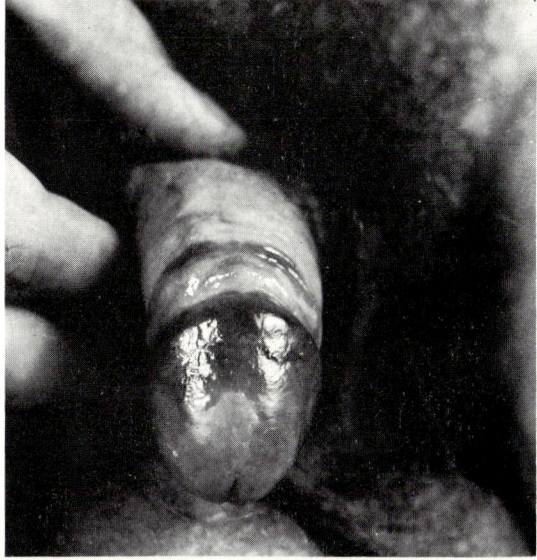

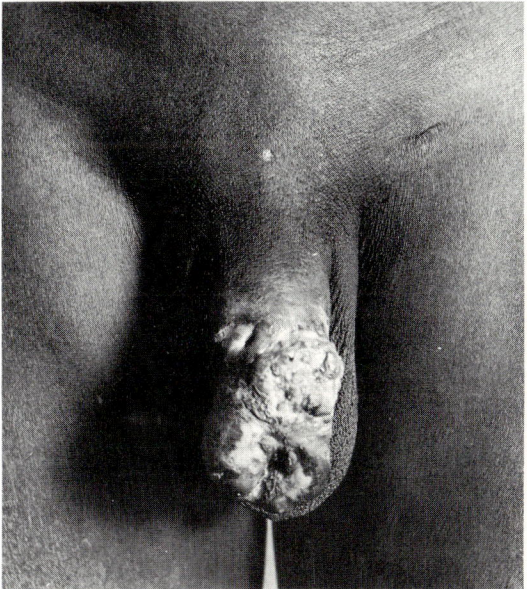
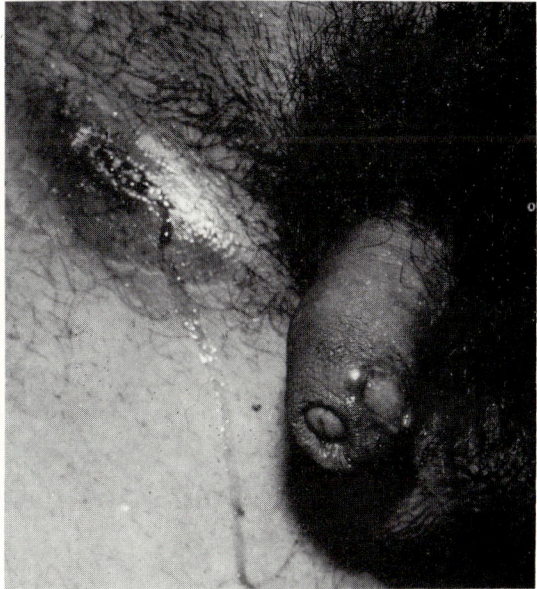

Fig. 3–69

Fig. 3–70

Figure 3–67   Characteristic annular lesion of lichen planus of glans penis.
Figure 3–68   Erythroplasia of Queyrat. Malignant changes may occur in this lesion.
Figure 3–69   Advanced squamous cell epithelioma of penis occurring in a young adult patient.
Figure 3–70   Chancroidal ulcer of penis with associated draining bubo.

Fig. 3–71

Fig. 3–72

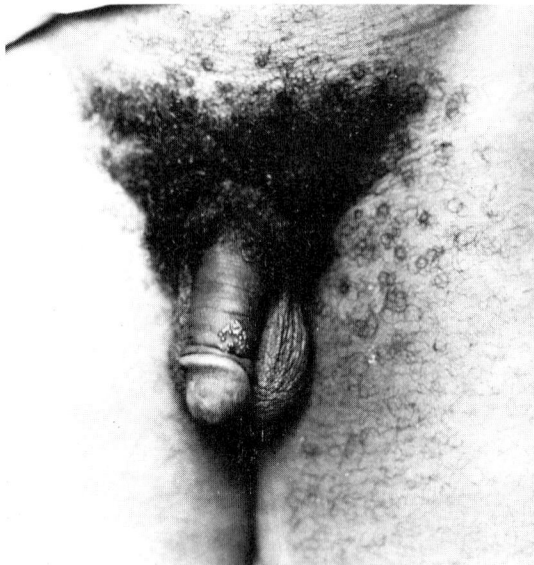
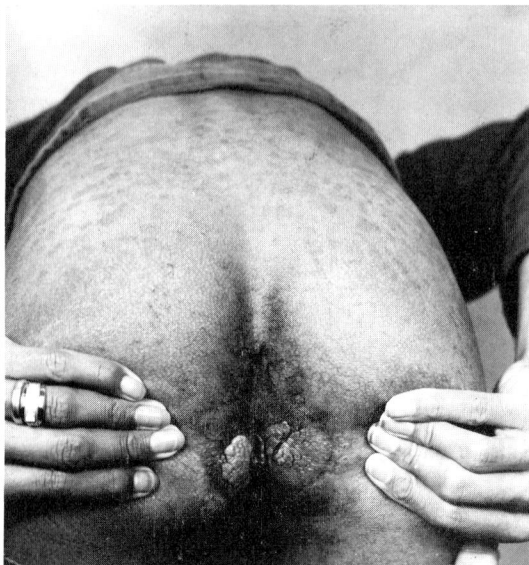

Fig. 3–73

Fig. 3–74

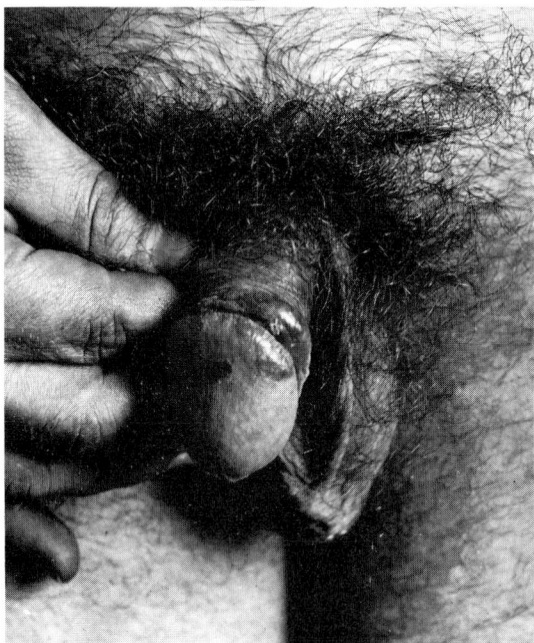
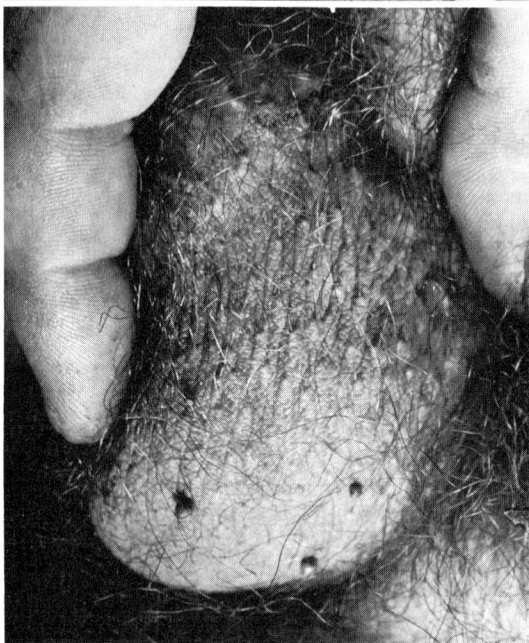

Figure 3–71   Characteristic group lesions of herpes simplex on genitalia (herpes progenitalis).
Figure 3–72   Granuloma inguinale of perianal region.
Figure 3–73   Recurrence of chancre at site of initial lesion, after inadequate treatment.
Figure 3–74   Small angiomatous lesions of scrotum, a common lesion of middle age.

Legs

Dermatoses of the feet and legs have many features in common with those of the hands and arms. There are, however, several affections of the legs, especially the lower legs, that are related in full or in part to peripheral vascular disease, nodular vasculitis, peripheral arteritis, and venostasis. The legs are subject to a considerable amount of exposure, especially in women, and this may lead to marked dryness (ichthyosis). The lower legs inevitably sustain a considerable amount of sharp physical trauma, and this may lead to localized cutaneous or subcutaneous lesions.

In addition to most of the conditions which have been listed as occurring with some frequency on the arms, the following dermatoses, some of them rare, found principally on the lower legs, may be listed:

Dermatitis

Contact dermatitis is common on the legs, distributed to the entire lower leg and lower thigh in women, but usually to the ankles in men, because of differences in type of clothing and the varying degrees of protection afforded by it. The legs are commonly the site of lesions of *nummular dermatitis.* The popliteal space is a characteristic localization of *atopic dermatitis.* The legs are also a fairly frequent site of *localized neurodermatitis.* But far exceeding all these in frequency is dermatitis related to venostasis and edema. This characteristically appears first on the inner lower legs just above the ankle but may be a factor in persistent patches of dermatitis elsewhere. The skin of areas which are the site of venostasis is often *more easily sensitized* than skin in other areas. In topical therapy in such regions, vigilant watch for any evidence of irritation or sensitization should be maintained.

Psoriasis

The prepatellar region is a very common site of localization of psoriasis, probably incident to the trauma to which this region is constantly subjected. Not infrequently, the patches become extremely thick. The buttocks and lower legs are frequently involved as well.

Lichen Planus

While the legs are probably not as frequently involved as some other sites in this disease, it is worthy of note that the lesions on the lower legs are commonly hypertrophic. They may occur as thick large papules which lose the characteristic morphology of a typical lichen planus lesion. In particular, the lower legs may be the site of lichen planus–like (lichenoid) reactions to drugs; for example, antimalarials, gold, phenothiazide, and chlorothiazide.

Infections

Ecthyma, secondarily infected dermatitis.

Lesions Related to Vascular System

The phylogenetic progress of man has not sufficiently advanced to allow him to walk upright without paying a considerable price for this privilege. The most convincing evidence of this is in relation to the bones and joints, wherein a wide variety of physiologic and anatomic changes arise due to the stresses and strains of man's upright position. The vascular system likewise suffers and, secondarily to it, the skin and subcutaneous tissues. The most common manifestation of this is seen as a direct result of venous dilatation and valvular incompetence induced by the steady pounding of columns of blood. In addition, there are other conditions, some of infectious or allergic origin and of considerable medical significance, in which the localization seems in part due to the stresses and strains to which the vascular system of the lower legs is subject. These include, in part, the following:

STASIS DERMATITIS AND ULCERATION. PURPURA, acute and chronic, mild and severe. In an ambulatory patient who develops acute purpura, dependent portions, especially the lower legs, are usually first involved. Not infrequently, the area of purpura about the ankles terminates sharply at the level of the shoe tops.

CHRONIC PURPURIC STATES OF THE LOWER LEGS. These are common. In persons above middle age it is almost always possible to find evidence of hemosiderin deposits which have resulted from prior deposition of red blood cells in the cutis. These may be quite extensive and at times assume rather bizarre patterns in association with various overlying skin lesions. These varying patterns have stimulated observers to describe a variety of different dermatologic syndromes, some

(Text continued on page 168.)

Fig. 3–75

Fig. 3–76

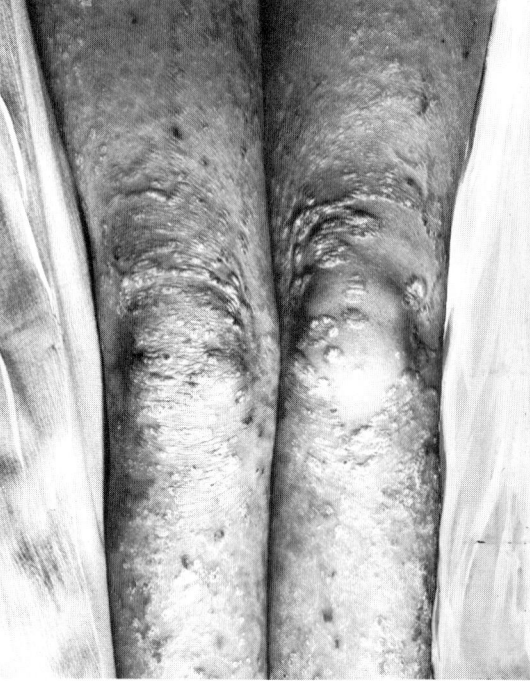
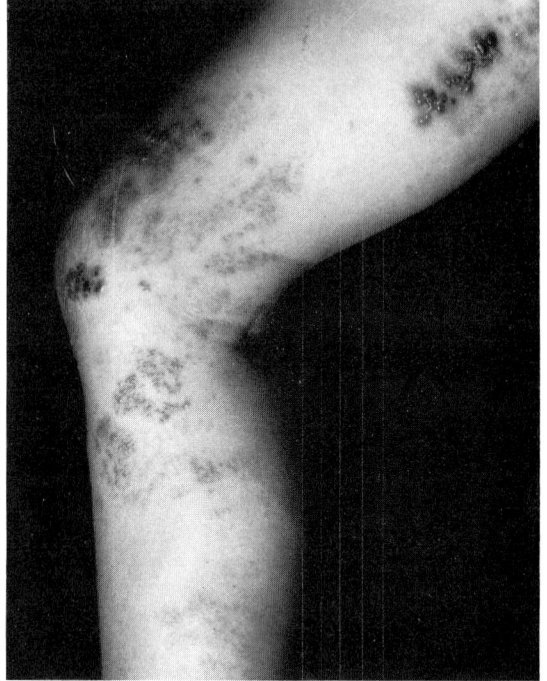

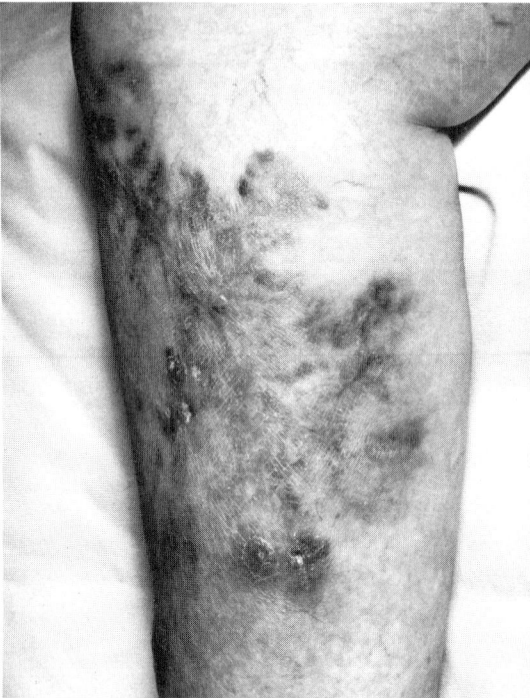
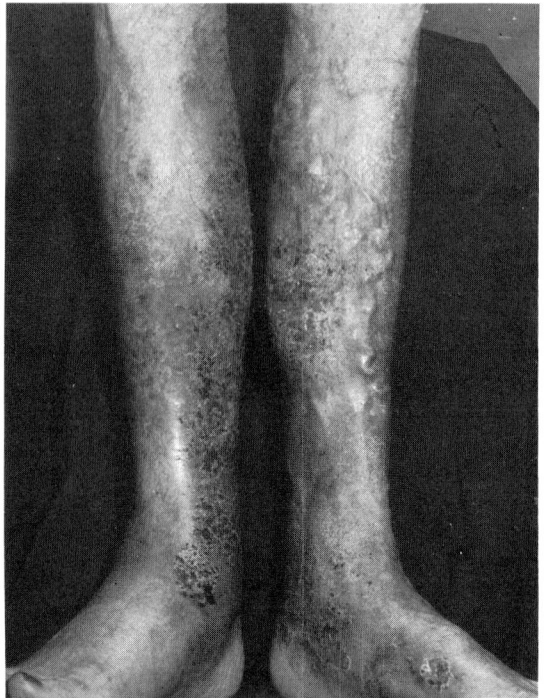

Fig. 3–77

Fig. 3–78

Figure 3–75   Extensive annular and papular lesions of psoriasis of lower legs. Many of the lesions are undergoing confluence, with formation of large plaques.

Figure 3–76   Characteristic grouped inflammatory lesions of herpes zoster of lower leg.

Figure 3–77   Annular lesions of late syphilis of lower leg. Some of the nodules have healed spontaneously, with resultant pigmentation and scarring. Note characteristic annularity.

Figure 3–78   Stasis dermatitis and varicosities of lower legs.

Fig. 3–79

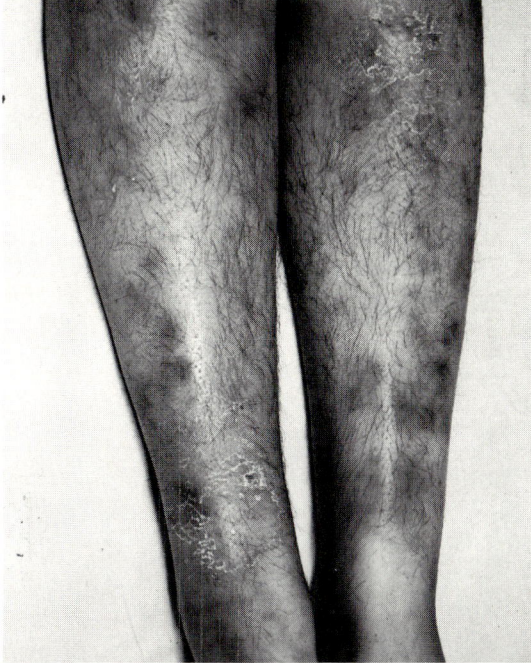

Fig. 3–80

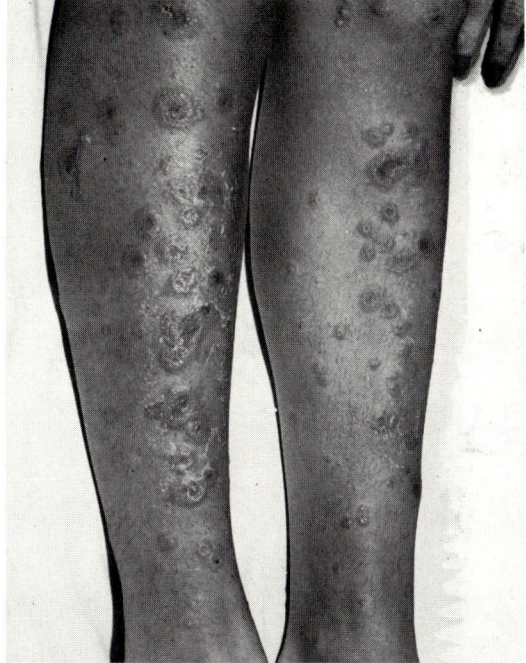

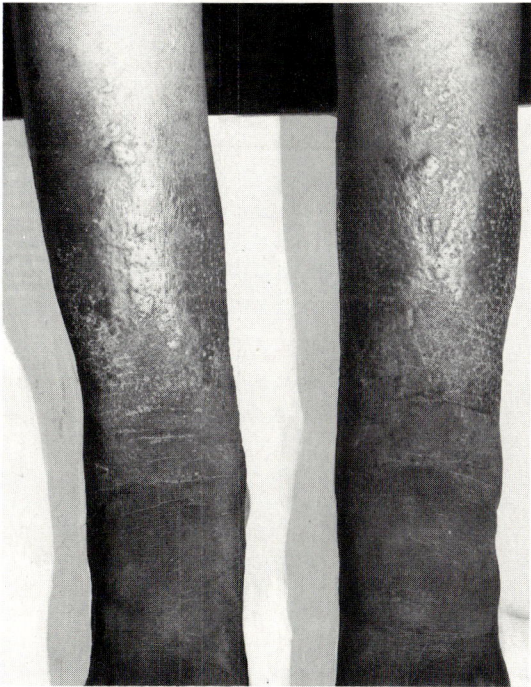

Fig. 3–81

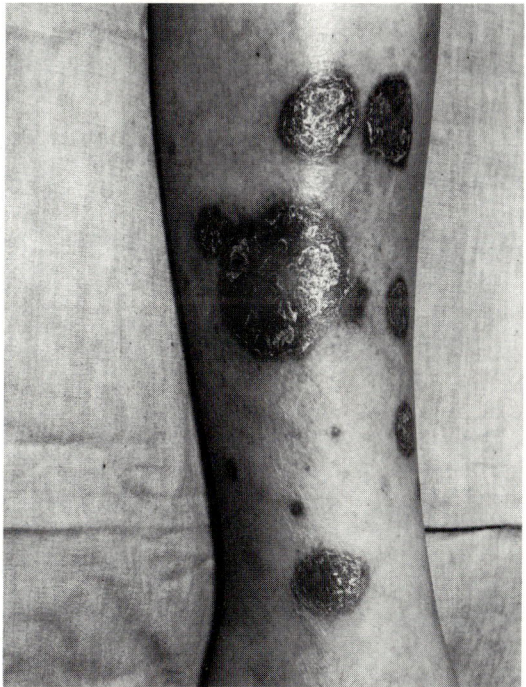

Fig. 3–82

Figure 3–79 Extensive lesions of erythema nodosum of lower legs. This is an important cutaneous sign of possible sytemic disease.

Figure 3–80 Urticarial and beginning bullous lesions of erythema multiforme.

Figure 3–81 Localized myxedema of lower legs, associated with toxic hyperthyroidism.

Figure 3–82 Necrobiosis of lower legs. The condition is frequently associated with diabetes, though not necessarily so. There may be evidences of disturbances of lipid metabolism.

of which even experts find indistinguishable. No specific cause is determinable, as a rule.

ERYTHEMA NODOSUM. This characteristic syndrome may be an exceedingly important sign of early invasive systemic infections, and *must never be regarded lightly.* Its most characteristic localization is over the pretibial surfaces.

Interesting and Significant Rarities

The localization of circumscribed myxedema and of cutaneous amyloidosis to the lower legs is of interest. Necrobiosis (more common in diabetics) is found almost solely in this area.

Feet

The skin of the feet is probably subjected to a greater variety and intensity of trauma than any other portion of the body. The only exception is in exposure to sunlight. The effects of mechanical trauma are numerous. The sole of the foot has a remarkable capacity to respond precisely to the optimal point of thickening in response to the trauma of walking. However, this trauma is sometimes so unevenly distributed by the effects of shoes or by underlying bone and joint abnormalities that it leads to a wide variety of inflammatory and hyperkeratotic responses. Occasionally, vesiculation may result from very moderate mechanical stimulus ("acquired" epidermolysis bullosa, rare). Or there may be an inborn tendency to keratosis of the palms and soles (in mild to moderate forms not uncommon). In patients with abnormal reaction patterns of the skin to trauma, such as in psoriasis, lesions of this disease may be quite sharply localized on the skin of the foot.

Man has had only a comparatively few generations in which to become adapted to the wearing of shoes. The occlusive, traumatic, and potentially sensitizing environment induced by civilized footwear has exacted a considerable toll, dermatologically and orthopedically. Conditions for the growth of bacteria and fungi are ideal, especially in persons with hyperhidrosis. In addition, footwear of modern design includes a wide variety of materials capable of sensitizing the skin, including particularly cements and glues, dyes, plastics, and various chemicals used in the preparation of leather. Reactions produced by these are ordinarily diagnosed initially as fungal infections.

All in all, the lot of the skin of the feet is not a happy one; the diseases affecting it are numerous, and adequate treatment often is impossible if the patient is ambulatory and "on his feet." The chief regional diagnostic considerations in dermatoses of the feet are as follows:

Superficial Inflammatory Conditions

A number of seemingly distinct affections are grouped under this heading, because, though they are frequently quite easily differentiated elsewhere on the skin surface, they do not commonly exist in "pure" uncomplicated form on the feet.

SUPERFICIAL RINGWORM INFECTIONS. Though rarely seen in children, infections of this type are common in young adults. They have a reasonably characteristic distribution on the foot (see p. 639). In most patients with chronic, subacute, or acute fungal infections of the feet, it is an error to consider the invasion of the dead stratum corneum by fungi as the only precipitating factor. There is, variably, some abnormality of sweating, some degree of associated bacterial invasion, some trauma from walking and scratching, and frequent irritation or sensitization from treatment.

BACTERIAL INFECTIONS. The bacterial count of the normal skin of the feet is very high. Pathogenic bacteria may gain a foothold quite easily. Moreover, the opportunities for invasion of these bacteria into and below the skin are numerous through inflammatory vesicles, traumatic blisters, and fissures. An overt bacterial infection which produces marked localized cellulitis and involvement of lymphatics is ordinarily promptly recognized, and the treatment of it presents no great problem. Less invasive bacterial infections are, however, common and frequently overlooked.

EFFECTS OF MOISTURE. Patients vary greatly in the amount of perspiration from the feet. In addition, most persons are careless about drying the feet thoroughly after bathing. As a result, sodden epider-

Fig. 3–83

Fig. 3–84

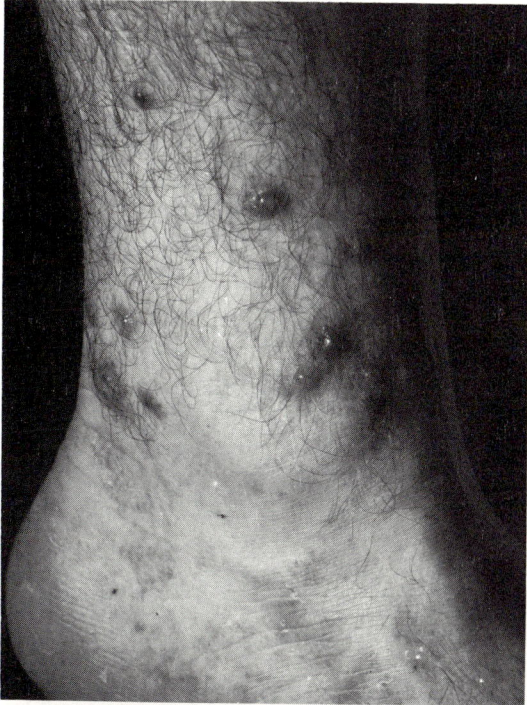

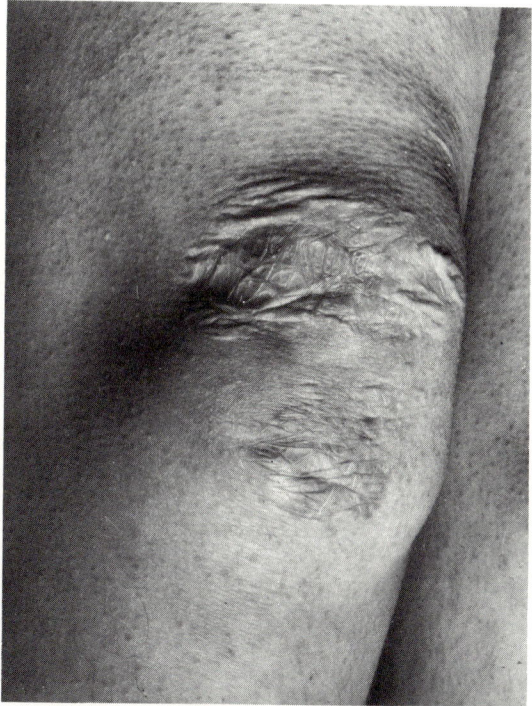

Fig. 3–85

Fig. 3–86

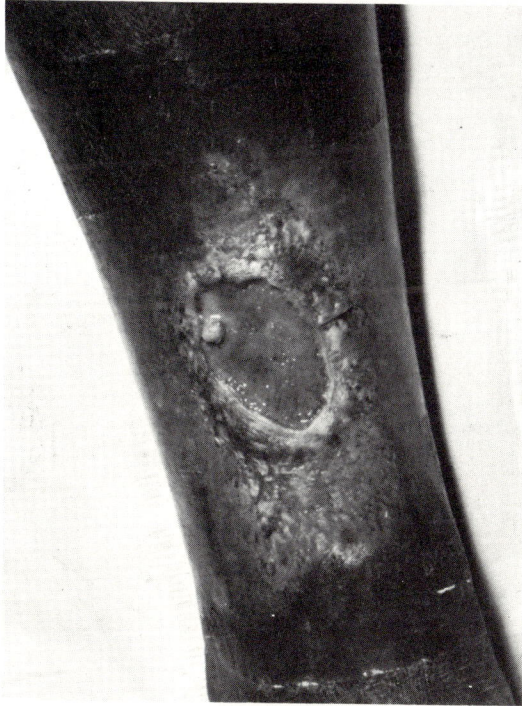

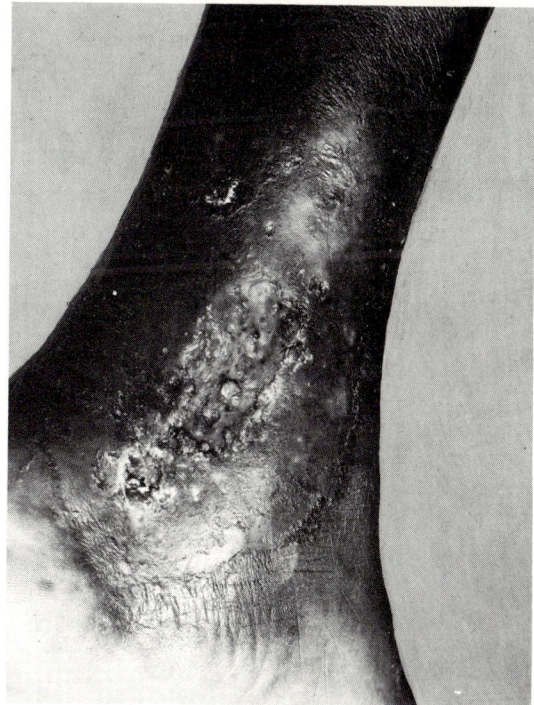

Figure 3–83 Vesicular and inflammatory reaction to insect bites. Type of insect not established.
Figure 3–84 Characteristic fragility and scarring of the skin of prepatellar region in association with Ehlers-Danlos syndrome.
Figure 3–85 Long-standing ulcer associated with stasis.
Figure 3–86 Ulceration of inner lower leg in a patient with sickle cell anemia.

Fig. 3–87

Fig. 3–88

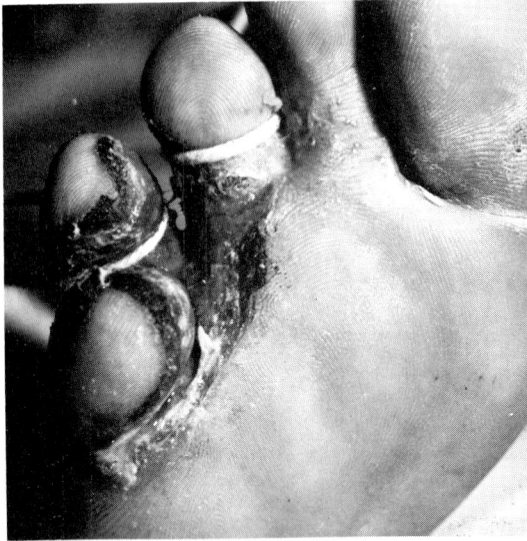
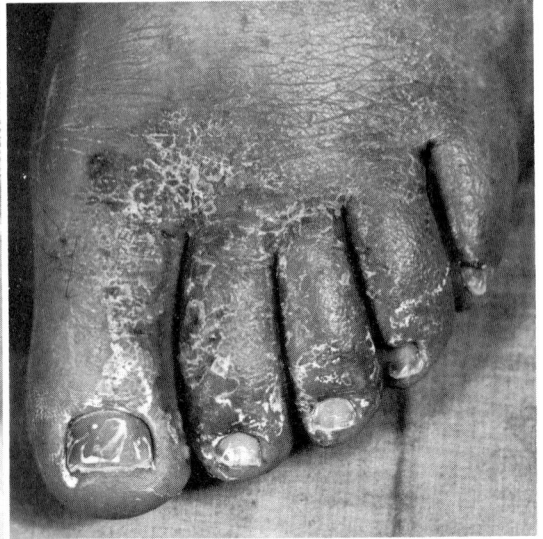

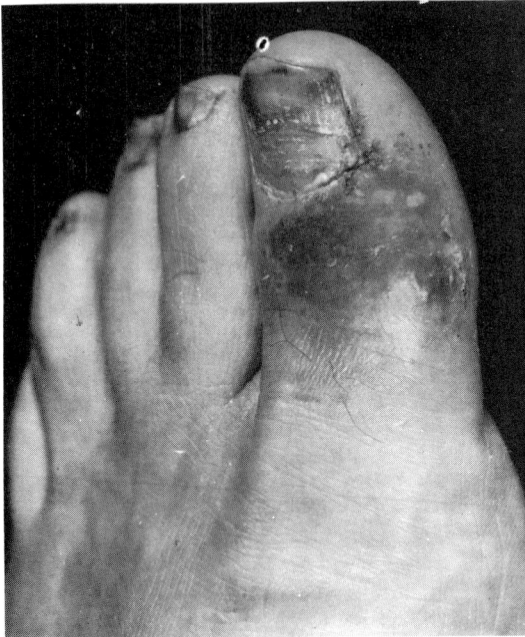
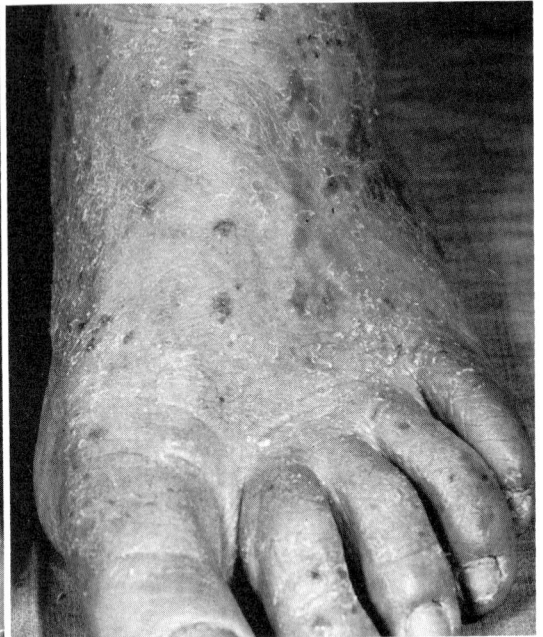

Fig. 3–89

Fig. 3–90

Figure 3–87   Severe intertriginous inflammatory reaction and fissuring of toes. This condition is not necessarily fungal in origin.

Figure 3–88   Secondary intertrigo and treatment reaction in patient with chronic *T. rubrum* infection.

Figure 3–89   Chronic inflammation at site of rubbing on great toe. Beta-hemolytic streptococci were recoverable. A combination of antibacterial therapy and prevention of trauma was curative.

Figure 3–90   Lesions of atopic dermatitis on feet; to be differentiated from contact dermatitis.

mis and debris are common, especially between the toes, furnishing an excellent starting point for all types of superficial infection and for the development of fissures.

VIRAL INFECTIONS.   Of these, plantar warts are by far the most common. Herpes simplex and zoster on the feet are uncommon. Warts are decidedly contagious, both to the patient's own skin and to that of

Fig. 3–91

Fig. 3–92

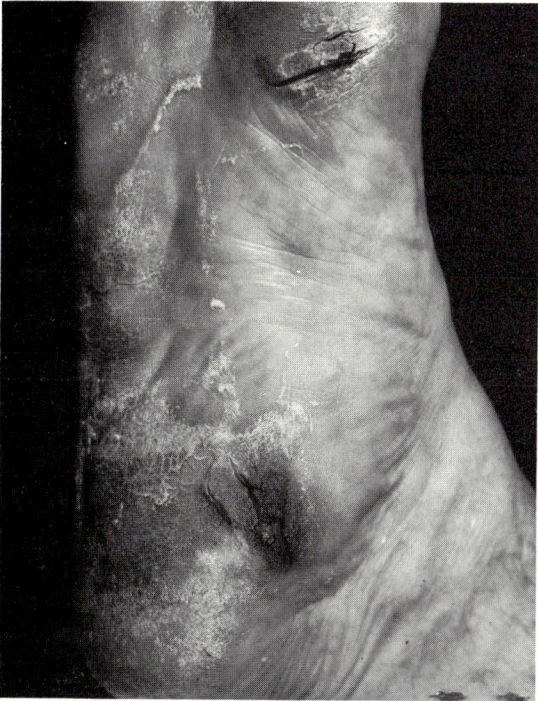

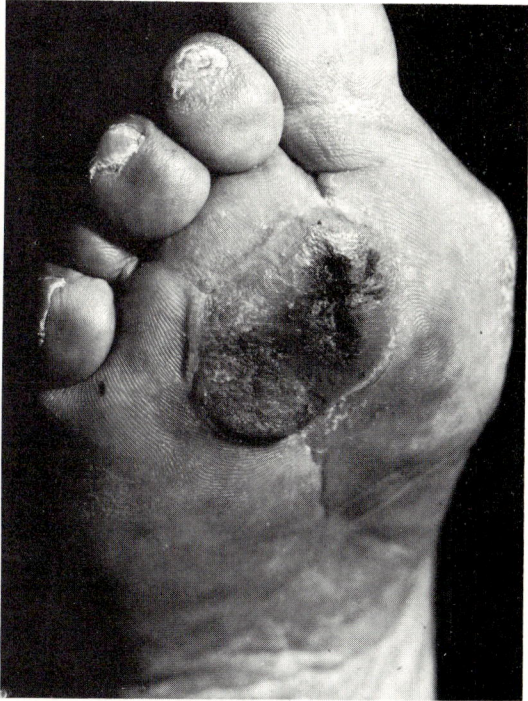

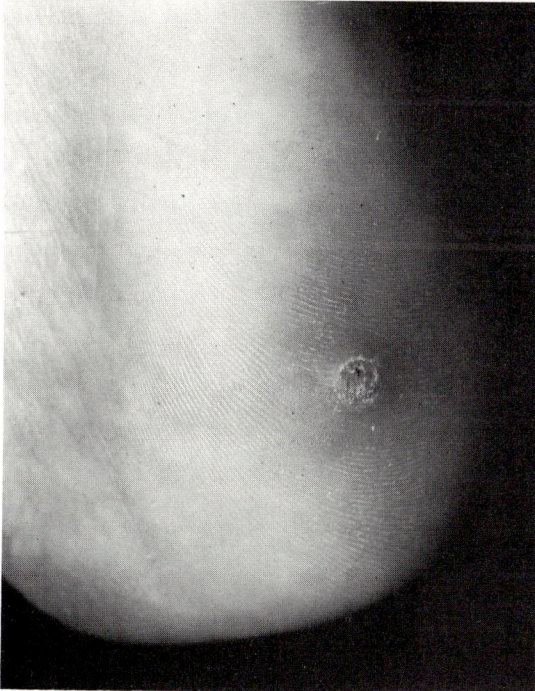

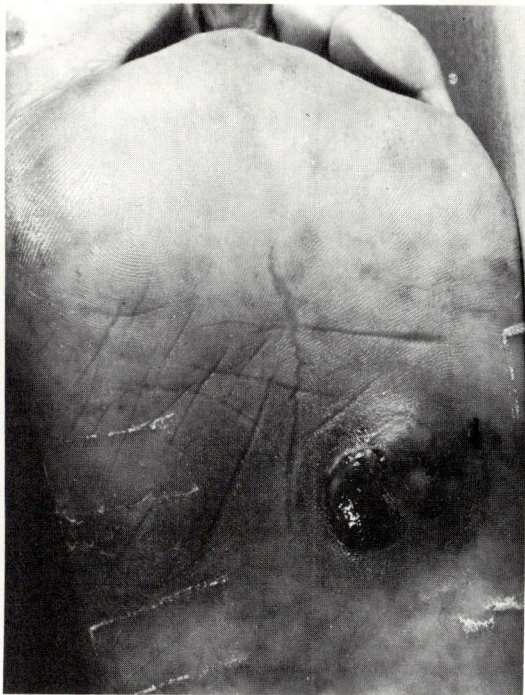

Fig. 3–93

Fig. 3–94

Figure 3–91 Sharply outlined keratotic and fissured lesions of psoriasis of the sole.
Figure 3–92 Trophic ulcer (malum perforans) of sole.
Figure 3–93 Typical single plantar wart on inner side of heel.
Figure 3–94 Melanoma of sole developing at site of junction nevus. The lower legs and feet are a vulnerable area for the development of melanoma.

others. Plantar warts differ from warts elsewhere on the body in that they produce pain. Any method of removal of warts on pressure points which results in deep scarring may substitute an incurable painful lesion for a potentially curable one.

MISCELLANEOUS. The papules of secondary syphilis frequently occur on the soles, in association with the palms. The feet are a not uncommon site of reactions to medicaments taken internally, and again there may be coincident involvement of the hands. Such rare affections as keratosis blennorrhagica may be seen on the feet.

Tumors

Tumors of the skin arising from the adnexal structures are uncommon on the feet. *Melanoma* frequently arises on the feet and lower legs. Assessment of nevi on the feet may offer a difficult problem, especially since excision of the nevus from a weight-bearing surface may produce a painful scar. Kaposi's sarcoma, though an uncommon disease, is much more frequently seen on the feet than anywhere else.

Ulcers

These frequently offer much difficulty in diagnosis; they may result from peripheral arterial disease, repeated trauma, neurologic disorders or various types of infection.

TYPES OF SKIN LESIONS

The diagnosis of a disease affecting the skin is dependent upon accurate morphologic classification of the individual skin lesions. In those diseases in which the skin is the only organ involved, in which there is no systemic disturbance nor any decisive information obtainable by laboratory studies, the morphologic characteristics of the lesions themselves furnish the only diagnostic clues.

The presenting skin lesions of a dermatosis are describable in straightforward, simple terms. There is no need to use an obsolescent or esoteric terminology. The essential facts to be noted are:

1. The distribution or special localization of lesions.
2. Physical characteristics.
   a. Solid or containing fluid (serum or pus).
   b. Size, shape, and color.
   c. If palpable, any special characteristics (but avoid aimless and indiscriminate "pawing" of lesions).

Many conditions of the skin, especially chronic ones, present a variety of lesions. With few exceptions, however, a skin disease in the individual patient is usually characterized initially by a single type of lesion, and this may be pathognomonic. It is the mark of the expert, in any field of medicine or surgery, that he is able to sort out the presenting signs and symptoms in a complicated pathologic condition and to determine which finding is basically most representative of the disease. This faculty is particularly helpful in classifying diseases of the skin. Among the mélange of presenting skin lesions, papules, pustules, crusts, and so forth, it is ordinarily possible to determine which type of lesion came first and gave rise to the chain of secondary or consequential lesions. Among the debris of a chronic dermatosis, the characteristic primary lesion represents true diagnostic treasure.

In the following sections, the essential morphologic groups of skin lesions are defined briefly and illustrated by common examples. Some lesions are pathognomonic. For others, a differential diagnostic list becomes the starting point for unraveling the diagnostic puzzle. A word of warning is essential. Too great dependence upon the morphologic skin changes alone in arriving at a diagnosis may, with many diseases, lead to neglect of the patient as a whole and to erroneous interpretations. One must study the patient as well as the skin.

Macule

This is simply a flat circumscribed *change in the color* of the skin. The term ordinarily connotes lesions of relatively small size, up to 1 or 2 cm.; larger than this, changes in color are ordinarily re-

(Text continued on page 177.)

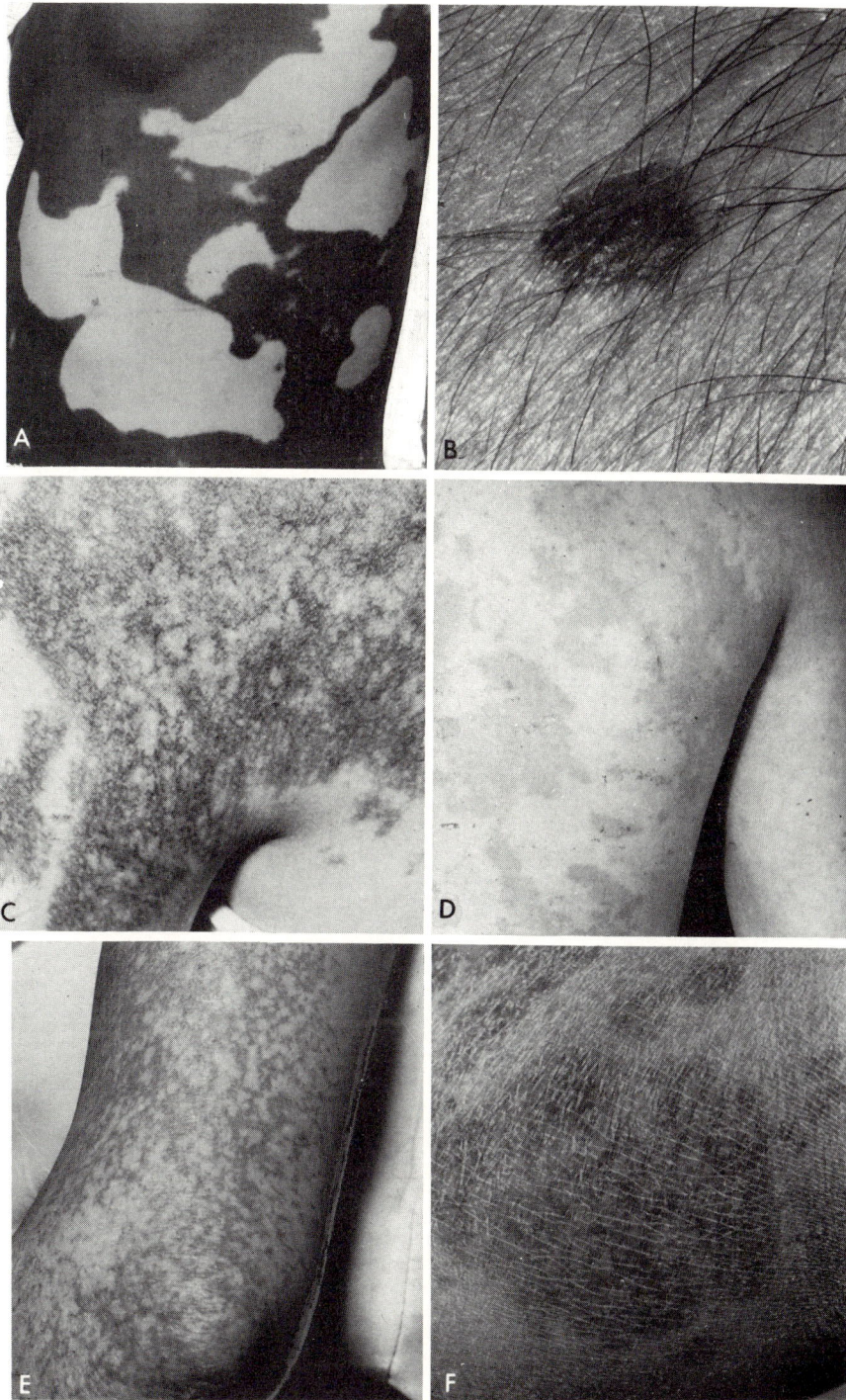

Figure 3–95 Representative macular and flat patchy lesions. *A*, Bizarre disfiguring patches of vitiligo. *B*, Flat pigmented nevus. Probably the single most common skin lesion; few individuals have none. *C*, Extensive flat angioma (portwine mark). *D*, Macular, slightly scaling pigmented patches of tinea versicolor. *E*, Extensive macular reaction to drug (aspirin). Differentiate from infectious disease. Look for other "shock sites," especially bone marrow, in drug eruptions. *F*, Residual pigmentation of fixed drug eruption (phenolphthalein). Erythema and increased residual color after each dose.

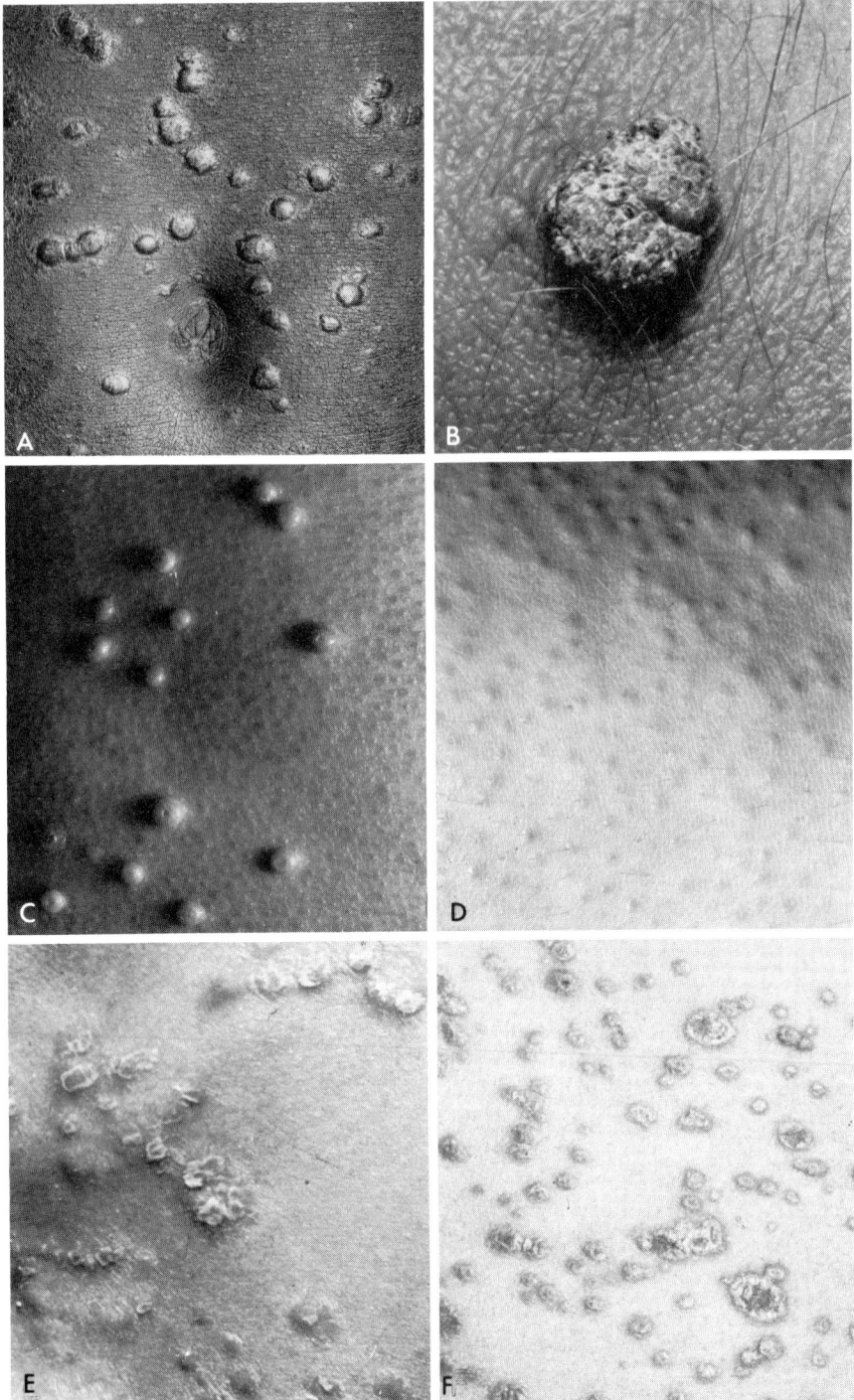

Figure 3–96   Examples of papules. *A*, Profuse papular eruption of early syphilis. Rather indurated lesions, suggestive in character, but dependent on confirmative clinical and laboratory evidence for diagnosis. *B*, A fairly large common wart. Diagnosis ordinarily obvious. *C*, Molluscum contagiosum. A highly characteristic viral infection. *D*, Miliaria profunda. Due to obstruction of sweat ducts deep in skin. *E*, Characteristic, almost pathognomonic, papules of psoriasis. Note typical scaling and also tendency to annular arrangement. *F*, Lichen planus. Usually a highly characteristic papule. Note flat tops, angularity, and tendency for papules to form a circle.

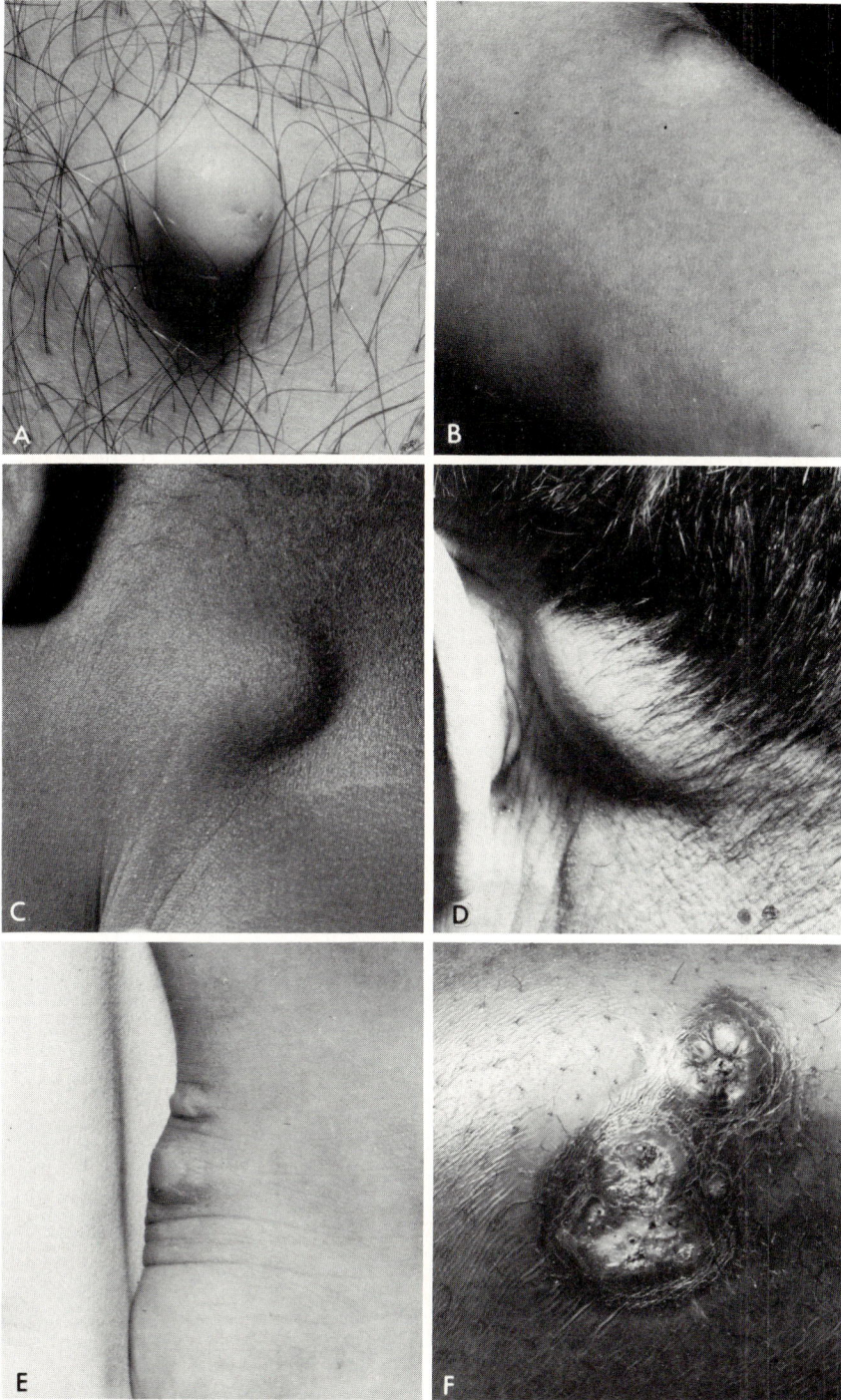

Figure 3–97 Examples of nodules. *A*, Typical superficial keratinous cyst. Often multiple. In scalp, called a wen. *B*, Soft nodules of neurofibromatosis (von Recklinghausen's disease). *C*, Large nontender lymph node in association with primary inoculation tuberculosis of skin. Typical of chancre-bubo (primary) complex. *D*, Lipoma. Often multiple; sometimes huge. *E*, Xanthoma tuberosum. Typical location over tendon. Usually yellow. *F*, Portion of chain of sporotrichotic nodules which are beginning to break down.

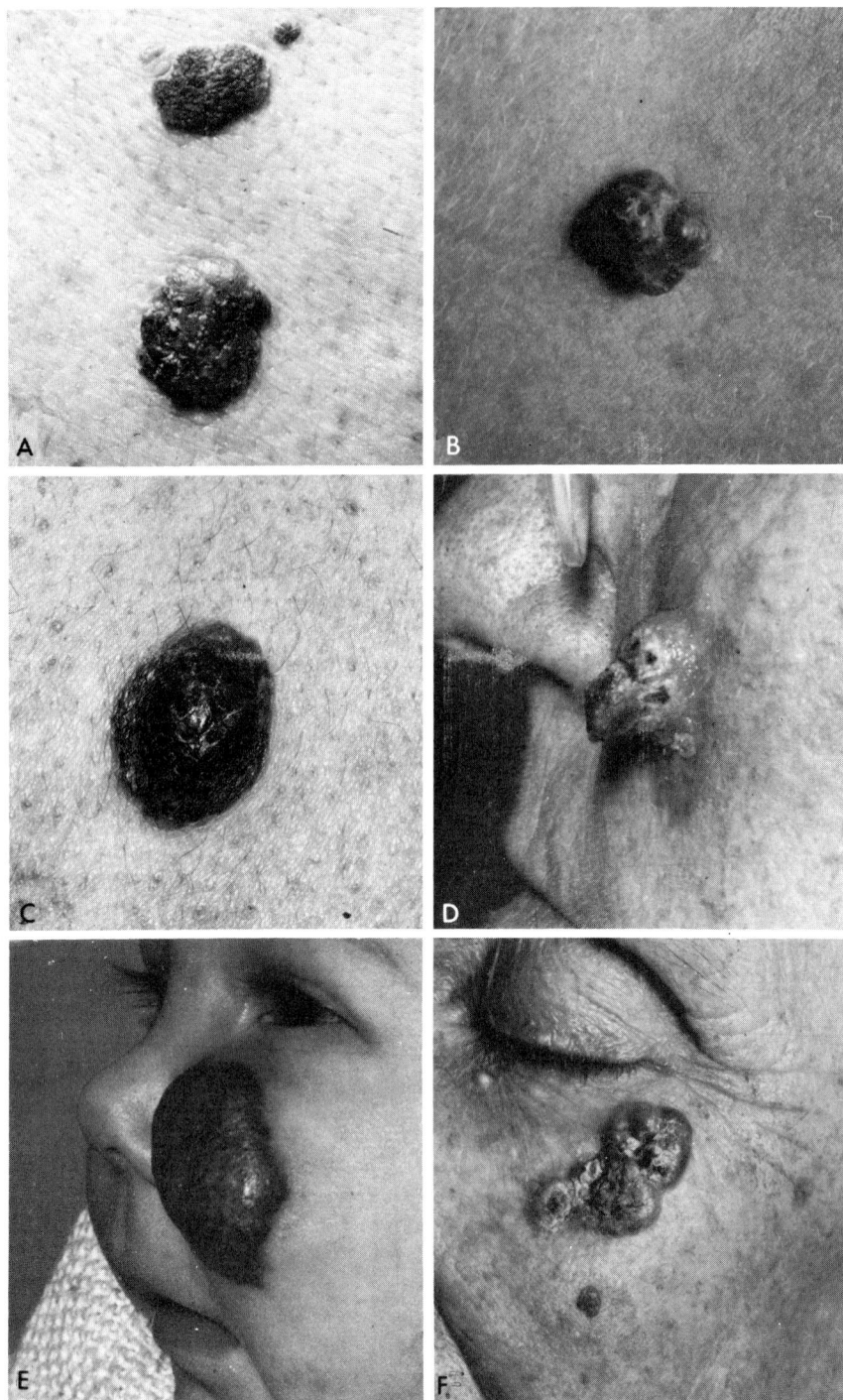

Figure 3–98 Examples of tumors. *A*, Seborrheic keratoses. Very characteristic common benign lesion. Light to very dark in color. Often greasy scale. *B*, Pyogenic granuloma. Common lesion, often misdiagnosed. Extremely vascular; may bleed profusely on injury or at time of removal. *C*, Melanoma (nodular type). The most unpredictable and vicious of all malignant lesions of skin. *D*, Cutaneous horn on top of squamous cell cancer. *E*, Cavernous hemangioma. *F*, Pigmented basal cell (nonmetastasizing) epithelioma. Slow-growing, but relentlessly invasive.

ferred to as patches or areas. Macular processes are of three general types:

Due to Extrinsically Derived Colored Materials. Tattoo marks, imbedded material from lacerations or explosions.

Intrinsically Derived Pigment. Flat moles, freckles, petechiae and hemorrhages, localized increase or absence of melanin.

Erythematous Reactions to a great variety of pathogenic agents and stresses. In the presence of systemic reaction, or if there are purpuric changes in the lesions, macules may be an extremely important sign of systemic disease.

Papules, Nodules, and Tumors

These are solid lesions of the skin which differ in size and in their location within the skin and subcutaneous tissue.

Papules are circumscribed elevations of the skin, varying roughly from a millimeter to a centimeter in size. Larger infiltrated areas are often called plaques.

Nodules are circumscribed, usually solid lesions which are often deeper in the skin or subcutaneous tissues. The term is frequently applied to inflammatory processes, for example, erythema nodosum, but often refers to tumors. Among the nodular lesions which are painful to the touch are neuroma, leiomyoma, eccrine spiradenoma, glomus tumor, and chondrodermatitis chronica helicis.

Tumor. The term tumor ordinarily designates larger and deeper circumscribed infiltrations of the skin or subcutaneous tissue. It is also commonly used to describe lesions which are obviously neoplastic, regardless of size or location.

Wheals (Hives)

A wheal is a special type of papule. It is usually sharply circumscribed, as in a mosquito bite, though sometimes it involves a wide area (angioneurotic edema). It is usually evanescent, white to pink in color, and often has a "pigskin" appearance due to upward swelling of skin about hairs which are firmly anchored below. Hives are often a part of many inflammatory eruptions; for example, erythema multiforme, drug eruptions, and dermatitis. If the marked tissue edema overflows and becomes intercellular, vesicles or bullae

may form. In unusual forms of low-grade erythema multiforme (erythema perstans), the wheal may persist for long periods, often progressing slowly in an annular fashion.

Vesicles and Bullae

These are sharply circumscribed collections of free fluid. A bulla is a large vesicle. Common examples of diseases with vesicles are contact dermatitis, pompholyx, and herpes simplex. Large vesicles or bullae represent a very marked reaction of the skin, in effect a vigorous effort to counteract the effects of physical trauma or to dilute or drown a noxious agent. Bullae may be evidence of severe skin injury or of serious systemic disease. Careful study to determine their origin is always indicated.

Pustules

A pustule is a circumscribed collection of free pus—in essence, a very superficial abscess of the skin. Combinations of vesicles and pustules in lesions are quite common; hence, the term vesiculopustular. As do vesicles, pustules vary in size from tiny (miliary) to the equivalent of bullae. However, larger pustules ordinarily rupture promptly. The presence of cloudy fluid in a pustule does not necessarily signify infection; many pustular lesions are sterile. Pustules are sometimes confined almost entirely to the hair follicles (follicular impetigo or pustular folliculitis) or to the sweat glands, as in pustular miliaria. The latter relation is often not apparent from superficial examination, however. Certain dermatoses such as subcorneal pustulosis, pustular psoriasis, Reiter's disease, and acrodermatitis continua have pustules as their primary lesions.

Pustular lesions of the skin cover a wide range of conditions from banal unimportant eruptions to extremely chronic dermatoses and to manifestations of systemic disease. Representative pustular conditions are illustrated in Figure 3–101.

Certain skin lesions are not part of the primary changes of a dermatosis, but are *evolutionary*—for example, crusts from drying of serous oozing or *scars* from the replacement of destroyed tissue; others are *added* or *complicating* lesions—for example, alteration produced by scratching

(Text continued on page 180.)

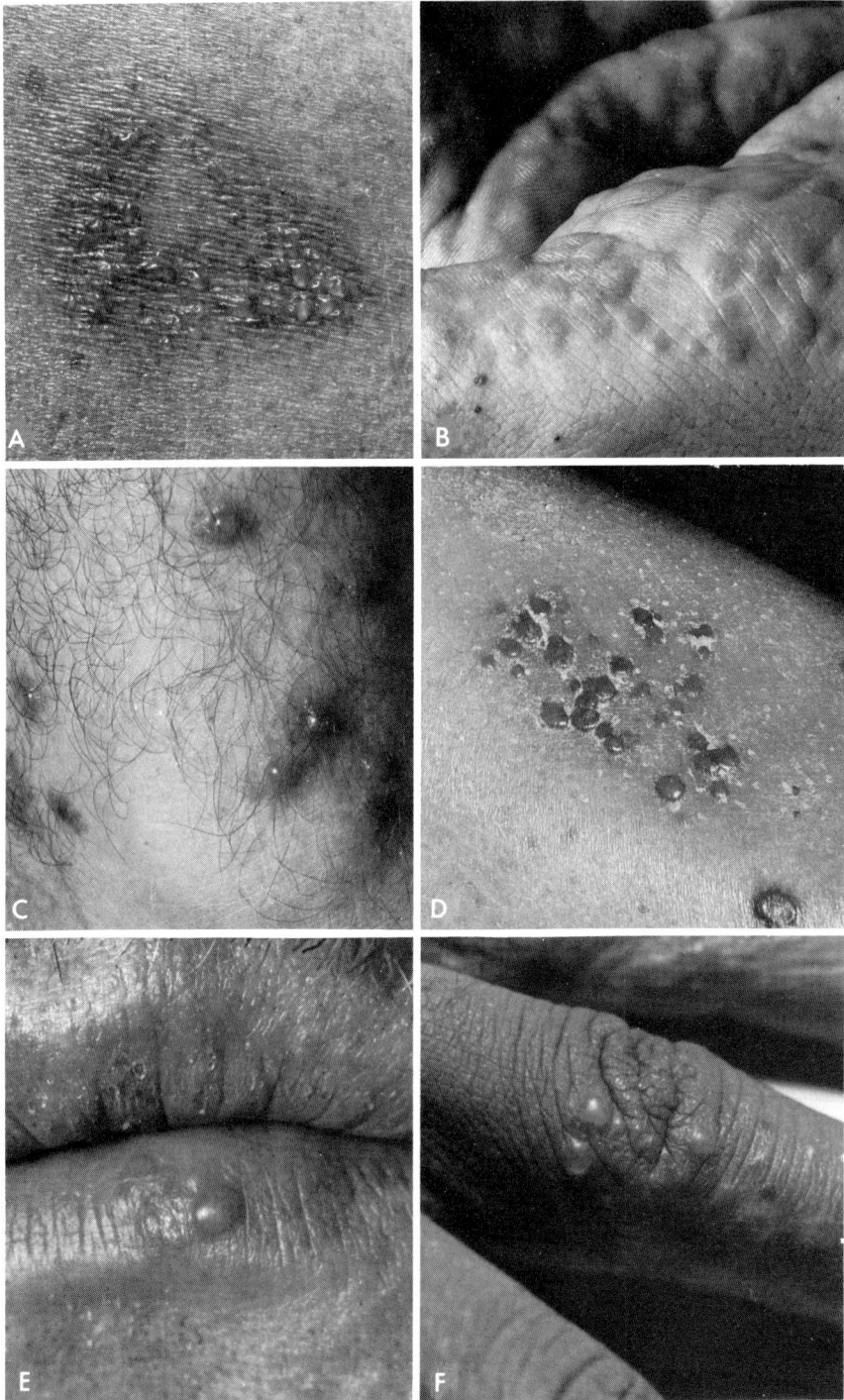

Figure 3–99 Examples of vesicles. *A,* Erythema and minute vesicles at site of positive patch test reaction (penicillin). *B,* Diffuse dyshidrosis of hands. A morphologic pattern which is poorly understood in respect to causation. *C,* Vesicles with inflamed bases at sites of insect bites, probably fleas. Usual reaction is a wheal, but degree of response is dependent upon the sensitivity to the host. Some individuals do not react at all. *D,* Typical grouped vesicles of herpes zoster, a highly characteristic sign. Remains of a drying shake lotion are seen. *E,* Very early herpes simplex. Prodromal tingling and slight burning. *F,* Vesicles of fingers occurring in patient with severe reaction to hair dye.

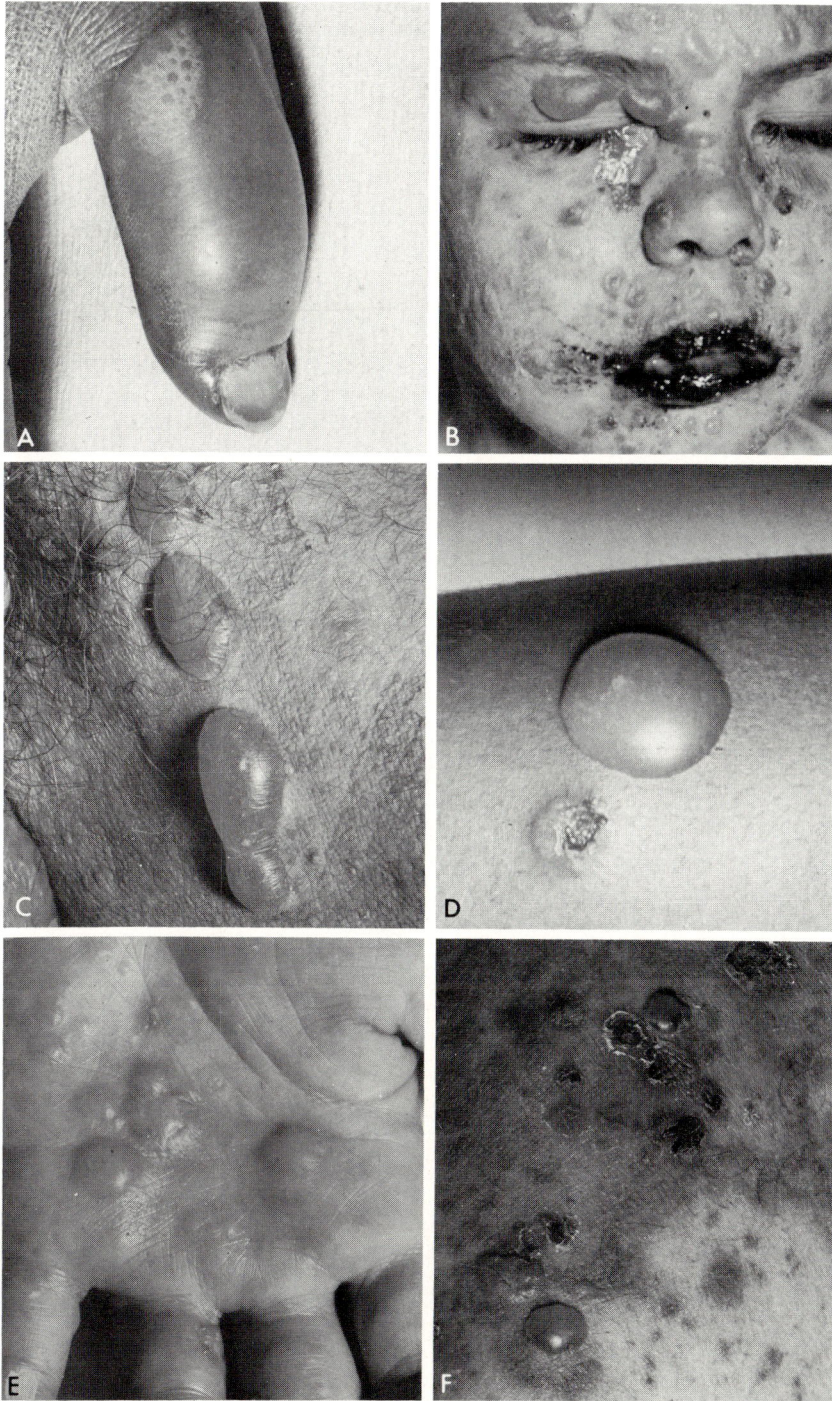

Figure 3–100 Examples of bullous lesions. *A*, Bulla from second degree burn. Relieve symptoms by draining serous contents, but save keratinous wall. *B*, Vesicles, bullae, and mucous membrane involvement in severe erythema multiforme (Stevens-Johnson type). *C*, Bullae of pemphigus. No inflammation at base. Diagnosis accurately establishable by cytologic or histologic examination. *D*, Bullous impetigo. Contents initially clear, but becoming purulent within a few hours. *E*, Bullae of palm due to "id" reaction. Vesicles often coalesce into larger lesions. *F*, Bullous lichen planus. An example of a marked deviation from the standard pattern of a disease.

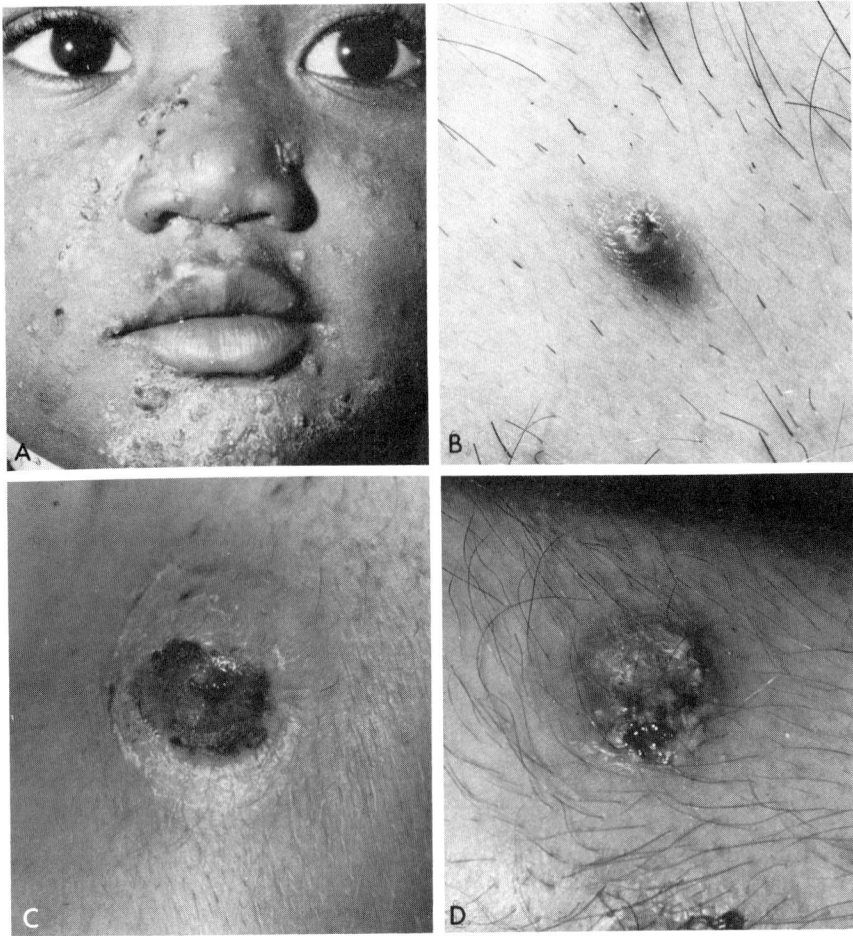

Figure 3–101   Examples of pustular dermatoses. *A*, Diffuse impetigo in child. Some lesions new and pustular, others older and crusted. *B*, Acneiform pustule due to industrial contact with paraffin oils. Usually confined to exposed areas or to sites of contact with oil-soaked clothing. *C*, Typical furuncle; some spontaneous drainage has already occurred. Often multiple and recurrent. *D*, Bromoderma. A granulomatous pustular drug eruption. Iodides may produce same picture.

(excoriation) or fissures over joints in areas of dermatitis or infection. These lesions should not be considered as something separate or distinct but rather as signs which are of aid in interpreting the *dynamic* pathologic forces involved in the disease. They are of great aid in judging whether or not a particular process is acute or chronic, and if the latter, how long it has been present.

Evolutionary changes include:

Scales

These are simply accumulations of loose, horny fragments of stratum corneum. Certain types of scales are quite characteristic —for example, the greasy, rather yellowish scales of the seborrheic state, or the silvery, piled-up scales of psoriasis—but it is not possible to interpret the underlying disease very closely on the basis of varying appearances in this end stage of keratinization.

Ulcers

A destructive process which removes the epidermis and extends into the dermis results in an ulcer. Ulcers vary from small, very superficial erosions of the epidermis to deep and sometimes widespread destructive lesions in which the underlying tissues, even adjacent bone, may undergo (*Text continued on page 185.*)

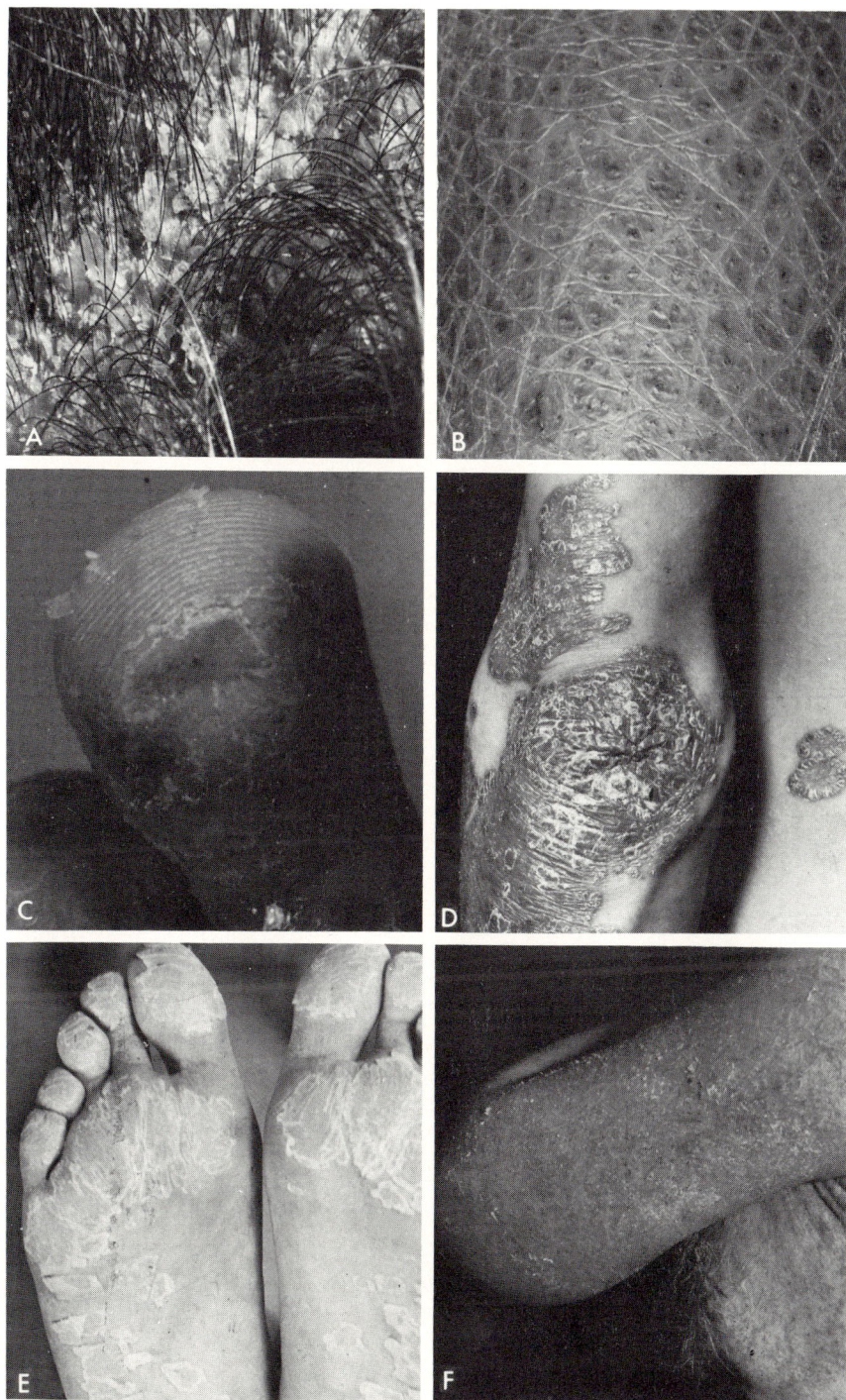

Figure 3–102 Various types of scaling. *A*, Heavy seborrheic scaling of scalp. *B*, Characteristic "fish skin" appearance of adherent scales of ichthyosis on legs. *C*, Scaling of chronic dermatophytosis of feet. Between toes, scales may become a sodden adherent mass. *D*, Characteristic lesions and scaling of psoriasis. *E*, Diffuse scaling after scarlet fever. Often very marked and prolonged on palms and soles. *F*, Scaling following contact dermatitis from antihistaminic ointment.

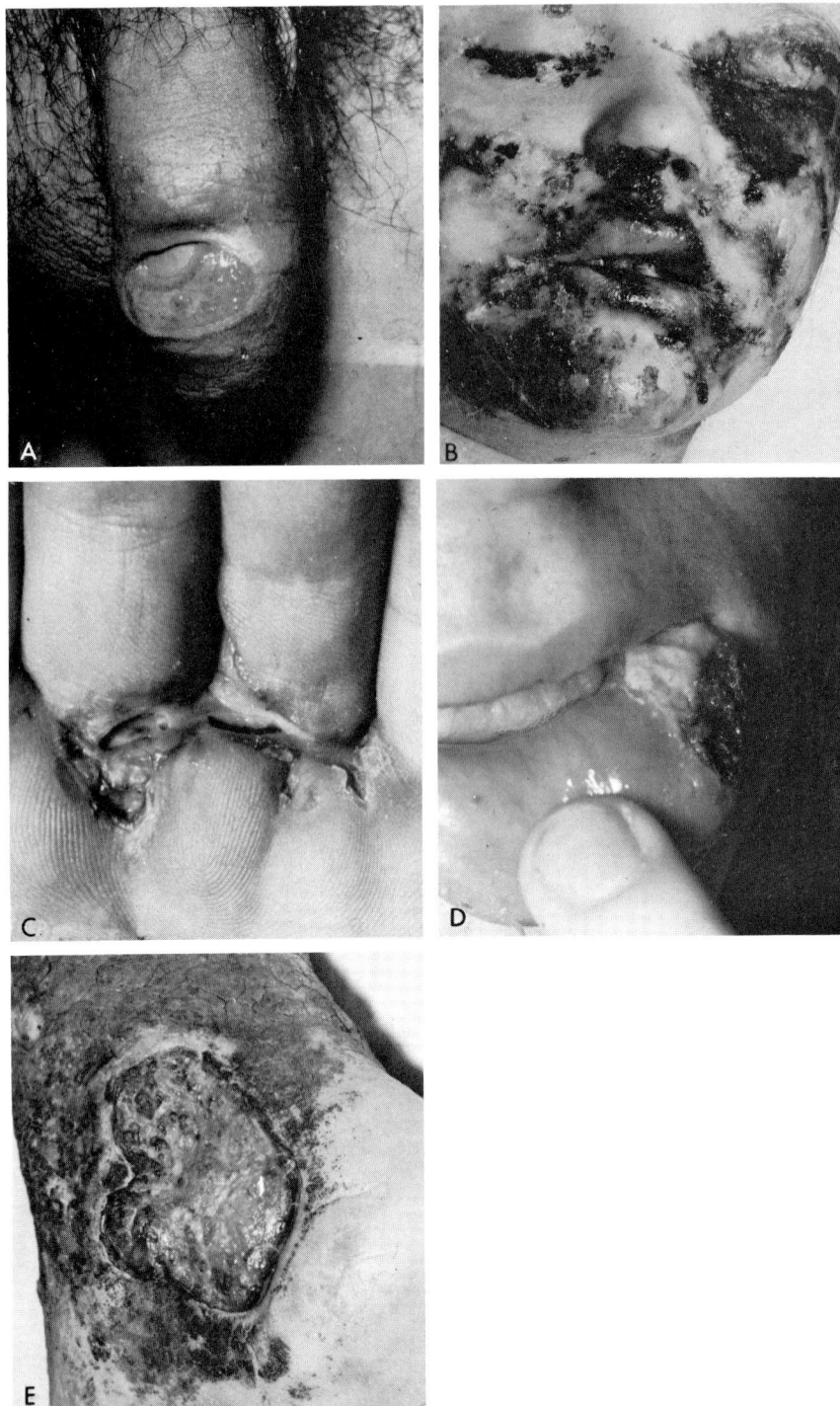

Figure 3–103   Examples of ulcers. *A*, Large late healing ulcer of chancroid. Still a common disease, especially among overseas military personnel. *B*, Hemorrhagic crusting disseminated herpes simplex of the face in a patient with terminal leukemia. *C*, Severe chronic infected fissures at proximal joint of fingers. *D*, Chancre of syphilis on lip. Large associated bubo. *E*, Highly anaplastic squamous cell carcinoma at site of "stasis" ulcer; basal cell carcinoma is a more frequent malignant complication.

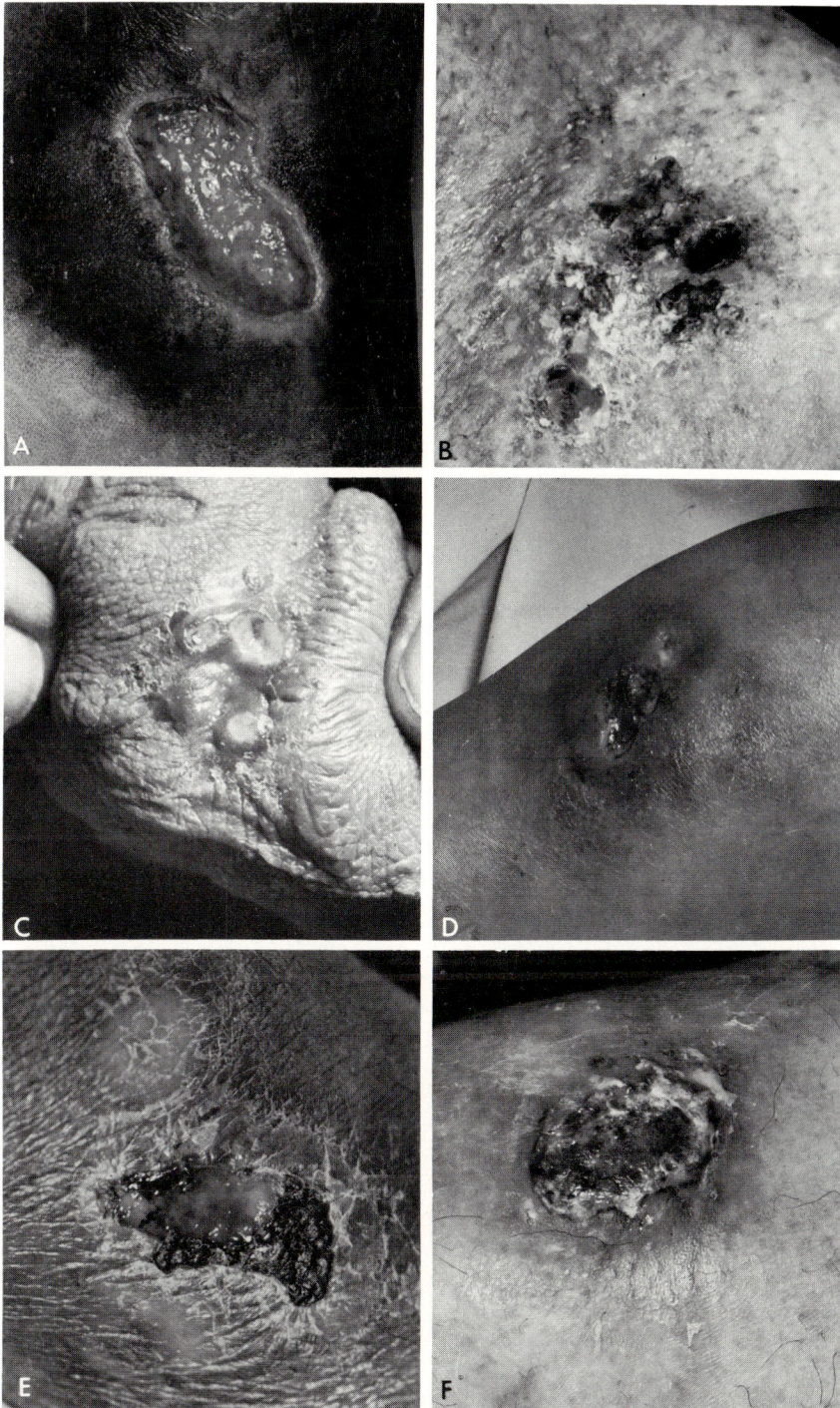

Figure 3–104 Examples of ulcers. *A,* Very chronic ulcer of inner ankle in area of scarring and hyperpigmentation, in patient with hypertensive cardiovascular disease. *B,* Multiple ulcers (cancer?) in area of x-ray atrophy. The time for medical therapy has passed. Surgical excision and repair essential. *C,* Early multiple ulcers of chancroid in sulcus of penis. *D,* Ulcers of calf due to breakdown of syphilitic gummas. A very characteristic lesion. *E,* Persistent ecthymatous ulcer. *F,* Ulcer of erythema induratum (tuberculous panniculitis).

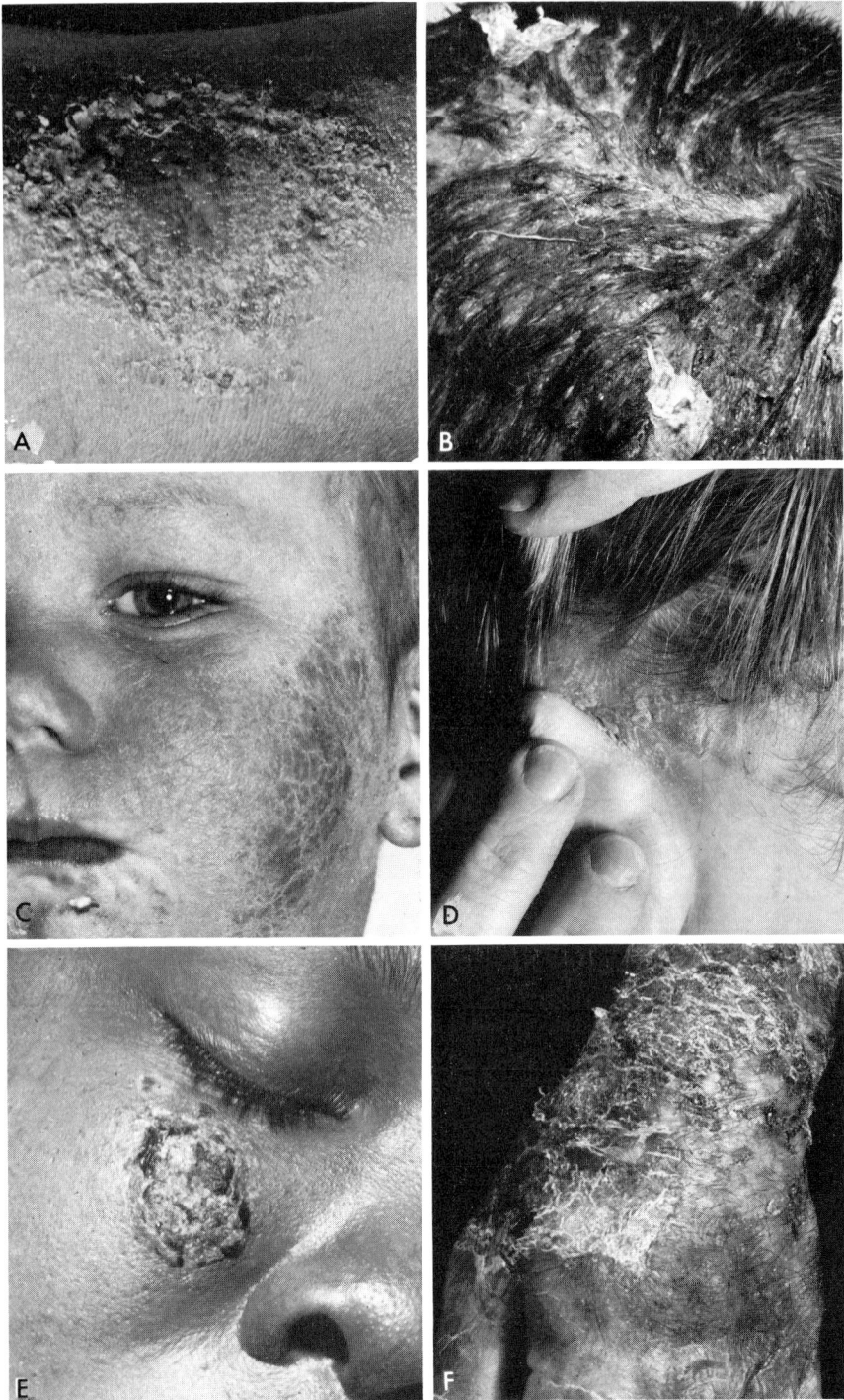

Figure 3–105   Examples of crusts and scales. *A*, Crusting and scaling in patch of subsiding contact dermatitis. *B*, Diffuse crusted inflammatory reaction in tinea capitis. *C*, Crusting and scaling in atopic dermatitis. *D*, Seborrheic dermatitis with crust of subsiding infected fissure at upper retroauricular fold. *E*, Crusting of lesion of pemphigus of the erythematosus type superficially simulating lupus erythematosus. *F*, Crusted subsiding primary irritant dermatitis.

destruction. To destroy tissue, the pathologic forces involved must be powerful or the physiologic status of the area very poor. Any process of the skin in which there is persistent ulceration deserves the most thorough study. The cause of the ulcer is at times readily apparent, but in some instances the factors concerned may be multiple and obscure. Ulcers generally heal with scar formation.

Crusts (Scabs)

Crusts are the dried remains of exudate from erosive or ulcerated skin lesions. They may consist of dried blood, as after an injury; dried serum, as after an oozing dermatitis; or dried pus from a cutaneous infection. In "pure" form, the appearance of each of these is somewhat different. Varying admixtures of the three may occur, or the scab may be mixed with scale and the ingredients of topical medicaments, especially shake lotions. Possibly the most important diagnostic consideration in regard to crusts is to recognize the dirty gray to green crust sometimes resulting from infection; it is always advisable to remove this and see what lies underneath. Crusts may at times become extremely thick and assume bizarre appearances. This is particularly common in the scalp where the material is anchored by the hair.

Scars

Scars are the permanent skin changes seen following damage to the corium; like ulcers, they always demand an explanation. They vary from slight superficial atrophy, with some loss of pigment and of some of the accessory glands, to processes in which the epidermis, cutis, and subcutaneous tissues have been completely destroyed. Scar formation may be exuberant (hypertrophic scar). It is important to distinguish between fresh scars which are temporarily accentuated, in a keloidal-like fashion, and true keloids, in which progressive hypertrophy of the scar may be expected. Some supposedly excellent results in the treatment of "keloids" really represent the spontaneous healing of what were in the first place hypertrophic scars. Subjective symptoms such as pain from scars, especially early ones, are not un-

common. While scars ordinarily contract with the passage of time, some of them characteristically do not; for example, those following the gummas of syphilis.

Configurations of Lesions

Three characteristics of the configuration of multiple lesions, among others, have wide usefulness.

GROUPING. The most characteristic grouped lesions are those which are herpetiform; that is, distinct aggregations of vesicles. These include herpes simplex, zoster, and dermatitis herpetiformis. Skin reactions to generalized infections are sometimes grouped as well; for example, grouped follicular and papular lesions of early syphilis. Representative lesions are seen in Figure 3–108.

ANNULARITY. A great many dermatoses assume annular shapes, either characteristically or occasionally. This is true of many bacterial and mycotic infections, of urticarial reactions, erythema multiforme, and many invasive and destructive processes. Some of the more common dermatoses are so characteristically annular as to make this a useful aid in diagnosis.

LINEAR ARRANGEMENT. Several diseases affecting the skin are characterized by the arrangement of lesions in linear fashion. This may come about as part of the basic pattern of the disease, as a result of a peculiar reaction to trauma (Koebner phenomenon), or as a result of the inoculation of infectious material along a scratch or cut. Examples of diseases which are characteristically linear include linear localized scleroderma, linear nevi, and herpes zoster. In some diseases, the skin reacts to trauma in a characteristic pattern, and lesions may be very precisely arranged along a scratch; for example, lichen planus and psoriasis. Keloids are often linear, depending upon the type of trauma which initiated them. Viral infections such as warts and, less commonly, molluscum contagiosum may show a linear arrangement due to inoculation with the virus through a scratch or cut. Superficial infections, such as impetigo, may occasionally show a linear arrangement. Reactions to contactant allergens are frequently and characteristically linear, depending upon

(*Text continues on page 191.*)

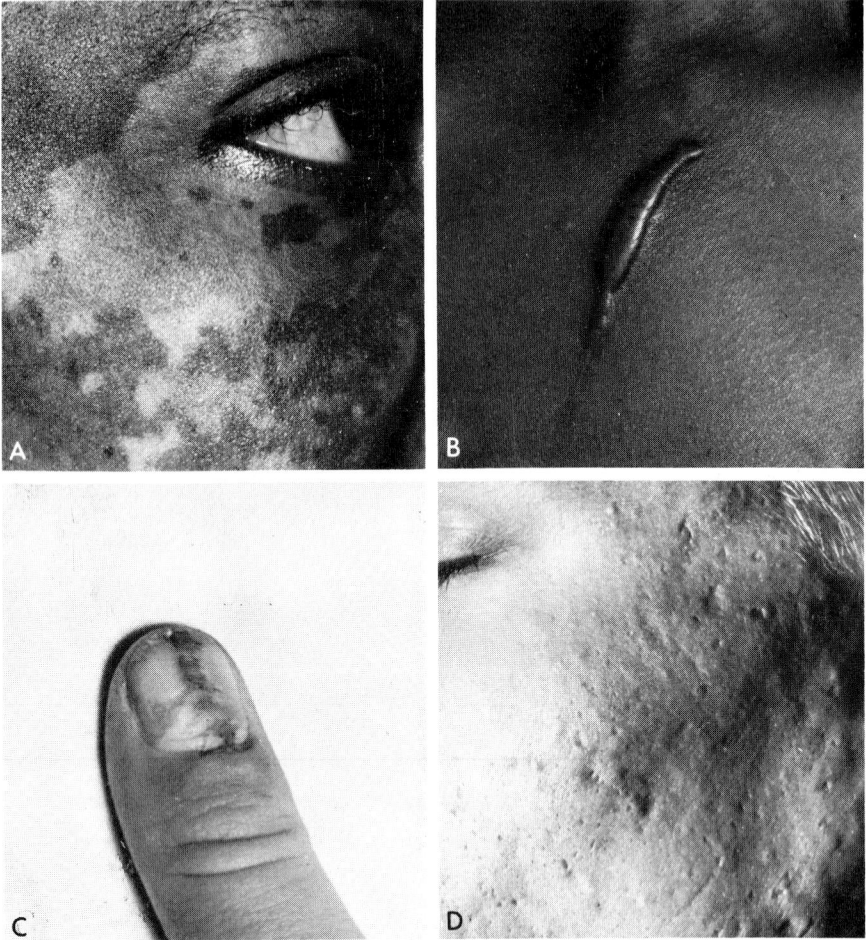

Figure 3–106   Examples of scars. *A,* Superficial atrophy and depigmentation following lupus erythematosus, now quiescent. *B,* Linear keloid of upper chest following cut. *C,* Linear nail dystrophy produced by chronic factitial (tic) injury to nail matrix. *D,* Typical pitted scarring following grade III acne.

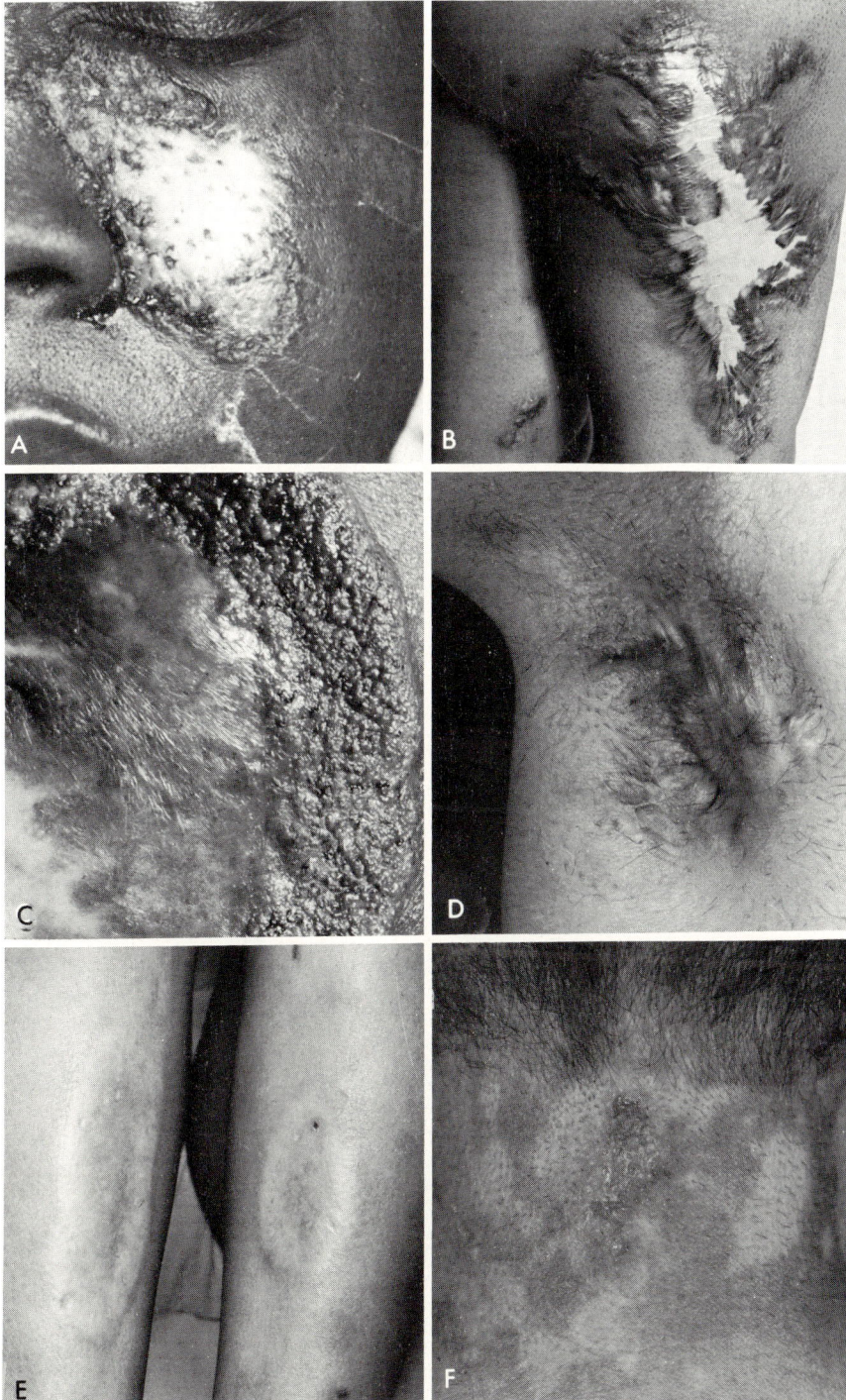

Figure 3–107 Types of scarring. *A,* Deep scarring of long-standing lupus vulgaris (tuberculosis). Some activity still present. Possibility of later malignant degeneration. *B,* Deep scarring and peripheral keloid formation from 3rd degree burn. *C,* Destruction produced by slowly advancing blastomycosis of face. *D,* Scarring of hidradenitis suppurativa (chronic inflammation of axilla with involvement of apocrine sweat glands). *E,* Circumscribed scleroderma, pretibial surface. Difficult to distinguish from pretibial necrobiosis sometimes seen in diabetics. *F,* Scarring from factitial ulcers.

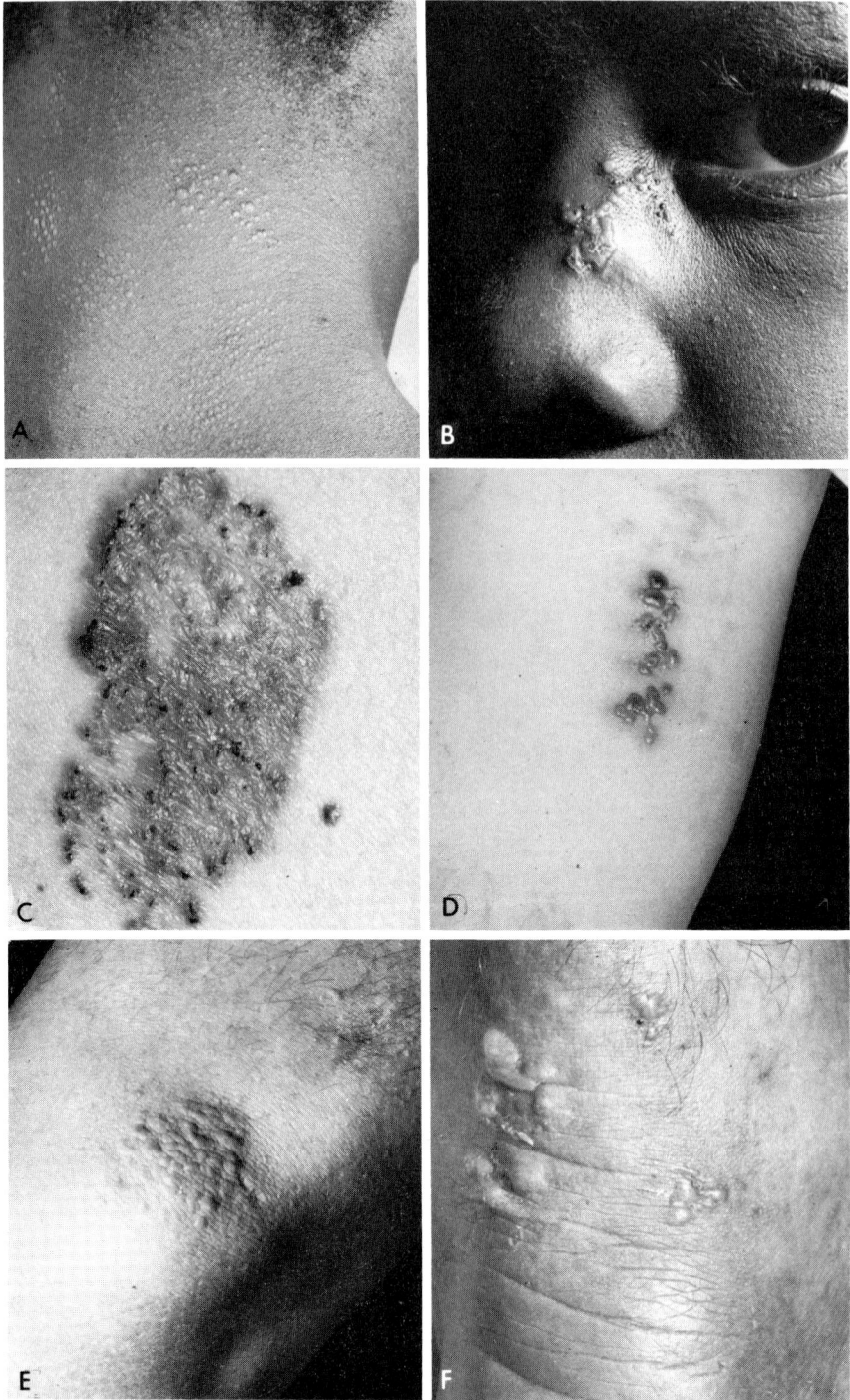

Figure 3–108 Examples of grouped skin lesions. *A,* Lichen scrofulosorum. Associated with extreme sensitivity to tuberculin; to be differentiated clinically from lichenoid sarcoid or follicular lichen planus. *B,* Grouped vesicles of herpes simplex. Often recurrent at exactly the same site. *C,* Superficial epitheliomatosis. Grouped multicentric foci of basal cell epithelioma. *D,* Herpes zoster. *E,* Groups of xanthoma papules. *F,* Grouped poison ivy vesicles.

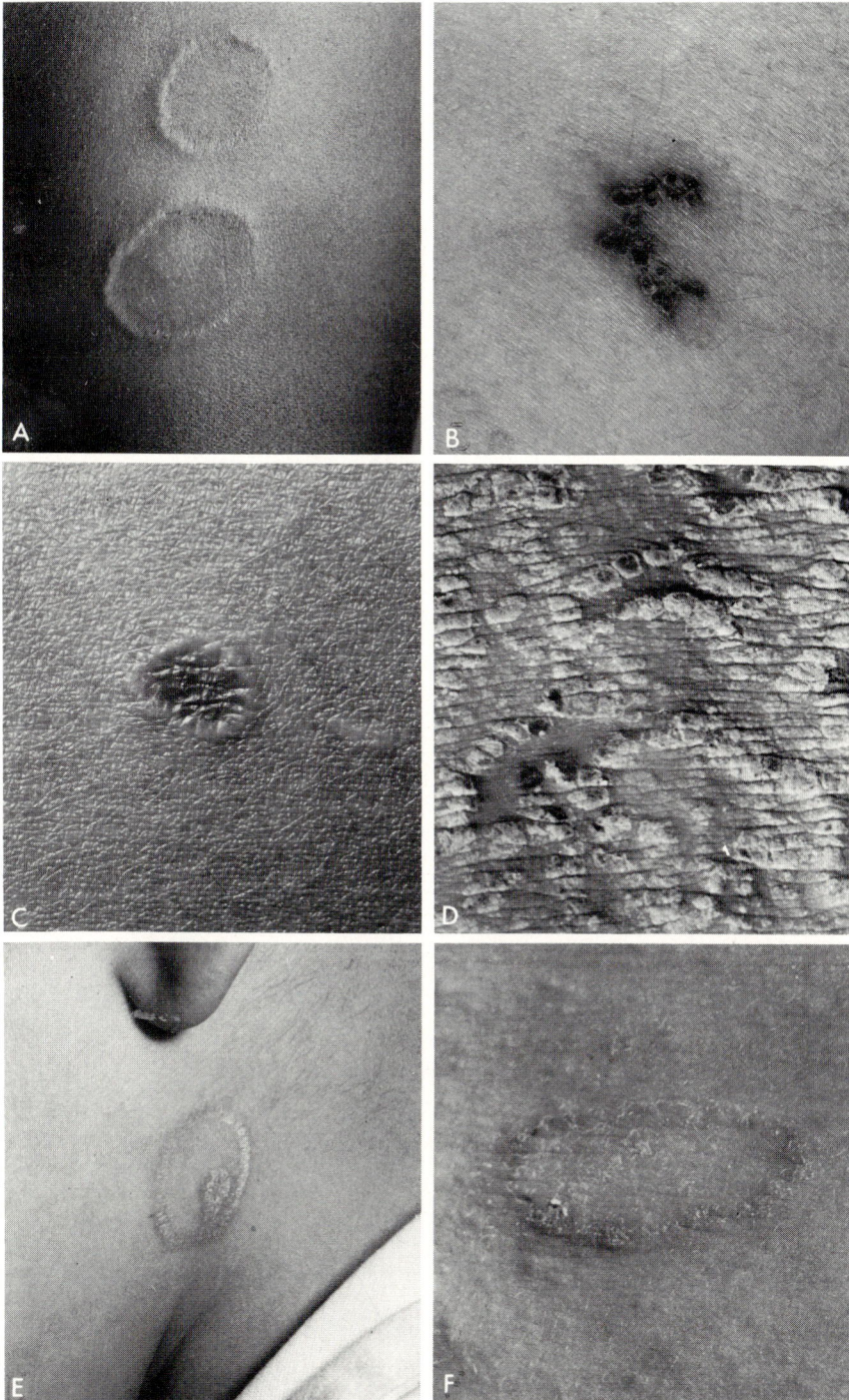

Figure 3–109 Representative annular lesions. *A,* Granuloma annulare. As the term indicates, the well developed lesion is annular. *B,* Ring shaped herpes simplex. *C,* Advancing annular lesion of lichen planus, with hyperpigmentation in center. *D,* Irregular annular patterns in psoriasis. *E,* Ringworm. Tinea circinata. Another lesion is starting within the old one. *F,* Typical annular lesion of pityriasis rosea.

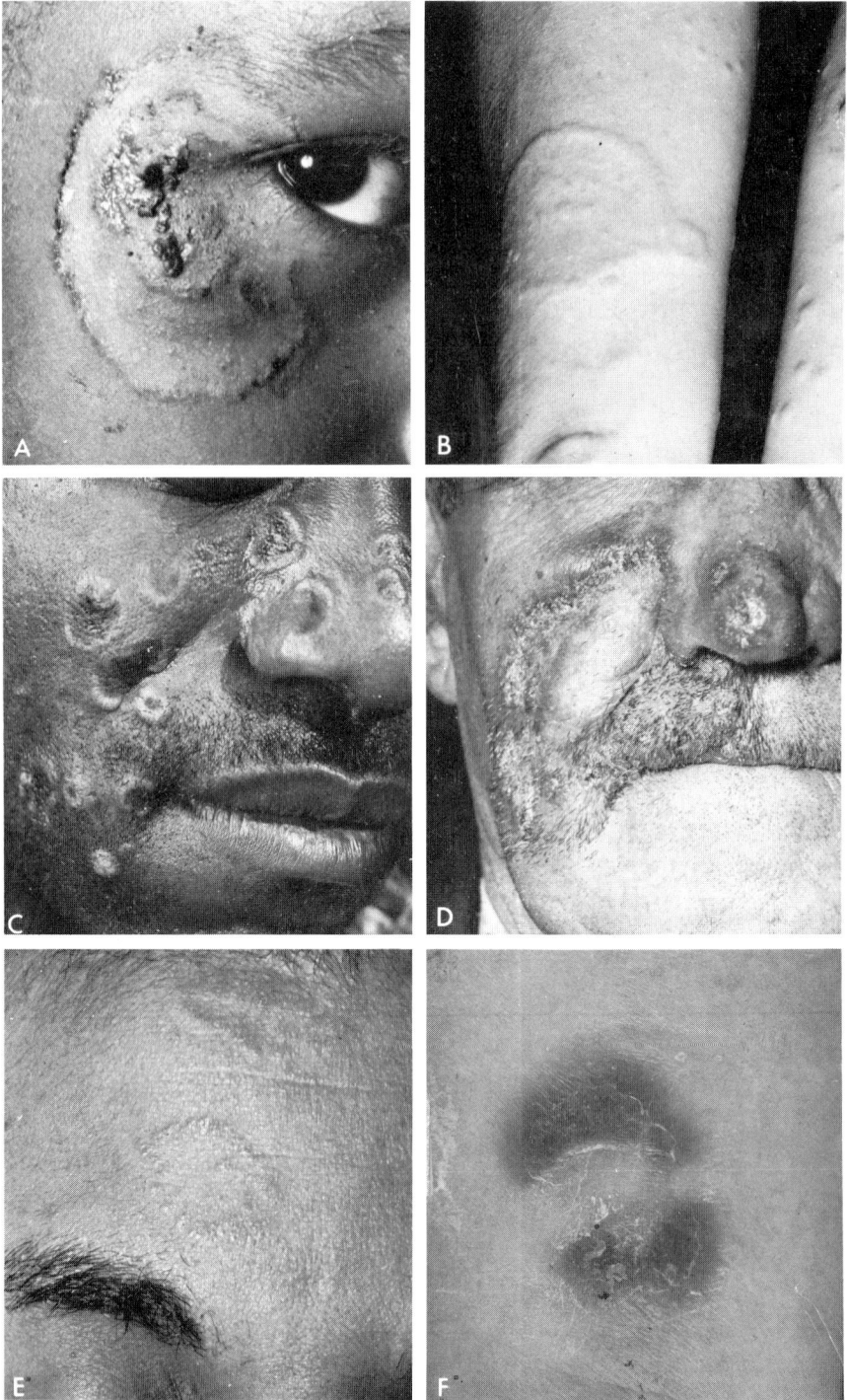

Figure 3–110   Representative annular lesions. *A*, Low-grade impetigo in concentric ring. *B*, Erythema multiforme of the forearm. Lesions principally urticarial, some papular, some annular. *C*, Annular lesions of early syphilis on face. A highly characteristic lesion of florid mucocutaneous syphilis in the Negro. *D*, Gumma. Long-standing. *E*, Annular lesions of forehead due to sarcoid infiltration of skin. *F*, Nodules of mycosis fungoides.

the mode of deposition of the offending material.

The development of lesions within the skin or subcutaneous tissue following primary inoculation of the skin is frequently in linear fashion. A wide variety of infections may show this pattern, including streptococcal and staphylococcal, tuberculous, syphilitic, and sporotrichotic. Metastasis of a malignant lesion, such as melanoma and carcinoma of the breast, along the lymphatics may sometimes be linear.

DISTRIBUTION PATTERNS AS AN AID TO DIAGNOSIS

The pattern in which skin lesions are distributed over the body is often a useful aid in arriving at a diagnosis. In some diseases, the distribution is so characteristic as to be almost pathognomonic; in others, while one distribution pattern may be most characteristic, variations from it are frequent. The more typical distribution patterns of several dermatoses are indicated in the following pages. The dermatoses concerned vary from common to rare.

Acne

The distribution of the lesions of acne is highly characteristic. Since acne is a disease in which the follicular orifices and sebaceous glands are affected, the lesions are concentrated where these structures are most abundant, large, and active. The face is the most frequently involved site, but lesions appear on the shoulders, chest, upper back, neck, and upper arms in more severe types of the disease. The lack of involvement of the scalp is striking; even in extremely severe acne, only the scalp margins are involved, as a rule. An even more extensive distribution may be noted in so-called tropical acne, in which the entire trunk may be affected, with lesions on the buttocks and thighs as well.

Rosacea

The lesions of rosacea occur in a highly characteristic pattern. In severe and long-standing examples, diffuse involvement of the face may be noted, but the flush areas are the sites affected initially. Rosacea frequently occurs in middle-aged persons. Pustules occur in association with rosacea in the more severe forms (acne rosacea), but these do not characteristically arise from comedones. There is frequently an associated seborrheic dermatitis. The eyes should always be examined for evidence of rosacea keratitis, though fortunately this is not a frequent complication.

Seborrheic Dermatitis

This is the third member of a common triad, acne and rosacea being the others. In seborrheic dermatitis of moderate severity, the chief, often the only, site of involvement is the scalp, with the following areas affected in approximate order of frequency: eyebrows, skin above bridge of nose, sides of nose, ears (especially the external auditory canals and the retro-auricular region), presternal and interscapular region, eyelid margins (a frequent source of blepharitis), and folds or creases of the face and neck. In some patients, intertriginous regions over the body may become extensively affected, especially the axillae, the anogenital region (particularly the gluteal cleft and crural folds), under the breasts in women, and all intertriginous sites in obese patients. Associ-

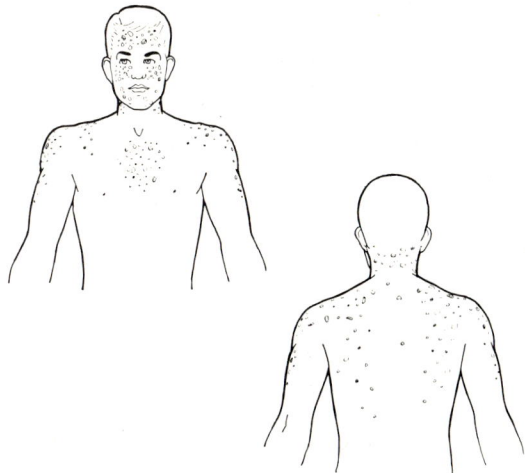

Figure 3–111 The characteristic distribution of lesions in a grade IV acne.

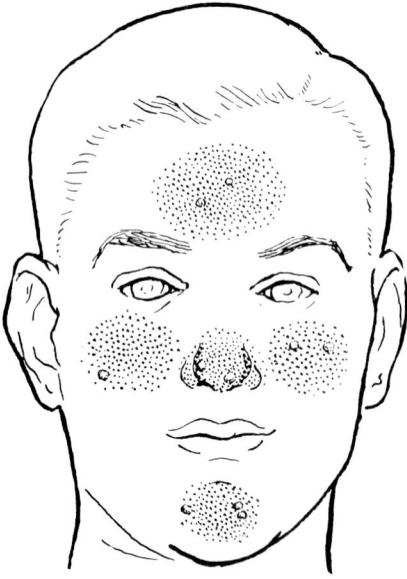

Figure 3–112 Characteristic sites of involvement in rosacea.

ated acute or chronic secondary bacterial infection is very common.

Psoriasis

The tendency to involve the scalp, the knees, the elbows, and the back is characteristic of at least 75 per cent of all cases of psoriasis. Misdiagnosis is particularly prone to occur in involvement of the nails (confusion with ringworm), the feet and hands (confusion with ringworm and with syphilis), and the genitalia (confusion with venereal disease and precancerous dermatoses). The most common "aberrant" distribution of psoriasis is to the "seborrheic" areas, and seborrheic dermatitis and psoriasis often exist coincidentally. It is probable that a prime factor in the localization of lesions is the fact that the skin of a person with psoriasis tends to react to trauma or chronic superficial inflammation in a characteristic psoriasiform pattern.

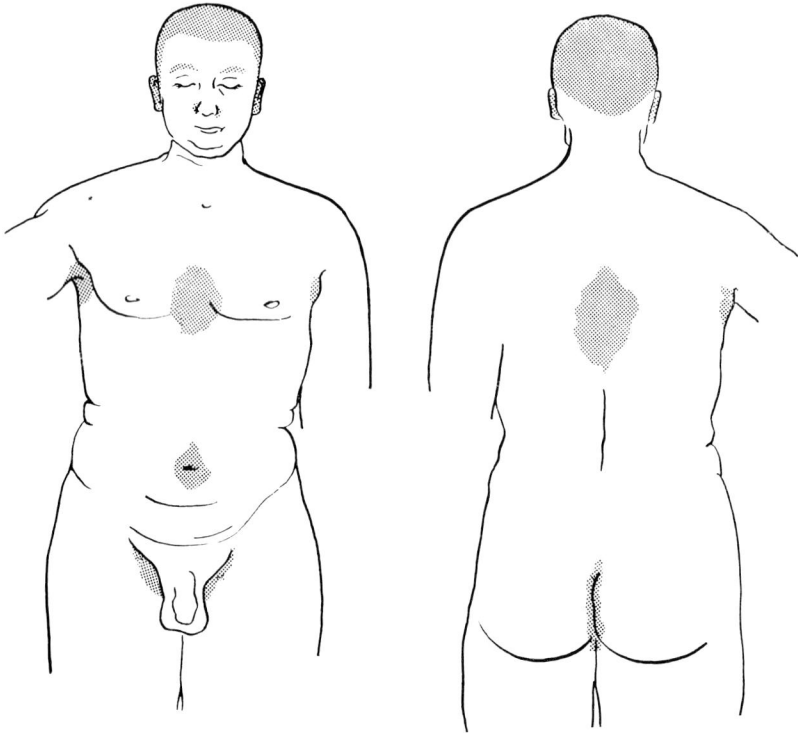

Figure 3–113 Common sites of involvement in extensive seborrheic dermatitis. Intertriginous lesions on the body occur principally in infants and in obese middle-aged patients.

This may explain the localization of lesions on the elbows, knees, and pretibial surfaces (trauma), the sharply localized areas on the palms and soles (trauma), and localization in the scalp, axillae, and anogenital region (maceration, seborrheic dermatitis, and so on.).

Pityriasis Rosea

The diagnosis in pityriasis rosea ordinarily offers no difficulty; it is one of the most characteristic of all dermatologic diseases. The distribution pattern indicated in Figure 3–115 will be noted in at least 75 per cent of all cases, though the number of lesions may be more sparse. A so-called inverse distribution sometimes occurs, in which the distribution may be most markedly to the extremities, especially the distal portions thereof, with few lesions on the trunk. Involvement of the face is uncommon. The appearance of the individual lesions is usually characteristic.

Early Syphilis

The distribution of lesions in early syphilis sometimes follows a characteristic pattern. Eroded moist papular lesions in the anogenital region or dry nonvesicular papules of the palms and soles should be regarded as syphilitic until proved otherwise. *The lesions of early syphilis, especially if eroded, are highly infectious.*

Scabies

This disease has a highly characteristic distribution. The extent of the involvement is directly proportional to the lack of good bathing hygiene. The face is almost never involved in adults. Aside from the characteristic burrow, the most pathognomonic lesion of scabies is an itching papule of the penis. In females, involvement of the areola of the breast is characteristic. Early diagnosis will result in prompt easy cure; delay invites a variety of persistent and disabling sequelae.

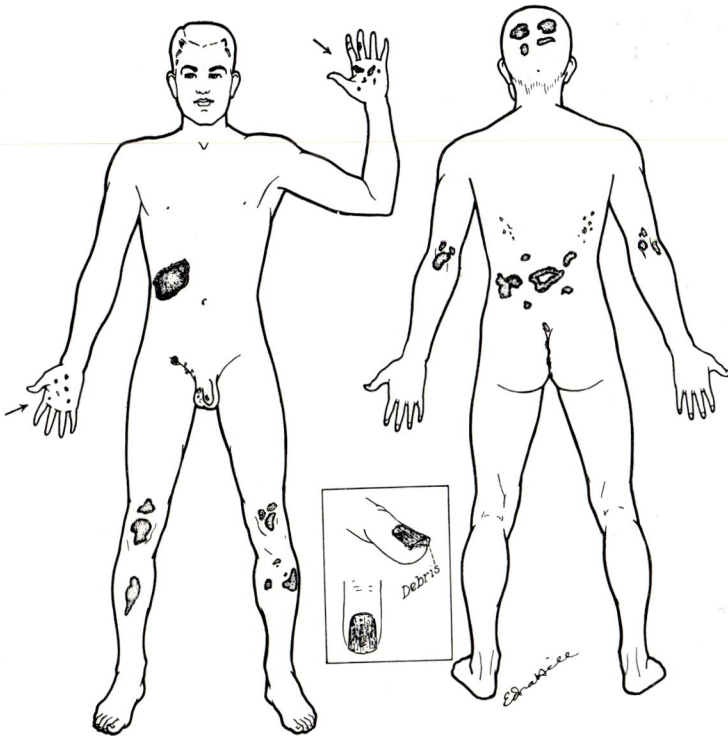

Figure 3–114 The most common sites of involvement in extensive psoriasis. An alternate distribution pattern may be seen in the seborrheic areas (Fig. 3–113).

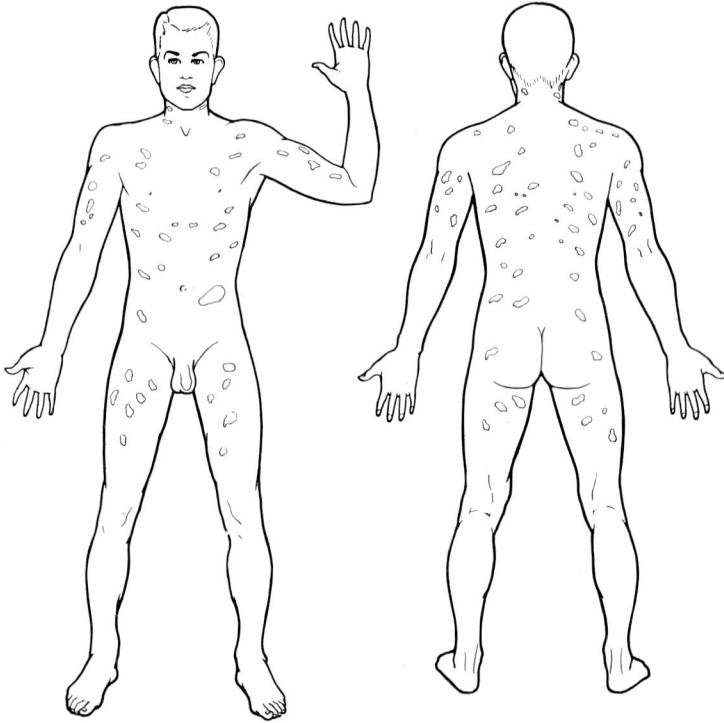

Figure 3–115   Distribution of lesions in pityriasis rosea. This pattern is seen in some 75 per cent of all instances of the disease. The large lesion to the left of the umbilicus represents the "mother" or primary plaque.

Atopic Dermatitis (Disseminate Neurodermatitis) in the Postinfantile Phase

This has an extraordinarily characteristic distribution pattern, especially in late childhood, adolescence, and early adult life. The distribution of atopic dermatitis in infants is erratic and it may occur anywhere, though the face is almost always

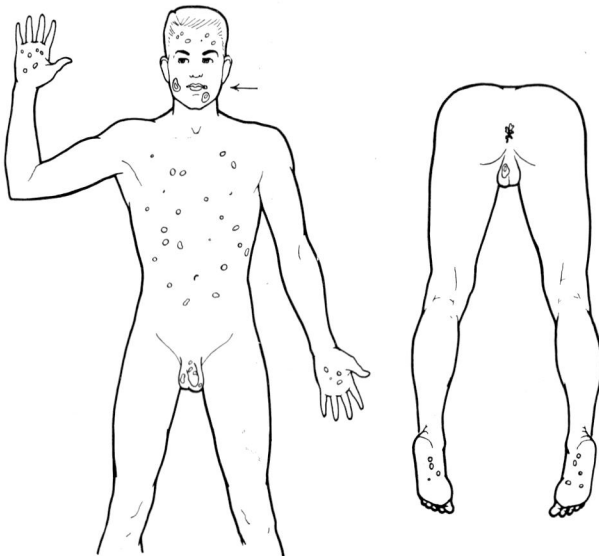

Figure 3–116   Common sites of mucocutaneous lesions in early syphilis. The mouth is often involved.

involved. In middle age, the disease ordinarily subsides, but recurrent lesions, often only on the face or hands, may be seen.

Erythema Multiforme

In a broad sense, erythema multiforme is a reaction pattern of the skin rather than a specific disease, with considerable variation in the types of lesions and the severity and extent of the process. The distribution pattern is fairly characteristic for all types, the face, lower portions of the extremities, and the genitalia being the most common sites. There may be extreme involvement of the mucous membranes, including the conjunctiva (Stevens-Johnson syndrome). Reiter's syndrome (urethritis, conjunctivitis, arthritis, and skin lesions) and Behçet's disease (oral and genital lesions, uveitis or iridocyclitis, plus occasional skin lesions)

at times must be considered in the differential diagnosis of erythema multiforme. In some types the course is explosive and may be fatal; in others the disease is benign and mild.

Chronic Discoid Lupus Erythematosus

Lesions of this disease have a marked predilection for exposed sites of the head, neck, and hands, and there is ordinarily evidence of photosensitivity. It is important that this process be differentiated as promptly as possible from systemic acute lupus erythematosus. The chronic discoid type involves only the skin and mucous membranes and is essentially a benign disease, though its course may be very prolonged, and the lesions often produce much scarring and cosmetic disfigurement. The disease may sometimes be confused with other diseases in which there is a

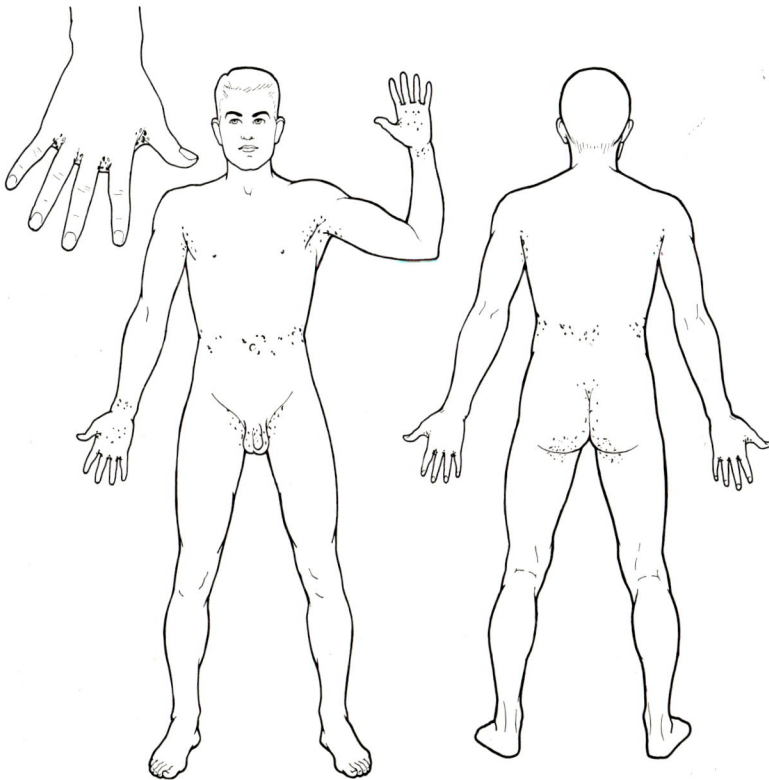

Figure 3–117 Scabies occurs in a highly characteristic distribution. In persons of good hygiene, the lesions may be very sparse; in those of poor hygiene, much more extensive.

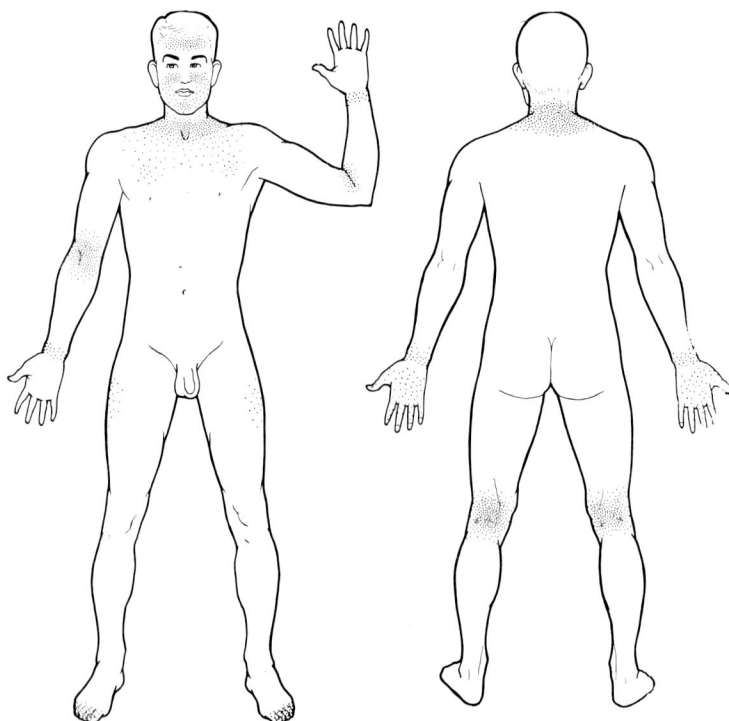

Figure 3–118 Very characteristic distribution of sites of involvement in atopic dermatitis in older children and young adults.

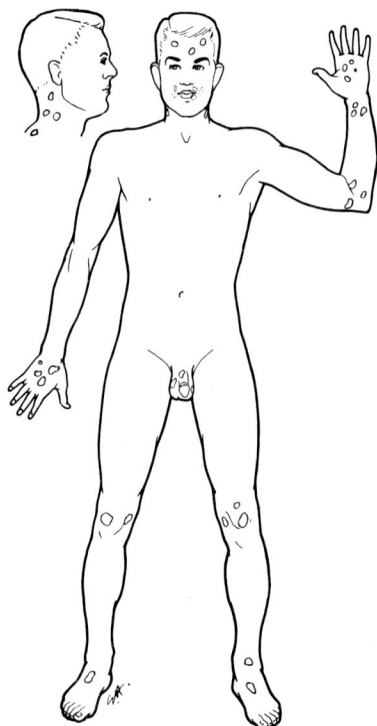

Figure 3–119 The most typical distribution of lesions in erythema multiforme of moderate severity. The process may be more extensive in severe types of this syndrome.

photosensitization factor; for example, polymorphous light eruptions and pellagra.

Erythema Nodosum

This is an acute or subacute perivascular subcutaneous reaction in which the lesions are chiefly seen on the distal portions of the extremities; the most common site of involvement is the pretibial area. The syndrome may be precipitated by a wide variety of agents, including drugs, and a large number of systemic infections during their early invasive phases; for example, tuberculosis, streptococcal infections, viral infections (cat-scratch fever, lymphopathia venereum, and measles), coccidioidomycosis, and histoplasmosis.

Lichen Planus

The extent of the papular lesions in this disease varies greatly. In mild to moderate form, the principal sites of involvement are the mouth, especially the buccal surfaces of the cheek, the genitalia, the flexor surfaces of the wrists, and the trunk. In the

Figure 3–120 Chronic discoid lupus erythematosus. Characteristic sites of involvement on head and neck.

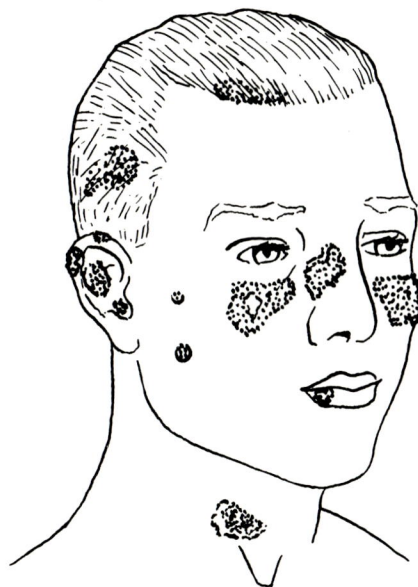

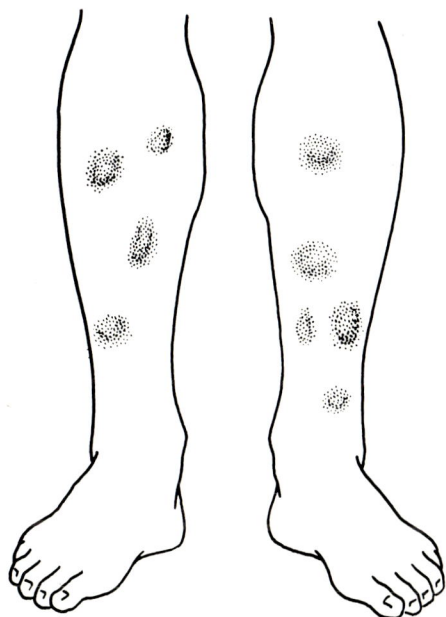

Figure 3–121 The most common site of involvement in erythema nodosum.

Figure 3–122 Sites most frequently involved in extensive lichen planus. The leg inset represents the hypertrophic lesions which sometimes are seen in this region.

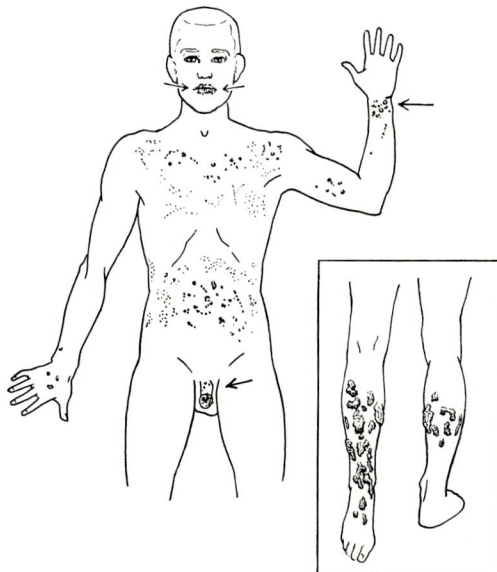

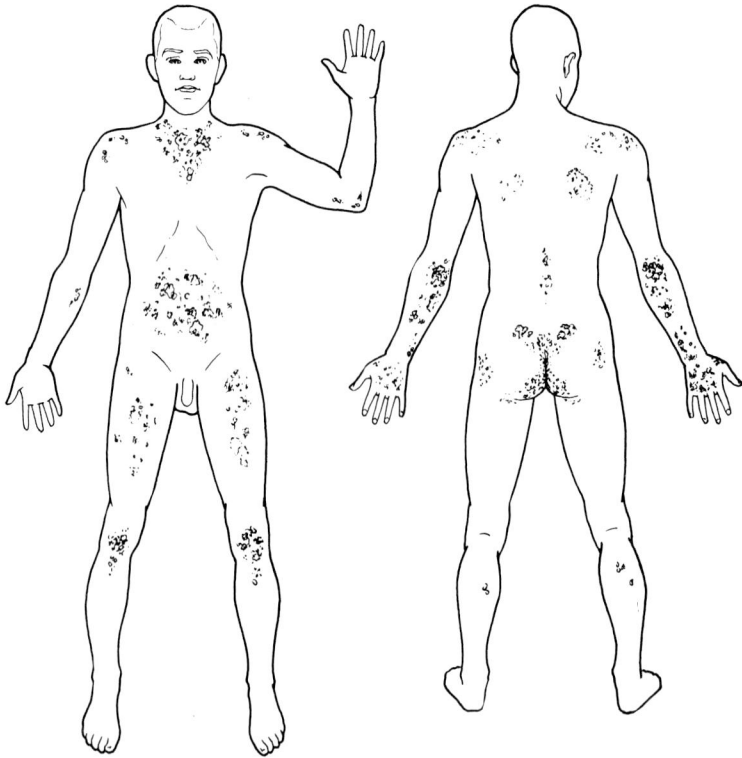

Figure 3–123 Most common sites of involvement in dermatitis herpetiformis. Lesions are seen occasionally on the face in this disease and commonly on the scalp.

hypertrophic form of the disease, the most marked lesions may be found on the lower legs.

Dermatitis Herpetiformis

This is an uncommon but exceedingly chronic disease, in which the rather poly-morphic grouped lesions and their distribution are ordinarily characteristic. The extremities are almost always involved, often in areas which receive the most rubbing and trauma. The lesions are roughly symmetric. The scalp, the region over the scapulae, and the lower back are commonly involved.

DISORDERS OF IMMUNITY, HYPERSENSITIVITY, AND INFLAMMATION

Section I

CLINICAL IMMUNOLOGY
John M. O'Loughlin

Most individuals have experienced one or more allergic reactions. The skin may be one of the involved systems and is used to detect, investigate, and study allergic phenomena. Consequently, it is important to understand the basic principles of allergy and immunology in order to increase diagnostic acumen, to appreciate the cause of some diseases, and to render effective therapy.

Immunologic development begins in utero and, by the end of the first year, this defense system is a well-functioning entity. A primary stem cell is responsible for development of the humoral antibody system and the cell-mediated functions. De-

ficiencies of either or both of these divisions are found in congenital disorders and in neoplastic and non-neoplastic diseases. Diagnosis of these deficits can be made when there is a high index of suspicion.

The two basic types of immunologic processes are those that are cell mediated and those that involve the secretion of humoral antibody. Thymus-controlled lymphocytes (T cells) are involved in cellular immunity, and lymphocytes believed to be independent of thymus control (B cells) are primarily responsible for humoral antibody release (Fig. 4-1). T cells and B cells are believed to originate

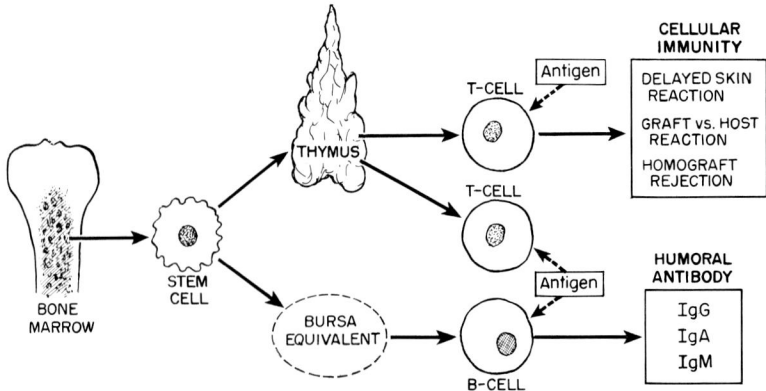

Figure 4–1 T cells from the thymus recognize foreign antigenic determinants such as those found on cells of transplantation organs; they multiply and attack these foreign cells, resulting in a cell-mediated response. B cells from the bone marrow detect these same antigens and, with or without communication with T cells, multiply and produce cells (plasma cells) that make antibodies to specific antigens. (From O'Loughlin, J. M.: Lahey Clin. Found. Bull. 22:69, 1973.)

from a common stem cell in the embryo and differentiate during the first trimester of gestation by passing through the thymus. T cells remain under control of the thymus, and B cells are influenced by a human analogue of the animal's bursa of Fabricius. If this analogue exists in human beings, it probably is located somewhere in the gastrointestinal tract or near Peyer's patches. T cells, in general, are longer lived, are constantly recirculating through the thoracic duct and systemic circulation, and are susceptible to irradiation. B cells are generally shorter lived, and their proliferation may be controlled effectively by immunosuppressive agents. The ratio

of T cells and B cells circulating at any one time is approximately 4 to 1.

IMMUNOGLOBULINS

Among the humoral immunologic factors are serum proteins which, in general, separate electrophoretically as gamma globulins. These antibodies can combine directly with antigens and belong to the group of serum proteins known as immunoglobulins. The five classes of antibodies are designated as IgG, IgA, IgM, IgD, and IgE. Table 4–1 lists some of the properties that distinguish these different classes of antibodies. Figure 4–2 reviews

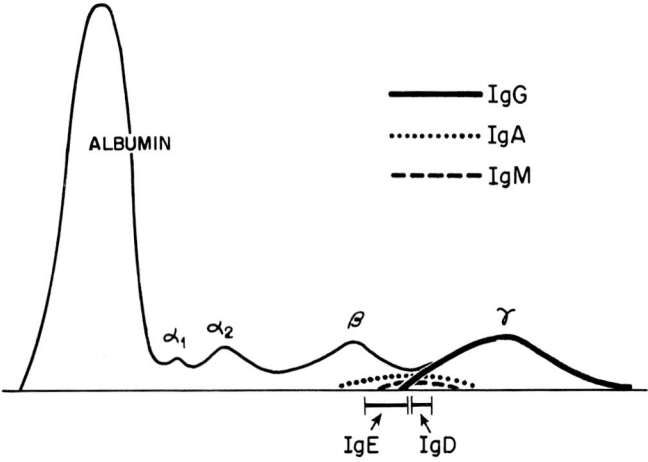

Figure 4–2 Protein-electrophoretic pattern superimposed over electrophoretic mobility. (From O'Loughlin, J. M.: Lahey Clin. Found. Bull. 22:70, 1973.)

TABLE 4–1 PROPERTIES OF SPECIFIC ANTIBODIES*

	IgG (γG)	IgA (γA)	IgM (γM)	IgD (γD)	IgE (γE)
Concentration in normal human serum, gm. per cent	1.2	0.24	0.12	0.003	0.000,01
Molecular weight	160,000	170,000 (serum) 390,000 (secretory)	900,000	160,000	200,000
Sedimentation coefficient	7S	7S, 11S	19S	7S	8S
Electrophoretic mobility	γ	Slow β	Between β and γ	Between β and γ	Slow β
Nomenclature heavy chains (subclasses)	γ (1,2,3,4)	α (1,2)	μ (1,2)	δ	ε
Number of heavy chains	2	2	10	2	2
Number of light chains	2κ or 2λ	2κ or 2λ	10κ or 10λ	2κ or 2λ	2κ or 2λ
Bind complement	+	−	+	−	−
React with rheumatoid factor	+	−	−	−	−
Carbohydrate, per cent	2.5	5–10	5–10	...	10
Synthetic rate, gm./day/70 kg.	2.3	2.7	0.4	0.03	
Half-life, days	25	6	5	3	2–3 (serum) 9–10 (skin)

*From O'Loughlin, J. M.: Lahey Clin. Found. Bull. 22:70, 1973.

the familiar protein-electrophoretic pattern of each class of antibodies described in Table 4–1.

Figure 4–3 is a schematic representation of IgG structure and demonstrates disulfide linkage between heavy and light chains as well as between heavy chains. At one end of the molecule, a variable portion exists in both the light and heavy chains that accounts for the specificity of each antibody.

Ordinarily, the fetus is supplied with maternal IgG so that, at birth, cord serum IgG concentration closely approximates maternal concentration. Practically no maternal IgA or IgM crosses the placental barrier. Passage of gamma globulin begins about the fourth month of gestation and appears to involve an active transport system. The fetus synthesizes varying amounts of IgM antibodies in utero, and levels usually rise rapidly after birth, reaching about 75 per cent of adult level by the end of the first year of life. IgA synthesis begins a few weeks after birth and reaches 75 per cent of adult level by the end of the second year. The newborn's maternal IgG is rapidly catabolized so that by the third month of life a period of physiologic hypogammaglobulinemia

Figure 4–3. The structure of IgG molecule. (From O'Loughlin, J. M.: Lahey Clin. Found. Bull. 22:70, 1973.)

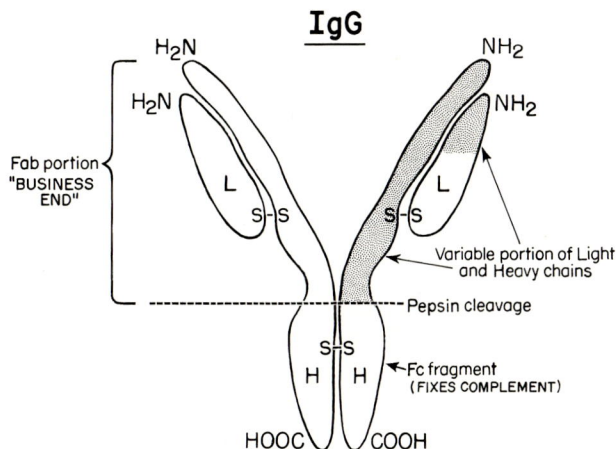

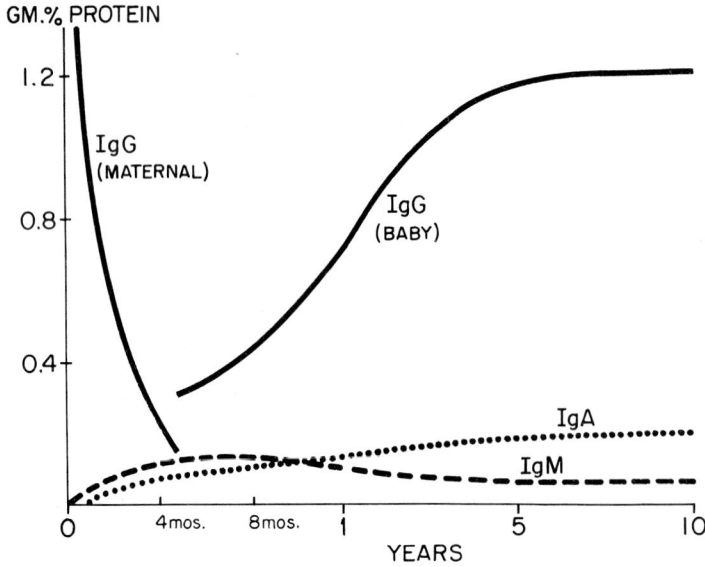

Figure 4–4 Antibody production in early life. (From O'Loughlin, J. M.: Lahey Clin. Found. Bull. 22:71, 1973.)

exists. However, the infant's production rate of IgG rises rapidly and approximately achieves adult levels by the end of the first year. A diagrammatic representation of antibody production in the first few years of life is shown in Figure 4–4.

The immunoglobulins are synthesized by B lymphocytes that have differentiated into plasma cells. It is believed that one cell makes only one type of antibody with a single specificity. Ordinarily, few or no plasma cells can be found in the normal newborn; however, as the child matures immunologically, maturation of the lymphoid tissue occurs with the organization of follicles and the appearance of plasma cells during the third month of life.

Studies have been performed on age-matched control groups to determine normal levels. Table 4–2 reviews these findings and gives approximate adult values that might be found when ordering studies for quantitative immunoglobulins.

CELL-MEDIATED IMMUNOLOGIC MECHANISMS

Cellular immunity is manifested in vivo by delayed hypersensitivity skin test responses that occur when antigen is fixed in tissues, such as a solid tissue homograft, or when it is a modified part of the body's

TABLE 4–2 LEVELS OF IMMUNE GLOBULINS IN SERA OF NORMAL SUBJECTS BY AGE°

	IgG		IgM		IgA		Total Immunoglobulin	
Age	mg./100 ml.	% of Adult Level	mg./100 ml.	% of Adult Level	mg./100 ml.	% of Adult Level	mg./100 ml.	% of Adult Level
Newborn	1,031±200	89±17	11±5	11±5	2±3	1±2	1,044±201	67±13
1–3 mo.	430±119	37±10	30±11	30±11	21±13	11±7	481±127	31±9
4–6 mo.	427±186	37±16	43±17	43±17	28±18	14±9	498±204	32±13
7–12 mo.	661±219	58±19	54±23	55±23	37±18	19±9	752±242	48±15
13–24 mo.	762±209	66±18	58±23	59±23	50±24	25±12	870±258	56±16
25–36 mo.	892±183	77±16	61±19	62±19	71±37	36±19	1,024±205	65±14
3–5 yr.	929±228	80±20	56±18	57±18	93±27	47±14	1,078±245	69±17
6–8 yr.	923±256	80±22	65±25	66±25	124±45	62±23	1,112±293	71±20
9–11 yr.	1,124±235	97±20	79±33	80±33	131±60	66±30	1,334±254	85±17
12–16 yr.	946±124	82±11	59±20	60±20	148±63	74±32	1,153±169	74±12
Adults	1,158±305	100±26	99±27	100±27	200±61	100±31	1,457±353	100±24

°From Stiehm, E. R., and Fudenberg, H. H.: Pediatrics, 37:715, 1966.

TABLE 4–3 CHARACTERISTICS OF CELL-MEDIATED AND HUMORAL REACTIONS*

	Arthus Reaction *(Humoral Antibody)*	*Tuberculin Reaction* *(Cell Mediator)*
Systemic manifestations	Deposition of immune complexes in organs	Fever
Time to maximum response	4–8 hours	24–48 hours
Gross appearance	Hemorrhage, edema	Erythema induration
Microscopic appearance	Polymorphonuclear infiltrate	Mononuclear infiltrate

*From O'Loughlin, J. M.: Lahey Clin. Found. Bull. 22:73, 1973.

own tissues, for example, skin treated with a sensitizing agent—2,4 dinitrofluorobenzene (2,4 DNFB). Lymphocytes passing through tissue are sensitized in the periphery and pass to the paracortical area of local lymph nodes. These sensitized cells differentiate into large cells, reaching peak concentration three to four days after sensitization, and then divide into a new population of lymphocytes, some of which leave the local lymphatic tissue and proceed to other lymph nodes. The cell-mediated response is dependent upon the integrity of the thymus during embryonic and early neonatal life. If the thymus is removed in animals in early neonatal life, cellular immunity will be unable to develop.

Some of the major characteristics distinguishing reactions involving cellular and humoral immunity are shown in Table 4–3. Familiar humoral antibody reactions are listed in Table 4–4, while common cell-mediated immune reactions are outlined in Table 4–5.

IMMUNOLOGIC DEFICIENCY DISORDERS

What happens should nature fail in the proper development of either or both of these immune systems? The clinician must deal with the very rare, disabling, and often fatal immunologic deficiency diseases that have recently been reclassified by the World Health Organization (Fudenberg et al., 1970; Table 4–6).

The Swiss type or combined type of immune deficiency disease is characterized by defects in both cell-mediated immunity and immunoglobulin synthesis. A defective immunoblast stem cell line or absence of this cell is believed responsible

TABLE 4–4 HUMORAL ANTIBODY REACTIONS*

1. Passive sensitization (Prausnitz-Küstner reaction)
2. Anaphylactic antibodies
   a. Mild reactions, i.e., conjunctivitis, rhinorrhea secondary to pollens, animal dander
   b. Systematic anaphylaxis, i.e., drug injection (penicillin), foreign sera, stinging insect
   c. Blocking antibodies: Desensitization of anaphylactic individuals by regular and repeated injections of antigen; results in formation of blocking antibodies (IgG)
3. Arthus reaction: Takes 2–8 hours to begin, lasts 12–24 hours; occurs in walls of small blood vessels as a result of antibody from the circulation meeting antigen diffusing inward from the extravascular space
4. Serum sickness: Reactions occurring are due to IgG or IgM; however, if antibodies are mainly anaphylactic, IgE; the symptoms will be mainly anaphylactic because of reactions taking place on the cell surface

*From O'Loughlin, J. M.: Lahey Clin. Found. Bull. 22:73, 1973.

TABLE 4–5 CELL-MEDIATED IMMUNE REACTIONS*

1. Delayed hypersensitivity to heterologous serum proteins (foreign serum, i.e., horse serum)
2. Delayed hypersensitivity to microbial antigen
   a. Tuberculin
   b. Vaccinia—"reactions of immunity"
   c. Diphtheria toxoid—"pseudo" Schick reaction
   d. Fungal antigen—coccidioidal mycosis, histoplasmosis
   e. Protozoal antigens—leishmaniasis (Montenegro test)
3. Insect bites
4. Chemical contact sensitivity
5. Homograft reaction
6. Skin reactions to homologous tissue in allergic auto-immune states

*From O'Loughlin, J. M.: Lahey Clin. Found. Bull. 22:74, 1973.

TABLE 4–6 Classification of Primary Immunodeficiency Disorders[*]

Infantile X-linked agammaglobulinemia
Selective immunoglobulin deficiency (IgA)
Transient hypogammaglobulinemia of infancy
X-linked immunodeficiency with hyper-IgM
Thymic hypoplasia (pharyngeal pouch syndrome, DiGeorge)
Episodic lymphopenia with lymphocytotoxin
Immunodeficiency with normal or hyperimmunoglobulinemia
Immunodeficiency with ataxia-telangiectasia
Immunodeficiency with thrombocytopenia and eczema (Wiskott-Aldrich)
Immunodeficiency with thymoma
Immunodeficiency with short-limbed dwarfism
Immunodeficiency with generalized hematopoietic hypoplasia
Severe combined immunodeficiency
  a. Autosomal recessive
  b. X-linked
  c. Sporadic
Variable immunodeficiency (largely unclassified)

---

[*]From Fudenberg, H. H., et al.: N. Engl. J. Med. 283:656, 1970. Reprinted by permission from the New England Journal of Medicine.

for this dual disease. It is an autosomal recessive or X-linked trait. Children are sick from early life, and death frequently occurs within the first two years. Generally, the lymphocyte count is less than 1500 cells per cubic millimeter, and all the immunoglobulins are absent. Lymphoid tissue is virtually absent in the body. The thymus is underdeveloped and difficult to find at postmortem examination because it usually weighs less than 1.0 gm. Patients readily accept skin grafts and cannot be sensitized to produce contact sensitivity to 2,4 DNFB. They suffer repeated bacterial, viral, and fungal infections. These patients are much more vulnerable than patients with defective immunoglobulin synthesis only because the latter can deal with viral infections and their defense mechanisms can be brought to near normal range by replacement gamma globulin therapy. Intractable diarrhea with Salmonella and pathogenic *Escherichia coli* strains, together with thrush and pyoderma, is a frequent clinical manifestation. Infections from Pseudomonas and pneumonia from *Pneumocystis carinii* are frequent causes of death.

Defective immunoglobulin synthesis, described in 1952, is characteristic of Bruton's disease found in boys and is in-

herited as an X-linked recessive characteristic. Because of the presence of maternal immunoglobulin, symptoms begin during the second year of life, when IgG levels are generally less than 100 mg. per 100 ml. Pyogenic infections with staphylococci, streptococci, pneumococci, and *Hemophilus influenzae* frequently occur. Responses fail to develop to tetanus toxoid, pertussis, and diphtheria. Anti-A and anti-B isohemagglutinins are low or absent. The ability to reject homografts is maintained. Antigenic stimulation of lymph nodes fails to produce plasma cells therein. Disabling collagen disorders, such as rheumatoid arthritis and dermatomyositis, occur frequently. Treatment consists of gamma globulin regularly in sufficient doses. Patients have delayed reactions to mumps, Candida, streptokinase-streptodornase, and 2,4 DNFB. In vitro, lymphocyte transformation and proliferation induced by phytohemagglutinin are normal.

Rare cases have been reported of congenital deficiency in cell-mediated immunity only, in which thymic dysplasia, lymphoid tissue depletion, and lymphopenia are found. As expected, these patients can neither reject homografts nor become sensitized to 2,4 DNFB. DiGeorge's syndrome, a variant of this syndrome, is characterized by a defect in the third branchial arch and absence of the parathyroid glands.

There are many forms of dysgammaglobulinemia with variable differences in IgG, IgA, and IgM (Janeway et al., 1967). Recently, a group of patients with selective IgA deficiency who were followed for a long period were shown to have a greater incidence of auto-immune disease, especially rheumatoid arthritis, systemic lupus erythematosus, thyroiditis, and pernicious anemia (Amman and Hong, 1971). Many of these patients had recurrent sinus and upper respiratory tract infections.

About 80 per cent of patients with hereditary ataxia-telangiectasia lack both serum and secretory IgA. Earliest signs may begin in infancy with choreo-athetoid movements. Telangiectasia starts between the ages of 6 and 14 and involves the conjunctivae and exposed areas of the body—mainly the face, arms, and eyelids. Frequent and severe infections of the sinuses, middle ear, and lungs occur, and death usually results from overwhelming infection or lymphoreticular malignancy. The relationship between low IgA levels and respiratory tract infection is unclear.

ACQUIRED HYPOGAMMAGLOBULINEMIA

In addition to the congenital deficiencies, a multitude of acquired forms of hypogammaglobulinemia exist. The commonest form is found in adults, and levels of IgG are usually less than 500 mg. per 100 ml. It affects both sexes, and there is an associated high incidence of systemic lupus erythematosus, hemolytic anemia, and thrombocytopenia. This is the commonest immune deficiency disease and has been reclassified by the World Health Organization as "idiopathic hypogammaglobulinemia of variable duration" (Fudenberg et al., 1970).

Secondary acquired hypogammaglobulinemia occurs in diseases when loss of protein is excessive, such as in exfoliative dermatitis and in renal and gastrointestinal disorders. Diseases of the reticuloendothelial system, such as Hodgkin's disease, chronic lymphatic leukemia, and lymphosarcoma, are responsible for a large portion of this group.

Levels of immunoglobulins vary in certain diseases and are, therefore, of prognostic value, since usually the more severe the disease, the lower the level. Infection by certain organisms is more frequent in specific deficiency states, as noted in Table 4–7. Table 4–8 lists some of

TABLE 4–8 Causes of Secondary Hypogammaglobulinemia*

1. Physiological: Both of these can be distinguished from hereditary hypogammaglobulinemia since levels of IgA and IgM are normal
   a. Premature babies
   b. Delayed maturity
2. Catabolic: Increased turnover of protein; affects IgG but not IgM or IgA
   a. Nephrotic syndrome
   b. Protein-losing enteropathy
   c. Malnutrition
   d. Dystrophia myotonica
   e. Thoracic duct fistula
3. Marrow disorders: IgM antibodies present against IgG antigens
   a. Hypoplasia
   b. Bony metastases
   c. Myelosclerosis
   d. Paroxysmal nocturnal hemoglobinuria
4. Toxic factors
   a. Renal failure
   b. High levels of steroids
   c. Cytotoxic therapy
   d. Gluten-sensitive enteropathy (IgM deficiency)
   e. Thyrotoxicosis
   f. Diabetes mellitus without proteinuria
   g. After severe infections
   h. Congenital heart disease

*From Hobbs, J. R.: Sci. Basis Med. 106–127, 1966.

the causes of secondary hypogammaglobulinemia (Hobbs, 1966). Tumors associated with defective humoral deficiency states are listed in Table 4–9.

As the immunoglobulin level may be affected in certain neoplasms, so too may be the degree of cell-mediated response. Hodgkin's disease can range from total anergy to normal cell-mediated response. It has been shown that patients who have a negative tuberculin response and become tuberculin sensitive when vaccin-

TABLE 4–7 Infections*

Cell-Mediated Deficiency	Humoral Deficiency
Tuberculosis	High-grade encapsulated
Atypical mycobacteria	pyogenic pathogen
Listeria	i.e.; Pneumococcus
Salmonella	Hemophilus
Vaccinia	Streptococcus
Rubeola	Meningococcus
Cytomegalic inclusion	Pseudomonas
disease	No trouble with recurrent
Fungi (esp. Candida)	viral or fungal infections; very susceptible to hepatitis virus

*From O'Loughlin, J. M.: Lahey Clin. Found. Bull. 22:75, 1973.

TABLE 4–9 Primary Reticuloendothelial Tumors*

Reticulum cell sarcoma
Mycosis fungoides
Hodgkin's disease
Lymphosarcoma
Giant follicular lymphoma
Chronic lymphatic leukemia
Thymoma
Malignant paraproteinemia
  macroglobulinemia

*From O'Loughlin, J. M.: Lahey Clin. Found. Bull. 22:76, 1973.

ated with Calmette Guérin bacillus (BCG) have a better prognosis (Sokol and Aungst, 1969). However, previous anergy can be lost during remissions. The loss of cellular immunity is therefore reversible, but in the end stage of the disease it is usually irreversible.

DIAGNOSTIC PROCEDURES

How does one diagnose these experiments of nature? Suspicion should be aroused when an infant fails to thrive and has frequent infections and diarrhea. Initial studies should include a Schick test, which measures IgG neutralizing antibody to diphtheria toxin and should give negative results after one or two diphtheria immunizations. Total gamma globulin levels can be determined by paper electrophoresis, and the value should be more than 400 mg. per 100 ml. Saline isoagglutinin titers of anti-A or anti-B or both are a measure of IgM antibodies. Titers should be more than 1 to 4 to A or B erythrocytes or both (depending on ABO group) at six months and higher at one year. Except for patients with an AB blood type, low or absent isoagglutinin titers indicate poor IgM function.

When any of the above tests are abnormal, quantitative immunoglobulin levels should be determined. Measurement of IgA, IgG, and IgM can be performed with commercially available agar radial diffusion kits. Values are determined in milligrams per 100 ml. and compared with age-matched controls.

To evaluate cell-mediated deficiency for diagnosing a congenital problem or a tumor-related deficiency, or for rendering prognosis, one should perform tuberculin, histoplasmin, coccidioidin, blastomycin, mumps, streptokinase-streptodornase, and Candida skin tests. These will show no delayed skin reactions. Direct lymphocyte count is usually less than 1500 cells per cubic millimeter, and the response of peripheral lymphocytes to stimulation with phytohemagglutinin has generally shown a diminished or absent response. Poor or no sensitization to 2,4 DNFB is seen. A summary of the diagnostic workup is shown in Table 4–10.

TABLE 4–10 STUDIES TO DIAGNOSE IMMUNOLOGIC DEFICIENCY SYNDROMES[*]

Humoral Deficiency
  Schick test
  Total gamma globulin level
  Isoagglutinin titers of anti-A or anti-B
  Quantitative immunoglobulin determination
  Recurrent severe bacterial infections

Cell-Mediated Deficiency
  Lymphopenia
  Severe viral infections
  Skin tests: Negative (PPD, histoplasmin, Candida, Coccidioides immitis, blastomycosis, streptokinase-streptodornase)
  2,4 DNFB skin test—No response after sensitization dose

[*]From O'Loughlin, J. M.: Surg. Clin. North Am. 56:755, 1973.

TREATMENT

In the combined form of deficiency, gamma globulin is of no help, but bone marrow transplants have occasionally been successful. In congenital or acquired hypogammaglobulinemia, gamma globulin can be lifesaving. Bacterial infection can usually be prevented by raising the level to 200 mg. per 100 ml. A loading dose of 1.8 ml. per kilogram of body weight in three divided doses (0.6 ml. or 100 mg. per kilogram) is given. Since the half-life of gamma globulin is 25 to 30 days, a monthly injection of 0.6 ml. per kilogram is needed to maintain an approximate 200 mg. per 100 ml. serum level. Antibiotic therapy is given only for specific infections. Great caution must be taken not to give the gamma globulin intravenously, since severe pyrogenic and cardiovascular problems can occur. Injections have been given for years to patients without isosensitization. Severe reactions to intravenously administered gamma globulin have been attributed to aggregations of small amounts of globulin during preparation of the product. Commercial gamma globulin contains only trace amounts of IgA and IgM and is made from a pool of donor plasmas so that antibodies to many infectious agents will be present in adequate titer. Not more than 5.0 ml. should be given in any one site.

Among the diseases that have an immunologic derangement and are associated with cutaneous or mucocutaneous disorders are Wiskott-Aldrich syndrome and mucocutaneous candidiasis.

Wiskott-Aldrich Syndrome

The Wiskott-Aldrich syndrome is characterized by a clinical triad of eczema, thrombocytopenia, and recurrent cutaneous and respiratory infections. Patients with this condition are frequently incapable of being sensitized to 2,4 DNFB and have an immunoglobulin deficiency mainly of IgM, but any combination can be present. Baldini (1969) has demonstrated that the platelet deficiency is caused by accelerated destruction secondary to an inherent platelet defect. The syndrome appears early in life and is usually fatal; the cause of death is sepsis or hemorrhage. The eczema, which favors the scalp, face, flexures, and buttocks, may resemble atopic or seborrheic dermatitis and may become purpuric. Superimposed bacterial infections and, reportedly, Kaposi's varicelliform eruption occur (Palmgren and Lindberg, 1963; Valdimarsson et al., 1970). As in other immunoglobulin deficiency states, there is a high incidence of lymphoreticular malignancy. Treatment consists of appropriate antibiotics. Bone marrow transplantation, transfer factor (Levin et al., 1970), and thymic transplant have recently been successful.

Mucocutaneous Candidiasis

Mucocutaneous candidiasis is found when the usual saprophytic organism, *Candida albicans,* becomes a pathogen. Chronic mucocutaneous candidiasis is a rare infection of children who have an underlying endocrinopathy or immunologic deficiency (Kirkpatrick et al., 1971). Usually, the body can defend itself against this organism when the cell-mediated immune system is intact and the opsonins are functioning properly, facilitating phagocytosis. Defective performance of either of these defense systems, whether due to a genetic disorder or the result of being iatrogenically produced or secondary to underlying disease, may permit severe and often fatal systemic candidiasis.

Candida accounts for from 5 to 10 per cent of clinical infections in normal children during the neonatal period. By one year of age, 80 per cent of children have positive delayed hypersensitivity reactions to challenge. Of children older than six months, 80 to 90 per cent have immunofluorescent antibody titers greater than 1 to 16. Clinically, the child presents with Candida infection of the skin on the face and oral mucosa, weight loss, and failure to grow. While the incidence of severe pulmonary opportunistic infections is great, primary pneumonia caused by Candida is infrequent.

Either sex may be affected. The involved mucous membranes usually have white adherent plaques on the buccal mucosa and tongue, and there is loss of papillae of the tongue. The corners of the mouth, when involved, may become ulcerated or fissured. Laryngeal involvement may cause hoarseness, but candidal esophagitis rarely produces dysphagia. Skin involvement is usually superficial and affects particularly the nail (chronic paronychia), nasolabial folds, ears, and occasionally the groin and trunk. Involvement of the hairline and scalp also occurs.

The diagnosis is confirmed by demonstrating the responsible organism and the associated underlying endocrinopathy, such as hypoparathyroidism and Addison's disease, or defective cellular immunity. The immunologic deficit is appreciated by the demonstration of a decreased absolute lymphocyte count, negative intradermal tests, and the failure to produce migration inhibitory factor. These patients have impaired humoral antibody production, especially of IgA.

Therapy has been successful utilizing appropriate doses of amphotericin B for longer than one month at a time, since therapy must be continued beyond the usual one-month turnover time of skin and the treatment of the underlying disease. Success has been reported with the use of transfer factor (Levin et al., 1970).

THE COMPLEMENT SYSTEM

The complement system consists of nine distinct serum proteins reacting sequentially with each other, producing a variety of biological effects. Its components interact in a cascade type of sequence similar to that of the blood coagulation mechanism. While intermediate steps produce products that have certain biological effects, the end result of the system's activation is cell membrane damage. An alternate pathway exists in which the first three reactions are by-passed, and the last six proteins are activated. This involves the properdin system (Götze and Müller-Eberhard, 1971); congenital absence of control of these proteins can result in clinical disease, such as hereditary angioneurotic edema or an increased susceptibility to infection. Levels of certain of the proteins are lowered in inflammatory processes such as C3. CH50 is the sum of the components of hemolytic complement, and its measurement can be useful in following the course of clinical disease.

The complement system is activated when an antibody with a complement-fixing ability (IgG and IgM) unites with a specific antigen. The complex of C1 (C1qrs) attaches to the Fc fragment. C1q has the binding site for antibody and by the actions of C1r, C1s is activated to form C1 esterase. Activated C1 activates C4 and

C2, from which is formed an enzyme, C3 convertase, which then splits C3 into two fragments. C3a has anaphylatoxic and chemotactic activity, while C3b stays on the cell surface, allowing interaction of the next three components. The C5, C6, and C7 complexes have chemotactic activity for polymorphonuclear leukocytes. C8 is added, resulting in a partially damaged cell and, with the addition of C9, membrane lysis occurs. A summary of the cascade reactions is shown in Figure 4–5.

Because of the potent biological effects in the complement system, nature has provided controls. There is usually rapid deterioration and loss of their binding capacity. Loss of enzyme activity controls the system as well. Inhibitors from outside the system control the reactions, as evidenced by lack of inhibitor of C1 esterase with the resultant disease, hereditary angioneurotic edema.

Hereditary angioneurotic edema is a rare disorder transmitted as a Mendelian dominant trait. Clinically, it presents as localized transient swelling of the skin and mucous membrane of the throat and intestinal mucosa. There is often severe, sudden abdominal pain and swelling of any part of the skin. Laryngeal edema re-

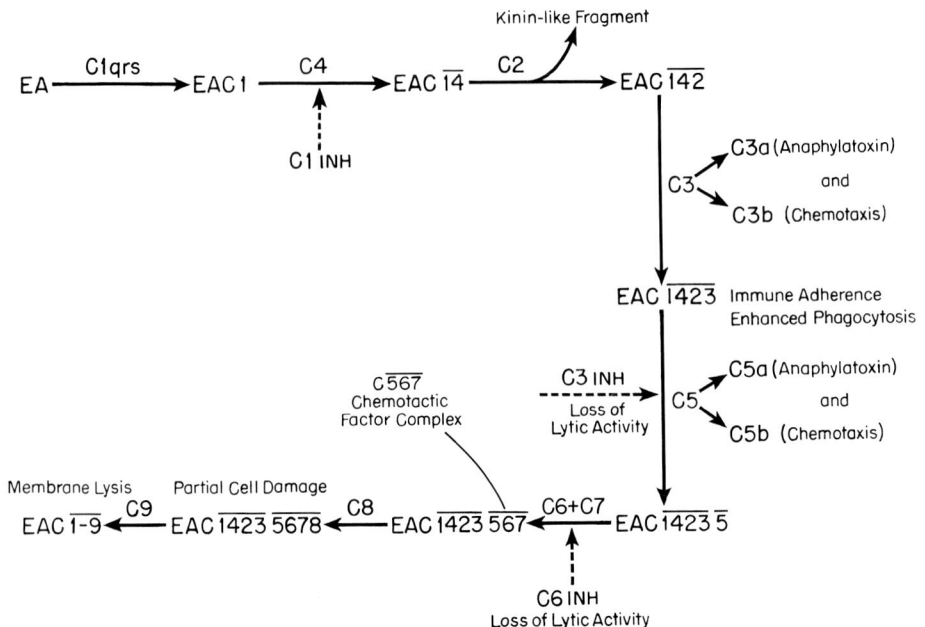

Figure 4–5 Complement cascade. (Modified from Schur, P. H., and Austen, K. F.: Bull. Rheum. Dis. *22*:667, Nos. 5 and 6, 1971–72 Series.)

curs in 20 to 25 per cent of patients and is a frequent cause of death. Symptomatology usually begins in the first two decades but may occur later. The cutaneous swelling, which is rarely preceded by or associated with a serpiginous erythema, is localized, pale, nonpruritic, and nonpitting. The lesion appears on the face and extremities and is usually precipitated by trauma which sometimes may be minimal. The mucocutaneous swellings may occur independently of abdominal symptoms, which often require surgical intervention. In some patients, the attack occurs at regular intervals. The second and fourth components of complement are substrates for C1 esterase, and with lack of the latter's inhibition, levels of these complement components are low. Hence, measurement of the fourth component of complement (B1E) is a useful screen to diagnose this order. Epsilon aminocaproic acid (Frank et al., 1971) and an analogue, tranexamic acid (Sheffer et al., 1972), are being used and evaluated for therapy.

Inherited deficiencies of the complement system in addition to hereditary angioneurotic edema include C3 deficiency associated with increased susceptibility to pyogenic infections, C5 deficit manifested by impaired phagocytosis, and decreased C1q characterized by defective IgG synthesis.

Levels of complement vary in inflammatory states. Decrease in blood levels is found with excessive utilization (antigen-antibody complexes) in systemic lupus erythematosus, acute glomerulonephritis, and auto-immune hemolytic anemia, and in connective-tissue disorders such as rheumatoid disorders with joint effusion. Decreased synthesis, which is found in severe liver disease, proliferative glomerulonephritis, and lupus erythematosus, also results in lowered blood levels.

IMMUNE REACTIONS

The types of immune reactions which can be injurious are the immediate hypersensitivity reactions, such as anaphylaxis, cytolysis, soluble antigen-antibody complexes, and delayed hypersensitivity (Table 4–11).

Anaphylaxis

Anaphylaxis is a hypersensitivity state that may be acute (response within seconds) or subacute (response within hours) and is characterized by an antigen-antibody reaction. Mast cells, when exposed to antigen, release mainly histamine and other vasoactive peptides, bradykinin, serotonin, eosinophilic chemotactic factor of anaphylaxis (ECF-A; Kay et al., 1971), and a lipoprotein called slow-reacting substance of anaphylaxis (SRS-A). The last is thought, by some, to be a product of the polymorphonuclear leukocyte and is an acidic lipid whose structure is still unknown.

The clinical manifestations of the syndrome vary and are discussed in detail in section II of this chapter. It characteristically affects smooth muscle and small blood vessels. The offending antibody is reagin, immunoglobulin IgE, and has the following characteristics: it is present in extremely small concentration in serum; it persists at the skin site for up to six weeks; it cannot be transferred across the placenta; it is inactivated by heat and sulfapyridine; it moves electrophoretically as slow beta globulin; and it cannot passively sensitize guinea pigs. The complement system is not involved in anaphylaxis. In experimental animals, the three types of anaphylaxis that can be produced are systemic (usually resulting in acute, fatal shock), local cutaneous anaphylaxis, and organ anaphylaxis. The local cutaneous reaction can be produced by intradermal injection of antigen into actively sensitized guinea pigs with the production of a wheal and flare response or by passive cutaneous anaphylaxis.

Cytolysis

Although complement is usually necessary for injury or death of a cell, lysis can result when cytophilic anaphylactic antibodies react with extrinsic antigen at the cell surface or within it. These cytolytic antibodies are almost always IgG with the exception of IgM agglutinins, which require complement. The penicillin-induced immunohemolytic anemia is an example of this complement-associated cytolysis. It appears that IgG renders the coated cells

TABLE 4–11 COMPARISON OF HARMFUL IMMUNE REACTIONS

	Anaphylaxis	*Cytolysis*	*Soluble Antigen-Antibody Complexes*	*Delayed Hypersensitivity*
Response mediated by	IgE (antibody)	IgG and IgM	IgG and IgM	Sensitized lymphocytes and macrophages; question of special class of high affinity antibodies
Complement	Absent	Usually absent except with cold hemagglutinins	Present	Absent
Effector cells	Mast cells and leukocytes	Mononuclear and macrophages	Polymorphonuclear leukocytes (opsonin)	"Inflammatory cells"
Passive transfer	Serum		Serum	Transfer factor (extract of human WBC)
Inhibited by	Antihistamine, not by steroids unless high enough to inhibit antibody formation	None	None; Arthus except urticaria of serum sickness	No
Skin test	Immediate wheal and flare		Infiltration 12 to 48 hours; wheal and flare	Delayed tuberculin-type response
Clinical syndrome	Urticaria, angioneurotic edema, hay fever, asthma	Several types of hemolytic anemia, i.e., newborn, penicillin-induced immunohemolytic anemia, neutropenia, thrombocytopenia	Arthus syndrome, serum sickness, acute poststreptococcal glomerulonephritis, lupus nephritis, allergic nodular vasculitis	Contact dermatitis, homograft rejection

susceptible to damage by macrophages and mononuclear cells.

Soluble Antigen-Antibody Complex (Aggregate Anaphylaxis)

In contrast to the cytotropic anaphylaxis, which requires a latent period for the attachment of the antibody to cell receptors, the reaction in aggregate anaphylaxis occurs within minutes after injection of antigen. The size of insoluble immune aggregates results in their removal by the reticuloendothelial system, which makes them harmless. The soluble immune complexes persist intravascularly and permeate the vascular system. Since the kidneys filter the blood, deposition of the complexes in the basement membrane can be anticipated. The complement system is activated with the generation of the chemotactic product. The polymorphonuclear cells appear and phagocytize the deposits. The lysosomal granules of these cells rupture, and their lytic enzymes are released. The antigen must be in slight to moderate excess of equivalence to antibody in the region of the reaction, and then the severity depends upon the concentration of the precipitating antibody.

The duration and amount of production of soluble immune complexes govern the type of disease, prognosis, and the lesion that may develop in the kidney. If it is transient, acute serum sickness or acute poststreptococcal glomerulonephritis can occur and heal. When these complexes are continually formed, a membranous glomerulonephritis can result by deposition of antigen, antibody, and complement in the subepithelial area of the glomerulus. The renal deposition of soluble complexes of DNA and anti-DNA results in lupus nephritis. In the diseased glomerulus of patients with poststreptococcal glomerulonephritis, bacterial antigenic and antibacterial antibodies have been demonstrated.

In animals, the Arthus reaction is an experimentally induced example of a localized, immediate hypersensitivity precipitated by soluble immune antigen complexes and mediated in part by complement. Biopsy of the site of injection reveals hemorrhage, capillary thrombosis, and necrosis. Mild and severe Arthus reactions following cutaneous injection of various serums, vaccine, and antibodies can cause extensive local necrosis of skin and muscle of man. The vasculitides associated with the administration of drugs and foreign serum are probably caused by the Arthus reaction.

Serum Sickness

Serum sickness syndrome develops 8 to 12 days after the therapeutic administration of foreign serum protein, usually horse antitoxin, and is characterized by fever, lymphadenopathy, splenomegaly, urticarial rash, arthralgias or arthritis, and nephritis. Before the onset of symptoms, unbound protein can be detected in the serum. Leukopenia, hypocomplementemia, and albuminuria are present. The immunologic mechanisms have not been identified. The syndrome appears to be an expression of both Arthus and anaphylactic responses. The presence of focal vascular lesions, antigen-antibody aggregates, and hypocomplementemia suggests that serum sickness is a disseminated form of Arthus reaction. The skin eruption is probably the result of antibodies of the Prausnitz-Küstner type. If a patient becomes sensitized to horse serum by contact with horse dander or by the previous administration of horse antiserum, he can experience anaphylaxis and immediate serum sickness upon reexposure. After recovery has occurred, intradermal injection of the foreign protein results in an immediate wheal and flare response.

Delayed Hypersensitivity

Delayed hypersensitivity is an immunologic reaction which occurs on exposure to the antigen and results in an inflammatory reaction apparent in the first few hours but normally appreciable in 24 to 48 hours. The tuberculin reaction is a dermal hypersensitivity reaction in appropriately sensitized persons or animals occurring 12 to 48 hours after intradermal injection of tuberculoprotein. The reaction is regularly transferable to sensitized subjects with cells but not with serum. The mediators important in immediate hypersensitivity, histamine and kinins, are not needed for delayed hypersensitivity. It can be induced with infectious agents, certain chemicals, and foreign animal cells. The induction of delayed hypersensitivity is favored by the use of agents such as Freund's adjuvants.

Cellular immunity is playing an increasing role in biological phenomena and in the pathogenesis of several diseases. Among these are the defense against bacterial and viral infections, allograft rejections, immunologic responses against malignant diseases, graft versus host reactions, and the pathogenesis of some autoimmune diseases. Among the diseases with absent delayed hypersensitivity are congenital thymic dysplasia and the Swiss type of agammaglobulinemia. Depressed delayed hypersensitivity occurs in Hodgkin's disease, chronic lymphatic leukemia, sarcoidosis, certain viral infections (measles, influenza), lepromatous leprosy, chronic mucocutaneous candidiasis, ataxia-telangiectasis, and Wiskott-Aldrich syndrome.

CHEMICAL MEDIATORS

At the present time, it is believed that antigen-antibody reactions involve several chemical substances such as histamine, serotonin, bradykinin, SRS-A, and the recently described ECF-A (Kay et al., 1971), each having the potential for mediating the responses of smooth muscle contraction or increasing vascular permeability—hallmarks of immediate hypersensitivity. Failure of an antihistamine drug to relieve all the symptoms of an allergic reaction could be attributed to the number of substances involved in the reactions.

Evidence implicating another substance

appeared in 1940 when Kellaway and Trethewie (1940) demonstrated that sensitized guinea pig lung tissue could slowly contract guinea pig ileum. It was termed slow-reacting substance. Brocklehurst (1960) proved this reaction when he duplicated it on an isolated guinea pig ileum in the presence of a potent antihistamine, thereby suggesting a compound other than histamine. He named the substance slow-reacting substance of anaphylaxis, SRS-A, to distinguish it from other materials that also could produce such contractions in the presence of antihistamine but that were not formed or released as a result of an immunologic event. Beraldo, in 1950, demonstrated that the plasma of a dog undergoing active system anaphylaxis contained bradykinin, a blood-pressure lowering and a smooth muscle contracting substance.

Of the mediators, histamine has been studied the most intensively. In mammals, it is found mainly in the granules of mast cells located in the perivascular connective tissue. It is stored by electrostatic binding to a heparin-protein complex, and its release is accomplished by interaction of human reaginic antibody with its specific antigen at cell surfaces. This form of immunologic release of histamine from either the human polymorphonuclear leukocyte or the rat mast cell is a process unaccompanied by the discharge of other intracellular molecules.

Presently, there is no strong evidence that serotonin contributes to the immediate hypersensitivity reaction in man. It, too, is present in rat mast cells. It is found abundantly in platelets of some species of animals as well as in the enterochromaffin cells of their gastrointestinal tracts. Like histamine, serotonin in its final form exists in the primary target cell and is released as a result of a relevant immunologic event.

Kinins are peptides formed by the enzymatic action of kallikrein on the alpha globulin plasma substrate, kininogen. Plasma kallikrein elaborates the nonapeptide, bradykinin, and tissue kallikrein, the decapeptide, kallidin. The latter is rapidly degraded to bradykinin by plasma aminopeptidase. Hence, enzyme activation is necessary for the kinin system to be operable. The enzyme system is set off by any change in surface charge because the first protein triggering the pathway is the Hageman factor, which also starts the clotting sequence. Whenever the kinin cascade is begun, it is necessary to determine whether such activation is primary (the result of an immunologic event) or secondary to nonspecific tissue injury. In either event, it may aggravate the response and contribute to further tissue injury. Newer methods for more refined assays of bradykinin and kallikrein may eventually allow determination of whether the presence of kinin in an anaphylactic reaction is caused by a specific immunoglobulin or is the result of a secondary response.

The structure of SRS-A, an acidic lipid, is unknown. Its biologic significance in man comes from the following: it is released from the lungs of allergic humans on challenge with specific pollen antigen; human bronchiolar smooth muscle is very sensitive to the contracting activities of SRS-A preparations; and antihistamines are of limited benefit in controlling allergic bronchospasm. Diethylcarbamazine, an antifilarial agent, has been shown to decrease the severity of asthma. It has been demonstrated to be an active inhibitor of immunologic release of SRS-A in the rat without being an end-organ antagonist of SRS-A. Altounyan (1967), a British pharmacologist who had allergies, stimulated studies to find substances to block SRS-A release. Challenged with methacholine, histamine, and antigen, he observed that khellin protected him against antigen challenges but not against histamine or methacholine. Colleagues then were persuaded to synthesize structurally related compounds. From this research was developed disodium cromoglycate (Intal), shown to be effective against aerosol challenge tests in man, presumably by stabilizing mast cell wall membrane and inhibiting the release of SRS-A and histamine.

It has been shown that IgE mediates the direct release of both SRS-A and histamine, and that diethylcarbamazine blocks the pathways leading to the release of SRS-A and histamine. Studies (Lichtenstein and Margolis, 1968; Lichtenstein and Norman, 1969) suggested that beta-ad-

ISUPREL or EPINEPHRINE ←———————————————— ? STEROIDS

←- - - - - - - - - - - *β* BLOCKERS (Propanolol)

ADENYLCYCLASE IN CELL MEMBRANE

ATP $\xrightarrow{Mg^{++}}$ CYCLIC 3'5' AMP $\begin{pmatrix} \downarrow \text{SRS-A} \\ \downarrow \text{HISTAMINE} \end{pmatrix}$ $\xrightarrow{\text{Phosphodiesterase}}$ 5'AMP

XANTHINE
? STEROIDS

Figure 4–6 Catecholamines stimulate formation of cyclic-AMP by stimulating adenylcyclase. Theophylline derivatives block breakdown of cyclic-AMP by inhibiting phosphodiesterase. Steroids: ? enhance effect of epinephrine; ? overcome beta blockade.

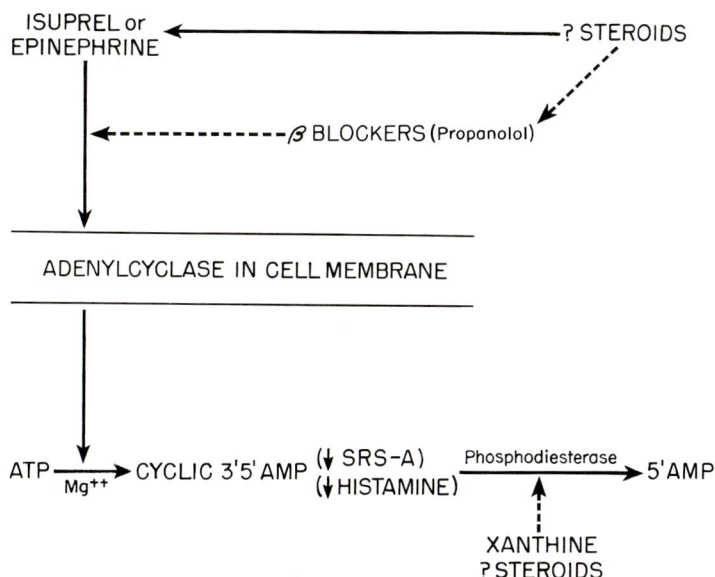

renergic agents inhibit the IgE-mediated release of histamine from human peripheral leukocytes. Evidence indicates that agents capable of increasing the intracellular level of cyclic-AMP also inhibit the release of SRS-A and histamine. Methylxanthine derivatives, such as theophylline, which block the phosphodiesterase-mediated catabolism of cyclic-AMP, are inhibitory. The synergism between methylxanthines and beta-adrenergic drugs accounts for their efficacy in asthmatic patients (Fig. 4–6).

CYCLIC-AMP

Cyclic-AMP (adenosine-3',5'-[cyclic]-monophosphate) is formed by the action of adenylcyclase on adenosine triphosphate (ATP). The effects of cyclic-AMP occur without its being destroyed. However, it is rapidly inactivated by a phosphodiesterase, which opens the phosphate-ribose ring to yield 5'-AMP.

During the past several years, cyclic-AMP has been implicated in the actions of a wide variety of hormones. Most of these hormones, including epinephrine, glucagon, thyroxine, ACTH, and others, have a significant effect on target organs by either increasing or decreasing cyclic-AMP. For

instance, increased cyclic-AMP levels in the liver acted on by glucagon cause increased glycogenolysis and gluconeogenesis. Catecholamine effect on the heart with elevated cyclic-AMP results in an increased inotropic effect. Conversely, decreased levels of cyclic-AMP in fatty tissue when thus acted on by insulin result in decreased lipolysis.

PROSTAGLANDINS

Another group of substances whose action is only partially known at this time but which probably have a role in anaphylaxis are prostaglandins. Chemically, they consist of two hydrocarbon chains connected by a cyclopentane ring. They are synthesized mainly from essential fatty acids, which are both lipid soluble and water soluble. The four different groups of prostaglandins that are known by differences in the pentane ring are PGE, PGF, PGA, and PGB. The biological properties vary depending on the structure and include vasodilation and constriction, contraction or relaxation of smooth and cardiac muscle, water and salt diuresis, fever, and wheal and flare skin reactions. The mechanism of action and release of these compounds is complex and probably involves adenylcyclase as well as the membrane binding of calcium. It has been postulated that many properties of prostaglandins, as well as their formation from precursors, can be inhibited by salicylates and indomethacin (Vane, 1972). Because of their probable relationship to adenylcyclase and certain biologic properties, prostaglandins probably have a role in immediate hypersensitivity and the pathophysiology of asthma.

INFLAMMATION

Nature's response to the injury or destruction of cells is called inflammation. Foremost of the causes of this process are such agents as bacteria and viruses; however, heat, cold, radiation, chemicals, or mechanical trauma can provoke the response of inflammation. The inflammatory response is often aided by necrotic products released from dead cells when necrosis occurs. Regardless of the injurious agent or the involved area, a certain number of tissue adjustments that involve mainly blood vessels and fluid and other cellular components of the blood as well as the surrounding connective tissue occur. Arteriolar dilation causes an increased rate of blood flow through the arterioles, capillaries, and venules and an increased permeability that permits the outpouring of the inflammatory fluid into the injured tissue. Red cells are concentrated in the capillaries, causing slowing of the blood flow, sometimes to a standstill. Peripheral movement of the white cells in the capillaries results in the ultimate migration of white blood cells from the vessel walls to the inflammatory focus. It is believed that polymorphonuclear leukocytes migrate first and are then followed by mononuclear cells, including monocytes, lymphocytes, and plasma cells. To be a true acute inflammatory reaction, vascular dilation, fluid exudation, and an accumulation of inflammatory white cells must be present.

To the clinician, inflammation is characterized by redness, which is a result of increased vascularity in the injured areas. Exudation of fluid and production of edema cause localized swelling. Pain results from the involvement of nerve fibers in the inflammatory area, either by pressure of edema or by chemical irritation by at least some of the substances. Loss of function is probably secondary to the involvement of the nerve fibers. Electron microscopy indicates that capillaries and venules are actually sieves rather than intact tubes. The existence of local pores leading into the lining cells suggests a means of transfer from the lumen to extracellular spaces. Venules now are thought to be the first set of minute vessels that show increased vascular permeability when a tissue is injured. As long as the basement membrane area is intact, only filtered plasma can form the exudate of inflammation.

The idea has evolved that injury compels cells to discharge their components or to manufacture during their dissolution endogenous substances that guide the events of inflammatory origin. It is possible to locate chemical mediators, such as histamine and serotonin, and other mediators in certain regions of the cells, especially in the mitochondrial lysosomes. It is generally accepted that the chief chemical mediator is histamine, and while it probably initiated, it does not sustain the vascular response. Histamine is found in two types of cells—basophilic leukocytes and mast cells. Changes in permeability occurring after injury are divided into two stages—an early stage caused by histamine liberation and a later sustained interval independent of histamine action.

Some inflammations are short lived and are completed within hours or days, while others are maintained for weeks. Some chemicals held to be responsible for the sustained vascular reaction are polypeptides and kinins. Bradykinin is one of the most active vasodilating substances in man. It is formed by the action of plasma kinin-forming enzymes (kallikrein) on plasma globulins; this reaction probably occurs in the interstitial tissue spaces. Cellular injury occurs and probably exerts its effects on the closest blood vessels. The epinephrine precursors are inactivated by enzymatic mechanisms, especially that of monoamine oxidase. After inactivation, the vessels dilate, and the raised hydrostatic capillary pressure consequent to the greater blood flow through their distended lumina leads to exudation of plasma.

It is probable that the destruction of leukocytes at the site of injury might yield other substances that would help to maintain altered permeability. During normal cellular life, leukocytes pass from the smallest vessels to tissue spaces; however, this migration is greatly accelerated during injury. Microscopically, large numbers of leukocytes can be seen at the site of damage, especially when necrosis has occurred. Since the cells at these places are phagocytic, it is believed that migration and tendency toward aggregation are defense mechanisms aimed at destroying and neutralizing the agents responsible for injury. As circulation slows in the injured area, the process known as pavementing occurs wherein leukocytes cling to the endothelial lining and soon attach themselves firmly. Leukocytes then appear to leave the small blood vessels by pseudopods that protrude into the endothelial cells and wiggle through the wall by amoeboid movement.

Chemotaxis has been defined as a positive directional response to a chemical stimulus. The stimulus appears to direct the leukocytes and monocytes toward the injurious agent and damaged cells. The stimulus may come from the agent itself or may be produced by the cells after injury. The early stage of almost all inflammation is marked by the predominance of the polymorphonuclear leukocytes, especially if the inflammation is caused by bacterial infection. When this response subsides, mononuclear cells then far outnumber the polymorphonuclear leukocytes. However, in some bacterial infections, especially brucellosis, typhoid, and tuberculosis, monocytes have the primary contact, but polymorphonuclear leukocytes appear to be transiently present in the early stages of infection.

Phagocytosis

The first line of defense in pyogenic infection is mobilization of the polymorphonuclear leukocytes with back-up by the monocyte and mononuclear phagocytes. Phagocytosis is the ingestion and immobilization of foreign material whether it be bacterial, parasitic, or necrotic tissue from a foreign material. Phagocytosis is largely accomplished by polymorphonuclear leu-

kocytes. Gamma globulin and the third component of complement (C3) opsonize microbes, rendering them more susceptible to phagocytes. The phagocyte then ingests the opsonized microorganism. Degranulation follows these steps, and finally the generation of hydrogen peroxide by the phagocytes causes microbial death. Failure of any of these steps (chemotaxis, opsonization, ingestion, degranulation, and peroxidation) causes the patient to experience an increased frequency of severe pyogenic infections, many of which would ordinarily be well handled by the host. Two diseases with defective phagocytosis and dermatologic manifestations are chronic granulomatous disease of children and Chediak-Higashi syndrome.

Chronic Granulomatous Disease of Children

Chronic granulomatous disease of childhood is an X-linked, inherited, fatal disorder characterized by frequent infections and septic granulomatous lesions in the skin, lymph nodes, and lungs (Good et al., 1968). The nitroblue tetrazolium test (NBT) can be utilized to identify defective cellular functions that lead to low levels of hydrogen peroxide production (Baehner and Nathan, 1968). (See also page 780.)

Chediak-Higashi Syndrome

Among the clinical entities associated with a marked susceptibility to pyogenic infections is the Chediak-Higashi syndrome. It is a rare disease inherited as an autosomal recessive trait. Manifestations of the disorder, in addition to frequent infections, include defective pigmentation and abnormal granulation of leukocytes. The pigmentary disturbances of the skin and its appendages consist of partial albinism, lack of pigment in the areola and genital areas, and frosted gray hair. Pigmentary changes are also found in the uveal tract and fundus. While phagocytosis is quantitatively normal, defective postphagocytic degranulation and diminished intracellular bactericidal ability occur.

Patients frequently have pyoderma, ulcerations of the mouth, and fever. Many patients die within the first few years of life. The terminal phase is not unlike that of lymphoma, as hepatosplenomegaly, lymphadenopathy, and pancytopenia develop.

Generally, both cell-mediated and humoral antibody production are normal. Large lysosomal inclusion bodies can be identified in circulating granulocytes, and lymphocytic inclusions have been found in relatives of patients. These giant inclusion bodies illustrate the functional derangement that leads to poor handling of normal lysosomal enzymes and probably involves an accelerated turnover of sphingolipids in leukocytes (Kanfer et al., 1968). Large melanin granules and cytoplasmic granules within neurons may explain the many neurologic manifestations associated with this disorder, such as cranial and peripheral neuropathy, drop foot, and electroencephalographic abnormalities. Treatment consists of appropriate antibiotics as indicated. Antibiotics appear to be ineffective prophylactically (Wolff, 1972).

IMMUNOLOGIC PROCESSES IN INFECTION

Much immunity against infection is innate, but immunity to certain microorganisms and toxins occurs following contact with the antigens in the microorganism. Immunity at any one time will depend on environmental factors.

Innate resistance varies among races and species. For example, certain genetic traits, such as those of sickle cell anemia, hemoglobin C, glucose-6-phosphate dehydrogenase deficiency, and thalassemia, are associated with resistance to malaria.

Natural immunity to certain organisms is present at birth as a result of the transplacental passage of these organisms from the mother. Immunity occurring after infection may be permanent or temporary.

Humoral antibodies play a major role in the body's defense against bacteria by influencing phagocytosis, neutralizing toxins, or by inhibiting the organism. Antibodies against viruses are effective by means of neutralization of the virus-infecting cells. Antibody can only be effective outside the cell and cannot interfere with intracellular duplication. Immunity to viruses is almost always lasting. An important feature of helminthic infections is the increased frequency of IgE antibodies against parasites, which can be demonstrated by immediate wheal and flare reactions to intradermal extracts of the worms. Peripheral eosinophilia is present in most helminthic infections.

The interaction of cellular immunity and humoral antibodies can be shown by demonstrating their relative roles in leprosy at different stages. The leprosy bacillus is not eliminated by humoral antibodies but rather by cellular immune mechanisms. While not killed by humoral antibody, it can stimulate humoral antibody against its constituent antigens. In the tuberculoid form of leprosy, the bacillus growth and proliferation are controlled. The skin is characterized by red inflammatory lesions with mononuclear cells. During this phase of the disease, there is a high degree of a specific cell-mediated immune activity to the bacillus. In the downgrading to the lepromatous form, there is complete failure of this specific cell-mediated immune reaction, and skin biopsy shows uncontrolled bacillus proliferation. At this time, there is no failure of humoral antibody production. A state of split tolerance is achieved, since the patient has become specifically unresponsive to cell-mediated immune responses but is still responsive to humoral antibody production. The lepromin reaction reflects the host's immunologic response to the infective organism. In the tuberculoid form, with a high degree of cell-mediated immunity, the reaction is positive. In lepromatous leprosy, with its aforementioned immunologic unresponsiveness, the reaction is negative. The test is performed by injecting killed whole leprosy bacilli intradermally.

FACTORS MODIFYING THE INFLAMMATORY REACTION

Modification of the inflammatory reaction is related to the strength of the noxious agent and the status of the host. The strength and amount of the noxious agent as well as duration of exposure to the attacking agent have relevance in regard to the severity of the reaction.

Generally, the amount of a bacteria involved will determine whether or not an infection will occur. Some bacteria and chemical agents are more virulent than others. The full-blown pattern of the inflammatory reaction often depends on the invading agent. Viruses rarely cause focal necrosis of tissue but rather an interstitial reaction that is evidenced by edema with a mononuclear infiltrate as opposed to polymorphonuclear response that is characteristic of pyogenic bacteria. Rickettsiae produce a hemorrhagic inflammation.

Spread of infection is enhanced by lowering the mechanical barriers. The ability of an offending agent to invade the tissue involved is dependent upon several factors, one of which is lymphatic blockage, which is characteristic of staphylococcal infections and which evokes fibrin thrombus formation. The converse is true, however, in streptococcal infections in which enzymes produce lysin (which dissolves ground substances and fibrin) and prevent organisms from being trapped. Blood vessel blockage, which is caused by clot formation, is another of nature's efforts to minimize the dissemination of infectious agents. Certain enzymes, such as the hyaluronidases, have been shown to hydrolyze the mucopolysaccharides of the ground substance of connective tissues, thereby making it more fluid and permeable, and they are elaborated by staphylococci, streptococci, and clostridia.

DEFENSE STATUS OF THE HOST

The ability of the host to counter the invading organism is very important in determining the extent of inflammation that may occur. The age, general health structure, and nutrition of the host are very important. In general, the younger the patient, the greater is the ability to withstand injuries and reduce damage. In older persons, preexisting diseases of blood vessel and dietary deficiencies are of great significance. Protein-depleted cells are more vulnerable to noxious agents. Antibodies, both naturally occurring and acquired, will modify the resistance of the host to infection. By coating bacteria, antibodies render them more susceptible to phagocytosis.

Certain metabolic diseases, particularly diabetes mellitus, make patients more prone to severe inflammatory reactions. Hormones, such as the glucocorticoids, influence the inflammatory reaction by their effect on lymphocyte response. An adequate blood supply renders the patient more resistant to infection and more capable of containing the offending agents. The location of injury may significantly modify inflammation, since compact tissues tend to resist spread of infection in contrast to loose tissues, such as lungs and subcutaneous fibrous tissues, whose cleavage planes allow spread of invasive agents.

CONDITIONS AND FACTORS THAT AFFECT HOST DEFENSE

In addition to the aforementioned deficiency syndromes and disease states in which there is either cell-mediated, humoral, or combined deficiency, predisposing conditions (Table 4–12) and factors (Table 4–13) make a patient more susceptible to opportunistic infections (Table 4–14). Generally, the preceding therapeutic modalities make the predisposed patient a candidate for these complications.

It has been shown in patients with leukemia (Gruhn and Sanson, 1963), lymphoreticular malignancies (Parkhurst and Vlahides, 1967), or neoplasms in general (Murray et al., 1966) that with increased use of immunosuppressive agents and steroids there has been an increase in opportunistic infections.

Many of the opportunistic pathogens normally inhibit man—that is, cytomegalovirus, which is found in almost 80 per cent of the population and only rarely causes disease in the patient with an intact immunologic system. Most persons who have had varicella infections harbor varicella/zoster the rest of their lives, but in the

TABLE 4–12 PREDISPOSING CONDITIONS FAVORING INFECTION

Immunoglobulin deficiency syndrome
Malignant disease
Connective tissue disorders
Burns

TABLE 4–13 PREDISPOSING FACTORS
FAVORING INFECTION

Antibiotics
Steroids
Cytotoxic drugs
Radiation
Organ transplantation

immunologically incompetent, severe and even fatal infections can occur. Likewise, *Toxoplasma gondii* is present in 35 to 50 per cent of the population but can cause disease especially in the patient who has received a transplant organ and whose defense mechanism has been altered by chemotherapy. *Pneumocystis carinii* can cause a rapidly progressive pneumonia in the immunosuppressed patient. In the lymphoproliferative and myeloproliferative disorders, there has been shown to be a reduced level of immunoglobulin and impaired phagocytosis, respectively increasing prospects for opportunistic infection and the rapid demise of the patient. The deleterious effect steroid therapy has on some patients is probably caused by the enhancement of lysosomal membrane stabilization. This prevents membrane rupture and consequent release of lytic enzymes. Antibiotics, by changing the endogenous flora, may encourage opportunistic organisms to flourish.

Specific antibiotics should be used, depending on sensitivity patterns. With the fungal infections, combination or single therapy with amphotericin B and 5-fluorocytosine is used. Infection with *Pneumocystis carinii* is treated with pentamidine isothionate or pyrimethamine and sulfadiazine combination when the former is unavailable.

TABLE 4–14 OPPORTUNISTIC PATHOGENS

Bacteria	*Viruses*	*Fungi*	*Protozoa*
Pseudo-monas	Herpes simplex	Candida	*Toxoplasma gondii*
Bacteroides	Varicella/zoster	Crypto-coccus	*Pneumocystis carinii*
Listeria	Cytomeg-alovirus	Aspergillus	
Serratia		Nocardia	

REFERENCES

Altounyan, R. E. C.: Inhibition of experimental asthma by a new compound—disodium cromoglycate "Intal." Acta Allergol. (Kbh) 22:487, 1967.

Amman, A. J., and Hong, R.: Selective IgA deficiency: presentation of 30 cases and a review of the literature. Medicine 50:223, 1971.

Baehner, R. L., and Nathan, D. G.: Quantitative nitroblue tetrazolium test in chronic granulomatous disease. N. Engl. J. Med. 278:971, 1968.

Baldini, M. G.: Platelet defect in Wiskott-Aldrich syndrome. N. Engl. J. Med. 281:107, 1969.

Beraldo, W. T.: Formation of bradykinin in an anaphylactic and peptone shock. Am. J. Physiol. 163:283, 1950.

Brocklehurst, W. E.: The release of histamine and formation of a slow-reacting substance (SRS-A) during anaphylactic shock. J. Physiol. (London) 151:416, 1960.

Frank, M. M., Sergent, J. S., Kane, M. A., et al.: Epsilon aminocaproic acid therapy of hereditary angioneurotic edema. A double-blind study. N. Engl. J. Med. 286:808, 1971.

Fudenberg, H. H., Good, R. A., Hitzig, W., et al.: Classification of the primary immune deficiencies: WHO recommendation. N. Engl. J. Med. 283:656, 1970.

Good, R. A., Quie, P. G., Windhorst, D. B., et al.: Fatal (chronic) granulomatous disease of childhood: a hereditary defect of leukocyte function. Semin. Hematol. 5:215, 1968.

Götze, O., and Müller-Eberhard, H. J.: The C₃-activator system: an alternate pathway of complement activation. J. Exp. Med. 134 (Suppl.):90, 1971.

Gruhn, J. G., and Sanson, J.: Mycotic infections in leukemic patients at autopsy. Cancer 16:61, 1963.

Hobbs, J. R.: Disturbances of the immunoglobulins. Sci. Basis Med. 106–127, 1966.

Janeway, C. A., Rosen, F. S., Merler, E., et al.: The Gamma Globulins. Boston, Little Brown & Co., 1967, pp. 83–86.

Kanfer, J. N., Blume, R. S., Yankee, R. A., et al.: Alteration of sphingolipid metabolism in leukocytes from patients with Chediak-Higashi syndrome. N. Engl. J. Med. 279:410, 1968.

Kay, A. B., Stechschulte, D. J., and Austen, K. F.: An eosinophil leukocyte chemotactic factor of anaphylaxis. J. Exp. Med. 133:602, 1971.

Kellaway, C. H., and Trethewie, E. R.: Liberation of slow-reacting smooth muscle-stimulating substance in anaphylaxis. Q. J. Exp. Physiol. 30:121, 1940.

Kirkpatrick, C. H., Rich, R. R., and Bennett, J. E.: Chronic mucocutaneous candidiasis: model-building in cellular immunity. Ann. Intern. Med. 74:955, 1971.

Levin, A. S., Stites, D. P., Spitler, L. E., et al.: Inductions of "delayed hypersensitivity" in a Wiskott-Aldrich patient by transfer factor. Clin. Res. 18:428, 1970.

Lichtenstein, L. M., and Margolis, S.: Histamine release in vitro: inhibition by catecholamines and methylxanthines. Science 161:902, 1968.

Lichtenstein, L. M., and Norman, P. S.: Human allergic reactions. Am. J. Med. 46:163, 1969.

Murray, J. F., Haegelin, H. F., Hewitt, W. L., et al.: The UCLA interdepartmental conference. Opportunistic pulmonary infections. Ann. Intern. Med. 65:566, 1966.

O'Loughlin, J. M.: Immunologic deficiency states. Med. Clin. North Am. 56:747, 1972.

Palmgren, B., and Lindberg, T.: Immunological studies in Wiskott-Aldrich syndrome. Acta Paediatr. Scand. [Suppl.] *146*:116, 1963.

Parkhurst, G. F., and Vlahides, G. D.: Fatal opportunistic fungus disease. J.A.M.A. *202*:279, 1967.

Sheffer, A. L., Austen, K. F., and Rosen, F. S.: Tranexamic acid therapy in hereditary angioneurotic edema. N. Engl. J. Med. *287*:452, 1972.

Sokol, J. E., and Aungst, C. W.: Response to BCG vaccination and survival in advanced Hodgkin's disease. Cancer *24*:128, 1969.

Valdimarsson, H., Holt, L., Riches, H. R., et al.: Lymphocyte abnormality in chronic mucocutaneous candidiasis. Lancet *1*:1259, 1970.

Vane, J. R.: Prostaglandins and the aspirin-like drugs. Hosp. Prac. *7*:61, 1972.

Wolff, S. M.: The Chediak-Higashi syndrome: studies of host defenses. Ann. Intern. Med. *76*:293, 1972.

Section II

ANAPHYLACTIC SYNDROMES

Harry Irving Katz

INTRODUCTION

The term anaphylactic syndrome (AS) encompasses a wide variety of disorders which may involve a number of organ systems (Austen and Sheffer, 1971; Valentine and Sheffer, 1969). In this section, the term will be limited to those clinical manifestations resulting from acute transient vascular permeability changes and smooth muscle contractions which occur in the host within minutes following a variety of types of challenge. This challenge may be either internal or external in its derivation, although its source is frequently unknown. The AS is solely a clinical, descriptive term, without implications as to etiology or the mechanism by which it comes about. It is the summation of the effects of one or more mechanisms which lead to the overt host response.

Depending upon the method of challenge and the susceptibility of the host, the clinical manifestations of the AS can

be either localized or generalized. In man, the clinical conditions included under the term AS are listed in Table 4–15. The local manifestations generally occur in the skin or mucous membranes. Increased vascular permeability leads to edema and localized swelling. The generalized manifestations may involve large areas of the skin and mucous membranes, but may also include the more vital respiratory and cardiovascular systems, with serious or even fatal outcome. In the past, such terms as anaphylaxis, anaphylactic shock, anaphylactic and anaphylactoid reactions, and others have been used to describe the overt clinical changes occurring after acute transient alterations of vascular integrity and smooth muscle contractility. However, these terms describe only the

The following physicians aided in the editing of this section: Kenneth P. Manick, M.D., Professor, Department of Dermatology, University of Minnesota; Patrick C. J. Ward, M.D., Associate Professor, Department of Laboratory Medicine and Pathology, University of Minnesota; and Stephen C. Weisberg, M.D., Clinical Instructor, Department of Medicine (Allergy), University of Minnesota.

TABLE 4–15 ANAPHYLACTIC SYNDROMES

Transient Vascular and Smooth Muscle Changes
  Localized Manifestations
    Angioedema (angioneurotic edema) and urticaria
    Asthma
    Gastrointestinal colic
    Rhinitis
  Generalized Manifestations
    Generalized angioedema and urticaria
    Respiratory distress
    Cardiovascular crisis

mechanism by which the host is producing the vascular and smooth muscle disturbance.

This section will discuss in detail urticaria, angioedema, and the generalized AS, as they are the major disorders of the anaphylactic syndrome with which dermatologists deal. The other manifestations, although of importance, will be discussed only as they relate to these three disorders. Other longer-lasting disorders, such as certain hemolytic anemias, persistent erythemas, purpuras, and drug reactions which may be produced by mechanisms analogous to those described below, but which do not involve transient vascular and smooth muscle reactivity, are not within the scope of this review.

The mechanisms resulting in vascular and smooth muscle changes are varied, and may be conveniently divided into allergic (anaphylactic reaction) and non-allergic (anaphylactoid reaction) mechanisms, as outlined in Figure 4–7. The challenge to the host, whether it is allergic or non-allergic, must either activate potent chemical mediators of inflammation or have a direct effect on the target cells of the host. The magnitude of the clinical response may be modified by physical, hormonal, or psychic factors, as well as by the previous response of the challenged host. Therefore, the discussions of the AS will be grouped for convenience under the various etiologies, chemical mediators, modifying host factors, and vascular and smooth muscle responses in the host leading to the overt signs and symptoms of the anaphylactic syndrome.

ETIOLOGY

The anaphylactic reaction (anaphylaxis) is, by definition, an immediate allergic reaction occurring within minutes of antigenic challenge by several different immunopathologic mechanisms. Anaphylaxis is perhaps the most spectacular and alarming of all allergic reactions. Anaphylactic reactions differ from anaphylactoid reactions only in method of production. The overt result of either anaphylactic or anaphylactoid reactions can be similar. Anaphylactoid reactions may share common pathologic pathways with, and activate similar chemical mediators as, the anaphylactic reaction. However, anaphylactoid reactions are initiated by non-allergic mechanisms. Anaphylactoid reactions are produced by chemical or physical stimuli that are capable of either direct cellular injury or release of the chemical mediators involved in the production of the anaphylactic syndrome. Some of the causes of the AS are listed in Table 4–16. It is readily apparent that the causes of the AS are varied and vast. Some causative agents act by as yet unknown mechanisms to produce the AS. It is evident that investigations into the causes of either the local or generalized manifestations of the AS must be of a broad scope.

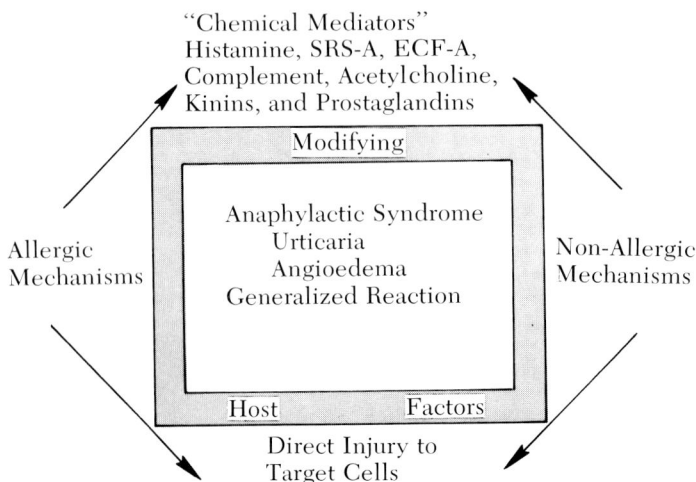

Figure 4–7 Mechanisms producing the anaphylactic syndrome.

TABLE 4–16 SUMMARY OF CAUSES OF THE ANAPHYLACTIC SYNDROME

Exogenous Causes
Allergic reactions
  Proteins—foreign serums, hormones, enzymes, venoms, blood products, pollens, and food extracts
  Polysaccharides—iron dextran, dextran
  Haptens—diagnostic agents, vitamins, analgesics, antibiotics, and anesthetics
Chemical mediator activators (See Table 4–19)
Physical factors
Internal Causes
Constitutional diseases
  Hereditary angioedema
  Urticaria pigmentosa (mastocytosis)
Internal diseases
  Hepatic, renal, collagen-vascular, and neoplastic
  Infectious

reactions in man. These include allergic rhinitis, allergic asthma, some cases of allergic urticaria, and some types of the generalized form of the AS following appropriate antigenic challenge (Sherman, 1971). The HAB in man is an immunoglobulin known as IgE. Synonyms include the skin sensitizing and reaginic antibodies (Sehon and Gyenes, 1971). IgE has unique characteristics which include heat lability, inability to cross the placental barrier, lack of complement fixing ability, and remarkable cytotropism. The latter accounts for the persistence of IgE for many weeks following its intradermal injection in the skin, a feature which distinguishes it from the other immunoglob-

ALLERGIC MECHANISMS (ANAPHYLACTIC REACTION)

The term anaphylaxis or the anaphylactic reaction implies an allergic mechanism of induction for the AS. Several immunopathologic pathways may be involved in the anaphylactic reaction reflecting different antibodies, target cells, or chemical mediators (Austen and Sheffer, 1971; Bloch, 1967a). Table 4–17 summarizes these pathways. Although there are a number of such immediate hypersensitivity pathways leading to anaphylactic reactions, the homocytotropic antibody (HAB) reaction may play the most important role in man. This HAB reaction refers to that type of anaphylaxis involving antigenic challenge of target cells passively sensitized by a homocytotropic antibody (Bloch, 1971). The HAB is a specialized immunoglobulin (Ig) that is attached to (cytotropism) certain target cells of the same species (see Table 4–17). Contact with antigen releases or activates pharmacologic agents from the target cells. Redefinition of this particular type of antibody is necessary because anaphylactic reactions may occur by immunologic mechanisms that do not necessarily involve either the passive sensitization of target cells or the release of chemical mediators from them. This is the case in two other described forms of anaphylaxis (see Table 4–17).

The atopic diathesis (atopy) classically reflects homocytotropic antibody-mediated

TABLE 4–17 ALLERGIC MECHANISMS INVOLVED IN PRODUCTION OF THE ANAPHYLACTIC SYNDROME

1. *Cytotropic Anaphylaxis*
  Chemical mediators are released by passively sensitized target cells after antigenic challenge. If the antibody is derived from the same species as the target cell, it is termed a homocytotropic antibody-mediated reaction; however, if the antibody is from a different animal species, it is termed a heterocytotropic antibody-mediated reaction. A latent period is required for antibody attachment to the target cell. Complement activation is not involved in the reaction. Atopic allergy is an example of a homocytotropic antibody-mediated reaction in man.

  i.e., target cells with cytotropic antibody + antigenic challenge → mediator release → increased vascular permeability and smooth muscle contraction

2. *Aggregate Anaphylaxis*
  Extracellular antigen-antibody reaction leading to the formation of antigen-antibody complexes that cause activation of chemical mediators. Complement is activated during this reaction; a latent period is not required. Serum sickness is an example of aggregate anaphylactic reaction in man.

  i.e., extracellular antigen-antibody + chemical complexes → activation of mediators → toxic vascular damage

3. *Cytotoxic Anaphylaxis*
  Antibody challenge of specific cellular antigen of the target cell leading to the activation of chemical mediators, resulting in lysis of the target cell. Complement activation is involved. Certain hemolytic anemias are examples of cytotoxic anaphylaxis in man.
  i.e., target cell + antibody to target cell antigen → activation of lytic complement → lysis of target cell

ulins. The non-antigen binding portion (Fc fragment) of IgE has the capacity to attach itself to specific receptors of both circulating and fixed cells (target cells) in the shock tissue of the host.

Following human HAB-antigen interaction, changes occur at the surface of the target cell which initiate enzyme activation and lead to the secretion of chemical mediators of inflammation involved in the production of the AS. The mediators released in the HAB reaction using human lung fragments include histamine, slow reacting substance of anaphylaxis (SRS-A), and eosinophil chemotactic factor of anaphylaxis (ECF-A; Kay and Austen, 1971; see Table 4–18). Specifically, the multivalent antigen bridges two or more IgE antibodies on the surface of the target cell. Complement activation is not required (Ishizaka, 1971). Instead, other enzymatic processes are activated that include serine esterase. Additionally, the intracellular concentration of cyclic adenosine-3′,5′-monophosphate (cyclic-AMP) may control the secretion of histamine from the target cell. It has been postulated that the amount of histamine secretion is inversely proportional to the intracellular level of cyclic-AMP (that is, high levels of cyclic-AMP favor reduced secretion of histamine; Austen, 1971). The tissue mast cells and circulating basophils are probably the most important target cells of the HAB type of anaphylactic reaction.

Eosinophils may provide a modifying influence in HAB reactions (Litt, 1964). Eosinophils are attracted to the site of an HAB-mediated reaction by ECF-A (Kay and Austen, 1971). These cells may protect the host by absorbing antigenic material or by liberating an inhibitor of further histamine release from the target cell (Nilzen, 1970).

Since the HAB-mediated reaction is not detected by the usual or routine laboratory procedure, direct wheal and flare scratch or intradermal testing of the patient is sometimes necessary. Under some circumstances skin testing with drugs may be indicated but is not recommended routinely. Alternatively, IgE can be detected by the Prausnitz-Kützner (PK) test, which involves the injection of the suspected allergic serum into the skin of a non-allergic individual, followed by intracutaneous challenge with the suspected antigen 24 hours later (Ishizaka, 1971). A positive PK test is indicated by a wheal and flare reaction. Other less widely available methods for the detection of IgE include radioimmunoassays and the basophil/mast cell degranulation or histamine release assay (Osler et al., 1968). These techniques are of limited practical usefulness and are presently available only in the experimental research laboratory.

The ability to form HAB is a universal phenomenon in man. The elaboration of this antibody routinely follows helminthic

TABLE 4–18 CHEMICAL MEDIATORS THAT MAY BE INVOLVED IN THE ANAPHYLACTIC SYNDROME

Mediator	Source	Major Effect
Histamine	Mast cells Basophils Platelets	Transient increased vascular permeability and vasodilation
Slow reacting substance of anaphylaxis (SRS-A)	Sensitized lung and other tissue	Prolonged slow smooth muscle contraction; slow smooth muscle relaxation
Eosinophil chemotoxic factor of anaphylaxis (ECF-A)	Sensitized lung and other tissue	Attraction of eosinophils to the site of challenge
Kinin system	Plasma	Increased vascular permeability, vasodilatation, smooth muscle stimulation, leukotaxis; causes pain
Complement	Plasma	Increased vascular permeability, immune lysis, leukotaxis, release of histamine through the generation of anaphylatoxin
Prostaglandins	Various tissues	Vasodilatation, vasoconstriction, smooth muscle stimulation, increased vascular permeability, may cause release of histamine
Acetylcholine	Nerve tissue	Smooth muscle contraction, vasodilatation

infection. Individuals or families with the atopic diathesis, however, seem to have an increased ability to form this unique Ig following exposure to naturally occurring antigens (Sherman, 1971). Hence, anaphylactic reactions are more likely to occur in individuals with the atopic diathesis. Such individuals form IgE in response to both natural and synthetic antigens, such as pollens, dust, fungi, sera, and drugs. Other members of an atopic family have an increased incidence of HAB reactions. This may be due to a genetically controlled increased permeability of the mucous membranes to certain antigens or to a greater tendency to form IgE. Patients with atopic dermatitis also have an increased ability to form IgE (Juhlin et al., 1969). However, the roles of IgE and atopic allergy in the production of atopic dermatitis are yet to be established.

Anaphylactic reactions have occurred following antigenic challenge by either complete antigens such as foreign sera and polysaccharides or incomplete antigens such as haptens, including drugs and chemicals (Austen and Sheffer, 1971; Boston Collaborative Drug Surveillance Program, 1973; see Table 4–16). The haptens or their degraded products combine with tissue protein to form complete antigens. Patients with a prior history of an immediate allergic reaction (however mild) or a strongly suggestive history of atopic disease should be given known anaphylactogens, such as penicillin and foreign sera, with extreme caution, if at all. Anaphylactic reactions may also occur in individuals without a previous allergic background, however.

NON-ALLERGIC MECHANISMS (ANAPHYLACTOID REACTIONS)

Non-allergic mechanisms are triggered by stimuli which either liberate or activate the mediators of acute inflammation, or which have a direct toxic effect on target cells. Antigen-antibody interaction is not involved. These stimuli include such agents as heat or cold, trauma, sunlight, emotional disturbances, and exercise. In addition, many chemicals may trigger this type of reaction (Table 4–16). The clinical

and pathological picture may be indistinguishable from that following an anaphylactic reaction—indeed, similar pathophysiologic pathways are shared.

There are a number of examples of non-allergic precipitants of the AS (Baughman and Jillson, 1963; Miller et al., 1968; Thompson, 1968). The following are a few of them:

1. The simplest form of non-allergic process producing a miniature AS is that which follows direct trauma to the skin. Simple scratching of the skin causes the triple response of Lewis. This consists of the red line, wheal, and flare reactions deriving from both axon and histamine-mediated vascular dilation and increased permeability after direct injury to the microvasculature of the skin.

2. Dermographism or factitious urticaria is an exaggeration of the normal physiologic triple response of Lewis and occurs in about 5 per cent of the normal population.

3. Abnormal whealing may also occur in conditions in which the threshold for the release of histamine and other mediators from target cells is allegedly lowered (that is, thyroid disease, diabetes, infections, and the post-menopausal state).

4. The non-allergic process occurs in conditions in which there are increased numbers of target cells, in certain lymphomas, urticaria pigmentosa, and other forms of mastocytosis. The latter state is characterized by local wheal formation over the lesions following a gentle scratch (Darier's sign). Urticaria pigmentosa and mastocytosis may also give rise to systemic signs and symptoms following release of histamine. Hence, it is important to avoid the use of aspirin, codeine, morphine, and other liberators or potentiators of histamine in such patients.

5. Complement activation may also precipitate the AS. Complement activation occurs in a cascade, each step depending on a preceding product. In normal individuals the first component of complement (C1) is converted to C1 esterase in a rate-limiting reaction, with feedback enzymatic inhibition. C1 esterase can provoke increased vascular permeability. In certain abnormal individuals the inhibitor of C1 esterase is deficient or

functionally inactive, and the production of C1 esterase may proceed unchecked, as occurs in hereditary angioedema. The macromolecular proteins frequently present in infectious disease, multiple myeloma, systemic lupus erythematosus, lymphoma, and in neoplasia may also initiate the complement cascade with the generation of a histamine-releasing substance known as anaphylatoxin. This substance causes the release of histamine from mast cells without cellular lysis. Certain venoms may also generate the formation of anaphylatoxin from complement.

6. Heat and cold may initiate nonallergic AS. Exposure to cold may cause cryoglobulins, cryofibrinogens, and cold hemolysins to fix complement and trigger the complement cascade, with resultant alterations of vascular permeability. Urticaria may be an important clinical sign in many disease states associated with circulating cryoproteins.

7. Solar energy may cause acute transient vascular reactivity in solar urticaria and erythropoietic protoporphyria. The phototoxic effects in these conditions, however, may involve the release of mediators of inflammation other than histamine (for example, kinins).

8. Several classes of drugs and chemicals may cause the direct release of histamine without initiating the complement cascade. The prototype is compound 48/80, which has a direct degranulating effect on basophils and mast cells. Other materials having a presumably similar direct effect include the opiates, some broad-spectrum antibiotics, strawberries, certain citrus fruits, and vitamins.

HOST FACTORS

A variety of host factors may modify the observable manifestations of both allergic and non-allergic mediated AS reactions in man (Miller et al., 1968; Thompson, 1968). The susceptibility of the individual, as well as the accessibility, number, and responsiveness of the target cells, may modify the severity of the reaction. Genetic influences (for example, atopic diathesis) may determine susceptibility to certain environmental allergens. The previous response of the target cells or depletion of the mediators of inflammation can lead to a temporary refractory state in which the host does not respond to a challenge. This can occur after a severe generalized AS reaction. Psychogenic and infectious factors may also influence the expression of the AS by unknown mechanisms. Dry skin in a patient with dermographism or urticaria may cause pruritus, precipitating or aggravating the symptomatology. Other host factors have been alluded to in section I of this chapter.

CHEMICAL MEDIATORS

A number of chemical mediators of acute inflammation are involved in the production of the increased vascular permeability, smooth muscle contractility, and heterogenous symptomatology found in the overt expression of the AS in man (Austen, 1971; Austen and Sheffer, 1971; Thompson, 1968). These are of either cellular or plasma origin. A list of the mediators involved and a summary of their sources and roles in the induction of the AS appear in Table 4–18.

Histamine is the principal vasoactive amine responsible for many of the signs and symptoms observed in angioedema, urticaria, and upper respiratory tract obstruction following appropriate challenge. Its pharmacologic actions are transient. Histamine is also responsible for a group of immediate symptoms that include flushing, headaches, hypotension, tachycardia, and wheezing. Histamine causes increased vascular permeability, probably by the production of gaps between adjacent vascular endothelial cells in the postcapillary venules. Fluid escaping from the leaking venules causes edema.

Histamine is stored in mast cells and basophils. Mast cells are located strategically around blood vessels within the connective tissue stroma of such vital shock organs as the skin, mucous membranes, respiratory and gastrointestinal tracts, and the cardiovascular system. Basophils, commonly regarded as circulating mast cells, constitute about 1 per cent of the white cells in the blood stream. Histamine is bound to the acid mucopolysaccharides in the metachromatic granules of both mast cells and basophils and is secreted after appropriate challenge. In the depleted state (post-histamine release), the target cells may be temporarily unresponsive to further stimulation. Following reestablishment of histamine levels, the mast cells or basophils may then again participate in further reactions. Both mast cells and basophils are presumably the principal target cells in the HAB-mediated reaction in man, but they also have a similar role in many non-allergic reactions in which symptoms follow histamine release. The effects of histamine may be minimized or reversed either by blockage of the histamine release mechanism or by the use of histamine antagonists. Histamine release from mast cells can be blocked by disodium cromoglycate and possibly by material elaborated by eosinophils. Antihistaminic drugs are competitive antagonists of histamine and compete with histamine at the receptor sites on effector cells (endothelial, smooth muscle) surfaces. Antihistamines occupy these histamine receptor sites without eliciting a detectable response.

Slow-reacting substance of anaphylaxis (SRS-A) causes prolonged and severe bronchoconstriction in man. SRS-A is an acidic lipid substance which is either released from preexistent inactive precursors or formed de novo in sensitized tissue by antigen/antibody interaction or experimentally by compound 48/80. It causes smooth muscle contraction in human bronchioles which is slower in onset but of longer duration than histamine. SRS-A may be responsible for the bronchioconstriction of asthma. Diethylcarbamazine (Hetrazan) has been demonstrated to be an antagonist of SRS-A.

Eosinophil chemotactic factor of anaphylaxis (ECF-A) is released from sensitized tissue following the HAB-mediated reaction (Kay and Austen, 1971). Eosinophils are thereby attracted to the site of histamine elaboration, exerting a protective and possibly neutralizing influence upon further reactivity.

Kinins are a group of peptides known to be active in the symptomatology of the AS. Kinins are formed directly from the precursor plasma globulins. Their pharmacologic actions include vasodilation, increased vascular permeability, production of pain, smooth muscle contraction, and leukotaxis. Kinin activation may occur during both allergic and non-allergic reactions and may be suppressed by steroid therapy. Aspirin may antagonize kinins, thereby reducing their bronchoconstrictive effects.

The complement system may act directly or indirectly through the activation of other mediators of inflammation in triggering the AS. Complement is discussed in section I of this chapter.

Other mediators such as prostaglandins and acetylcholine may play a role in the production of AS. Prostaglandins are a group of potent vasoactive proteins which have been shown to cause prolonged wheal and flare reactions following intradermal injection (Solomon et al., 1968). They also induce histamine release. Acetylcholine has an acknowledged role in the expression of autonomic nervous system activity. Following neural transmission, acetylcholine is released from terminal parasympathetic nerve fibers, where it is hydrolyzed (and hence inactivated) by acetylcholine esterase. Acetylcholine causes smooth muscle contraction and increased capillary permeability. In certain individuals, either defective inactivation or exquisite sensitivity to acetylcholine results in cholinergic urticaria, which is discussed below (Miller et al., 1968; Moore-Robinson and Warin, 1968; Thompson, 1968).

While serotonin is known to play an important role in the induction of the AS in rodents, it has not been shown to have this role in man (Austen, 1971).

CLINICAL MANIFESTATIONS

URTICARIA AND ANGIOEDEMA

Urticaria is a vascular reaction pattern characterized by the appearance of transient erythematous or whitish swellings in the skin or mucous membranes (Champion, 1968; Pillsbury et al., 1956; Sheffer and Austen, 1971). These swellings represent localized areas of edema and are called wheals. The edema is due to the extravasation of protein-rich fluid from small blood vessels and is a reflection of increased permeability of vessel walls. Serum proteins aggregate in the dermis in abnormally large quantities. Resorption is slow because of abnormal osmotic pressures in the extravascular space. Gradually, however, absorption occurs and the wheal slowly resolves, generally within several hours. The major feature of urticaria, therefore, is edema; as a result, the lesions involute without any of the sequential changes which can be seen in a dermatitis. However, severe urticaria may induce bullous or even purpuric changes. These latter findings are infrequent and occur most often in children.

Clinically, wheals vary from pinpoint to palm sized or larger and enlarge by peripheral extension to become confluent, with resultant bizarre geographic configurations (Fig. 4–8). Some urticarial lesions

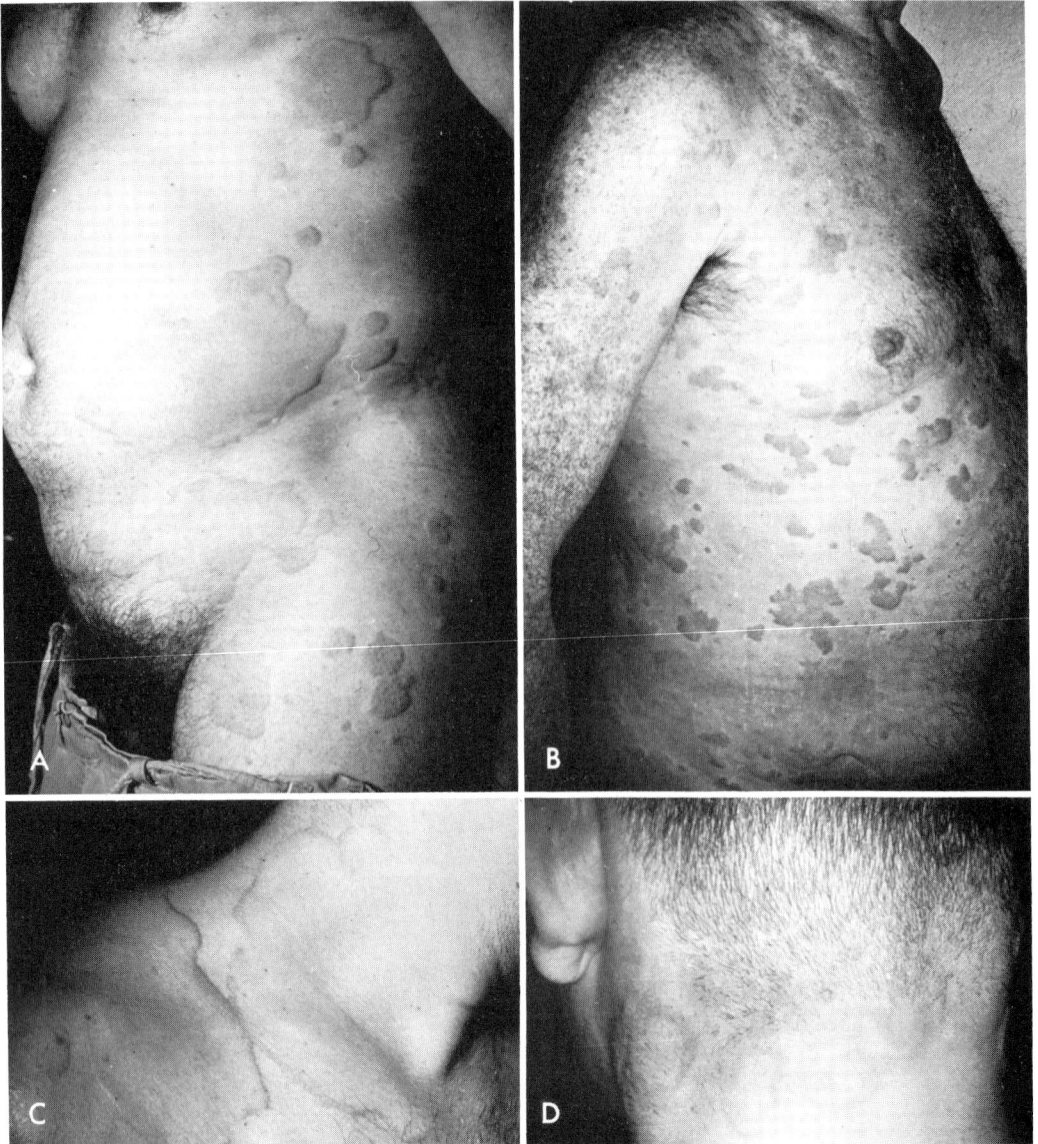

Figure 4–8   Urticaria—various clinical presentations. *A*, Patient who had a penicillin reaction characterized by erythematous pruritic wheals. *B*, Small, multiple wheals resulting from allergic reaction to sulfamethoxazole (Gantrisin). *C*, An unusual geographic configuration is seen in a patient who was taking diazepam (Valium). *D*, An annular edematous pruritic eruption appeared in a youngster who was taking a cough syrup.

may be surrounded by an erythematous areola or halo. Individual wheals rarely persist longer than 12 to 24 hours, a feature distinguishing the wheal from the other primary lesions of the skin. However, multiple stages in the evolution of wheals may lead to a more or less constant eruption in a localized area, stimulating a more protracted skin reaction. The crucial fact remains that the individual lesion or wheal is of transient duration. Urticarial lesions are usually pruritic and stinging. Prickly sensations commonly precede the actual development of the wheal. Symptoms are present only in the early phase of wheal formation. Wheals may occur in any area of the body. They may be localized to one small area or may become so extensive and generalized as to cover almost the entire skin surface. The reaction is not limited to the skin, since the mucosal surfaces may be involved, with related symptoms including coryza, respiratory distress, abdominal pain, and hoarseness. The latter symptom is serious, since edema of the larynx may lead to grave respiratory embarrassment and, as in the generalized AS, require immediate therapy.

Angioedema is the term used to describe giant wheals, or wheals involving mucous membrane surfaces (Fig. 4–9). Angioedematous swelling, in which the subcutaneous tissue is involved rather than the superficial skin, may occur over the face (Fig. 4–10A), an entire extremity (Fig. 4–10B), or within a vital organ system, such as the upper respiratory tract. Lesions of urticaria and angioedema differ only in terms of degree and often coexist in the same patient. Hereditary angioedema is considered a separate entity and merits further discussion (see below).

The etiology of urticaria is as diverse as the causes and mechanisms outlined for production of the AS. Wheal formation, the cardinal feature of urticaria, implies the action of histamine, the kinins, or other mediators of inflammation on the microvasculature of the skin. The major effect of the mediators are vasodilatation and increased permeability. It is interesting to compare urticaria to the persistent erythemas and purpuras. The fundamental difference between these disorders is one of degree. In the persistent erythemas (toxic erythemas, erythema multiforme, and erythema annulare centrifugum), the individual lesions last longer than the evanescent urticarial wheal. Histologically, the persistent erythemas are characterized by fixed perivascular infiltrates, contrasting with the relatively spare and transient infiltrates and edema in the wheal. Purpuric conditions resulting from either coagulopathies or vasculitides are characterized by dermal extravasation of red cells.

For convenience, urticaria may be classified as acute or chronic, depending on duration. Acute urticaria evolves over a

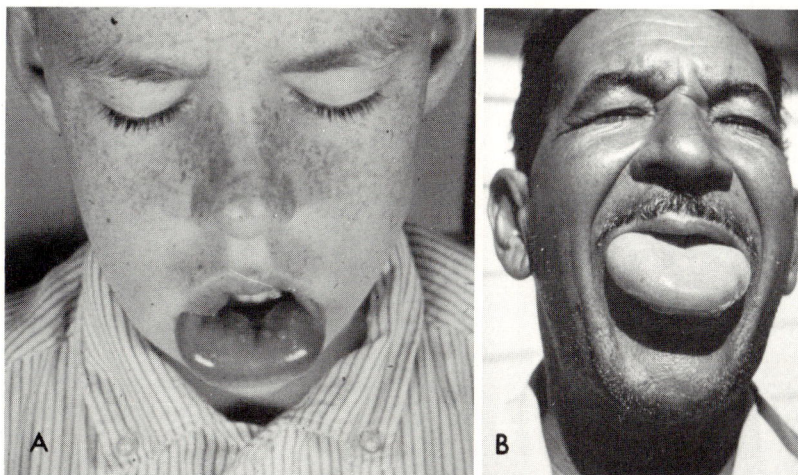

Figure 4–9 Angioedema. *A*, Youngster had unexplained recurrent acute angioedema of lower lip. *B*, Acute angioedema of tongue in a patient who is sensitive to fish.

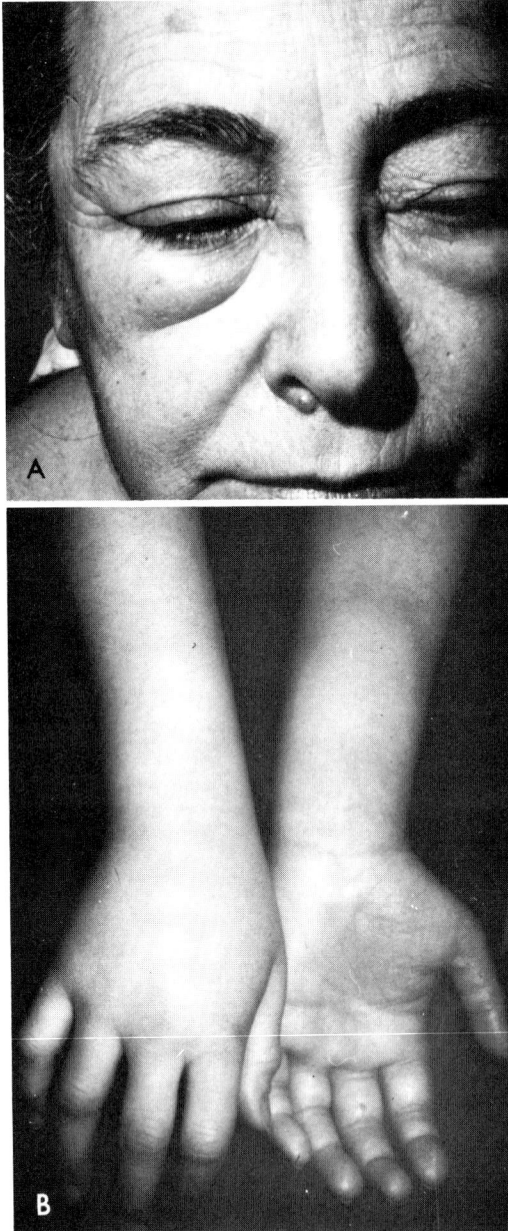

Figure 4–10 Angioedema. *A,* Angioedematous swelling of periorbital skin which invited the differential diagnosis of dermatomyositis, trichinosis, localized myxedema, and scleredema. *B,* Angioedema swelling in a child who was taking prophylactic penicillin.

period of days or several weeks. Following this short duration, there is complete involution and no further occurrence. Chronic urticaria persists for at least two months and sometimes for years, or it may be episodic.

Causes of Urticaria and Angioedema

The exact mechanism producing urticaria in a particular patient is generally unknown, especially in chronic forms. In addition, such factors as dry skin, wool clothing, mechanical irritation, and aspirin ingestion may aggravate or perpetuate urticaria (Miller et al., 1968). The role of aspirin as a direct or contributory cause of urticaria deserves mention. Aspirin may function as an antigen and participate in the allergic mechanism producing the AS (James and Warin, 1970). In addition, it may affect peripheral receptor sites and enhance the effect of the mediators involved in the production of the AS.

A functional or operational classification, using known precipitating causes (irrespective of the mechanism involved), will be used to categorize the various types of urticaria. There may be more than one etiologic factor underlying the production of urticaria. Urticaria can be thought of as a symptom complex in which multiple factors can cause and perpetuate the condition (Miller et al., 1968). This is especially true in cases of chronic urticaria. The more common precipitating causes of urticaria are listed in Table 4–19.

Allergic Urticaria

Allergic urticaria is due to injectables, inhalants (Fig. 4–11*A*), ingestants (Fig. 4–11*B*), and contactants, and is seen usually in individuals with either a personal or family history of atopy (Beall, 1964; Champion et al., 1969; Miller et al., 1968; Zamm, 1973). The antigenic challenge may come from many sources, as shown in Table 4–19. Diagnosis depends upon a thorough history. The occurrence of symptoms coincidental with a particular season or geographic location should raise the possibility of inhalant allergy (Derbes and Coleman, 1972). Wheal and flare skin testing may be diagnostic in some cases. While food allergies are not generally amenable to such testing, an elimination or rare food diet (rice, rye, lamb, turkey, and duck) may offer the only method to detect this condition (Zamm, 1973). Allergic factors may also be involved in the production of urticaria in many drug and

TABLE 4–19 A SUMMARY OF THE ETIOLOGIC CLASSIFICATION OF URTICARIA

Allergic Urticaria
Inhalants—pollens, animal danders, mold spores, feather down, aerosols, smoke, dust, and volatile chemicals.
Injectants—drugs, diagnostic agents, vaccines, insect stings, serums, and blood.
Ingestants—drugs, chocolate, eggs, nuts, shellfish, pork, vegetables, coffee, grapes, bananas, strawberries, tomatoes, cow's milk, cheese, wheat, foods derived from yeast fermentation and mushrooms, and occult additive materials found in foods, beverages, and medications.
Infections—foci of bacterial, fungal, viral and parasitic infections.
Contactants—animal products, plant materials, cosmetics, plastic, and other chemicals.
Drugs—penicillin, aspirin, quinine, sulfonamides, insulin, and many others.
Exogenous (Obligate) Urticaria due to Urticariogenic Materials
Aquagenic
Chemicals—compound 48/80, Tween 80, and acacia.
Drugs—cocaine, morphine, codeine, atropine, quinine, thiamine, pilocarpine, polymyxin B, *d*-tubocurarine, dextran, dehydrocholate sodium (Decholin), and other drugs.
Foods—certain citrus fruits, strawberries, and certain fish.
Toxins—cobra venoms, jellyfish toxin, and certain plant and insect toxins.
Physical Urticaria
Dermographic—immediate and delayed
Heat
Cold
Light
Secondary Urticaria
Infections—infectious mononucleosis, serum hepatitis, malaria, cystitis, sinusitis, prostatitis, cholecystitis, dental abscesses, dermatophytosis, rheumatic fever, trichinosis, and other parasitic infections.
Collagen vascular diseases—lupus erythematosus, rheumatoid arthritis, dermatomyositis, and angiitides.
Neoplasia—internal malignancy, lymphoma, and leukemia.
Psychogenic
Other conditions
  Dermatologic—pemphigoid, dermatitis herpetiformis, amyloidosis, urticaria pigmentosa (mastocytosis), and scabies.
  Systemic—thyrotoxicosis, hypothyroidism, polycythemia vera, uremic states, pregnancy, and serum sickness.
Cholinergic Urticaria
Hereditary Angioedema

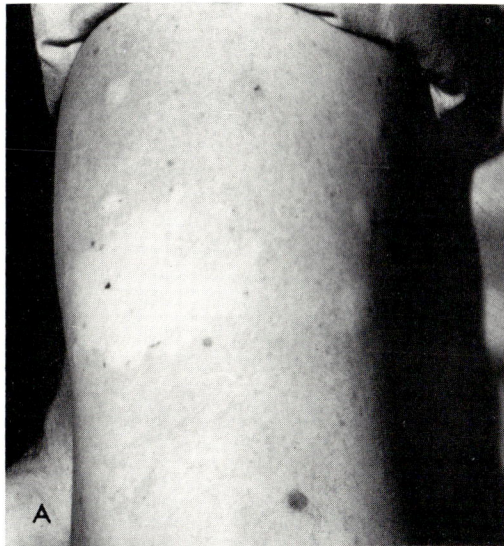

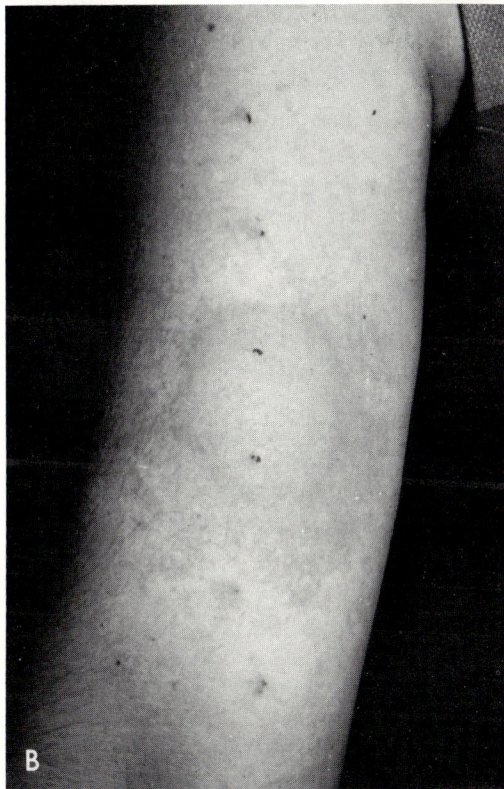

Figure 4–11 Allergic urticaria. *A,* One very strongly positive and two other positive reactions to inhalant skin tests in an atopic patient who had asthma and eczema. *B,* Another markedly positive skin test to the tested ingestant, soybean, in a patient with allergic rhinitis and bronchitis.

transfusion reactions, as well as in serum sickness.

Mold allergy has been implicated in many cases of chronic urticaria (James and Warin, 1971). The *Candida albicans* indigenous to the gastrointestinal tract of many individuals may be an important contributory source of mold allergen. A favorable response to nystatin and/or avoidance of foods derived from mold fermentation (for example, mushrooms, cheese, buttermilk, mayonnaise, vinegar, fermented and malted products, and spicy dressings) may be both diagnostic and therapeutic in cases of mold hypersensitivity.

It is well known that some dairy products contain penicillin contaminants; therefore, patients with a history of penicillin reaction, or of onset of urticaria following penicillin administration, should be given a diet free of dairy products (milk, butter, ice cream, cheese, creamed foods, and baked goods). Other contaminants found in foods, drinks, and medications include preservatives, stabilizers, and coloring agents that are thought to be innocuous but may not be in certain patients with allergic urticaria (Juhlin et al., 1972; Lockey, 1971).

Avoiding the antigenic challenge is of paramount importance in the treatment of allergic urticaria. Antihistamines are of use in the symptomatic management if the etiology cannot be eliminated. Some of the more commonly prescribed antihistamines include chlorpheniramine (Chlor-Trimeton, 2 to 8 mg. q. 6 h.), diphenhydramine (Benadryl, 50 to 100 mg. q. 6 h.), and promethazine (Phenergan, 25 to 50 mg. q. 6 h.). Other useful drugs include cyproheptadine (Periactin, 4 mg. q.i.d.) and hydroxyzine hydrochloride (Atarax, 10 to 50 mg. q. 6 h.).

Urticariogenic Materials

Primary urticariogenic substances which do not act as antigens can be ingested or injected, or may otherwise come in contact with the host, causing wheal formation (Thompson, 1968). Some of these substances present in, for example, strawberries, fish, and certain drugs may also act as antigens, as seen in Table 4–19. The net effect of this type of challenge is histamine release or activation of the other mediators of acute inflammation. Morphine and codeine are well-known histamine liberators. They may in this way cause pruritus and urticaria. Other histamine liberators include atropine, quinine, thiamine, and pilocarpine. The dose necessary for the induction of urticaria varies with these compounds, but all of them in optimal concentration are obligate whealing agents. In addition, histamine itself may be introduced into the skin or the blood stream and cause urticaria by direct action on blood vessel walls. A continuing cycle may develop, since exogenous histamine also causes a release of endogenous histamine from the mast cell. Leeches and jellyfish are examples of living forms which can induce urticaria by contact with surface toxins. Plants such as nettles may also induce urticaria. Finally, a small, beadlike urticaria (aquagenic urticaria) following exposure to water has been described (Shelley and Rawnsley, 1964). Presumably, the action of water on sebum produces a substance which results in mast cell degranulation and histamine release.

Physical Urticaria

Physical agents, such as mechanical pressure and exposure to heat, cold, and light, may also induce urticaria. The mechanisms of induction are largely unknown.

Immediate dermographic urticaria is an exaggerated triple response of Lewis (Fisher and Schwartz, 1953; Ostrov, 1967; Fig. 4–12A). It occurs in about 5 per cent of the normal population. Although dermographism is usually idiopathic, it occasionally follows an infection, systemic illness, or emotional upset. Dermographism may recur for months or years. This condition does not occur more frequently in the other types of urticaria than that which is seen in the non-urticarial population. Dermographic wheals characteristically follow the lines of injury or trauma and may be quite dramatic in response to gentle scratching. Sometimes this phenomenon manifests itself as swellings at friction points of tight-fitting clothing, usually around the waist, ankles, or feet. Delayed dermographism is a rare form of dermographia in which whealing occurs several hours after the initial immediate effects of direct skin trauma have faded (Baughman and Jillson, 1963). Pressure urticaria is a variant of dermographism in which the wheals occur several hours after trauma but are not preceded by an immediate dermographic whealing phase (Ryan et al., 1968; Fig. 4–12 B). Hydroxyzine (Atarax) has been a successful thera-

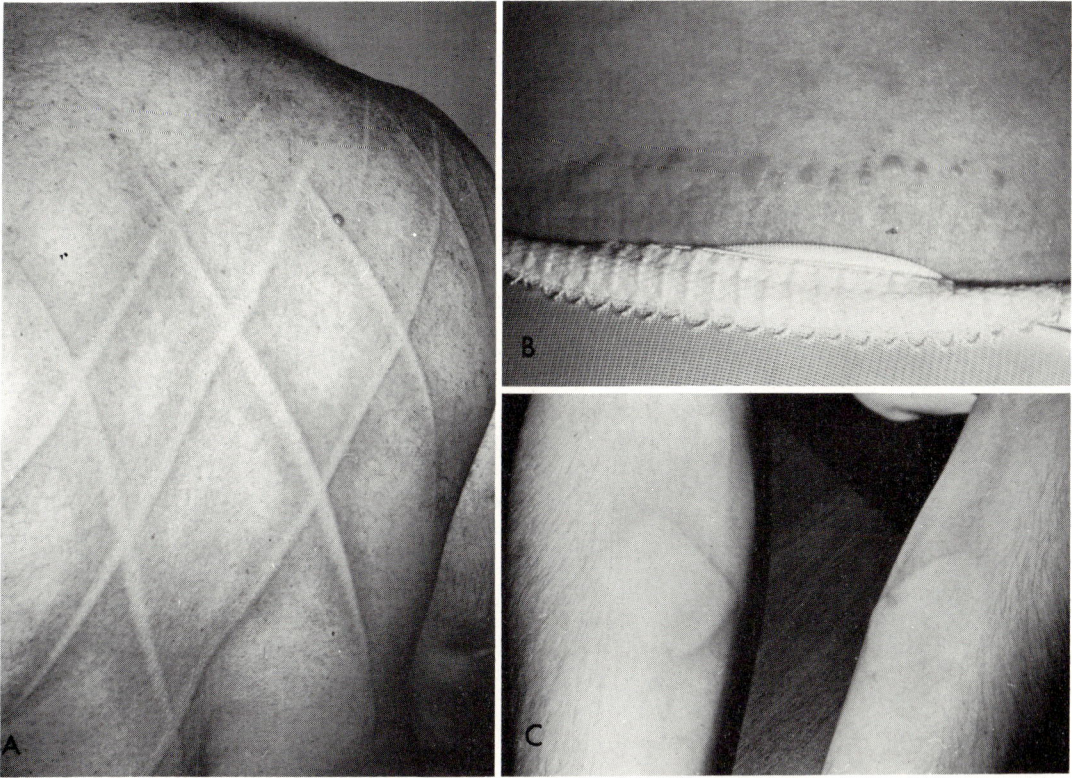

Figure 4–12   Physical urticaria. A, Chronic dermographism of two years' duration in an American prisoner of war. B, Pressure urticaria in a patient who was free of an immediate dermographic whealing phase. C, Wheal formation following application of ice in a patient with cold urticaria.

peutic agent in many cases of dermographic urticaria.

Thermal factors may precipitate urticaria. Heat urticaria is a rare form in which the swelling is produced by the local application of heat (Jillson, 1956). This is a localized form of urticaria and is not related to the more common cholinergic urticaria. Heat application or immersion of an extremity in water at 38° C. for several minutes may cause a sudden appearance of this form of urticaria. Cold urticaria may be divided into several classes (Houser et al., 1970; Tindall et al., 1969). The rare familial cold urticaria has its onset in infancy. The wheals are not pruritic. It is associated with fever, leukocytosis, arthralgia, and cannot be passively transferred. Certain types of cold urticaria are acquired, and about 50 per cent can be passively transferred. In many cases, the cause is not apparent (idiopathically acquired). Some forms are related to the presence of cold hemolysins or other cryoproteins. They may be associated with a variety of systemic disorders, including infectious disease and other underlying diseases. Syphilitic paroxysmal cold hemoglobinuria may be associated with cold hemolysins in the serum. The occurrence of cold urticaria and red or smokey-colored urine should suggest the diagnosis of paroxysmal cold hemoglobinuria. Cryoproteins, including cryoglobulins or cryofibrinogens, may be important clues to underlying disease states (Thompson, 1968). Cryoproteins have been found in patients with dysglobulinemia, collagen-vascular disease, leukemia, liver disease, a variety of infections, and malignancies.

Cold urticaria may be symptomatic or latent. In the latter instance, it is precipitated by the application of ice (Fig. 4–12C) or exposure to cold air. The patient will often relate a history of the urticaria occurring upon rewarming after cold exposure. The diagnosis of cold urticaria is suggested by the history and occurrence of wheals primarily limited to exposed areas. The diagnosis may be confirmed by controlled exposure of the skin to cold. This may be performed simply with an ice cube held to the skin of the face, neck, or forearms for three minutes or by cold air exposure for 10 minutes. The diagnostic wheal should appear following rewarming; however, some cases are difficult to reproduce artificially, and the specific environmental precipitating challenge may be necessary. The patient should be further investigated for an underlying disease state if cryoproteins are found. Therapy should be directed towards the instruction of the patient in avoidance of exposure to the cold. Furthermore, patients with cold urticaria should be warned of the hazard of accidental drowning while swimming. Finally, an antihistamine such as cyproheptadine (Periactin 4 mg. q. 6 h.) has been used in this condition.

See Solar Urticaria in Chapter 6 for a discussion of light urticaria.

Symptomatic Urticaria

Urticaria and angioedema may occur as components of diseases of the skin or in conjunction with a variety of general medical disorders (Braverman, 1967; Beall, 1964; Miller et al., 1968; Thompson, 1968). Urticaria is a significant sign in mastocytosis (urticaria pigmentosa) and in such skin disorders as bullous pemphigoid and dermatitis herpetiformis. It may be seen in hepatic disease, carcinomatosis, and lymphoma. It has also been reported in malaria, hyperthyroidism, hypothyroidism, rheumatoid arthritis, lupus erythematosus, rheumatic fever, leukemia, and renal disease. Focal infections, such as periapical dental abscesses, tonsillitis, sinusitis, cystitis, and chronic infections of the gastrointestinal tract, the kidney, and the gallbladder, have also been associated with urticaria. It may occur in association with acute bacterial disease or be the first sign of such viral infections as hepatitis or infectious mononucleosis. Intestinal parasites occasionally cause urticaria.

Finally, trichophytids may give rise to an urticarial skin response. A trial of either a systemic antibiotic or an antihelmintic medication may be indicated in some forms of chronic urticaria where a focus of infection is suspected. A thorough internal medical examination plus laboratory studies may be necessary to establish the diagnosis in many of the conditions listed under the causes of secondary urticaria.

Psychogenic factors are considered to be a secondary or underlying cause of urticaria. Psychogenic urticaria is of nebulous character, in that the urticaria may be related to various tension states or fatigue. The mechanism underlying psychogenic urticaria is unknown, although there is little question that in certain individuals emotional stress can precipitate it. In certain patients, minor psychic distress may be the sole cause of the urticaria. In other individuals, psychogenic stresses may contribute to the exacerbation of urticaria due to other causes. An awareness of the possible dual roles that stress may play is important in successful therapy. A mild tranquilizer, such as diazepam (Valium), or a medication combining both antihistaminic and tranquilizing effects, such as hydroxyzine (Atarax), may be helpful therapeutically when tension states are present.

Cholinergic Urticaria

Discussed in Chapter 30.

Hereditary Angioedema

Hereditary angioedema is a type of angioedema transmitted by a Mendelian dominant gene (Fromer, 1967; Sheffer and Austen, 1971). It was described by Osler (1888) as a rare inherited familial form of edema. The disorder affects the skin and mucosa of different target organs. It is characterized by acute recurrent episodes of transient edema involving the skin and the mucosa of the gastrointestinal and respiratory tracts. Cutaneous involvement is usually localized and is manifested by nonpitting, nonpruritic swelling of an extremity or the face; it may frequently be preceded by trauma. Abdominal crisis with severe colic, simulating an acute surgical emergency, may occur. The most serious and life-threatening aspect of this disorder, however, is acute laryngeal edema necessitating immediate intubation or tracheotomy. Asphyxiation as a result of laryngeal involvement is the leading cause of death in patients with hereditary angioedema.

Patients and relatives with hereditary angioedema have either deficient or functionally absent serum alpha-2 globulin inhibitor of C1 esterase (Rosen and Austen, 1969). Normal individuals have functional active alpha-2 globulin inhibitor present in the serum. The lack of an inhibitor of the activated first component of complement allows for a rational explanation of hereditary angioedema. Unchecked C1 esterase activity may bring about increased vascular permeability. The diagnosis of hereditary angioedema is suggested by the family history, episodic recurrence of nonpruritic swellings involving the skin, and by symptomatology of the gastrointestinal and upper respiratory tract involvement. The diagnosis is established by the laboratory demonstration of absent or functionally inactive defective alpha-2 globulin inhibitor of C1 esterase. Indirect confirmation can be obtained by demonstrating diminished amounts of C1 naturally occurring substrates, such as the second (C2) and fourth (C4) components of complement.

Treating hereditary angioedema with the conventional drugs used in urticaria or in other forms of angioedema is of little value. Definitive therapy should be directed towards the administration of a functional inhibitor of C1 esterase. Patients with hereditary angioedema should seek immediate medical aid if upper respiratory tract swelling occurs. Since conventional therapy is generally ineffective in this form of laryngeal edema, a tracheotomy may be lifesaving and a permanent tracheotomy may be necessary. Sublingual testosterone has been used in some cases with success (Spaulding, 1960). Epsilon-aminocaproic acid and its analogue, trans-4-(amino ethyl)cyclohexanol-1-carboxylic acid (tranexamic acid), have, in preliminary studies, prevented attacks of angioedema in several patients with hereditary angioedema (Sheffer et al., 1972). Fresh normal plasma may also be beneficial in an emergency situation (Pickering et al., 1969).

Diagnosis

The most important clinical aspect of urticaria is determination of the cause.

Urticaria and angioedema are both reaction patterns occurring in the skin and mucous membranes and are always secondary to an underlying process. In the clinical investigation of acute urticaria, the history cannot be too detailed. In acute urticaria, there is generally a history of a recent illness, drug therapy, or dietary indiscretion. Most cases of acute urticaria are not seen by physicians because of their evanescent and banal course. The remainder of the discussion on the diagnosis of urticaria will, therefore, be directed primarily to the chronic variety.

A prerequisite in the investigation of urticaria is the establishment of a pattern of occurrence (Zamm, 1972). Patterns are documented in terms of time (season), place (immediate home/work environment), or activity (ingestion of foods or drugs, physical activity, and so forth). A random or varying pattern of onset suggests that the source of the challenge to the individual is from some external factor, such as is found in the allergic, exogenous, and physical causes of urticaria. A constant pattern of onset suggests habitual exposure to an exogenous challenge, such as common foods, or a cause within the patient, as occurs in certain underlying infectious disease, malignancy, collagen-vascular disease states. A history of arthralgia or arthritis suggests underlying viral hepatitis, collagen-vascular disease, serum sickness, or rheumatic fever associated with urticaria.

The question of drugs requires particular scrutiny, and the patient should be questioned thoroughly regarding drug usage. The physician should make a detailed review of systems, including a list of all home, proprietary, and prescription remedies which were employed for the treatment of minor symptoms (Lockey, 1971). Less obvious precipitants, including foods, toothpastes, and cosmetics, should be reviewed. In some instances, drugs or chemicals are ingested accidentally when used as preservatives, antioxidants, or artificial coloring agents (Juhlin et al., 1972; Lockey, 1971).

An example of an allegedly innocuous additive is tartrazine (a yellow azobenzene dye used commonly as an approved food and drug coloring agent). Cross-reactivity between tartrazine and aspirin has been described. Urticaria has resulted from tartrazine ingestion by patients with aspirin hypersensitivity. Such patients should therefore avoid challenge with this occult additive that may be found in some foods and drugs (certain antihistamines, antibiotics, birth control pills, and soft drinks among others). A diary may be of value in determining the chronologic occurrence of wheals and will document the types of exposure a patient experiences during the day.

The dermatologic examination may reveal evidence of the atopic diathesis (boggy nasal mucosa, atopic dermatitis), dermographism, and cutaneous manifestations of other diseases. Clinically, most cases of urticaria look alike regardless of etiology. However, there are subtle variations in the physical appearance of the wheal which may be of diagnostic aid. Bizarre gyrate hives have been associated with internal malignancy and drugs. Wheals which lack pseudopods are more characteristic of physical urticaria. A small wheal (1 to 2 mm. in diameter) and a large erythematous flare are typical of cholinergic urticaria. The swelling of angioedema can be confused with inflammatory edema. However, compared to the latter, angioedema is nonpitting and transient.

Several simple provocative tests can be performed, including stroking of the skin (dermographism), application of ice cubes (cold urticaria), and Mecholyl skin test (cholinergic urticaria; Akers, 1972; Miller et al., 1968). Brief physical exercises may also precipitate the latter condition. Further investigative studies are outlined in Table 4–20 for each of the listed categories. Extensive laboratory and x-ray examination may be necessary in some cases of chronic urticaria. At the very least, a patient with chronic urticaria should have a complete blood count, urinalysis, sedimentation rate, fluorescent antinuclear antibody test, liver battery, cryoprotein determination, and chest x-ray. More than one cause is frequently found in cases of chronic urticaria (Akers, 1972).

Treatment

One of the most important aspects of therapy in urticaria is elimination of the cause. When this has been accomplished, the urticaria will usually resolve either partially or completely. Antihistamines are the drugs of choice in most forms of urticaria. The maintenance of adequate dosage is of paramount importance. The choice of antihistamine may depend upon the type of urticaria; those antihistamines more commonly used have been discussed previously. Sympathomimetics such as ephedrine sulfate (25 mg. q. 6 h.) or epinephrine injection USP (0.2 ml. subcutaneously q. 2 h. p.r.n.), if not medically contraindicated, may be used in addition to antihistamines in severe exacerbations of urticaria. A short course of systemic corticosteroids may be considered in refractory acute urticaria, but these agents are not recommended in chronic cases. Tranquilizers may be used to treat patients with an emotional or stress component. A trial of elimination diets (no vegetables, fruits, sea foods, chocolate, and so forth), rare food diets, and antibiotic, antifungal and, antihelmintic drugs where indicated in certain cases of chronic urticaria may be diagnostic as well as therapeutic. Avoiding ingestion of aspirin and exogenous urticariogenic materials may help to control urticaria. Prevention and treatment of dry skin and avoidance of wool and other pruritic stimuli can help alleviate irritating factors which might perpetuate urticaria. Hyposensitization may be useful in those select cases due to inhalant allergy (pollens, dust, molds, and so forth).

GENERALIZED ANAPHYLACTIC SYNDROME

Diagnosis

The clinical manifestations of the generalized AS reaction are usually easily recognized after the condition is well established. However, for therapy to be effective, early recognition is most important. The signs and symptoms of such reactions may be as varied as the chemical mediators producing them. The generalized AS may begin with one or more of the localized manifestations previously described. Progression to the potentially

TABLE 4–20 DISTINGUISHING CHARACTERISTICS OF THE SIX CATEGORIES OF URTICARIA

	History	*Physical Examination*	*Studies or Tests*
Allergic urticaria	Varying pattern— inhalant allergies Constant pattern—with food allergies Atopic diathesis Drug exposure	Boggy nasal mucosa Wheezing Eczema	Eosinophilia Inhalant allergen skin tests Elimination and rare food diets Nystatin trial
Exogenous urticaria	Varying pattern Urticariogenic materials	Lesions may follow line contact with material	Thorough history
Physical urticaria	Varying pattern Cold, light, or heat precipitants Welts following trauma	Wheals on exposed sites Wheals lack pseudopods Dermographism	Cold, heat, or light exposure and skin trauma Cyroproteins, STS, and tests to rule out symptomatic causes
Symptomatic urticaria	Constant pattern with underlying disease Foci of infection Positive review of systems Precipitation by tension states	Dental disease Sinus disease Tinea infection Ichthyosis Lymphadenopathy Vasculitis Neoplasia Presence of other skin lesions (vesicles, bullae, purpura, and so forth) Bizarre gyrate wheals with malignancy Darier's sign	Antifungal, antibiotic, and antihelmintic trial CBC, sedimentation rate Cryoproteins Complement Urinalysis and culture STS, fana, LE prep, renal, thyroid, and liver function tests Rheumatoid factor Heterophile antibody Stools for ova and parasites X-ray studies of the teeth, sinuses, lung, G-U and gastrointestinal tract where indicated If a primary skin condition is present, a biopsy is indicated Nitroblue tetrazolium dye test
Cholinergic urticaria	Varying pattern Small welts Precipitation by sweating, exertion, and tension states May have symptoms of anxiety reaction	Tiny wheals with a large red axon flare Spares palms and soles	Reproduction with exercise Mecholyl skin test
Hereditary angioedema	Varying pattern Precipitated by trauma Family history Abdominal distress Respiratory distress Lack of pruritus Relatives die at an early age	Nonpruritic edema Nonpitting swelling Laryngeal edema	Absent or functional lack of alpha-2 globulin inhibitor of C1 esterase Low levels of C2 and C4

life-threatening systemic reaction may follow within minutes. Usually one of three clinical patterns involving the skin or respiratory or cardiovascular systems is recognized (Austen, 1971; Austen and Sheffer, 1971). However, combinations may also occur. The effects of increased vascular permeability in the skin and mucous membranes are manifested by diffuse urticaria or angioedema. Early symptoms in the skin include pruritus and a feeling of generalized warmth. However, the most frequent sign of impending danger may be upper respiratory angioedema leading to airway obstruction; this occurrence will require immediate treatment if the patient's life is to be saved.

Swelling in the upper respiratory tract manifested as laryngeal edema causes tightness in the throat, hoarseness, or even stridor. Bronchial wheezing is not a feature of this type of angioedema and should not be a prerequisite to either making the diagnosis or instituting therapy in this form of the generalized AS. Tightness in the chest associated with pulmonary hyperinflation manifested by expiratory wheezing may herald another type of clinical presentation of the generalized AS due to severe bronchospasm. Either angioedema of the upper respiratory tract or severe bronchospasm of the lower respiratory tract may lead to respiratory failure, cyanosis, hypotension, and death. A third clinical presentation may be that of cardiovascular collapse with dizziness, hypotension, loss of consciousness and, if the condition is not reversed, death. Other possible clinical features of these severe reactions include loss of sphincter control, gastrointestinal colic, and seizures. The generalized AS must be distinguished from other acutely occurring medical emergencies such as syncope, seizure disorders, and cardiovascular catastrophes (myocardial infarction, cardiac arrest, and cerebral vascular accident).

Causes

The frequently cited causes of the generalized AS are listed in Tables 4–16 and 4–19 (Austen and Sheffer, 1971; Boston Collaborative Drug Surveillance Program, 1973). Although the challenge precipitating the generalized AS is usually administered parenterally (especially intravenously), some cases have occurred following other routes of access, including ingestion and contact with the skin or mucous membranes. The more common causes of this type of reaction include insect stings, antibiotics (especially penicillin), blood products (foreign sera), diagnostic agents (iodine-containing radiographic materials), certain foods (sea foods and strawberries), and various antigens used in the course of hyposensitization procedures.

Prevention

Prevention of the generalized AS is most important. In patients with increased numbers of target cells (urticaria pigmentosa), or heightened target cells susceptibility, aspirin, opiates, macromolecular substances, and other mediator releasing agents should be avoided. Preventive measures include directing patients with increased susceptibility to immediate allergic reactions to avoid potential anaphylactogens. Penicillin and foreign sera are examples of potent antigens. A history of either a previous immediate allergic reaction or atopy may mitigate the administration of such strong antigens, and the use of non–cross-reacting substances may be considered.

In addition, there are other methods that may prevent the allergic mechanisms which produce the generalized AS. Blockage of antigen-antibody union on the target cell may occur during specific host hyposensitization procedures. Repeated injections of small amounts of antigen over a period of time have resulted in the production of blocking antibodies. Circulating blocking antibodies presumably combine with antigen and thereby reduce the quantity of antigen that is available to react with the HAB present on the target cell. Prevention may be induced by the inhibition of the release or activation of the chemical mediators that are involved; this may be done by using such experimental agents as diethyl carbomazine (Hetrazan) or disodium cromoglycate. Diethyl carbomazine inhibits the release of SRS-A. Disodium cromoglycate inhibits the immunologic release of both histamine and SRS-A. Both of these agents need further study, but they may offer a new and fertile field of selective preventive therapy of the AS.

Finally, the use of antagonists of the chemical mediators, such as the antihistamines, is probably the most practical albeit not the ideal method of prevention. Antihistamines are not completely effective and frequently produce undesirable side effects. Specific antagonists are not available for many of the other chemical

TABLE 4–21 TREATMENT OF SYSTEMIC SHOCK STATES

I. General Measures
  A. Start an intravenous infusion of 5 per cent dextrose in water.
  B. Eliminate or reduce absorption of offending material (tourniquet proximal to site of challenge for several minutes, ice application, or local epinephrine).
  C. Supine position with clear airway.
  D. Maintain observation for 30 to 60 minutes.
  E. Administer oxygen.
  F. Have resuscitation equipment available.
  G. Observe vital signs.
II. Generalized Urticaria and Angioedema
  A. Aqueous epinephrine (0.3 to 0.5 ml., 1:1000 dilution) injection subcutaneously; may be repeated in 15 minutes.
  B. Antihistamine [diphenhydramine (Benadryl) 20 to 50 mg. I.M. or I.V.].
III. Respiratory Distress
  A. Aqueous epinephrine in above II-A.
  B. Antihistamine as above II-B.
  C. Maintain airway (intubation) or with tracheotomy (surgically or with large bore needle) for severe laryngeal edema.
  D. Aminophylline, 500 mg. in 1000 ml. of 5 per cent dextrose in water given over one hour for bronchospasm.
IV. Cardiovascular Collapse
  A. Aqueous epinephrine as II-A or 0.5 to 1.0 ml., 1 to 10,000 dilution, given intravenously or with cardiac needle injected directly into a ventricle in case of cardiac arrest (the latter only as a last resort). External chest wall cardiac massage can be done as a life-saving measure if there is complete cardiac standstill.
  B. Levarterenol bitartrate (Levophed) intravenous infusion—4 ml. of .2 per cent solution to 1000 ml. 5 per cent dextrose in water given 2 ml. per minute for hypotension.
  C. Hydrocortisone hemisuccinate (Solucortef) 100 mg. intravenously as a direct push and then an additional 100 mg. given in 1000 ml. 5 per cent dextrose in water intravenously to reduce late effects from generalized reaction.

---

mediators involved in the production of the AS.

Treatment

The cardinal rules in treatment of the generalized AS are to reduce or eliminate if possible the offending agent(s), maintain adequate ventilation, and sustain a normal blood pressure (Austen and Sheffer, 1971; Valentine, 1973). The outline of treatment for these reactions is shown in Table 4–21. The drug of choice for all clinical patterns is aqueous epinephrine. The epinephrine injection USP is parentally administered, the route depending upon the severity of the reaction. At the site of challenge, 0.2 ml., 1:1000 dilution, of aqueous epinephrine may be administered subcutaneously to retard the absorption of the offending agent. Epinephrine and other catecholamines promote the intracellular accumulation of cyclic-AMP, which reduces the amount of histamine secreted from mast cells and basophils. If bronchospasm is present, aminophylline may be of benefit. Hypotension is best treated by intravenous levarterenol bitartrate (Levophed). Systemic corticosteroids and antihistamines may be of some therapeutic usefulness for the later effects in generalized AS.

REFERENCES

Akers, W. A.: Chronic urticaria: Seek at least two causes. Cutis 10:591, 1972.

Austen, K. F.: Histamine and other mediators of allergic reactions. In Sampter, M., (ed.): Immunological Diseases. Boston, Little, Brown and Company, 1971, pp. 332–355.

Austen, K. F., and Sheffer, A. L.: The anaphylactic syndrome. In Fitzpatrick, T., Clark, W., Van Scott, E., et al., (eds.): Dermatology in General Medicine. New York, McGraw-Hill Book Co., 1971, pp. 1244–1261.

Baughman, R. D., and Jillson, O. F.: Seven specific types of urticaria. Ann. Allergy, 21:248, 1963.

Beall, G. N.: Urticaria: A review of clinical and laboratory observations. Medicine 43:131, 1964.

Bloch, K. J.: The anaphylactic antibodies of mammals including man. Progr. Allergy 10:85, 1967a.

Bloch, K. J.: Hypersensitivity due to antigen antibody interaction. Postgrad. Med. 42:28, 1967b.

Boston Collaborative Drug Surveillance Program: Drug-induced anaphylaxis. J.A.M.A. 224:613, 1973.

Braverman, I. M.: Urticaria as a sign of internal disease. Postgrad. Med. 41:450, 1967.

Champion, R. H.: Urticaria. In Rook, A., Wilkinson, D. S., and Ebling, F. J. G., (eds.): Textbook of Dermatology, Philadelphia, F. A. Davis Company, 1968, pp. 412–418.

Champion, R. H., Roberts, S. O. B., Carpenter, R. G., et al.: Urticaria and angioedema: A review of 554 patients. Br. J. Dermatol. 81:588, 1969.

Derbes, V. J., and Coleman, W. P.: Urticaria due to inhalants. Cutis 9:847, 1972.

Fisher, A. A., and Schwartz, S.: Low incidence of dermographism in subacute and chronic urticaria. Arch. Dermatol. 68:553, 1953.

Fromer, J. L.: Atopic urticaria and angioneurotic

Edema. *In* Criep, L. H., (ed.): Dermatologic Allergy: Immunology, Diagnosis and Management. Philadelphia, W. B. Saunders Co., 1967, pp. 279–297.

Hegedus, S. I., and Schorr, W. F.: Urticaria diagnostic workup and management. Postgrad. Med 52: 132, 1972.

Houser, D. D., Abesman, C. E., Ioto, K., et al.: Cold urticaria. Am. J. Med. 49:23, 1970.

Ishizaka, K.: Experimental anaphylaxis. *In* Sampter, M., (ed.): Immunological Diseases. Boston, Little, Brown and Co., 1971, pp. 202–219.

James, J., and Warin, R. P.: Chronic urticaria: The effect of aspirin. Br. J. Dermatol. 82:204, 1970.

James, J., and Warin, R. P.: An assessment of the role of Candida albicans and food yeasts in chronic urticaria. Br. J. Dermatol. 84:227, 1971.

Jillson, O. F.: Hypersensitivity to heat. *In* Baer, R. L., (ed.): Allergic Dermatoses. Philadelphia, J. B. Lippincott Co., 1956, pp. 69–78.

Juhlin, L., Johansson, S. G. O., Bennich, H., et al.: Immunoglobulin E in dermatoses. Arch. Dermatol. 100:12, 1969.

Juhlin, L., Michaelsson, G., and Zetterstrom, O.: Urticaria and asthma induced by food and drug additives in patients with aspirin hypersensitivity. J. Allergy Clin. Immunol. 50:92, 1972.

Kay, A. B., and Austen, K. F.: The IgE-mediated release of an eosinophil leukocyte chemotactic factor from human lung. J. Immunol. 107:899, 1971.

Litt, M.: Eosinophils and antigen-antibody reactions. Ann N.Y. Acad. Sci. 116:964, 1964.

Lockey, S. D.: Reactions to hidden agents in foods, beverages, and drugs. Ann. Allergy 29:461, 1971.

Mathews-Roth, M. M., Pathak, M. A., Fitzpatrick, T. B., et al.: Beta-carotene as a photoprotective agent in erythropoietic protoporphyria. N. Engl. J. Med. 282:1231, 1970.

Miller, D. A., Freeman, G. L., and Akers, W. A.: Chronic urticaria. Am. J. Med. 44:68, 1968.

Moore-Robinson, M., and Warin, R. P.: Some clinical aspects of cholinergic urticaria. Br. J. Dermatol. 80:794, 1968.

Nilzen, A.: The antihistaminic effect of human eosinophils. Allerg. Asthma (Leipz.) 16:24, 1970.

Osler, A. G., Lichtenstein, L. M., and Levey, D. A.: In vitro studies of human reaginic allergy. Adv. Immunol. 8:183, 1968.

Osler, W.: Hereditary angio-neurotic edema. Am. J. Med. Sci. 95:362, 1888.

Ostrov, M. R.: Dermographia: A critical review. Ann. Allergy 25:591, 1967.

Pickering, R. J., Kelley, J. R., Good, R. A., et al.: Replacement therapy in hereditary angioedema. Successful treatment of two patients with fresh frozen plasma. Lancet 1:326, 1969.

Pillsbury, D. M., Shelley, W. B., and Kligman, A. M.: Dermatology, 1st ed. Philadelphia, W. B. Saunders Co., 1956, pp. 771–778.

Rosen, F. S., and Austen, K. F.: The neurotic edema (hereditary angioedema). N. Engl. J. Med. 280: 1356, 1969.

Ryan, T. J., Shim-Young, N., and Turk, J. L.: Delayed pressure urticaria. Br. J. Dermatol. 80:485, 1968.

Sehon, A. H., and Gyenes, L.: Antibodies in atopic patients and antibodies developed during treatment. *In* Sampter, M., (ed.): Immunological Diseases. Boston, Little, Brown and Company, 1971, pp. 785–811.

Sheffer, A. L., and Austen, K. F.: Vascular responses: Urticaria and angioedema. *In* Fitzpatrick, T., et al., (ed.): Dermatology In General Medicine. New York, McGraw-Hill Book Co., 1971, pp. 1261–1274.

Sheffer, A. L., Austen, K. F., and Rosen, F. S.: Tranexamic acid therapy in hereditary angioneurotic edema. N. Engl. J. Med. 287:452, 1972.

Shelley, W. B., and Rawnsley, H. M.: Aquagenic urticaria. Contact sensitivity reaction to water. J.A.M.A. 189:895, 1964.

Sherman, W. B.: The atopic diseases—introduction. *In* Sampter, M., (ed.): Immunological Diseases. Boston, Little, Brown and Company, 1971, pp. 767–774.

Solomon, L. M., Juhlin, L., and Kirschenbaum, M. B.: Prostaglandin on cutaneous vasculature. J. Invest. Dermatol. 51:280, 1968.

Spaulding, W. V.: Methyltestosterone therapy for hereditary episodic edema. Ann. Intern. Med. 53: 739, 1960.

Thompson, J. S.: Urticaria and angioedema. Ann. Intern. Med. 69:361, 1968.

Tindall, J. P., Beeker, S. K., and Rosse, W. F.: Familial cold urticaria. Arch. Intern. Med. 124:129, 1969.

Valentine, M. D., and Sheffer, A. L.: The anaphylactic syndromes. Med. Clin. N. Am. 53:249–257, 1969.

Valentine, M. D.: Anaphylaxis. *In* Conn, H. F., (ed.): Current Therapy. Philadelphia, W. B. Saunders Co., 1973, pp. 530–531.

Zamm, A. V.: Chronic urticaria: A practical approach. Cutis 9:27, 1972.

Zamm, A. V.: Chronic urticaria, Part 3: The role of food allergy. Cutis, 11:670, 1973.

CHAPTER
5

DERMATITIS AND ECZEMA

Section I

CONTACT DERMATITIS
Edmund D. Lowney

All inflammations of the skin can be divided into two categories: those of internal and those of external origin (see Table 5–1). The former includes most eruptions due to systemic diseases and drugs, while the external group includes all dermatoses caused by agents which act upon the skin surface. When those external agents are alive, we are dealing with infectious dermatoses such as impetigo and tinea; if they involve radiation, we are dealing with the radio- or photo-dermatoses; when inflammation is caused by external heat, we are dealing with a burn. The preceding categories of disease are discussed elsewhere in this volume. The term *contact dermatitis* includes those inflammations due to all remaining external agents — the chemical allergens, toxins, and irritants, and the mechanical

irritants. [An excellent text on this subject is that of Fisher (1973)].

TABLE 5–1 CLINICAL FEATURES OF CONTACT DERMATITIS VERSUS THOSE OF SYSTEMIC ERUPTIONS

	Contact	*Systemic*
Localization of lesions	Localized to area of contact	Unrelated to exposure
	"Sensitive" skin involved; "tough" skin spared	Unrelated to sensitivity of skin
Shape of lesions	Lesions may be linear, angular, etc., depending on exposure pattern	Lesions round, oval or multicentric
Surface texture	Eczematous often	Erythematous often

239

MORPHOLOGIC FEATURES

It is often very helpful to be able to determine from clinical features alone whether an eruption is due to internal or external causes. Externally produced lesions have certain features in common which help to distinguish them from eruptions of systemic origin. Some of these features are summarized in Table 5–1.

Lesions of contact dermatitis tend to begin in the area of contact, and the shape of the lesions will reflect the localization of the exposure. For example, poison ivy dermatitis usually involves whichever extremity was exposed to the leaf, and often appears as linear streaks, which are produced as the plant brushes over the skin. In contrast, a systemic eruption (such as one due to a drug) usually appears in the form of symmetrically located lesions which "pop out" anywhere. Such lesions tend to be round, and are never square or linear. Another characteristic of contact dermatitis is that the topographic features of the skin determine to some extent the location and intensity of the dermatitis. An ointment which causes a contact dermatitis, for instance, is likely to accumulate in creases of the skin, or under a ring, producing an intense dermatitis there while sparing exposed surfaces from which it is readily removed. A solid contactant, however, will produce the opposite pattern, as the creases will be protected from contact. Clothing and hair may protect against some contactants, while forming a trap in which others may accumulate to intensify their effect. A drug or other systemic eruption, on the other hand, would appear from within at any location without regard to structures on the surface of the skin.

Regardless of exposure, certain areas of skin are more readily affected by contact irritants than others. The periorbital area and the dorsa of the hands are relatively sensitive, while it is more difficult to induce a dermatitis on the scalp, palms, or soles. The unusual sensitivity of the periorbital area is illustrated in Figure 5–2.

Another aspect of contact dermatitis which may differentiate it from a systemic eruption is the nature of the eruption itself. Most contact dermatitides are ec-

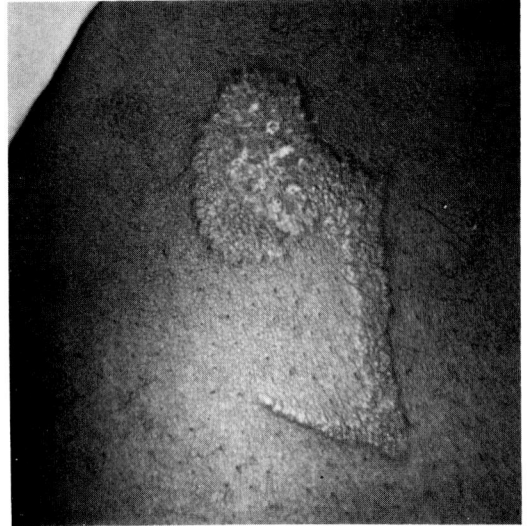

Figure 5–1 Contact dermatitis due to allergy to Merthiolate, applied to a trivial folliculitis. The fine, superficial vesicles and the linear and angular nature of the lesion are typical of contact dermatitis.

zematous and superficial, with epidermal involvement appearing relatively early. Fine, superficial, erythematous papules and vesicles are often the first evidence of an acute contact dermatitis (such as is seen in Figures 5–1 and 5–8). Most systemic eruptions, however, begin as a deep erythema, which produces scale only several days later. This distinction between an eczema and a toxic erythema is a very

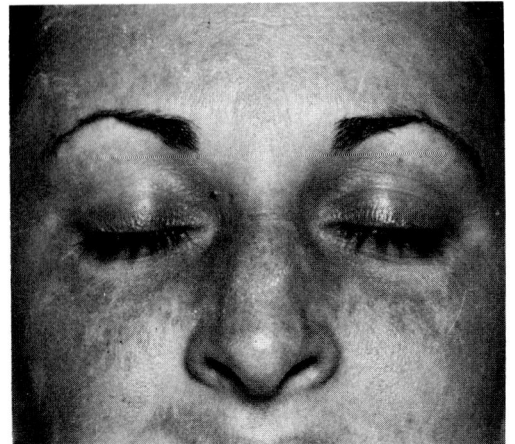

Figure 5–2 This patient was allergic to a nail polish, but the dermatitis was seen in the periorbital region because of the great sensitivity of this area.

meaningful one, but unfortunately requires some experience to be appreciated.

Even with the use of these principles, appearance alone cannot always be relied upon to establish a diagnosis of contact dermatitis. Dermatomyositis, for instance, may mimic a generalized contact dermatitis by producing an eczematoid dermatitis on exposed areas and on the periorbital skin.

Another confusing feature of contact dermatitis is that an allergen may be absorbed from the site of contact and produce a generalized systemic eruption. Such "auto-eczematization" is a systemic eruption superimposed on a contact dermatitis.

CLASSIFICATION OF CONTACT DERMATITIS

Contact dermatitis is classically broken down into two categories: *irritant* contact dermatitis (which includes all non-immunologic mechanisms) and *allergic* contact dermatitis (due to an acquired immunologic response). These two types are also cross-categorized according to the kind of reaction produced. Most allergic contact reactions are of the classic eczematous type, but urticarial and granulomatous reactions can occur. Irritant reactions may take these forms also, but, in addition, may be manifested in many other ways (pustular reactions, follicular hyperplasia, papules, blisters, dryness, redness, and scaling.

IRRITANT CONTACT DERMATITIS

Many substances are capable of irritating the skin if they are applied in high concentration, with occlusion, and for a long enough period of time. Even pure water, by producing maceration and washing away some "protective" skin lipids, becomes an irritant under special circumstances.

Potential Irritants

Manufacturers of cosmetics and soaps are understandably concerned lest a new compound incidentally included in their products turn out to be a significant irritant, and they often employ extensive testing in animals and in human volunteers to determine the irritancy of a proposed ingredient. As pointed out by Kligman and Wooding (1967), a compound can be assigned an L.D.$_{50}$, the dose which causes irritation in 50 per cent of subjects in a standard patch testing situation. Although most compounds can be shown to be potential irritants, relatively few are actually irritating in the usual encounter. For instance, many soaps will irritate skin almost 100 per cent of the time when applied in high concentration under an occlusive patch, but only a small fraction of the population has difficulty from casual use of soap at any one time.

Mechanical Irritation

The skin can be inflamed by mechanical factors, without mediation by soluble chemicals. The clearest example of this is dermatitis due to fiberglass particles. Generalized itching is occasionally produced when clothing becomes contaminated with fiberglass particles. (This can happen when the clothing is washed in the same tub with fiberglass fabric). Studies by Heisel and Hunt (1968) have shown that the inflammation is due to purely mechanical factors—particles of certain large sizes cause itching while small particles of the same substance do not.

WOOL. The most common mechanical irritant of clinical significance is wool. Wool clothing may cause itching in a large number of people, and is an especially common cause of itching and dermatitis in patients with atopic dermatitis (see p. 262). Although one occasionally encounters a patient with a specific allergy to wool alcohols or to lanolin, most wool dermatitis appears to be due to the mechanical "scratchiness" of the fabric.

Chemical Irritants

WATER. Although water is not an irritant per se, exposure to water can cause irritation of the skin in several ways.

1. When the thick, horny layer of the sole is soaked in water for a number of

days, a painful maceration known as *immersion foot* is produced. The callus becomes shriveled, or folded and fissured, turns white, and becomes exquisitely tender (Taplin et al., 1967). Immersion foot (also known as "paddy foot") was a major cause of disability to troops in Viet Nam.

2. The skin of most areas of the body loses some of its barrier function when macerated by water for several hours. This is the basis for the use of plastic occlusion to enhance penetration of topical steroids; however, exposure to water can also be associated with increased penetration of chemical irritants (such as soaps), and in this way water can act as a co-irritant.

3. Intermittent exposure to water, with intervening periods of dryness, often produces so-called dry skin or "xerotic eczema," which is described on page 291. The mechanism of this dermatitis is not understood. It is generally presumed that this intermittent exposure to water washes away lipids or other humectant substances which serve to maintain the smoothness and turgor of the epidermis, contributing to barrier function.

4. Chronic exposure to water promotes yeast and other intertriginous infections, especially in the paronychial area.

SOAPS AND DETERGENTS. These common surface-active agents enhance the drying and irritating actions of water, amplifying the xerotic eczema described above. Many soaps are mildly irritating, in part because of the alkalinity of soap solutions, and in part because of inherent qualities of the fatty acids and detergent molecules which are contained in soap. Commercial powders made for washing clothing are continually being altered by the addition of enzymes, fabric softeners, brighteners, germicides, and bleaches. Some of these additives are irritants, and a few are also allergens or photoallergens. For obvious reasons, soaps and detergents are especially likely to cause dermatitis of the hands. However, soaps sold for routine use on the skin are of necessity much less irritating, and seldom cause difficulty except in association with xerosis or some other dermatitis or under conditions of excessive use. (The exceptions to this statement are some deodorant soaps, which contain germicides that are both mild irritants and photosensitizers).

OTHER CHEMICALS AND MEDICATIONS. Chemical and medicinal substances of many sorts may cause an irritant dermatitis. These include a number of acids, alkalis, solvents, and oils. Such compounds are used as cleaning solutions and insecticides, or as reagents in industrial or chemical processes. The chemical irritants are commonly encountered in industrial situations or by the "do it yourselfer" who undertakes to carry out industrial processes at home; these problems are discussed in detail in Chapter 31.

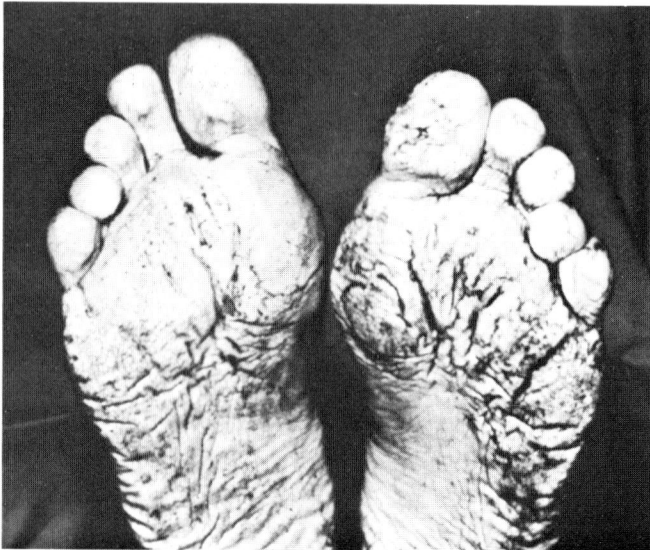

Figure 5–3 Immersion foot (or "paddy foot"), due to prolonged immersion in warm water. This is disabling because of tenderness.

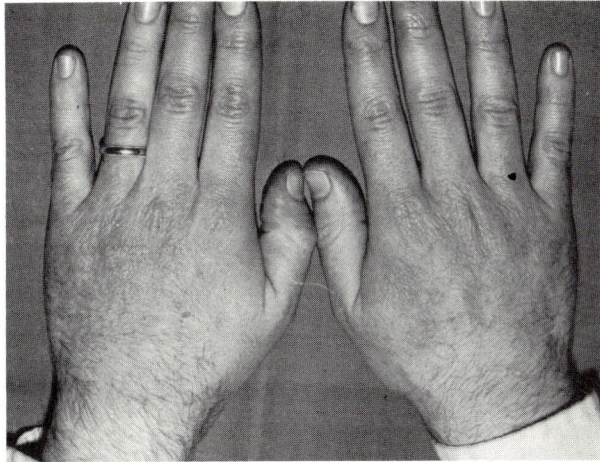

Figure 5–4 Irritant contact dermatitis due to exposure to a solvent (paint thinner).

Hand Eczema

The majority of cases of hand dermatitis are not due to the use of irritants but are caused by atopic dermatitis, dyshidrosiform eczema, allergic contact dermatitis, psoriasis, or fungal infection. Any dermatitis on the hands, however, can be exacerbated by contact with irritants. Hence, the patient with hand dermatitis, regardless of cause, should be cautioned to avoid exposure to potentially irritating compounds.

Irritant dermatitis of the hands is more likely to involve the tender dorsal skin rather than the palms. Irritant hand dermatitis typically is a chronic and relatively mild phenomenon, evolving into a dry, cracking, reddened, and often hyperpigmented eczema. When the case is mild, it may resemble the chapping of hands which is often seen in winter (and is an irritant dermatitis). On the other hand, an irritant dermatitis may occasionally be acute and severe, and may appear as a red, oozing, bullous lesion, resembling a thermal burn. Chronic vesiculation of the hands, however, is more likely to be due to dyshidrosis than to an irritant dermatitis.

The most common causes of irritant hand dermatitis are soaps and cleaning compounds, although the number of other irritants the hands can contact is legion.

Treatment consists primarily in avoidance of the irritant; in the typical case of housewives' hand eczema, this means avoidance of cleaning solutions. If this cannot be done, the hands should be protected from the cleaning solution by water-impermeable gloves worn over white cotton gloves.

Hand dermatitis is commonly exacerbated by use of irritating soaps, especially in the compulsive or guilt-ridden patient who tries to "wash away" his dermatitis. This source of irritation can be minimized by washing only when necessary and by using less irritating soaps. There are a number of bland soaps on the market, which, presumably, are made less irritating by increasing the fat content of the bar (for example, Basis, Oilatum, and others) or decreasing the pH of the solution they make (for example, Lowila, Dove, and others).

Symptomatic treatment of hand eczema is similar to that of any other eczema (see p. 318).

Biological Irritants

DIAPER DERMATITIS. Human excrement is the constant companion of the skin in infancy, and it is amazing that we do not see more irritant diaper dermatitis than we do. Parental negligence affects personal hygiene and facilitates the occurrence of this condition. Dermatitis of the diaper area is often attributed to the formation of ammonia from urine; this is a reasonable hypothesis, but has not been proved. Many mothers know that fecal material will be more irritating at certain times than at others, irritation often being associated with intestinal disturbance. A great deal of diaper dermatitis is not due to direct irritation by urine and feces but to infection with yeast or bacteria and to irritation from ill-advised medication and over-zealous cleaning. The papuloerosive type of eruption can resemble condylomata lata.

Treatment of diaper dermatitis involves three questions: Is it a yeast infection? Is it a bacterial infection? Is it being mistreated? At times, it is difficult to determine the cause of the dermatitis. The mother can usually tell the physician what potential irritants and allergens she has been applying.

In a previously untreated case of diaper dermatitis, which is not obviously due to one of the three factors described above, therapy should be directed toward several possible causes at once. The following program is often useful:

1. Stop all previous medication.
2. Change diapers as frequently as possible. (Disposable diapers are helpful.)
3. Expose area to air whenever possible.
4. Wash with plain water without soap.
5. Use absorbent diapers and apply talcum powder.
6. A nystatin-neomycin-gramicidin-triamcinolone cream (Mycolog) may be given as shotgun therapy in some cases. Vioform cream (3 per cent) may also be used for a similar purpose (it will stain diapers a yellowish-brown color). Ointment bases may be macerating and should be specifically avoided.

FISTULA DERMATITIS. In the adult with contamination of the skin due to incontinence or gastrointestinal or urinary fistula, the relative incidence of dermatitis is much greater than in the infant. Fistulae may drain liquid feces of high pH or enzymatic activity, and the surrounding skin may be additionally insulted by application of adhesives and rubber or plastic collection devices. Consequently, as McNamara and Farber (1964) point out, the patient with an ileostomy is especially prone to difficulty. As in the case of diaper dermatitis, fistula dermatitis is often complicated by infection and dermatitis medicamentosa.

Treatment of fistula or stomal dermatitis is similar to that of diaper dermatitis but is clouded by the necessity of using appliances, the deteriorating condition of the patient, and the lack of any real prospect of eventual remission. The principles of avoiding irritants and moisture, outlined in the preceding section, are applicable. It is important to perform a patch test on the patient, with all medications and adhesives being used, in order to eliminate specific irritants or allergens. Even in the absence of positive patch tests, a change to a new adhesive or medication is often helpful. Any measures which can decrease the frequency of bowel movements should be taken. An acute dermatitis may be relieved by compressing the skin with dilute Burow's solution (1:40) for 15 minutes twice a day, followed by dusting with karaya powder (as an absorbent). Often the patient and physician must cooperate in a long series of trials and errors before the optimal regimen is found.

OTHER BIOLOGICAL IRRITANTS. The number of chemical substances manufactured within the animal and plant kingdoms which are capable of causing inflammation of human skin is undoubtedly as great as the number of potential irritants in industry. In addition to excreta, saliva and tears produced by the human body may incidentally be irritating to its surface. Many animals make specific toxins for purposes of defense or aggression: Caterpillars, beetles, and other insects produce agents which cause dermatitis or vesication; sea nettles and many other aquatic animals and plants produce toxins which affect the skin. Cowage produces itching by means of a protease.

A number of infectious agents also produce toxins which affect the skin. Maibach and Kligman (1962) have shown that *Candida albicans* causes a contact dermatitis by means of toxic compounds liberated by the organism. A specific toxin elaborated by certain strains of Group II staphylococci has been shown by Melish et al. (1972) to be responsible for bullous lesions seen in the scalded skin syndrome in children and in bullous impetigo.

Unusual Irritant Reactions

The typical irritant produces a dermatitis—erythema, burning or itching, and, when more severe, weeping. Dermatitis caused by an irritant usually appears sooner than that due to an allergen (see below). However, there is great variety in the time of onset, symptoms, and appearance of an irritant dermatitis, for there are undoubtedly many mechanisms by which irritation may be produced. In addition, some chemicals characteristically produce nondermatitic reactions of various sorts, some of which are described below.

COMEDONES. Comedones due to keratinous hyperplasia of the follicles are produced by prolonged application of hexachloronaphthalene and many other related acne-causing substances. Industrial oils often contain these compounds, producing so-called oil acne (see p. 1476).

HYPERKERATOSIS. Hyperkeratosis and callus formation are produced by repeated application of dilute solutions of formaldehyde, as well as by a number of other low-grade irritants.

BULLAE. Bullae are readily produced by the cantharidin and other vesicants.

ERYTHEMA. Erythema without corresponding inflammation can be produced by topical application of vasodilators, such as histamine, Trafuril, and so forth. Conversely, *vasoconstriction* can be caused by topical application of some sympathomimetic compounds.

DEPIGMENTATION. Depigmentation may result from contact with rubber products containing monobenzyl ether of hydroquinone (Agerite alba), and from certain phenolic antiseptic compounds.

CONTACT URTICARIA. Contact urticaria results from application of many simple irritants in the susceptible patient.

FOLLICULITIS. Folliculitis is produced by a number of tars and oily compounds upon application to the skin.

ONYCHOLYSIS. Onycholysis, or separation of the nail from its bed, has been reported with application of nail hardeners. The cause of this reaction may be formaldehyde. 5-Fluorouracil may cause nail separation when applied to periungual warts.

Hardening

Repeated application of an irritant sometimes causes the dermatitis to become progressively worse; in other cases, the reaction of the skin decreases with repeated exposure. The latter phenomenon, which is known as "hardening," is sometimes seen in industrial dermatitides. When the hardened worker returns from a vacation, the dermatitis characteristically recurs in its original intensity. We have no explanation for hardening, although it has been suggested that chronically inflamed skin rids itself of irritant compounds by exfoliation of the epidermis to the outside, and by increased phagocytosis and blood flow, removing the irritant which penetrates into the dermis from the dermatitic area. (In the case of *allergic* contact dermatitis, hardening may be due to a hyposensitization mechanism; see Hyposensitization below).

ALLERGIC CONTACT DERMATITIS

Dermatitis may be produced by irritants in many ways, but in allergic contact dermatitis the mechanism is always the same.

Delayed Hypersensitivity

With the exception of allergic contact urticaria, which is quite unusual in adults, all allergic contact dermatitis is presumed to be mediated by delayed hypersensitivity. Allergic contact dermatitis thus finds itself in company with the tuberculin reaction, the homograft reaction, and certain drug reactions considered to be manifestations of this form of allergy.

Mechanism

The precise mechanisms of delayed hypersensitivity and the essential ways in which they differ from those of other immunologic reactions are currently the center of much new research, speculation, and controversy. [For a more detailed discussion, see a review of delayed hypersensitivity, such as that of David (1968).]

The balance of the evidence, however, permits agreement on some of the most salient features of allergic contact dermatitis.

THE ANTIGEN. Typical causes of allergic contact sensitivity include the poison ivy antigens, many industrial chemicals (for example, mercaptobenzothiazole, chromates), many drugs (for instance, sulfanilamide, penicillin, Merthiolate), and some metals (especially nickel and chromates). Other chemicals, such as

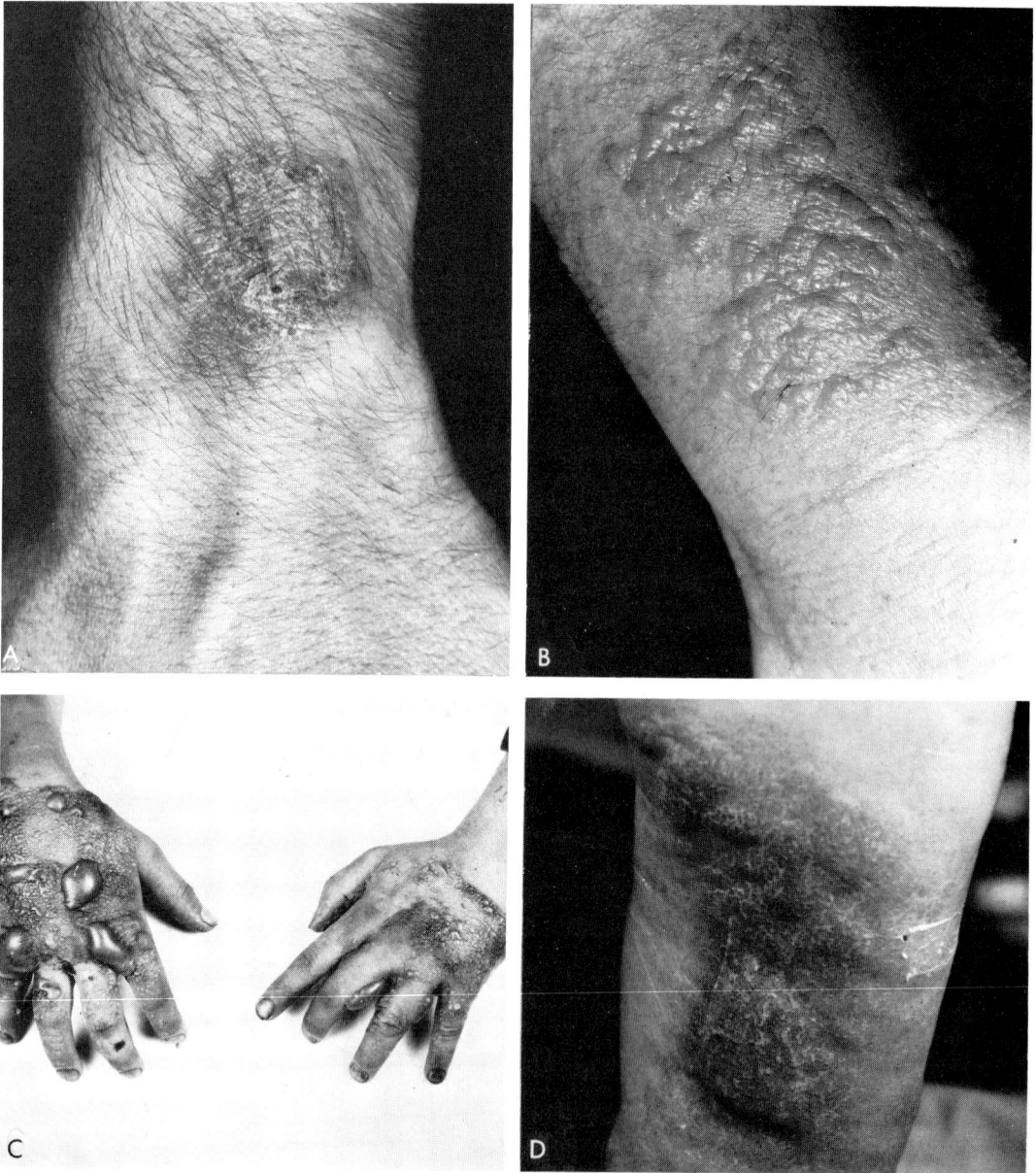

Figure 5–5 Variations in contact dermatitis. *A*, From wrist watch (nickel). *B*, From chlorpromazine solution. *C*, From organic mercurial solution applied to warts. *D*, From insole of sneaker shoe, after immersion in water.

dinitrochlorobenzene (DNCB), picryl chloride, and oxazolone, are commonly used to study the phenomenon in the laboratory.

Study of the sensitizing potential of a wide range of compounds has shown that, while some compounds are excellent sensitizers, a much larger number of compounds are weaker sensitizers, capable of sensitizing under special circumstances. Even hydrocortisone has caused contact dermatitis on very rare occasions.

An antigenic determinant of fairly large size is required to induce allergic contact sensitivity. Large protein molecules are antigenic but cross the epidermal barrier with great difficulty and, perhaps for this reason, rarely induce or elicit contact sensitivity. Most of the compounds which are good sensitizers are small enough to cross the stratum corneum, but also have the ability to combine with protein (or perhaps with other larger molecules) within the skin to produce a new molecule or complex which is large enough to be antigenic. In this situation, the sensitizing chemical is called a haptene, and the resulting sensitizing molecule is a *haptene-protein* or *haptene-carrier complex.*

The *antigenic determinant* responsible for contact sensitivity embraces an area larger than the haptene itself, and includes an adjacent portion of the carrier protein. An animal sensitized to one haptene-protein complex often will not respond when tested with the same haptene combined with a different protein. The same specificity has also been observed in man. This phenomenon is referred to as *carrier specificity.* In many cases, carrier speci-

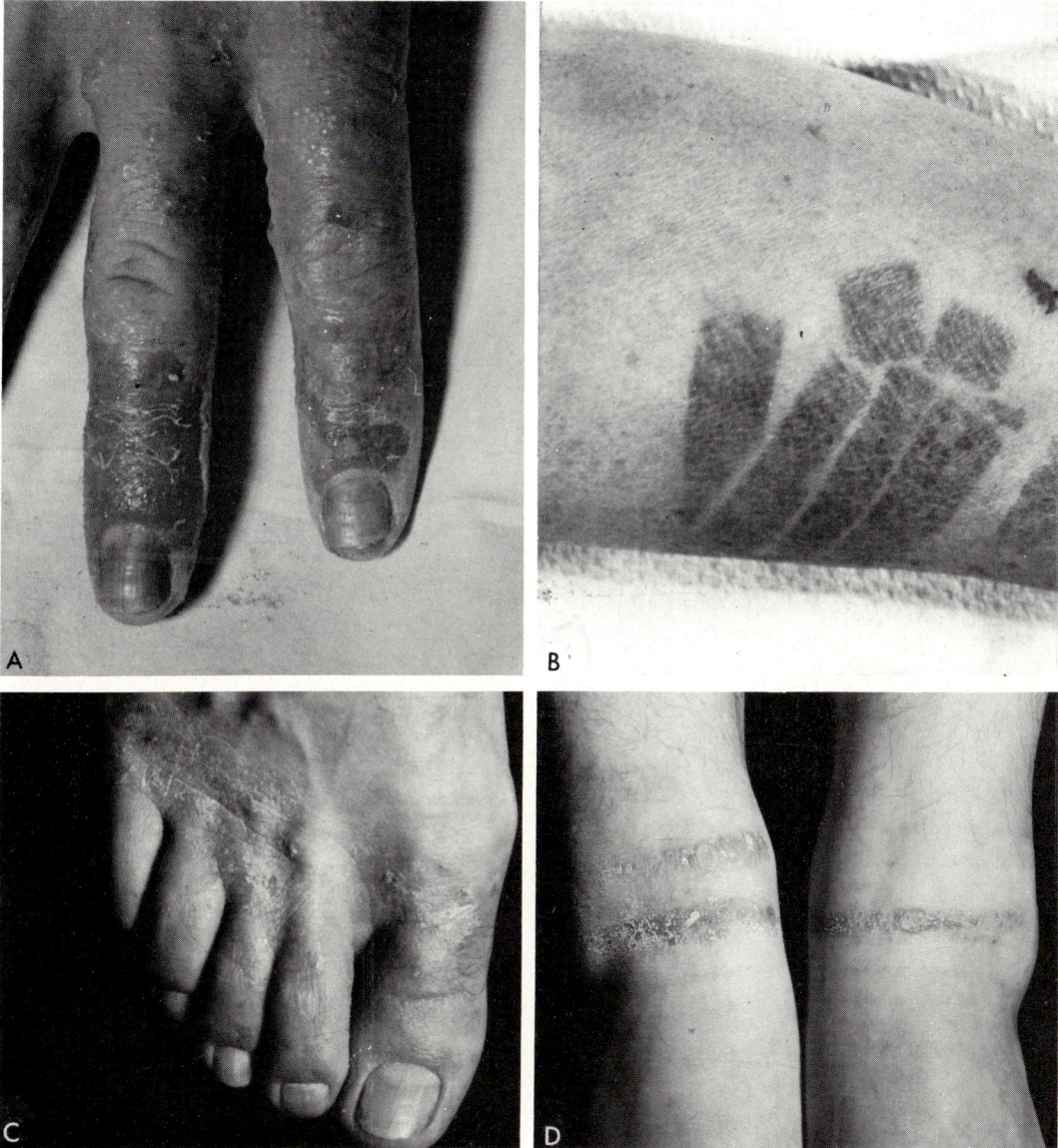

Figure 5–6 Various sources of contact dermatitis. *A*, Procaine dermatitis in typical site in dentist. *B*, Reaction to adhesive tape. *C*, Sensitivity to shoe leather. *D*, Sensitivity to leather shoe strap. Such patterns of dermatitis are often seen with "buffalo-hide" sandals of Indian origin.

ficity is seen in delayed, but not in immediate, reactions to the same haptene.

Obviously, when a very reactive sensitizing chemical is put on the skin, it must combine with quite a number of proteins of epidermal, dermal, and vascular origin, so that many contact sensitivities to a whole family of haptene-protein combinations may be induced. It is probable that different sensitizers tend to react with different proteins or at different locations in the skin so that not all contact sensitizers produce exactly the same pattern of dermatitis.

SENSITIZATION. Allergic contact dermatitis can be induced readily in man, in the guinea pig, and in the monkey, but only with difficulty in most other animals. The simplest way to induce contact sensitivity is by direct application of the haptene to the surface of the skin, or, in the guinea pig, by injection of the haptene mixed with Freund's complete adjuvant into the footpad.

Kligman (1966) has shown that, in certain situations, the incidence and degree of sensitivity produced is proportional to the amount of sensitizer given at a single time, and to the amount applied per unit surface area of skin. A large amount of a sensitizer spread over a large area of skin in a very dilute solution is likely not to sensitize as effectively as would the same amount concentrated onto a small site. Application of the sensitizer to a mucous membrane is less likely to sensitize than the same amount of sensitizer put on a small area of skin. When a series of small, subsensitizing doses of a sensitizer are applied to the skin, sensitivity may eventually be induced, but the intensity of the dermatitis produced is likely to be low. We do not know as much as we would like about the effects of conditions of exposure to the haptene or the degree of sensitivity which ultimately develops.

Not all people can be sensitized to a contact antigen with equal facility. Whenever a series of normal subjects are exposed experimentally to a sensitizer such as dinitrochlorobenzene (DNCB), varying degrees of sensitivity will result; and a small percentage of subjects will not be sensitized at all. Patients with impairment of delayed hypersensitivity (such as those with advanced Hodgkin's disease, other lymphomas, sarcoidosis, and so forth) often cannot be sensitized to DNCB. It has recently been suggested that resistance to sensitization by DNCB may be a sign of aggressive malignancy, but, as Johnson et al. (1971) have pointed out, this relationship may be spurious.

Contact sensitizers can be given to guinea pigs by mouth or intravenously in such a way that the animals are not sensitized, and are made tolerant, so that they then cannot be sensitized even by methods which are usually effective. This phenomenon in the guinea pig is known as the *Sulzberger-Chase* effect. A somewhat similar phenomenon has been shown to occur in man following administration of DNCB to the buccal mucosa. It has been suggested that some degree of tolerance is produced whenever a sensitizer is administered, and that the level of clinical sensitivity resulting from a given exposure to a sensitizer reflects algebraically the degrees of tolerance and sensitization induced. The phenomena of tolerance in animals and the prospects of their reproduction in man have been reviewed by De Weck and Frey (1966) and by Lowney (1970).

Little is known about the cellular metabolism of the haptene-protein conjugate which induces contact sensitivity. When a sensitizer is injected into the skin, sensitivity may result, even though the sensitizing molecule may not be detected in regional nodes. From this it has been suggested that the sensitizing conjugate may be processed in the skin so as to "instruct" an information-bearing "messenger" compound or cell which in turn gives rise to the sensitization process elsewhere (presumably in the proximal lymph node). This concept, developed by Macher and Chase (1969), is often referred to as "peripheral sensitization."

The thymus apparently plays a permissive role in contact sensitization, since neonatally thymectomized animals often fail to develop delayed hypersensitivity. This permissive effect may be hormonally mediated.

The mechanisms by which tolerance is produced are poorly understood, and there may be several varieties of tolerance.

TRANSFER. Allergic contact sensitivity can be transferred from one animal to another with white cells from a sensitive donor, but not ordinarily with serum. Hence, circulating immunoglobulins are presumed to play no role in elicitation of the reaction. In a number of experiments, acellular transfer factors have been observed to transmit various forms of delayed hypersensitivity. Some of the factors identified are actually sensitizing agents (inducing sensitivity which becomes apparent a week or so later) rather than true mediators of preexisting sensitivity. However, Lawrence and Landy (1969) have described a human cell extract which can transfer specific tuberculin sensitivity within a short period of time. Compounds with somewhat similar activities can be released from sensitive cells by exposure to antigen or by large doses of x-ray. Whether such transfer factors circulate and play a role in elicitation of human contact sensitivity in vivo is not known. In any event, there is little evidence that contact sensitivity can be transferred by a circulating immunoglobulin, and the view that sensitive cells or products which diffuse into their immediate vicinity are responsible for mediation of contact sensitivity still predominates.

ELICITATION. About 10 days after a sensitizing exposure has occurred, another application of a small amount of the sensitizer will elicit an eczematous, dermatitic reaction, demonstrating that a state of sensitivity has been induced. Contact dermatitis is commonly elicited experimentally in routine patch testing. This reaction characteristically begins to appear several hours after application of the chemical, and usually reaches its peak about three days later. The smaller the eliciting dose, the weaker the reaction and the more time required for it to appear. Severe reactions may be vesicular; weak reactions may consist only of faint erythema. Itching does not necessarily appear, but it is usually present in a reaction of moderate intensity. Once induced in a human subject, allergic contact sensitivity, as measured by epicutaneous tests, most often lasts for a number of years, although the intensity of the reaction may show a gradual decline.

What is the mechanism by which a contact sensitizer elicits a dermatitic reaction? Once again we must be vague because of conflicting concepts. It is believed that the chemical must combine with a protein (or proteins) very similar to those used to sensitize in order for elicitation to occur. Once this conjugate forms in the skin, it presumably interacts with a "sensitive" lymphocyte, which supposedly releases various substances which lead to the inflammatory response. One substance which may be involved is MIF (migration inhibition factor), which may retain monocytoid cells in the area of the reaction by preventing their further migration. A number of other substances capable of mediating inflammation are also released by the antigen-stimulated cell. Some theorists have speculated that the process of elicitation recapitulates that of sensitization. According to this concept, the elicitation differs from the original sensitization only in the increased number of sensitive cells which have become available to react with the antigen.

Hyposensitization

There is good evidence in both man and animals that the level of contact sensitivity can be decreased in a quantitative way by exposure to excessive amounts of the antigen. This is shown by a decline in the intensity of epicutaneous test reactions. This phenomenon, best described by Kligman (1958b), is the basis for the clinical use of poison ivy antigen given by mouth to depress the severity of the dermatitis resulting from subsequent exposure. In some cases, the depression produced appears to be permanent, but it is often transient.

Complete desensitization (with completely negative patch tests) is rarely produced without administration of prohibitively massive amounts of the sensitizer. Systemic administration of a sensitizer to a sensitized individual can also produce a generalized dermatitis if an adequate amount of the sensitizer reaches the skin.

The mechanism of hyposensitization is not understood, although the process behaves as a quantitative neutralization phenomenon. The mechanism may have much in common with that which induces tolerance; in both cases the antigen acts to block rather than to stimulate sensitivity.

Cross-Reactivities

Few contact sensitizers are chemically unique; most are related to other compounds with which cross-reaction may occur. Cross-reacting compounds may act as contact sensitizers when put on the skin or may cause systemic allergic reactions when ingested as drugs. Cross-reactivity does not always occur, however; two related compounds may cross-react in one patient, while the next patient may react to only one. A common example of this is the many compounds which cross-react with poison ivy (see below). Other common "families" of cross-reacting sensitizers include the halogenated salicylanilides used as germicidal agents in soaps, and the para-amino compounds.

Clinical Features of Allergic Contact Dermatitis

Severe, acute dermatitis appears as a very itchy, superficial eruption consisting of small vesicles surrounded by redness. Milder degrees of the same dermatitis may consist simply of redness, or of redness with varying degrees of swelling or papulation.

The distribution and other aspects of allergic contact dermatitis are similar to those of other forms of contact dermatitis (see p. 241). Each contact sensitizer, however, may present special features of distribution because of the way in which the compound is encountered. A few of the more common distribution patterns encountered are described in Table 5–2.

TYPES OF CONTACT DERMATITIS

Poison Ivy Dermatitis

By far the most common cause of contact dermatitis, and probably the most common cause of acute eczema of all forms (in the United States), is poison ivy. In the eastern and central parts of the United States, this dermatitis is caused by contact with a common weed, *Rhus radicans*. This plant with its characteristic three leaves

TABLE 5–2 COMMON CAUSES OF CONTACT DERMATITIS OF DIFFERENT AREAS

Area	Cause
Face	Cosmetics; hair sprays; hair dyes; airborne contactants
Ears, lobes	Nickel
Ears, pinnae	Photosensitizers
Ears, canals	Medications
Eyelids	Cosmetics. Any sensitizer on hands and any airborne sensitizers may be transferred to periorbital area
Nose, bridge	Metal or plastic spectacle supports
Lips or surrounding area	Toothpaste; lipstick
Neck	Perfumes; clothing (especially wool)
Axillae	Deodorants; clothing; perfumes
Scapular area	Nickel in clasps on straps
Breasts	Elastic and other brassiere material
Waist	Elastic
Perianal area	Dibucaine (Nupercaine) and other medications; excessive use of cleansers
Arms and legs	Poison ivy and other plants
Wrists	Nickel, etc. in watch bands
Hands	Detergents and other cleansers; gloves
Feet	Medication for "athlete's foot"; shoes

(Fig. 5–7) is found in woods and in many inhabited areas as well. In the western states, and occasionally elsewhere, a closely related group of antigens is found in the poison oak (*R. toxicodendron*). The poison sumac plant (*R. vernix*) also belongs to this group. It is commonly found in swampy areas.

The same group of antigens may also be found in the shell of the cashew nut, in the mango rind, in Japanese lacquer, and in a number of other sources; hence, people from the Tropics and the Orient may become sensitized to poison ivy without exposure to the plant itself. Europeans, however, seldom develop sensitivity to poison ivy before coming to the United States.

Poison ivy dermatitis is more apt to be vesicular than many other forms of contact dermatitis. The plant is most commonly encountered by young people out of doors; hence, the rash is commonly seen on legs and arms. It may be carried by the hands to the face, genitals, and other parts of the body not directly

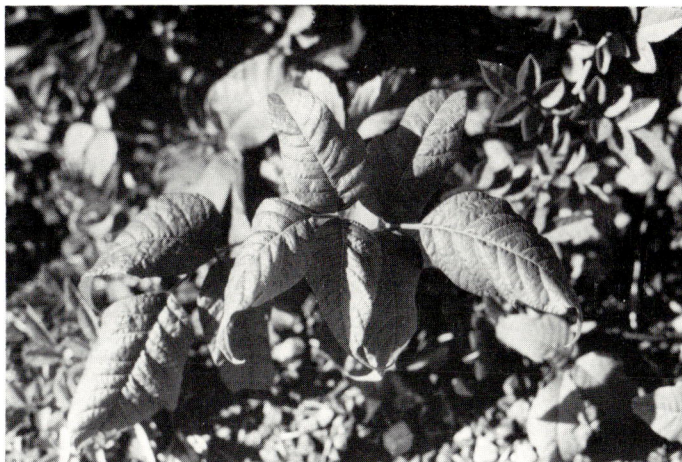

Figure 5–7   The poison ivy plant.

touched by the plant. The most characteristic lesion is a linear one (Figs. 5–8 and 5–9), appearing on an extremity which has brushed past the leaf. If such a linear lesion can be found, it may clinch the diagnosis.

The poison ivy antigen has been the object of intensive biochemical and biological study, reported by Dawson (1954, 1964) with several collaborators, and by Kligman (1958a). It appears that poison ivy actually contains a family of four sensitizing compounds, historically known as "urushiols." The most active of the urushiols now appears to be the di-unsaturated or diolefin form of 3-*N*-pentadecylcatechol. One concept of its structure is presented in Figure 5–10. The other three members of the family are the mono- and tri-unsaturated forms, as well as saturated 3-*N*-pentadecylcatechol itself. Contrary to previous belief, recent evidence indicates that the fully saturated "hydrourushiol" is one of the less active antigenic components.

Similar compounds have been found to make up the Japanese lacquer antigens, which cross-react with poison ivy. At least one of the urushiols of Japanese lacquer differs from those found in poison ivy, however. Of greater local interest are

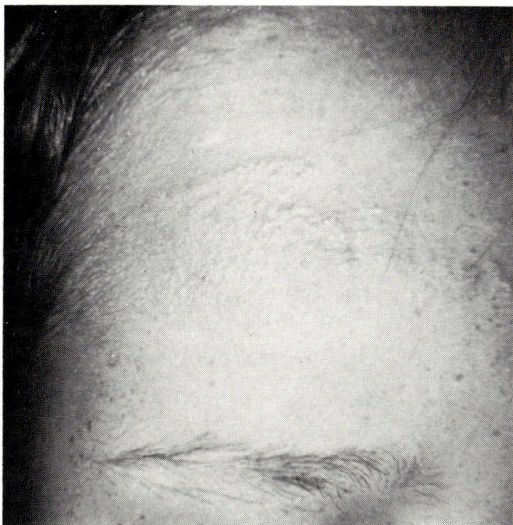

Figure 5–8   Poison ivy dermatitis. The presence of a linear vesicular lesion is highly suggestive.

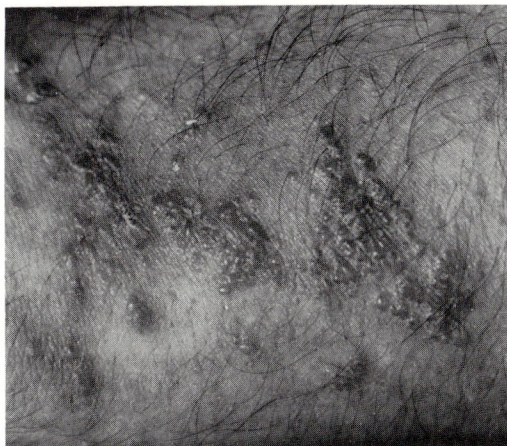

Figure 5–9   Acute poison ivy dermatitis.

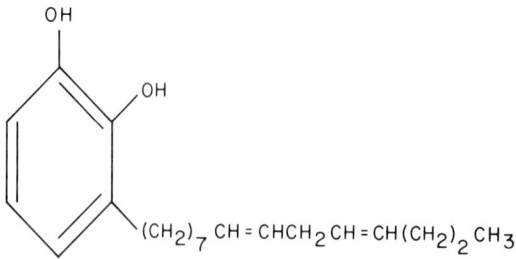

$$OH$$
$$OH$$
$$(CH_2)_7 CH = CHCH_2 CH = CH(CH_2)_2 CH_3$$

Figure 5–10   The diolefinic urushiol of poison ivy (After Symes and Dawson, 1954).

recent observations that some of the urushiols of Western poison oak may differ from those of poison ivy in at least one structural detail.

Nickel Dermatitis

Perhaps as common as poison ivy dermatitis is the dermatitis due to acquired sensitivity to nickel. This sensitivity manifests itself most commonly as dermatitis from nickel-containing costume jewelry and from metal clasps found on feminine underclothing. The dermatitis is therefore seen on the ear lobes (from earrings), on the wrists (from watch bands or bracelets) on the thighs (from garter clasps), and in other locations. The dermatitis is seldom severe, and the patient is often able to determine the cause without medical advice. Occasionally, however, nickel dermatitis arises from unexpected sources, such as metal trays, counters, tools, and so forth.

Shoe Dermatitis

Although almost any dermatitis of the feet can be made worse by wearing close-fitting, occlusive shoes in hot weather, many patients suffer from a specific contact sensitivity to a compound found in shoes (Epstein, 1969). The most common sensitizers are antioxidants and accelerators used in the manufacture of rubber, such as monobenzyl ether of hydroquinone, or dimethylthiuram, which may be found in rubber parts of the shoe or in rubber-based cement used to glue the shoe together.

The dermatitis most often involves the dorsum of the foot, but usually spares the space between the toes which does not contact the shoe. This helps distinguish this dermatitis from tinea pedis, which often is prominent between the toes. However, many cases of shoe dermatitis persist for years, being diagnosed as athlete's foot, dyshidrosis, or neurodermatitis before the real cause is found.

Diagnosis is made by screening patch tests with a series of common sensitizing chemicals found in shoes and, equally important, with pieces cut from various parts of the shoe itself.

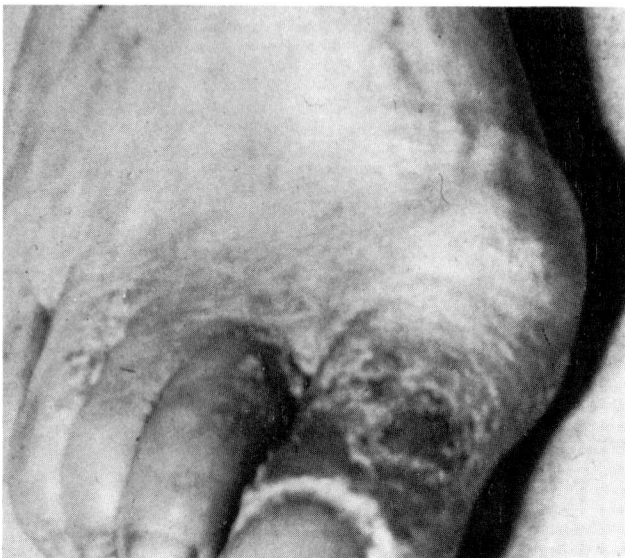

Figure 5–11 Contact dermatitis from shoes. The patient was allergic to 2-mercaptobenzothiazole, an accelerator used in the manufacture of rubber and rubber-based glues. (Courtesy of Dr. M. H. Samitz.)

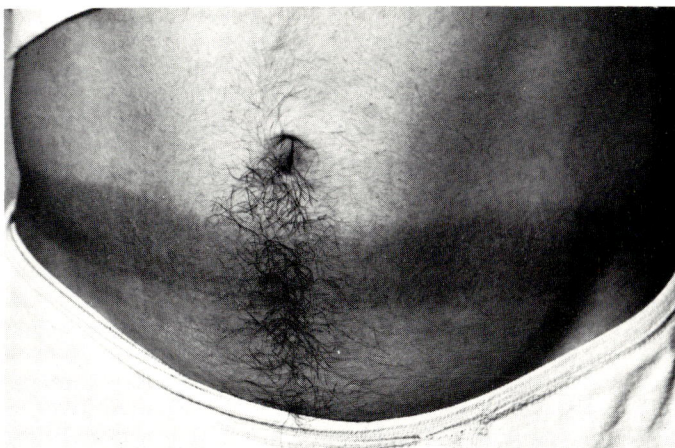

Figure 5–12 Contact dermatitis due to elastic sensitivity.

Clothing Dermatitis

Contact dermatitis due to clothing is not a common occurrence, since most manufacturers have learned to avoid the use of sensitizing compounds. Dermatitis from nickel clasps and from shoes has already been discussed. Rubber sensitivity may manifest itself as a dermatitic reaction to apparel containing *elastic,* and leather sensitivity may result in a dermatitis from leather objects, such as hatbands. Some processes used to make fabrics crease-resistant involve treatment of the cloth with formaldehyde, which can cause dermatitis in a patient with formaldehyde sensitivity. After several washings, the formaldehyde may be washed out of the material, leading to improvement in the dermatitis. Other, newer, "wash and wear" processes occasionally cause dermatitis by means of residual, unpolymerized reagents. Dermatitis from dyes is not common, but is occasionally seen when a sensitizing dye is poorly "fixed" to the fabric. The classic sensitizing dye, *p*-phenylenediamine, is now seldom used to dye clothing, but does occasionally cause clothing dermatitis from its use in furs and leather. Other agents to be suspected in clothing dermatitis include cleaning solutions and chemical finishes of various sorts.

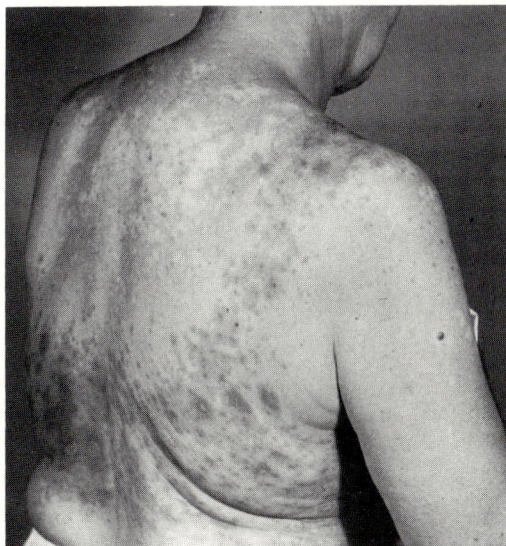

Figure 5–13 Reaction to "Spandex" elastic.

The fabric itself is rarely responsible, except in the case of irritant dermatitis due to wool.

The clinical picture seen in clothing dermatitis obviously varies with the article of clothing involved. Anatomic factors also influence the location of the dermatitis. Warm, sweaty areas, such as the axillae and inguinal creases, are frequently involved when the clothing is in contact with the vault of the crease but are often spared from contact with more loosely fitting garments. Surfaces to which pressure is applied are also likely to be affected. The typical case of dermatitis due to a pair of pants, for instance, involves the posterior thighs in a person who sits a great deal.

Dermatitis Medicamentosa

Whenever a dermatosis fails to improve with proper treatment, one must suspect contact allergy to the topical medication which has been applied. Common causes of contact dermatitis include neomycin, dibucaine (Nupercaine), benzocaine, Merthiolate, ammoniated mercury, and many other medications. Stabilizers and preservatives (for example, paraben, ethylenediamine) used in the manufacture of cream and ointment bases may be unsuspected allergens. Dermatitis medicamentosa often presents a confusing diagnostic picture because one is dealing with two diseases, and some insight is required to realize that a new dermatosis has been superimposed upon an old one.

Airborne Contactants

When a contact sensitizer is diffused in the air in fine particles, a generalized dermatitis of exposed parts is produced. A common example of this is elicitation of a generalized dermatitis in very sensitive persons exposed to smoke from burning poison ivy plants. In the midwest farmlands, sensitivity to the oleoresin of ragweed pollens occasionally produces a similar picture. This dermatitis resembles a photodermatitis in that exposed parts are involved, but differs from it in the involvement of the shaded areas (such as the underside of the chin). Cosmetic and medicinal aerosols can cause allergic dermatitis in exposed areas in sensitive individuals.

Photocontact Dermatitis

Photosensitizing compounds can reach the skin from within, as in the case of photosensitizing drugs or porphyria, or they may be applied to the surface of the skin. In both instances, either a phototoxic or a photoallergic mechanism may be in play (see Chap. 6). Historically, the best known phototoxic contact dermatitis is that due to oil of bergamot, which is used occasionally in the formulation of perfumes. This produces a streaky, pigmented dermatitis when the perfume is applied to sun-exposed areas, such as the neck. This particular entity is known as Berlock dermatitis.

Salicylanilide Photodermatitis

Certain antibacterial agents of the salicylanilide group commonly added to soaps are capable of inducing a photoallergic dermatitis. These compounds include tetrachlorosalicylanilide and tribromsalicylanilide (TBS). The latter compound is widely distributed in a number of commercial deodorant soaps. Occasionally, bithionol and hexachlorophene cross-react with members of this group. Fortunately, only a minute fraction of persons exposed to these compounds develop the photoallergy.

This photodermatosis presents as a generalized pruritic dermatitis on sun-exposed areas, and often there is a history of exacerbation by sunlight. Such exacerbations may be more common in the spring than later in the sunny season. Since the action spectrum of salicylanilide photodermatitis is in the area of 3600 Å, symptoms can be produced by sunlight passing through window glass (which usually does not transmit light below 3200 Å).

Although many patients with soap-induced photodermatitis improve when the soap is avoided, some continue to react to sunlight for many years.

The mechanisms of photoallergic contact dermatitis are not clear, although it has been suggested that sunlight may de-

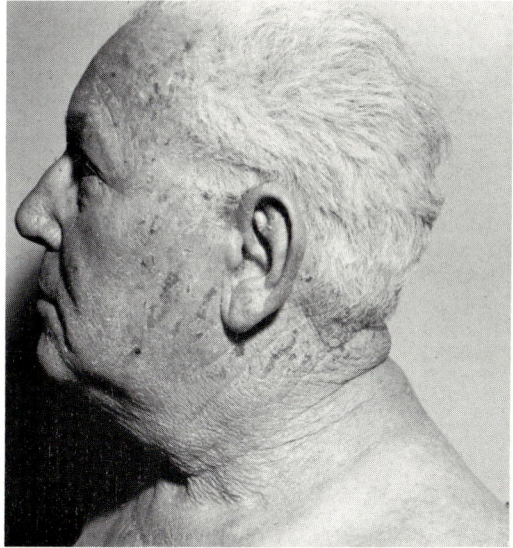

Figure 5-14 Photoallergic contact dermatitis due to an antibacterial soap containing a brominated salicylanilide.

grade the "photosensitizing" agent to another compound which is itself an active contact sensitizer. The degradation product then induces a simple contact dermatitis.

TREATMENT OF
CONTACT DERMATITIS

Find The Sensitizer

There are several rather obvious approaches which can be used to find the cause of a suspected contact dermatitis.

HISTORY. Often the patient already suspects the cause of his problem. If not, careful attention to the circumstances in which the process had occurred and improved in the past may lead to an answer. It is often helpful to ask if the eruption was aggravated following changes in employment or during vacations away from the usual environment. It is very important to obtain a detailed history of all topical medications and cosmetics which have been used.

PATCH TESTING. Experimental elicitation of the dermatitis by application of the sensitizer may demonstrate its probable cause.

Patch tests may be used in two ways. When one has no leads as to the cause of

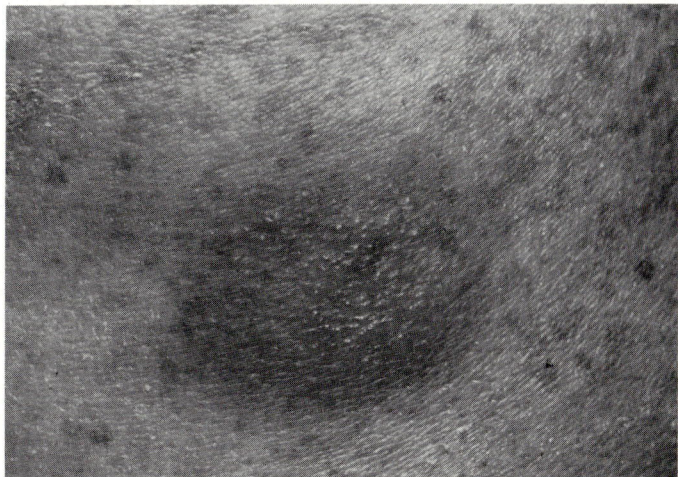

Figure 5-15 Positive patch test.

the eruption, a series of common sensitizers may be applied in the hope of detecting one to which the patient is sensitive. Sometimes, it is then possible to explain the eruption. Compounds generally used in such a *scout tray* are described in Table 5–3. Patch tests may also confirm the etiologic role of an agent which is already suspected. For example, if it is believed that a dermatitis is caused by a shoe allergy, bits of lining from the shoe, or samples of sensitizers commonly found in shoes, can be used for patch testing in order to demonstrate that such an allergy does indeed exist.

Method. Although patch tests have been performed in many ways under special circumstances, a standard method has come into common usage. The test material is applied to a small square (about .6 cm.) of cotton cloth or gauze which is in turn kept in place by adhesive tape. For this purpose, a Band-Aid may be used, or the patch can be improvised. A small number of patches can be applied to the upper arm, but the back should be used for larger numbers of patches. The patch should be kept in position for 48, or preferably 72, hours before it is removed, and the test

TABLE 5–3 COMPOUNDS COMMONLY USED FOR PATCH TESTING

Common Sensitizers—Used as Scout Battery When No Particular Contactant is Suspected

Benzocaine	5% in petrolatum
Epoxy glue resin	1% in acetone
Formaldehyde	.8% aqueous solution
Lanolin	As is
Mercaptobenzothiol	1% in petrolatum
Mercuric bichloride	.1% aqueous solution
Neomycin sulfate	20% in petrolatum
Nickel sulfate	5% aqueous solution
Paraphenylenediamine	2% in petrolatum
Potassium dichromate	.025% aqueous solution
Tetramethylthiuram disulfide	1% in petrolatum
Turpentine	25% in olive oil

Battery of Tests for Shoe Dermatitis (in Petrolatum)

Basic chromic sulfate	0.2%
Bismark Brown	5%
Formaldehyde	.8%
Hydroquinone monomethyl ether	1%
Mercaptobenzothiazole	1%
Paraphenylenediamine	2%
Potassium dichromate	0.5%
Tetramethylthiuram disulfide	1%

site is observed. However, the patient must be instructed to remove the patch at once from any site which demonstrates pain or burning, as some reactions may be unduly severe.

Interpretation. The interpretation of patch test reactions involves the following questions:

1. Is this an irritant reaction? Patch tests with substances which are inherently irritating are useless for demonstration of allergic contact sensitivity, for they will elicit positive tests in everyone. To avoid this problem, irritant concentrations of most of the common sensitizers have been determined, and concentrations known to be below the irritant threshold of the normal person can be used for testing. Commonly used concentrations of a number of sensitizers are described in Table 5–3.

2. Was the result of the test obscured by a reaction to the tape?

3. Was the reaction truly eczematous, and not due to occlusion, folliculitis, or pressure?

4. If the patch tests were negative, was the test properly applied, and was occlusion maintained for the proper period of time?

5. Finally, one must ask if a positive patch test is a reasonable explanation of the clinical picture. Many patients have "incidental" sensitivities to common sensitizers (nickel or poison ivy, for instance), while suffering from a dermatitis of an entirely different etiology.

Care must be taken to avoid test applications of irritating concentrations, and it must be remembered that a chemical which is only slightly irritating when applied openly to the skin may cause a severe burn when put on the skin and occluded with a bandage. It is usually unwise to apply patch tests to a patient suffering from an acute contact dermatitis, as a positive reaction is very likely to exacerbate and prolong the eruption. The problems of patch testing have been described in further detail by Shelley (1967) and Epstein (1967).

USE TEST. Sometimes dangers of severe irritation from patch testing can be avoided by a use test, in which the patient is instructed to use a suspected agent in a routine way in order to determine if the agent in question will evoke the dermatitis. Such use tests can detect the cause of an irritant as well as an allergic contact dermatitis.

Environmental Manipulation. Another detective method which can be helpful is environmental manipulation. For instance, a patient with a chronic unexplained dermatosis can be sent out of town (or away from his work) for a few weeks to see if improvement occurs. While this approach occasionally leads to rewarding observations, it is seldom practical.

In vitro tests for detection of contact sensitivity by observing reactions of the patient's peripheral leukocytes are very badly needed but have not yet been developed for practical clinical use. Since the antigenic determinant includes a portion of the carrier protein, hapten-protein conjugates presumably would be required as reagents for such a test.

Symptomatic treatment of allergic contact dermatitis is similar to that of other acute eczemas. In the presence of secondary infection, topical compresses and, if necessary, systemic antibiotics should be used. For the weeping but uninfected eczema, topical compresses (for example, Burow's solution, 1:40, for 20 minutes q.i.d.) may be useful. They should be discontinued as soon as the lesion is dry.

Dry dermatitic areas are best treated with topical corticosteroid creams. When large areas are involved, dilute creams must be used because of the expense. Occasionally, dry areas can be treated by steroid creams with clear plastic film (for example, Saran) occlusion.

Contact dermatitis *of known cause* is almost always an affliction of short duration, and hence can be quite safely treated with short courses of systemic corticosteroids. Systemic steroids should not be used to treat a mild contact dermatitis which will respond to topical therapy. However, in a perfectly healthy person, prednisone, given in doses decreasing from 40 to 5 mg. a day over a week's time rarely if ever does any harm. Sedatives such as diphenhydramine (Benadryl), phenobarbital, or hydroxyzine (Atarax, Vistaril) are also useful in controlling itching, especially at night. Further remarks on the nonspecific treatment of eczematous dermatitis will be found later in this chapter.

Hyposensitization to poison ivy or poison oak is occasionally of value in the patient with severe rhus sensitivity who cannot avoid exposure to the plant. A series of increasing amounts of the oleoresin must be given orally over a period of several months before the start of the poison ivy season. This program is helpful if enough oleoresin is given, but effective doses often produce uncomfortable side effects, such as pruritus ani, generalized itching, and hives. Oleoresin should never be given to the patient who already has active poison ivy dermatitis.

REFERENCES

David, J. R.: Delayed hypersensitivity. *In* Miescher, P. A., and Muller-Eberhard, H. J., (eds.): Textbook of Immunopathology. Vol. 1, New York, Grune and Stratton, 1968, p. 111.'

DeWeck, A. L., and Grey, J. R.: Immunotolerance to simple chemicals. Monogr. in Allergy *1*:1, 1966.

Epstein, E.: Simplified patch test screening with mixtures. Arch. Dermatol. 95:269, 1967.

Epstein, E.: Shoe contact dermatitis. J.A.M.A. *209*: 1487, 1969.

Fisher, A. A.: Contact Dermatitis. 2nd ed. Philadelphia, Lea and Febiger, 1973.

Heisel, E. B., and Hunt, F. E.: Further studies in cutaneous reactions to glass fibers. Arch. Environ. Health *17*:705, 1968.

Johnson, M. W., Maibach, H. I., and Salmon, S. E.: Skin reactivity in patients with cancer. N. Engl. J. Med., *284*:1255, 1971.

Kligman, A. M.: Poison ivy (rhus) dermatitis. Arch. Dermatol. 77:149, 1958.

Kligman, A. M.: Hyposensitization against rhus dermatitis. Arch. Dermatol. 78:47, 1958.

Kligman, A. M.: The identification of contact allergens by human assay. J. Invest. Dermatol. 47:369, 375, 393, 1966.

Kligman, A. M., and Wooding, W. M.: A method for the measurement and evaluation of irritants on human skin. J. Invest. Dermatol. 49:78, 1967.

Lawrence, H. S., and Landy, M.: Mediators of Cellular Immunity. New York, Academic Press, 1969.

Lowney, E. D.: Dermatologic implications of immunological unresponsiveness. J. Invest. Dermatol. 54:355, 1970.

Macher, E., and Chase, M. W.: Studies on the sensitization of animals with simple chemical compounds. J. Exp. Med., *129*:81, 103, 1969.

Maibach, H. I., and Kligman, A. M.: The biology of experimental human cutaneous moniliasis (Candida albicans). Arch. Dermatol. 85:233, 1962.

Markiewitz, K. H., and Dawson, C. R.: On the isolation of the allergenically active components of the toxic principle of poison ivy. J. Org. Chem. 30:675, 1964.

McNamara, R. J., and Farber, E. M.: Circumileostomy skin difficulties. Arch. Dermatol. 89:675, 1964.

Melish, M. E., Glasgow, L. A., and Turner, M.D.: The staphylococcal scalded-skin syndrome: isolation and partial characterization of the exfoliative toxin. J. Infect. Dis. *125*:129, 1972.

Shelley, W. B.: The patch test. J.A.M.A. *200*:874, 1967.

Symes, W. F., and Dawson, C. R.: Poison ivy "urushiol," J. Am. Chem. Soc. 76:2959, 1954.

Taplin, D., Zaias, N., and Blank, H.: The role of temperature in tropical immersion foot syndrome. J.A.M.A. *202*:546, 1967.

Section II

ATOPIC DERMATITIS

Lawrence M. Solomon

Atopic dermatitis is a highly specific, easily diagnosed disease which results from a hereditarily determined lowered cutaneous threshold to pruritus and is characterized by intense itching. When the skin of individuals with this condition is chronically scratched, the result is eczema and lichenification. Eczema is a generic term which identifies a type of cutaneous reaction pattern having many causes. The word *atopy* was first coined by Coca in 1923 to describe the hereditarily determined predisposition to hay fever, asthma, urticaria, and the distinctive dermatitis with which it is sometimes associated. The eruption is often responsible for prolonged discomfort and disability and embarrassing cosmetic disfigurement.

Atopic dermatitis has been referred to in the past by a host of names, but those most widely used today are atopic dermatitis, Besnier's prurigo diathèsique, and neurodermatitis. When seen in the infant, it is also called infantile eczema and the differentiation from less serious forms of eczema may be difficult. None of these terms is truly adequate, but atopic dermatitis is probably the most useful.

CLINICAL FEATURES

INCIDENCE

Atopic dermatitis is a common disease which causes much physical suffering, disability, and anguish for the patient and his family. It is responsible for a large segment of dermatologic practice. The reported incidence of atopic dermatitis in the general population ranges from 0.25 to 20 per cent (Carr, 1964). There are many variables which may account for this discrepancy, among them being the inconsistencies from study to study in the criteria used to make the diagnosis, the types of populations studied, and the geography. The incidence in the United States may range from 3 to 5 per cent. The true incidence is very difficult to determine, since it requires a large scale prospective study which would include the examination of many neonates, with long term follow-up.

DIAGNOSIS

The diagnosis of atopic dermatitis may be made with reasonable certainty in most cases from family history, past personal history, and examination of the skin. Occasionally, some laboratory procedures and skin testing with a few pharmacologic agents may add useful information.

Genetic Inquiry (Family History)

About 70 per cent of patients with atopic dermatitis have a family history of atopic dermatitis (Fig. 5–16), asthma, or hay fever. The mode of transmission of the disease is not clear. Some have felt that a single dominant gene is responsible (Cooke, 1916), but the evidence at present favors more than one autosomal recessive gene. A difficulty which might intervene in determining the Mendelian inheritance is

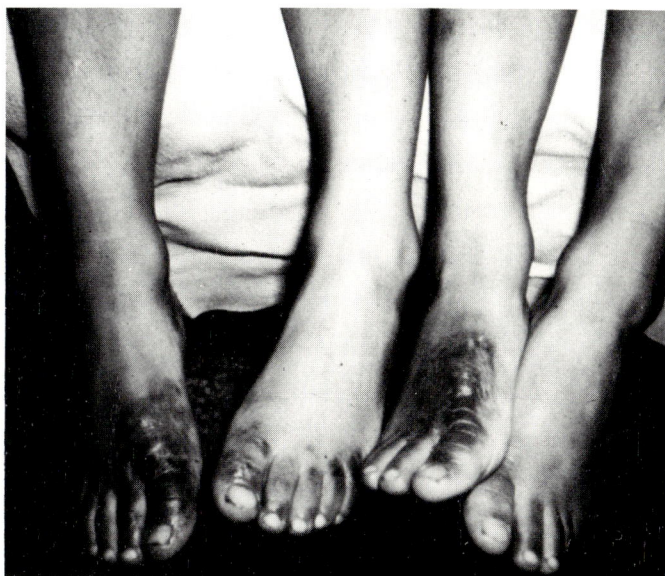

Figure 5–16 Atopic dermatitis in identical twins.

the fact that what is inherited is not a skin lesion but a tendency to pruritus, which becomes evident on exposure of the skin to a stressful internal or external environment. The pruritus threshold in atopic dermatitis may vary from patient to patient or indeed from day to day in the same person. This is best illustrated by Rajka's (1960) studies with identical twins, in which the course of the disease was not similar in both twins. In spite of the uncertainty of the mode of genetic transmission, the evidence for its genetic nature is very convincing, and a positive family history of atopy is good supportive evidence for the diagnosis.

Morphology

Atopic dermatitis is, as Jaquet has noted, an itch that rashes rather than a rash that itches. The primary lesion, if it can be dignified by that name, is a small papule, not unlike a goose pimple (Baer, 1959). The changes which may result from scratching include erythema, weeping, scaling, and lichenification. The presence of lichenification alone is not enough to permit a diagnosis of atopic dermatitis, but it is the characteristic result of scratching and should be found somewhere at some time for the diagnosis to be made with confidence.

Atopic dermatitis may arbitrarily be divided into four stages, according to the age of the patient. In the infant, atopic dermatitis is the most common type of eczematous change. Many believe that atopic dermatitis may be differentiated from seborrheic dermatitis in the young infant. Since a seborrheic component is frequently part of the picture of atopic dermatitis, this differentiation may be impossible to make (Rostenberg and Solomon, 1968). Patients who are initially diagnosed as having seborrheic dermatitis frequently develop classic atopic dermatitis later. It is extremely difficult to rule out atopic dermatitis in the infant, even if it presents primarily with a seborrheic picture. Atopic dermatitis usually appears in the infant about the third month (Hellerstrom and Rajka, 1967), ordinarily in the form of moderately erythematous dry or oozing patches which may coalesce.

The distribution of the lesions in the infantile phase is not characteristic, often affecting extensor and flexor areas but almost always involving the face, particularly the cheeks (Fig. 5–17). The dermatitis may disappear or become much less severe at the age of 2 to 3 years. In a high proportion of such patients, the disease recurs in late childhood (Fig. 5–18 A), adolescence, or even early adult life. At this time, the lesions in their torpid stage

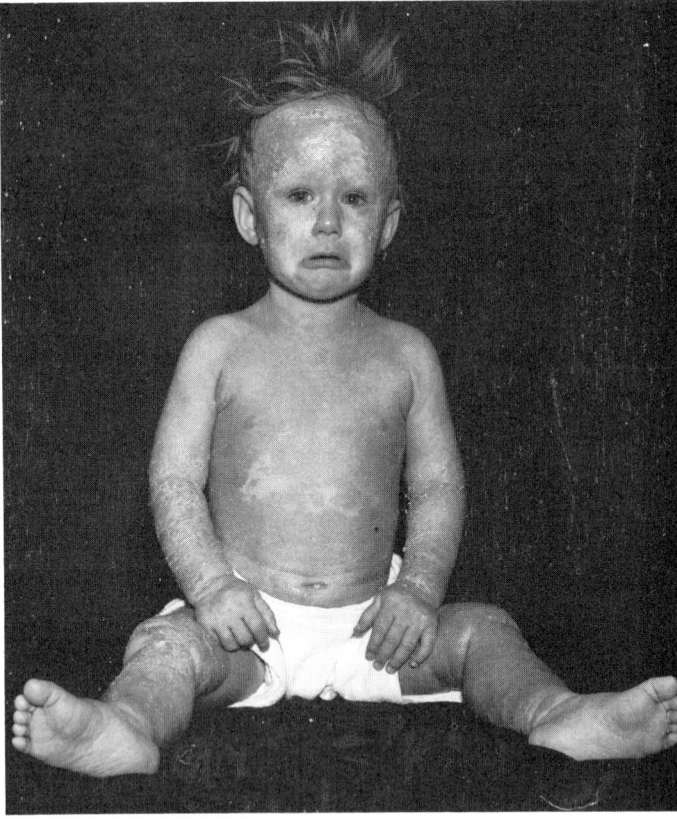

Figure 5–17 Atopic dermatitis. The considerable unhappiness of infants with extensive forms of this disease is well shown. (Children's Hospital of Philadelphia.)

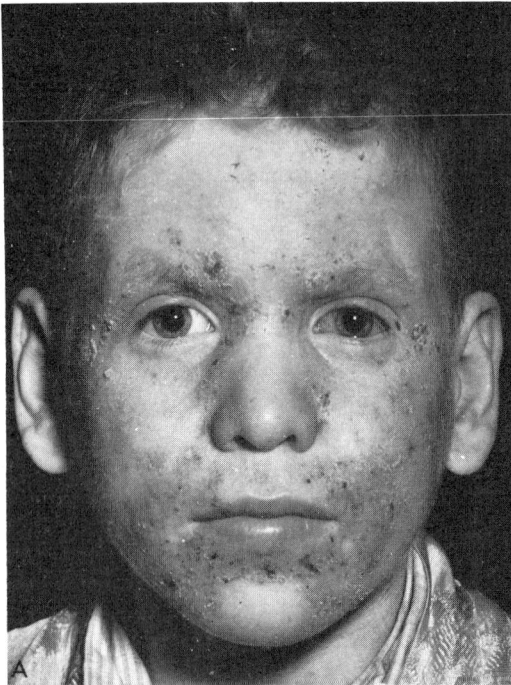

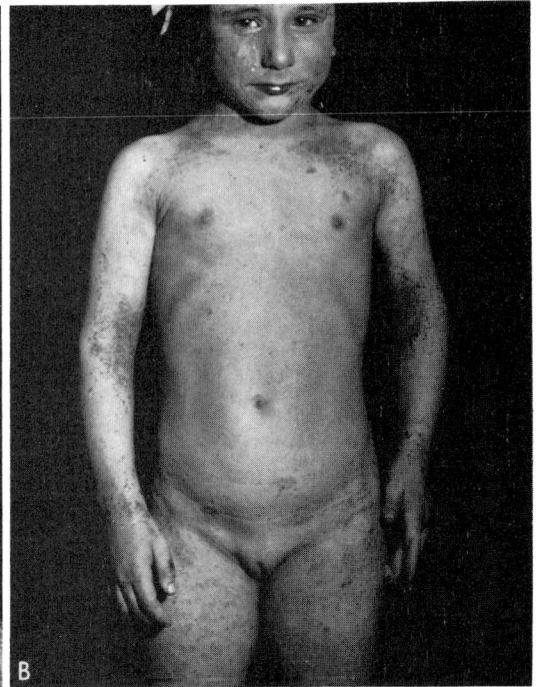

Figure 5–18 Atopic dermatitis. *A*, Characteristic facial appearance, chronic excoriated dermatitis, and "sad" and "strained" look. *B*, Female child with characteristic facies and predominantly flexural involvement.

tend to localize in the flexural areas (Fig. 5–18 *B*), namely, the neck, antecubital spaces, popliteal folds, the eyelids, behind the ears, and the wrists. Seborrheic changes in the scalp and extreme itching often precede the eruption. At times, the eruption may become generalized in a patchy way or be accompanied by secondary infection. The areas of eczema are duskily erythematous and streaked with excoriations. The more chronic areas may reveal excoriations and infection (Fig. 5–19 *A*); they become deeply lichenified and hyperpigmented (Fig. 5–19 *B*). In time, the chronic inflammatory process may lead to destruction of melanocytes, with permanent depigmentation in the flexures. At about 30 years of age, the disease abates in some patients, to recur as a chronic hand or foot eczema (particularly in women). In some patients, the disease remains chronic and widespread late into the fifth decade.

Patients with atopic dermatitis also have a strong tendency to a mild form of dominant ichthyosis vulgaris (Wells and Jennings, 1967), as well as the previously mentioned seborrhea, and keratosis pilaris. The incidence of psoriasis in these patients seems (to the author) to be less than

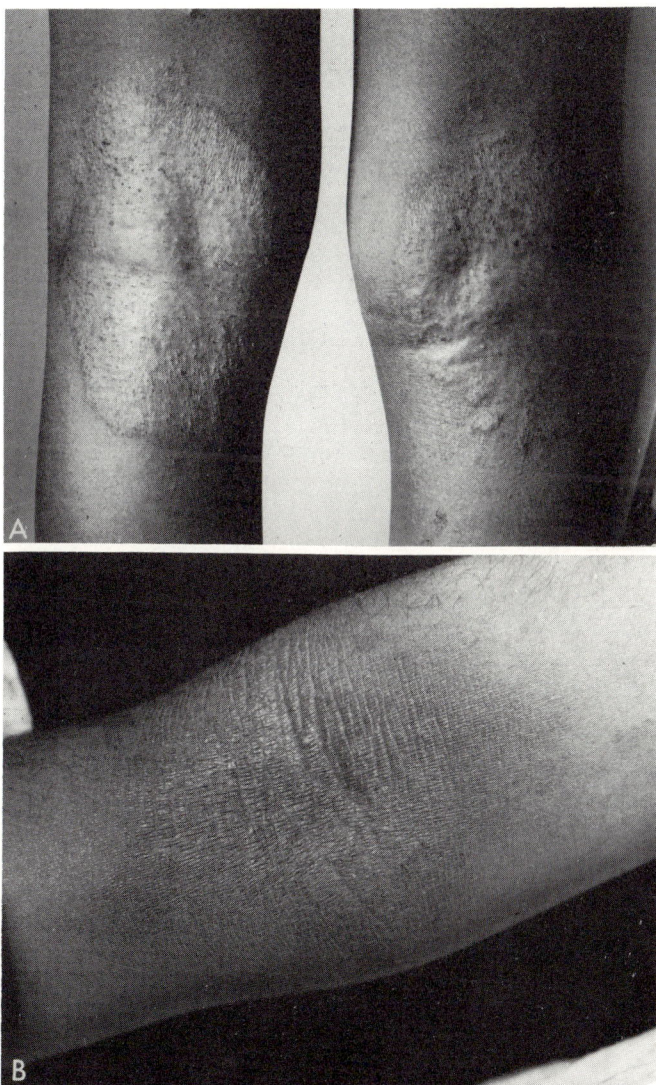

Figure 5–19 Atopic dermatitis — characteristic lesions. *A*, Sharply marginated excoriated lesions of popliteal spaces. *B*, Lichenification and thickening—antecubital fossa.

one would expect to find in the population as a whole.

Routine Laboratory Studies

There are no laboratory tests available at this time which establish a diagnosis of atopic dermatitis. Eosinophilia is a frequent finding in patients with this condition (Sulzberger, 1955) but is not specific nor essential (Roth and Kierland, 1964) for the diagnosis. Serum IgE levels (see below) may be elevated in atopic dermatitis (Juhlin et al., 1969), but high levels have also been found in other diseases (Heiner and Rose, 1969), and some patients without IgE (those with agammaglobulinemia) may have atopic dermatitis (Peterson, 1965) so that this test is of limited diagnostic value. The histopathologic changes in atopic dermatitis are not specific for that disease, so that a biopsy may not be useful in establishing the diagnosis. It may, however, be informative in the diagnosis of some diseases in which an atopic-like dermatitis may be a prominent feature (for example, histiocytosis X and ectodermal dysplasia).

EXACERBATING FACTORS

A number of factors exacerbate the pruritus of atopic dermatitis. This has led some to consider a cause-and-effect relationship between these factors and the dermatitis. The number and type of events and substances which are said to cause atopic dermatitis should lead to the suspicion that, rather than causing the dermatitis, the provoking events are all acting by way of a common underlying pathway, and are etiologically unrelated.

Patients with atopic dermatitis are often highly intolerant to sudden changes and extremes of temperature and humidity. As a result, the pruritus is most intense in the dry winter and humid summer months. It is worse after undressing or leaving a bath; these actions lead to a sudden lowering of skin temperature. These patients also tolerate exercise poorly because their cutaneous vessels are unable to adapt quickly to the changes in skin temperature induced by sweating. Ironically, many patients relieve their pruritus by taking a hot shower or bath. The heat replaces the itch sensation by causing a more tolerable sensation of pain. Unfortunately, hot water causes intense vasodilation and increases the inflammatory component, leading to aggravation of the dermatitis, greater pruritus, and more scratching—the vicious scratch-itch cycle.

Patients are almost unanimous in their belief that psychological stress may contribute to a flare-up of the dermatitis. The relationship between a parental or marital conflict and a bout of intense pruritus is commonplace. The dermatitis itself may induce feelings of inadequacy which in turn may lead to anxiety, depression, and aggravation of the need to scratch. While psychogenic factors are obviously important in the course of atopic dermatitis, there is much disagreement about their role in the genesis of the disease.

The patient with atopic dermatitis has a highly sensitive skin and many substances will cause pruritus when placed in contact with it. This is particularly true of wool, furs, and, to a lesser degree, of nylon. The pruritus caused by these substances is not due to an allergic contact dermatitis but simply reflects the increased tactile sensitivity of these patients. Some subjects are intolerant of substances having oil and ointment bases and others prefer them. Direct contact with detergents, primary irritant chemicals, perfumes, and colognes may be an aggravating factor in some patients, precipitating a bout of intense pruritus.

The question of the immunologic nature of atopic dermatitis will be discussed later in this chapter. At this point, it should be acknowledged that atopic patients may rarely become allergic to systemically administered drugs as well as to topically applied agents, but with no greater frequency than non-atopic individuals (Cronin et al., 1970). When an immediate or delayed type of allergic reaction does occur, the skin will also become more pruritic. Food allergy, particularly to cow's milk, has been incriminated as both cause and aggravating circumstance in infantile atopic dermatitis. There is no convincing evidence for, and considerable evidence against this empiric notion. Milk or any other food is probably not a primary cause of atopic eczema.

Patients frequently complain of dry skin and inability to sweat, and state that sweat-inducing stimuli, such as exercise, provoke itching. Whether these patients sweat normally or not is still a subject of controversy (Sulzberger, 1954; Rovensky and Saxl, 1964). The "dryness" the patients complain of is usually due to scaling which results from chronic, subacute inflammation. The pruritic effect of exercise may be related not only to sweating problems but also to the demands exercise makes on their cutaneous vasculature.

SYSTEMIC MANIFESTATIONS

Patients with atopic dermatitis have been a source of intensive study in recent years and a number of observations have been made which suggest that more than the skin may be involved in the disease process. The following paragraphs describe some of these observations.

Congenital Anomalies

Atopic dermatitis is a frequent component of anhidrotic ectodermal dysplasia (Reed et al., 1970); phenylketonuria (Jervis, 1937); Netherton's disease (Wilkinson et al., 1964), which consists of congenital ichthyosiform erythroderma, trichorrhexis invaginata, and atopic diathesis; long arm 18 deletion syndrome (Smith, 1970); and the Wiskott-Aldrich syndrome (Krivit and Good, 1959). It also occurs with surprising frequency in ataxia telangiectasis (Reed et al., 1966), sex-linked agammaglobulinemia (Peterson, 1965), and ahistidinemia (Snyderman et al., 1963). When a random group of patients with atopic dermatitis were studied for the presence of congenital defects, they were found to have twice as many as a control group (Torsney and Blumstein, 1966).

Carbohydrate Metabolism

It has been observed by several independent investigators that patients with atopic dermatitis tend to have a flat oral glucose tolerance curve, lacking the normal glycemic response (Kierland, 1955).

Eosinophilia

Not only do patients with atopic dermatitis tend to have eosinophilia in a stressful environment (such as a hot room) but they also lack the expected eosinopenic response to an exogenously administered epinephrine load as well as the eosinopenic response to an alarm reaction (endogenous epinephrine) (Sternberg and Zimmerman, 1952).

Thyroid Function

Thyroid dysfunction has been seen in an unusually high frequency by a number of authors; however, this finding has been disputed by others (Raffle and Hall, 1967).

Blood Pressure and Cardiovascular Function

Atopic individuals were found to have a more rapid resting heart rate by one group of investigators (Varonier and Hahn, 1966). Low blood pressure has also been observed by some (Baer, 1952) but not found to be present by others (Varonier and Hahn, 1966).

Central Nervous System

Russell and Last (1955), among others, reported a high incidence of electroencephalographic abnormalities resembling those found in epilepsy among patients with atopic dermatitis.

Personality

The personality of the patient with atopic dermatitis has been a source of interest and controversy among dermatologists for many years (Stokes, 1930). One group (Sulzberger, 1955) believes that these patients have no consistent personality traits, and another (Fiske and Obermayer, 1954) describes the patient with atopic dermatitis as a repressed individual whose anxieties and hostility are communicated by scratching. The pitfalls and unaccountable variables which intervene in making personality evaluations leave the question undecided (Solomon and Beerman, 1966).

Menstrual Cycle Relationships

It has been noted that female patients tend to have a flare-up of pruritus prior to menstruation. This is unrelieved by progesterone or estrogen (Garell, 1964). It is possible that the pruritus experienced may reflect another nonspecific stressful situation rather than a specific endocrine effect.

DIFFERENTIAL DIAGNOSIS

The differential diagnosis of atopic dermatitis includes two classes of diseases (Rostenberg and Solomon, 1968; Solomon and Esterly, 1973): (1) those which are systemic diseases but have an eruption very similar to or indistinguishable from atopic dermatitis, and (2) those cutaneous eruptions which are clearly not atopic dermatitis but bear some resemblance to it. In the first category are phenylketonuria, Aldrich's syndrome, congenital ectodermal dysplasia, ataxia telangiectasia, sex-linked agammaglobulinemia, ahistidenemia, the long arm 18 deletion syndrome, and gluten-sensitive enteropathy. In Hartnup's syndrome, histiocytosis X, acrodermatitis enteropathica, and Hurler's syndrome, there may exist an eczematous dermatitis which resembles the infantile phase of atopic dermatitis. It should be noted that most of these entities fall into three major categories: metabolic diseases, immunodeficiency diseases, and ectodermal dysplasias. The diagnosis of an underlying systemic disease depends on the physician's awareness that atopic dermatitis may be part of such a condition. Appropriate laboratory tests will help to discover a chromosomal abnormality, a metabolic abnormality, or an immunologic defect. A cutaneous biopsy may uncover a genodermatosis or infiltrate of abnormal histiocytes.

In the group of diseases which are primarily cutaneous and which may resemble atopic dermatitis, the most prominent are seborrheic dermatitis, lichen simplex chronicus, chronic eczematous allergic contact dermatitis, dermatitis medicamentosa, nummular dermatitis, and chronic exfoliative dermatitis. The situation may be quite complex, since seborrhea, lichenification, nummular lesions, exfoliation, and localized patches of lichenification are often present in atopic dermatitis. Frequently, the situation cannot be resolved immediately but must await an evolutionary process which would allow one disease or another to declare itself. Some helpful points are as follows: seborrheic dermatitis has no lichenification and demonstrates a distribution somewhat different from that of atopic dermatitis. Lichen simplex chronicus lacks a genetic background, is usually localized to one or two extensor areas, and tends to stay localized. The diagnosis of an eczematous contact dermatitis requires skill in history taking and appropriate patch testing. A drug eruption should improve with abstention from the drug.

When the eruption presents as a chronic, idiopathic, exfoliative dermatitis, it must be differentiated by history, clinical examination, and histopathologic and immunologic studies from other potentially generalized exfoliative dermatitides, such as contact dermatitis, seborrheic dermatitis, drug eruptions (for example, those due to gold compounds, sulfas), psoriasis, pityriasis rubra pilaris, lymphomas, acute lichen planus, ichthyoses (ichthyosis vulgaris dominant, icthyosiform erythroderma), and pemphigus foliaceus.

COMPLICATIONS

Atopic patients are heir to a number of complications which result from the dermatitis or from its underlying cause.

Viral Infections

Certain viruses, notably vaccinia virus (Copeman and Wallace, 1964), herpes simplex virus (Wenner, 1944), and molluscum contagiosum virus (Solomon and Telner, 1966) tend to spread more extensively and may result in a more serious disease in patients with atopic dermatitis as a result of T-cell deficiency. Infection with vaccinia virus (Fig. 5–20) or herpes simplex virus may, in the *presence or absence* (Mailman et al., 1964) of active dermatitis, give rise to a widespread vesiculopustular eruption accompanied by high fever and significant mortality (Copeman and Wallace, 1964). This erup-

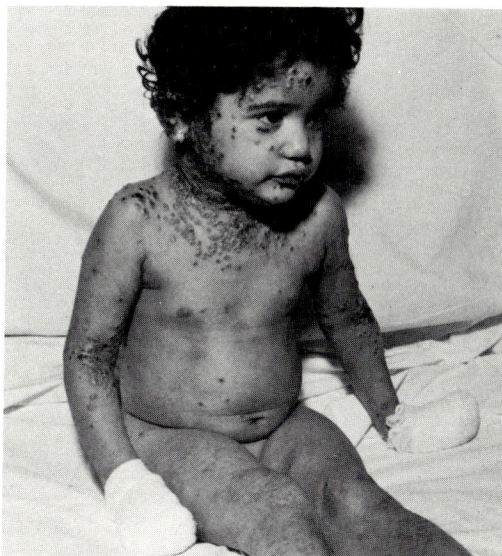

Figure 5–20 Eczema vaccinatum. This complication developed after vaccination in a child with relatively mild atopic dermatitis. The systemic reaction was moderate. Note gauze "boxing gloves" to restrict scratching.

tion, first described by Kaposi (1899), is called Kaposi's varicelliform eruption. For this reason, it is contraindicated, at this time, to vaccinate patients with atopic dermatitis, and it is imperative to segregate these patients from other vaccinated individuals until the contagious phase has passed. In an increasing number of countries with an almost nonexistent incidence of smallpox, routine vaccination is being discontinued, and this complication will undoubtedly be seen with much less frequency.

Bacterial Infections

Patients with atopic dermatitis who chronically excoriate themselves are prone to pyoderma due primarily to *Staphylococcus aureus* and beta-hemolytic streptococci. It is not certain whether these patients suffer from as many infections as would be predicted by the extent and duration of their dermatitis, but they do acquire pyoderma not infrequently (Sedlis and Prose, 1955) and if untreated, the pyoderma may in fact smolder and increase pruritus. It is imperative to culture and to treat cutaneous infections appropriately when they occur.

Fungal Infections

The incidence of chronic dermatophytic infections in atopic subjects was found, by Jones et al. (1973), to be about three times more frequent than in a nonatopic population. Furthermore, half of the chronically infected subjects manifested no evidence of delayed allergy to the infection, although some of them manifested immediate hypersensitivity. Jones and his colleagues suggested that there may be a relationship between atopy, chronic tinea infection, decreased cell-mediated immunity, and IgE.

Most recently, Luckasen and his co-workers (1974) have demonstrated a decrease in the T-cell population of patients with atopic dermatitis, confirming a defect in cell-mediated immunity in these patients and perhaps explaining their difficulty in handling and eliminating viral and fungal infections.

Ocular Complications

The eyelids are a frequent area of intense pruritus which leads to scratching, eczematization, swelling, and hyperpigmentary changes (Karel et al., 1965). The lower lid often shows a double fold near the medial epicanthus (Morgan's fold, Dennie's fold, or Mongolian fold; Fig. 5–21) which, together with the often pallid facies, gives a characteristic facial appearance. The eyes themselves may develop complications, the most common of which

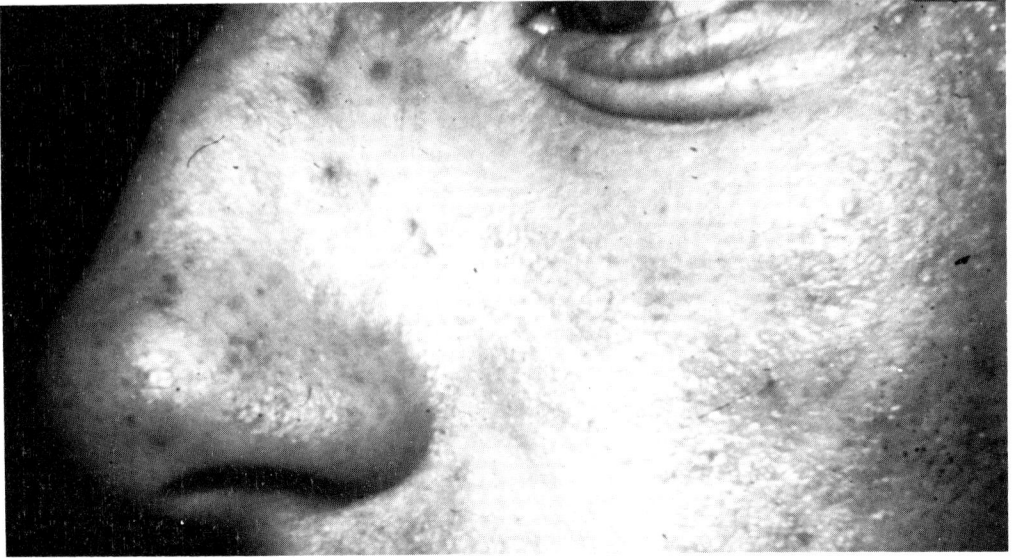

Figure 5-21   There is a double fold under the eye, illustrating Morgan's fold, Dennie's fold, or Mongolian fold, in a patient with atopic dermatitis.

is atopic cataract (Fig. 5–22). First described in 1914 by Andogsky, the incidence of atopic cataracts was found by Brunsting et al. (1955) to be about 8.5 per cent in a large series of cases. The cataracts may be minimal to totally occlusive, and occur most frequently in the second to third decade. Patients who have atopic dermatitis of such a degree that it requires continuous dermatologic care may develop cataracts which limit vision significantly, but the incidence of cataracts in all patients with atopic dermatitis is probably less than the reported incidence of 5 to 10 per cent. When cataracts develop they are usually bilateral, shield-shaped, anterior, subcapsular, and preceded by small opacities (Rosen, 1959). Other rare reported ocular complications include keratoconus, uveitis, retinal detachment, iris pathology, glaucoma, and phthisis bulbi (Rosen, 1959). Patients with longstanding severe atopic dermatitis should have an ophthalmologic examination periodically starting at about age 16 years.

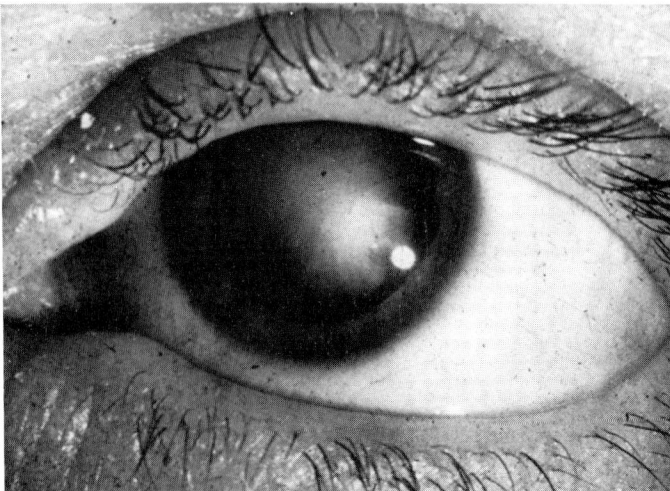

Figure 5-22   The atopic cataract.

Allergic Contact Dermatitis

Patients who have atopic dermatitis where scratching is frequent are exposed to many topical agents, some of which may cause allergic contact dermatitis. It should be noted, however, that these patients are no more prone to the development of allergic contact dermatitis than anyone else (Cronin et al., 1970) and, in fact, develop cutaneous allergic contact reactions much less frequently than those with stasis dermatitis of the legs (Wereide, 1970).

In studying rhus dermatitis, Jones, Lewis, and McMarlin (1973) found that 3 per cent of patients with atopic dermatitis gave a clinical history of sensitivity to poison ivy, whereas 35 per cent of nonatopic healthy individuals did so. Similarly, only 6 per cent of previously nonsensitive atopics could be sensitized to rhus oleoresin, whereas 31 per cent of a nonsensitive normal control group was sensitized by the first patch test.

Urticaria

Patients with asthma, hay fever, or atopic dermatitis may occasionally have urticaria. The relationship of urticaria to atopic dermatitis is not clear (Sulzberger, 1955), neither as to its incidence nor its significance. An urticarial eruption in these patients should be managed as urticaria in any other subject, and a search for a responsible antigenic stimulus should be made.

Adenopathy

Patients with longstanding eczematous changes in the skin often develop enlargement of the lymph nodes which drain the affected sites. The resultant pathologic change in the nodes is due to lymphoid hyperplasia and a deposit of melanin in the macrophages within the nodes. The importance of this occurrence lies in recognizing the benign and often static nature of these nodal enlargements (also called dermatopathic lymphadenitis).

Pigmentary Changes

Chronically affected areas may show hyperpigmentation and ultimately permanent depigmentation in an area of constant rubbing and inflammation. Areas of mild subacute eczematous change on the face in the Negro may appear as somewhat scaly hypopigmented areas. This has been called pityriasis alba, but it is probably nothing more than a mild chronic dermatitis. Patients with atopic dermatitis have a higher incidence of vitiligo (Muller and Winkelmann, 1963) than the general population. The reason for this is as obscure as the etiology of vitiligo.

Hair Changes

These are of three types: (1) areas of chronic dermatitis in the scalp may give rise to sparse, lusterless hair which is broken by rubbing and scratching; (2) alopecia areata (Penders, 1968), which occurs more frequently in atopic subjects; and (3) trichorrhexis invaginata, a structural hair defect in Netherton's disease, of which the atopic diathesis is part.

Socioeconomic Complications

The patient's disease may lead to stressful overprotection alternating with resentment by the parents in early childhood. The frequent relapses, added to the parents' attitude, cause a certain amount of hostility in the patient. In addition, the cosmetic changes which may occur at a most sensitive time in life, together with loss of time from school and later from work, may lead to anxiety and depression. The high cost of the necessary topical medications, the need for an environment controlled for temperature and humidity, and the inability to engage in strenuous physical activity (atopic dermatitis is a reason for exclusion from active military service) make this disease a personal and national financial burden of great significance.

HISTOLOGIC FEATURES

The histologic features of atopic dermatitis are those common to all the eczemas. Nothing distinguishes it from seborrheic dermatitis, contact dermatitis, or chronic allergic eczematous drug eruption (Lever, 1967). Nor, unfortunately, are there any histologic characteristics which can help to distinguish the infantile form of weeping atopic dermatitis from the acute phase of the adult version. The acute stage may show certain histologic changes which differentiate it from the chronic lichenified stage, but these differences can readily be seen with the naked eye.

The section subjected to microscopic study usually shows regular acanthosis and spongiosis, but few intra-epidermal vesicles. The parakeratotic stratum corneum has an adjacent keratohyalin layer. The epidermis shows a varying amount of glycogen deposit in the affected areas (Sedlis and Prose, 1959) which may represent an epidermal response to injury (Miura and Lobitz, 1964). The dermis has a perivascular infiltrate, which is denser in the subpapillary layer, consisting mainly of lymphocytes but also containing some eosinophils and mast cells. There may be a decrease in active sebaceous glands in involved areas. The sweat glands, reported as plugged by some (Sulzberger and Herrmann, 1954) were found to be essentially normal by others (Prose, 1965). The more acute the lesion, the greater the intradermal edema, the greater the epidermal hyperplasia and parakeratosis, and the less prominent is the granular layer (Prose, 1965).

The electron microscope can differentiate more clearly between the acute and chronic eczematous process. Prose (1965) found that the corium in the acute phase had much edema, young collagen, and dilated capillaries with marked pinocytotic infoldings of their endothelium. The epidermis showed a thinned basement membrane, large basal cells with irregular nuclei, and disturbed tonofibril architecture. There was dispolarity of the cells in the prickle layer. Fluid appeared in the granular layer, with polymorphism of the keratohyaline granules becoming marked. The stratum corneum showed changes consistent with imperfect keratin formation and parakeratosis. The changes found in the lichenified areas were less conspicuous, but desmosomal attachments were more prominent in the epidermal layers. Lysosomal bodies may be seen in the upper layers of the epidermis in atopic dermatitis but these are not found consistently (Prose et al., 1965).

PATHOGENESIS

There have been three major theories about the cause of atopic dermatitis and, although the issue is still unsettled, there has accumulated a body of experimental evidence to which one may turn for guidance. These three theories, the inborn-error-of-metabolism (diathetic, constitutional) theory, the allergic (immunologic, atopic) theory, and the psychiatric theory, are examined on the following pages in the light of the available evidence.

INBORN-ERROR-OF-METABOLISM THEORY

When Besnier first recognized atopic eczema as an entity distinct from the other eczemas, he thought it to be due to some inborn constitutional peculiarity of the patient and, therefore, called it "prurigo diathèsique" (itching due to a constitutional defect). This belief was also accepted by Brocq, Ingram, and others who viewed the skin of these patients as having an innate abnormality which results in excessive itching. In recent years, the center of interest has been focused more specifically on the sympathetic portion of the autonomic nervous system and its organ receptors as possible loci for the abnormality. The reasons for considering the sympathetic nervous system are based on two sets of observations, one dealing with the cutaneous and systemic reactions to environmental stress and trauma, and the second dealing with a multitude of unusual reactions to pharmacologic agents which the skin of these patients displays.

The systemic abnormalities have already been enumerated earlier in this chapter.

The cutaneous abnormal reactions were recently reviewed by Sly and Heimlich (1967) and are as follows: (a) the peripheral cutaneous small blood vessels appear to be in a semipermanent hypertonic constricted state (Bystryn and Hyman, 1969), so that the patients appear pale; (b) the vessels respond poorly to small changes in environmental temperature (Abrams and Farber, 1963), dilating slowly in a warm atmosphere and constricting rapidly in a cold one; (c) the basal digital skin temperature is persistently lower in these patients (Johnson and Winkelmann, 1965); (d) on stroking the affected skin firmly with a blunted point, there appears an immediate linear pallor followed (inconstantly) in about five seconds by the usual red line which, in the next 10 seconds or so, is followed by a white line wider than the area of stroking (Whitfield, 1938; Fig. 5–23). This white reaction (white dermographism, the white line response) lasts about five minutes. There is no wheal. This reaction should be contrasted to the normal histamine-mediated triple response of Lewis (red line, flare, wheal). The blanching has been thought by most investigators to indicate vasoconstriction, but some (Davis and Lawler, 1958) believe it may be due to the effect of increased intradermal pressure due to edema. Whatever its cause, the white streak which results from scratching an area of dermatitis gives a striking picture. Though not found exclusively in atopic dermatitis, it is very characteristic of that disease.

Abnormal Pharmacologic Responses

Acetylcholine

When injected intradermally, acetylcholine (or its analogue, methacholine) normally produces a vasodilatory flare, seen as an area of erythema, as well as sweating and pilomotion. This normal response to acetylcholine can be blocked by local anesthetics but not by atropine and is therefore attributed to an axon reflex. When introduced into the skin of a patient with atopic dermatitis, acetylcholine or methacholine produces a paradoxical vascular response of blanching (the delayed blanch) which may last up to 60 minutes (Fig. 5–24). It may be preceded by a short-lived flare (Lobitz and Campbell, 1953). The delayed blanch is blocked by atropine and iontophoretically introduced guanethidine but not by procaine (Lobitz et al., 1957). This abnormal reaction occurs in affected skin but may also be found in 48 per cent of unaffected relatives of patients with atopic dermatitis (West et al., 1962). Here again the cause of the blanching has been thought by many to be due to vasoconstriction, but some authors believe it may be due to edema (Ramsay, 1969). The water content of acetylcholine-treated skin remains unchanged or decreases as compared to untreated skin (Lobitz, 1958). If a dye is introduced into the skin together with acetylcholine, no spreading of the dye takes place (Kalz and Fekete, 1960). At present, the body of evidence seems to favor the theory that the delayed blanch phenomenon is due to vasoconstriction (Champion, 1963), but the issue has not been settled in a convincing manner.

Not only does the skin in atopic dermatitis react abnormally to exogenously administered acetylcholine but it may also

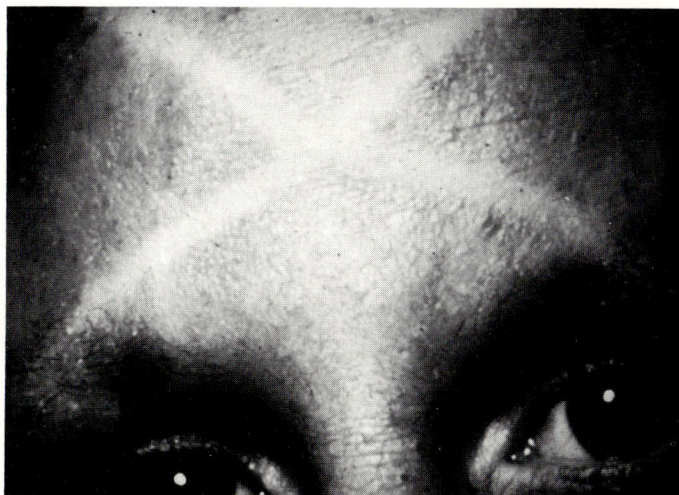

Figure 5–23 The white line response.

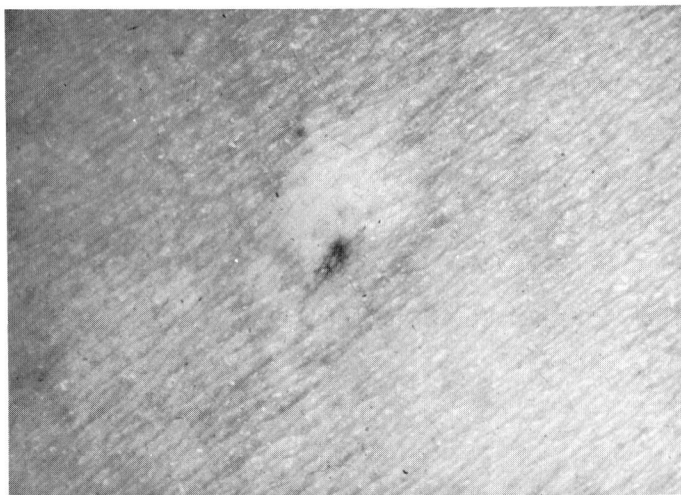

Figure 5–24   The delayed blanch phenomenon.

contain up to 60 times as much acetylcholine as skin from non-atopic dermatoses (Scott, 1962), as well as an excess of acetylcholinesterase (Scheidegger, 1966). The sweat glands of patients with atopic dermatitis show an increased sensitivity to acetylcholine (Warndorff, 1970), not unlike that produced by partial beta receptor blockade (Hemels, 1970).

Nicotinic Acid Esters

The topical application of nicotinic acid esters to the skin of patients with atopic dermatitis does not produce, in a high percentage of cases, the expected erythema and, instead, may result in blanching (Illig, 1952). The relationship of this phenomenon to atopic dermatitis is not clear, since the same abnormal response is found in a wide variety of other disease processes.

Histamine, Serotonin, Bradykinin

These three endogenous vasodilators, on introduction into the affected skin, do not cause the expected vasodilation (Clendenning et al., 1959; Eyster et al., 1952; Michaelsson, 1970) but, instead, may result in a reduced erythema reaction, in no change at all, or in blanching. The histamine content of affected skin is increased (Johnson et al., 1960), and the serum of atopic patients has been reported

as containing a globulin capable of binding and inactivating histamine.

Prostaglandin E₁

This vasodilator distinguishes itself by the normalcy with which atopic skin reacts to it. The expected intense, long-lasting vasodilation is found in atopic dermatitis as well as in normal skin and a few other dermatoses tested (Solomon et al., 1968).

Catecholamines

The catecholamines are a group of naturally occurring vasoactive substances the most important of which are norepinephrine, epinephrine, and dopamine. Patients with atopic dermatitis show a series of abnormalities of norepinephrine and epinephrine disposition which may be summarized as follows: (a) the cutaneous vasculature is excessively sensitive to norepinephrine and epinephrine when introduced iontophoretically into the skin; these substances cause blanching with doses lower than those required in other dermatoses (Juhlin, 1961); (b) injected intravenously, a lesser amount of isotopically labeled norepinephrine is excreted in the urine in 24 hours than in control dermatoses (Solomon et al., 1964); (c) the skin has an affinity for norepinephrine and stores intravenously or intracutaneously administered norepinephrine for a prolonged period (Solomon et al., 1964); (d) more norepinephrine is produced by inflamed skin (Moller, 1964) than normal skin, as is catechol-o-methyl transferase, one of the enzymes responsible for norepinephrine degradation (Bamshad, 1969); (e) isotopically labeled norepinephrine injected intracutaneously is found, 24 hours later, to accumulate in the arrector pili muscle, in the epidermis and, less markedly, around blood vessels (Solomon and Nadler, 1967); (f) endogenously produced norepinephrine and its metabolites are excreted in the urine of patients with atopic dermatitis in amounts equal to control subjects; (g) the "grainy" skin of patients with atopic dermatitis probably represents a state of permanent piloerection (the arrector pili muscle is an organ mediated only by norepinephrine).

The consolidation of these and other findings into a comprehensive hypothesis subject to experimental verification would explain the causative genetic defect and could lead to specific therapy for the disease, but this has not yet been achieved. However, it is very tempting to think of atopic dermatitis as a disease in which there is an inherited defect in the production, storage, or degradation of norepinephrine, in the ability of norepinephrine to act at the receptor level, or a defect in the receptor system itself. Since it has been shown that there is no abnormality in the production of catecholamines in atopic dermatitis (Hingerty and Meehan, 1964), a defect in the storage and turnover time of norepinephrine must come under serious consideration. The primary defect may be in the disposition of norepinephrine or may reflect a receptor organ deficit. Catecholamine receptor sites have been called Alpha and Beta. One of these, the Beta receptor, may be adenyl cyclase. In this regard, Szentivanyi (1968) has suggested that the primary defect in atopic asthma may be a "partial beta blockade" or deficiency in adenyl cyclase:

The theory postulates that the atopic abnormality in asthma lies in the reduced functioning of the beta adrenergic system, irrespective of what the triggering event may be in a particular case (immunological, infectious, psychic, etc.). In this situation, the adrenergic neurotransmitters are released in the face of a relatively unavailable beta effector system, and the resultant imbalance deprives the bronchial tissue from its normal counter-regulatory adjustment.

The most critical component of this malfunctioning effector system, the beta adrenergic receptor, is currently being identified with an enzyme, adenyl cyclase. It follows, therefore, that the fundamental abnormality common to all asthmatic persons may be an inherited or acquired enzyme deficiency, that is, a relative unavailability of the enzyme because of its reduced synthesis, partial blockade, or production of defective enzyme molecules incapable of binding the adrenergic neurotransmitter.

Adenyl cyclase combines with magnesium—magnesium has variously been reported as elevated (MacCardle et al., 1941) and decreased (Lipkin et al., 1964) in atopic dermatitis—and adenosine triphosphate to form cyclic 3'5' adenosine monophosphate (cyclic AMP). This has been called part of a "second messenger" (Robison et al., 1968) system necessary for the maintenance of a proper balance between alpha and beta adrenergic function. Recent studies (Mier and Urselmann, 1970) have not shown any decrease in adenyl cyclase activity in the skin of patients with atopic dermatitis but there are other substances which follow in the cascade of events leading to the ultimate effect of catecholamine-induced cyclic AMP stimulation. Among these are activation of a number of phosphorylating enzymes, the protein kinases. These protein kinases appear to be tissue-specific (Rajkumar et al., 1972). Mier et al. (1972) have studied their content in atopic dermatitis. Although these authors found no quantitative differences in the cutaneous content of these enzymes, the entire story leaves much to be explained (Carr, 1973).

The relationship of the metabolic peculiarities found in these patients to their demonstrated T-cell abnormality may contain the long-sought elusive key to understanding the nature of this disease. The studies of Bourne et al. (1974) have suggested that a metabolic chain of events, perhaps generated by a particular cell, may regulate the relationships between T- and B-cell functions.

ALLERGIC THEORY

The theory that atopic dermatitis is allergic in origin rests on some or all of the following observations. Atopic dermatitis is one of the conditions commonly found in association with hay fever and bronchial asthma. These patients frequently give immediate urticarial reactions to skin tests with common antigens (foods and pollens) and demonstrate the ability to transfer passively this cutaneous urticarial reaction to another subject by the serum (the Prausnitz-Kustner test.) This test is positive in almost all cases of hay-fever, most cases of non-seasonal allergic rhinitis, and about two-thirds of patients with bronchial asthma (Sherman, 1965). The serum substance responsible for the Prausnitz-Kustner reaction has been called reagin or skin sensitizing antibody and has recently been identified as a distinct immunoglobulin and designated IgE (Ishizaka et al., 1967). It was postulated around 1930 that reagin fixed to cutaneous tissues resulted in the cutaneous analogue of hay fever and asthma. Feinberg, et al. (1960) felt that in an individual with a particular constitutional background, following exposure to a specific antigen such as food, the specific reagin developed and attached itself to the tissue. On re-introduction of the antigen, this caused an antigen-antibody reaction with subsequent development of inflammation of the skin. In vitro studies with lymphocyte transformations (Girard et al., 1967) tend to confirm this view.

This seemed a reasonable hypothesis, but several troublesome inescapable facts intervened: (a) not all patients with atopic dermatitis have atopy (between 20 and 30 per cent do not); (b) patients with agammaglobulinemia with presumably little or no IgE may have atopic dermatitis (Peterson, 1965); (c) patients without the ability to form delayed allergic reaction (that is, those with ataxia-telangiectasia) have an incidence of atopic dermatitis at least equal to that of the general population (Reed et al., 1966); (d) Lobitz et al. (1972) described two patients with life-long atopic dermatitis and depressed cell-mediated immunity; (e) Jones and colleagues (1973) found that patients with atopic dermatitis are much less capable of developing poison ivy dermatitis than normal individuals; (f) immunoglobulin deficiencies (particularly IgA) were found in 79 per cent of patients with atopy (an incidence 35 times that found in a normal control group; Kaufman, 1970) (g) the highest incidence of atopic dermatitis is found in two hereditary diseases, phenylketonuria (Jervis, 1937) and anhidrotic ectodermal dysplasia (Reed et al., 1970), underscoring its hereditary nature; (h) the injection of an antigen into the skin of a patient who is sensitive by the criterion of a wheal reaction does not induce dermatitis at the site, in marked contrast to the tests for epidermal sensitization with which, in many instances, a localized dermatitis may be induced which is similar in every respect to the dermatitis which the patient has; (i) exposure of the patient with atopic dermatitis to materials to which he is demonstrably sensitive on scratch testing will rarely precipitate flare-ups of the dermatitis. The instances of occurrence of such precipitation are so uncommon as to make it appear that they are coincidental. The rare exception to this rule is contact with pollens; (j) in patients with atopic dermatitis in whom the eruption is assumed to be due to inescapable contactants and inhalants, the dermatitis may clear entirely following a change in climatic environment, even though the contact with the supposedly responsible contactants and inhalants may be the same or even increased; (k) the treatment of atopic dermatitis with attempts at hyposensitization or diet control ends so frequently in failure as to make it appear that the occasional seemingly good results are due to chance; (l) the atopic dermatitis will subside in an area of anesthesia caused by paraplegia.

What then remains of the allergic theory which bears further examination? It is undoubtedly true that many patients with atopic dermatitis have hay fever and/or asthma. Also, some patients with atopic dermatitis may have excessive serum levels of IgE. IgE is a thermo- and cryo-labile protein with a weight intermediate between 7S and 11S. It may be found in tears, nasal secretions, and saliva of atopic individuals but cannot cross the placental membrane. The normal serum level of IgE is usually under 200 mg. per ml. in the non-atopic individual. Juhlin and colleagues (1969) found serum IgE levels to be significantly greater than normal in 23 of 28 patients with atopic dermatitis. But there is little correlation between the serum levels and the severity of the dermatitis (Clendenning et al., 1973). Ogawa et al. (1971) did find a positive correlation between the serum level of IgE and the severity of the dermatitis. But, extremely high serum IgE levels have also been found in a variety of non-atopic conditions (Spitz et al., 1972; Winkelmann and Gleich, 1973).

The injection of rabbit or guinea pig anti-IgE serum into human skin containing IgE produces a wheal and flare reaction in 15 minutes (reversed passive cutaneous anaphylaxis or reversed P-K reaction). The amount of anti-IgE required to elicit a standard wheal and flare reaction did not differ in the atopic dermatitis and non-atopic groups (Newcomb and Ishizaka, 1969; Ogawa et al., 1971).

IgE appears to be neither necessary for the presence of the disease nor sufficient to cause it. Yet, there seems little doubt that elevated IgE seems to occur with increased frequency in these patients. Some authors (Jones et al., 1973) have suggested that IgE elevation depresses T-cell function. It is equally plausible that as T cells are depressed and when B cells are capable of reacting, the elevation of IgE may represent an attempt by the organism to compensate for the deficiency in cell-mediated immunity by overactivity of the B-cell (humoral) system.

Other findings which may relate to the allergic theory include the discovery of a significantly higher serum complement (beta 1C) level in infants with atopic dermatitis than in normal infants (Kaufman et al., 1968). Other authors (Fontana et al., 1962) found normal serum complement titers in atopic dermatitis. There has also been some evidence to support the concept that atopic dermatitis has some qualities of an autosensitization phenomenon (Hashem, 1965), but this last hypothesis, as well as an autoimmune hypothesis (Lorincz, 1965), needs further investigation.

PSYCHOSOMATIC THEORY

The psychiatric theory holds that atopic dermatitis is *caused* by an unresolved neurosis which results in chronic abnormal vegetative responses, such as itching.

The unresolved neuroses may be due to the influences of anxiety, hostility, frustration, guilt feelings, and so forth. These emotions, according to one theory, cause a regression to infantile (lower order) autonomic function and a preponderant activity of the parasympathetic nervous system (Szasz, 1951). Another theory specifically names rejection of the infant by its mother (Rosenthal, 1952) as the causal factor in atopic dermatitis. Unfortunately, there is no precision in these theories. Patients with the same conflicts have different diseases, or no disease at all. Patients with no apparent psychological conflicts or with a loving mother-child relationship do have the disease (Kuypers, 1968). Patients with marked mental retardation and little intellectual perception have the disease; identical twins raised under quite different emotional environments have the disease. It seems evident that the psychosomatic (or emotional-cause) theory is unacceptable (Rostenberg, 1959). What is undoubtedly true is that, in individuals born with the defect in the skin, emotions may precipitate itching, aggravate the dermatitis, and lead to feelings of anxiety, frustration, and inferiority. Until further evidence is brought forth, these feelings must be considered a complication rather than the cause of atopic dermatitis.

TREATMENT

From the foregoing discussion it is quite apparent that the management of certain individuals with atopic dermatitis may offer considerable difficulty. The majority of patients, however, may be treated effectively in a palliative sense by carefully controlling or reducing exacerbating influences and by reducing inflammation and pruritus so that the dermatitis becomes a bearable one, permitting the patient to maintain a normal living pattern. Because the underlying defect is not known, all therapy must be preventive or symptomatic.

The main symptom is itching and all efforts must be directed toward relieving it. If the physician does not think of atopic dermatitis as a disease which flares under a variety of exacerbating causes, he will fail the patient. For the purpose of clarity, therapy will be discussed under a variety of headings, but an integrated approach is advised. It is also important when seeing a patient for the first time to obtain a careful review of previous medication and to avoid those drugs which the patient has found irritating or which the patient dislikes.

Topical Therapy

The application of cool compresses (the so-called active ingredients, such as aluminum acetate and potassium permanganate, do little to add to the effectiveness of water alone) is sometimes indicated while weeping exists. Most of the time, even for a mildly weeping acute dermatitis and for the subacute and lichenified lesions, the mainstay of therapy is a corticosteroid in a cream or ointment base. In the adult with localized lesions, the fluorinated corticosteroids provide greater activity, but there is little to choose among the various commercial products available. For children or in widespread dermatoses, 0.5 to 1 per cent hydrocortisone in hydrophilic ointment may be adequate. In adults with extremely lichenified localized areas, polyethylene wrap occluding the steroid ointment may increase the penetrative effectiveness of the steroid. The complications of such prolonged local steroid therapy are folliculitis from bacterial and candidal infections, atrophy and striae, Trichophyton infections of the skin, and miliaria.

The type of vehicle is often indicated by the patient's wishes. Some patients prefer greasy bases, some cream bases, and a few prefer propylene glycol. Ointment is best applied after a bath. Another useful topical agent is tar, in the form of 2.5 per cent crude coal tar or 1 to 5 per cent ichthammol ointment in hydrophilic petrolatum. Topical antibiotics are rarely necessary, but a widely excoriated dermatitis in an adult may benefit from a hexachlorophene wash (where this is tolerated) every 24 hours. Hexachlorophene should not be used on widespread dermatoses in infants because it may be absorbed and cause central nervous system excitation. Shake lotions, powders, topical antihistaminics, and topical anesthetics should not be used

because they are poorly tolerated, potentially sensitizing, or not effective. A water-dispersible oil added to the bath water is often soothing.

Systemic Therapy

Systemic therapy should be reserved for patients who are not pregnant. There are no agents which are specifically antipruritic, but there are a variety of substances acting on the central nervous system, and perhaps peripherally as well, which may help some patients better tolerate the acute episodes of intense pruritus. Antihistamines, for the most part, are mildly sedative. The drowsiness they cause may be undesirable in working people, or those who must drive. Occasionally, they may paradoxically cause excitation in the very young and old. In general, antihistamines are limited in their usefulness for the treatment of atopic dermatitis. Of the antihistaminic substances available, probably the most effective are the phenothiazines, particularly chlorpromazine. Chlorpromazine has, unfortunately, numerous side effects, including cholestatic jaundice, which limit its usefulness. In the face of intractable pruritus, 25 to 50 mg. of chlorpromazine three times a day for one week may give some relief. Patients with chronic skin disease may have associated anxiety and depression which aggravate the cutaneous problem. Nortriptyline or amytriptyline in combination with perphenazine given in appropriate doses may help the associated psychiatric condition and the skin.

Certain patients present primarily a picture of extreme agitation and hostility. These patients may best respond to a norepinephrine-depleting agent, such as reserpine or guanethidine, but the side effects from the doses necessary to achieve a therapeutic response limit its usefulness. Care should be taken not to prescribe some of these drugs simultaneously, since they may be mutually antagonistic.

A relatively safe sedative useful in many patients is chloral hydrate. Antibiotics are indicated when a specific bacterial agent has been cultured and identified, and sensitivity studies done. Infection is relatively common and antibiotics may be required several times a year.

Penicillin and erythromycin stearate or ethyl succinate may be used for beta-hemolytic streptococci and *Staphylococcus aureus.*

Corticosteroids

The corticosteroid tablet is the Lorelei of therapy for atopic dermatitis. It is tempting to the physician and often not understood by the patient. Atopic dermatitis is a chronic disease with exacerbations and it would seem reasonable to use systemic steroid to see the patient through a crisis. But once systemic corticosteroid therapy is started it is extremely difficult to stop, and its side effects are such that their use must be deprecated. A detailed account of the dangers inherent in such treatment should be made to the patient (Siegel, 1965) so that the caution for which his comfort is being sacrificed will be understood. Occasionally, one finds a patient whose disease is of such severity that nothing but corticosteroids will suffice.

Psychotherapy

Formal psychotherapy is rarely required in patients with atopic dermatitis. It is wise to refer those patients who ask for psychiatric help. Almost all patients (those who are old enough to understand) will require considerable attention from their physician, and supportive psychiatric help should be a routine part of the patient's management.

Preventive Care

These patients tolerate poorly changes in environmental temperature and humidity; therefore, room temperatures and humidity should be kept fairly constant. Bedroom air conditioners in the summer and vaporizers in the winter are helpful. Bath water should be at skin temperature. When coming out of their baths or taking their clothes off, patients will experience pruritus, but, if they understand this, many choose to tolerate it than to be prohibited from bathing. Baths are preferable to showers, and the patient should hydrate the skin by remaining in the water for 20 to 30 minutes. Detergents and excessive use of soap are to be avoided. Nonperfumed, water-dispersible oil may be added to the bath water. Frequent shampooing is de-

sirable, and after bath or shampoo a steroid cream or ointment may be applied. Wool, nylon, and scratchy textured clothes should be avoided. The patients and their families should be counseled concerning the prognosis. Patients should avoid occupations which require strenuous outdoor physical activity or exposure to harsh chemicals. Those individuals whose occupational activity inhibits their improvement or whose dermatitis makes work unbearable should be rehabilitated. A change in climate during the height of winter's cold or summer's heat is advisable, if possible. A stay at the seashore during the summer often has markedly beneficial effects, as does residence in a nonhumid, warm environment.

Other Forms of Management

Several forms of treatment used in former days but for which there is little justification today must be mentioned in order to be condemned.

X-ray therapy, deep or superficial, has no place in the treatment of atopic dermatitis because of the patient's age (often in the reproductive years), the cumulative noxious effects of radiation, as well as its inconstant and short-lived benefits.

Atopic patients show positive intradermal reactions to many substances. There is no evidence that desensitization to any of them has been beneficial. In fact, there is no reason to do intradermal testing in these patients.

Similarly, there is no evidence that patients treated by some form of diet control have had any advantage over those in whom diet has been ignored. Food allergy probably plays an insignificant role in atopic dermatitis. Carried to excess, malnutrition may result from overzealous parents wishing to avoid presumed dietary allergens.

PROGNOSIS

The prognosis of atopic dermatitis may be considered from several points of view: How long will the dermatitis last? What are the chances for developing hay fever and asthma? What are the chances for other complications?

The studies which have attempted to answer these questions are few in number, differing in approach and giving a fairly wide range of answers. In general, patients with atopic dermatitis tend to have the disease a long time (approximately 30 years for about 50 per cent of the patients (Roth and Kierland, 1964). The exacerbations become less frequent after adolescence in most patients and tend to localize on the extremities. The chronicity of the disease does not appear to be related to its severity (Brereton et al., 1959). Asthma occurs in approximately 50 per cent of patients affected by atopic dermatitis (Bono and Levitt, 1964). Other complications depend on the severity of the dermatitis, the presence of asthma, and the type of therapy administered. Atopic patients have a greater frequency of cutaneous and pulmonary infections, associated congenital diseases, and ocular complications, all of which lead to a greater risk from unwanted side effects to medications. Vowles et al. (1955) found that 6 of 84 severely affected atopic children had died of infection in infancy, a figure of slightly higher than the 5 per cent mortality found by Torsney (1966) among 200 severely atopic children. Atopic dermatitis may therefore be a mild recurrent nuisance or a life-threatening affliction.

REFERENCES

Abrams, G., and Farber, E.: Peripheral vascular responses in atopic dermatitis. Arch. Dermatol. 88:554, 1963.

Andogsky, N.: Cataracta dermatogenes: Ein betrag zur aetiologie der linsentrubung. Klin. Monatsbl. Augenheilkd. 52:824, 1914.

Baer, R. L.: In discussion of paper by Eyster, W. H., Jr., Roth, G. M., and Kierland, R. R.: Studies on the peripheral vascular physiology of patients with atopic dermatitis. J. Invest. Dermatol. 18:37, 1952.

Baer, R. L.: Atopic dermatitis. Med. Clin. North Am. 43:765, 1959.

Baer, R. L.: Conference on infantile eczema: history, definitions, concepts. J. Pediatr. 66:153, 1965.

Bamshad, J.: Catechol-o-methyl transferase in skin of patients with atopic dermatitis. J. Invest. Dermatol. 52:100, 1969.

Bono, J., and Levitt, P.: Relationship of infantile atopic dermatitis to asthma and other respiratory allergies. Ann. Allergy 22:72, 1964.

Bourne, H. R., Lichenstein, L. M., Melmon, K. L., et al.: Modulation of inflammation and immunity by cyclic AMP. Science 184:19, 1974.

Brereton, E. M., Carpenter, R. G., Rook, A. J., et al.: The prevalence and prognosis of eczema and asthma in Cambridgeshire School children. The Medical Officer, Dec. 18, 1959, p. 317.

Brunsting, L. A., Reed, W. B., and Baer, R. L.: Occurrence of cataracts and keratoconus with atopic dermatitis. Arch. Dermatol. 72:237, 1955.

Bystryn, J. C., and Hyman, C.: Skin blood flow in atopic dermatitis. J. Invest. Dermatol. 52:189, 1969.

Carr, R. D., Berke, M., and Becker, W. S.: Incidence of atopy in the general population. Arch. Dermatol. 89:27, 1964.

Carr, R. H.: Failure of catecholamines to inhibit epidermal mitosis in vitro. J. Allergy Clin. Immunol. 51:254, 1973.

Champion, R. H.: Abnormal vascular reactions in atopic eczema. Br. J. Dermatol. 75:12, 1963.

Clendenning, W. E., Clack, W. E., Ogawa, M., et al.: Serum IgE studies in atopic dermatitis. J. Invest. Dermatol. 61:233, 1973.

Clendenning, W. E., De Oreo, G. A., and Stoughton, R. B.: Serotonin. Its effect in normal and atopic skin. Arch. Dermatol. 79:503, 1959.

Cooke, R. A., and Vander Veer, A.: Human sensitization. J. Immunol. 1:216, 1916.

Copeman, P. W. M., and Wallace, H. J.: Eczema vaccinatum. Br. Med. J. 2:906, 1964.

Cronin, E., Bandmann, H. J., Calnan, C. D., et al.: Contact dermatitis in the atopic. Acta Derm. Venereol. 50:183, 1970.

Davis, M. J., and Lawler, J. C.: Observations on the delayed blanch phenomenon in atopic subjects. J. Invest. Dermatol. 30:127, 1958.

Eyster, W. H., Jr., Roth, G. M., and Kierland, R. R.: Studies on the peripheral vascular physiology of patients with atopic dermatitis. J. Invest. Dermatol. 18:37, 1952.

Feinberg, S. M., Durham, D. C., and Dragstedt, C. A.: Allergy in Practice. 2nd ed. Chicago, Year Book Medical Publishers, Inc., 1960.

Fiske, C. E., and Obermayer, M. E.: Personality and emotional factors in adult atopic eczema. Arch. Dermatol. 68:506, 1954.

Fontana, V. J., Sedlis, E., Prose, P. H., et al.: Complement titer, C-reactive protein, and electrophoretic serum protein patterns in eczematous children. N. Y. State J. Med. 1:2801, 1962.

Garell, D. C.: Atopic dermatitis in females during adolescence. Am. J. Dis. Child. 107:350, 1964.

Girard, J. P., Rose, N. R., Kunz, M. L., et al.: In vitro lymphocyte transformation in atopic patients induced by antigens. J. Allergy 39:65, 1967.

Hashem, N.: The possible role of autosensitization in eczema, as demonstrated by a new experimental technique. J. Pediatr. 66:248, 1965.

Heiner, D. C., and Rose, B.: Elevated levels of IgE in conditions other than classical atopy. J. Allergy 43:183, 1969.

Hellerstrom, S., and Rajka, G.: Clinical aspects of atopic dermatitis. Acta Derm. Venereol. 47:75, 1967.

Hemels, H. G.: The effect of propranolol on the acetylcholine-induced sweat gland response in atopic and non-atopic subjects. Br. J. Dermatol. 83:312, 1970.

Hingerty, D., and Meehan, F. O. C.: Catecholamine excretion in children with atopic eczema. Ir. J. Med. Sci. 6:71, 1964.

Illig, L.: Derm. Wochenschr. 127:753, 1952, as quoted by Rajka, G. in Acta Derm. Venereol. 40:285, 1960.

Ishizaka, K., Ishizaka, T., and Hornbrook, M. M.: Allergen-binding activity of gamma-E, gamma-G and gamma-A antibodies in serum from atopic patients: In vitro measurement of reaginic antibody. J. Immunol. 98:490, 1967.

Jervis, G. A.: Phenylpyruvic oligophrenia: Introductory study of 50 cases of mental deficiency associated with excretion of phenylpyruvic acid. Arch. Neurol. Psychiat. 38:944, 1937.

Johnson, H. H., Jr., De Oreo, G. A., Lascheid, W. P., et al.: Skin histamine levels in atopic dermatitis. J. Invest. Dermatol. 34:237, 1960.

Johnson, L. A., and Winkelmann, R. K.: Cutaneous vascular reactivity in atopic children. Arch. Dermatol. 92:621, 1965.

Jones, H. E., Lewis, C. W., and McMarlin, S. L.: Allergic contact sensitivity in atopic dermatitis. Arch. Dermatol. 107:217, 1973.

Jones, H. E., Reinhardt, J. H., and Rinaldi, M. G.: A clinical, mycological, and immunological Survey for Dermatophytosis. Arch. Dermatol. 108:61, 1973.

Juhlin, L.: The fate of iontophoretically introduced epinephrine and norepinephrine in patients with atopic dermatitis and normal skin. J. Invest. Dermatol. 37:257, 1961.

Juhlin, L., Johansson, G. O., Bennich, H., et al.: Immunoglobulin E in dermatoses. Arch. Dermatol. 100:12, 1969.

Kalz, F., and Fekete, Z.: Studies on the mechanism of the white response and the delayed blanch phenomenon in atopic subjects by means of coomassie blue. J. Invest. Dermatol. 35:135, 1960.

Kaposi, M.: Pathologie und therapie der Hautkrankheiten. 5th ed. Berlin, Urban und Schwartzenberg, 1899.

Karel, I., Myska, V., and Kvicalova, E.: Ophthalmological changes in atopic dermatitis. Acta Derm. Venereol. 45:381, 1965.

Kaufman, H. S.: Immunoglobulin deficiencies in an atopic population. Lancet 2:1061, 1970.

Kaufman, H. S., Frick, O. L., and Fink, D.: Serum complement (beta 1C) in young children with atopic dermatitis. J. Allergy 42:1, 1968.

Kierland, R. R.: Certain stigmata associated with atopic dermatitis. In Baer, R. L., (ed.): Atopic Dermatitis. Philadelphia, J. B. Lippincott Co., 1955.

Krivit, W., and Good, R. A.: Syndrome of Aldrich. Am. J. Dis. Child. 97:137, 1959.

Kuypers, B. R. M.: Atopic dermatitis: Some observations from a psychological view point. Dermatologica 136:387, 1968.

Lever, W. F.: Histopathology of the Skin. 4th ed. Philadelphia, J. B. Lippincott Co., 1967.

Lipkin, G., March, C., and Gowdey, J.: Magnesium in epidermis, dermis and whole skin of normal and atopic subjects. J. Invest. Dermatol. 42:293, 1964.

Lobitz, W. C., Jr.: In discussion of article by Davis, M. J., and Lawler, J. C.: Observations on the delayed blanch phenomenon in atopic subjects. J. Invest. Dermatol. 30:127, 1958.

Lobitz, W. C., Jr., and Campbell, C. J.: Physiologic studies in atopic dermatitis (disseminated neurodermatitis). I. Arch. Dermatol. 67:575, 1953.

Lobitz, W. C., Jr., Heller, M. L., and Dobson, R. L.: Physiologic studies in atopic dermatitis (disseminated neurodermatitis). II. Arch. Dermatol. 75:228, 1957.

Lobitz, W. C., Jr., Honeyman, J. F., and Winkler, N. W.: Suppressed cell-mediated immunity in two

adults with atopic dermatitis. Br. J. Dermatol. 86:317, 1972.

Lorincz, A. L.: Autoimmune disease—possible mechanisms. J. Pediatr. 66:245, 1965.

Luckasen, J. R., Sabad, A., Goltz, R. W., et al.: T and B lymphocytes in atopic eczema. Arch. Dermatol. 110:375, 1974.

MacCardle, R. C., Engman, M. F., Jr., and Engman, M. F., Sr.: Spectrographic analysis of neurodermatitic lesions. Arch. Dermatol. 44:429, 1941.

Mailman, C. J., Miranda, J. L., and Spock, A.: Recurrent eczema herpeticum. Arch. Dermatol. 89:815, 1964.

Marten, R. H., and Sarkany, I.: Atopic eczema in European and Negro West Indian infants in London. Br. J. Dermatol. 73:410, 1961.

Medical Letter, The: Interactions of Drugs. 12:93, 1970.

Michaelsson, G.: Decreased cutaneous reactions to kallikrein in patients with atopic dermatitis and psoriasis. Acta Derm. Venereol. 50:37, 1970.

Mier, P. D., and Urselmann, E.: The adenyl cyclase of skin. II. Adenyl cyclase levels in atopic dermatitis. Br. J. Dermatol. 83:364, 1970.

Mier, P. D., Van Den Hurk, J., Holla, S. W. J., et al.: Cyclic 3'-5' adenosine monophosphate-dependent protein kinase of skin. II. Levels in atopic dermatitis and psoriasis. Br. J. Dermatol. 87:577, 1972.

Miura, Y., and Lobitz, W. C.: Histochemical studies in atopic dermatitis: Responses following controlled strip injury. J. Invest. Dermatol. 42:115, 1964.

Moller, H.: On catecholamines of the skin. Acta Derm. Venereol [Suppl] 55:7, 1964.

Muller, S. A., and Winkelmann, R. K.: Alopecia areata. Arch. Dermatol. 88:290, 1963.

Newcomb, R. W., and Ishizaka, K.: Skin reactions to anti-gamma-E antibody in atopic, nonatopic and immunologically deficient children and adults. J. Allergy 43:292, 1969.

Ogawa, M., Berger, P. A., McIntyre, O. R., et al.: IgE in atopic dermatitis. Arch. Dermatol. 103:575, 1971.

Orange, R. P., Ishizaka, T., Ishizaka, K., et al.: Pharmacologic inhibition of the release of the chemical mediators elicited by the interaction of IgE antibodies with specific antigen. Clin. Res. 18:534, 1970.

Penders, A. J. M.: Alopecia areata and atopy. Dermatologica 136:395, 1968.

Penrose, L. S.: Genetic background of common diseases. Acta Genet. 4:257, 1953.

Peterson, R. D. A.: Immunologic responses in infantile eczema. J. Pediatr. 66:224, 1965.

Prose, P. H.: Pathologic changes in eczema. J. Pediatr. 66:178, 1965.

Prose, P. H., Sedlis, E., and Bigelow, M.: The demonstration of lysosomes in the diseased skin of infants with infantile eczema. J. Invest. Dermatol. 45:448, 1965.

Raffle, E. J., and Hall, R.: Atopic eczema and thyroid autoimmunity. Lancet 1:981, 1967.

Rajka, G.: Prurigo Besnier (atopic dermatitis) with special reference to the role of allergic factors. Acta Derm. Venereol. 40:258, 1960.

Rajka, G.: Itch duration in the uninvolved skin of atopic dermatitis (Prurigo Besnier). Acta Derm. Venereol. 48:320, 1968.

Rajkumar, T., Tao, M., and Solomon, L. M.: Adenosine 3'-5' cyclic monophosphate stimulated protein from human skin. II. Isolation and properties of multiple forms. J. Invest. Dermatol. 59:196, 1972.

Ramsay, C.: Vascular changes accompanying white dermographism and delayed blanch in atopic dermatitis. Br. J. Dermatol. 81:37, 1969.

Reed, W. B., Epstein, W. L., Boder, E., et al.: Cutaneous manifestations of ataxia-telangiectasia. J.A.M.A. 195:746, 1966.

Reed, W. B., Lopez, D. A., and Landing, B.: Clinical spectrum of anhidrotic ectodermal dysplasia. Arch. Dermatol. 102:134, 1970.

Robison, G. A., Butcher, R. W., and Sutherland, E. W.: Cyclic AMP. Annu. Rev. Biochem. 37:149, 1968.

Rosen, E.: Atopic Cataract. 1st ed. Springfield, Charles C Thomas, 1959.

Rosenthal, M. J.: Psychosomatic study of infantile eczema. I. Mother-child relationship. Pediatrics 10:581, 1952.

Rostenberg, A., Jr.: Psychosomatic concepts in atopic dermatitis — a critique. Arch. Dermatol. 79:692, 1959.

Rostenberg, A., Jr., and Solomon, L. M.: Infantile eczema and systemic disease. Arch. Dermatol. 98:41, 1968.

Roth, H. L., and Kierland, R. R.: The natural history of atopic dermatitis. Arch. Dermatol. 89:209, 1964.

Rovensky, J., and Saxl, O.: Differences in the dynamics of sweat secretion in atopic children. J. Invest. Dermatol. 43:171, 1964.

Russell, B., and Last, S. L.: Besnier's Prurigo: Observations on abnormal cutaneous and central nervous reactions. Br. J. Dermatol. 67:65, 1955.

Scheidegger, J. P.: Acetylcholinesterasegehalt normaler und neurodermatischer haut. Arch. Klin. Exp. Dermatol. 226:265, 1966.

Scott, A.: Acetylcholine in normal and diseased skin. Br. J. Dermatol. 74:317, 1962.

Sedlis, E., and Prose, P.: Infantile eczema with special reference to the pathologic lesion. Pediatrics 23:802, 1959.

Settipane, G. A., Connell, J. T., and Sherman, W. B.: Reagin in tears. J. Allergy 36:92, 1965.

Shelley, W. B., and Arthur, R.: The neurohistology and neurophysiology of the itch sensation in man. Arch. Dermatol. 76:206, 1957.

Sherman, W. B.: Atopic hypersensitivity. Med. Clin. North Am. 4:1607, 1965.

Siegel, S. C.: ACTH and the corticosteroids in the management of allergic disorders in children. J. Pediatr. 66:927, 1965.

Sly, R. M., and Heimlich, E. M.: Physiologic abnormalities in the atopic state: A review. Ann. Allergy 25:192, 1967.

Smith, D. W.: Recognizable Patterns of Human Malformation. Philadelphia, W. B. Saunders Co., 1970.

Snyderman, S. E., Boyer, A., Roctman, E., et al.: The histidine requirement of the infant. Pediatrics 31:786, 1963.

Solomon, L. M., and Beerman, H.: Atopic dermatitis. Am. J. Med. Sci. 252:478, 1966.

Solomon, L. M., and Esterly, N. B.: Neonatal Dermatology. Philadelphia, W. B. Saunders Co., 1973, p. 125.

Solomon, L. M., and Nadler, N.: Radioautography of noradrenaline-^{14}C in atopic dermatitis. Can. Med. Assoc. J. 96:1147, 1967.

Solomon, L. M., and Telner, P.: Eruptive molluscum contagiosum in atopic dermatitis. Can. Med. Assoc. J. 95:978, 1966.

Solomon, L. M., Juhlin, L., and Kirschenbaum, M. B.: Prostaglandin on cutaneous vasculature. J. Invest. Dermatol. 51:280, 1968.

Solomon, L. M., Wentzel, H. E., and Tulsky, E.: The physiological disposition of C^{14} norepinephrine in patients with atopic dermatitis and other dermatoses. J. Invest. Dermatol. 43:193, 1964.

Spitz, E., Gelfand, E. W., Sheffer, A. L., et al.: Serum IgE in clinical immunology and allergy. J. Allergy Clin. Immunol. 49:337, 1972.

Sternberg, T. H., and Zimmerman, M. C.: Stress studies in the eczema-asthma-hayfever diathesis. Arch. Dermatol. 65:392, 1952.

Stokes, J. H.: The eczema problem. Am. J. Med. Sci. 179:69, 1930.

Sulzberger, M. B.: Atopic dermatitis: Its clinical and histologic picture. In Baer, R. L., (ed.): Atopic Dermatitis. Philadelphia, J. B. Lippincott Co., 1955.

Sulzberger, M. B., and Herrmann, T.: Clinical significance of disturbances in the delivery of sweat. Springfield, Charles C Thomas, 1954.

Szasz, T. S.: Oral mechanisms in constipation and diarrhea. Int. J. Psychoanal. 32:196, 1951.

Szentivanyi, A.: The beta adrenergic theory of the atopic abnormality in bronchial asthma. J. Allergy 42:203, 1968.

Torsney, P., and Blumstein, G. I.: Atopic dermatitis. J. Allergy 38:41, 1966.

Varonier, H. S., and Hahn, W. W.: Cardiac and vascular reactivity in atopic and nonatopic children. J. Allergy 38:352, 1966.

Vowles, M., Warin, R. P., and Apley, J.: Infantile eczema: Observations of natural history and prognosis. Br. J. Dermatol. 67:53, 1955.

Warndorff, J. A.: The response of the sweat gland to acetylcholine in atopic subjects. Br. J. Dermatol. 83:306, 1970.

Wells, R. S., and Jennings, M. C.: X-linked ichthyosis and ichthyosis vulgaris. J.A.M.A. 202:485, 1967.

Wenner, H. A.: Complications of infantile eczema caused by the virus of herpes simplex. Am. J. Dis. Child. 67:247, 1944.

Wereide, K.: Neomycin sensitivity in atopic dermatitis and other eczematous conditions. Acta Derm. Venereol. 50:114, 1970.

West, J. R., Johnson, L. A., and Winkelmann, R. K.: Delayed-blanch phenomenon in atopic individuals without dermatitis. Arch. Dermatol. 85:227, 1962.

Whitfield, A.: On the white reaction (white line) in dermatology. Br. J. Derm. 50:71, 1938.

Wilkinson, R. D., Curtis, G. H., and Hawk, W. A.: Netherton's Disease. Arch. Dermatol. 89:46, 1964.

Winkelmann, R. K., and Gleich, G. J.: Chronic acral dermatitis associated with extreme elevations of IgE. J.A.M.A. 225:378, 1973.

Worth, R. M.: Atopic dermatitis among Chinese infants in Honolulu and San Francisco. Hawaii Med. J. 22:31, 1962.

Section III

ECZEMA

Donald M. Pillsbury

DERMATITIS AND ECZEMA

Acute and chronic dermatitis constitute a major segment of all clinical dermatology. While the changes in the skin follow a basic pattern which is reasonably constant, the factors which may initiate a dermatitis are extraordinarily numerous. The precise cellular and enzymatic changes which occur are as yet not determined fully, though an approach to a more clear understanding is being revealed in the case of contact dermatitis (see Section I of this chapter). The various factors which become operative secondarily in many cases of dermatitis are becoming better understood. Such factors often supplant the original excitant as the principal etiologic agent, and produce a chronic inflammatory process.

The material contained in this chapter represents some oversimplification of a very large aspect of dermatology. This approach has seemed advisable for several reasons. The varied morphologic patterns which dermatitis and eczema may assume have brought about an accumulation of diagnostic and descriptive terms which are overwhelming. Well over one hundred terms containing the words "dermatitis," "dermatitic," "eczematous," or "eczematoid" are in more or less current use. Many of these represent duplications based on minor morphologic variations, and some designate conditions which are not really dermatitic. The word "eczema" has never been satisfactorily defined clinically, has different interpretations in different countries, has gradually lost its medical significance, and has become a catch-basket for many types of chronic dermatitis.

The morphologic changes of acute and chronic dermatitis are clear cut and not easily confused with other gross changes of the skin. The signs of dermatitis in the order of their evolution are as follows:

1. Erythema and swelling of the skin.
2. Oozing and/or vesiculation.
3. Crusting and scaling.
4. Thickening and evidences of repeated excoriation.
5. Hyperpigmentation, "scratch papule" formation, and/or lichenification.

The first three changes are those of acute dermatitis. The latter two are seen only if the process persists for several weeks or longer.

The microscopic changes in acute dermatitis are those which might be expected from the gross changes, namely, intercellular and intracellular edema, the formation of intra-epidermal vesicles, and a minimal infiltration of inflammatory cells into the epidermis. In the dermis there are edema, vascular dilatation, and beginning perivascular cellular infiltration. If the dermatitis persists, the epidermis thickens (acanthosis), some of the stratum corneum cells may retain their nuclei (parakeratosis), and there is usually an abundant cellular infiltrate in the upper dermis consisting mostly of lymphocytes, but also of histiocytes and fibroblasts. Capillary proliferation may be prominent. Vesicles are absent. Grossly, the skin is usually thickened, and has an infiltrated feel. The various types of chronic dermatitis cannot be differentiated on the basis of the histopathologic changes alone.

While there is no completely satisfactory classification which will include all variants of the dermatitis-eczema group of diseases, a certain amount of categorization is helpful. No single criterion of differentiation is possible. Separate classification of a particular group is justified if one or more of the following criteria are satisfied: (1) that it is a type in which a definite cause can be determined, (2) that it occurs in a fairly definite pattern which, (3) is helpful in determining the prognosis in the individual patient, or gives clear indication for more or less specific treatment, or indicates the need for further medical studies.

Using these criteria, dermatitis and eczema may be divided into the following main groups.

Acute Contact Dermatitis (Section I of this Chapter)

There are two major causes: (1) allergic sensitization to a wide variety of contactant materials, and (2) primary irritation from toxic substances. Contact dermatitis is the prototype of all dermatitic reactions and the most satisfactory to manage therapeutically. In a very high proportion of patients, the responsible substance may be determined accurately and the cause removed.

Atopic Dermatitis (Section II of this Chapter)

This is a chronic dermatitis which possesses distinctive features in respect to localization of lesions, personal and familial evidence of allergy, and a characteristic though often erratic course.

Seborrheic Dermatitis

This is a clear-cut type in respect to localization of lesions, frequent association with evidences of sebaceous dysfunction, increased vulnerability to secondary bacterial infections, and a fairly characteristic course.

Nummular Dermatitis

This type of dermatitis has a distinctive morphologic pattern (nummular, coinlike). The basic etiologic factors are unknown. The diagnosis carries certain definite implications as to the type of treatment which is most likely to be satisfactory, though none is completely so.

Lichen Simplex Chronicus

Itching is the initial symptom of this distinctive disorder which at first has no objective manifestations. The various subsequent evidences of chronic dermatitis are entirely the result of excoriation of infection or of reactions to topical treatment.

Stasis Dermatitis

This is another clear-cut form of dermatitis in which the basic etiologic factors are peripheral venous disease and tissue edema.

Although the above six forms of dermatitis are reasonably clear-cut and important types, two other less well-defined large groups are as follows:

Infantile Eczema of all Types

This is a classification based entirely on age and the dermatitic patterns of the infantile skin, which vary considerably from those of the adult. An increasing number of concomitant systemic diseases are being recorded. See Tables 5–4 and 5–5.

Chronic Dermatitis of Hands and/or Feet

This is a classification based upon regional involvement, but it is justified because it is such a common problem. Several of the main causes of dermatitis may, variously, participate in this complex, and certain etiologic factors are more responsible than others, as a rule.

Certain more or less well-defined subdivisions of this group may be recognized, including:

POMPHOLYX. A vesicular eruption, usually of the hands, non-inflammatory, which may come and go for no apparent reason.

DERMATITIS REPENS. A distinctive inflammatory eruption of the digits, palms and/or soles characterized by a thin annular vesiculopustular border which gradually extends and recurs, leaving inflamed, mildly exfoliating skin and is probably an expression of the so-called "dyshidrotic" eczema.

"ID" REACTIONS. A vesicular sensitization reaction caused by absorption of an allergen, usually fungal, derived from an inflammatory focus elsewhere on the skin. No fungi are demonstrable in the hand lesions.

"HOUSEWIVES' HANDS." This syndrome is so common and resistant to etiologic analysis as to deserve a separate colloquial designation. While the original cause is usually a contactant, other factors may become predominant, and result in prolonged chronicity.

CHRONIC PUSTULAR ERUPTIONS OF THE HANDS AND FEET ("BACTERID," PUSTULAR PSORIASIS). This condition consists of miliary, grouped pustular lesions of the palmar and plantar surfaces which come and go, endlessly at times. The pustules are often sterile. The differentiation between pustular psoriasis and secondarily infected dyshidrotic eczema is frequently difficult to make. (See Table 5–6, p. 316.)

Before proceeding with a discussion of each of these types of dermatitis in terms of individual characteristics, the principal etiologic factors, and prognosis and treatment, certain general statements which apply variously to all types of dermatitis must be made. These relate to the fact that many have a complexity of etiologic factors from their onset, and that in any dermatitis which persists for two or three weeks, certain secondary factors become either actively or potentially operative.

Factors common to all types of dermatitis are as follows:

ITCHING. Itching is a frequent symptom. It may be noted only in certain phases of the disease, as in seborrheic dermatitis, but in other types (for example, atopic dermatitis and lichen simplex chronicus), itching is a predominant feature and the beginning of almost all that follows. The effects of excoriation are, therefore, important in all types of dermatitis, and these may vary from simple rubbing of the skin to extreme trauma produced in many ways. In addition to mechanical injury, dermatitis is frequently subjected to the irritant and sensitizing effects of topical medication.

SWEAT RETENTION. Following any dermatitis, however brief in duration, blockage of a small to large proportion of the sweat ducts in the area occurs. This is innocuous if the sweat gland is not stimulated. If a large number of sweat ducts are occluded and the environment is warm, severe itching, increased scratch dermatitis, and frank inflammatory or pustular miliaria may develop. If the stimulus to sweating is continuous, as in a tropical climate or in some psychoneurotic pa-

tients, the sequelae of sweat duct retention become pyramided and may be responsible for very persistent inflammatory changes.

SECONDARY BACTERIAL INFECTION. In an area of skin affected by a persistent dermatitis, marked change in the superficial bacterial flora always occurs. The micrococcic species which are normally found in large numbers on the skin surface disappear and are displaced by coagulase-positive *M. aureus,* sometimes by beta-hemolytic streptococci, and sometimes by pseudomonas and other bacteria.

SECONDARY CONTACT DERMATITIS FROM APPLIED MEDICATION. In the midst of an acute dermatitis, the skin is highly vulnerable. The loss of some of its normal protective capacity is readily demonstrable by the stinging and burning which often occur following the application of some chemical which might produce no sensation whatever if applied to normal skin. The stratum corneum of dermatitic skin is often partially or completely lost, and the basal portion of the epidermis, and even the dermis or subcutaneous tissues, may be easily accessible to substances applied to the surface.

In addition to this break in the mechanical barrier, the patient with a dermatitis (excepting atopic dermatitis) is often a more likely candidate for induced sensitization than a patient with, for instance, acne or psoriasis. A chemical which has been shown to have a low sensitizing index on hundreds of normal skins may show a higher incidence when used on patients with acutely dermatitic skins. The failure to recognize irritant or sensitization reactions from applied medication is an extremely common error in the management of any type of dermatitis. It is unfortunately assumed by the patient who is having such a reaction that, because the dermatitis is becoming worse, more frequent application of the substance which is actually producing the exacerbation is indicated.

During the past three decades, an increasing number of endogenously or exogenously administered chemicals have been found to be capable of producing a variety of inflammatory reactions in the skin. These are considered in detail in Chapter 7.

SEBORRHEIC DERMATITIS

Seborrheic dermatitis has several distinct characteristics, including the distribution of the eruption, frequent association with an oily type of skin, frequent increased vulnerability to secondary infection by bacteria and Candida, and a responsiveness to treatment methods which vary somewhat from those applicable to other types of dermatitis. Seborrheic dermatitis is basically a constitutional diathesis which affects usually certain areas and rarely the entire skin and is often regarded as an inborn physiologic trait which usually can be controlled but not "cured."

Diagnosis

The distinctive features of seborrheic dermatitis are as follows:

1. Scaling patches, the margins of which are ordinarily rather indistinct, with only slight to moderate erythema of the base, and scaling which is frequently oily and slightly yellow.

2. The distribution of lesions occurs in a fairly regular pattern. In mild seborrheic dermatitis, or ordinary "dandruff," the scalp may be the only area of involvement. The scaling tends to be rather diffuse, and this is an important distinguishing point from psoriasis involving the scalp. In moderately severe seborrheic dermatitis, the other sites of involvement include the eyebrows, the portions of the forehead above the bridge of the nose, the nasal folds, the retroauricular areas and, on the trunk, the presternal and interscapular regions. Mild to marked blepharitis is a common finding and may be accompanied by styes. In seborrheic dermatitis of increasing severity, the portions of the skin near the scalp hairline become increasingly affected, extension from the special sites noted above occurs, and involvement of intertriginous folds of the trunk is noted (that is, the axillae, under the breasts in women, the umbilicus, and the anogenital region, particularly the crural folds and the gluteal cleft). In obese patients, all pendulous folds on the neck and trunk may become involved. In addition, isolated patches may appear on the face, trunk, and upper portion of the extremities, usually as erythematous scaling patches which sometimes assume an annular shape (seborrhea petaloides). Seborrheic dermatitis, which may rarely undergo intractable dissemination, is one of the causes of chronic generalized exfoliative dermatitis.

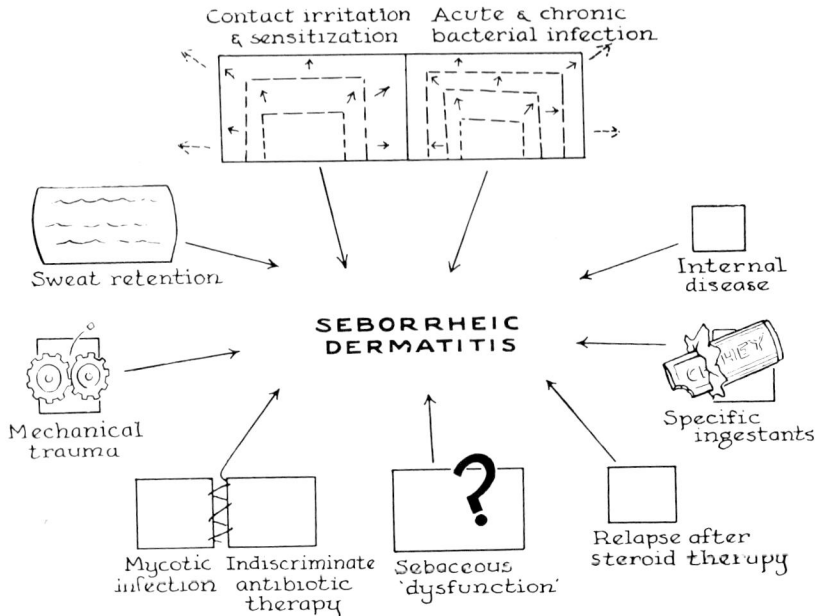

Figure 5–25 Factors contributing to exacerbations and persistence of seborrheic dermatitis.

The reasons for the particular localization of lesions are not completely understood, though they are found in areas of high sebaceous gland concentration and in areas which are not likely to be thoroughly washed in ordinary bathing. Moisture and maceration of the skin also play a distinct role, and some degree of chronic secondary bacterial infection is almost always operative at this phase.

3. General medical background. Certain general diseases are associated with seborrheic dermatitis frequently enough to deserve comment. Some types of mental defectives and patients with Parkinson's disease present oily skins with varying degrees of seborrheic dermatitis. Although this is in part due to poor hygiene, it cannot be attributed to this alone. Endocrine states associated with obesity appear to favor seborrheic dermatitis. One of the physiologic effects of corticosteroid therapy is an increase in greasiness and seborrheic scaling of the skin, although this is less prominent than the acneiform changes. Obese diabetics frequently have seborrheic dermatitis with intertriginous involvement, although to what extent this is due to the obesity and the diabetes, respectively, is difficult to determine. In any event, the proneness to secondary infection in these areas constitutes a distinct hazard in the diabetic. Psychosomatic influences undoubtedly play a role; through mechanisms which are not understood, chronic worry and tension and loss of sleep frequently appear to aggravate seborrheic dermatitis. The cutaneous reactions to broad-spectrum antibiotics, from the sites in which Candida may be recovered in profusion, may be particularly severe and persistent in seborrheic patients.

4. The association of seborrheic dermatitis with certain other diseases affecting the skin is striking. Severe acne is almost always accompanied by some seborrheic dermatitis. The same may be said for rosacea. Seborrheic dermatitis and psoriasis are seen not infrequently in the same patient as to excite notice. In the scalp and sometimes in intertriginous areas, the same patient may show lesions which might be diagnosed as "pure" seborrheic dermatitis and which later might be distinctly those of psoriasis. Whether or not there is some single basic etiologic factor can only be conjectured. Although patients with premature male-type baldness frequently have or have had evidence of seborrheic scaling of the scalp, there is no indication that seborrheic dermatitis of and by itself causes alopecia. Miliaria is a frequent complication of seborrheic dermatitis in hot climates, and in such patients it is sometimes difficult to determine whether small punctate lesions on the trunk are those of "follicular" seborrheic dermatitis or of sweat retention. Such patients seem somewhat more vulnerable to ordinary impetigo or to the widespread tropical variety.

The factors which are chiefly contributory to seborrheic dermatitis are outlined in Figure 5–25.

Treatment

Potent topically applied corticosteroids are effective in the treatment of seborrheic dermatitis. Nevertheless, particularly in the treatment of milder cases, less expensive compounds are often quite effective. Furthermore, the number and variety of proprietary compounds available, and the vigor with which they are promoted, induce an enormous amount of self-treatment, which often is adequate.

The patient with oily seborrheic scaling of the scalp must shampoo regularly. However, differentiation must be made between seborrheic dermatitis and the dry, diffuse scaling which is noted in patients with generalized dryness of the skin or ichthyosis; in the latter condition, excessive shampooing may increase the amount of scaling. The type of detergent used does not make much difference; choice will depend upon advertising propaganda and upon individual preference and prejudices. Nonsoap detergents for shampooing are widely used; they are generally good and occasionally seem somewhat less irritating than soap. It is essential that, when soap is used, the hair and scalp be rinsed thoroughly.

For moderate scaling and itching of the scalp, a "hair tonic" may be indicated for application once or twice a day. Such a tonic will ordinarily be in a vehicle containing 20 to 40 per cent ethanol or propanal and variously including 1 to 3

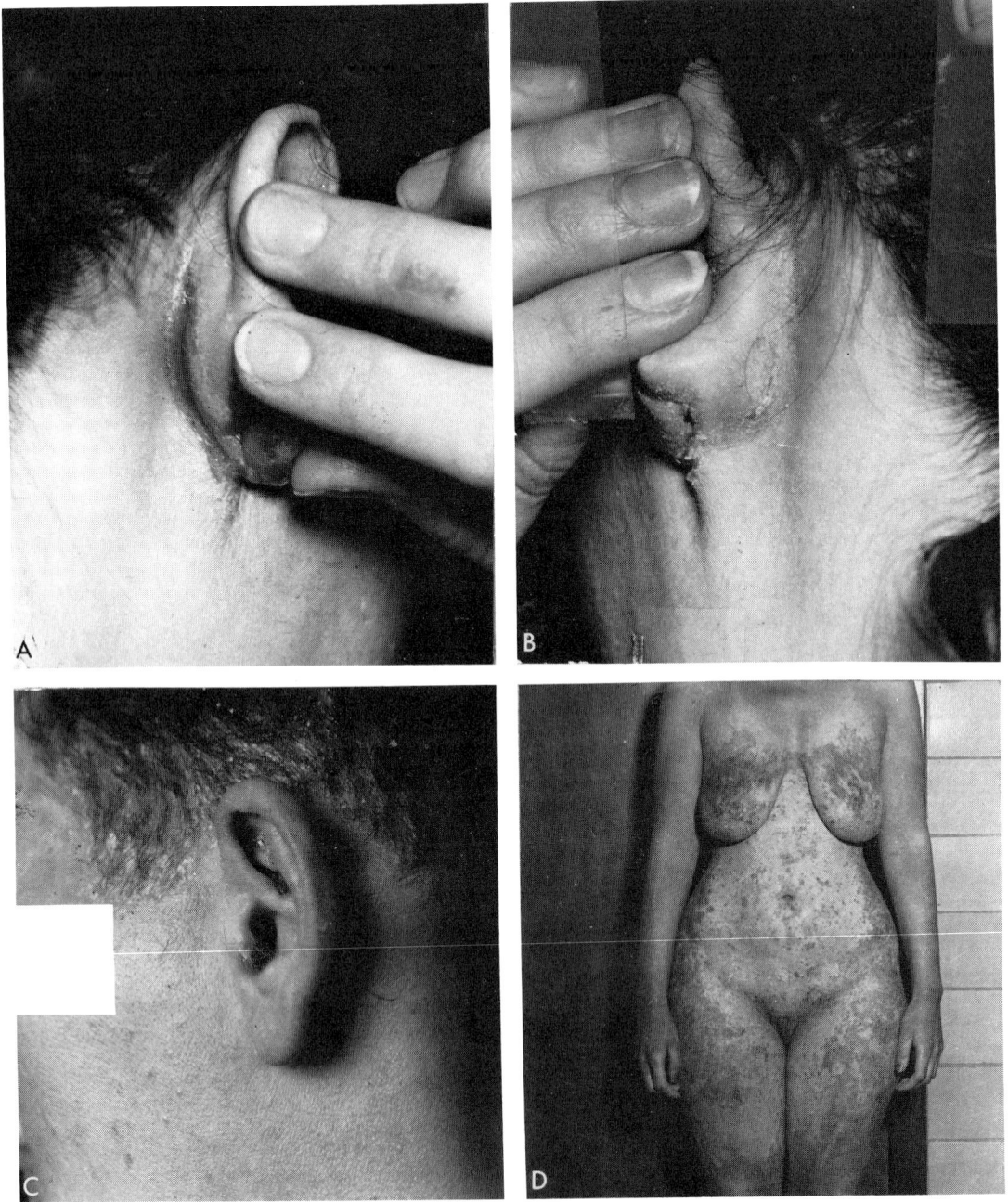

Figure 5-26 *A* and *B*, Retroauricular seborrheic dermatitis. Same patient. *C*, Heavy seborrheic scaling of the scalp. *D*, Extensive chronic seborrheic dermatitis. Severe exacerbations occurred regularly in warm weather.

per cent salicylic acid, 0.5 to 1 per cent resorcinol monoacetate, and a dash of camphor (0.5 to 1 per cent) if an antipruritic effect is desired. If the hair is naturally "dry," the addition of 1 to 3 per cent castor oil furnishes a satisfactory amount of oil. The number of hair tonic formulae available is legion.

A shampoo containing selenium sulfide (Selsun) has achieved considerable popularity. It is generally agreed that with weekly use it has good temporary suppressive effects on seborrheic scaling of the scalp. An alternate form of treatment is the application of an ointment containing 3 per cent each of sulfur and salicylic acid in a washable base in small amounts to all portions of the scalp on retiring and then shampooing the next morning. If desired, a small amount of the preparation may be rubbed into the hair as it is drying. It is essential to use a preparation with a base which is easily washable; bases such as lanolin or petrolatum prove unacceptable.

Not infrequently, the seborrheic scaling is so thick and adherent as to justify stronger preparations. In this general "mange cure" group, the following ointment is representative:

Oil of cade...........................20%
Sulfur.................................10%
Salicylic acid...................... 5%
Aquaphor q.s.

Such a preparation is not suitable for frequent use because of its odor and diffi-

culty in removal, but application twice weekly at night, followed by shampooing the next morning, is not too arduous a regimen if the seborrheic dermatitis is severe.

When there is a moderate to severe amount of seborrheic dermatitis present, topical corticosteroid therapy is the treatment of choice. The least expensive hydrocortisone creams, ointments, and lotions are probably worthy of an initial trial. *A concentration of at least 1 per cent of hydrocortisone should be employed;* weaker concentrations appear to have little more effect than the vehicle alone. Locally compounded preparations are often of uncertain effectiveness because of varying release of the steroid from the vehicle. Preparations distributed by reputable manufacturers are preferable. In many instances, the use of fluorinated corticosteroid creams which are more potent than hydrocortisone becomes necessary; in some of the most resistant cases, betamethasone valerate lotion has

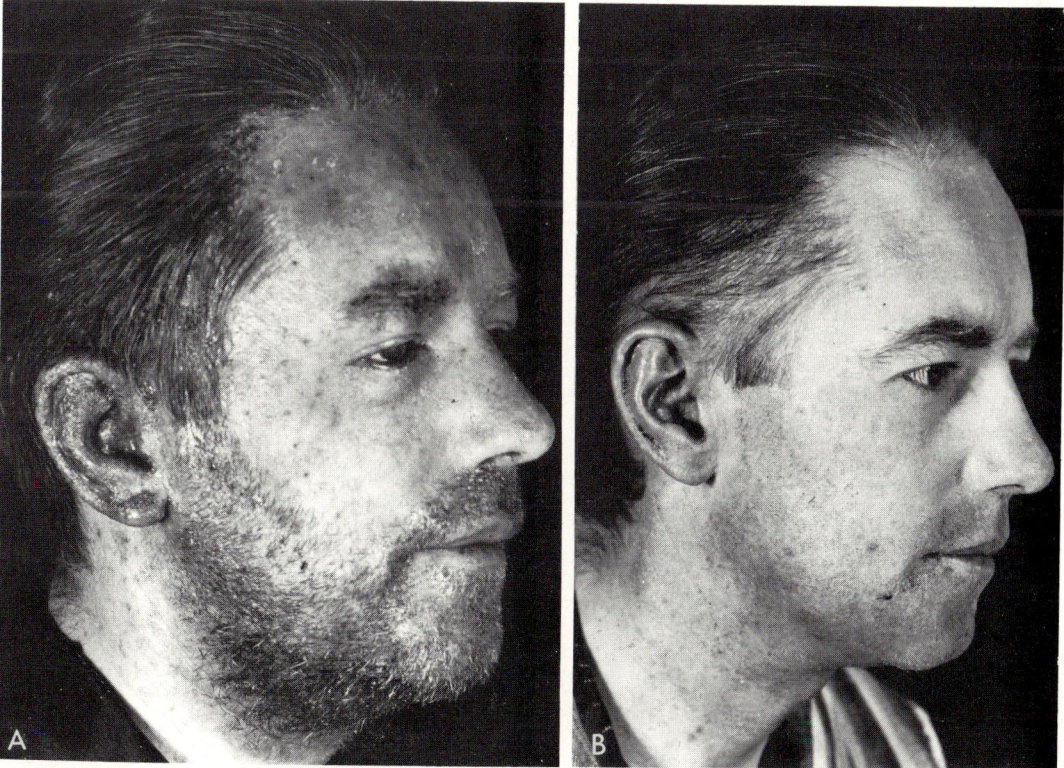

Figure 5–27 *A,* Secondarily infected extensive seborrheic dermatitis. Note otitis externa and blepharitis. *B,* Three weeks later.

been most helpful. Creams to which neomycin has been added show no clearly superior therapeutic effect, and carry a definite risk of inducing neomycin sensitivity. They are not recommended.

Seborrheic dermatitis may sometimes persist in special localized forms which offer difficulties in respect to both diagnosis and treatment. The more common of these are:

DERMATITIS OF THE EXTERNAL EAR AND ADJACENT AREAS. Seborrheic dermatitis of the external ear, particularly in the external auditory canal, is the most common underlying factor in otitis externa.

OTITIS EXTERNA. Otitis externa is in a diagnostic twilight zone between the territories of the dermatologist and the otolaryngologist. Various authorities hold divergent views of causation. Much of the disagreement and confusion arises from failure to recognize that this condition is not a disease; it is a syndrome of varying origin. The term has no more etiologic meaning than "eczema," about which there has been equal contention.

A list of the diseases affecting the external ear canal would include many of the diseases of the glabrous skin, such as seborrheic dermatitis, psoriasis, contact dermatitis, neurodermatitis, furunculosis, and so forth. The ear involvement may simply be part of a more generalized condition, or it may be a localized expression of such a condition. The anatomic construction of the external ear, which is the only blind cul-de-sac in the body lined with stratified squamous epithelium, accounts for the peculiarities of pathogenesis. Its architecture is highly variable, and in many individuals the canal is tortuous and may be occluded to a variable degree by abnormal accumulation of cerumen. This peculiarity, above all others, favors persistent lesions in this area by reason of the failure of exudates and inflammatory products to drain away readily and the inaccessibility of the region for everyday cleansing. Moisture retention and maceration are inevitable and, whatever the initial cause of irritation, healing is impaired. Swelling further narrows the canal. Serous exudate provides a culture milieu which is highly inviting to the growth of bacteria and possibly of fungi. In acute inflammations, therefore, bacterial prolifera-

tion is greatly enhanced, and the results of this may obscure the original condition, especially if there is much pus formation. In less acute conditions, particularly if there is a ceruminous retention, saprophytic fungi may colonize the debris and accumulate in the form of a plug of fungal elements.

The robust growth of saprophytic fungi has impressed many observers and the term "otomycosis" has come to be almost synonymous with otitis externa in many quarters. Otomycosis is a rare disease; the fungi commonly found in diseased external ears are not different from ordinary saprophytes and are apparently not capable of initiating disease. They are secondary colonists, vegetating on retained products, usually a mixture of cerumen and inflammatory debris; they may grow so well in this highly favorable situation that a plug largely made up of fungal filaments may be more or less a cast of the canal. Whether any injurious effect should be credited to the fungal growth is debatable, though it is possible that exotoxins produced by Aspergillus species, the commonest of all the ear molds, might be harmful. Of course, the fungi add to occlusion of the canal, an effect which is undesirable in respect to healing. However, use of the term "otomycosis" as a loose designation for many types of inflammation of the external ear is inaccurate and has been responsible for much misdiagnosis and harmful mistreatment.

Similar misconceptions prevail about the role of bacteria, though they are much more contributory to disease of the external ear than are fungi. The real problem is to evaluate the etiologic role played by the variety of organisms recoverable in abundance from diseased ears. The issues are not different from those which are presented when bacteria are encountered in any kind of diseased skin. Dermatitic skin is practically always colonized by nonresident organisms, particularly if there is much exudate or crust. Mere isolation of coagulase-positive staphylococci and beta-hemolytic streptococci, however, does not necessarily indicate that they are playing a pathogenic role even in a secondary sense.

The normal flora of the external ear is much more varied than that of normal skin.

In particular, the growth of gram-negative organisms which require moisture for survival on the skin's surface is greatly favored by local conditions in the inflamed ear. Coliform bacteria, Pseudomonas, and Proteus species are found much more frequently than in lesions of the glabrous skin. When present in abundance and when accompanied by suppuration, their injurious effects cannot be doubted. It is unlikely that they initiate the disease process with any frequency. However, once they have a foothold in the external canal which is already the site of some disease, even though it be trivial, the manifestations of secondary infection may eclipse the original process completely. Pus formation in particular tends to focus the observer's attention on the bacterial infection, to the exclusion of antecedent pathogenic events. A search for the primary cause is always in order and, in fact, unless the primary condition can be resolved, recurrence is likely even though the infection may be controlled.

The diseases which make up the syndrome of otitis externa may be divided into acute and chronic types.

Acute Otitis Externa may be mild or severe. In the severe form, pus formation is prominent, and *Pseudomonas aeruginosa* is recovered in pure culture in some cases. In milder inflammations, this organism often dominates but is frequently accompanied by a variety of other microorganisms.

Chronic Otitis Externa is divisible into two groups: (1) suppurative, and (2) eczematous. The causes of the eczematous conditions are varied and ill defined. Many different microorganisms are recoverable and these do not appear to play either a primary or a secondary role. The ear canal generally shows varying degrees of scaling and erythema. Pruritus is the chief symptom and is the principal reason why patients apply for treatment. The condition fluctuates in intensity, remissions occurring spontaneously. Quite often the primary condition is a localized neurodermatitis. Seborrheic dermatitis often involves the ear and here, too, emotional factors are commonly a significant etiologic force.

Chronic otitis externa, however, may be suppurative when secondary infection supervenes and, again, *P. aeruginosa* is the predominant organism. Maltreatment and overtreatment are perpetuating causes.

The treatment of otitis externa cannot be

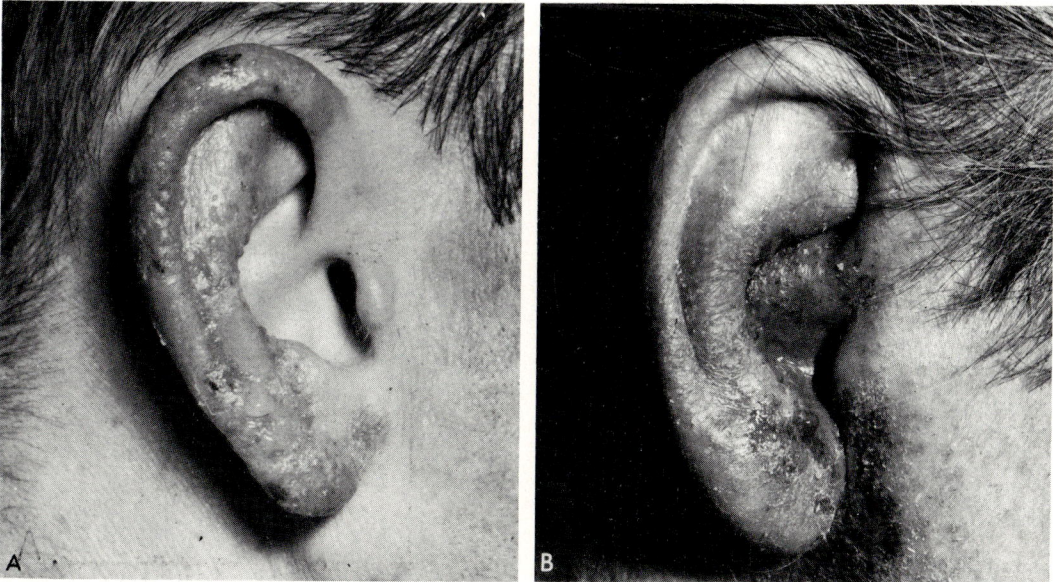

Figure 5–28 Types of otitis externa. *A*, Chronic eczematous dermatitis with infection. No involvement of external auditory canal. Prognosis excellent. *B*, Sequelae of chronic middle ear infection. Prognosis doubtful.

standardized, considering the diversity of operative causes. The single most important objective in all instances, however, is to provide an optimal opportunity for the skin to repair itself. The reversal of the disease process involves more than suppressing bacterial and fungal contaminants. Any obvious factor which interferes with recuperation must be corrected. In suppurative conditions this means two procedures: removal of exudate, an objective which can be hastened by the proper use of antibiotics, and, secondly, the maintenance of dryness within the ear, mainly by appropriate cleansing. In the acute stage, antibiotics which are sufficiently stable to be prepared in solution should be employed. Polymyxin, in particular, is active against most strains of *P. aeruginosa* and is the antibiotic of choice in otitis externa, although it has a limited spectrum otherwise.

Chronic eczematous eruptions of the ear are managed in the same way as corresponding lesions on the smooth skin. Locally applied corticosteroid preparations are quite useful in the management of neurodermatitis and seborrheic dermatitis of the ear canal.

Low-grade seborrheic dermatitis of the external ear is a common instigator of neurodermatitis. Scratching of the ear is a common habit tic. Some patients develop great facility in scratching the external auditory canal, either vigorously with a finger, or with objects such as paper clips or hairpins. In addition to the trauma involved, there is always a risk of contact dermatitis from something transferred by the fingers (fingernail polish) or from the objects used (lacquer on hairpins). Furunculosis of the external auditory canal is an occasional complication and an extraordinarily painful one.

SPECIAL FORMS OR COMPLICATIONS OF SEBORRHEIC DERMATITIS. *Localized Neurodermatitis of the Occipital Area of the Scalp* (so-called nuchal or suboccipital dermatitis) may have its onset with seborrheic dermatitis. The two conditions are frequently seen together, and sometimes with psoriasis as well.

Chronic Dermatitis and Fissuring of the Umbilicus may have its genesis in seborrheic dermatitis. The area is one which is rarely cleansed thoroughly, and it sometimes collects a surprising amount and variety of debris. When it is involved by seborrheic dermatitis, bacterial infection and fissuring occur almost inevitably, and this may be annoyingly recurrent. The cellulitis may be severe and persistent; infection of urachal cysts sometimes occurs, and excision may be necessary in rare instances.

Dermatitis of the Areolar Area of the Breasts in women may be a manifestation of seborrheic dermatitis or atopic dermatitis. It may offer some anxiety at times in relation to differentiation from a possible Paget's disease, particularly if the process tends to be unilateral.

Seborrheic Dermatitis Frequently Involves the Anogenital Region. The localization in the crural folds and gluteal cleft in both males and females has been mentioned. In males, seborrheic dermatitis may persist in localized patches on the penis, particularly on the glans or under the prepuce.

Blepharitis and Dermatitis of the Upper Eyelids may be a manifestation of seborrheic dermatitis. With involvement of this type, it is important to examine the scalp and other areas, and it may occasionally be associated with a severe and resistant folliculitis of the beard. In blepharitis particularly, treatment of the seborrheic dermatitis of the scalp is essential if the inflammation of the lid margin is to be brought under control.

NUMMULAR DERMATITIS

Nummular dermatitis is a distinctive member of the dermatitis-eczema group principally by reason of its characteristic round nummular (coinlike) lesions. While the extent of the dermatitis may be minimal at times, as with two or three patches on the hands, numerous lesions are the rule, and these ordinarily have a characteristic distribution to the extensor surfaces of the extremities (especially on the arms), the posterior portion of the trunk, the buttocks, and the lower legs.

Diagnosis

The individual lesions of nummular dermatitis are usually distinctly annular, the diameter of lesions measuring from one to several centimeters. The lesions characteristically appear quite suddenly in the involved site, on skin which had previously appeared quite normal or was asteatotic. The size of the lesion remains the same, as a rule, though in occasional instances there may be some peripheral extension but without any evidence of clearing of the lesions at the center. The lesions frequently ooze from their onset, often itch severely, and rapidly become crusted and scaling. A purulent exudate is frequently seen.

As indicated in Figure 5–29, the basic cause of nummular dermatitis is quite unknown, and the separate classification of it is on morphologic grounds. Patients with nummular dermatitis may sometimes give a history of a recent contact dermatitis, or there may be some skin changes of the lower legs related to stasis. Under such circumstances, the process may be regarded as an "id" due to a reaction to materials absorbed from a primary eczematous patch. Nummular dermatitis is seen more frequently in middle-aged to older patients than in young persons. An atopic history is present in some patients, and it seems entirely possible that nummular dermatitis may in some persons be a later manifestation of atopic dermatitis, though the morphology of the two conditions is quite different. In many patients with nummular dermatitis, however, there is no history whatever of a preceding contact dermatitis or any allergic history.

The course of the dermatitis varies greatly. It may remain for some time as a few small scaling patches which are not particularly bothersome. In some patients, gradual relentless appearance of new lesions occurs, particularly in persons with dry skin and during cold winter weather. Excessive soap and water bathing is definitely harmful in such patients.

Nummular dermatitis may at times appear suddenly with an extensive shower of lesions. This is especially true in patients who have had some form of chronic dermatitis of the lower legs, stasis dermatitis, a scratch dermatitis resulting from insect bites, or a contact dermatitis from a plant or other material which has become persistent. It has frequently been observed that such a shower of lesions may follow the application of an irritating or sensitizing topical medicament to the original dermatitis of the legs. Or it is sometimes noted when evidence of low-grade secondary infection becomes more marked. In some instances, the sudden appearance of extensive lesions can be related to the ingestion of a drug, for example, sulfonamides. It is a characteristic feature of nummular dermatitis that as the process remits

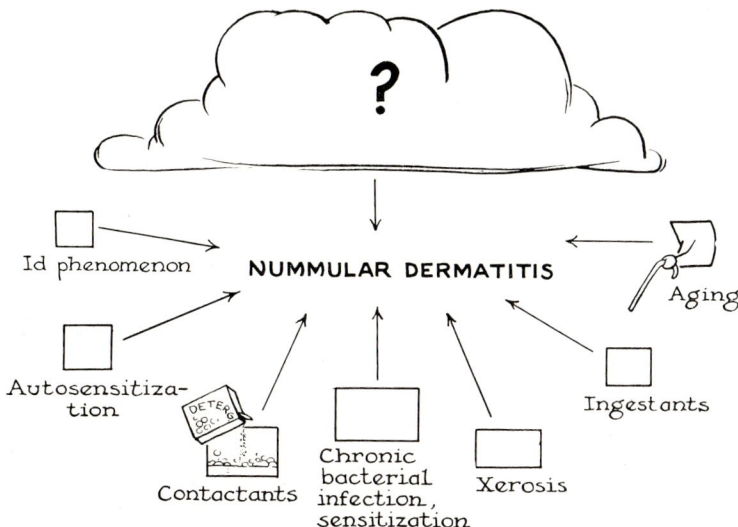

Figure 5–29 The unknown and the known in nummular dermatitis. The marked psychosomatic factors in nummular dermatitis have not been included in this figure.

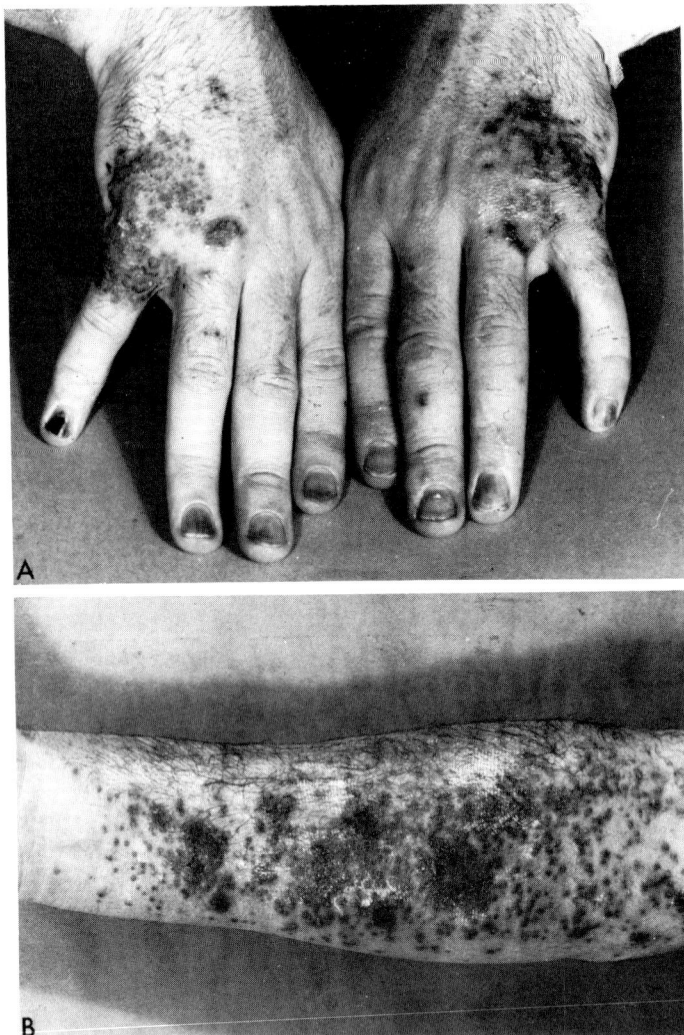

Figure 5–30 Nummular dermatitis. *A,* Characteristic grouped patches on the hands. *B,* Extensive coalescing lesions on the forearm.

and recurs, almost all of the sites previously involved are affected during each recurrence. The reasons for this are not clear, but the patches are obviously a locus minoris resistentiae. Another finding encountered with some regularity is the recovery of large numbers of hemolytic coagulase-positive *Micrococcus aureus* or *M. albus* from the surface of active lesions. This may be the case even when there is no definite gross evidence of bacterial infection. In an occasional patient with nummular dermatitis, the author produced a dermatitis with the intradermal injection of vaccines or toxins from these micro cocci; a subcutaneous injection may incite a flare-up of all the existing lesions.

This has led to the hypothesis that nummular dermatitis may be essentially a superficial chronic bacterial infection of the skin, with sensitivity to the bacteria themselves or to toxins combined with skin proteins. The administration of the usual effective antibiotics has a variable effect on the lesions in the absence of gross evidence of bacterial infection, and attempts at producing hyposensitization to the bacteria or their toxoids have been disappointing and may even be harmful.

The prognosis in nummular dermatitis is toward eventual involution, though this may require several months to two or three years and may not occur at all if secondary etiologic factors are still active.

Treatment

From the foregoing discussion it will be seen that the etiology of nummular dermatitis is so uncertain as to make specific therapeutic approaches difficult. Nevertheless, a great deal can be done for such patients.

"PASSIVE" TREATMENT. It is important to protect the skin of the patient from various agents which regularly or occasionally appear to have a bad effect in this disease. These are as follows:

Overdrying (Xerosis). This is a fairly constant feature of the skin of such patients, particularly among older ones. Overbathing, either in the form of very frequent baths or too prolonged exposure to hot soap and water, must be avoided. It is necessary to restrict general bathing to not more than twice weekly and sometimes even once weekly in cold winter weather. The patient must learn to be satisfied with "spot" bathing in the interim. Thorough greasing of the skin after a bath is helpful in preserving the hydration of the stratum corneum. Humidification of overheated houses or flats during the winter months sometimes seems worthwhile.

Primary Irritants are poorly tolerated by the skin of these patients. For this reason, in addition to precautions as to bathing, special care should be exerted to avoid undue contact with detergents, gasoline, furniture polish, and many other household and industrial irritants.

As in atopic dermatitis, exposure to natural sunlight, particularly in conjunction with a relaxing environment, is often extremely helpful in nummular dermatitis.

LOCAL THERAPY. Topically applied

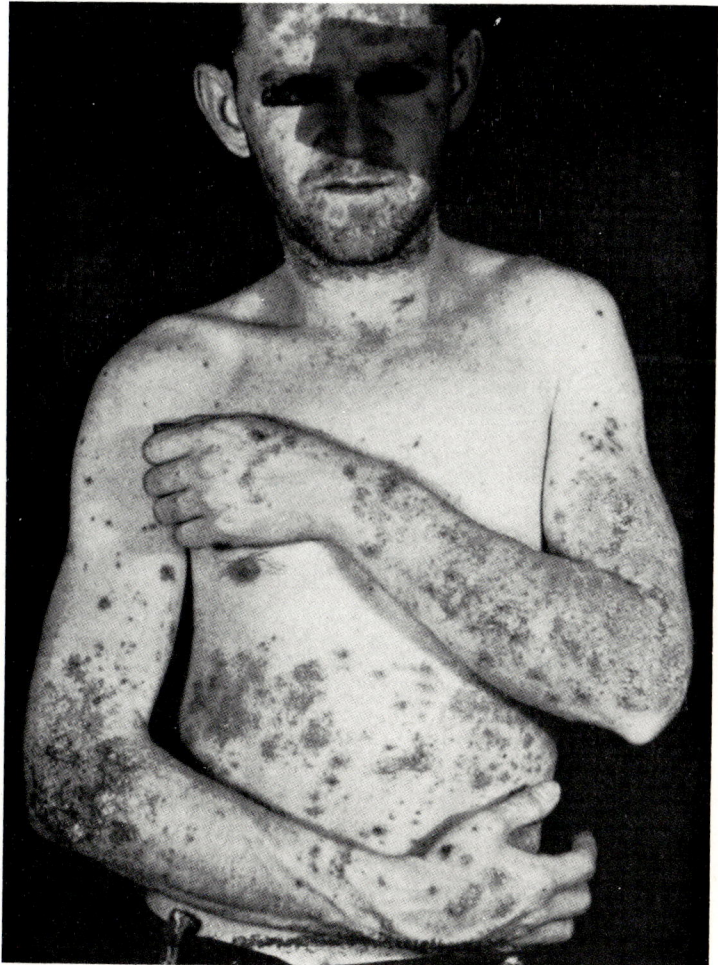

Figure 5-31 Extensive nummular dermatitis of sudden onset. Usually associated with an eczematous focus elsewhere on the skin. May follow chigger bites or contact dermatitis from weeds or clothing. May herald onset of chronic nummular dermatitis.

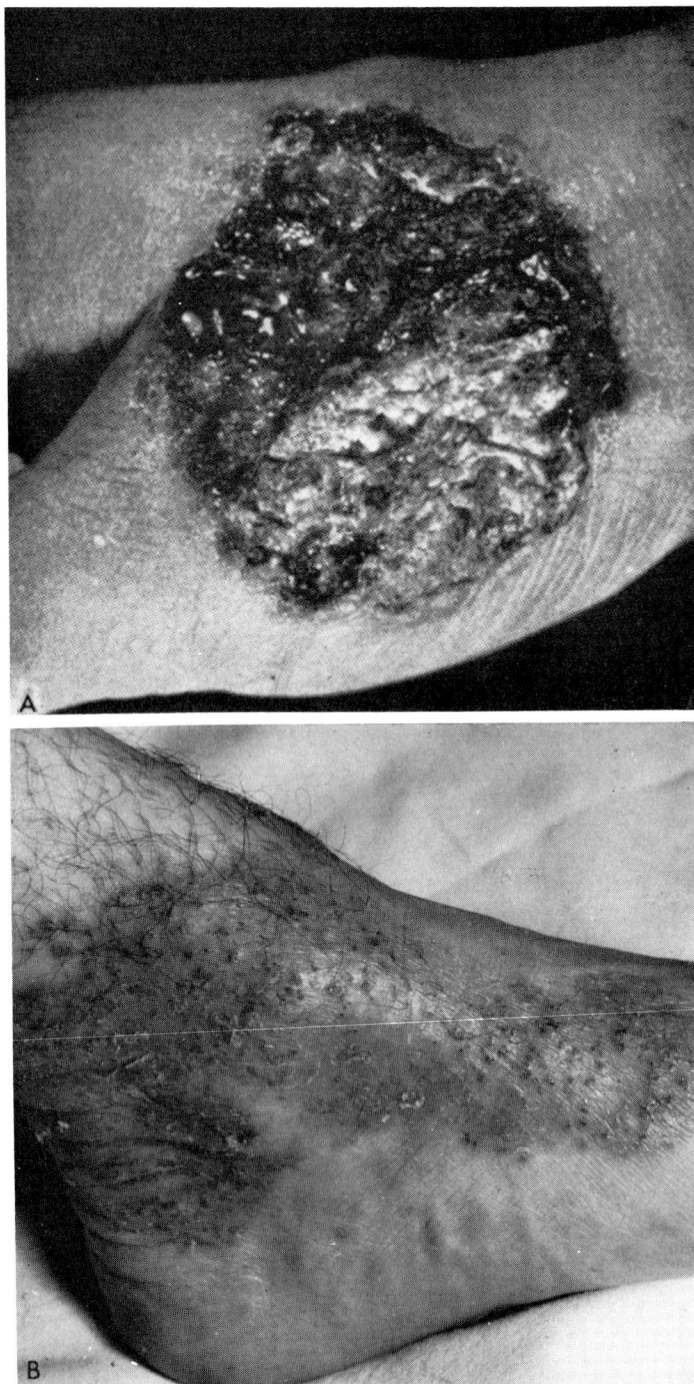

Figure 5–32 *A*, Infected nummular dermatitis of the hand. *B*, Nummular dermatitis of the ankle and foot.

corticosteroid preparations are the initial treatment of choice in nummular dermatitis, though they are erratic in their effectiveness. In oozing lesions, lotions are usually best, and if dryness is prominent, ointment compounds rather than creams often seem more effective. In extensive nummular dermatitis, the expense of corticosteroid preparations becomes significant.

Several older type preparations may prove useful. In dry lesions, a paste containing 2 to 3 per cent ichthammol in equal parts of Lassar's paste and Aquaphor may be tried. On individual oozing lesions, Castellani's paint often has a good drying and antibacterial effect. Preparations containing coal tar (2 to 5 per cent) are preferred by some. Vioform cream is sometimes useful.

Ultraviolet therapy is occasionally useful in nummular dermatitis and as part of the Goeckerman treatment in severe disseminated cases. In isolated areas, a short series of grenz ray exposures may be helpful.

ANTIBIOTIC THERAPY. In many cases of nummular dermatitis, bacterial infection is playing a more or less contributory role, and systemic antibiotic therapy (for example, erythromycin 1 gm. daily) is worthy of trial for a week or two, and then continued in smaller doses for several weeks, if effective. Topically applied antibiotic creams are, on the whole, disappointing in comparison with systemic therapy.

SYSTEMIC CORTICOSTEROID THERAPY. The corticoids are usually so rapidly effective in nummular dermatitis as to offer a constant temptation to use them too readily and too long. Nevertheless, in extensive symptomatic involvement of the skin, such therapy becomes entirely justified in the absence of compelling contraindications. The author prefers initial and/or interrupted intramuscular injections of a slowly absorbed corticosteroid, depending on the response of the patient.

PERSISTENT SEARCH FOR PRECIPITATING AGENTS. In some patients with nummular dermatitis, it will be apparent that the disseminated lesions have arisen as an aftermath of a chronic eczematous dermatitis, usually of the lower legs. It is particularly important that this "primary focus" be treated to complete involution if possible. In occasional patients, flare-ups of the nummular dermatitis may be traced to topical allergic reaction such as that to nickel, ingestion of drugs or, less commonly, to foods, which is often very difficult to establish.

GENERAL MEASURES AND INTERNAL THERAPY. There are no systemic disturbances which accompany nummular dermatitis with any regularity. The disease is possibly seen more frequently in nervous patients with too many responsibilities, real or fancied, and some attention to psychosomatic factors may be helpful. The patient should be studied for foci of infection, but treatment or attempted removal of such foci should be carried out only upon the most clear-cut grounds.

LICHEN SIMPLEX CHRONICUS

Lichen simplex chronicus (circumscribed neurodermatitis) is a characteristic syndrome in the dermatitis group. The individual lesion is a circumscribed scaling patch which is entirely the result of repeated scratching or rubbing of the skin. The margins are ordinarily fairly sharp. The features of acute dermatitis, namely, marked erythema and vesiculation, are not observed as an inherent part of the syndrome of circumscribed neurodermatitis, though they may occur secondarily as a result of topical medication. Thickening of the skin is always present in well-established lesions, and the papule formation in response to scratching varies from the mosaic pattern known as lichenification to more discrete raised papules which are often dry and keratotic, and to the uncommon discrete "giant" scratch papules of the type known as prurigo nodularis.

In most patients a single area is affected, but in others the sites may be multiple. The favorite areas are those which are subject to minor irritations of one sort or another and which may be reached easily. The disease is rarely encountered in children. Women are more frequently affected than men, and the occipital region of the scalp in women (so-called nuchal or suboccipital dermatitis; Figure 5–33) is a predominant site. It is very common among Chinese Americans. Areas about the face and neck and in the external auditory canals are frequently involved. The process may occur in the scalp as single lesions which appear verrucous — the so-called Picker's nodules which may be seen elsewhere. The trunk is not commonly involved, but lesions are frequently seen on the extremities, especially about the

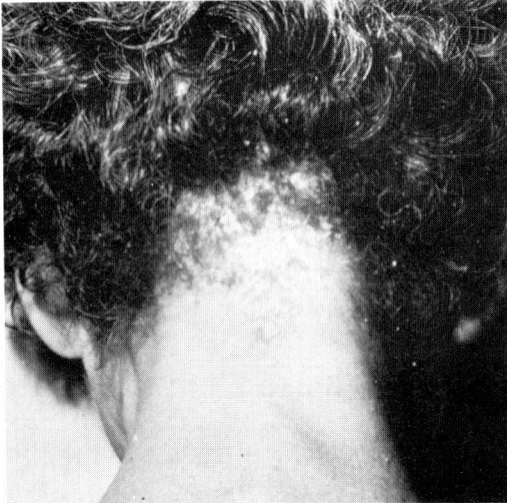

Figure 5–33 Nuchal dermatitis.

wrists, on the extensor surface of the fore-arm, near the elbow, or on the thighs and lower legs. The outer lower portion of the lower legs is a favorite site, since it is easily reached and may be scratched unobtrusively during periods of tension and concentration. Lesions of the lower legs are particularly prone to exhibit a hypertrophic papular response. It is probable that many cases of anal and vulvar pruritus are localized neurodermatitis; frequently the inflammatory changes are marked.

Localized neurodermatitis may be initiated by or may exist coincidentally with other dermatoses, particularly seborrheic dermatitis, psoriasis, and lichen planus.

Scalp involvement in women is especially prone to be psoriasiform, and the scaling may be very obvious and thickened. In this area, as well, the lesion may coincide quite sharply with the "physiologic birthmark," a patch of nevus flammeus which is frequently noted in the occipital area.

Secondary bacterial infection of circumscribed neurodermatitis occasionally occurs, but not as frequently as might be expected. Secondary sensitization dermatitis is very common. This may occur as a result of the wide variety of materials which are transferred to the patch by the fingers, or through topical applications in an effort to relieve the intense itching.

The prognosis in lichen simplex chronicus is variable. If scratching can be prevented, prompt cure ordinarily results. However, this is sometimes extremely difficult to accomplish and, indeed, a patient may sometimes substitute another more vital organ as the target of his psychosomatic outlet.

The morphologic response of the skin to prolonged vigorous scratching and pinching varies greatly in some individuals. These variations have led to a variety of names, many of them rarely employed at the present time. The following are some examples.

LICHEN RUBER MONILIFORMIS is, in our opinion, a variant of lichen simplex chronicus; the supposed beaded arrangement of the papules, reflected in the designation "moniliformis," is nothing more than the prominent alveolar pattern

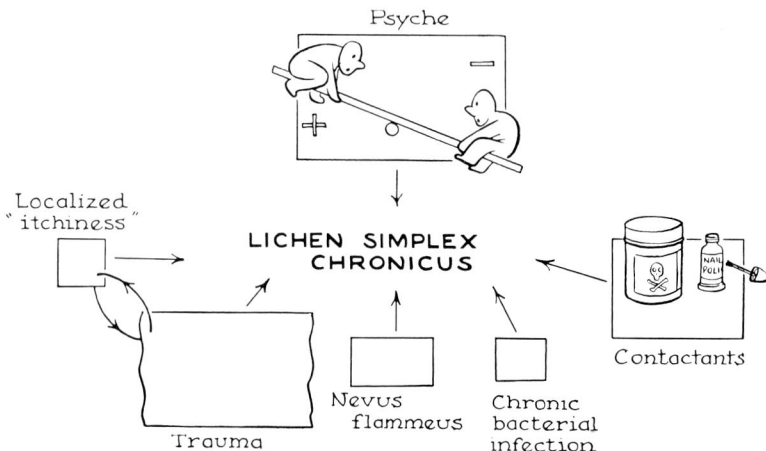

Figure 5–34 Factors contributing to lichen simplex chronicus.

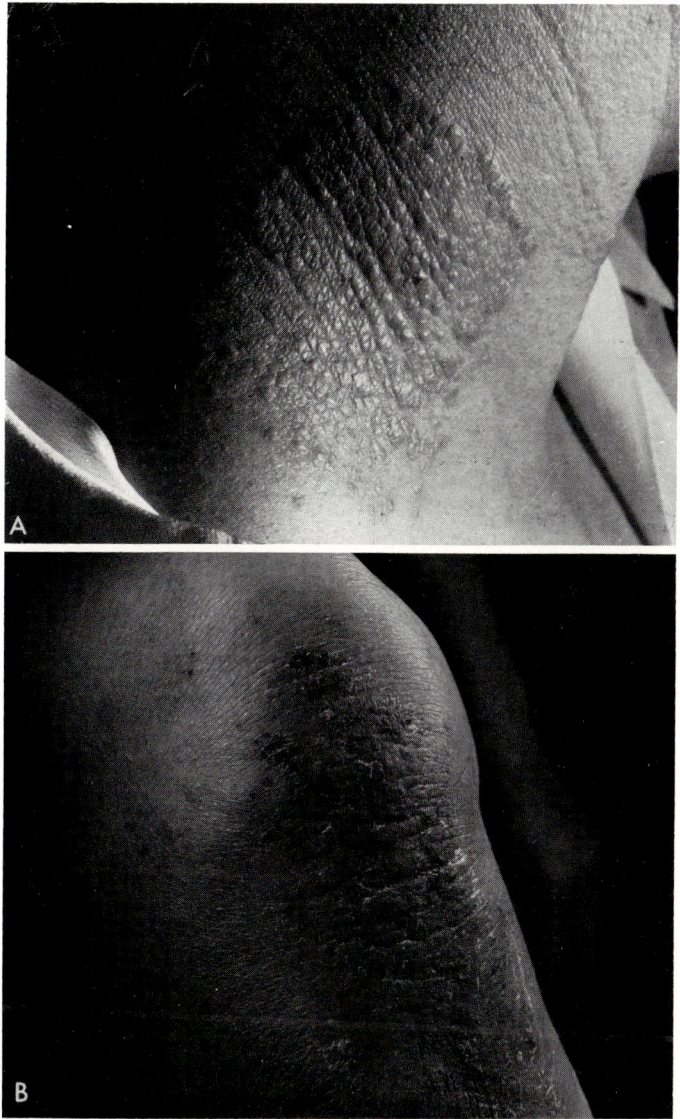

Figure 5–35 Typical circumscribed neurodermatitis of (*A*) neck, (*B*) prepatellar region.

of the skin lying between the deepened furrows.

LICHENIFICATIO GIGANTEA is another variant of lichen simplex chronicus. Thick, verrucous patches are formed which generally show some features of ordinary lichenification at the periphery. The predilected regions are the legs and groin.

POLYMORPHIC NEURODERMATITIS (POLYMORPHIC PRURIGO). Originally a nerve abnormality was presumed to be the basis of neurodermatitic lesions, but modern concepts of psychogenesis have brought about a revision in meaning, making some reclassification mandatory. Older

entities, considered distinct, may now be consolidated as natural relationships become evident. The term "polymorphic neurodermatitis" encompasses an extremely variable syndrome of possible psychic origin, having the potentiality of producing different types of lesions at the same or different times, and varying in extensiveness, course, and morphologic expression in different patients. The prototype of this syndrome is the "exudative discoid and lichenoid dermatitis" of Sulzberger-Garbe (oid-oid disease). Nowhere is there a better example of the protean and mutable nature of psychocutaneous expression. The manifestations include lesions typically encountered in other separately classified disorders, namely, exudative neurodermatitis (nummular eczema), disseminated neurodermatitis, lichen simplex chronicus, and even lichen planus.

Oid-oid disease provides the opportunity to see these different psychocutaneous components in ensemble and reveals the connections and close relationships among the members of this group. Individual patients vary greatly in respect to how many of these components are present at the same or different times and to what degree. The generic term polymorphic neurodermatitis has the advantage of including all the variations, of which oid-oid disease may be regarded simply as the ultimate type. In the classic form of the latter, more or less distinct phases can be recognized, though this should not be taken too literally. The first phase is mainly exudative, with weeping discoid and oval patches scattered irregularly over the body surface, save the scalp, palms, and soles. Many of the lesions are of the nummular eczema type, erythematous, oozing patches, ordinarily containing many tiny vesicles and subsequently becoming crusted. Eventually, these may undergo lichenification. Many of the discoid patches acquire an infiltrated feel and the picture at times strongly suggests mycosis fungoides. In the next phase, the exudative lesions regress or at least stop oozing and become dry and lichenified. Discrete lichenoid papules, many of them follicular, are present; some resemble lichen planus. In progressive cases, a generalized, lichenified, scaling eruption develops, has characteristics of an exfoliative dermatitis, and is indistinguishable from disseminated neurodermatitis. Showers of urticarial lesions occur from time to time throughout the evolution of the disorder. The itching is maddening. The course is chronic with partial remissions. Oid-oid disease, in full flower with its various phases, is rather uncommon. It is not limited to Jews, but seems to be far more prevalent in them.

The older term "prurigo" has variable meanings to different clinicians, and has attracted a wide variety of qualifying terms, many of them obsolete. Though some of these terms may have hidden underlying factors, the pervading one is a response to trauma by the patient.

Prurigo nodularis is seen in the form of persistent, violently pruritic nodules, principally on the extremities in middle-aged women (Fig. 5–36). Probably as the result of trauma, schwannomas are seen histologically in the dermis and result from the accelerated turnover rate of nerve fibers and Schwann cells. In some patients, a psychosomatic factor appears to be operative, but it is difficult to determine whether this is a cause or the result of constant itching and, often, much loss of sleep. Furious scratching may produce fissures, hemorrhagic crusts, or markedly verrucous changes. The disorder is extremely resistant to treatment. Intralesional injections of a corticosteroid are often effective in prurigo nodularis.

Treatment

The only thing which needs to be accomplished to cure circumscribed neurodermatitis is the prevention of scratching. This may be produced very simply in some patients; in others, it defies all measures. It is particularly important that this suppression of the impulse to scratch

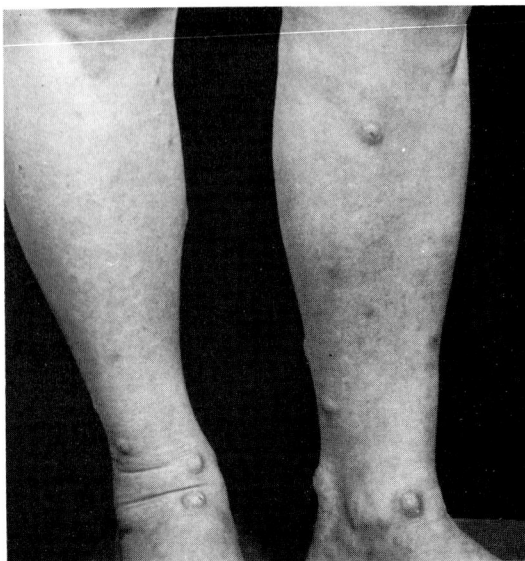

Figure 5–36 Prurigo nodularis. Persistent pruritic nodules of the lower extremities in a 50-year-old neurotic woman. The pruritus and nodules are temporarily reduced by intralesional steroid.

be without further irritation of the affected patch, because irritation will only serve to re-initiate the scratch-itch-scratch cycle.

The following methods of treatment of circumscribed neurodermatitis are listed in approximate descending order of importance:

EXPLANATION TO PATIENT. When the diagnosis of circumscribed neurodermatitis is made, and this is not difficult, it is of the utmost importance to explain the condition to the patient. He must understand clearly that if he does not scratch the area, the skin changes will disappear. It should be pointed out that even moderate occasional light rubbing of the skin may be sufficient to perpetuate the changes, and also that rubbing and scratching may be done quite unconsciously, even while the patient is asleep. It must be understood by the patient that it is essential that he bring the excoriation to the level of a conscious, known movement.

THERAPY. The availability of potent topically applied corticosteroid preparations has revolutionized the treatment of lichen simplex chronicus. Inunction of a small amount of the cream or ointment twice daily is often sufficient, particularly if it relieves the itching. This failing, occlusion of the affected area with Saran Wrap or similar film at night increases the therapeutic effect. In small, nonhairy areas this may conveniently be accomplished by corticosteroid-mediated tape (Cordran tape). A more intensive measure is the intralesional injection of a corticosteroid suspension. With this method, care must be exercised in respect to the amount and concentration of the steroid, lest atrophy of the skin be produced.

For temporary relief of episodes of pruritus, application of very hot or very cold compresses may afford considerable relief. The topical use of benzocaine or related compounds is unwise because of the risk of inducing sensitization.

Since neurodermatitis is initiated by a number of other dermatoses, treatment appropriate for them may be necessary if recurrences are to be prevented. Examples of this are the treatment of seborrheic dermatitis associated with localized neurodermatitis of the scalp, of an associated psoriasis, of tinea cruris which may be the progenitor of lichen simplex chronicus in the groin, and of various precipitating factors in anal and vulvar pruritus.

FIXED DRESSINGS. When the localization of a patch of circumscribed neurodermatitis makes such treatment feasible, the application of a fixed dressing which will prevent scratching may cause very rapid involution of the dermatitis. The application of adhesive directly over the area often produces reactions, however, and some other type of dressing such as Plastex gauze or even an Unna's boot type of dressing may be better tolerated. If this produces improvement, it will ordinarily become evident within three or four days and be associated with a reduction or cessation of itching.

STASIS DERMATITIS

Dermatitis of the lower legs related to stasis following peripheral venous disease constitutes a clear-cut condition. If neglected by the patient in its earlier phases, and it usually is, it may progress to inflammation and persistent ulceration for which there is no entirely satisfactory treatment. While edema and evidence of venous incompetency are the most common preliminary warnings of stasis dermatitis, they are by no means always present. In many patients, the edema and varicosities are not striking. Hemosiderin deposits in the skin are almost invariably noted. The pathologic changes are not confined to the veins but may involve arterioles. Recurrent localized thrombophlebitis is frequently present. A characteristic brawny low-grade cellulitis is typical of long-standing stasis dermatitis.

The favorite initial site of involvement is on the inner lower leg just above the internal malleolus. In patients with obese or edematous lower legs, a characteristic dimpling, due to attachment of the subcutaneous tissues, is noted in this region. It is a highly vulnerable area, in which the vascular supply and nutrition of the skin and subcutaneous tissues are less adequate than elsewhere on the lower legs.

Initial evidence of inadequacy of the vascular system of the lower legs is frequently a deposit of hemosiderin following diapedesis of red cells. This may be quite extensive and may assume rather varied patterns. While extensive hemosiderin deposition may be seen on the lower legs in younger persons as a result of allergic purpura or other causation, it is overwhelmingly more common in persons of middle age or above. It is sometimes accompanied by itching and a lichenoid eruption. These varied patterns have led to descriptions of a variety of cutaneous syndromes to which several long and complicated terms have been applied, but which are essentially similar.

The prodromal phases of stasis dermatitis are usually prolonged and fairly clearcut. It is of importance that these early signs be recognized promptly and simple measures taken to combat progression of the disease. Moderate restriction of physical exercise, particularly in respect to prolonged standing, may easily prevent the development of changes which are not completely reversible. The prevention of thrombophlebitis as a complication of major surgical procedures, of fractures, of pregnancy, of various systemic infections and other diseases is of the greatest importance. In many patients with severe stasis dermatitis in which the precipitating anatomic and physiologic derangements are irreversible, the onset may be traced to a failure to recognize and deal with evidences of beginning thrombus forma-tion. The "milk leg" of Victorian medicine is now largely preventable by adequate anticoagulant therapy and the application of sound general medical and surgical principles in any patient who has been severely traumatized by injury or disease.

The onset of active stasis dermatitis and ulceration may take one of several forms. The usual one is the development of an area of rather cyanotic erythema which frequently itches. The initial site of involvement is the area of the lower leg immediately above the internal malleolus of the ankle. A scratch dermatitis may be produced. Local topical treatment may induce a primary irritant or sensitization reaction; the lower legs in patients with stasis dermatitis are exceedingly susceptible to such reactions. This complication may involve the entire lower legs or portions thereof, and the development of patches elsewhere on the body as an apparent result of absorption from the primary focus on the legs is common.

Ulceration may develop rapidly, but more often only after some degree of stasis dermatitis has been present for years. It may appear at the site of a superficial localized vasculitis which breaks down in an exquisitely painful ulcer with a "trophic" appearance, not particularly inflammatory, sharply marginated, and relatively superficial. The lesion heals

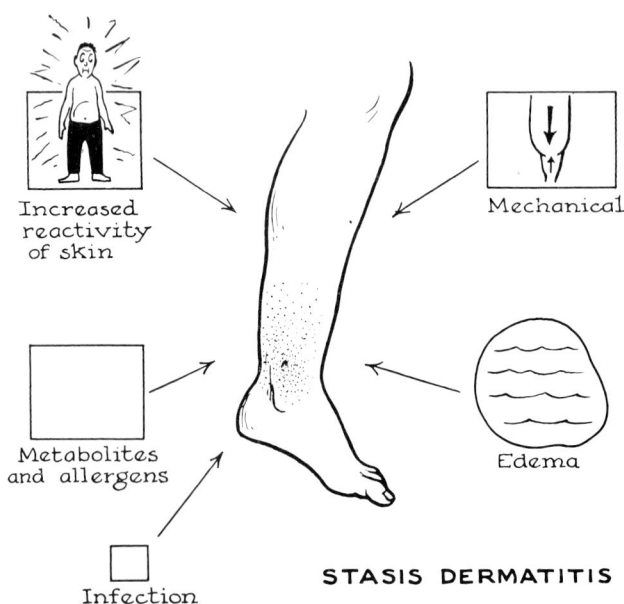

Increased
reactivity
of skin

Mechanical

Metabolites
and allergens

Edema

Infection

STASIS DERMATITIS

Figure 5–37.

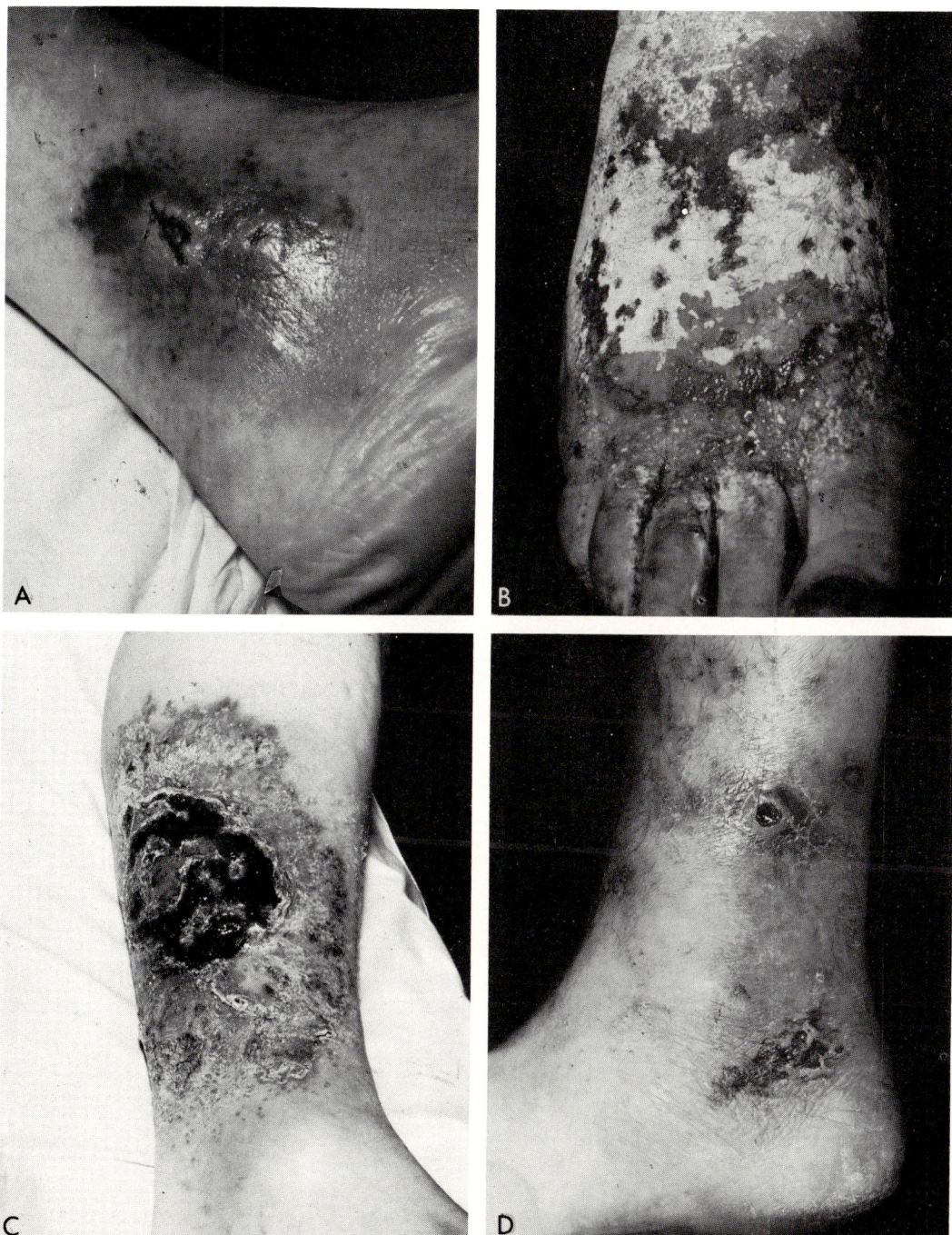

Figure 5-38 Types of ulcerative lower leg lesions. *A*, Hemosiderin, hyperpigmentation, and "traumatic" ulcers in a patient with hypertensive cardiovascular disease. No gross evidence of stasis. *B*, Contact sensitization reaction to nitrofuran. Patch test positive. *C*, Stasis, varicosities, dermatitis, and ulceration. *D*, Multiple, punched-out ulcers in a patient with moderate evidence of stasis.

with formation of ivory-white telangiectatic sclerotic plaques with a surrounding hyperpigmentation; the condition has been described as atrophie blanche. In other cases, an area of indurated low-grade cellulitis may develop which goes on to ulceration. At times there is a definite history of moderate injury which simply fails to heal or in which there is evidence of secondary bacterial infection.

When stasis dermatitis becomes well established, particularly if there is ulceration and evidence of contact sensitization of the skin, effective management becomes exceedingly difficult in some patients, and restoration to normality may be impossible.

In the management of stasis dermatitis, the following therapeutic aspects are emphasized.

Prevention

Since a considerable proportion of patients with stasis dermatitis give a history of preceding thrombophlebitis following an operation, pregnancy, or an acute infection, it is obviously of importance that this complication be prevented insofar as possible at the time of acute trauma or illness and treated promptly and vigorously if it occurs.

In individuals who have never sustained a clear-cut thrombophlebitis of the iliofemoral vein, the prodromal signs indicating the eventual development of stasis phenomena are often just as clear-cut. Obese persons or those with congenitally large lower legs, particularly women, are highly susceptible. Persistent slowly developing edema which is present on retiring but disappears by morning is well worthy of thorough investigation as to cause. In other persons, marked "primary" superficial varicosities may develop, and these are worthy of attention prior to the onset of secondary inflammatory changes. In other patients, gradually increasing deposition of hemosiderin subcutaneously may be the only sign, and this is sometimes accompanied by small areas of whitening or even definite superficial atrophy of the skin. The preceding changes are obviously much more likely to occur in persons whose occupations involve much standing. In such patients, a change in work habits

to obviate long periods of standing may be possible. Patients with stasis are well advised to acquire the habit of placing the feet at body level or above as often as possible while sitting. This may not be a particularly dignified posture, but it is a physiologic one if stasis and lymphedema are present.

Persons who have had erythema nodosum, erythema induratum, nodular vasculitis, or recurrent chilblains may often anticipate the development of increasing evidences of stasis in future years. In part, each of these conditions may to some extent have originally been associated with moderate preexistent stasis.

Supportive dressings are useful and are undergoing constant improvement from both physiologic and cosmetic standpoints. Ace bandages, if properly applied, are helpful, though unsightly on women. By and large, the use of supportive bandages not containing rubber is to be preferred if there is any significant degree of dermatitis. A very effective modality of treatment is the application of a gelocast boot which is covered and thereby reinforced by an elastic dressing (3M Coban elastic bandage) which is worn for at least 10 days to two weeks. Excessively heavy surgical stockings are now being replaced to some extent by lighter materials made of nylon impregnated with an elastic. It is particularly important that such supportive stockings be carefully fitted, because otherwise there may be areas which receive no support whatever, or folds in the elastic stocking may inflict considerable trauma to the skin. Inflated supportive devices (for example, Jobst stocking), in which gentle even pressure can be maintained by air pressure, are receiving increased use, though the expense of such "air boots" is a limiting factor. They must be expertly fitted by specially trained technicians.

These supportive dressings should be applied in the morning before the patient gets out of bed. It may be advisable to give support well above the knee in some patients.

Active Therapy

In the presence of definite stasis dermatitis or ulceration, the measures for improving blood and lymphatic return should be intensified. It may be necessary for the patient to rest in bed for an hour in the afternoon and early evening, if possible. Prolonged inactivity in bed is not advised, however, because this sometimes seems to increase the tendency to local or extensive thrombophlebitis.

TOPICAL APPLICATIONS. In reviewing the experience of many patients with stasis dermatitis, it is difficult to avoid the conclusion that the topical therapy employed has often done more harm than good. It is certainly true that topical treatment will be of little or no value if measures to combat the stasis are not taken. The skin of the lower legs in stasis dermatitis is exceedingly susceptible to sensitization reactions, and measures which may be used with reasonable impunity elsewhere on the body may be contraindicated here. Care should be taken in respect to possible sensitivity to adhesive tape in applying dressings. It would appear that bacterial infection is not as common a factor in stasis ulcers as is supposed, and the overuse of antibacterial compounds may be harmful. Simple nonirritating ointments, such as 2 per cent ichthammol in zinc oxide ointment or Burow's paste, are often as good as anything else. The use of nitrofuran ointment and of ointments containing antibiotics is not advised. Corticosteroid ointments may be very helpful in reducing the superficial inflammation and itching, but they also have variable vasoconstricting effects.

In acute exudative stasis dermatitis, elevation of the leg and wet compresses become advisable. If the reaction is truly severe, and particularly if there is evidence of patches of dermatitis appearing elsewhere on the body, the systemic administration of a corticosteroid may be justifiable for a short time, provided that no significant contraindications exist.

UNNA'S BOOT. Supportive therapy by means of the zinc gelatin dressing commonly known as Unna's boot is a very useful measure. While it should not be applied when there is extensive acute oozing, the presence of some degree of active dermatitis or of ulceration is not a contraindication. If there is doubt as to the presence of active infection, a window may be cut in the boot to observe the area in question. The type of boot used may be that originally recommended, or one of the prepared commercial dressings with or without an added elastic bandage for reinforcement. It is preferable to apply the boot after the leg has been raised and the edema allowed to subside for a time. Evenness of application is essential; otherwise, rubbing may prove troublesome. The boot is ordinarily allowed to remain in place for at least a week, though an earlier replacement may be necessary if there is much oozing or ulceration.

Continuous even pressure is essential to the healing of stasis ulcers. A useful device for obtaining this is a piece of sponge rubber, a centimeter or more thick, cut with a liberal margin to overlap the skin surrounding the ulcer. Theoretically the rubber should be sterilized, but practically it makes no difference. To avoid undue pressure at the margin of the sponge rubber, some beveling of it is advisable. The sponge rubber may be kept in place with an ordinary dressing or under an Ace bandage or gelatin boot. Occasional instances of sensitivity to sponge rubber will be encountered, but these are uncommon.

While bacterial infection is not frequently a predominant factor in stasis ulcers, there will be occasional instances when this will be the case. It may be suspected if there is excessive gross purulent exudate, a markedly inflammatory zone about the ulcer, rapid extension of the ulcer, or a tendency to an undermined overhanging border. Bacteriologic study of such lesions is worthwhile, and it is of importance to obtain adequate smears. Culture for anaerobic organisms may be useful. When these are present, greater opportunity for aeration of the ulcer may be advisable; the use of a zinc peroxide paste may be helpful. The latter may be made by mixing zinc peroxide with water to form a paste and applying it to the ulcer under a dressing. Activation of the zinc peroxide by heating will increase the release of oxygen, but this is not essential. Zinc peroxide is particularly effective in reducing the odor of stinking ulcers.

If the ulcer persists or enlarges in spite of good therapy, biopsy of the margin should be done to diagnose the unusual complication of a basal or squamous cell epithelioma.

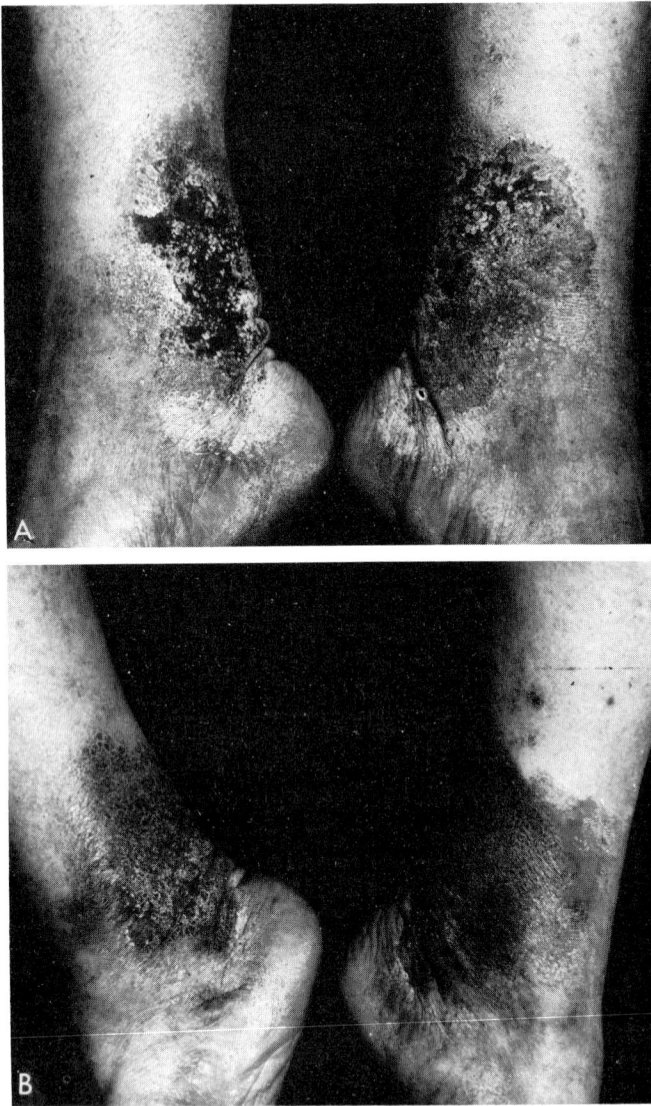

Figure 5-39 *A*, Bilateral stasis dermatitis in a patient who had sustained a bilateral thrombophlebitis many years previously. No marked edema. Severe itching. *B*, One month later. Slow improvement with hydrocortisone and 2 per cent ichthammol ointments, plus regulation of exercise regimen. Occasional relapses almost inescapable.

SURGICAL THERAPY. Since dermatitis and ulceration due to stasis are basically caused by disturbances in the dynamics of return blood flow, the condition is sometimes susceptible of relief by well-selected surgical therapy. This is particularly true if the disturbance is recognized early in its course and the indicated surgical therapy carried out. It is outside the scope of this discussion and the experience of the author to discuss surgical therapy in any detail. It may be remarked, however, that surgical therapy is by no means always indicated and may be detrimental. During the past twenty years, there have been successive waves of enthusiasm for various surgical methods. The therapeutic injection of sclerosing solutions for varicosities in lieu of surgery has been almost completely abandoned except for unusual and local conditions. High ligation of the saphenous vein is sometimes helpful and is a relatively simple procedure in the hands of a competent surgeon. As of now, it would appear that multiple ligations and the stripping of veins is the more popular procedure in the presence of severe varicosities.

It is obvious that any decision as to correction of varicosities of superficial veins must be preceded by the most careful study to determine the competence of the deep venous system. It also seems reasonable to insist that surgical therapy be undertaken by surgeons with experience in peripheral vascular diseases.

CHRONIC ECZEMATOUS DERMATITIS

This very large segment of the dermatitis-eczema group, which is in some respects a catch-all for dermatitis which cannot otherwise be classified, has been designated by a number of names. It may be regarded as a type of dermatitis in which secondary factors have largely or completely superseded the original instigator of the inflammation. Not infrequently it will be found that the process started originally as a contact dermatitis, either of primary irritant or sensitization type, with prolonged exposure and the development of more or less "irreversible" inflammatory changes in the skin. This has led to the use of the term "contact-type." Because of occasional evidences of infection in such chronic dermatitis, the term chronic infectious eczematoid dermatitis has come into wide use, though this often places undue weight upon the bacterial factor in the process.

In chronic eczematous dermatitis there is no set pattern of distribution of lesions nor a characteristic course which would place it in one of the six better defined groups. All the clinical phases of dermatitis may be seen, from the acute inflammatory to the chronic thickened types. Lesions may be single or multiple. One portion of the body, such as the face, the hands or feet, or the anogenital region, may be the sole site of involvement for long periods. The most characteristic site of involvement may clear entirely for many months until a sudden relapse occurs through forces which are often difficult to determine. Many of the chronic industrial dermatitides behave in this manner.

Chronic eczematous dermatitis constitutes a significant public health problem. It is by no means under adequate control; in fact, it is a constantly expanding area of clinical dermatology. The constant increase in this problem is attributable to the continuous and increased exposure of the public to new and old therapeutic and cosmetic drugs and preparations, as well as to industrial hazards.

Following the production of a chronic dermatitis by repeated application of a compound, the secondary additive factors or "collaborators" assume the burden of perpetuating the dermatitis. Figure 5–40 indicates the principal factors which contribute to chronicity. These have been discussed in connection with certain of the more basic patterns of dermatitis. The role of trauma, both physical and chemical, is often marked, for example, the rubbing of a shoe or continued irritation from a strong industrial cleanser. Disturbances in the bacterial and fungal flora of the skin are frequently noted. The micrococci which are normally present in abundance ordinarily disappear completely. More or less marked evidence of secondary bacterial infection may be present. A marked change in the fungal flora may be seen, as in the presence of an abundance of Candida in some reactions to broad-spectrum antibiotics.

Patients with chronic eczematous dermatitis are often prone to marked sensitivity to topical medicaments. During acute flare-ups of the process, the skin may be unable to tolerate even very bland common preparations. It is of particular importance that the possibility of further contact sensitization be kept in mind in connection with all new topical medicaments. The use of known potent sensitizers should be avoided, and the patient must be instructed to use any new local preparation on only a small area initially and then to observe this site for 24 hours before applying it more widely.

The factor of possible photosensitization in a dermatitis must not be neglected. It would appear to be increasing. Among the chemicals which may induce photosensitive reactions are sulfonamides, para-aminobenzoic acid, sulfonylurea, chlorthiazides, phenothiazides, antibiotics (demethylchlortetracycline and chlortetracycline, griseofulvin), furocoumarins, coal tar and its derivatives, halogenated salicylanilides, and artificial sweeteners.

Regardless of the limited extent or ap-

THE ORIGINATORS

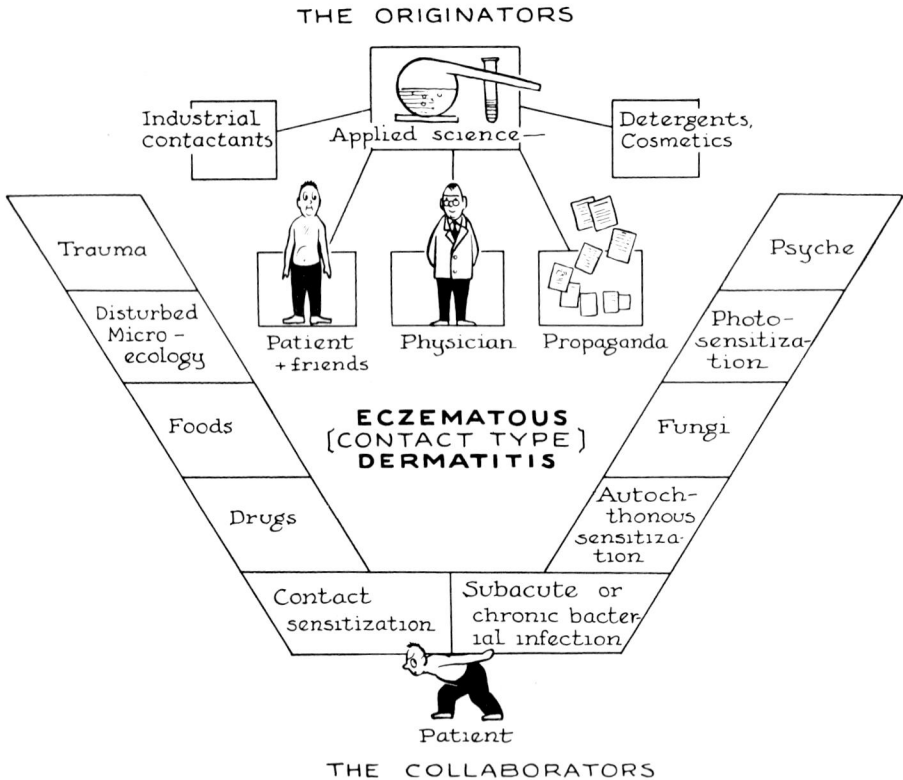

Figure 5–40   The pattern of origination and perpetuation of chronic eczematous dermatitis.

parent initial cause of a chronic eczematous dermatitis, the possibility of perpetuation of the process by drugs must be kept in mind. Trial interdiction of all drugs, including such common household ones as aspirin, vitamins, barbiturates, and tonics, should be carried out for at least two weeks. In many chronic eruptions related to drug sensitivity, the dermatitis may not disappear promptly on cessation of the medication. It is a well-established fact that a contact dermatitis which has been originally produced by topical application of a compound, for example, a sulfonamide, may be reactivated by internal administration. It has also been shown that certain "certified" dyes of the azo group may induce sensitization on local application, and this may be reactivated by ingestion of the dyes in food stuffs or by the administration of chemical compounds of similar molecular structure. There are many examples of cross group sensitization to compounds having an amino group in the para position on the benzene ring, such as quinones, azo dyes, sulfonamides, PABA, and procaine.

Reaction to Foods

The role of ingested foods in the production of dermatitis is a point of considerable disagreement as to relative importance. While it is not to be doubted that in occasional instances a particular food can be shown to be capable of producing dermatitis, this is regarded as a rarity by some and as an important causative or contributory factor in from 5 to 10 per cent of all cases of chronic eczematous dermatitis by others. Part of this difference of opinion may lie in the great difficulty of proving the presence or absence of food sensitivity in the individual patient. Scratch and intradermal tests with food extracts are not, in our experience, of any value in determining this. The possible role of foods may be ascertained only on the basis of various types of trial elimination diets, which are sometimes exceed-

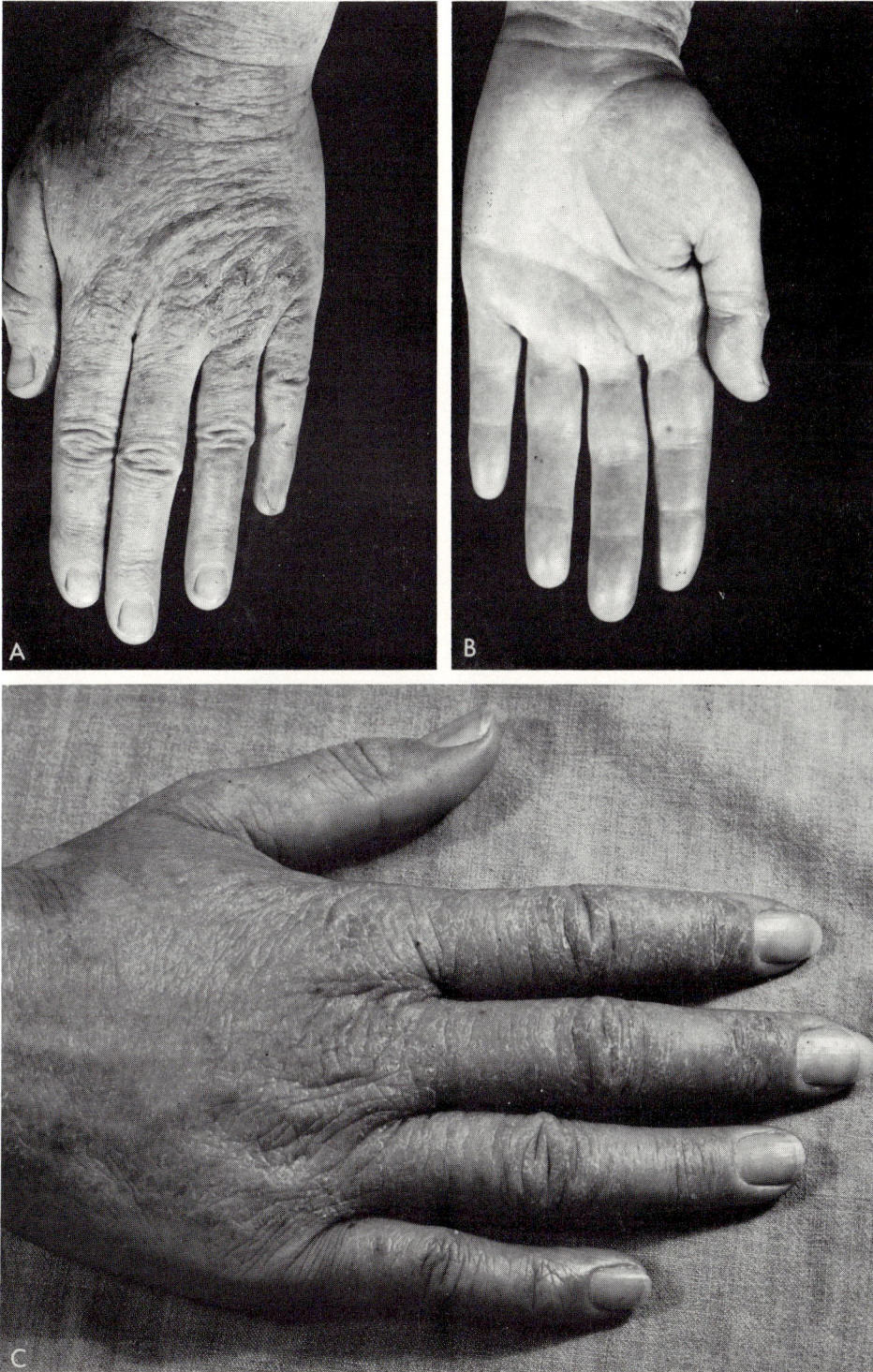

Figure 5–41 Chronic eczematous dermatitis. "Housewives' hands." *A* and *B* show the absence of involvement of the palm seen early in this dermatitis. *C*, Thickening, scaling, and fissuring in chronic phase.

ingly tedious to both patient and physician. It is easy to misinterpret the results of such diets, and the effects, at best, are often far from clear-cut.

Treatment

The treatment of chronic eczematous dermatitis is very similar to that outlined for contact and nummular dermatitis. Hydrocortisone and antibacterial ointments are frequently of value. If the dermatitis is of limited extent, it is difficult to justify the administration of steroids internally.

For purposes of convenience, the problems of infantile eczema and of chronic dermatitis involving the hands and feet receive separate consideration. Both types present peculiarities in course and special problems in treatment, though they do not constitute truly separate dermatologic entities.

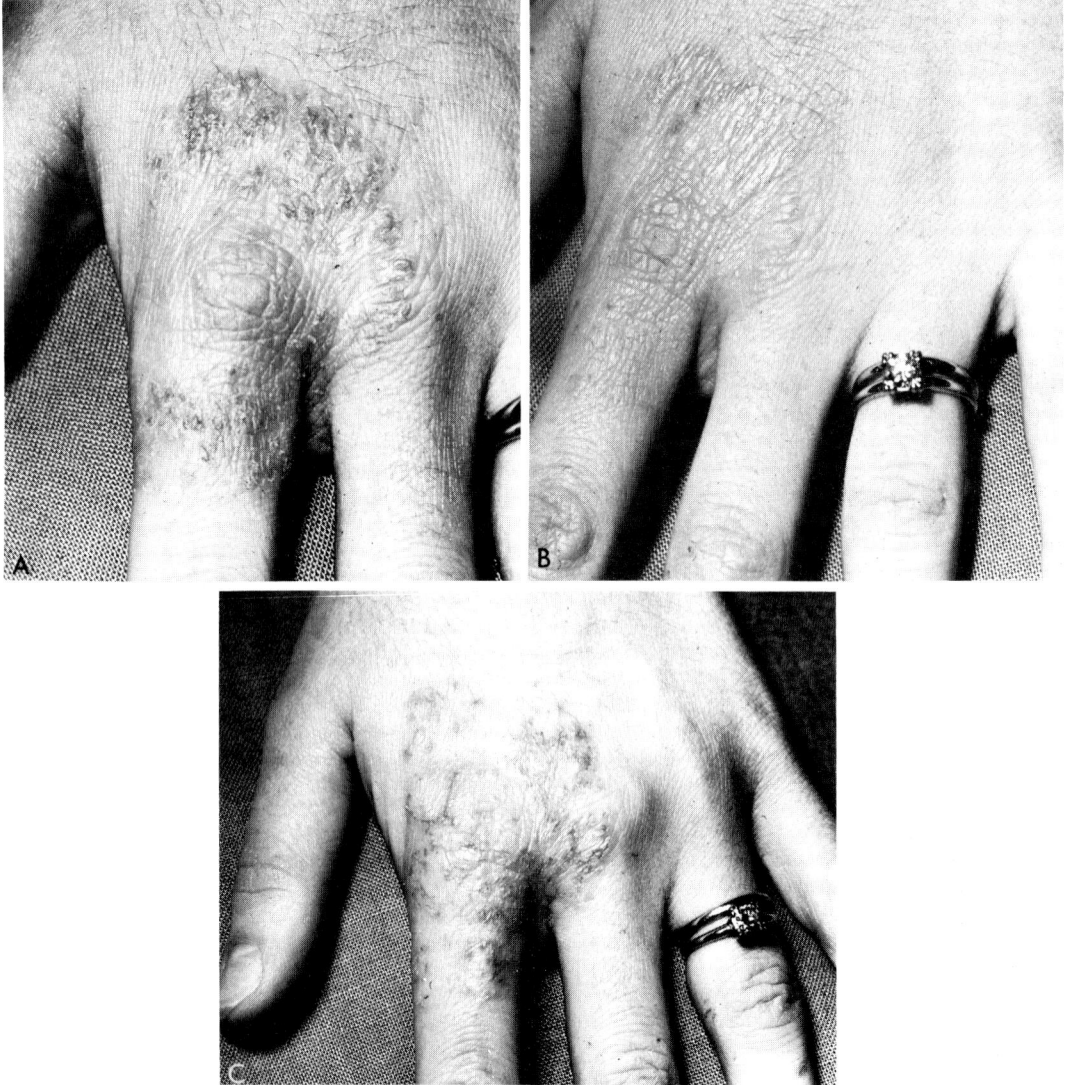

Figure 5-42   Nummular eczema type of lesion on dorsum of hand of eight months' duration. Failed to respond to local treatment and four x-ray treatments. *A*, December 11, 1950—appearance on original visit. *B*, December 15, 1950—improvement after four days of low allergen diet. No local treatment. *C*, December 27, 1950—exacerbation following the breaking of diet over Christmas. Sensitivity to tomatoes was demonstrable. (Courtesy of Dr. James R. Flood, Guthrie Clinic, Sayre, Pennsylvania.)

INFANTILE ECZEMA

The problem of infantile eczema is a continuing enigma. It is difficult to classify the dermatitis changes accurately in many instances or to determine the principal etiologic factors. The most common type of infantile eczema, atopic dermatitis, is one of the most difficult of all chronic diseases to control. Its course is capricious and uncertain, the affected infant highly uncomfortable, and the parents often overwrought and concerned. In contrast to atopic dermatitis, there is an additional variety of eczematous changes of the infant's skin which are relatively evanescent and which respond promptly to appropriate treatment.

The skin of the infant is more susceptible to primary irritation than that of the adult; subacute or acute superficial bacterial infection is more prone to develop; and the vasomotor responses in the form of erythema and localized swelling are often more marked in the infantile skin than in older children and adults. In any individual instance of infantile eczema, it is usually impossible to predict whether or not the condition will eventually develop into characteristic atopic dermatitis. The following conditions are the various clinical expressions of infantile eczema.

Contact Dermatitis in Infants

Contact dermatitis based upon a true sensitization reaction is rare in infants. On the other hand, primary irritation is very common. The areas affected are often bright red, swollen, and sharply marginated. The most frequently involved area is the face, and foods which have only mild primary irritant properties in the adult may be responsible. Orange and tomato juices are examples. The infant's face may be continuously irritated by the constant moistening of the skin with saliva and regurgitated feedings; the resultant dermatitis may be further aggravated by the child's rubbing of the affected area against the bed linen. Other common sites of primary irritant dermatitis include the elbows and knees, rubbed on sheets or carpets, and areas which are constricted and moist from clothing and diapers. In some instances, the changes seen are very similar to chapping seen in adults, though often more sharply localized. These changes may become particularly marked upon exposure to cold or wind. The healthy appearing "apple cheeks" of some infants and young children often actually represent moderate dermatitic changes which deserve simple preventive treatment.

A specialized and very common form of contact dermatitis in infants is that occurring in the diaper region (diaper or napkin dermatitis, erythema of Jacquet). In spite of the most scrupulous maternal care, the diaper region of infants is inevitably exposed to prolonged contact with feces and urine and to variable bacterial flora and decomposition products. With such exposure, blockage of sweat ducts is an inevitable sequel, and all types of sweat retention may be seen as components of diaper dermatitis. A long accepted explanation of the etiology of diaper dermatitis is that it is the result of irritation of the skin by the ammoniac decomposition products of urine. We are not aware of any absolute proof of this theory, attractive as it may be, insofar as the specific effects of a higher pH and of any decomposition product are concerned. The folds of skin about the buttocks in overweight infants furnish an excellent starting point for irritation, since they are difficult to cleanse thoroughly and are often incompletely dried after bathing. Whether or not application of special antibacterial rinses to the diapers has any effectiveness may be debated, though it is now standard practice in diaper washing services.

Seborrheic and Intertriginous Infantile Eczema

This is a distinct type of eczema seen most frequently in young infants. If it is recognized early and properly treated, the prognosis is good. If neglected, however, it may progress to extensive intertriginous involvement with secondary bacterial and candidal infection, or to an extensive exfoliative form of seborrheic dermatitis known as Leiner's disease. A type of fatal familial Leiner's disease associated with a deficiency of the opsonic activity of serum complement has been described (Jacobs

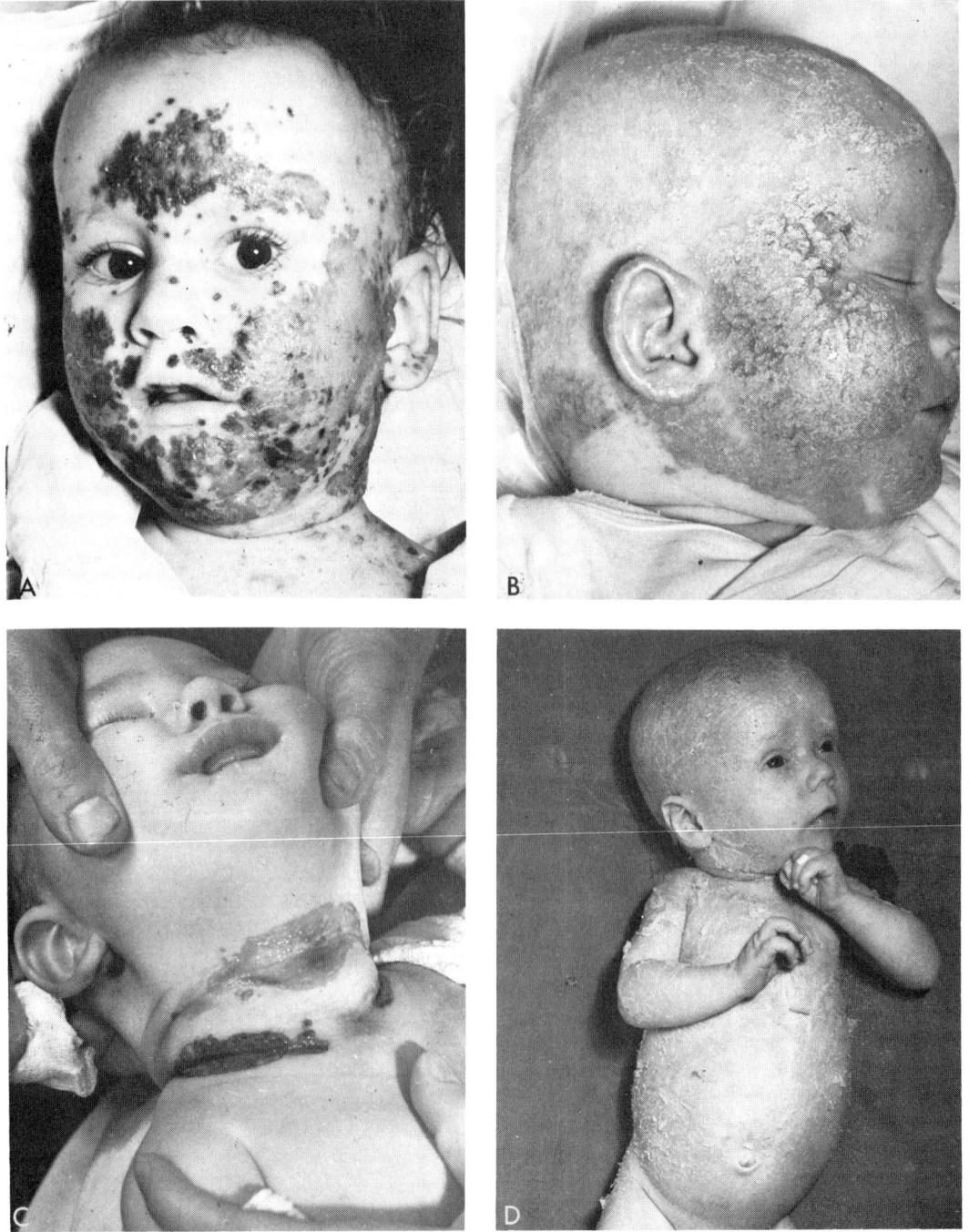

Figure 5–43   Variants of infantile eczema. *A*, Secondary inoculation with virus of herpes simplex (eczema herpeticum). *B*, Seborrheic eczema in overweight infant. *C*, Intertriginous seborrheic eczema with erosive escharotic reaction to 2 per cent gentian violet tincture. *D*, Diffuse exfoliative seborrheic eczema.

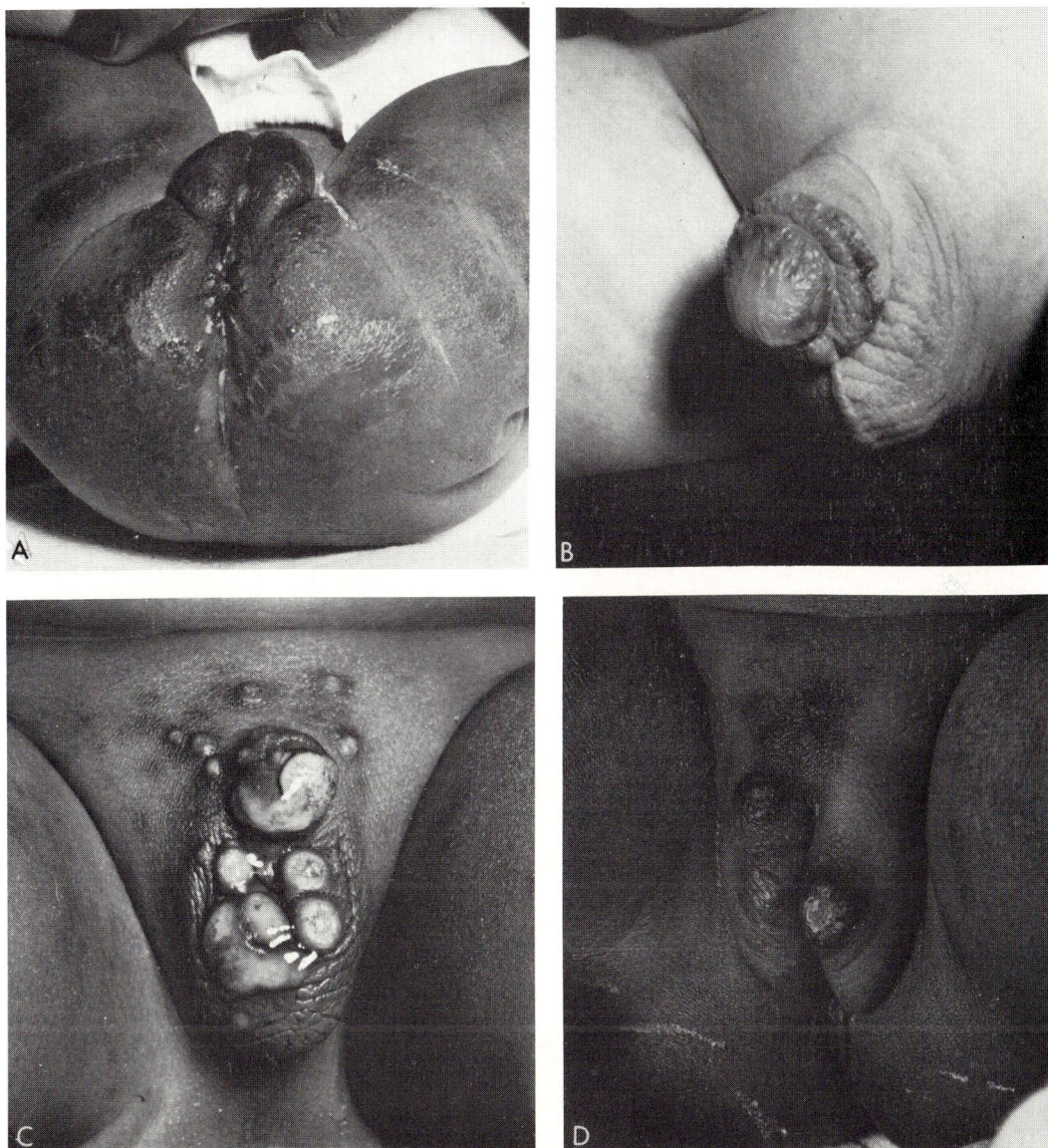

Figure 5–44 Variations of diaper dermatitis. The papular erosive type requires prolonged neglect for development. The mild cases present with a mild scaling dermatitis of the anogenital area. However, in more severe cases, vesicles and papules with superficial erosions or ulcerations are seen.

and Miller, 1972). Neonates with this condition have a severe generalized eruption with intractable diarrhea, local and systemic infection, and wasting. They have a functional C5 deficiency. Other members of the family also exhibit a defective opsonizing activity in the plasma. Fresh plasma as a source of C5 can be lifesaving.

The simplest evidence of seborrheic dermatitis is ordinary "cradle cap." This is seen most frequently over the vertex of the scalp in infants whose skin sometimes appears grossly oily and in whom milia and comedones may be present on the face. The scale on the scalp is often rather adherent and greasy, without any evidence of underlying inflammation at its onset. It frequently accumulates through the young mother's fear of washing the scalp over the open fontanelle.

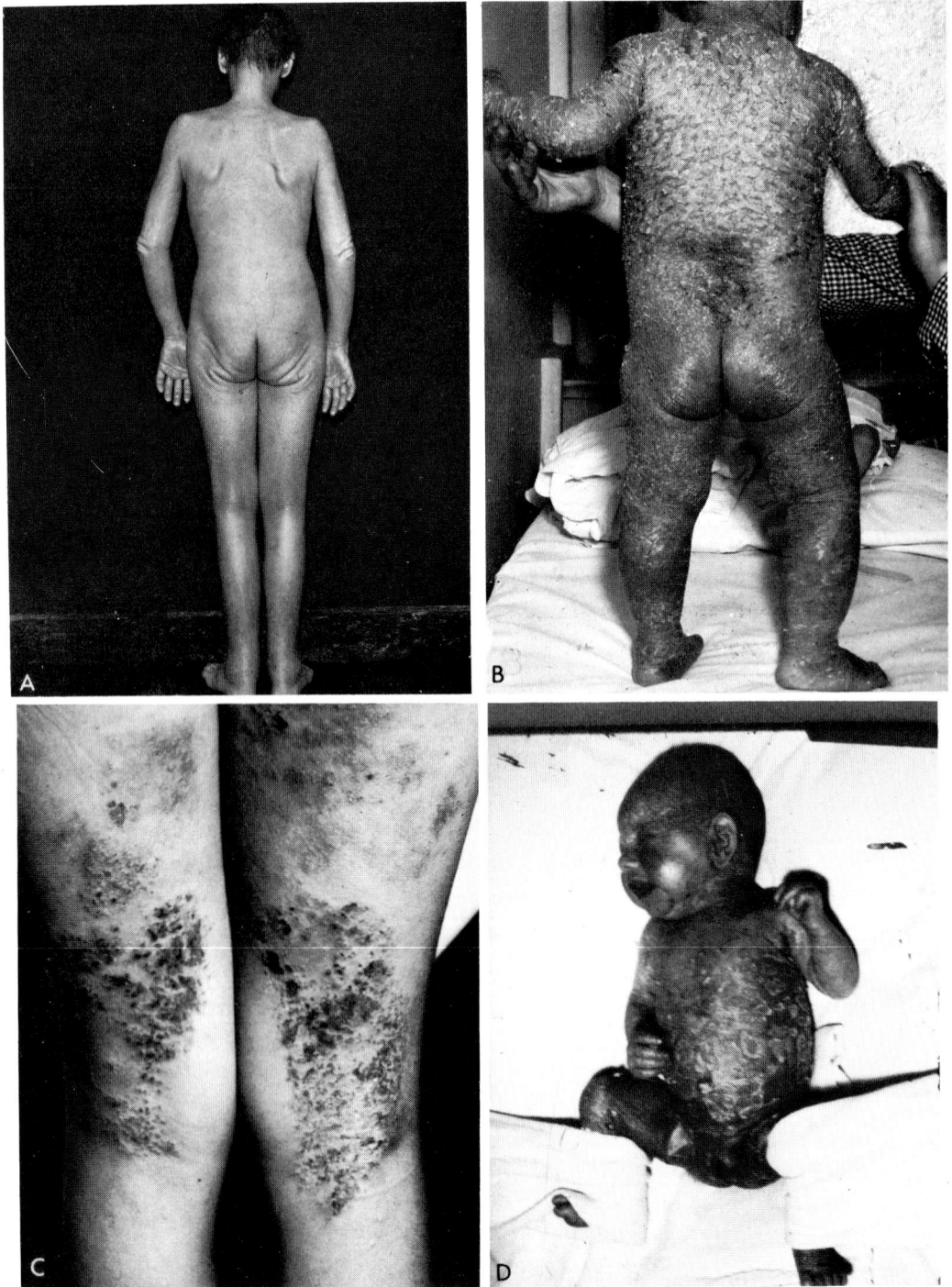

Figure 5–45 *A*, Diffuse erythroderma in atopic teen-ager. Generalized lymphadenopathy. Edema of lower legs. *B*, Diffuse severe atopic dermatitis in infants with congenital ichthyosis. *C*, Patchy extensive atopic dermatitis. *D*, Seborrheic dermatitis (Leiner's syndrome?) in sick, underweight infant.

A definite form of seborrheic eczema is seen in the development of sharply marginated, usually symmetric, eczematous plaques on the cheeks, which may appear swollen and angry. In its well-developed form, this variant of eczema may be striking in appearance, but control of it at this phase is ordinarily fairly simple. If it is allowed to persist, however, bacteria become established easily, and gross evidence of bacterial infection may be seen. Coincident with this, fissures and inflammation of the retroauricular fold and of the intertriginous areas of the neck often occur, especially in infants who are overweight. More extensive involvement of all body folds may then occur and frequently present the clinical picture which is ordinarily associated with moniliasis, that is, macerated scaling on an erythematous sharply marginated base, with fissuring. The bacteria flora of such regions is varied, and beta-hemolytic streptococci may be recoverable. It is particularly important that adequate treatment be instituted at this phase, because the eczema may otherwise become very chronic.

The exfoliative dermatitis known as Leiner's disease is fortunately rare. It may present a serious general pediatric problem and is best managed in a hospital. Secondary infection may be extensive, heat regulation may be much disturbed, and protein losses from excessive exfoliation may be significant.

Infantile Atopic Dermatitis

The principles underlying the interpretation and management of atopic dermatitis in general have been summarized in Section II of this chapter. These apply fully to infantile atopic dermatitis as well. There are, however, marked differences of localization of the lesions of atopic dermatitis in the infant, as compared with the older child and adult. There is, also, much greater emphasis in medical literature upon the role of foods in the genesis of atopic dermatitis in the infant than in the disease in children and adults. Some of this emphasis would appear to be adherence to tradition rather than founded upon sound clinical evidence.

Certain different or even unique characteristics of atopic dermatitis in the infant are as follows:

The localization of the lesions is haphazard, though the face is almost always involved. There is no tendency to select the anticubital and popliteal fossae to the exclusion of other areas. The process may remain fairly localized, or it may become disseminated to all portions of the cutaneous surface in the form of large or small patches and even generalized exfoliative dermatitis. The palms and soles ordinarily remain clear.

Itching, which often seems constant, is an almost invariable feature of atopic dermatitis in infants. The evidences of excoriation are marked. The characteristic heightened reactivity of the infant's skin is often striking in the form of considerable erythema and swelling of the involved patches. These patches are often well marginated. This reactivity may be most evident in well-fed infants, possibly because of the degree of hydration of the skin in infants who are on fairly high carbohydrate intakes. In thin and semimarasmic infants, the patches of eczema often have a tendency to be more diffuse and less well marginated.

In the infant with atopic dermatitis, there is no conscious inhibition of scratching; the response to itching is prompt and often surprisingly versatile and athletic. Infants scratch and rub with any convenient portion of the hands, forearms, feet, or lower legs. This may be carried out in tireless and vigorous fashion, even after the infant is asleep from exhaustion. In addition, the infant uses any available resistant object for a base against which to rub the skin. The sheets of the bassinet or crib are most convenient, but infants will also employ the headboard and sides of the bed to best advantage, or even objects which may be placed in the crib.

Atopic dermatitis occurs more commonly during the first two years of life than at any other period. The majority of adult patients with atopic dermatitis have a history of infantile eczema. Atopic dermatitis is not often seen in the first few weeks after birth, though seemingly unrelated disturbances of the skin in newborns may eventuate in characteristic atopic dermatitis. As a rule, the lesions of atopic dermatitis appear prior to six months of age, and there is a definite tendency for the infantile phase of the eczema to subside at approximately age two. It is frequently stated that atopic dermatitis develops much more frequently in babies who are bottle-fed, or who receive supplementary feedings, than in infants who are wholly breast-fed; this statement deserves re-evaluation.

The serious general direct pediatric complications of atopic dermatitis are not common, but the number of associated systemic diseases is being expanded constantly (Rostenberg and Solomon, 1968). In spite of widespread involvement and marked excoriation, scarring from uncomplicated atopic dermatitis is extremely rare. Strong assurance may be given to the mother on this score. Regional adenopathy in association with atopic dermatitis is common, but this does not appear to be primarily or solely the result of bacterial infection of the skin. In spite of wakefulness and increased motor activity, children with infantile eczema usually remain quite well, provided that the general pediatric management is adequate. In some instances, however, weight loss may be noted, and difficulty may be encountered in getting the infant to take its feedings. It would almost seem, in some infants with atopic dermatitis, that the urge to scratch is so all-pervading as to make it difficult to arouse interest in anything else. Even the short time required for feeding may be constantly interrupted by the movements of scratching.

Acute secondary bacterial infection is less common in atopic dermatitis than in other forms of infantile eczema. When it does occur, it deserves prompt attention, because widespread impetigo in the infant or child may be the starting point of infectious glomerulonephritis. Under such circumstances, a combination of internal and external antibacterial therapy seems advisable, and dependence should not be placed solely on topical therapy if the bacterial infection is at all extensive. Secondary viral infection with the virus of herpes simplex or vaccinia is a very real danger of infantile eczema and may produce alarming cutaneous and systemic symptoms. This is discussed more fully in Section II of this chapter. The evidence is clear that it is not advisable to vaccinate a child with active or inactive atopic dermatitis against smallpox or to expose such a child to others who have been recently vaccinated. We are equally convinced of the validity of keeping adults with active herpes simplex away from a child with eczema. Recently, Coxsackie A-16 has been described as producing Kaposi's varicelliform eruption.

As with any other chronic disease occurring in an infant, there is necessity for repeated reassurance of the parents and an explanation to them of the probable outcome of the disease. Mothers are inclined to be greatly concerned about babies with infantile eczema, particularly as to whether or not a permanent change in the skin will result and whether or not the infant will have the condition all its life. This tension is accentuated by the constant nursing care and loss of sleep resulting from the responsibility for an infant with eczema. This frequently sows the seeds of resentment and hostility between mother and child. Such mothers not infrequently compare the eczematous child unfavorably with a sibling who "has always had a beautiful fair skin—never gave me any trouble." Aside from concern as to the prognosis in the infant itself, mothers frequently regard any chronic condition of the skin as something loathsome and a possible source of danger to siblings or playmates by reason of infectiousness. Feelings of guilt or resentment may be aroused by the uncovering of an atopic history in the mother or father. All these sources of tension are increased by the fact that relatives, friends, and playmates almost invariably make inquiries and express concern if an infant or child has conspicuous evidence of eczema. It is worthwhile to discuss these matters frankly with the parents as far as may seem necessary, and to give the strong reassurance which is justified. Such reassurance may have a good effect on the patient, because the parent, who is continuously concerned, obviously disappointed, or even resentful regarding flare-ups of eczema which occur in the child, would soon transmit tension and hostility.

PREVENTION OF VARIOUS TYPES OF INFANTILE ECZEMA

To what extent a hygienic and sensible regimen of normal skin care will contribute to the prevention of atopic dermatitis is unknown, but certain measures are logical and worth trying. In other forms of eczema (that is, those due to irritant contactants, to seborrhea and infection, or to dry skin), sensible day-to-day preventive measures are of unquestionable value and may be sufficient to ward off a chronic extensive eruption.

The Newborn: Care of the Skin

There is now little disagreement among competent pediatricians that in the transfer from a bland and physiologic intrauterine environment, the skin of the infant should not be assaulted with unnecessary cleansing by chemical and mechanical means. Meconium should, of course, be wiped off gently, and it is probable that aesthetic reasons will demand some removal of the vernix caseosa from the face. Elsewhere on the body, however, it should be left in place; it is the most physiologic of all ointments and mitigates the numerous chemical and mechanical shocks to which the skin of the newborn must become adjusted in his new environment. The vernix gradually comes away on successive changes of clothing, within two or three days. There is no justification for the application of ointments or lotions containing antiseptics at this time, unless there has recently been an outbreak of impetigo in the nursery. Under such circumstances, bathing with a detergent is probably as good a measure as any. The routine daily use of hexachlorophene-containing cleansing agents has been discredited because it may produce central nervous system changes (Blank, 1972).

The differentiation of the various types of infantile eczema, and the various systemic diseases associated with them (fortunately rarely) have been well summarized by Solomon and Esterly in the following tables.

TABLE 5–4 FEATURES OF ATOPIC DERMATITIS, PRIMARY IRRITANT DERMATITIS, AND INFECTIOUS DERMATITIS IN THE NEWBORN*

	Atopic Dermatitis	*Primary Irritant*	*Infectious Dermatitis*
Age of onset	Usually not before 3 months, rarely at end of first month, not at birth	Any time during first month	Any time
Family history	High incidence of respiratory allergy, hay fever, atopic dermatitis	None	May have bacterial carrier in family
Skin lesions	Weeping, vesicular, scaling; little lichenification before 4 months. Extensor surfaces, cheeks, ears and scalp. Symmetrical. Rarely diaper area alone	Bright red, weeping. Less scaling. Any site may be involved but mostly diaper area, perianal area. May not be symmetrical	Weeping, much crusting. Perioral, nasal, umbilical and diaper areas. Punched out ulcers frequent on buttocks, perineum
Pruritus	Marked, precedes lesion	May be variable—follows lesions	Little
Culture	Often negative	Often negative	Positive—*Staphylococcus aureus* Streptococci Enterococci *Candida albicans* Pseudomonas
Other skin lesions	Associated "seborrheic" lesions, ichthyosis vulgaris frequent. Not seen until after 3 months of age	Usually none	Usually none. May be a complication of congenital defects. Bullous lesions frequent
Consequence of delay in treatment	May improve spontaneously	Usually gets worse locally	Usually gets worse locally; satellite lesions develop nearby and at a distance
Incidence	Very rare	Very common	Common

*From Solomon, L. M., and Esterly, N. B.: Neonatal Dermatology. Philadelphia, W. B. Saunders Co., 1973, p. 125. By permission.

TABLE 5–5　Causes of Eczema in the Newborn*

Exogenous		With the cutaneous process predominant	**Cutaneous process secondary to a systemic process
Primary irritant	Contact dermatitis	With the cutaneous process predominant	**Cutaneous process secondary to a systemic process
Allergic		Infantile eczema, atopic seborrhea, "cradle cap"	Wiskott-Aldrich syndrome Congenital sex-linked agammaglobulinemia Leiner's disease with C_5 dysfunction
Bacteria	Infection	Desquamative erythroderma	Ataxia-telangiectasia Chronic granulomatous disease
Fungi		Ritter's disease	Phenylketonuria Ahistidinemia
Light			Mucopolysaccharidoses
Cold	Physical agents	Congenital ichthyosiform erythroderma	Hartnup disease Acrodermatitis enteropathica Gluten-sensitive enteropathy
Heat		"Diaper dermatitis"	Anhidrotic ectodermal dysplasia Histiocytosis X
Allergic component	Insect bites		Long arm 18 deletion syndrome Hereditary acrokeratotic poikiloderma

*From Solomon, L. M., and Esterly, N. B.: Neonatal Dermatology. Philadelphia, W. B. Saunders Co., 1973, p. 126. By permission.

**This list is not all-inclusive. Many additional reports exist wherein an eczematous process forms part of a syndrome.

DERMATITIS OF FEET AND HANDS

Chronic inflammatory dermatoses affecting the feet and hands are among the most difficult of all dermatologic therapeutic problems. In persons whose livelihood depends upon work which involves much walking or use of the hands, this group of diseases may be occupationally disabling.

The following diagnostic possibilities apply principally to any inflammatory condition which may be a true dermatitis or which may be confused with such a condition.

CONTACT DERMATITIS DUE TO PRIMARY IRRITANTS OR SENSITIZERS. This is the most common instigator or source of perpetuation of inflammatory processes affecting the hands and feet. It may rapidly be replaced by chronic eczematous dermatitis.

DYSHIDROSIFORM ERUPTIONS. These represent another common primary or contributory source of hand and foot eruptions. They are discussed in some detail in Chapter 24.

SUPERFICIAL FUNGAL INFECTIONS. The role of superficial ringworm infections in inflammatory processes of the feet and hands, particularly the latter, has been overemphasized. The most characteristic type of superficial fungal infection affecting the hands and feet is that caused by *Trichophyton rubrum*, and it is principally in this type that chronic changes are clearly and undubitably seen. The phenomenon of dermatophytid affecting the hands rests on secure clinical and experimental grounds, but here again such a diagnosis should not be made or accepted too readily.

ATOPIC DERMATITIS AND NUMMULAR DERMATITIS may sometimes be confined entirely to the hands and feet. This is particularly true in middle-aged patients in whom the more disseminate type of atopic dermatitis has long since abated.

BACTERIAL INFECTIONS. The bacterial flora of the hands and feet is high. The resistance of the normal skin of the hands and feet to bacterial infection is extraordinary, but constant breaching of the normal defenses in these regions is the rule rather than the exception. Acute primary bacterial infections are ordinarily easily overcome by suitable topical or systemic therapy. The principal exceptions to this rule are various bacterial infections occurring around the paronychial margin or in the nail bed. Such infections, even when recognized early, may sometimes become chronic.

The role of chronic secondary infection occurring in areas of repeated trauma or patches of dermatitis is difficult to assess.

PSORIASIS. Psoriasis often masquerades under the appellation of chronic dermatitis if it affects the hands and feet. It most frequently occurs in the form of dry, sharply marginated plaques, principally on pressure points or about the nails.

UNCOMMON CONDITIONS AFFECTING THE HANDS AND FEET. Confusion as to the diagnosis of an inflammatory change affecting the hands and feet may arise from a number of uncommon to rare conditions, as follows:

Acrodermatitis Perstans Continua (Dermatitis Repens, Pustular Acrodermatitis). This condition has a characteristic clinical presentation. It frequently occurs as a single patch, though there may be several; the disease is very chronic, resistant, and persistent. The condition has its onset with a group of deep vesicles and/or pustules and moderate inflammation, and it affects one or more digits. Local trauma and infection are precipitant factors. Extension may occur peripherally by separation of the stratum corneum and upper layers of the epidermis or by the appearance of satellite lesions. The stratum corneum

may be curetted off very easily, revealing some serous or seropurulent exudate and a moderately inflamed base. This material may yield large numbers of coagulase-positive micrococci, but the role of these in the perpetuation of the disease is uncertain. The process may cause atrophy of the skin and destruction of the nail and digit. Antibacterial therapy is disappointing in its effects, as are most other methods of treatment. Hydrocortisone ointment and Castellani's paint are worth a trial and at most give only a temporary, if any, response. Systemic corticosteroid therapy may cause dissemination of the disease which then resembles generalized pustular psoriasis. Every effort to prevent trauma, occlusion, and chemical irritation of the involved site must be made. The condition may persist for many years, and some degree of atrophy may result.

Pustular Psoriasis (Pustular Bacterid). As mentioned above, attempts to dissociate this condition from psoriasis have resulted in much controversy. That a clinical syndrome exists which fits into this pattern cannot be doubted. It has many similarities to dermatitis repens. The onset oc-

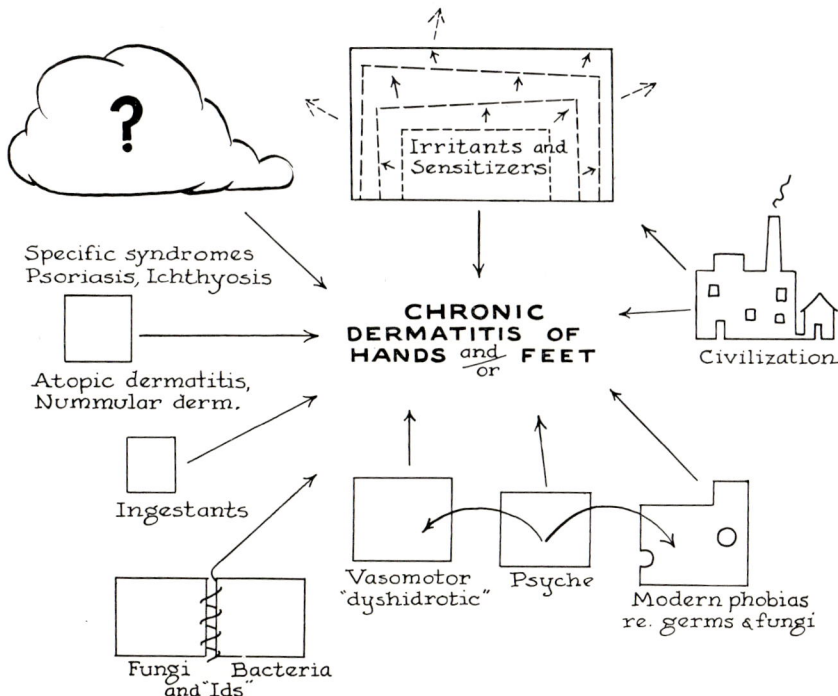

Figure 5–46 Diverse mechanisms in dermatitis of the hands and feet.

TABLE 5–6　Uncommon Conditions Affecting the Hands and Feet

Names	*Synonyms*	*Histopathology*	*Clinical Picture*	*Treatment*
Acrodermatitis perstans continua	Dermatitis repens Pustular acrodermatitis	Psoriasiform changes with spongiform pustule	Follows local trauma or infection. Affects digits. Sterile pustules. Atrophy of skin and destruction of digits and nails can occur. Long course. Rarely generalized, resembling generalized pustular psoriasis.	Ineffective
Pustulosis palmaris et plantaris	Pustular psoriasis Pustular bacterid	Large intra-epidermal unilocular pustule; no psoriasiform changes	Sterile pustules involving symmetrically thenar, hypothenar, soles, and sides of heels. Glazed erythema with purpuric pustules and brown scales. Protracted course. Occasionally, psoriasis develops later.	Ineffective. Intralesional steroid gives temporary response
Dyshidrosis with pustules	Pompholyx with secondary infection	Intra-epidermal spongiotic vesiculation and pustulation	Acute recurrent or chronic eruption of deep-seated ("sago-like") vesicles involving digits, palms, and soles. Scrapings for fungi and bacterial culture of pus are unrewarding.	Treatment for eczema plus antibiotics for secondary infection

curs with the appearance of a group of deep vesicles and, more characteristically, hemorrhagic vesicopustules involving thenar and hypothenar eminences and the soles and heels of the feet. On the extremely thick skin of the palms and soles, these may originally seem to be papules. The lesions may be bilateral and symmetric. Crops of vesicopustules occur, often with moderate to marked itching at their onset. Some hyperkeratosis may develop. These pustules are invariably sterile at their onset if the culture is carefully taken. The condition is extraordinarily chronic, and may have an up and down course for many years. Bacterial sensitization resulting from a focus of infection as the causal mechanism for the dermatitis is controversial and has been debated. Some patients with this condition may subsequently develop typical psoriasis.

Herpes Simplex and Zoster. These viral infections may occur on the hands and feet. It is an uncommon localization for recurrent herpes simplex, but, when it occurs, the correct diagnosis may not be immediately obvious and can be substantiated by Tzanck test of an intact vesicle.

Dermatitis Herpetiformis. This condition may affect the hands and feet principally, and the diagnosis may be difficult when this is the case. Ordinarily, however, characteristic lesions will be found elsewhere.

Dyshidrosis (Pompholyx)

Dyshidrosis (pompholyx, dyshidrotic eczema) is an eczematous reaction pattern which appears on the palms or soles and in the interdigital spaces. Clinically it is distinctive in that erythema is minimal or absent, and the vesicles are deep below the thick stratum corneum of this area. In the strict sense of the term, dyshidrosis is defined as an acute, recurrent, noninflammatory, vesicular eruption strictly limited to the palms and/or the soles. The eruption is not seen elsewhere, except as an extension onto the lateral surfaces of the fingers and toes, but palmar and plantar dyshidrosiform eruptions commonly occur as a part of a generalized eczematous reaction. In such instances, the dyshidrosiform pattern is part of the generalized eczematous reactions. It is only when the palmar or plantar vesicular eruption is the sole change that the label dyshidrosis is employed and not infrequently leads to terminologic quibbling.

The normal course of dyshidrosis is one of sudden onset and rapid evolution, followed by complete spontaneous involution in about three weeks. Scaling marks the terminal phase. The striking difference between dyshidrosis and eczematous patterns elsewhere is the fact that the dyshidrotic vesicles do not rupture and exude serum. Involution occurs as a result of intradermal absorption of the vesicular fluid. Dyshidrosis usually occurs in the summer. Almost invariably there is accompanying hyperhidrosis of the palms and soles.

Dyshidrosis may show secondary changes and complications. These include secondary infection and irritation by topical medication. Under these circumstances the physician may see the patient in a stage in which the primary dyshidrosis is no longer discernible.

From the histopathologic standpoint, dyshidrosis presents superficial epidermal vesiculation. The corium does not show marked inflammatory changes. It is interesting to correlate the superficial histologic location of the vesicles with their clinical appearance. Apparently the thick stratum corneum is responsible for the "sago grain" type of vesicle which appears in dyshidrosis, and it may also account for the fact that rupture does not occur.

At present there is no convincing evidence that the sweat gland plays a primary role in the pathogenesis of dyshidrosis. It is true that secondary sweat retention does occur in the dyshidrotic vesicles, as it may in any vesicle of the skin. Secondary sweat retention may cause an exacerbation of dyshidrosis. Because of this secondary factor of sweat retention, it may be possible to ameliorate dyshidrosis by the administration of systemic drugs which inhibit sweating. On the other hand, some observers have noted the occurrence of dyshidrosis after a sympathectomy which effectively suppressed sweat gland activity. The sympathectomy ameliorated but did not dismiss the dyshidrosis.

Clinical observation supports the view that dyshidrosis is a nonspecific reaction pattern of the palmar and plantar skin. The epidermis of these two sites is apparently more responsive than skin elsewhere, and as a result may be the only area which responds to an allergen or toxin within the blood stream or to neural stimuli. The more common occurrence of dyshidrosis in the summer months may be a manifestation of a heightened sensitivity of the epidermal cells during this season. Secondary sweat retention may also be more prominent in the summer, bringing latent examples of dyshidrosis up to the clinical level. The relationship of the amount of sweating on the palms and the seasons is not a simple one, however, since palmar sweating generally is under cortical control and is unrelated to environmental temperature.

PREVENTIVE METHODS IN DERMATITIS OF THE HANDS AND FEET

In a very large proportion of chronic dermatitis affecting the hands or feet, the factors involved at the beginning of the process are fairly clear-cut. It is reasonably certain that if some patients had been more careful regarding the normal hygiene of the hands and feet, the chronic disabling eruption would not have occurred, though this is by no means, always true. The varieties of unphysiologic trauma to which the skin of these areas is subjected are numerous and are constantly increasing. Such eruptions furnish a very significant source of disability in many useful segments of the population. For instance, inflammatory eruptions of the feet have disabled many military personnel for unrestricted duty. We have observed a considerable number of surgeons, dentists, and nurses who become more or less completely disabled occupationally because of dermatitis of the hands. Such eruptions often reduce greatly the efficiency and happiness of housewives, who find it impossible to carry out routine maternal and household tasks without chronic discomfort and disability.

Washing and Drying of the Skin

Many persons wash their hands far more frequently than is necessary. This may be done hurriedly, without adequate rinsing off of soap and without sufficient drying, particularly under rings or between the fingers. In persons with compulsive phobias against germs or fungi, the hands may be washed dozens of times daily. In the case of medical, dental, and nursing personnel, there may, indeed, be a necessity for washing far more than is desirable. In many industrial occupations, the removal of conspicuous or irritant materials from the hands at the end of the day is necessary, but it is too frequently carried out with harsh agents such as very strong soaps, turpentine, or strong lipid solvents.

In many individuals, the skin of the hands will tolerate almost unlimited washing. In others, effects in the form of small warning signals of irritation are present long before any significant inflammation results. Individuals with a dry skin and tendency to chapping of the hands ordinarily learn very quickly the necessity of reducing the number of washings. Persons who are sustaining mild primary irritation from detergents under rings and between the fingers often neglect the warning signals for many months. Under such circumstances, reduction of washing to an absolute minimum is indicated. It may be found that a superfatted soap or a soap substitute may be better tolerated, though this must be determined by trial. Rings should be removed before prolonged immersion of the hands. Thorough rinsing of the skin, particularly around the nails and between the fingers, is important. Simple creams are helpful in maintaining a proper degree of hydration of the stratum corneum and also in facilitating later washing; the dirt does not have an opportunity to become so firmly adherent and imbedded in the skin surface.

Adequate drying of the skin is likely to be neglected after washing the feet. The interdigital spaces of the toes are rarely dried sufficiently, and this leads to maceration and a foothold for bacteria, fungi, and yeast.

CHRONIC ANAL AND VULVAR PRURITUS

Various diseases affecting the skin and mucous membranes of the anogenital region have been alluded to previously in various sections. A number of these are capable of producing itching which is a relatively common problem in general medical, dermatologic, gynecologic, and proctologic practice. It is not surprising that occasional itching of the anogenital region should be almost physiologic. The area is one of obvious psychoerotic significance, and the nerve endings are easily alerted. The physiologic conditions for normality of the skin and mucous membranes are less than optimal, by reason of urinary and fecal contamination, intertriginous folds, overvigorous cleansing, occlusive clothing and sports gear, and lack of exposure to light and air.

Certain dermatologic syndromes (see Table 5–7) commonly affect the anogenital region and produce varying degrees of itching, as follows below.

Localized Neurodermatitis or "Essential" Pruritus

This is by far the most common type of chronic anogenital itching. Its genesis is entirely comparable to that of circumscribed neurodermatitis seen elsewhere, and the sources of irritation which initiate paroxysms of itching are more numerous. In such patients, the only changes seen are excoriation, thickening, and lichenification. When the anal or vulvar mucosa are scratched, the thickening is of a white

TABLE 5–7 ANOGENITAL CONDITIONS WHICH MAY BE ASSOCIATED WITH PRURITUS

Skin diseases	Contact dermatitis, psoriasis, seborrheic dermatitis, lichen planus, lichen sclerosis et atrophicus, epithelioma, idiopathic pruritus ani
Infections	
Bacterial	Pyodermas, hidradenitis suppurativa, erythrasma
Fungal	Tinea, candidiasis
Treponemal	Condylomata lata
Viral	Verruca accuminata, molluscum contagiosa, herpes progenitalis
Parasitic infestation	Scabies, pediculosis pubis, pinworm, larva currens
Anorectal and genital diseases	Vaginal and rectal discharge of vaginitis or proctitis, malignancy of the cervix or rectum or colon, fissures, fistulas, hemorrhoids, polyps, enlarged anal papillae, rectal or vaginal prolapses
Associated general diseases (so-called metabolic pruritus)	Diabetes mellitus, gout, uremia, Hodgkin's disease, polycythemia, carcinomatosis

Diagnostic Procedures
Health scan (lab blood and chemistry profile) and to include also chest plate and urinalysis.
Scrapings for fungi.
Scotch tape examination for pinworm.
Wood's light examination for erythrasma.

macerated character which may simulate leukoplakia. In fact, there can be little question that leukoplakia may supervene after prolonged excoriation of the vulvar mucous membrane, just as irritation of other types is a source of leukoplakia in the buccal mucous membrane. Circumscribed neurodermatitis may succeed some other itching dermatosis which has long disappeared. It is particularly important that the psychic or neurodermatitic component in any itching process of the anogenital region be recognized and that visible organic changes not be accepted as the sole source of such itching.

Seborrheic Dermatitis

Seborrheic dermatitis of the anogenital region is most commonly seen in folds, such as the gluteal cleft or crural region, but may be follicular, especially in the pubic hair. Other evidences of seborrheic dermatitis will ordinarily be seen elsewhere, almost always in the scalp and frequently in the usual sites on the trunk.

Psoriasis

Psoriasis commonly involves the anogenital region. The lesions are usually quite sharply marginated. In intertriginous folds they may simulate seborrheic dermatitis or candidiasis. Confusion with premalignant conditions, such as erythroplasia or leukoplakia, may occur, and biopsy is often helpful.

Contact Dermatitis

This is an ever present possibility in the anogenital region, regardless of the primary nature of the itching. The male genitalia are particularly susceptible to irritation or sensitization. Topical medication is a frequent source of such irritation, and cosmetics also play a role.

Physical Irritation: Moisture and Friction

The presence of folds and decreased opportunity for evaporation produce a normal increase in the surface moisture of the anogenital region. To this may be added hyperhidrosis of psychic origin. The anal area of both sexes and the vulvar region in females may be subjected to constant moistening from discharges, sometimes of irritant or infected character.

Lichen Planus

The lesions of lichen planus are characteristic at their onset and are not easily confused with other conditions. If present for a long period of time, they may become hypertrophic and simulate leukoplakia or clear, with a residual post-inflammatory hyperpigmentation. It is exceedingly uncommon to encounter lichen planus distributed solely to the anogenital region, though it can occur. If not seen on the glabrous skin surface, lesions may be present in the mouth. Biopsy is sometimes essential. There is no more futile and unnecessary procedure than vulvectomy for lichen planus, but we have observed this in patients who did not have an antecedent biopsy.

Parasitic Infestations

"Crabs" (pediculosis pubis) in the anogenital region are large animals and not easily missed if the inspection is at all thorough. Nevertheless, they may be responsible for very prolonged pruritus and are particularly liable to be missed in persons of good hygiene. Kwell (gamma benzene hexachloride) is an effective treatment, usually applied on only two occasions one week apart. Scabies commonly affects the male genitalia, rarely the female genitalia.

Pinworm Infestation

Pinworms must always be considered as a possible cause of chronic pruritus ani. This condition is less common in adults.

TREATMENT OF ANOGENITAL PRURITUS

The diverse and varied origin of this characteristic pruritus is indicated in the preceding paragraphs. It is particularly important that the underlying disease of the skin or mucous membranes be classified as accurately as possible and any associated underlying condition be found. If any gynecologic or proctologic changes are present, they must be carefully assessed. Adequate study and treatment of these patients may sometimes depend upon two or three specialty disciplines.

Though the methods of treatment of inflammatory processes affecting the anogenital region and methods of combating itching are similar to methods used elsewhere, there are special features of the region which render some methods of management more satisfactory than others. In general, topical therapy must be milder than that used elsewhere on the skin, and this is particularly true in eruptions of the male genitalia. Topical antipruritic compounds are somewhat more effective at the mucocutaneous junction than on skin elsewhere.

It is particularly important to keep the possible factor of circumscribed neurodermatitis in the forefront in relation to any itching eruption of the anogenital region. If the itching is not due to this syndrome at the onset, it frequently is later in the course. The prevention of scratching is invariably a basic goal in the treatment. In connection with this, it must be kept in mind that many methods of treatment act strongly through suggestion in anal and vulvar pruritus, including changing topical medicaments, x-ray, or other physical therapy, and surgical procedures. The effects of such suggestion therapy are, however, more often evanescent than permanent.

Acute inflammatory involvement, whether frank dermatitis due initially to a fungal infection or to some dermatosis such as psoriasis, is treated as any acute process elsewhere. Sitz baths are often very soothing and frequently give prompt temporary response to acute exacerbations of itching. Topical hydrocortisone therapy may be helpful in this phase, and a lotion is often more effective than an ointment if the inflammation is acute. In very acute processes which give the prospect of being self-limited, systemic corticosteroid therapy may be justifiable.

Anal hygiene is of first importance in the control of pruritus ani. Cleansing after a bowel movement should be particularly thorough, though as bland as possible. Moistened facial tissue rather than ordinary toilet tissue may be helpful. The use of a soap substitute may be found less irritating. If soap is used, it is particularly important that it be thoroughly removed. It is often worthwhile to apply a small amount of a fairly occlusive paste, such as zinc oxide ointment, to the area after a bowel movement.

Constipation or diarrhea, especially the latter, may cause exacerbation of pruritus ani. Constipation apparently acts by increasing the distention and edema of the tissues, or by widening or extending small external or internal fissures. Severe diarrhea, even in patients with normal skin, is always followed by irritation and itching if the diarrhea is long continued. Chemical changes in the stool will sometimes be noted to be more productive of itching and irritation, though the exact nature of these is unknown. In certain instances, patients may note that the taking of particular foods will be followed by anal itching at a bowel movement several hours later, and this may occasionally be due to a true epidermal sensitization. In attempts at hyposensitization to poison ivy by administering the extract by mouth, for instance, it is commonplace to note perianal itching due to a reaction from portions of the extract which pass through the gastrointestinal tract unabsorbed.

It would appear that hydrocortisone ointments in adequate strength will produce temporary relief of itching and inflammation in a very high percentage of patients with pruritus ani, certainly over 75 per cent. Very small applications are sufficient, preferably three or four times daily.

There can be no question that some patients with severe chronic pruritus ani are relieved by operations designed to correct some well-defined abnormality. A persistent fissure which does not respond to conservative therapy may serve as the trigger mechanism of pruritus. Definite crypts with inflammation and retention of fecal material in them also may act as a cause, and these may occasionally require surgical obliteration. Exuberant external hemorrhoids or anal warts and other perianal tissue prevent thorough cleansing and may be the chief source of itching. Internal hemorrhoids are not commonly a source. Chronic anal fistulae which produce constant soiling and maceration obviously may contribute to pruritus. Though these and some other proctologic difficulties may at times be responsible for itching, surgical correction of these problems does not always guarantee a cure for the pruritus ani; consequently, an attitude of conservatism is desirable and protective. Patients sometimes and unfortunately undergo a succession of operations for the relief of another proctologic condition which may have been relatively inconsequential at the beginning and was assumed to be significant and responsible for the pruritus.

Vulvar pruritus is an exceedingly common gynecologic problem. Classification as to the underlying dermatosis is sometimes fairly easy, though the causes may be obscure (Table 5–8). The majority of patients will be found to fall into the essential pruritus or neurodermatitis group. In these, any source of irritation may be sufficient to set off prolonged paroxysms of itching. The changes associated with seborrheic dermatitis, psoriasis, or lichen planus are ordinarily quite characteristic to the experienced eye. In vulvar pruritus associated with sclerotic or atrophic changes, classification may be difficult, and biopsy is often helpful in such instances.

Gynecologic examination is essential in any patient with persistent pruritus vulvae. An amount of discharge which might be regarded as hardly more than normal may be sufficient to perpetuate the itching. Excessive discharge inevitably increases the maceration and irritation, and it is frequently impossible to produce any relief of the itching until this is brought under control. Though the diagnosis of itching related to vaginal trichomonads or candida is frequently made, it is often difficult to attribute the itching to this source. However, the topical therapy for both of these "infections" is relatively satisfactory, but overtreatment with the necessary therapy or the prolonged use of irritant or sensitizing intravaginal medication frequently does more harm than good insofar as the itching is concerned.

The sources of irritation and sensitization of the vulvar skin and mucous membranes should be carefully investigated in relation to cosmetics, douches, pads and inserts and chemicals incorporated in them, particular items of underclothing, and contraceptives. When such patients are first seen, suspension of any long used topical agent for a few days is ordinarily advisable. Routine urinalysis is essential, though the only abnormal finding which is associated with vulvar inflammatory changes with any regularity is glycosuria.

Aside from the irritating effects of discharges, the gynecologic changes which may be factors in pruritus vulvae are extremely variable. Any abnormality which may produce edema or significant discomfort may well be contributory, though this requires careful and expert assessment. Exacerbations of the itching before, during, or after the menses may be noted, and may be related to nervous tension, edema, contactants, or other factors. Pregnancy has variable effects on pruritus vulvae, sometimes relieving it completely, sometimes producing exacerbation.

In postmenopausal women or those who have had oophorectomy, atrophy of the external genitalia may occur. There is shrinkage and dryness of the external genitalia (labia minora, frenulum, and inner aspects of the labia majora). The

TABLE 5–8 PRURITUS VULVAE

Dermatologic conditions	Essential or idiopathic pruritus, contact allergic or irritant dermatitis, lichen simplex, lichen sclerosis et atrophicus, psoriasis, seborrheic dermatitis, lichen planus, nonviral blistering diseases (anogenital aphthosis, erythema multiforme, pemphigus), Fox-Fordyce disease, leukoplakia, Bowen's disease, Paget's disease
Vulvovaginitis	Non-infective (senile vaginitis, secondary reaction to intravaginal foreign bodies); infective (gonorrhea and streptococcal, staphylococcal, trichomonal and candidal infections)
Vulvar infections or infestations	Herpes simplex, verruca accuminata, molluscum contagiosa, scabies, pediculosis pubis, enterobius (oxyuris) vermicularis
Gynecologic conditions	Cervicitis, cystocele, rectocele, vaginal sinuses and fistulae
General diseases and states	Pellagra, liver disease, lymphoma, polycythemia, diabetes mellitus, pregnancy

area may become pruritic. Although the associated senile vaginitis responds to estrogens, the genitalia are not affected but improve with emollients.

Various hormones, usually estrogens, have been used systemically and topically for pruritus vulvae, particularly when atrophic changes are present. While such treatment would appear to have a sound rationale, the author has not been impressed with its effectiveness in many cases, and it should be administered with sound endocrinologic judgment.

In acute vulvitis, sitz baths or simple douches, or both, are sometimes the only medication which is helpful and well tolerated. Topical hydrocortisone therapy is less effective in vulvar itching than in perianal itching. In the presence of seborrheic dermatitis, a mild regimen, as for this condition in the scalp, may be helpful. As with pruritus ani, variation in the type of ointment used may be necessary for actual or psychosomatic reasons, but it is particularly important that these ointments be selected carefully for their blandness and low sensitizing capacity. Thick paste-type preparations are not well tolerated on the vulva, and shake lotions are almost unusable. In the presence of intertriginous inflammation and fissuring, Castellani's paint or 2 per cent silver nitrate may be helpful.

In candidiasis of the vagina, the possibility of conjugal infection must be kept in mind. This may produce a "ping-pong" sequence in which cure of the yeast infection in the patient is promptly followed by reinfection by the sexual partner.

PITYRIASIS ALBA

Many chronic inflammations or injuries of the skin tend to produce increased melanin production and clinical pigmentation. However, the reverse may be true, as in pityriasis alba. The same phenomena may occur at times in atopic and seborrheic dermatitis, tinea versicolor infection, or in reactions to agarite alba.

Pityriasis alba is a common, quite distinctive disease consisting of round or oval, slightly scaling patches with distinctive depigmentation which at times may lead to confusion with vitiligo. The lesions most commonly involve the face, especially the cheeks and about the mouth. However, scattered lesions may occasionally be seen on the neck, upper arms, and elsewhere.

Pityriasis alba is seen most commonly in young children and adolescents. At the onset, a slight erythema may be noted, but inflammation is a very minor feature. The scaling is always finely exfoliative. The lesions are understandably more marked in tanned or dark-skinned children. The supposed increased incidence in spring and summer months may be due to the increased contrasting tanning occurring at these times.

Pityriasis alba has been designated by a variety of names which serve only to confuse. The cause of this condition is unknown, though superficial bacterial infection has been suggested. Although it has been described more frequently in atopic patients, it has no relation to atopic dermatitis; it has been suggested that it might be a variant of seborrheic dermatitis.

If the condition is mild and relatively inconspicuous, no treatment is necessary, and spontaneous involution may be anticipated. A corticosteroid cream may be tried, but the effect is not striking as a rule, and a simple emollient cream, plus avoidance of excessive soap and water washing, is probably as effective as anything.

REFERENCES

Abrahams, I., McCarthy, J. T., and Sanders, S. L.: 101 cases of exfoliative dermatitis. Arch. Dermatol. 87:96, 1963.

Bereston, E. S.: Use of selenium sulfide shampoo in seborrheic dermatitis. J.A.M.A. 156:1246, 1954.

Blank, 1972. Personal communication.

Blohm, S. G., and Lodin, A.: Eczema of the hands in women. Acta Derm. Venereol. 48:7, 1968.

Fowle, L. P., and Rice, J. W.: Etiology of nummular eczema. Arch. Dermatol. 68:69, 1953.

Friedman, M., and Hare, P. J.: Gluten-sensitive enteropathy and eczema. Lancet 1:521, 1965.

Fry, L., Shuster, S., and McMinn, R. M. H.: D-xylose absorption in patients with eczema. Br. Med. J. 1:967, 1965.

Glickman, F. S., and Silvers, S. H.: Hand eczema and atopy in housewives. Arch. Dermatol. 95:487, 1967.

Illig, L. (Marburg): Importance of nervous system to manifestation of neurodermatitis. Hautarzt 5:408, 1954.

Jacobs, J. C., and Miller, M. E.: Fatal familial Leiner's disease: a deficiency of the opsonic activity of serum complement. Pediatrics 49:225, 1972.

Laymon, C. W.: Dermatitis of the hands. Minn. Med. *53*:687, 1970.

O'Quinn, S. E., Cole, J., and Many, H.: Problems of disability and rehabilitation in patients with chronic skin disease. Arch. Dermatol. *105*:35, 1972.

Petrozzi, J. W.: Infectious mononucleosis manifesting as a palmar dermatitis. Arch. Dermatol. *104*:207, 1971.

Rostenberg, A., Jr., and Solomon, L. M.: Infantile eczema and systemic disease. Arch. Dermatol. *98*:41, 1968.

Shaffer, B., and Beerman, H.: Lichen simplex chronicus and its variants. Arch. Dermatol. *64*:340, 1951.

Shuster, S., and Marks, J.: Dermatogenic enteropathy. Lancet *1*:1367, 1965.

Vowles, M., Warin, R. P., and Apley, J.: Infantile eczema: Observations on natural history and prognosis. Br. J. Dermatol. *67*:53, 1955.

Zackheim, H. S., Arnold, J. E., Farber, E. M., et al.: Topical therapy of psoriasis with mechlorethamine. Arch. Dermatol. *105*:702, 1972.

CHAPTER

6

PHOTOSENSITIVITY

Isaac Willis

The phrases "photosensitivity reaction" and "photosensitivity disorder" are generally used to denote either a quantitative or a qualitative abnormality in the skin's response to sunlight or artificial light exposure. To date, nearly 40 etiologically different types of photosensitivity reactions have been described (Fig. 6–1). Since many of these reactions will have similar clinical morphologic characteristics, it is difficult to institute specific therapy and an appropriate prophylactic regimen until one has obtained a patient history regarding participating environmental and genetic factors, the results of laboratory, histologic, and histochemical studies, and knowledge as to what specific wavelengths are responsible for inducing the reaction. This chapter is devoted to describing the various photosensitivity disorders and the methods of diagnosis, treatment, and prophylaxis.

PHYSICAL AND ENVIRONMENTAL FACTORS

Radiant energy emanates from the sun as a result of its internal thermonuclear

reactions (Deutsch, 1955). That portion of energy reaching the earth's outer atmosphere is composed of wavelengths that range from the very short, highly energetic x-ray spectrum to the very long, low-energy radio wavelengths. Fortunately, we are protected from the very short, more potentially lethal wavelengths by the filtering action of oxygen and ozone layers in the outer atmosphere. As wavelengths shorter than 240 nm.* reach the earth's outer atmosphere, they convert oxygen to ozone; and as the latter continually absorbs up to 290 nm., the ozone is reconverted to life-sustaining oxygen. Under these conditions, less than 1 per cent of the sun's radiation that reaches the earth's surface is composed of ultraviolet (UV) wavelengths (290–400 nm.). Under optimal conditions, only about 0.2 per cent of this UV is of the type (290–320 nm.) that causes sunburn in human skin. Thus, the major portion (>99 per cent) of solar radiation that reaches our immediate environment is composed of visible, infrared, and longer wavelengths.

This relative percentage distribution of

---

*nm = nanometer = 10^{-9} meter

324

Xeroderma Pigmentosum
Bloom's Syndrome
Cockayne's Syndrome
Rothmund-Thomson Syndrome
Disseminated Superficial Porokeratosis
Aminoacidurias

Genetic

SUN

Herpes Simplex
Lymphogranuloma
Venereum
Varicella

Infectious
(Mainly Viral)

Acute

DIRECT

Sunburn

INDIRECT

Endogenous Factors

Biochemical
Metabolic
Nutritional
Hormonal
Enzymatic

Porphyria(s)
Pellagra
Hartnup Disease
Phenylketonuria
Hypopituitarism
Hypogonadism
Albinism

Chronic

+

Exogenous
Factors

+

Premature Aging
Premalignant Lesions
Malignant Lesions

Miscellaneous,
Primarily
Cutaneous
(Koebner's
Phenomena)

Immunologic

Systemic
Drugs

Topical
Agents

Psoriasis
Lichen Planus
Keratosis Follicularis
Pityriasis Rubra
Pilaris
Erythema Multiforme
Sarcoid
Lymphocytoma
Atopic Dermatitis
Rosacea
Hailey-Hailey Disease
Granuloma Annulare
Seborrheic Dermatitis

Lupus Erythematosus
Pemphigus Erythematosus
Solar Urticaria
Scleroderma
Dermatomyositis
(?) Polymorphic Light
Eruption
(?) Actinic
Reticuloid
(?) Vitiligo

Phototoxicity

Photocontact
Allergy
+
Phototoxicity

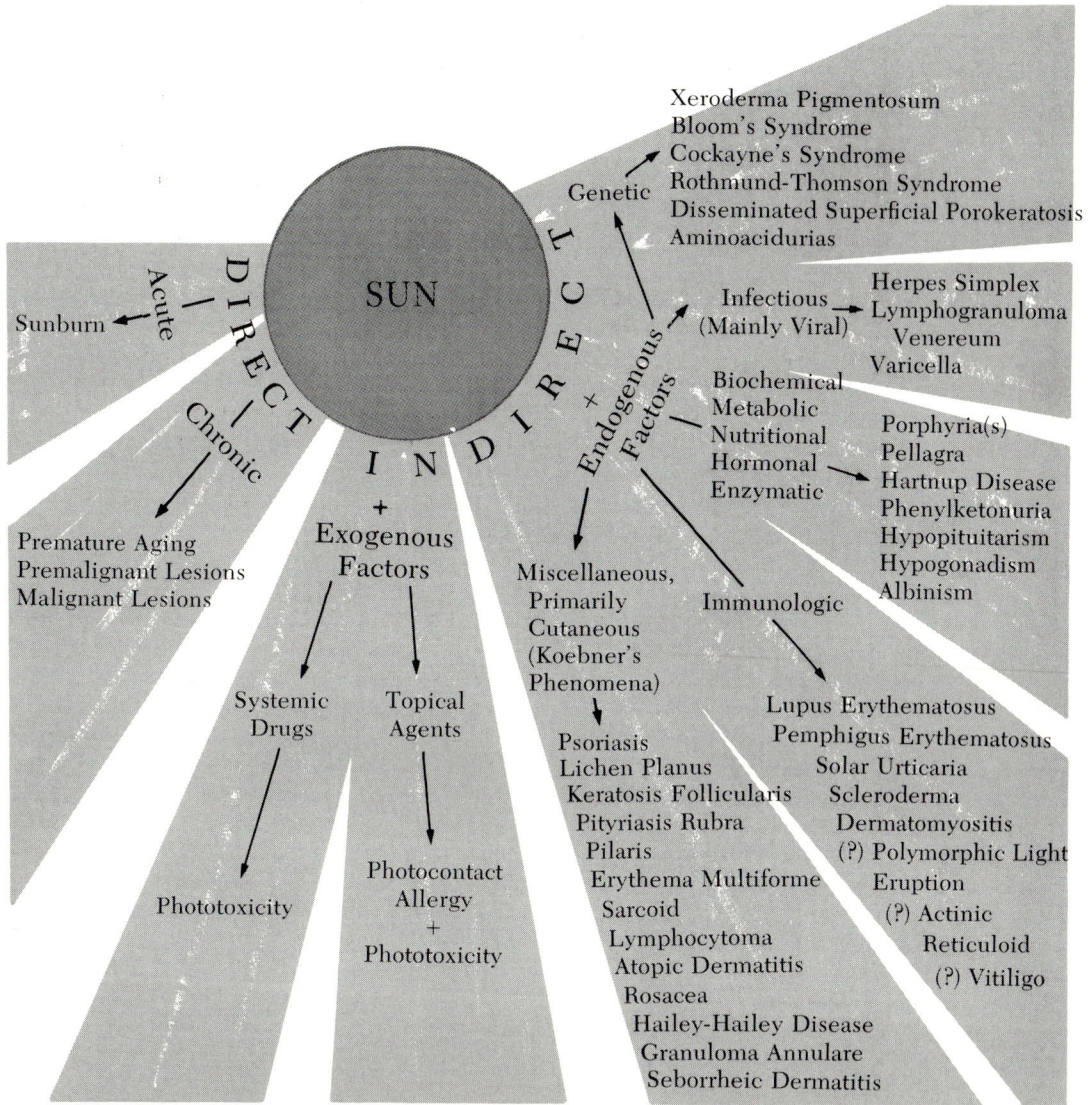

Figure 6–1   Sunlight-related disorders. (After Willis, J.: J.A.M.A. *217*:1089, 1971.)

wavelengths is ideal for healthy existence, except when, by personal habits and desires, indiscriminate prolonged sun exposures are obtained. It is important to note that human skin has neither a neural nor a humoral system that can immediately alert one as to when an overdose of harmful UV radiation is being received. However, if one heeds the warnings of intense brightness and heat from the sun, due to its concomitant great output of visible and infrared rays, dangerous overdoses of UV can be avoided.

The amount of harmful UV radiation that reaches skin at any given time is dependent upon latitude, season, time of day, and the conditions of one's immediate environment (Daniels, 1962; Fitzpatrick et al., 1963; Norins, 1969; Urbach et al., 1966). The most consistent of these factors is latitude. The lower the latitude (for example, 30° North in New Orleans, La. vs. 40° North in Philadelphia, Pa.), the greater will be the risk of sun damage to skin per hour, per day, and per season. The time of greatest risk at all latitudes occurs in midsummer between the hours of 10:00 A.M. and 2:00 P.M. solar time.

Several factors in one's immediate environment have been found to significantly increase the total dose of radiation that one receives. These include white beach sand; concrete; snow; and shiny, metallic, glazed, and painted surfaces. Contrary to common belief, a water surface does not greatly enhance one's risk of sun damage during the critical hours of the day. A lower angle of incidence (past 20° and approaching 0°) is necessary for significant UV reflection by water (Urbach et al., 1966). Although one's clothing will generally reflect or absorb UV, it is important to note that certain white fabrics, when wet, will transmit large amounts of UV to the skin (Daniels, 1962). An overcast or light fog which may not allow one to appreciate sunshine will scatter sufficient UV rays to cause serious skin damage. On the other hand, airborne pollutants, such as dust and smoke, will absorb a significant amount of UV rays on even the sunniest day, and therefore lessen one's chances of receiving sun damage.

Knowledge of these factors is not only useful in educating the population as to hazardous environmental conditions but is also particularly helpful in forming the basis of successful prophylaxis and therapy for the photosensitive patient. Simple avoidance of direct sunlight exposure during the hours of its peak irradiance, and of indirect exposure to the solar-enhancing environmental conditions described above, will significantly decrease the need for prophylactic and therapeutic measures.

PHOTOBIOLOGICAL EVENTS

The first law of photochemistry (Grotthuss-Draper Law) requires that in order for a photochemical or photobiological reaction to proceed, radiant energy must be absorbed (Norins, 1969). Under normal conditions, molecules in the skin are continuously absorbing light; thus, photochemical and biological reactions occur almost continuously both day and night. The wavelengths that are absorbed by a particular molecule when examined spectrophotometrically are referred to as the molecule's absorption spectrum.

The absorption spectrum of each molecule is unique since it is determined by the types and arrangements of its basic atoms. Absorption involves a transfer of energy to the molecule, and once the transfer has occurred the molecule may be raised to an excited or activated "singlet state" in which an electron within the molecule is excited to one of the unoccupied orbitals of the molecule but without change in its direction or orbital spin. This activated state is extremely short-lived (approximately 10^{-8} sec), and its decay is manifested by fluorescence. The singlet state may be converted to a triplet state if the spin of one of the electrons is inverted or becomes parallel. This state may last from 10^{-4} to 1 second. Phosphorescence occurs when the molecule is converted to the triplet state and then decays to the ground state. The triplet state molecule is important in transferring energy and in the initiation of biochemical reactions in vivo. The absorbing molecule may also become so energized that it loses an electron. In this free radical state the molecule is extremely reactive chemically.

Molecules normally found in skin which absorb light include the proteins of keratin, blood, hemoglobins, porphyrins, carotene, nucleic acids, melanin, lipoprotein, peptide bonds, and aromatic amino acids such as tyrosine, tryptophan, and histidine (Fitzpatrick et al., 1963). Such molecules are referred to as chromophores.

PHOTOSENSITIVITY REACTIONS

Distribution

The single common denominator which leads to recognition of all photosensitivity disorders resides in the distribution of lesions. It is important to find not only dermatitis on exposed skin areas but also *uninvolvement* of certain skin sites within these areas. The areas of greatest involvement include the forehead, nose, malar eminences, superior portion of the ears, cheek, lateral and posterior neck, "V" area of the chest, extensor surfaces of the forearms, and dorsal surfaces of the hands. Those sites that remain uninvolved, although they are located on exposed body regions, include the hair-covered areas, such as the scalp, eyebrow, and moustache skin, and those areas that are anatomically shaded from light, namely, the folded portions of the upper eyelids, the recessed portions of the optic orbits, the retro-auricular and nasolabial folds, the upper lip just beneath the nose, the indented portion of the lower lip, the submentum, the upper portion of the anterior neck, and the creases of the lateral neck. These areas quite often remain unaffected in even the most exquisitely photosensitive patient.

In exquisitely photosensitive patients, eruptions are more likely to occur on clothed body skin, where light may penetrate depending upon the type of fabrics worn, rather than on skin covered with dense hair or shaded by anatomic barriers. When the latter areas are involved, it is usually because of the patient's exposure to reflected or scattered light, his assumption of a vulnerable position while exposed to light (namely, lying in a prone, supine, or Trendelenburg position), or the concomitant development of another cutaneous or systemic disorder (for example, contact allergy, seborrheic dermatitis, lupus erythematosus, and so forth). Thus, the involvement of areas that should be spared may be a serious sign of either failure on the part of the patient to avoid hazardous physical and environmental factors or the presence or onset of some other cutaneous or systemic disease.

Classifications of Disorders

Once photosensitivity is suspected, the clinician must establish a specific diagnosis in order to initiate proper therapy and prophylaxis. In narrowing the range of diagnostic possibilities, it is useful to have some systematic classification of the various types of disorders. These disorders may be grouped morphologically, as either quantitative or qualitative abnormalities in reactivity; evolutionarily, as either immediate or delayed responses; mechanistically, as either direct or indrect effects of sunlight; spectrally, as either short or long ultraviolet to visible light-induced; and etiologically, as either endogenously or exogenously induced.

In this chapter, disorders will be di-vided into two basic types (see Fig. 6–1): (1) *direct disorders*, to denote those reactions that simply follow an overexposure or chronic exposure to sunlight alone, and (2) *indirect* disorders, to denote reactions that require endogenous or exogenous photosensitizing factors along with sunlight exposure for manifestation. Both types of disorders will be subdivided on the basis of evolutionary (immediate vs. delayed), genetic, and environmental factors.

DIRECT DISORDERS

Direct photosensitivity disorders can be subdivided into two types: (1) immediate, or acute sunburn reactions, and (2) delayed, or chronic sun damage (senile degeneration, premalignant and malignant lesions). Both types of disorders are due to a direct damaging effect of the sun's rays on skin. More specifically, this damage has been attributed mainly to the short UV rays (290–320 nm.) which penetrate into the epidermis and cause detrimental photochemical changes within viable cells (Everett et al., 1965; Fitzpatrick et al., 1963; Freeman, et al., 1966; Johnson et al., 1968). The most significant alterations occur in purine and pyrimidine bases of DNA; in proteins which undergo rupture of hydrogen and disulfide bonds; in vital enzymes which lead to inhibition of glucose oxidation, glycolysis, transamination, acid maltase inhibition, and lactic acid dehydrogenation; and in a variety of other vital cellular activities, namely, lysosomal labilization and rupture, decrease in phospholipid content, alterations in urocanic acid isomerization and in lipid peroxidase formation (Daniels et al., 1968; Ippen, 1969; Johnson and Daniels, 1969; McLaren and Luse, 1961; Smith, 1969; Yeargers, 1969). The less energetic long UV rays (320–400 nm.) penetrate deeper into the epidermis and down to the mid- and lower dermis. Although little or no evidence of the kinds of changes described above has been noted following this type of radiation exposure, direct damage to capillaries with necrotic changes produced in vascular endothelium have been found (Miescher, 1957; Terus, 1946). Visible rays (400–700 nm.) penetrate into the epidermis, dermis, and subcutis. Aside from their potential damaging thermal effects, studies have shown these wavelengths to cause destruction of cytochrome A3, riboflavin, and flavin enzymes (Smith, 1971). Infrared rays (> 700 nm.) penetrate throughout the skin and are known to cause coagulation necrosis of the skin (thermal burn).

Although direct disorders have been thought to be due mainly to the effects of short UV exposure, more recent experimental studies have shown that longer wavelengths play a significant role in their development. It has been found that exposure to so-called harmless doses of long UV rays, either before or after full-spectrum sunlight exposure, results in a marked increase in the degree of sunburn damage to skin. Although when massive doses of long UV are given alone erythema responses can be obtained, the type of enhancement described above can be seen after small doses of long UV, and the response is far greater in intensity than what one would expect from a simple additive effect of long UV and short UV exposures (Willis et al., 1972).

Another type of short UV enhancement has been previously described in mice when exposed to a combination of short UV and infrared radiation. The carcinogenic effects of short UV were found to be increased owing to the presence of heat (Freeman and Knox, 1964).

The degree of damage produced by sunlight exposure depends not only upon the physical and environmental factors described up to this point but also upon host defenses. Host defenses are mainly inherited qualities of skin manifested in terms of skin color (melanin content) or race, and to some extent, the thickness of the stratum corneum (Claesson, 1959; Fitzpatrick, 1965). The latter is of approximately the same thickness in different races but differs in thickness (and thus in its UV scatter, reflection, and absorption capabilities) on different body areas (Kligman, 1964; Thompson, 1955). Melanin serves not only to reflect, absorb, and scatter light but also to capture free radicals that may produce detrimental photochemical reactions in the skin. Therefore, those most susceptible to developing direct disorders are the less melanized, lighter complexioned individuals of any race or group, the rufous (red-haired) and blond individuals being symbolic of this type. The high susceptibility of rufous persons to cutaneous sun damage may be due to a qualitative difference in melanin as well as quantitatively less melanin. Negro or black individuals are the least susceptible of all races, regardless of skin color; however, even though endowed with greater solar defenses, they are not exempt from the deleterious effects of prolonged sun exposure.

Immediate Reactions (Sunburn)

This type of reaction results from a single overexposure to sunlight or a short UV-emitting artificial light source. Reactivity may range in severity from a mild, asymptomatic erythema to a more intense erythema, accompanied by tenderness, pain, edema, and sometimes vesiculation or bulla formation. Mild reactions begin approximately 6 to 12 hours from the beginning of exposure, reach a peak intensity within about 24 hours, begin to decline gradually over the next three to five days, and generally end in an "appealing" tan that reaches its maximum approximately two to three weeks after exposure. Intense reactions begin similarly except that signs and symptoms continue to progress, reaching their peak in about 48 hours. Within another 24 to 48 hours, necrosis and sloughing of the skin may occur. This type of reaction will lead to uneven pigmentation and sometimes permanent scarring.

When a large portion of the body's surface has been severely sunburned, cutaneous signs and symptoms may be followed approximately 12 hours later by systemic signs and symptoms of toxicity (namely, fever, chills, nausea, delirium, and prostration). Therapeutic requirements, morbidity, and mortality in these cases are similar to cases of extensive first and second degree thermal burns. All intense sunburn reactions should be viewed with suspicion for the possible presence of some underlying, abnormal, sunburn-enhancing etiologic factor (for example, photosensitizing drug or disease) unless circumstances and exposure time clearly justify the reaction.

The histologic features of sunburn damage may be present in biopsy specimens (hematoxylin and eosin–stained sections) as early as 8 to 12 hours after sun exposure. Within 18 to 24 hours, one can usually find the "characteristic" epidermal cells with homogeneous eosinophilic cytoplasm and pyknotic nuclei ("sunburn cells"). Further evidence of epidermal injury can be seen in the form of glycogen deposition and lysosomal enzyme release detected by histochemical staining with the Hotchkiss-McManus (PAS) and acid phosphatase techniques, respectively. The dermis shows very little change except for mild to moderate vascular dilatation and the presence of perivascular mononuclear and polymorphonuclear cells.

Autoradiographic studies have added much to our understanding of cellular biochemical changes and kinetics following sunburn damage (Epstein et al., 1968, 1969, 1970; Fukuyama and Epstein, 1966; Tan, et al., 1970; Willis et al., 1972). Studies using tritiated thymidine (TdR-H³) have shown evidence of DNA damage through its repair ("unscheduled" DNA synthesis) as early as 15 minutes after light exposure. This type of repair continues to occur for approximately six hours. The number of epidermal cells that are ordinarily in a stage of "scheduled" DNA synthesis is initially suppressed after sunburning UV exposure. This suppression continues for approximately 48 hours, depending upon the dose of light received, after which, a marked increase in synthesis occurs which may last as long as 5 to 10 days. Tritiated histidine (histidine-H³) studies have shown that protein synthesis becomes depressed within one hour post-exposure and may last for 96 hours or more, depending upon the severity of the sunburn reaction.

At the same time the above events are taking place, the cutaneous pigmentary system also undergoes certain changes (Bachem, 1955; Breit and Kligman, 1969; Pathak and Stratton, 1969; Willis et al., 1973). The "immediate pigment darkening phenomenon" (IPD) is the first event to occur; that is, the skin immediately becomes darker owing to the oxidation of colorless (reduced) melanin already present in the skin. This darkening is temporary and fades within a few hours. The major pigmentary change in skin begins two to three days after sun exposure and reaches maximum intensity in about two to three weeks. The melanocyte number and size are usually increased in a DOPA-incubated and/or Fontana silver stained specimen.

Within approximately three weeks after a moderate sunburn reaction, the skin will appear quite normal; however, it is known that impaired vasomotor tone can be detected in skin more than a year after it has been sunburned (Holti, 1955).

Electron microscopic studies of skin following sunburn radiation exposure have revealed additional findings (Epstein, 1971; Miescher, 1957; Pathak and Epstein, 1971). The earliest change (that is, a decrease in the malpighian and granular cell keratinosomes) occurs about two hours post-exposure. Soon afterwards, other cytoplasmic, nucleolar, and nuclear changes can be seen. These include the appearance of electron-dense bodies beginning in the basal cell layer about six hours post-exposure and their eventual appearance throughout the epidermis by 72 hours, alterations in lysosomes, and more specific features of sunburned cells that include clumping of their tonafilaments, reduction in their desmosomes, cytoplasmic vacuolization, nuclear and nucleolar fragmentation, and an absence of keratinosomes.

Delayed Reactions (Premature Aging, Premalignant and Malignant Changes)

These conditions result from repeated, prolonged exposure to sunlight. Although the total amount of sun exposure required to produce these effects in man is unknown, there is evidence to indicate that some degree of irreversible damage to skin occurs with each prolonged exposure. Cumulative damage eventually results in the clinical and histologic changes characteristic of senile skin (Howell, 1960; Kligman, 1969). Clinically, there is a change in the skin's texture with varying degrees of uneven atrophy and hyperplasia, yellowish thickened plaques and nodules (solar elastotic changes; Fig. 6–2), erythema, telangiectasias, and brown macular irregular pigmented lesions (benign keratoses). Histologically, this skin generally shows

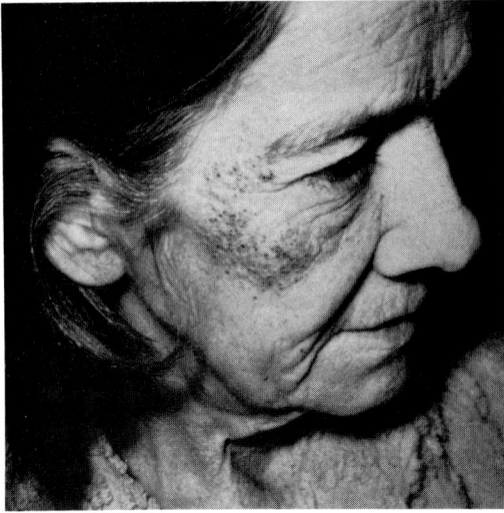

Figure 6–2 Nodular elastosis (Favre-Racouchot syndrome). This 67-year-old widow demonstrates nodular elastotic changes with comedones and follicular cysts.

ment transfer from melanocytes to keratinocytes. Although one can observe an increase in the number of melanocytes and alterations in Langerhans' cells after repeated acute sunburn exposures, these changes are not seen in chronically damaged skin (Epstein, 1971; Pathak and Epstein, 1971).

The above changes commonly precede, and even seem to create, the milieu for development of premalignant and malignant lesions. The principal premalignant lesion is an actinic or solar keratosis. It usually begins as a telangiectatic area of less than one-half centimeter in size and progresses to develop an adherent yellowish brown scaly surface, while its base remains erythematous (Fig. 6–3). Lesions are usually multiple, localized to sunexposed areas, and are in different stages of development. Histologically, lesions may be one of three types—atrophic, hypertrophic, or Bowenoid. Microscopic examination of any of the types will reveal a disorderly arrangement, abnormality and dyskeratotic change in the malpighain cells, and collagen degeneration and monocytic infiltration in the dermis.

Approximately 25 per cent of individuals with multiple actinic keratoses have been reported to develop squamous cell carcinomas in one or more of the lesions (Lever, 1967). Malignancy developing in an actinic keratosis usually presents as a shallow central ulceration covered by a crust with a widely elevated and indurated border, although occasionally no signifi-

progressive degenerative changes in collagen with its replacement by elastic fibrils, and finally, homogenization and elastosis of the dermis, vascular dilation or ectatic vessels, and thinning of the overlying epidermis with abnormal malpighain cells arranged in a disorderly manner. Basal layer clefts and increased pigmentation are also prominent features. Electron microscopy reveals degenerative features in epidermal cells, including decreases in endoplasmic reticulum, ribosomes, tonafilaments, and keratohyalin. There appears to be an impairment of pig-

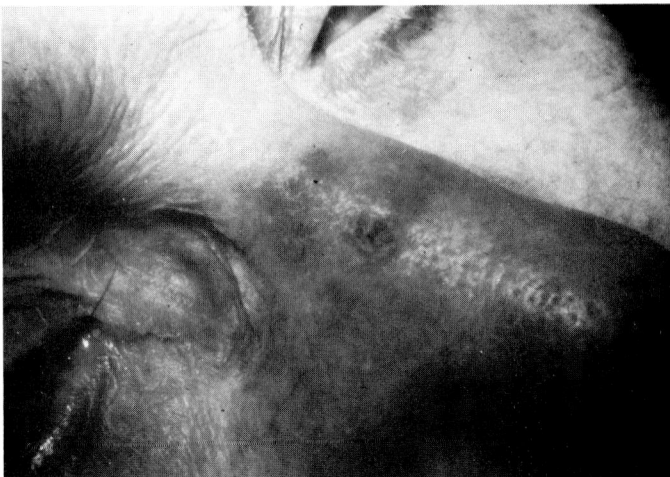

Figure 6–3 Actinic keratoses in 70-year-old retired sailor; the lesions appeared on the diffusely thin skin of the face accompanied by telangiectases and erythematous patches with adherent, "dirty" appearing, heaped-up scales.

cant changes except induration will be observed. When the malignancy presents as a fungoid or verrucoid growth, it is considered to be somewhat less aggressive than the ulcerated type. It is generally felt that squamous cell carcinomas arising in sun-damaged skin are less apt to metastasize than those arising in other types of lesions (for example, x-ray dermatitis, burn scars, and so forth); however, treatment will be the same, depending upon the tumor's grade and stage, regardless of etiologic factors.

It is to be noted that while malignancies such as basal cell cancers and melanomas are not as directly related to sun damage as are squamous cell cancers, they do tend to occur with greater frequency in sun-damaged skin.

For the treatment of multiple premalignant lesions (keratoses) on sun-damaged skin, good results can be obtained through the use of topical fluorouracil (Fluoroplex, Efudex). This chemotherapeutic agent not only removes the majority of premalignant and superficial malignant lesions that can be seen but also will uncover and destroy clinically undetectable lesions of this type (Fig. 6–4). Lesions that persist after treatment with fluorouracil and those that are obviously invasive when seen initially should be treated by surgical methods.

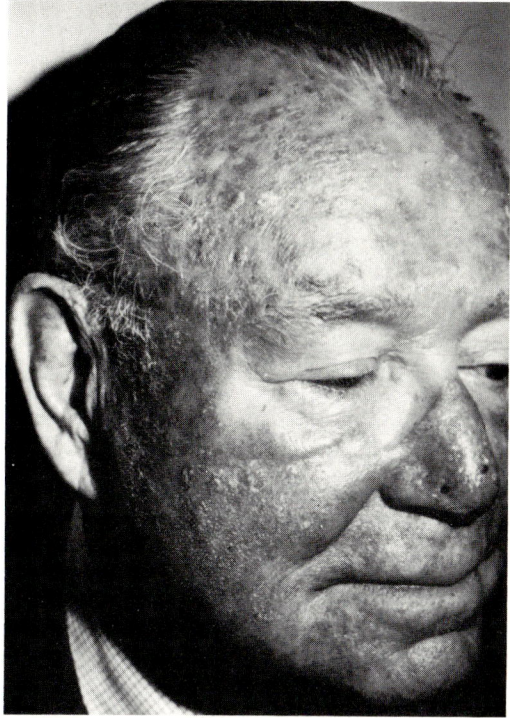

Figure 6–4 Retired businessman who exhibits the anticipated inflammation resulting from use of topical fluorouracil which not only destroys the premalignant and superficial malignant lesions but also uncovers and treats lesions which were not initially appreciated clinically.

INDIRECT DISORDERS

Indirect photosensitivity disorders may be subdivided into two types, depending upon the origins of their underlying etiologic factors: (1) photosensitivity of exogenous origin, in which reactions are due to drugs or agents that reach the skin via topical contact or systemic administration (see Table 6–1), and (2) photosensitivity of endogenous origin, in which reactions are due to an underlying disturbance in biochemical, metabolic, nutritional, hormonal, enzymatic, or immunologic functions; genetic disorders; infectious processes; or an abnormality in cutaneous responsiveness (isomorphic or Koebner reactivity) due to an underlying disease (see Fig. 6–1).

Although many of these disorders are activated primarily by sunburn rays (290–320 nm.), the majority require exposure to radiation in the long UV to visible light range (320–700 nm.) for manifestation. In many instances, the characteristic lesions for a particular indirect disorder due to long UV or visible light or both may not be apparent upon clinical examination because of superimposed sunburn and/or thermal effects from natural simultaneous overexposure to short UV and infrared rays from the sun. For this reason, phototest and photo patch test procedures (to be described later) are available for local elicitation of the unaltered dermatitic process in order to arrive at an accurate action spectrum and diagnosis.

Photosensitivity of Exogenous Origin

Reactions of this type can be divided into two kinds: (1) phototoxicity and (2) photocontact allergy. These reactions account for perhaps the largest number of indirect disorders that will be seen. Their

TABLE 6–1   Common Photosensitizing Drugs and Agents

	Common Uses	*Photosensitivity Reactions*
Tetracyclines (mainly demeclo-cycline HC1)	Antibiotics	Ptx°
Sulfonamides	Antibacterials	Ptx; may induce PCA
Nalidixic acid	Antibacterial	Ptx
Griseofulvin	Antifungal	Ptx
Halogenated salicylanilides, halogenated carbanilides halogenated phenols	Antibacterials in deodorant bar soap, antiseptics, cosmetics	PCA; mild Ptx
Phenothiazines	Sedatives, tranquilizers, antiemetics, antihistaminics, analgesic potentiators	Ptx; may induce PCA
Chlorothiazides	Diuretics	Ptx; may induce PCA
Sulfonylureas	Hypoglycemics	Ptx; may induce PCA
Furocoumarins	Melanogenics and in cosmetics	Ptx; may induce PCA
Coal tars, wood tars, and petroleum products	Antipsoriatics and in cosmetics	Ptx; may induce PCA
Aminobenzoates	Sunscreens	PCA; ? mild Ptx

°Ptx signifies phototoxic reaction; PCA, photocontact allergic reaction.

steady increase in incidence over the past few years has been in direct proportion to the increase in production and use of unsuspected photosensitizing chemicals in antibacterial bar soaps, antiseptics, cosmetics, drugs, and numerous other commercial, industrial, and environmental chemical products.

The induction, elicitation, and severity of reactions depend not only upon the environmental and host factors previously outlined but also upon the following factors in particular (Pathak, 1969): (1) the age, integrity, degree of hydration, temperature, pH, and physiologic and immunologic responsiveness of skin, (2) the spectral absorption, structural characteristics, and stability of the etiologic chemical, that is, its inherent photosensitizing potentiality, (3) the solubility and penetrability of the chemical, (4) the chemical's vehicle, and the latter's effect on the rate and type of photochemical reactivity, (5) the level at which the chemical is located or its distribution in skin, (6) the total dose or concentration of the chemical received, (7) the time lag between chemical administration and light exposure, (8) the absorption and penetrability of skin to wavelengths required for chemical activation, (9) the intensity of both indirect and direct impinging light from the sun or artificial light source, and (10) the total dose of activating light received.

In neither phototoxicity nor photo-allergy is sunburn necessary for the reactions to take place, since the primary activating rays have been found to reside in the range of 320 to 425 nm. (Cripps and Enta, 1967; Freeman and Knox, 1968; Harber et al., 1966; Jillson, 1969; Willis and Kligman, 1968).

PHOTOTOXICITY. This type of photosensitivity is generally referred to as a chemically induced exaggerated sunburn response. However, except when induced by psoralen-type chemicals, these responses are quite different from sunburn in both their evolution and histology. The mechanisms of each response is based upon the type of direct toxic effect which results from each particular kind of photochemical reaction that the chemical is capable of causing. Phototoxicity occurs independent of any known type of immunologic mechanism.

Based upon clinical evolution and underlying mechanism, there are two types of phototoxic reactions: (1) the immediate type, commonly referred to as a photodynamic reaction, and (2) the delayed type, which more closely mimics an exaggerated sunburn reaction.

The immediate type of reaction is most commonly seen in persons receiving systemic antibacterial drugs (Declomycin and sulfonamides), certain dyes, (for example, acridine, methyl violet, eosin; Fig. 6–5), psychotherapeutic drugs (phenothiazines), sulfonylurea hypoglycemic agents, thiazide diuretics, and antifungal griseofulvin. Upon exposure to intense light, there is a rapid onset of a burning sensation followed by erythema (Fig. 6–6A), edema (Fig. 6–6B), and sometimes vesiculation (Fig. 6–6C). A mild to moderate reaction will be acutely urticarial within two to six hours, followed by erythema and tenderness resembling a sunburn at 24 hours. This inflammation resolves over the next two to four days, resulting in hyperpigmentation and desquamation. More severe reactions may reach maximum acute intensity within a shorter period of time followed by vesiculation and bulla formation within 12 to 24 hours post-exposure (Fig. 6–6C). Such reactions tend to have a slower decline in inflammation and often result in mottled hypo- and hyperpigmentation and varying degrees of scarring. In some cases, an intense violet erythema or lichenoid changes or both (Jones et al., 1972) may persist for weeks.

Microscopic examination of biopsy specimens obtained from immediate phototoxic reactions at 12 to 24 hours after light exposure will reveal reactions ranging from vascular dilatation and slightly increased lymphocytic perivascular infiltrate to more severe changes of subepidermal bulla formation, upper dermal edema, vasodilation, and dense perivascular

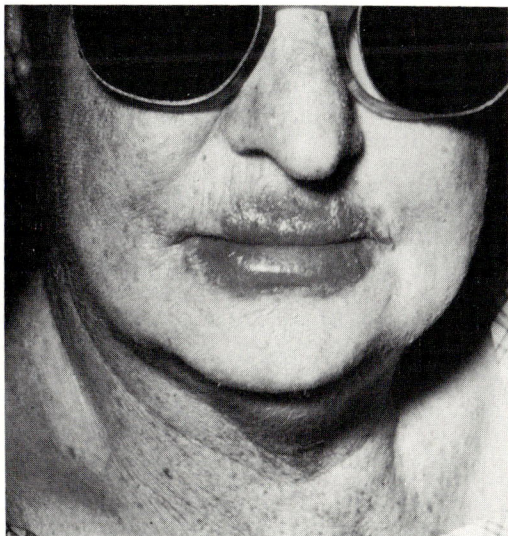

Figure 6–5 Patient developed acute cheilitis which resulted from use of lipstick containing eosin; this was confirmed by photo patch testing.

lymphocytic infiltration. Epidermal cell necrosis with subsequent increased cellular proliferation and hyperpigmentation will be seen in biopsy specimens obtained 48 to 72 hours post-exposure.

The mechanism of the immediate phototoxic reaction (due to dyes) was originally shown to depend upon the presence of molecular oxygen (Blum, 1941). The complete mechanism may include the absorption of light by a chemical with subsequent release of energy as intense heat and fluorescence and in some cases the formation of free radicals with subsequent damage to vital cell components and cell membranes.

The delayed type of phototoxic reactions, in some cases, may be due to the presence in skin of high concentrations of natural furocoumarins found in plants (for example, of the Rutaceae and Umbelliferae families—parsley, celery, lime, and citrus fruits). However, the majority of these reactions are due to therapeutically administered synthetic or natural psoralen chemicals. The cutaneous response that one sees following the use of psoralens for repigmentation in vitiligo typifies this type of phototoxicity (Fig. 6–7). The furocoumarin chemicals were commonly present in perfumes in the past. Skin exposed to light after the application of these perfumes would develop mild to moderate erythema followed by hyperpigmentation (Berlock dermatitis; Fig. 6–8). More severe reactions following contact with concentrated plant juices resulted in bulla formation confined to the areas of contact and light exposure (phytophotodermatitis).

The earliest signs of furocoumarin phototoxicity usually do not occur until approximately 6 to 12 hours post-exposure to light and do not reach a peak until almost 48 hours after light exposure, at which time erythema, edema, and vesiculation will be present. Unlike the symptoms that occur as a result of the immediate type of phototoxicity, the patient does not experience burning, tingling, and so forth, during or shortly after exposure. Symptoms eventually appear after about 24 hours and consist mainly of tenderness in the area of inflammation. Mild to moderately inflamed reactions tend to decline over the next 7 to 14 days, and end in mild desquamation and hyperpigmentation.

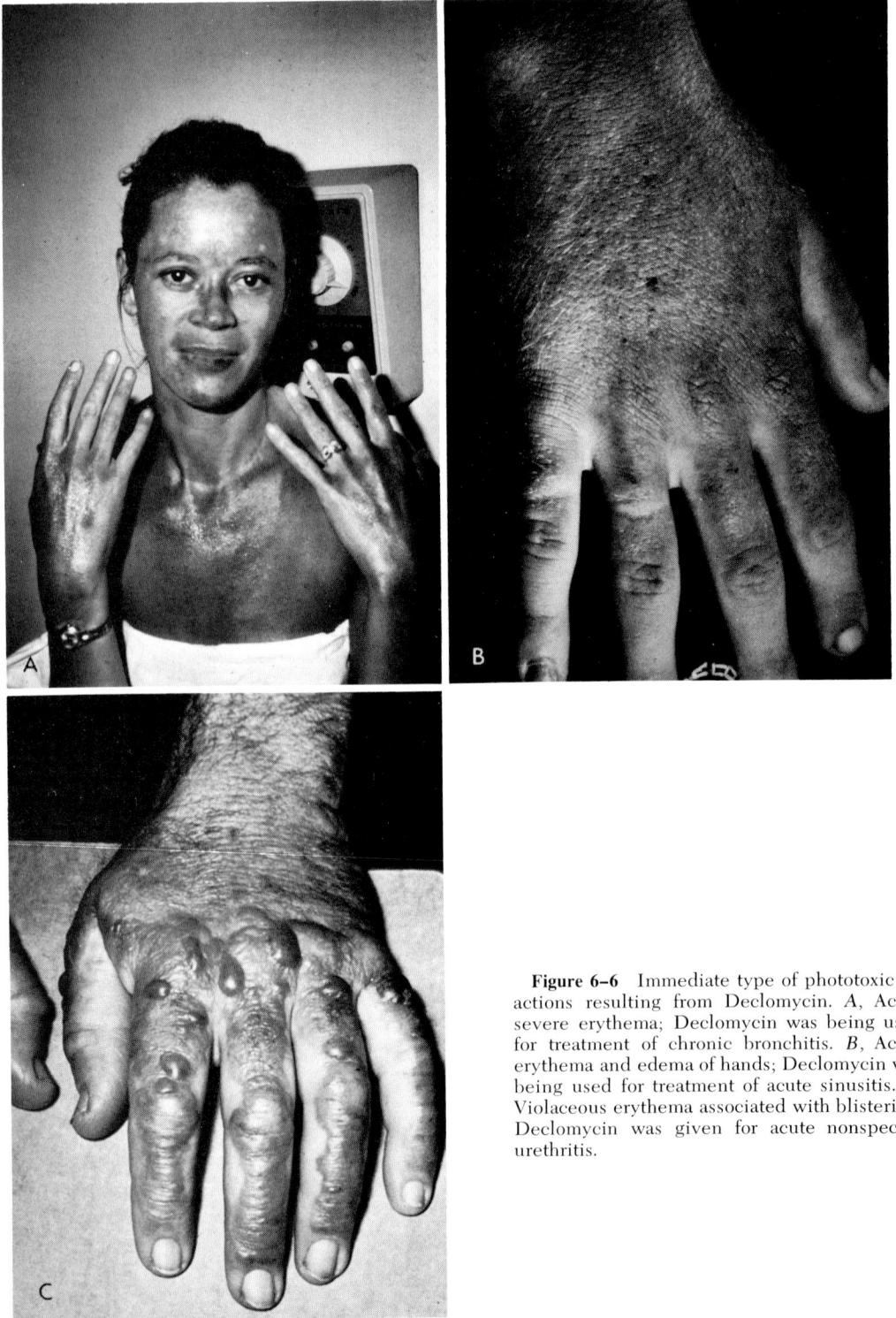

Figure 6-6 Immediate type of phototoxic reactions resulting from Declomycin. *A,* Acute severe erythema; Declomycin was being used for treatment of chronic bronchitis. *B,* Acute erythema and edema of hands; Declomycin was being used for treatment of acute sinusitis. *C,* Violaceous erythema associated with blistering; Declomycin was given for acute nonspecific urethritis.

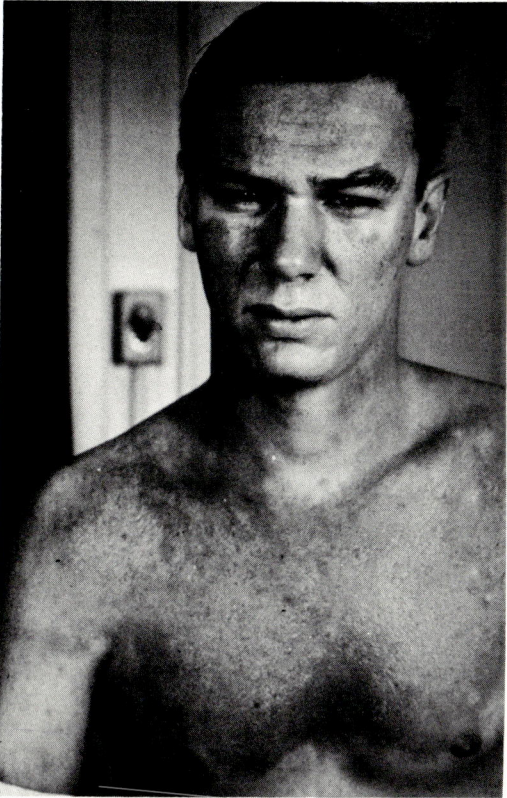

Figure 6–7 Patient developed phototoxic reaction induced by use of 8-methoxypsoralen for vitiligo of trunk.

layer and epidermis of these individuals will effectively filter out the potential activating rays, and perhaps it may also serve as a free radical trap. Immediate phototoxic reactions generally require far more energy for elicitation than do the delayed reactions.

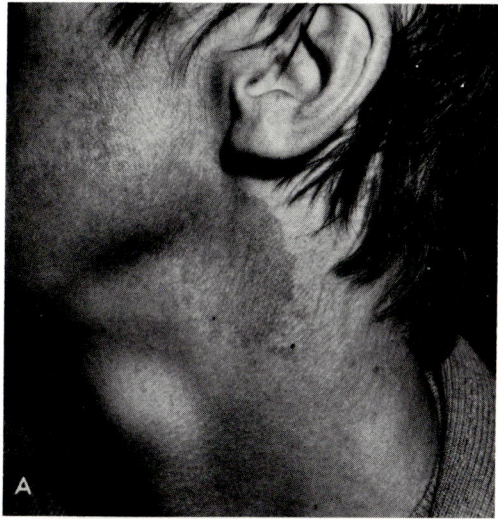

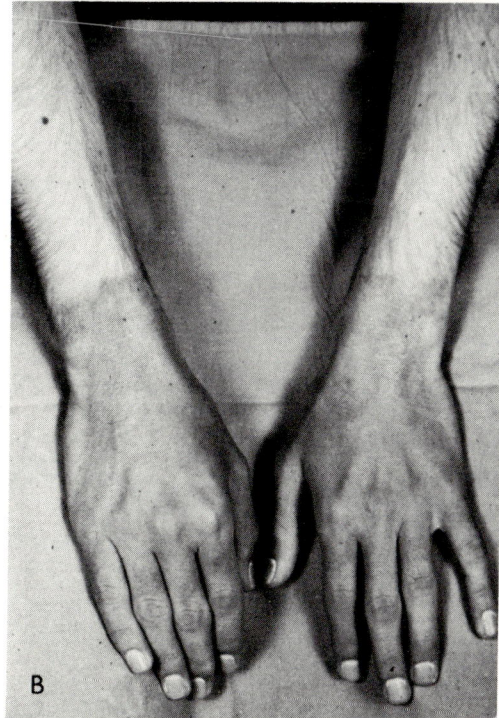

In contrast to the immediate phototoxic reaction, in which photochemical damage occurs mainly within the upper part of the dermis, furocoumarin photochemically induced damage occurs chiefly in the epidermis. The long wavelength ultraviolet light (320–400 nm.) induces free radical formation in psoralens and in this state the psoralen causes lethal photochemical changes in cell constituents, the most critical of which is DNA. Pyrimidine dimerization in DNA, damage to proteins, and so forth cause the sunburn type of epidermal cellular death, dyskeratosis, and desquamation that is seen (Epstein and Fukuyama, 1970; Nizuno and Freeman, 1969; Pathak and Epstein, 1971).

An important point in the differential diagnosis of photosensitivity reactions is that phototoxicity reactions will rarely occur in dark-skinned or black individuals, except for very mild reactions of the delayed furocoumarin type. Presumably the dense melanin present within the horny

Figure 6–8 Berlock dermatitis. *A,* Usual location with cologne users and the residual pigmentation. *B,* Unusual location resulting from accidental spilling of the mother's cologne.

When the diagnosis of phototoxicity is suspected, one may choose to either determine the etiologic substance by appropriate photo tests and photo patch tests or simply withdraw the most likely causative drug or agent from use by the patient. If a particular drug or dose of drug is necessary for the treatment of a patient despite its known high phototoxic potentiality, then the physician must warn the patient not to expose himself to intense light of any type and to use appropriate full-spectrum sunscreening agents (to be described later) when light exposure cannot be avoided. Although the possibility of inducing photoallergy after repeated phototoxic insults exists, the incidence of this development is extremely low. The prescription of a potentially phototoxic drug or agent for use by an individual who already has a photosensitivity disorder should be strictly prohibited, except under circumstances of very close physician supervision, because of the potentially severe consequences.

PHOTOALLERGY. Aside from a few isolated case reports in which systemically administered drugs were thought to be etiologic, the vast majority of cases of photoallergy has developed following contact with photosensitizing chemicals (Harber et al., 1966; Sidi et al., 1955; Wilkinson, 1961). The preferred terminology for describing the latter reaction is "photoallergic contact dermatitis." The most common etiologic chemicals are found in deodorant bar soaps and cosmetics. Following sufficient exposure to the chemical agent and 320 to 425 nm. wavelength light, there is an initial refractory period of 5 to 10 days, after which, subsequent exposure to the chemical and light results in a cell-mediated immune response that is identical to that of ordinary delayed hypersensitivity of the contact allergic type (Burckhardt, 1941; Harber et al., 1966; Willis and Kligman, 1968). The induction of photoallergic contact dermatitis can be accomplished in any normal individual; however, the incidence of the naturally occurring disease is highest in middle-aged and elderly males.

Two basic mechanisms to explain the induction of this disease have been proposed: (1) that light acts upon the chemical to form a stable haptene which then binds to protein to form a complete antigen (Burckhardt, 1941; Willis and Kligman, 1968), and (2) that light acts upon the chemical to form an unstable (free radical) haptene which binds to protein to form an antigen (Harber et al., 1966; Jenkins et al., 1964).

It is significant to note that all known photoallergic drugs and agents are also phototoxic (see Table 6–1). However, photoallergy may be elicited in its severest form without the coexistence of phototoxicity because very low energy is required to bring about photoallergic reactions (Willis and Kligman, 1969) and the phototoxic potentialities of most photoallergenic agents are not great. All phototoxic drugs, however, are not photoallergenic; for example, demethylchlortetracycline is a potent phototoxic agent but photoallergy has not been seen (Willis, 1968).

Photoallergy, unlike phototoxicity, may occur in any race or color of individual (Fig. 6–9). In Caucasian or very light-skinned individuals who sunburn easily or are susceptible to phototoxicity, photoallergic reactions may be enhanced by sunburn and phototoxicity reactions.

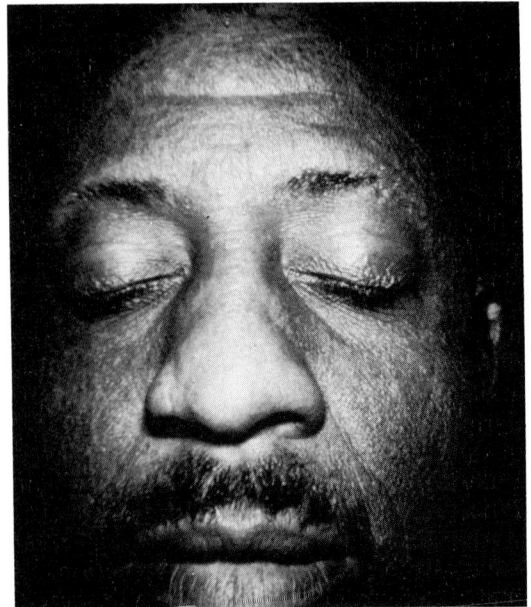

Figure 6–9 This 39-year-old Negro male had a persistent light reaction for at least five years and had to reverse his life style, working at night under nonfluorescent lighting.

Photocontact allergy is one of the most distressing of dermatologic disorders. Initial signs and symptoms consist of intense pruritus and acute eczema with oozing, weeping, and crusting of affected areas which begin within 24 to 48 hours after combined chemical and light exposure. Areas of involvement and sparing include those described earlier concerning photosensitivity distribution; however, clothed areas frequently show mild to moderate eczematous dermatitis since the activating long UV–visible rays can penetrate clothes (Willis and Kligman, 1969). Maximum inflammation is usually reached by 72 hours after light exposure and regresses over the next 10 to 14 days. Some reactions may continue in a subacute stage for a much longer period because of the patient's inadvertent contact with the sensitizer or when use of a related chemical is continued. The skin may eventually become lichenified as a result of chronic inflammation, scratching, and rubbing of pruritic skin.

The level of photosensitivity in some cases may be so great that minute amounts of the residual chemical in the skin plus light are sufficient to maintain a persistently active disease state (Willis and Kligman, 1968). This type of patient is referred to as a "persistent light reactor" (Jillson and Baughman, 1963; Fig. 6–10).

Many of these patients have been reported to manifest a lowering of the UV dose requirement for sunburn (that is, a decreased minimal erythema dose) on uninvolved skin surfaces. It is to be noted, however, that in exquisitely hypersensitive patients with widespread active eczema, nonspecific hypersensitivity reactions to a variety of inflammatory chemical and physical stimuli, including sunburn, can occur, and may be likened in a sense to a Koebner reaction. As previously noted, sunburn, phototoxic reactions, or both may significantly enhance the inflammation of the mildest photoallergic reactivity.

Histologically, the 24- to 48-hour-old, uncomplicated, moderately severe photoallergic reaction shows marked epidermal spongiosis, intra-epidermal vesiculation, infiltration of the epidermis by lymphocytes (exocytosis), and moderately dense perivenular infiltrates of mononuclear cells. Intensely severe reactions with

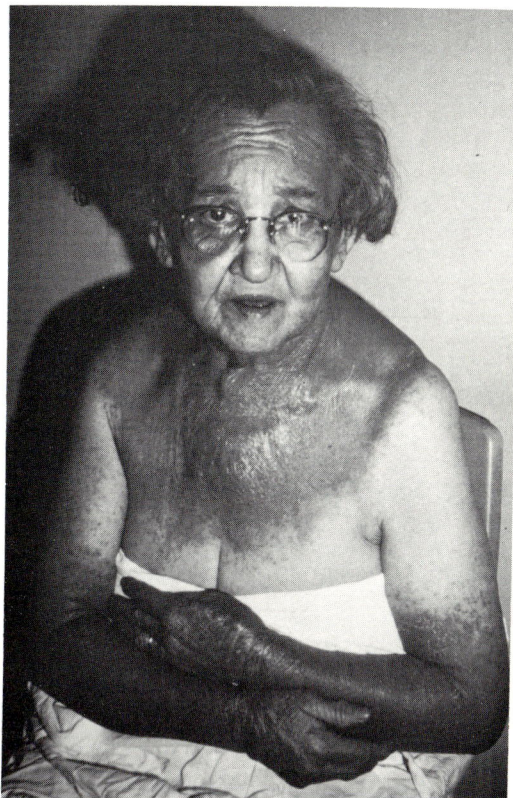

Figure 6–10 Patient has been a persistent light reactor; the eruption was initiated by the use of an antiseptic soap, halogenated salicylanilide.

marked epidermal destruction may show eosinophils and polymorphonuclear leukocytes in both the dermis and epidermis. The mildest reactions may show only perivascular mononuclear cell infiltrates. All of the above reactions are identical histologically to reactions or ordinary contact dermatitis (Willis and Kligman, 1968).

It is sometimes difficult to establish a diagnosis of photocontact allergy because of an unconvincing history of contact with a potential photosensitizing chemical, an atypical distribution of the eruption, or the presence of only very mild and transient clinical dermatitis. In these instances, establishment of the diagnosis will depend upon the results of photo test and photo patch test procedures.

Once the diagnosis has been suspected or established, it is of utmost importance to instruct the patient to avoid all soaps, cosmetics, and other products which contain potential photosensitizing chemicals, as

well as any known products which contain
chemicals related to the suspected sensitizing chemical. In addition, these patients
should minimize their exposure to natural
sunlight and avoid unnecessary exposure
to lamp sources with high irradiance in the
UV or visible light spectrum, such as
movie projector lamps, fluorescent lights,
sun lamps, and very intense incandescent
light.

The photoallergic contact dermatitis
should be managed as an ordinary contact
allergic dermatitis, that is, on the basis of
the stage of the dermatitic process.

As soon as the acute dermatitis has resolved, a suitable sunscreening agent
should be added to the therapeutic regimen. Full-spectrum screens, to be described later, will be of greatest prophylactic benefit to patients with this condition.

Photosensitivity of Endogenous Origin

Disorders of this type can be thought of
as "photocutaneous manifestations of systemic disease." The cutaneous response is
the result of some underlying disease or
abnormality. The photosensitivity can be
expected to be suppressed or cured if the
underlying abnormality or disease is controlled, corrected, or cured.

When an underlying abnormality or disease has been in remission rather than
cured, excessive sun exposure may provoke not only a cutaneous eruption but
also, in some cases, renewed manifestations of the underlying disease (as in lupus
erythematosus).

These photosensitivity eruptions will be
discussed in five different groups based
upon their most common etiologic factors
and associated clinical features.

BIOCHEMICAL. The disorder may be
due to either acquired or inherited disturbances in specific enzymes, hormones,
metabolism, or nutrition.

The most common of these disorders are
the porphyrias (excluding the acute intermittent type). Photosensitivity is due to
the presence of circulating porphyrin
molecules that are strongly absorbent in
the visible wavelength spectrum of sunlight. Peak absorption by these chromophores occurs in the violet blue light region of 400 to 410 nm. and in the orange
500 to 600 nm. range (Magnus, 1968;

Schmid, 1966). Except for the acquired
type of porphyria (that is, cutanea tarda),
these disorders are due to autosomal dominant inheritance of disturbances in porphyrin metabolism or the normal biosyn-
thetic pathway which leads to heme formation.

In the case of erythropoietic protoporphyria, signs and symptoms begin in early
childhood and closely resemble those
previously described for the immediate
type of drug phototoxicity. Burning pain
and edema may occur upon exposure to as
little as 15 to 20 minutes of intense sunlight. Repeated exposures may result in
eczematization, linear crustations, purpura, and permanent scarring. This condition is also characterized by the laboratory
finding of increased fecal protoporphyrin,
and by the finding of fluorescing erythrocytes upon fluorescent microscopic examination of peripheral blood. The latter feature is most helpful diagnostically; however, erythrocyte fluorescence can also be
found in patients with erythropoietic coproporphyria, Günther's porphyria, and
coproporphyria. The diagnosis can be
more specifically confirmed by fecal and
urinary porphyrin levels. Both levels are
normal in erythropoietic coproporphyria,
and only the urine porphyrins are increased in Günther's porphyria. Coproporphyria patients excrete increased urinary porphyrins and sometimes increased
porphobilinogen.

Günther's erythropoietic porphyria
manifests during childhood, and sun exposure results in far more destructive
changes than in any of the other porphyrias. Acute lesions are followed by extensive scarring of the eyelids and eyes and
severe mutilation with loss of ear and nose
cartilages, as well as terminal phalanges.

Porphyria variegata and porphyria cutanea tarda (either acquired or inherited)
begin in adult life and present similar
cutaneous features of hypertrichosis and
skin fragility. Sun-induced changes include vesicles that may become hemorrhagic, atrophic scarring, thickened hypertrophic scleroderma-like plaques, pellagra-
like pigmentation and desquamation, and
other changes seen in aged skin. The
photosensitivity of variegate porphyria is
more variable in its manifestation. Lesions tend to occur mainly during the

summer and spring. Patients with this condition, particularly the females, may also be plagued with symptoms of the type that occur in acute intermittent porphyria.

The rare hereditary coproporphyria may symptomatically resemble acute intermittent porphyria but presents with photosensitivity.

A second group of disorders that resemble drug-induced phototoxicity in their clinical manifestations includes the aminoacidurias, namely, Hartnup disease, hydroxykynureninuria, and tryptophanuria, and the nutritional-vitamin deficiency condition called pellagra. Patients with these disorders develop erythema, edema, sometimes vesiculation, and subsequently desquamation in exposed body areas. Lesions also occur in clothed pressure areas. Pigmentation and varying degrees of scarring and atrophy may follow repeated inflammatory reactions. The exact mechanisms of these reactions have not been fully elucidated. Another aminoaciduria, phenylketonuria, and hormonal-enzymatic disorders, including hypopituitarism, hypogonadism, and albinism, manifest inadequate pigmentation that leads to an increased sunburn susceptibility.

IMMUNOLOGIC. Various mechanisms have been proposed to explain these photosensitivity reactions. However, most tend to incriminate sunlight as causing photochemical reactions in skin that lead to tissue destruction and the formation of antigenic substances.

Lupus Erythematosus. Studies of patients with systemic lupus erythematosus (LE) indicate that more than 30 per cent will show evidence of photosensitivity (Epstein et al., 1965; Freeman et al., 1969). The primary activating wavelengths in these cases are mainly the short UV rays (290–320 nm.). The findings of persistent erythema, edema, urticaria, or vesiculobullous lesions on exposed skin following sun exposure may give an early clue to diagnosis in these cases.

Many patients with chronic discoid LE tend to develop new lesions (isomorphic responses) after prolonged sun exposures, and in some cases sunlight has been suspected of causing the disease to progress to a systemic form. The frequent occurrence of lesions on the scalp, through dense hair, and on covered skin of the body may be due to traumatic stimuli other than short UV light.

Immunofluorescent and ordinary light microscopic studies, along with other appropriate laboratory studies, can be used to establish the diagnosis and stage of the disease process. Management of photosensitive LE patients should include the use of appropriate short UV or full-spectrum sunscreening agents.

Polymorphic Light Eruption (PLE). This disease is mainly activated by sunburn rays in the 290 to 320 nm. range; however, longer wavelengths (>320 nm.) will elicit responses in some individuals (Baer and Harber, 1965). The mechanism of photosensitivity is thought to be based upon delayed hypersensitivity; however, the antigenic factor has not been identified (Laster et al., 1967). Although the histologic characteristics of these lesions often closely resemble lupus erythematosus, it is important to note that skin specimens from PLE lesions will not show the immunofluorescent antibody deposition at the dermo-epidermal junction that can be found in LE specimens (Charzelski et al., 1969; Fisher et al., 1970).

Following exposure to sunlight, the development of cutaneous lesions may be delayed from a few hours to several days. The lesions may be papular, papulovesicular, nodular, eczematoid, or plaquelike (Fig. 6–11). They may begin to appear at any age and tend to run a chronic course. Use of antimalarials and topical corticosteroids will help to control severe exacerbations, but the use of proper sunscreening agents (described later in this chapter) will be invaluable as a prophylactic measure against future exacerbations.

Solar Urticaria. This disorder usually does not manifest itself until the third or fourth decade of life. The action spectrum may be in either the UVB (290–320 nm.), UVA (320–400 nm.), or visible (400–700 nm.) light range. Based upon the action spectrum and the passive or reverse passive transferability of this condition, solar urticaria has been divided into five basic types (Harber et al., 1963). (On the basis of pathogenic mechanism, there are six types.) Signs and symptoms may begin either during or within seconds after intense sunlight exposure, with "burning" followed by erythema, wheal, and flare.

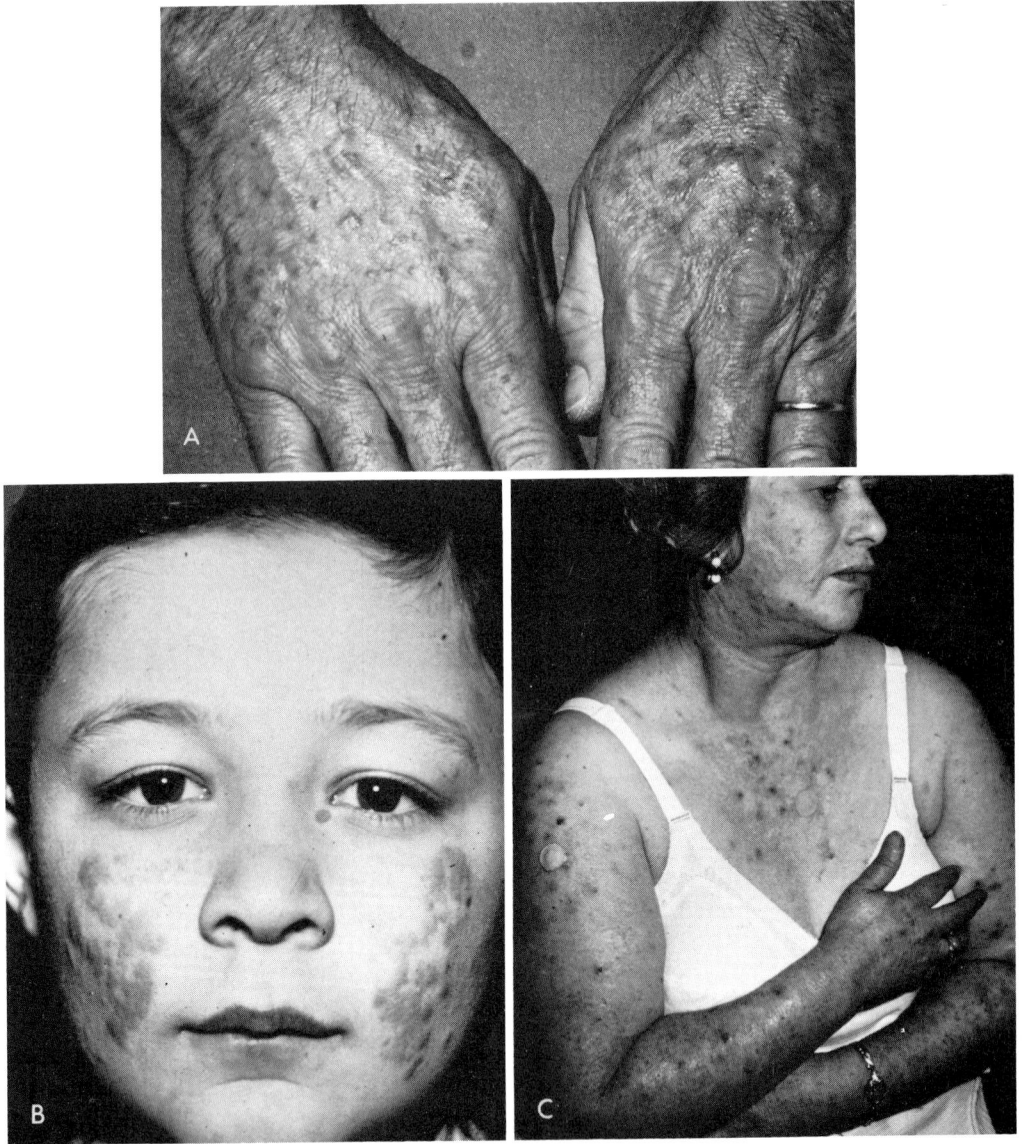

Figure 6-11 Polymorphic light eruption. *A,* Papular eruption of the hands; this lichenoid eruption involved the face and hands with no history of use of any potential photosensitizing agents or drugs. *B,* Recurrent seasonal (spring and summer) plaque eruption of the face and hands; no drug history or porphyrin disturbance. *C,* Recurrent idiopathic seasonal papulovesicular eruption of uncovered areas precipitated by sufficient exposure to sunlight.

The urticaria reaches a peak within 10 to 15 minutes and persists for one to two hours.

Studies have shown that this reaction can be blocked by injection of epinephrine but not by antihistamines. Recent electrophoretic and chromatographic studies of serum from certain affected patients have revealed the presence of a transfer factor which migrates as a globulin. The latter is thought not to be IgG or IgM, but it remains to be differentiated from IgA and IgE (Sams, 1967). Aside from the prophylactic effect obtained from avoidance of intense sunlight, some variable degree of benefit can be derived from systemic antimalarials, antihistamines, and corticosteroids. A sunscreening agent to block the specific activating rays will be the most consistently helpful modality in the management of these patients until more specific therapy is available.

Actinic Reticuloid. No definite evidence of an immunologic etiology has been established for this disorder, however, it resembles what is commonly known as the "persistent light reactor." The action spectrum extends from UVA into the visible spectrum. The eruption begins as a scaly erythema and extends rapidly over exposed areas, followed by edema, papules, and plaques (Fig. 6–12). Histologic findings are suggestive of a lymphoma; however, except for one case report of progression to a reticulosis, the disorder tends to remain benign and to clear when the patient avoids sunlight exposure (Ive et al., 1968; Jensen and Sheddon, 1970). Topical steroids, oral chloroquine, methotrexate, grenz-ray therapy, and even sunscreens appear to have little effect on this condition.

Four other conditions in which immunologic abnormalities exist and in which photosensitivity is associated deserve mention: pemphigus erythematosus and dermatomyositis, in which cutaneous lesions appear to worsen and the diseases sometimes exacerbate following intense sun exposure; scleroderma, in which there appears to be increased susceptibility to sunburn, particularly in poikilodermatous hypopigmented areas; and vitiligo, in which depigmented skin sunburns more easily because of the lack of protective melanin.

GENETIC. The disorders under this heading possess certain features that could permit their classification under other headings where photosensitivity of endogenous origin is based upon biochemical, metabolic, enzymatic, and immunologic defects. Clinical features of retardation in the physical and/or mental development of patients with these disorders, the tendencies to develop malignancies, and the development of degenerative and malignant changes in sun-exposed skin are predominant findings among these patients. Photosensitivity is due to an increased susceptibility to mainly short UV rays. Sunburn and subsequent premature degenerative, premalignant, and malignant changes develop at an early age. The increased susceptibility is generally unrelated to pigmentary deficiencies.

Xeroderma pigmentosum is an autosomal recessive disorder in which the increased tendency toward sunburn and toward the early development of cutaneous malignancies is most marked (Fig. 6–13). A most important finding in patients with this condition is the inability of their cells to repair normally the damage to DNA that is ordinarily caused by short UV light exposure. Studies of fibroblast cultures exposed to 254 nm. UVL reveal that the fibroblasts will not repair DNA damage if they are from patients with the severe De Sanctis-Cacchione syndrome, and that only 10 per cent of fibroblasts will show repair if they are from patients with simple

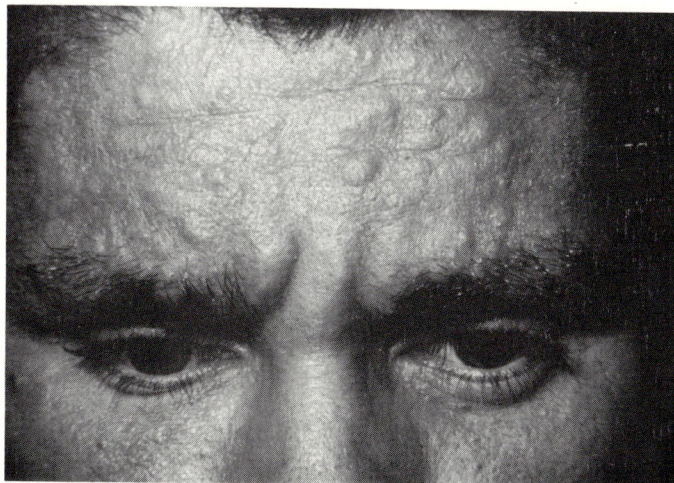

Figure 6–12 Actinic reticuloid. Twenty-eight-year-old male, a "persistent light reactor," whose eruption became more infiltrated with the formation of papules and plaques on exposed areas; the clinical and histopathologic picture suggested lymphoma cutis.

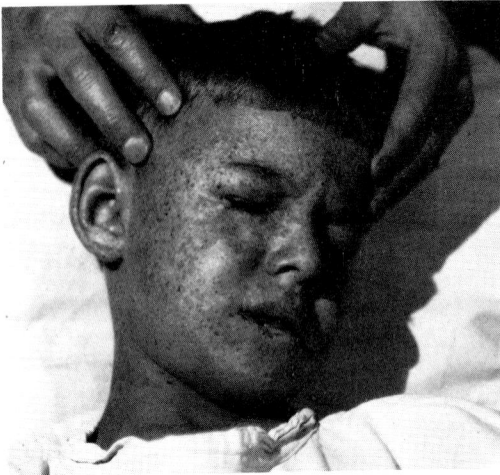

Figure 6–13 Xeroderma pigmentosum. Child, age 6. Freckling, keratoses, carcinoma of lower lip.

xeroderma pigmentosum (Cleaver, 1970). Fibroblasts from normal individuals showed 95 to 100 per cent repair under the same conditions. It has been postulated that the lack of repair is due to a defect in normal enzymatic excision of the damaged portion of DNA (pyrimidine dimer) in these patients (Epstein et al., 1970). Similar findings have been described in epidermal cells following in vivo exposures of skin to sunburning UVL (Epstein et al., 1970).

The earliest signs of light sensitivity in xeroderma pigmentosum include freckling, dryness of skin, and acute sunburn followed by persistent erythema. Repeated severe vesiculobullous sunburn responses may lead to poikilodermatous changes, severe scarring, and premalignant and malignant lesions as early as the third to fourth year of life. Since the disease is often fatal during the first two decades of life, owing to metastases of squamous cell cancer or melanomas, a vigorous and early prophylactic regimen consisting of the application of sunscreening formulations and the scrupulous avoidance of excessive sun exposure is of utmost importance. Antimalarials such as chloroquine, along with the diligent removal of premalignant and malignant lesions, have been helpful in the management of this disease. The best approach to the treatment of the premalignant and malignant lesions may be a combination of surgery or cyrosurgery and topical chemotherapy with fluorouracil.

Three other hereditary degenerative (autosomal recessively inherited) conditions of rarer occurrence that present with photosensitivity of the type in which there is increased sunburn susceptibility are Bloom's syndrome (Bloom, 1966; Landau et al., 1966), Cockayne's syndrome (Landau et al., 1966; Raub and Sonkup, 1968), and the Rothmund-Thomson syndrome (Franceschetti, 1953; Landau et al., 1966; Rook and Whimster, 1949). Only about 20 to 35 per cent of patients with the latter syndrome, however, show photosensitivity. Among the common clinical features of these syndromes are an onset in early life of repeated sunburn reactions ranging in severity from simple erythema to a vesiculobullous eruption, scarring, premature aging, and poikilodermatous changes in exposed skin. Avoidance of direct sun exposure and the use of sunscreens will be most helpful in the management of patients with these syndromes.

Although the condition called disseminated superficial actinic porokeratosis (Chernosky and Anderson, 1969) does not show the severe degree of cutaneous degenerative changes and the developmental defects seen in the above disorders, it is included here because of its suspected autosomal dominant inheritance and the fact that short UV exposure leads to the development of localized degenerative skin changes (Fig. 6–14). Since the lesions tend to involute to some degree in winter when less exposure to sun is obtained, an appropriate short UV sunscreen when properly used should be an effective prophylactic measure.

INFECTIONS. Certain viral eruptions have been suspected of being worsened or provoked by sun exposure since they appear localized and most severe on light-exposed areas, and occur mainly during the spring and summer months. However, satisfactory proof of a significant relationship between sun exposure and viral eruptions in general remains unestablished except in the cases of herpes simplex and lymphogranuloma venereum.

In the case of herpes simplex, there are numerous reports of indisputable clinical evidence which state that prolonged sunlight exposure can cause exacerbation of lesions. The exact action spectrum and mechanism of exacerbation, however, have not been fully elucidated. Studies of patients with lymphogranuloma venereum have shown that in approximately 60 per cent of chronic cases the patients develop eruptions following sunlight exposure (Carins, 1968). In subacute cases, 30 per cent of females and 12 per cent of males show photosensitivity eruptions. Pruritic papular, papulovesicular, urticarial, and plaquelike lesions on exposed skin areas characterize these eruptions. Treatment of the diseases and the use of sunscreening agents should be effective in controlling the photosensitivity problems.

MISCELLANEOUS-CUTANEOUS. The mechanisms of photosensitivity disorders in this group have not been fully elucidated; however, an underlying dermatologic disease exists in each case. The reactions resulting from sun exposure are not representative of photosensitivity in the same sense as those reactions previously described, since the types of lesions induced are neither unique to sunlight exposure nor elicited by every intense sun exposure received. The photosensitivity reactions in these cases are best referred to as isomorphic responses (Koebner phenomena). These sun-induced lesions are of the same type as those lesions that characterize the basic underlying skin disease.

Although the precise action spectra required for elicitation of the majority of these reactions have not been defined, it is generally agreed that short UV (290–320 nm.) radiation, sufficient in amount to elicit a moderate to severe sunburn reaction, is usually required. On the other hand, experimental studies have shown certain conditions, such as Hailey-Hailey disease, to be induced by exposure to non-sunburning long UV (Cram et al., 1967). In general, photosensitivity reactions in this group of disorders will appear within 24 to 96 hours after exposure to a sufficient amount of the proper activating light. Disorders in this group include: pityriasis rubra pilaris, Darier's disease, Hailey-Hailey disease, psoriasis, lichen planus, erythema multiforme, sarcoid, lymphocytoma, rosacea, atopic dermatitis, seborrheic dermatitis (light-sensitive seborrheid), and granuloma annulare.

The evolution of new lesions and the therapeutic requirements are usually the same as those described for the primary skin disease. However, when prolonged or repeated intense sun exposures are anticipated in a patient with one of the above diseases, the prescribing of an appropriate sunscreening agent should be included in the therapeutic regimen.

DIAGNOSTIC PROCEDURES

The choice of a diagnostic procedure or procedures for a given photosensitivity disorder will depend upon the patient's history and presenting clinical eruption. The physician should be aware of the pa-

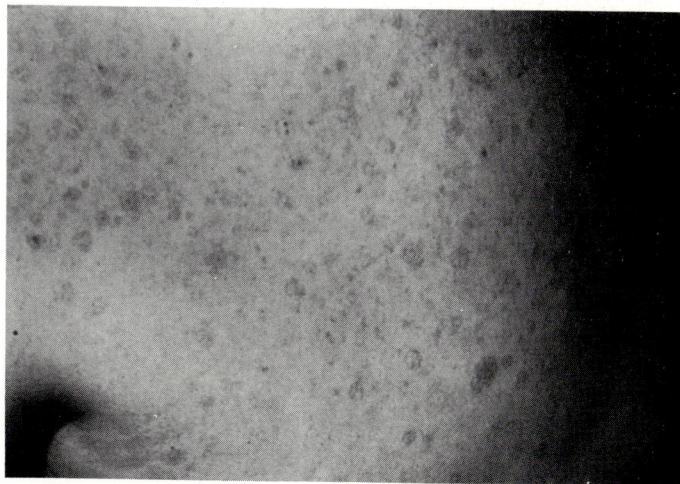

Figure 6–14 Disseminated superficial actinic porokeratosis (DSAP) in a 67-year-old female who spent a winter in Florida and acquired superficial papules with threadlike scaly borders on exposed areas, especially extensor surface of the lower extremities.

tient's past use of potential topical or systemic photosensitizers, the duration and conditions under which light exposure was obtained prior to the eruption, the time interval between light exposure and onset of cutaneous signs and symptoms, any previous personal or familial history of sunlight intolerance, and any history of other past or coexisting cutaneous disease.

Except in those cases in which there are clinical indications of abnormalities in porphyrins or there is suspected autoimmunity, the diagnosis and differentiation of photosensitivity disorders will depend mainly upon results obtained from *photo test* and/or *photo patch test* procedures. These procedures will allow one not only to produce locally the suspected photodermatitis for more accurate diagnosis but also to determine the wavelengths that are primarily responsible for eliciting the disorder. Results of the latter will be indispensable as a guide in selecting the most appropriate prophylactic regimen.

The source of light and the filters employed are perhaps the most important basic factors in designing efficient photo test and photo patch test procedures. Since the energy and spectrum of light from the sun are so variable from one time to another, the sun is obviously not the best choice of a light source for careful studies. However, the ideal source of light is one that emits a continuous spectrum of high intensity radiation that simulates mid-day, mid-summer, clear-day sunlight at the earth's surface. The light source that comes closest to meeting these criteria is the Xenon arc lamp based upon the model of Urbach and Berger (Urbach, 1969). Although many other artificial lamp sources can be used, the physician should realize their various advantages and disadvantages and properly interpret his results accordingly (Table 6–2). Filters of the Schott, Corning Glass, or other types must be employed with all lamps in order to obtain narrow wavelength bands of radiation that may precisely define the action spectrum for a particular photosensitivity reaction.

For any particular lamp source to be used, the physician must first know its energy output and/or exposure requirement in order to elicit a minimal erythema response in the average individual of a particular skin type, stock, or race. When the radiation from this lamp has been filtered to emit wavelengths only in the long UV to visible wavelength range (320–400 nm.), prolonged exposure should not cause a delayed (24-hour) erythema or sunburn response.

Photo Test Procedure

The test site should be skin that is not ordinarily exposed to sunlight (for examples, mid- to lower back). Sites of 1 square centimeter or longer should be demarcated in sufficient numbers (usually five or more) so that exposures can be given at doses both less and greater (in 25 per cent decrements and increments) than the average required for a minimal erythema dose (MED) response. Immediate and 24-hour observations of test sites exposed to full-spectrum (290–700 nm.) UV and visible light in this manner should reveal evidence of photosensitivity through either a decreased MED requirement (that is, the minimal amount of light exposure required to elicit a uniform redness extending to all margins of a test site at the 24-hour observation should be decreased) or a qualitative abnormality in the test response (for example, urticaria, edema, papules, plaques, vesicles, and so forth that appear either immediately or are delayed by one or more days). Using filters to progressively eliminate shorter wavelengths (for example, Schott WG345, 365, and so on to eliminate wavelengths < 320 nm., < 340 nm., and so on, respectively) and repeating the test exposures will more precisely reveal the action spectrum. In order to elicit an abnormal response to the longer wavelengths, the duration of exposure may have to be increased by two to three or more times the time required to induce an MED response.

Repeated exposures of the same site (Epstein, 1966) with radiation of less than 320 nm. may be necessary to elicit positive responses in patients with suspected polymorphous light reactions.

Photo Patch Testing

This type of procedure is designed primarily for establishing the diagnosis of

TABLE 6-2 Common Lamp Sources

Types	Characteristics	Advantages	Disadvantages
Xenon Arc	High intensity; continuous spectral emission; constant output; long life span; may be filtered to emit solar-simulating radiation in all important wavelength ranges.	All light effects can be accomplished using short exposure times.	High initial and moderately high maintenance costs. Small radiation field. Not portable.
Quartz-Iodine	Same as above except for a lack of high intensity UVB (290–320 nm.) radiation.	UVA (320–400 nm.) and visible (400–700 nm.) light effects can be accomplished using short exposure times. Portable.	Is not an adequate source for testing in the UVB range. High costs. Small radiation field.
Carbon Arc	High intensity; continuous but irregular spectral emission; variable output; short life span varies with carbons; may be filtered to emit radiation in all important wavelengths ranges.	Light effects can be accomplished using short exposure times. Low costs. Moderately large radiation field. May be portable.	Too much variability in energy intensity and spectral emission. Carbons are too short lived.
Fluorescent Sun Lamp (FS20T12 or FS40T12)	Moderate intensity; continuous spectral emission of 280–350 nm. radiation with a peak emission at 320 nm.; constant output; long life span.	UVB effects can be accomplished with moderately short exposure times. A reflecting bank containing several lamps may be used. Low costs. Large radiation field. Portable.	Is not an adequate UVA and visible light source.
Black-Light Fluorescent Lamp (24 in., 20 watt or 48 in., 40 watt B.L.)	Low to moderate intensity; continuous spectral emission of 320–420 nm. radiation with peak emission at about 360 nm.; constant output; long life span.	UVA effects can be accomplished. A reflecting bank containing several lamps may be used. Low costs. Large radiation field. Portable.	Moderately long exposure times are required for effects. Is not an adequate UVB and visible light source.
Hot Quartz (high pressure mercury arc lamp)	High intensity; linear spectral emissions in all wavelength ranges; constant output; long life span.	Many light effects can be accomplished with short exposure times if the desired action spectrum corresponds to emissions from the lamp. Large radiation field. Portable.	Many important photoactivating wavelengths are not emitted.
Cold Quartz (low pressure mercury arc lamp)	Linear spectral emission, approximately 90 per cent of which is at 253.7 nm.; constant output; moderate intensity; long life span.	None for routine photo testing.	Most important photoactivating wavelengths are not emitted.

photoallergic contact dermatitis and for specifically identifying the photosensitizer (Freeman and Knox, 1968; Harber et al., 1966; Willis and Kligman, 1968, 1969). The same general procedure can be used (investigationally) to detect potential phototoxic agents but is seldom used clinically for this purpose (Willis and Kligman, 1968).

Basically, the procedure consists of application of the potential photosensiters on the skin, irradiation of the site, and observation 24 to 96 hours later. In general, the suspected chemical may be prepared at 1 per cent or less concentration in petrolatum. If the suspected chemical is not available, then the commercial agent may be used, or, if it is soap, then it should be prepared as a 1 to 2 per cent soap solution. The main objective is to use a non-irritating concentration of the potential photosensitizer. The potential photosensitizer should always be applied in duplicate so that one site will serve as a non-irradiated control for contact allergy or nonspecific irritation. The conventional method is to apply the potential sensitizer and then to cover it with plastic occlusion and an opaque material (such as aluminum foil) for 24 hours prior to light exposure. An alternate method is to remove the horny layer by Scotch tape stripping (Willis and Kligman, 1968) prior to application of the potential sensitizer and then expose the site to light before covering it occlusively. The latter procedure enhances penetration of a photosensitizer, penetration of light, and thus the intensity of the test response.

Since the majority of drug-induced photosensitivity reactions are caused by wavelengths longer than 320 nm., and appropriate filter, such as window glass, a Schott WG345, or Myalar .005D, should be used to eliminate shorter wavelengths. The photo patch test site should receive an exposure equivalent to from 5 to 10 times that required to induce an MED response with most lamp sources. If a bank of four 24-inch, 24-watt Blacklites is used at a bulb-to-skin distance of 10 inches, the exposure should be about 20 minutes. A control site to which no drug has been applied should be exposed to the same dose of the same light to detect any abnormality in the skin's response to light alone.

Ordinarily, photo patch responses are read 24 to 48 hours after light exposure; however, positive responses may sometimes be delayed for up to 96 hours. Since responses at control sites will serve to eliminate spurious photo patch test interpretations due to chemical irritancy, allergy, or effects of light alone, the only remaining decision to make regarding a positive photo patch test response is to determine whether the response is phototoxic or photoallergic. The latter response is almost always pruritic and will persist for one to two weeks, while phototoxic responses are almost never pruritic, are often tender, will cause burning or painful sensation, and will usually regress rapidly over a period of 72 to 96 hours. It is possible for symptoms of phototoxicity to precede or occur simultaneously with photocontact allergy; this is rare, however. Potential photosensitizers are listed in Table 6–1.

PROPHYLAXIS AND THERAPY

Sunscreens

Since there are no known cures for the majority of photosensitivity disorders, the ideal approach in management is to prevent their exacerbations. In this regard, considerable investigational attention has been directed toward the development of sunscreens (Knox et al., 1957, Pathak et al., 1969; Stambovsky, 1968; Willis and Kligman, 1969, 1970). The majority of these are effective mainly against the development of ordinary sunburn reactions (short UV rays), although a few of these agents provide some degree of protection against longer wavelengths.

After the physician has determined the action spectrum for a particular photosensitivity reaction through photo tests and photo patch testing, as previously described, he may simply select the most appropriate sunscreen that is available or he may choose to repeat his photo test and photo patch tests, using different types of sunscreens to determine which one will be most effective. Sunscreens can be divided into three types, depending upon the range of light that they prevent from reaching the skin. These are the following:

1. Short UV sunscreens: This group of agents screen mainly in the UVB (290–320 nm.) spectrum of sunlight. The most effective agents in this group are formulations of para-aminobenzoic acid (for example, PreSun and Pabanol lotion) and its esters (for example, Block-out, Sea and Ski, and Pabafilm).

2. Full-spectrum UV sunscreens: These agents screen both UVB (290–320 nm.) and UVA (320–400 nm.) rays. The UVB screening effectiveness of these agents is not as great as that of the short ultraviolet sunscreens listed above. Their advantage is in preventing photosensitivity reactions that are due to UVA wavelengths. Agents in this group include the benzophenones (Sol-bar), and benzophenone sulfonic acid (Uval).

3. Full-spectrum UV and visible light sunscreens: These are light opaque formulations that are capable of screening all wavelengths between 290 and 700 nm. Such formulations as zinc oxide ointment, titanium dioxide formulations (RVPlus and A-Fil), and red petrolatum formulations (RVP, RVPaque, and RVPlus) are included in this group.

In addition to having a general knowledge of the above grouping of sunscreens, it is important to know particular advantages and disadvantages of sunscreens within each group. For example, opaque sunscreening formulations may appear to be ideal when tested in vitro or immediately after their applications to skin; however, their effectiveness is quickly abolished on skin by simple sweating. In addition, some of these formulations are not cosmetically acceptable and may be uncomfortably occlusive on skin. Although the long UV sunscreens are cosmetically acceptable, they also quickly lose their effectiveness under sweat-stimulating, warm environmental conditions. Under such circumstances it may be necessary to reapply the sunscreen as often as every 30 to 60 minutes in order to maintain a reasonably high degree of effectiveness. The sunscreens in the first group come closest to ideal in their qualities and in the accomplishment of their objectives. These agents are, in general, highly substantive to skin; that is, they are not easily removed by simply sweating, and they maintain some degree of protection even after immersion in water.

In order to achieve the best prophylactic effect in the majority of disorders described in this chapter, the author recommends the use of a combination of sunscreens in groups 1 and 2 above (for example, PreSun should be first applied and allowed to dry, followed by the application of Sol-bar or Uval). By this method one attempts to prevent not only the elicitation of the primary photosensitivity disorder but also the enhancing effects of reactions produced by other ultraviolet and near visible wavelengths.

Drugs

Systemic and topical drugs are often required in the management of photosensitivity disorders. These include corticosteroids, antihistamines (excluding those that are potential photosensitizers), and sometimes antimalarials.

In some cases of polymorphic light reactions and solar urticaria, the best therapeutic responses have been obtained with low-dosage chloroquine (Aralen phosphate, 250 mg. daily) or hydroxychloroquine (Plaquenil sulfate, 200 mg. daily); Brodthager, 1969; Epstein et al., 1963). However, it is essential to refer the patient for regularly spaced ophthalmologic examinations to detect signs of toxicity and to be aware of other possible serious side effects that may occur while these drugs are being used.

Recent studies (Mathews-Róth et al., 1970) have shown promising therapeutic effects of orally administered β-carotene in cases of erythropoietic protoporphyria. The exact mechanism of its protective action has not been fully elucidated.

Photosensitivity disorders of endogenous origin, in general, are best managed by treatment of the underlying disease and by prescribing the most appropriate sunscreen.

REFERENCES

Bachem, A.: Time factors of erythema and pigmentation produced by ultraviolet rays of different wavelengths. J. Invest. Dermatol. 25:215, 1955.

Baer, R. L., and Haber, L. C.: Photobiology of lupus erythematosus. Arch. Dermatol. 92:124, 1965.

Bloom, D.: The syndrome of congenital telangiectatic erythema and stunted growth. J. Pediatr. 68:103, 1966.

Blum, H. F.: Light absorption in photodynamic action. In Blum, H., (ed.): Photodynamic action and Diseases Caused by Light. Reinhold Publishing Corp., 1941, p. 53.

Blum, H. F.: Sunburn. In Hollaender, A., (ed.): Radiation Biology. Vol. 2, Chap. 13. New York, McGraw-Hill Book Co., Inc., 1955.

Breit, R., and Kligman, A. M.: Measurement of erythemal and pigmentary responses to ultraviolet radiation of different spectral qualities. In Urbach, F., (ed.): The Biologic Effects of Ultraviolet Radiation. Oxford, Pergamon Press, 1969, p. 267.

Brodthager, H.: Polymorphous light eruption. In Urbach, F., (ed.): The Biologic Effects of Ultraviolet Radiation. Oxford, Pergamon Press, 1969, p. 479.

Burckhardt, W.: Untersuchungen uber die photoaktivitat eininger sulfailamide. Dermatologica 83:63, 1941.

Burckhardt, W.: Photoallergic eczema due to blank sphores (optic brightening agents). Hantarzt 8:486, 1957.

Burry, N. J.: Photoallergies to fenticolor and multifungin. Arch. Dermatol. 95:287, 1967.

Carins, R. J.: Actinic and ionizing radiation-unexplained reactions to light. In Rook, A., et al., (eds.): Textbook of Dermatology. Oxford, Blackwell Scientific Publications, 1968, p. 349.

Charzelski, T., Jablonski, S., and Blaszczk, M.: Immunopathologic investigations in lupus erythematosus. J. Invest. Dermatol. 52:333, 1969.

Chernosky, M. E., and Anderson, D. E.: Disseminated superficial actinic porokeratosis: Clinical studies and experimental production of lesions. Arch. Dermatol. 99:401, 1969.

Claesson, S., Juhlin, L., and Wettermark, G.: Effects of ultraviolet rays on skin before and after removal of horny layer, effect of histamine liberator. Acta Derm. Venereol. 39:3, 1959.

Cleaver, J. E.: DNA damage and repair in light sensitive human skin disease. J. Invest. Dermatol. 54:181, 1970.

Cram, D. L., Muller, S. A., and Winkelman, R. K.: Ultraviolet-induced acantholysis in familial benign chronic pemphigus. Arch. Dermatol. 96:636, 1967.

Cripps, D. J., and Enta, T.: The action spectra of tribromosalicylanilide photosensitivity. Abst. Clin. Res., 15:248, 1967.

Daniels, F., Jr.: Physical factors in sun exposure. Arch. Dermatol. 85:358, 1962.

Daniels, F., Jr., van der Leun, J. C., and Johnson, B. E.: Sunburn. Sci. Am. 219:38, 1968.

Deutsch, A. J.: The sun. In The New Astronomy. New York, Simon and Schuster, Inc., 1955, p. 165.

Epstein, J. H.: Polymorphous light eruption. Ann. Allergy 24:397, 1966.

Epstein, J. H.: Adverse Cutaneous Reactions to the Sun. In Natkinson, F., and Pearson, R., (eds.): Yearbook of Dermatology. Chicago, Year Book Medical Publishers, 1971, p. 5.

Epstein, J. H., and Fukuyama, K.: A study of 8-methoxypsoralen (8-MOP) induced phototoxic effects on mammalian epidermal macromolecule synthesis in vivo. Abst. J. Invest. Dermatol. 54:350, 1970.

Epstein, J. H., Fukuyama, K., and Epstein, W. L.: UVL induced stimulation of DNA synthesis in hairless mouse epidermis. J. Invest. Dermatol. 51:445, 1968.

Epstein, J. H., Fukuyama, K., and Fye, K.: Effects of ultraviolet radiation on the mitotic cycle and DNA, RNA and protein synthesis in mammalian epidermis in vivo. Photochem. Photobiol. 12:57, 1970.

Epstein, J. H., Tuffanelli, D. L., and Dubois, E. L.: Light sensitivity and lupus erythematosus. Arch. Dermatol. 91:483, 1965.

Epstein, J. H., Vandenberg, J. J., and Wright, W. L.: Solar urticaria. Arch. Dermatol. 88:135, 1963.

Epstein, J. H., Fukuyama, K., Reed, W. B., et al.: Defect in DNA synthesis in skin of patients with xeroderma pigmentosum demonstrated in vivo. Science 168:1477, 1970.

Epstein, W. L., Fukuyama, K., and Epstein, J. H.: Early effects of UV light on DNA synthesis in human skin in vivo. Arch. Dermatol. 100:84, 1969.

Everett, M. A., Olsen, R. L., and Sayre, R. M.: Ultraviolet erythema. Arch. Dermatol. 92:713, 1965.

Fisher, D. A., Epstein, J. H., Kay, D., et al.: Polymorphous light eruption and lupus erythematosus: Differential diagnosis by fluorescent microscopy. Arch. Dermatol. 101:458, 1970.

Fitzpatrick, T. B.: In Bowen, E. J., (ed.): Recent Progress in Photobiology. Oxford, Blackwell Scientific Publications, 1965, p. 369.

Fitzpatrick, T. B., Pathak, M. A., Magnus, I. A., et al.: Abnormal reactions of man to light. In Annual Review of Medicine, Vol. 14, 1963, p. 195.

Franceschetti, A.: Les dysplasies ecrodermiques et les syndromes héréditaires apparentés. Dermatologica 106:129, 1953.

Freeman, R. G., and Knox, J. M.: Influence of temperature on ultraviolet injury. Arch. Dermatol. 29:858, 1964.

Freeman, R. G., and Knox, J. M.: The action spectrum of photocontact dermatitis. Arch. Dermatol. 97:130, 1968.

Freeman, R. G., Knox, J. M., and Owens, D. W.: Cutaneous lesions of lupus erythematosus induced by monochromatic light. Arch. Dermatol. 100:677, 1969.

Freeman, R. G., Owens, D. W., Knox, J. M., et al.: Relative energy requirements for an erythemal response of skin to monochromatic wavelengths of ultraviolet present in the solar spectrum. J. Invest. Dermatol. 46:586, 1966.

Fukuyama, K., and Epstein, W. L.: Epidermal keratinization: Localization of istopically labeled amino acids. J. Invest. Dermatol. 47:551, 1966.

Harber, L. C., Harris, H., and Baer, R. L.: Photoallergic contact dermatitis. Arch. Dermatol. 94:255, 1966.

Harber, L. C., Holloway, R. M., Wheatley, V. R., et al.: Immunologic and biophysical studies in solar urticaria. J. Invest. Dermatol. 41:439, 1963.

Holti, G.: Measurements of vascular responses in skin at various time intervals after damage with histamine and ultraviolet radiation. Clin. Sci. 14:143, 1955.

Howell, J. B.: The sunlight factor in aging and skin cancer. Arch. Dermatol. 82:865, 1960.

Ippen, H.: Topical Agents for Protection against Ultraviolet Radiation. Oxford, Pergamon Press, 1969, p. 681.

Ive, F. A., Magnus, I. A., Warin, R. P., et al.: Actinic reticuloid: a chronic dermatosis associated with severe photosensitivity and the histologic resemblance to lymphoma. Br. J. Dermatol. 81:469, 1968.

Jenkins, F. P., Welti, D., and Baines, D.: Photochemical reactions of tetrachlorosalicylanilide. Nature 201:827, 1964.

Jensen, N. E., and Sheddon, I. B.: Actinic reticuloid with lymphoma. Br. J. Dermatol. 82:287, 1970.

Jillson, O. F.: Testing for phototoxicity and photoallergy. In Urbach, F., (ed.): The Biologic Effect of Ultraviolet Radiation. Oxford, Pergamon Press, 1969, p. 533.

Jillson, O., and Baughman, R. D.: Contact photodermatitis from bithionol. Arch. Dermatol. 88:409, 1963.

Johnson, B. E., and Daniels, F., Jr.: Lysosomes and the reactions of skin to ultraviolet radiation. J. Invest. Dermatol. 53:85, 1969.

Johnson, B. E., Daniels, F., Jr., and Magnus, I. A.: Response of human skin to ultraviolet light. In Giese, A. C., (ed.): Photophysiology. Vol. 4. New York, Academic Press, 1968, p. 139.

Jones, H. E., Lewis, C. W., and Reisner, J. E.: Photosensitive lichenoid eruption associated with demeclocycline. Arch. Dermatol. 106:58, 1972.

Kligman, A. M.: The biology of the stratum corneum. In Montagna, W., and Lobitz, W., Jr., (eds.): The Epidermis. New York, Academic Press, 1964, p. 387.

Kligman, A. M.: Early destructive effect of sunlight on human skin. J.A.M.A. 210:2377, 1969.

Knox, J. M., Guin, J., and Cockerall, E. G.: Benzophenones: Ultraviolet light absorbing agents. J. Invest. Dermatol. 29:435, 1957.

Landau, J. W., Sasaki, M. D., Newcomer, V. D., et al.: Bloom's syndrome. Arch. Dermatol. 94:687, 1966.

Laster, R. S., Burnham, T. K., Fine, G., et al.: Immunologic concepts of light reactions in lupus erythematosus and polymorphous light eruptions. Arch. Dermatol. 96:1, 1967.

Lever, W. F.: Senile (solar) keratosis. In Lever, W. F., (ed.): Histopathology of the Skin. Philadelphia, J. B. Lippincott Co., 1967, p. 498.

MacDonald, W. B., Fitch, K. D., and Lewis, I. C.:

Cockayne's syndrome. An heredofamilial disorder of growth and development. Pediatrics 25:997, 1960.

Magnus, I. A.: The cutaneous porphyrias. Semin. Hematol. 5:380, 1968.

Mathews-Róth, M., Pathak, M. A., Fitzpatrick, T. B., et al.: β-carotene as photoprotective agent in erythropoietic protoporphyria. N. Engl. J. Med. 282:1231, 1970.

McLaren, A. D., and Luse, R. A.: Mechanism of inactivation of enzyme proteins by ultraviolet light. Science 134:836, 1961.

Miescher, G.: Zur histologie der lichtbedingten reaktinen. Dermatologica 115:345, 1957.

Mizuno, N., and Freeman, R. G.: Histologic and histochemical studies on 8-methoxpsoralen photosensitivity. Dermatologica 139:18, 1969.

Norins, A. L.: Immediate effects of light. In Urbach, F., (ed.): The Biologic Effects of Ultraviolet Light. Oxford, Pergamon Press, 1969, p. 31.

Pathak, M. A.: Basic aspects of cutaneous photosensitization. In Urbach, F., (ed.): The Biologic Effects of Ultraviolet Radiation. Oxford, Pergamon Press, 1969, p. 489.

Pathak, M. A., and Epstein, J. H.: Normal and Abnormal Reactions of Man to Light. In Fitzpatrick, T. B., (ed.): Dermatology in General Medicine. New York, McGraw-Hill Book Co., Inc., 1971, p. 989.

Pathak, M. A., and Epstein, J. H.: Normal and abnormal reactions of man to light-photodynamic action and photosensitization. In Fitzpatrick, T. B., (ed.): Dermatology in General Medicine. New York, McGraw-Hill Book Co., Inc., 1971, p. 1017.

Pathak, M. A., and Stratton, K.: Effects of ultraviolet and visible radiation and the production of free radicals in skin. In Urbach, F., (ed.): The Biologic Effects of Ultraviolet Radiation. Oxford, Pergamon Press, 1969, p. 207.

Pathak, M. A., Fitzpatrick, T. B., and Frank, E.: Evaluation of topical agents that prevent sunburn; The superiority of PABA and its ester in ethyl alcohol. N. Engl. J. Med. 280:1459, 1969.

Raub, J. L., and Sonkup, S. W.: Bloom's syndrome. Am. J. Dis. Child 116:409, 1968.

Rook, A., and Whimster, I.: Congenital cutaneous dystrophy (Thompson's type). Br. J. Dermatol. 61:197, 1949.

Sams, W. M., Jr.: Solar urticaria: Association of serum activity with an antibody other than IgG or IgM. Clin. Res. 17:277, 1969.

Schmid, R.: The porphyrias. In Stanbury, J. B., et al., (eds.): The Metabolic Basis of Inherited Disease. 2nd ed., New York, McGraw-Hill Book Co., Inc., 1966, p. 813.

Sidi, E., Hincky, M., and Gervias, A.: Allergic sensitization and photosensitization to Phenergan cream. J. Invest. Dermatol. 24:345, 1955.

Smith, K. C.: Biochemical effects of ultraviolet light on DNA. In Urbach, F., (ed.): The Biologic Effects of Ultraviolet Radiation. Oxford, Pergamon Press, 1969, p. 47.

Smith, K. C.: UV is dangerous, but is VIS light safe? Course on Photobiology at the Am. Acad. of Derm. Meeting, Chicago, 1971.

Stambovsky, L.: The suntan business. Drug Cosmetic Ind., 102:42, 1968.

Tan, E. M., Freeman, R. G., and Stoughton, R. B.: Action spectrum of ultraviolet light-induced damage to nuclear DNA in vivo. J. Invest. Dermatol. 55:439, 1970.

Tertus, W. S.: Inhibition of the erythema of sunburn by large doses of ultraviolet radiation. Am. J. Physiol. 146:96, 1946.

Thompson, M. L.: Relative efficiency of pigment and horny layer thickness in protecting the skin of Europeans and Africans against solar radiation. J. Physiol. 127:236, 1955.

Urbach, F.: Solar simulation for phototesting of human skin. In Urbach, F., (ed.): The Biologic Effects of Ultraviolet Radiation. Oxford, Pergamon Press, 1969, p. 107.

Urbach, F., Davies, R. E., and Forbes, P. D.: Ultraviolet radiation and skin cancer in man. In Montagna, W., (ed.): Advances in Biology of Skin-Carcinogenesis. Vol. 7, Chap. 12. Oxord, Pergamon Press, 1966.

Wilkinson, D. S.: Photodermatitis due to tetrachlorosalicylanilide. Br. J. Dermatol. 73:213, 1961.

Willis, I.: Action spectra and doses for elicitation of phototoxic and photoallergic reactions to topically applied drugs. Proc. 5th International Congress on Photobiology, 1968.

Willis, I., and Kligman, A. M.: Diagnosis of photosensitization reactions by the Scotch Tape provocative patch test. J. Invest. Dermatol. 51:116, 1968.

Willis, I., and Kligman, A. M.: The mechanism of photoallergic contact dermatitis. J. Invest. Dermatol. 51:378, 1968.

Willis, I., and Kligman, A. M.: The mechanism of the persistant light reactor. J. Invest. Dermatol. 51:385, 1968.

Willis, I., and Kligman, A. M.: Elicitation of photocontact allergic reactions by low doses of long wavelength ultraviolet light. Arch. Dermatol. 100:535, 1969.

Willis, I., and Kligman, A. M.: Evaluation of sunscreens by human assay. J. Soc. Cos. Chem., 20:639, 1969.

Willis, I., and Kligman, A. M.: Aminobenzoic acid and its esters. The quest for more effective sunscreens. Arch. Dermatol. 102:405, 1970.

Willis, I., Kligman, A. M., and Epstein, J. H.: The effects of long UV radiation on skin; photoprotective or photoaugmentative? J. Invest. Dermatol. 59:416, 1972.

Yeargers, E.: Ultraviolet effects on proteins. In Urbach, F., (ed.): The Biologic Effects of Ultraviolet Light. Oxford, Pergamon Press, 1969, p. 37.

DRUG ERUPTIONS (DERMATITIS MEDICAMENTOSA)

Herman Beerman and *Bernard A. Kirshbaum*

Drug eruptions are unwanted and unintended cutaneous or mucocutaneous reactions which occur upon the administration of any diagnostic or therapeutic agent reaching the skin through the general circulation and which are not characteristic of the desired pharmacodynamic effects of the drug. The eczematous reactions which result from a contact allergy to topical agents are not considered drug eruptions since the offending chemicals arrive at the skin by direct application and not via the blood vessels or lymphatics. Drug-induced contact dermatitis is discussed in Chapter 21.

Drug eruptions may result from ingestion, inhalation, injection by various methods (intradermal, hypodermic, intramuscular, intravenous) instillation, or inunction of medicaments given as liquids, aerosols, pellets, tablets, capsules, suppositories, and in various forms for application to the surface of the skin and mucous membranes. Absorption into the systemic circulation may follow the topical application of medication to the intact skin, mouth, nose, conjunctiva, vagina, rectum, and to deep open wounds, or the instillation of agents into the urinary bladder or respiratory tract. Other special avenues of entry, in the infant, are through ingestion of mother's milk and absorption across the placenta (Bleyer et al., 1970).

A *drug* is defined as any agent or combination of agents, organic or inorganic, which is used in medical diagnosis, prophylaxis, or therapy. In the broad sense this includes such diverse agents as adjuvants, antibiotics, chemical substances used in diagnostic procedures, disinfectants, dyes, coloring and flavoring agents, hormones, preservatives, serums, vaccines, vehicles, and vitamins, as well as chemicals that are used to induce specific physiologic-pharmacologic changes. In addition, cross-sensitization can occur with non-drug chemicals which are chemically or immunologically related to substances used medicinally.

In our present civilization the opportunities for exposure to drugs are legion and are often concealed. Moreover, the patient may be unaware of exposure. For example, many food products contain "drugs" used as preservatives, or as flavoring, coloring, or decolorizing (bleaching) agents; these products also contain antibiotics and hormones which have derived from animals treated before their products (milk or meat) have been processed. Other noteworthy sources include dental bridges and fillings, mouthwashes, toothpastes, disinfectants, cleansers, the ever increasing number of aerosols, sprays, and vapors, as well as chemicals used in the processing of clothing.

Until recent years an average of more than one new pharmaceutical prescription product was being introduced every day. In the decade between 1956 and 1966, this amounted to approximately 4000 new pharmaceutical products and does not include a host of proprietary medications available over-the-counter (Beerman et al., 1967). Of this number, several hundred were new chemical entities not previously known. The medical profession is continuously bombarded with additional new drugs, and it is almost impossible for the practicing physician to become thoroughly familiar with the nature of and reactions to all of these therapeutic agents. With the imposition by the Food and Drug Administration of more stringent regulations governing the development and production of drugs, there has been a sharp reduction in the number of new drugs appearing on the market in the past few years. However, since almost all of the currently available drugs are capable of producing one or more of a great variety of skin eruptions, drugs still loom large on the dermatologic scene as disease-producing agents.

Skin eruptions are probably the most common manifestations of drug sensitivity. Many minor eruptive reactions to drugs are easily overlooked so that the precise incidence of drug eruptions is difficult if not impossible to determine. There is, however, evidence that the incidence of drug eruptions is increasing. Some of the apparent reasons for this are the following: (a) the local and systemic administration of the same drug enhances allergic sensitization; (b) the intermittent use of drugs favors sensitization by re-exposure; (c) the administration of some drugs in repository or depot form tends to increase the possibility of sensitization, and (d) the use of more and more drugs which are strong sensitizers for relatively minor ailments also favors sensitization.

Drug eruptions are only one class of *drug reaction*, though a very conspicuous one. Virtually any tissue or organ may be affected in drug reactions. Drug eruptions are often associated with related changes in other organs, such as:

Central nervous system: "Drug fever," central hypothalamic derangement, psychoneuroses, or psychoses.

Hematopoietic system: Blood dyscrasias, leukopenia (even to agranulocytosis), hemolytic and aplastic anemia, thrombocytopenia.

Liver: Toxic hepatitis, bile "inspissation" type, usually benign or occasionally with parenchymal damage which may be extremely severe; also porphyria.

Kidney: Albuminuria, crystalluria; occasionally anuria due to tubule and lower nephron nephrosis.

Respiratory tract: Laryngeal edema; bronchial exudation and mucus plugs, "drug asthma," Loeffler's syndrome, pneumonitis and other pulmonary changes including alveolar rupture as may occur in anaphylactoid shock.

Gastrointestinal tract: Diarrhea, hemorrhage, gastritis, enterocolitis, proctitis, other gastric and colonic disorders, candidiasis.

Mucous membranes: Stomatitis, gingivitis, gingival hypertrophy, conjunctivitis, vaginitis, urethritis.

Vascular system: Vasospasm, shock (vascular collapse); vasculitides, including capillaritis, periarteritis nodosa; thrombophlebitis, nodular vasculitis, erythema nodosum, allergic cutaneous vasculitis.

Serum sickness, which produces a variety of manifestations in diverse tissues, including giant urticaria, angioneurotic edema, fever, and arthritis.

A number of predisposing or contributory factors may be operative in the development of drug eruptions. These include: an existing skin disease; other allergic processes (for example, atopy); functional states such as menses, menopause, and pregnancy; organic disease; the presence or absence of pigmentation;

blood type; nutritional states; and physical factors such as sunlight, heat, cold, and other vagaries of weather. Biochemical genetic factors influencing cellular enzyme systems may also play a role (LaDu, 1972).

Drug eruptions may simulate virtually every known cutaneous disease and may manifest themselves in a variety of clinical patterns which at times mimic common dermatoses. The following list of reactions illustrates the extraordinary diversity of cutaneous expressions which may be caused by drugs: acneiform, pustular, furunculoid, erysipelas-like; eczematous (with erythema, vesiculation, fissuring, weeping, crusting, and scaling); erythema multiforme-like; erythema nodosum-like; "fixed" eruptions, that is, recurrent localized (fixed) circumscribed, erythematous, edematous or bullous, and polychromatic pigmented eruptions; papulosquamous eruptions (pityriasis rosea-like, lichenoid and lichen planus-like); ulcerating and vegetating; purpuric; vesicular and bullous, (pemphigoid); scaling; purely erythematous, scarlatiniform, or morbilliform; exfoliative dermatitis; urticaria and angioneurotic edema; psoriasiform; hyperkeratotic lesions (keratoses); granulomatous lesions; pruritus (alone or in conjunction with other manifestations); hypopigmentation, and hyperpigmentation (melanoderma). Lupus erythematosus-like, lymphoma-like, and mycosis fungoides-like lesions (including fungating tumors) may also occur.

Other cutaneous manifestations observed after treatment with certain medicaments include: alopecia, hyperhidrosis, anhidrosis, cutaneous atrophy, stomatitis, glossitis, photosensitivity, seborrheic dermatitis-like eruptions, linear striae, hirsutism, and generalized xanthoma-like eruptions. Varying combinations of several of the foregoing also have been observed.

A single drug may produce a fixed eruption in one individual, erythema multiforme in another, purpura in another, and urticaria, exfoliative dermatitis, or other clinical manifestations in still other persons. It is true that certain drugs have a tendency to produce certain types of reactions, but in general the variety of possible expressions is so great that only in a few instances is there any advantage to linking cutaneous signs with specific drugs. Conversely, many different drugs may produce the same reaction pattern. In short, almost any drug can cause virtually any type of eruption.

Drugs have been known to produce tumors, activate viral infections, create functional changes in the skin, and cause permanent color changes: for example, keratoses and verrucoid lesions (arsenic, mercury), epitheliomas (arsenic, mercury, radiomimetic compounds); alopecia (thallium, heparin, and cytotoxic drugs), hyperhidrosis (pilocarpine), photosensitivity, (sulfonamides, chlorpromazine, demethylchlortetracycline, quinidine), and extraneous pigmentation (silver salts, other heavy metals, Atabrine).

PATHOGENETIC MECHANISMS OF DRUG ERUPTIONS

The pathologic dynamics of drug eruptions are still not completely understood. There is an unfortunate but very popular tendency to regard all drug reactions as allergic. It is important to recognize that there are many non-allergic mechanisms through which unintended responses to drugs may develop. To blame all sensitivity reactions on drug allergy impairs our understanding of this disease state and leads to unreasonable therapeutic practices, not to mention the diagnostic unsoundness of using this rationalization to explain all the drug reactions one encounters.

Many mechanisms have been proposed and the major ones which are operative are discussed below.

OVERDOSAGE (PHARMACOLOGIC-TOXIC MECHANISM). This implies an effect that would develop in anyone who took the drug in sufficient dosage for an adequate length of time. The reaction may actually be a normal pharmacodynamic action of the drug, but toxicity with cutaneous symptoms becomes apparent only when the drug is used in larger doses or for more prolonged periods than is normally permissible. For instance, the injection of too much ergot will produce gangrene; the prolonged ingestion of Atabrine results in a generalized yellowish discoloration; and argyria develops after the use of silver salts for a sufficient length of time.

SECONDARY EFFECTS OR SIDE EFFECTS. Secondary or side effects of the drug may occur as a part of its normal pharmacologic action, but they may not be the primary therapeutic objective. For example, somnolence or drowsiness may develop with the use of antihistaminic and antipruritic agents; alopecia may follow the use of cytotoxic drugs.

DIRECT TOXIC EFFECT (ENZYMATIC TOXICITY, INTERFERENCE OR COMPETITIVE PHENOMENON). Because of inherent toxicity, mercury, gold, arsenic, thallium, and other heavy metals always carry a risk when administered for a remedial effect, even when modest doses are given. These drugs have been found to alter enzymatic activity or compete for components of intracellular enzyme systems. They may have selective toxicity for one or more enzymes involved in the intermediary metabolism of the affected cell, thus producing cell damage. Cutaneous expressions of this toxicity, such as purpura, exfoliative dermatitis, and even keratoses leading to malignancy, are more likely to represent expressions of "poisoning" of certain essential cellular enzyme systems rather than true allergic reactions. On the other hand, in certain individuals, following the administration of a minute amount of these metals, (for example, 1 mg. of gold sodium thiosulfate), a severe cutaneous reaction may develop which may be properly ascribed to a state of allergic sensitization.

INTOLERANCE. This is a purely individual phenomenon related to a person's inability to tolerate even small amounts of a drug. Doses which evoke normal responses in the general population may cause an abnormal reaction in specific individuals. This is not due to allergic hypersensitivity but is probably related to an inherent susceptibility or predisposition to the action of a drug. Conceptually, it is a *quantitative* difference in reactivity. Individuals who are intolerant to a drug will develop symptoms with ordinary doses that are to be expected only with much larger amounts in most persons. For instance, ringing of the ears will develop in practically everyone who takes large amounts of quinine (overdosage or pharmacologic-toxic effect), but this sometimes occurs in people who take small doses (individual intolerance).

IDIOSYNCRASY. Idiosyncrasy to drugs denotes a *qualitative* abnormal response occurring without obvious reason, and not representing a reaction which can be produced in the majority simply by increasing the dosage given. It is possible that the vegetative lesions produced by iodides and bromides may represent idiosyncrasy rather than true allergy, despite the fact that the latter explanation is usually invoked and accepted without question. The factors underlying idiosyncrasy are undisclosed but are independent of immunologic mechanisms and may be due to genetically induced variations in enzyme systems (pharmacogenetic mechanism).

SANARELLI-SCHWARTZMAN PHENOMENON. This may be responsible for certain hemorrhagic and necrotic eruptions but it is unlikely that this mechanism is commonly operative in drug reactions. The Sanarelli-Schwartzman phenomenon is a two-stage process in which the initial step consists of preparing the skin locally by injection with a Schwartzman preparatory filtrate (usually bacterial products); the second stage (following an incubation period of 12 to 24 hours) consists of eliciting a reaction in the already prepared tissue, usually via intravenous injection. It has been shown that a wide variety of bacterial substances are capable of acting as skin preparatory factors. The Sanarelli-Schwartzman phenomenon apparently depends on the development of *local* hypersensitivity, yet it is not truly on the basis of an allergic mechanism. The incubation period is only 12 to 24 hours, not long enough for the development of true (allergic) antibodies; also the sensitizing agent ("skin preparatory factor") and the eliciting agent need not necessarily be the same, or even immunologically related. It is conceivable, therefore, that a patient may be given a medication to which he may be sensitive by virtue of previous exposure. If he has a "prepared" cutaneous site owing to bacterial infection or other similar process, a reaction may then ensue which could provoke hemorrhage and necrosis at that site, with intravascular coagulation playing a role in the patho-genetic process.

(JARISCH)-HERXHEIMER REACTION. The (Jarisch)-Herxheimer reaction refers to the exacerbation of existing lesions or development of new ones, along with fever and malaise, by an administered drug. It occurs when a drug too vigor-ously destroys the organisms for which it was intended, or because it affects such a wide bacterial spectrum that it kills many organisms besides the one for which it was administered. In either case, bacterial products are released which may be toxic or otherwise damaging to tissue, or to which the host may be allergically sensi-tive. Some of the dyshidrosiform eruptions seen after the use of penicillin ("peni-cillids") may fall into this category. It has often been observed that upon readminis-tration of penicillin these patients do not manifest the same eruption. It has been erroneously assumed that they have be-come "desensitized," but an allergic sensi-tivity to penicillin probably did not exist previously. The eruption apparently de-veloped in the first place because either the penicillin destroyed enough organisms to release bacterial products to which the host was allergically sensitive, or the re-leased materials were toxic enough to cause a reaction. In either case, the reac-tion did not arise because of an allergic sensitivity to penicillin. The absence of a reaction on readministration of penicillin may be explained by the absence or sub-stantial reduction of the same microbial flora. Thus, when the penicillin was again given the same bacterial products were either not released at all or appeared in in-adequate amounts. The (Jarisch)-Herx-heimer reaction was also seen in the days of arsenic-bismuth therapy of syphilis; it is not confined exclusively to penicillin.

ECOLOGIC IMBALANCE. Ecology is the study of the individual organism in rela-tion to the total environment; this includes interspecies competition. The term *eco-logic imbalance* in this case refers to the disturbance of the normal interrelation-ship of microorganisms. The concept of ecologic imbalance is used to explain cer-tain reactions seen after antibiotic therapy. Antibiotics may create ecologic imbalance by destroying certain organisms, thus making conditions more propitious for the growth of other organisms, on the skin as well as internally. There is a greater in-cidence of Candidiasis in patients who have received antibiotics, especially broad-spectrum antibiotics which destroy harmless, as well as pathogenic, micro-organisms. Some nonpathogenic bacteria are necessary for the well-being of the host, since they inhibit the "overgrowth" of Candida. When these "restraining" bac-teria are destroyed by the antibiotics, clinical candidiasis may result, seen in such forms as perleche, stomatitis, eso-phagitis, vaginitis, and proctitis; even fatalities due to overwhelming candidal infections are known.

In addition, many organisms can be found living essentially as saprophytes, but under conditions of unrestricted multi-plication they may assume a pathogenic role. The state of ecologic imbalance may also cause overgrowth of resistant staphy-lococcus, Proteus, and Pseudomonas or-ganisms by suppression of competing bac-teria. Virulent infections or super-infec-tions with antibiotic-resistant organisms may result. It has also been noted that aside from the direct effect of permitting overgrowth of certain microorganisms, the destruction by antibiotics of intestinal bacteria important in the synthesis of vitamin B factors may lead to hypovita-minosis, particularly riboflavin deficiency, as manifested by cheilitis and sore mouth and tongue. The simultaneous adminis-tration of vitamin B factors with antibiotics appears to minimize development of such lesions as well as diarrhea which fre-quently accompanies the skin and oral lesions. Change in pH as the result of alteration of gastrointestinal flora may also be responsible for the diarrhea sometimes noted after oral administration of anti-biotics. Not only is vitamin B metabolism interfered with by antibiotic therapy but there also may be disturbance in vitamin K synthesis, leading to certain types of purpura. Nicotinic acid deficiency follow-ing penicillin therapy may result in mel-anoglossia (black tongue).

BIOTROPIC MECHANISM. It has been postulated that bactericidal drugs may have a dual effect—necrotropic and bio-tropic. The necrotropic effect is the lethal action of a drug on certain microorganisms. The biotropic effect implies that this same drug may be stimulating to other micro-organisms. While many so-called bio-tropic effects are probably the result of an ecologic interference, some may be due to direct stimulation of the microorganisms themselves. Thus, by awakening a latent infection which produces an exanthem, a drug may cause an eruption. The ninth day erythema reactions following bismuth and arsenical treatment of syphilis are attributed to a biotropic mechanism of this type.

It has also been suggested that allergic or sensitizing factors may play a role in biotropic reactions, but in an indirect way. Erythema nodosum seen after the inges-tion of sulfathiazole may not necessarily be an expression of allergic reaction to the drug but may be due to sensitization to a latent microorganism that the drug has stimulated into activity.

ALLERGIC MECHANISMS. The subject of drug allergy is bewilderingly complex. Not only are there difficulties in definition but also an exposition of the characteris-tics of drug allergy is by no means simple because there is no consistently pathog-nomonic symptomatology, pathology, nor presently any single test which will re-liably and invariably detect such allergy. The confusion intrinsic in the subject has promoted much uncritical thinking, which consequently has made it still more diffi-cult to separate fact from fancy. Yet it is important to detect which drug reactions are allergic. The diagnostic criteria of drug allergy are by no means precise, and none of them is absolute in itself. More-over, drug allergy is the one category of allergy in which (with certain exceptions) antibodies can not be directly or indi-rectly demonstrated in many cases. This has hindered the development of useful clinical diagnostic test procedures; skin tests are ordinarily of little value, often responding when the individual is not systemically allergic to the drug ("false positive") or failing to respond when the individual is indeed allergic ("false nega-tive"). Thus, unlike contact dermatitis due to drugs, it is usually not possible to detect the allergic state and identify the responsi-ble drug by simple skin tests. The exist-ence of antibodies in drug allergy is as-sumed but is not often substantiated. Nevertheless, despite the lack of evidence

for an antigen-antibody reaction in many drug eruptions, some, perhaps the majority, of reactions are unquestionably allergic in nature.

Allergy may be defined as a specific, ac-quired alteration in the capacity of the individual to react to an antigen, which is mediated by circulating or cellular anti-bodies. This subject is more completely discussed in Chapter 4. However, in con-sidering drug allergy, it is well to remem-ber that allergic reactions may be classi-fied as Type I (anaphylactic), Type II (cytolytic or cytotoxic), Type III (Arthus reaction or toxic complex syndrome) and Type IV (delayed or tuberculin type sensi-tivity; Gell and Coombs, 1963). An addi-tional type of reaction, Type V, has been called late, delayed sensitivity and involves distinctive granulomatous reac-tions which are presumed to be allergic in nature (Hurley, 1974). The characteristics of these allergic reactions are summarized in Table 7–1. Because of inadequate knowledge it is impossible to precisely place all allergic drug eruptions in one or another of the above categories. The mechanisms involved may be any of the reactions Type I through Type V or may be a combination of these.

The characteristics of eruptions due to drug allergy have not changed significantly since they were originally stated; however, it is of value to re-emphasize certain points. The eruption may be produced and re-produced at any time thereafter by minute amounts of a drug which may have been previously well tolerated for years. There-for, successive attacks confer no immunity. While many drug eruptions do not itch, those of an allergic nature generally are marked by pruritus. In fact, pruritus may be the only symptom of a drug reaction, objective signs being entirely absent. In most persons, even after large dosage of a drug, allergic eruptions do not appear; yet once the allergic state has developed, the eruption is likely to recur upon subse-quent minute exposures to the offending drug or to a related compound (cross-reac-tion). In general, the clinical picture of the allergic response is entirely different from that produced by the pharmacologic or toxicologic action of the drug. Drugs with entirely different pharmacologic actions often produce identical allergic eruptions;

TABLE 7–1   CLASSIFICATION OF ALLERGIC REACTIONS°

	Type I	*Type II*	*Type III*	*Type IV*	*Type V*
Synonym	Anaphylactic, immediate	Cytolytic, cytotoxic	Arthus reaction; toxic complex syndrome	Delayed, tuberculin type	Late delayed, granulomatous
Mediating antibody	Serologic, tissue passive sensitizing	Serologic or cell-mediated	Precipitating	Cell-mediated	? Cell-mediated
Skin test	Immediate wheal and flare	Immediate wheal and flare. Also polymorphonuclear and granulomatous reaction	Arthus reaction with polymorphs in 2–4 hours, later may show necrosis	48–72 hour tuberulin response	Sarcoidal granuloma at 3–5 weeks
Clinical expression	Urticaria; angioneurotic edema	Purpura; ? SLE; homograft rejection	Serum sickness; allergic vasculitis; ? purpura; ? polyarteritis; ? Erythema multiforme; ? Erythema nodosum	Contact dermatitis	Zirconium and beryllium granulomas; ? Sarcoidosis; ? tuberculoid leprosy

°Modified from Gell and Coombs (1963).

moreover, the same drug is often capable of producing radically different manifestations in different individuals, or in the same individual at different times.

Drug sensitivity is often remarkably specific. Individuals sensitive to one drug may show no demonstrable sensitivity to isomers of that drug or to drugs with only slightly altered chemical constitution. However, just as has been demonstrated in sensitivity to other allergens, group specificity and cross-reactivity are features of drug allergy also.

Drug allergy shows many of the other general characteristics of other forms of allergy. Thus, in drug allergy, incubation periods, spontaneous flare-ups, and subsequent altered responses on re-exposure may be observed. Drug allergens can be rated as to relative sensitizing capacity, and in general tend to call forth characteristic clinical pictures. They tend to select certain tissues and sites, and their effects are influenced by variations in host susceptibility, environmental and dietary factors, and by fluctuations in sensitivity to drug allergen. Finally, some of the changes they produce may persist for long periods of time.

The significant features of drug allergy are as follows (Coombs, 1969):

Nature of the Allergen. No special class of substances is responsible or dominant throughout the various forms of drug allergy. Drugs may supply an antigenic chemical as simple as an inorganic ion, such as mercury, or as complex as a large organic derivative. For the most part, however, these substances are not highly antigenic in the immunologic sense; that is, antibodies (precipitating) are not readily formed in response to their injection. Drugs may form conjugates with body proteins and it is this combination which confers antigenicity or allergenicity. Drugs, therefore, are partial or incomplete antigens (haptens). The hapten or uncombined drug cannot ordinarily elicit the allergic response in a sensitized individual; only the complete antigen, namely the drug (hapten) conjugated with the body protein, can. Similarly, persons with drug allergy frequently do *not* react to skin tests using the very drugs to which they are sensitive. This is due to the fact that the drug alone is not the allergen and cannot elicit the response. The complete antigen must be formed by metabolic processes in the body to react with the antibody and produce the allergic reaction. Excluded from this consideration of the drug allergy are the allergic responses to proteins which are sometimes used as drugs, and which, being complete antigens, act in a different way (for example, serum sickness reactions).

Individual Sensitization. The factors which underlie the capacity to become sensitized are unknown. It is clear that the majority of individuals may take commonly used drugs indefinitely in ordinary doses without developing a cutaneous or other drug reaction. This is in contrast to what happens if a large number of subjects are exposed repeatedly to poison ivy leaves or other strong contact allergens, in which case a large percentage of exposed persons develop reactions. A constitutional factor, possibly one having to do with the capacity to form the proper conjugate, apparently determines which individuals will acquire drug sensitivity. The allergic state may develop at any time, except during the first 7 to 10 days after the initial administration of the drug (the incubation period), assuming that usage of the drug is continued. The patient's report that he has been taking a particular drug for many years without any sign of reaction is not a deciding factor for or against a diagnosis of drug allergy. A patient may be exposed to a drug for years before becoming sensitized to it, but nothing is known as to why one patient becomes sensitized within a few weeks after exposure while another may require as long as 20 years.

Testing Procedures in Vitro. While several laboratory tests have been devised (see discussion under Diagnosis below) there is no single test which will detect the various forms of drug allergy accurately and consistently. Indeed, there are few instances in which the responsible antibodies have been conclusively demonstrated in vitro. This reflects a host of factors, including inability to provide the complete (conjugated) antigen, an inadequate understanding of the nature of the antibody involved in the given response, and technical problems associated with duplication of the antigen-antibody reaction in the laboratory. It should be remembered that allergic reactions to drugs are varied and complex biologic responses which for the most part defy demonstration outside the body.

Skin Testing. As previously indicated, cutaneous tests are with rare exceptions, of little value in detecting drug allergy. Neither patch, scratch, nor intradermal injection techniques can be expected to yield a positive result in all cases. Certain positive reactions may have diagnostic import, but negative ones are meaningless. For instance, a positive reaction to an intradermal injection of penicillin in a patient with a suspected drug allergy to penicillin implicates this compound as the possible causal agent, but a negative reaction does not rule out such a causal relationship and does not provide any assurance of safety from untoward reaction if a suspect medication is to be readministered.

Specificity of Reaction Patterns. Certain drugs have a tendency to produce specific types of eruptions. This tendency is often of great aid in suspecting drug exposures which

the patient has concealed or of which he may not be aware. Notable examples are the acneiform eruption or fungating granulomas due to bromides and iodides, the fixed eruptions due to phenolphthalein, and the erythematous, bullous, and urticarial eruptions due to penicillin and barbiturates. Nonetheless, exceptions to the common eruptive patterns associated with a particular drug are well known. Practically every known type of cutaneous lesion may be reproduced in drug reactions. Thus, drugs must be considered in all types of eruptions for which no other explanation is apparent. Drugs not only cause manifestations in the skin, but may produce constitutional and other local manifestations which may occur independently or in association with the dermatosis, including fever, lymphadenopathy, bone marrow depression, conjunctivitis, mucous membrane lesions, and asthma. A possible reaction to drugs should be considered in the assessment of a great many systemic disturbances which do not fit into known patterns of disease.

Cross-Sensitization. This procedure may furnish important chemical proof of the allergic nature of the drug eruption. Exposure to related chemical substances may elicit the allergic response induced by the original substance; cross-sensitizations among different sulfonamides, certain barbiturates, and the procaine-group of anesthetics are well known. The cross-sensitizing spectrum, however, is not always the same, because an individual may become sensitized either to the whole molecule or to some moiety within the compound. If sensitization is to the latter, cross-reaction will be noted only with those substances which happen to contain that component; whereas, if it is the former, only a drug containing the entire structure will elicit the reaction. It is not always possible to predict which substances will cross-react, though it may be anticipated if there is a chemical relationship. Cross-reactions "make sense" chemically, but in different subjects the body may become sensitized to the same chemical in different ways. In one individual with a sulfonamide allergy, practically every other type of sulfonamide will cross-react and reproduce the allergic syndrome, whereas in another individual, only one or two other substances (or none) may cross-react, owing to sensitization to another part of the molecule. The sensitivity may extend to another class of substances altogether because of a common chemical component (for example, when a sulfonamide-sensitive patient cross-reacts to procaine, paraminobenzoic acid, and para-phenylenediamine because they all contain a para-aminophenyl group, the crucial allergen in this case).

Cross-sensitivity assumes clinical importance

in another phenomenon. Dermatitis due to external sensitization to an agent (allergic contact dermatitis) may become exacerbated through the administration, whether by ingestion or injection, of the same or related compound (for example, in an individual with a previous contact dermatitis to procaine). Eczema is usually a distinctive expression of contact dermatitis and not of drug allergy. However, once a person has acquired allergic contact sensitization, he may react with an eczematous response, not only when the allergen is put on his skin but also when it is ingested or injected. Drugs which are injected or ingested may elicit a reaction in an already established contact sensitization, but they cannot induce a contact allergic state by these routes.

Differentiating Allergic from Non-Allergic Reactions to Drugs

1. In allergic reactions, there must be an incubation period; that is, the individual does not react on first exposure unless, of course, there has been a previous exposure to an immunologically related compound. The incubation period is usually not less than 7 to 10 days. As in serum sickness, there may be sufficient traces of drug which persist from the initial administration, especially if injected, to bring out a reaction after sensitization has developed without any further administration of the drug. For instance, an individual may suddenly develop a dermatosis one to three weeks following a single injection of repository penicillin, although he has never before received penicillin and received none in the interim. The original injection serves both as the sensitizing and the eliciting dose. However, an eruption which appears within a day or two after the administration of a new drug for the first time either is non-allergic or may demonstrate that the individual has been previously sensitized to some related agent.

2. The allergic response is different from the pharmacodynamic reaction of the drug, or from any manifestation which represents simple accumulation.

3. Once sensitivity has occurred, minute amounts of the drug will cause exacerbation promptly. This is an extremely valuable and reliable diagnostic procedure; it is, in fact, the only really definitive one, but is often hazardous.

4. Withdrawal of the drug is generally followed by remission of the manifestations, although at variable rates depending on how rapidly the drug is removed from the body and the degree of sensitivity which has been produced. This is not surprising, because, in allergic states, extremely small residue may produce very large reactions. Following a single injection of penicillin, for example, patients have continued to react for many months.

In certain rare cases the eruption may persist for years following withdrawal of the drug, although this is ordinarily due to secondary factors in the chain of cutaneous changes originally initiated by the drug or to continued insidious exposure to a drug or a related chemical. It is a sound general rule, however, that in true drug allergy the symptoms and signs abate when there is no further exposure to the drug.

5. The sensitivity to the drug usually persists indefinitely. As with most generalizations, however, there are exceptions. Unaccountable fluctuations in sensitivity occur, and sometimes spontaneous desensitization takes place after many years. Unless the circumstances are compelling, however, no patient should be exposed to a drug to which he has reacted allergically in the past.

6. Hyposensitization is theoretically possible through the repeated administration of small quantities of the responsible sensitizing drug. This procedure is dangerous and time consuming and frequently does not provide a degree of hyposensitization which is clinically significant. Hyposensitization may be attempted in rare instances in which a patient absolutely requires a drug for which there is no adequate substitute. The effect is generally temporary, however, and attempts to induce this capricious phenomenon are rarely advisable.

7. Spontaneous flare-ups may occur at the site of injection of a drug to which an individual was previously not sensitive. When the sensitization develops, however, intense inflammatory reactions occur at all previous injection sites where sufficient antigen remains.

8. The fixed drug eruption (see below) is an extraordinary clinical phenomenon in which the eruption recurs precisely in the same areas whenever the drug is administered. It is a convincing demonstration that at times only certain portions of the integument become sensitized. The reasons for such localization are entirely unknown, but it is clear that in these cases the skin does not become sensitized as a whole. Curiously enough, a fixed drug eruption may be limited to a single lesion no larger than the fingertip, and there may be no other visible reaction to the responsible agent, no matter how much is administered.

FIXED DRUG ERUPTIONS. The term "fixed drug eruption" was introduced by Louis Brocq in 1894 to indicate an eruption in which the cutaneous manifestations appear as round or oval, apparently edematous plaques (one or more in number) varying in size from that of a small coin to that of a palm, appearing consistently at exactly the same sites on various parts of the body, and often accompanied by an itching or burning sensation. The patches are erythematous and dusky at their onset and have well-defined borders. At times the lesions progress to form bullae. Desquamation, or crusting following bullous lesions, appears as the eruption fades, leaving pigmentation of variable shade and duration (often remaining for months) in the affected areas. A special feature of the eruption is its tendency to relapse with recurrence of the lesions in the same pigmented sites which are the residual signs of the last exacerbation.

The mechanism of the production of fixed drug eruptions remains unknown. Details of the sensitization process have not yet been provided. Although specific antibodies can rarely be demonstrated, it is believed that an allergic hypersensitivity is the basis for the fixed drug eruption. Failure to recognize the fixed eruption and eliminate the cause will result in recurrence unless the drug is fortuitously stopped by the patient. The first drug known to produce this phenomenon was antipyrine (phenazone). Many additional drugs have since been incriminated in fixed eruptions (Savin, 1970). A list of such agents includes: acetanilide, acetylsalicylic acid, aminopyrine, antimony and potassium tartrate, arsenicals (Acetylarsan, arsphenamine, Mapharsen, Trisodarsen, tryparsamide), Atabrine, barbiturates, bismuth, bromides, chlordiazepoxide, cinchophen, Dilatin, emetine (ipecac), iodides, isoaminile citrate, mercury, oxyphenbutazone, penicillin, phenacetin, phenolphthalein, quinidine, quinine, salicylates, sulfonamides, and tetracycline (Delaney, 1970).

TOXIC EPIDERMAL NECROLYSIS (LYELL'S SYNDROME). In 1956, Lyell reported four patients with a toxic eruption closely resembling severe scalding of the skin. These patients did not exhibit surgical shock as may result from a severe and extensive thermal injury. Lyell called this necrosis of the epidermis "toxic epidermal necrolysis," which is described in Chapters 8 and 9 in greater detail. It has been induced by certain drugs in addition to other agents. Among the drugs which have been named as precipitants of this condition are aloin, Amytal, antipyrine, antitetanic serum, aspirin, atropine, dapsone, Dover's powder, formaldehyde, gold salts, hydantoin and its derivatives, oil of chenopodium, penicillin, promethazine, thorazine, sulfonamides, and tetracycline. In addition to drugs, however, bacterial and viral infection may also bring about this condition.

GENETICALLY INDUCED DRUG REACTIONS. An example of this type of reaction is the acute hemolytic anemia caused by administration of primaquine, para-aminosalicylic acid, phenacetin, sulfonamides, and nitrofurans to an individual whose red blood cells are deficient in glucose-6-phosphate dehydrogenase (LaDu, 1972). Another example is the prolonged apnea which develops in certain individuals unable to properly hydrolyze administered succinylcholine because of low serum cholinesterase. Anticonvulsant drugs may produce megaloblastic anemia due to a genetic disturbance of the metabolism of folic acid. Other examples include the peripheral neuritides produced by isonicotinic acid hydrazide and the intermittent porphyria caused occasionally by barbiturates. In individuals with these conditions apparently a genetic deficiency in a cellular or humoral enzyme system is responsible for the abnormal reaction.

PHOTOSENSITIZATION. This refers to the ability of certain agents to induce an alteration in the capacity of the skin to react to specific wavelengths of actinic radiation. An inflammatory response on the skin following exposure to light may be induced by porphyrins, certain plants and oils, sulfonamides, and some tranquilizers (mainly phenothiazine and chlorpromazine derivatives) (Harber and Baer, 1972).

Photosensitive eruptions characteristically involve the exposed skin areas and spare those sites usually covered by clothing or those receiving less radiation because of the natural protection afforded by skin folds or recesses (eyelids, infranasal skin, folds of the chin, submental skin). Photosensitive reactions may be of two types: phototoxic and photoallergic. Photo-onycholysis is the separation of the nail plate from the nail bed as a result of a phototoxic reaction in the nail bed skin. See Table 7–2 for a list of photosensitizing agents.

Photoallergic reactions may be differ-

TABLE 7–2   Photosensitizing Agents[*]

Drugs

Antidiabetic agents, oral: including carbutamide, tolbutamide, chlorpropamide (Nadisan, Diabinese, Orinase, Orabetic)

Anesthetics: the procaine group of local anesthetics

Antibiotics: including tetracyclines and their derivatives: chlortetracycline (Aureomycin), oxytetracycline (Terramycin), demethylchlortetracycline (Declomycin), and griseofulvin (a penicillium derivative)

Antihistaminics: including diphenhydramine hydrochloride (Benadryl), promethazine (Phenergan), tripyrathiazine hydrochloride (Pyrrolazote), isothipendyl (Therahistin)

Anticonvulsants: Tridione and Dilantin

Arsenicals

Barbiturates

Hormonal substances: including estrone and diethylstilbestrol

Topical antibacterial agents (antiseptics): bithional, tetrachlorsalicylanilide (TCSA), tribromsalicylanilide (TBS)

Phenothiazine derivatives: including chlorpromazine (Thorazine), prochlorperazine (Compazine), mepazine (Pacatal), perphenazine (Trilafon), trimeprazine (Temaril), triflupromazine (Vesprin), promazine (Sparine), thiopropazate dihydrochloride (Dartal)

Psoralens: Furocoumarin derivatives, including 5-methoxypsoralen, 8-methoxypsoralen, and others

Sulfonamides: including sulfacetamide, sulfadiazine, sulfaguanidine, sulfamerazine, sulfamethazine, sulfapyridine, sulfathiazole, sulfadimethoxine

Sulfonylureas: see oral antidiabetic drugs above

Thiazide diuretics (aromatic sulfonamide preparations): chlorothiazide (Diuril) and hydrochlorothiazide (Hydrodiuril)

Heavy metals: gold and silver salts

Porphyrins: hematoporphyrin (used to treat melancholia), chlorophyll

Miscellaneous: digalloyltrioleate, monoglycerol para-aminobenzoate, p-dimethylaminoazobenzene, phenylbutazone, quinine, stilbamidine, salicylates, Lantinin, Perloline, dicyanine-A, 5-fluorouracil, triethylene melamine (TEM), 9-aminoacridine

Dyes

Acridine dyes: acridine, trypallavine, and others

"Blankophores" (optical brighteners—mainly sulfa derivatives)

Dibenzypyran derivatives (eosin, fluorescein dyes, rose bengal and others)

Paraphenylenediamine

Phenothiazine dyes (methylene blue, toluidine blue, and others)

Phenoxazine dyes

Phenazine dyes

Trypan blue

Coal Tar Products and Petroleum Products

Crude coal tar and its derivatives (benzene, anthracene, xylene, nephthalene, toluene, phenanthrene, thiophene, phenolic compounds, pyridine, and others)

Pitch and pitch fumes

Essential Oils and Others

Oil of bergamot

Oil of cedar

Oil of citron

Oil of lavender

Lime oil

Vanillin oils

Other agents included in various perfumes and cologne water

Plants

Mainly members of the Umbelliferae family including: parsnips, carrots (wild and garden types), celery, yarrow, angelica, fennel, dill, and parsley

Members of the Rutaceae family (rue, bergamot and lime, wafer ash) meadow grass, clover mustards, agrimony, bavachi (corylifolia)

Agave lechiguilla: a perennial flowering plant of Amaryllis family, related to *A. belladonna*

Lantana: a shrub of the Verbenae family

Lady's thumb and smartweed: flower herbs of the buckwheat family

---

[*]Adapted from a list of photosensitizing agents prepared by Capt. James W. Young, USAF(MC), Bull. Assoc. Milit. Dermatol. *13*:33, 1964.

---

entiated from phototoxic drug reactions on the basis of the following criteria (Baer and Harber, 1961):

1. Photoallergic reactions occur only in a small percentage of those persons exposed to the drug plus sunlight, while phototoxic reactions can be elicited in virtually all or most of those individuals similarly exposed.

2. A phototoxic drug reaction can occur upon the first combined exposure to the drug and radiant energy, while a photoallergic drug reaction can occur only after an incubation period during which sensitization develops.

3. A phototoxic drug reaction usually has the appearance of an intensified sunburn. A photo-allergic drug reaction also may simulate a sunburn, but clinically and histologically it often resembles other forms of cutaneous reactions known to be associated with allergic phenomena.

4. In many cases of photoallergic drug reaction, a positive photo patch test or photo drug test which has the characteristics of an allergic reaction can be elicited.

5. In photoallergic drug reactions, flare-ups may occur in unexposed sites distant from the point of light exposure.

6. In photoallergic drug reactions, the phenomenon of photo–cross-sensitization to immunochemically related allergens may be demonstrated.

For a further discussion of the subject, the reader is referred to Chapter 6.

DIAGNOSIS AND CLINICAL FEATURES OF DRUG ERUPTIONS

The diagnosis of drug eruptions rests upon constant awareness of the capacity of drugs, like any other chemical, to produce disease. Drug eruptions are often marked by a sudden onset, symmetric and widespread distribution, pruritus, and bright red to dusky violaceous erythema. They may be accompanied by constitutional signs and symptoms of a toxic nature, especially fever. Only in certain of the allergic states are skin tests positive, and here they may be dangerous, sometimes leading to exacerbation and extension of the eruption, and even death.

Deliberate administration of a suspected drug to prove its causal relationship, while safe on occasion, is often fraught with danger and is categorically not recommended. It is contraindicated especially in any generalized or bullous eruption and in the immediate allergic reactions unless the patient is desperately in need of the drug under suspicion. If administered at all, the drug should be given in extremely minute initial test doses, although it is true that there is no precise stoichiometric dose-to-reaction–eliciting relationship. The test dose is best administered in the hospital where emergency measures are available in the event that a severe, life-threatening reaction develop. Moreover, the informed consent of the patient or his next of kin should be obtained.

The morphologic aspects of drug eruptions is protean and frequently bizarre. It includes every possible type of skin lesion and many reaction patterns. The most common lesions and drugs which may incite these eruptions are: maculopapular (morbilliform), erythematous pruritic eruptions of widespread distribution, usually symmetric (arsenic, belladonna, barbiturates, penicillin, sulfonamides); urticarial eruptions, including angioneurotic edema (penicillin); vesiculobullous eruptions (sulfonamides); pustular eruptions (bromides); purpuric eruptions (barbiturates).

In addition to these primary lesions which may occur in a generalized drug eruption, certain drugs may produce the following dermatologic reactions and disease patterns:

DYSHIDROTIC, ERYTHEMA MULTIFORME, ERYTHEMA NODOSUM, EXFOLIATIVE DERMATITIS, GRANULOMATOUS. The variable nature of drug reactions in the skin is further emphasized when one considers that drug eruptions may almost exactly mimic the following dermatoses: acne, erysipelas, exanthemata, lichen planus, disseminated lupus erythematosus, pemphigus, pityriasis rosea, psoriasis, seborrheic dermatitis (see Table 7–3).

DRUG ERUPTIONS AND L. E. CELL PHENOMENON. For some time, the lupus erythematosus (L. E.) cell phenomenon has been considered by some to be nonspecific. It can be found in a number of conditions other than lupus erythematosus; for example, in multiple myeloma, arthritis, leukemia, hemolytic anemia, pernicious anemia, dermatitis herpetiformis, generalized candidiasis, and other cutaneous processes including sensitivity to such drugs as penicillin, derivatives of hydantoin, sulfonamides, and especially Apresoline (hydralazine). Since 1953, a number of instances of acute systemic lupus erythematosus–like or rheumatic and febrile syndromes from hydralazine hydrochloride (Apresoline) have appeared in the literature. Many other agents have been reported to be responsible for this process, including the following: antihistaminics, antituberculous drugs (isoniazid, para-aminosalicylic acid), arsenicals, chlorpromazine, diphenylhydantoin, griseofulvin, gold, horse serum, penicillin, phenylbutazone, quinine, quinidine, prolonged steroid therapy, sulfonamides (for example, sulfadiazine, sulfamethoxypyridazine), tetracyclines, trimethadione, tuberculin, and typhoid-parathyphoid vaccine (Alarcon-Segovia, 1969; Alkalay and Ballard, 1971). The procainamide-lupus syndrome has also received much attention (Guss, 1970; Sheldon and Williams, 1970).*

---

*See also Arthritis Foundation Bulletin on the Rheumatic Diseases *20*:604, 1970 for extensive references.

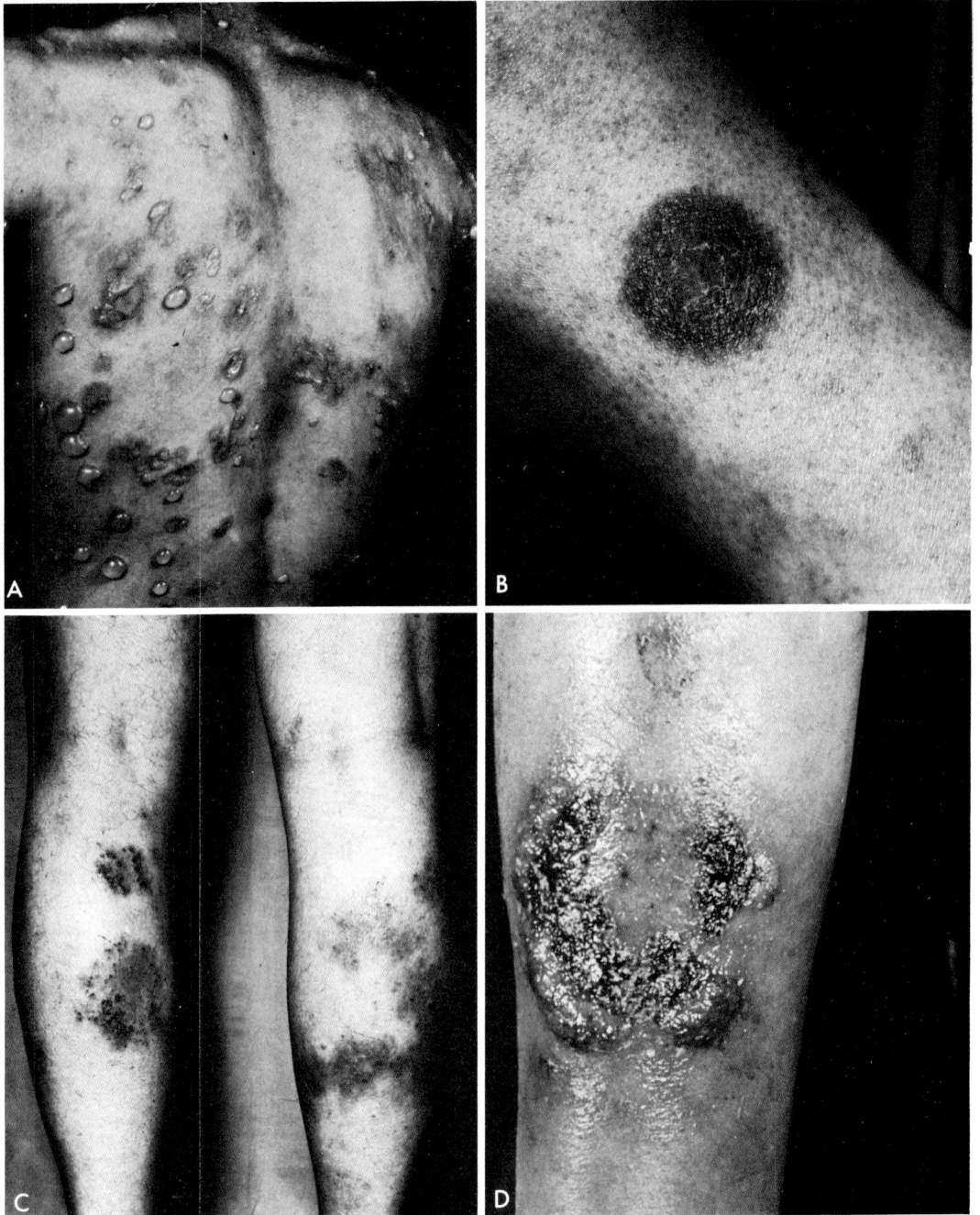

Figure 7-1 *A*, Bullous reaction appearing within a few hours after a single 0.5 gm. dose of sulfathiazole. The patient had been sensitized originally by topical application. *B*, "Fixed" eruption due to phenolphthalein. *C*, Patchy dermatitis induced by Atabrine therapy. A lichen planus–like eruption frequently results from prolonged suppressive therapy with this drug. *D*, Bromoderma.

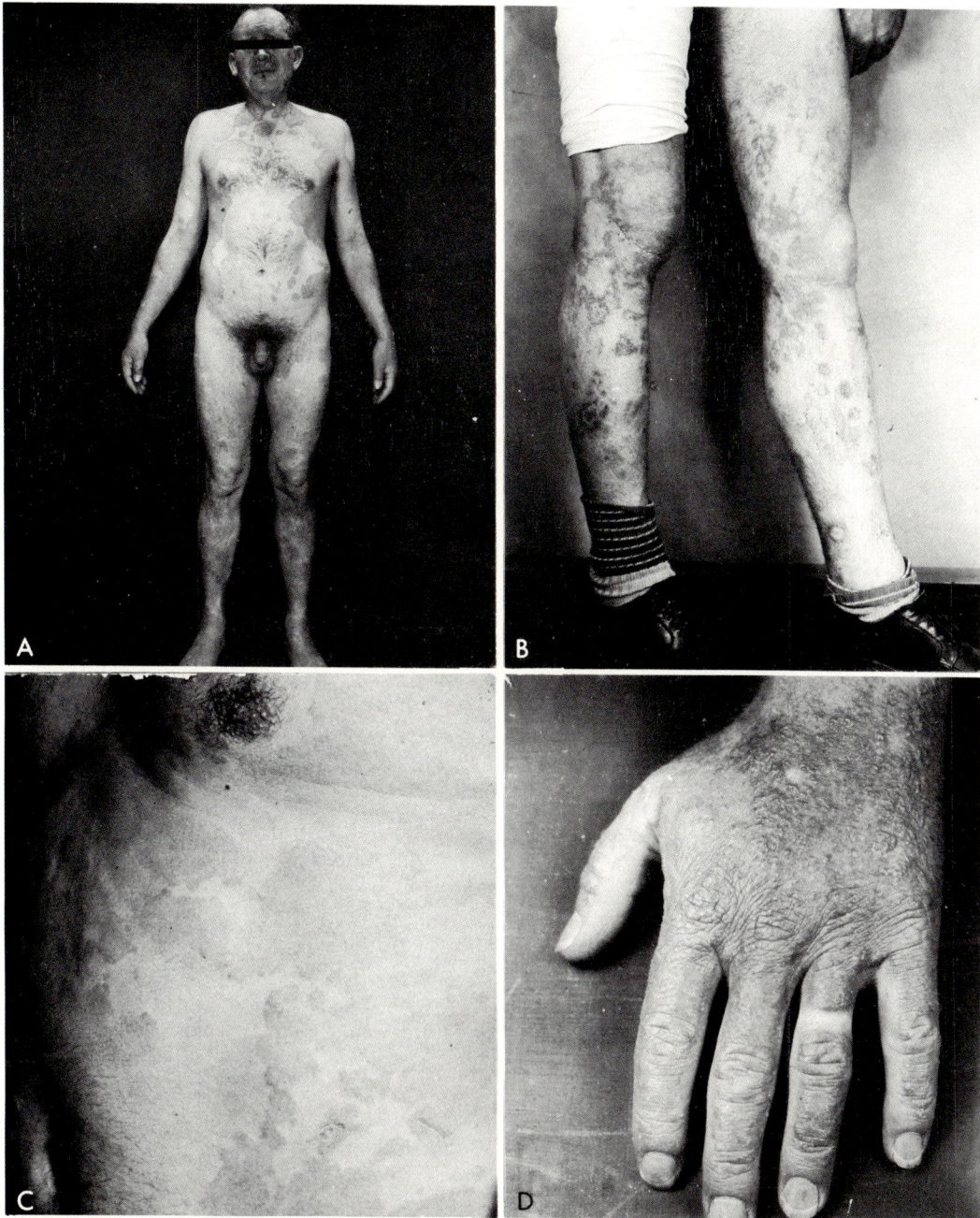

Figure 7-2 *A* and *B*, Urticaria following penicillin therapy. An exceedingly common type of reaction. *C,* Urticarial reaction to aspirin. *D,* Dermatitis due to Aureomycin given by mouth. Note lack of involvement of area compressed by ring.

The syndrome progresses from mild arthralgia to a clinical state compatible with rheumatoid arthritis. If there is continued administration of the drug, the classic symptoms of lupus erythematosus develop, including the typical "butterfly" eruption as well as other skin lesions. Usually the process regresses rapidly after the drug is stopped, but some of the findings may persist for years after the medication is discontinued. Readministration of the drug generally causes a prompt recur-

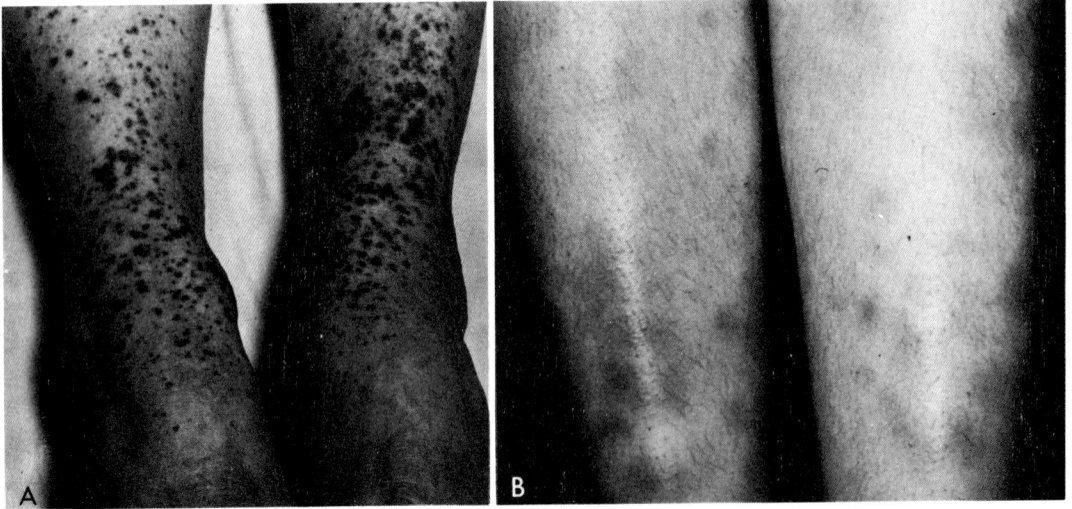

Figure 7-3   *A*, Purpuric eruption due to iodide therapy. *B*, Erythema nodosum, probably due to sulfonamide therapy.

rence of symptoms in most patients. The recurrent attack is more severe than the original. Wire loop–like deposits in the vessels of the skin, kidney, heart, spleen, and lung have been demonstrated by histologic methods and electron microscopy (Grishman and Churg, 1970). In some instances true systemic lupus erythematosus may exist in latent form but becomes "unmasked" by the action of certain drugs.

THROMBOCYTOPENIC PURPURA (Ackroyd, 1958; DeWeck, 1972). Thrombocytopenic purpura consists of widespread purpura and bleeding. There are purpuric spots and bullous hemorrhagic lesions of the oral mucosa. This condition may be induced by such drugs as antipyrine, chlorothiazide (Diuril), hydrochlorothiazide (Esidrix, HydroDiuril), iodine, propylthiouracil, quinine, quinidine, allylisopropyl-acetyl-carbamide (Sedormid), sulfamethoxypyridazine, and sulfisoxazole (Gantrisin). The platelets are reduced in number, and eosinophilia may be present. There is generally no splenomegaly. As a rule, the condition is transient, but it may become chronic. Thrombocytopenic purpura may well have an immunologic basis. The administration of a drug or the presence of infection or other factors may affect platelets in such a way that they become antigenic. The antibodies which are formed against the drug-platelet combina-

tion are incomplete antibodies. They become attached to the vascular endothelium so that readministration of the same drug causes vascular damage and subsequent purpura. However, drug-induced thrombocytopenic purpura occasionally may occur months after the original injection of the drug. This is particularly true when drugs are given by injection in depot form.

In most drug reactions no specific serologic changes or circulating antibodies can be discovered by available methods, nor does demonstration of the presence of a drug in the fluids or tissues of the patient constitute proof of the causal role of that drug; it proves only that the drug was encountered by the patient. Conversely, failure to demonstrate a drug in the fluids or tissues of the patient does not exonerate the drug as a possible causal agent. It proves only that the drug is not present in demonstrable quantity or form at the time of the examination.

From the foregoing statement of the principles of drug eruptions, it is obvious that the basic mechanisms of these phenomena are still little understood and much work remains to be done in order to elucidate their exact nature. Yet some basic advances are being made in the knowledge of the immunologic response to drugs (DeWeck, 1972). Illustrative of these advances are the immunochemical

TABLE 7-3 CHARACTERISTIC CLINICAL CUTANEOUS ERUPTIONS
AND THEIR MOST FREQUENTLY CAUSAL DRUGS*

Achromotrichia: Chloroquine (Aralen)

Acneiform and pustular:
ACTH	Cyanocobalamine
Bromides	Iodides
Corticosteroids	Tridione

Alopecia:
Antithyroid drugs	Allopurinol
Oral contraceptives	Hypocholesteremic drugs
Alkylating agents	Cytotoxic agents
Anticoagulants	Quinacrine (Atabrine)
Antimetabolites	Tribaranol
Vitamin A	Thallium

Dyshidrosis: Iodides

Eczematous:
Arsphenamine	Procaine (and other local anesthetics)
Chlorpromazine	
Ephedrine	Promethazine
Formaldehyde	Quinacrine (Atabrine)
Meprobamate	Resorcin
Neomycin	Streptomycin
Novobiocin	Sulfonamides
Penicillin	Thiamine

Erysipelas-like: Amidopyrine

Erythema multiforme:
Chlorpropamide	Sulfonamides
Penicillin	Thiazine derivatives
Phenothiazines	

Erythema nodosum: Iodides, sulfonamides

Exanthematic (Scarlatiniform, Morbilliform):
Aminosalicylic acid	Methaminodiazepoxide
Anticonvulsants	Novobiocin
Antihistaminics	Penicillin
Barbiturates	Phenothiazines
Chlorothiazides	Phenylbutazone
Chlorpromazine	Quinacrine (Atabrine)
Gold salts	Streptomycin
Griseofulvin	Sulfonamides
Insulin	Sulfones
Meprobamate	Thiouracil

Exfoliative erythroderma:
Aminosalicylic acid	Penicillin
Arsenicals	Phenothiazines
Chlorpropamide	Phenylbutazone
Gold compounds	Sulfonamides
Mercurials	

Fixed:
Antipyrine	Phenylbutazone
Barbiturates	Quinidine
Gold	Salicylates
Phenacetin	Sulfonamides
Phenolphthalein	Tetracyclines

Granulomatous: Bromides, iodides

Lichenoid and lichen planus–like
Arsenicals	Para-aminosalicylic acid
Chloroquine (Aralen)	Quinacrine (Atabrine)
Gold	Quinidine
	Thiazides

Lupus erythematosus–like
Aminosalicylic acid	Penicillin
Griseofulvin	Phenothiazines
Hydantoin	Phenylbutazone
Hydralazine (Apresoline)	Procainamide
	Streptomycin
Isoniazid	Sulfonamides
Mesantoin	Tetracycline
Methyldopa	

Pemphigus-like: Sulfonamides

Photosensitive:
Griseofulvin	Sulfonamides (chemo- therapeutics, anti- diabetics, and diuretics)
Phenothiazines	
Tetracycline	
Thiazides	

Pigmentary Changes: Chloroquine (Aralen), chlorpromazine

Pityriasis rosea–like: Barbiturates, bismuth

Porphyria (exacerbation):
Barbiturates	Griseofulvin
Chloroquine (Aralen)	

Psoriasis-like: Sulfonamides

Purpuric:
Barbiturates	Iodides
Carbamides	Quinidine
Chlorothiazide	Sulfonamides (chemotherapeutics, antidiabetics, and diuretics)
Chlorpromazine	
Gold salts	
Griseofulvin	

Seborrheic dermatitis: Gold

Urticarial:
ACTH	Penicillin
Barbiturates	Phenolphthalein
Chloramphenicol	Phenothiazines
Enzymes	Salicylates
Griseofulvin	Streptomycin
Insulin	Sulfonamides
Opiates	Tetracyclines

Vesiculobullous:
Aloin	Mercury
Arsenic	Phenolphthalein
Bromides	Salicylates
Iodides	

*Based in part on reports to the Section on Adverse Reactions of the Council on Drugs of the American
Medical Association; also Fellner, M. J., and Baer, R. L.: Cutaneous reactions from drugs. Med. Clin. North
Am. *49:*711, 1965, with additions and modifications.

studies of penicillin of the past decade which have stimulated qualitative investigation of the immune response to penicillin in man. These studies have shown that the incidence of an immune response after administration of a drug is considerably higher than would have been expected from the number of overt clinical allergic reactions. From serum antibody detectable by hemagglutination, it is apparent that a large percentage of patients receiving penicillin develop IgM antibodies. According to the sensitivity of the hemagglutination technique used, the number of such patients varies from 20 to 100 per cent. In any case, an immune response to a drug may not always be clinically manifested. Clinical data, such as the incidence of reactions to drugs which have not been immunochemically investigated, should be cautiously interpreted, particularly when suitable techniques for antibody detection are not available. It is also important to note that antibody formation per se is *physiologic* and does not neces-

sarily indicate allergy or hypersensitivity. With more refined methods of detection, many more antibody responses will eventually be revealed, even to drugs which do not cause clinical manifestations. Studies of immunologic response to penicillin in man also indicate that clinical manifestations of the hypersensitivity state are governed not only by the several types of antibodies formed but also by the relative proportion of the various immunoglobulins present at different times. The presence of IgM antibodies does not lead to clinical symptoms in most cases, and the presence of IgG antibodies sometimes appears to be protective. The disappearance of skin lesions in penicillin urticaria and the serum sickness syndrome often coincides with a marked rise of the IgG level in the serum. However, IgG is responsible for hemolytic anemia due to penicillin and also for the joint, lymph node, and kidney lesions found in the serum sickness syndrome. (See Table 7–4 for a summary of the immunoglobulins formed on adminis-

TABLE 7–4 CHARACTERISTICS OF "ANTIPENICILLIN" ANTIBODIES[*]

Characteristics	*Immunoglobulin M (IgM)*	*Immunoglobulin G (IgG)*	*Skin-Sensitizing Antibodies (IgE) "Reagins"*
Sedimentation coefficient	19S	7S	8S
Electrophoretic mobility	1—	2	1—
Thermostability	+	+++	—
Sensitivity to 2 mercaptoethanol	+++	—	+++
Agglutination of penicillin-incubated erythrocytes			
In saline	+++	+	(+)
In serum diluent	+++	+++	?
Hemolysis of penicillin-incubated erythrocytes	— to +	—	—
Passive transfer in man (Prausnitz-Kustner)	—	—	+++
Passive cutaneous anaphylaxis in guinea pigs	—	++	—
Specificity	Penicilloyl Other minor determinants?	Penicilloyl Other minor determinants?	Penicilloyl Penicillin Penicilloate and other determinants
Pathologic role	Some exanthems	Blocking antibodies Hemolytic anemia	Anaphylaxis Urticaria

[*]From DeWeck, A.: Drug reactions. *In* Samter, M.: Immunological Diseases. Boston, Little Brown, 1971.

tration of penicillin and their biologic and pathologic properties.)

It is quite likely that the findings with penicillin allergy will ultimately be applied to other drugs, when suitable conjugates for detection of antibodies and proper identification of the responsible antigenic determinants are established. The importance of delayed type hypersensitivity in clinical drug reactions is becoming more apparent. Drug fever and maculopapular exanthems seen in severe drug reactions may be an expression of delayed type hypersensitivity, although IgM has also been incriminated. The development of suitable test reagents and of methods of investigation for sensitized lymphocytes in vitro will probably bring new insights in the near future.

TESTING FOR DRUG SENSITIVITY

Sensitization Tests

There are no reliable sensitization tests which can infallibly predict the occurrence of the "immediate" type of reaction to a non-protein drug, nor is it safe to perform intracutaneous tests with suspected drugs, as this may sometimes cause severe and even fatal reactions. Sensitization tests include skin tests such as the scratch test, intracutaneous tests, and ophthalmic and nasal tests. The scratch test is safer but less reliable than the intracutaneous test (see below). It is not always possible to determine by skin testing, either by the scratch or by the intracutaneous test, whether the purpura or the dermatitis which the patient presents is due to a given drug. Only in exceptional instances, such as in true eczematous and occasionally in true urticarial drug eruptions, will the appropriate skin test prove valuable.

TESTS FOR PENICILLIN SENSITIVITY. *Skin Tests.* Aqueous dilutions of penicillin may be employed because they are helpful in scratch or intracutaneous testing and provide presumptive evidence of the presence of skin-sensitizing antibodies against penicillin. Positive reactions generally imply that the patient is actually allergic to penicillin. Potassium benzyl-

penicillin is an excellent antigenic substance to be employed for such tests. However, a positive skin test in itself does not indicate absolutely that the patient will develop a systemic reaction upon receiving penicillin, and a negative skin test does not mean that penicillin may be administered safely. The possibility that routine skin testing with penicillin may itself lead to sensitization must be mentioned. High aqueous dilutions are employed for skin tests. Thus, as a rule, one begins with the scratch test, employing a solution containing 100 units of penicillin per ml. The concentration of the drug is increased up to 5000 units per ml. In cases in which there is a history of a positive systemic reaction, one does not carry on the skin tests.

Penicilloyl-Polylysine (PPL) Test (Lentz and Nicholas, 1970). Conjugates consisting of penicilloyl groups coupled with amino groups of polylysine have been prepared in vitro. The penicilloyl group is a degradation product of penicillin. It is probably the most important antigenic determinant in penicillin allergy. The penicilloyl-polylysine (PPL) skin test has been used extensively and is accepted by many as a valid indication of penicillin sensitivity. However, patients who have positive skin reactions on being tested with penicilloyl-polylysine do not always show clinical systemic reactions upon receiving penicillin injections.

Hemagglutination Test (Ackroyd and Rook, 1968). Sensitization to penicillin may induce the formation of skin-sensitizing antibodies detectable by the passive hemagglutination technique. Hemagglutination (HA) tests are carried out with red cells that have been covered with benzylpenicillin or benzylpenicillinic acid and then exposed to dilutions of serum from a patient suspected of being allergic to penicillin. The hemagglutinating antibodies (HA) which may be found in some patients against benzylpenicillin belong to the 19S as well as 7S gamma globulins, the 19S being more frequent. There is some correlation, although it is not absolute, between the positive serum hemagglutination reactions and skin sensitivity to PPL. There is no universally satisfactory and accepted test today which may be used by the physician to predict which patients are allergic to penicillin. The indirect modified hemagglutination test using labeled sheep red blood cells has also been used to show antibodies against salicylate in aspirin-sensitive patients (Girard et al., 1969/70).

Histamine Release Test. Another test (suggested by Shelley and Comaish, 1965) for the determination of penicillin allergy consists of detection of the amount of histamine released from blood platelets of the rabbit as a result of the interaction of antibody in freshly drawn serum obtained from penicillin-sensitive individuals with the antigen which in this case is penicillin G used in various dilutions.

Basophil Degranulation Test (Shelley, 1963). Histamine is thought to be released from tissue mast cells and from the basophils in the blood as a result of a reaction involving antibody and the drug to which the patient is sensitive. These tests attempt to demonstrate the loss of granules from the basophils during this reaction (Kirshbaum et al., 1967).

The basophil degranulation test is usually negative if the patient's serum is withdrawn immediately after the reaction. The basophil test becomes positive several weeks after the reaction. In a similar way, the technique which determines the liberation of histamine from platelets in the rabbit is also more likely to be positive if human serum is withdrawn several weeks after the occurrence of the reaction. The reason for this is not altogether clear, but it is entirely possible that the factors or antibodies which are responsible for the test are depressed or used up by the antigen immediately after its injection. There are both direct and indirect forms of the basophil test, in which loss of granules from reacted basophils are compared with those seen in control preparations. However, the value and clinical application of the basophil degranulation test has not yet been clearly defined. It appears to be most useful in the detection of anaphylactic sensitivity.

OTHER IN VITRO TESTS FOR DRUG SENSITIVITY. Other in vitro tests for drug sensitivity include the red cell agglutination test and the antiglobulin test for hemolytic anemia; platelet agglutination and lysis tests, and inhibition of clot retraction for thrombocytopenic purpura; in

vitro stimulation of peripheral blood lymphocytes; blood counts, since they indicate the presence of drug sensitivity which may affect the formed elements of the blood (for example, eosinophilia); and immunofluorescence studies (Hicks et al., 1970). Unfortunately, most of the above techniques are so specialized and generally unavailable as to be of little practical value in the average clinical setting.

A drug eruption must be considered in a high percentage of all dermatologic patients. It is especially important to rule out this possibility (by history and diagnostic withdrawal of suspected drugs) in the following types of eruption: morbilliform-scarlatiniform, urticarial, vesiculobullous, purpuric, and exfoliative dermatitis, and in the following entities: erythema multiforme, erythema nodosum, and lichen planus.

In taking a history, careful direct and indirect questioning regarding medications must be employed. Repeated attempts must be made on successive visits. A simple question regarding "drugs" is often worthless, since the patient may interpret it in relation to narcotics. Specific questions should be asked concerning vitamins, tonics, proprietaries, special home remedies, even medicated chewing gum or mentholated cigarettes. A second line of approach is to question the patient regarding symptoms such as headache, dysmenorrhea, insomnia, and constipation. Following this, the patient's memory may be jogged regarding pet remedies for these specific complaints. A complete chronologic list of all of the drugs to which the patient has been exposed should be prepared. In this manner some if not the majority of the suspected medications can be excluded as possible causative agents. In addition, any and all drugs which could cross-react with the primary antigenic medication and produce otherwise inexplicable exacerbation of the reaction may be more easily identified.

COURSE AND PROGNOSIS

The extreme variability of the course of drug reactions makes the prognosis difficult in any individual patient. The reactions range from an evanescent morbilliform eruption lasting for a few hours to a protracted lichenoid (for example, post-Atabrine) dermatitis which may persist for many years. Prior to corticosteroid therapy, exfoliative dermatitis (for example, from an arsphenamine compound) frequently persisted for many months, though its beginnings were commonly manifested innocently in the form of slight erythema and pruritus.

Fundamentally the most important consideration is that drug eruptions usually improve promptly upon withdrawal of the drug and rapidly recur upon readministration. Even this rule has exceptions, however; the dermatitis to Atabrine, for example, may show no such correlation, probably because there are cutaneous depots of the drug which are slowly released. Another example is seen in urticaria due to the injection of penicillin, especially the depot-type, slow-release varieties. A supply of penicillin remains for months despite cessation of further therapy. It is significant that only trace amounts, far below those necessary for pharmacologic action, are needed for the intiation and continuance of a drug eruption. In addition, a large segment of the population may be rendered increasingly reactive to a drug by repeated exposure over a period of years. This occurred classically in the case of penicillin. When it was first administered in 1941–42, even the crude, impure forms then available produced only occasional moderate urticaria; in subsequent years penicillin has become capable of producing increasingly severe reactions and even death in some patients.

From the prognostic standpoint, generalized exfoliative dermatitis and widespread bullous eruptions have grave import. Occasionally these types of drug eruption are fatal. The reactions to the heavy metals are often serious and protracted, in part because of the persistence and slow excretion of the drug.

TREATMENT OF DRUG REACTIONS

The anaphylactic and atopic drug reactions must be treated promptly. Whenever possible, emergency treatment should be rendered in a hospital. If the drug was administered in a limb, a tourniquet is placed above the point of injection and 0.3 ml. of epinephrine hydrochloride (1:1000) is given subcutaneously in the other arm or leg. This is repeated every three to five minutes, if necessary. If the reaction is very severe, 0.2 ml. of epinephrine may be given intravenously. An antihistaminic such as chlorpheniramine or diphenhydramine hydrochloride may be given subcutaneously. Prednisone is given intramuscularly or intravenously in a dose of 100 to 300 mg. Corticosteroids may also be administered orally. Shock is controlled by keeping the patient warm and by administering levarterenol (Levophed). Blood or plasma transfusion, oxygen, and positive pressure breathing may be employed. Tracheostomy may be necessary if there are serious difficulties in breathing. Attacks of coughing, wheezing, or asthmatic breathing may be controlled by the intravenous administration of 0.25 to 0.5 gm. of aminophylline (theophylline ethylenediamine). Sedatives are also helpful.

Permanent resolution of a drug eruption is accomplished only by the elimination of the offending drug. With certain exceptions (Atabrine, heavy metals, and halogens), this leads to complete involution and cure in a reasonably short time. If any suspicion of drug eruption exists, prompt discontinuation of all drugs which are not essential to life is important.

Ordinarily, stopping the intake of a drug is followed by its prompt elimination from the skin. At times, however, persistence of the drug eruption is the rule. Arsenical and other heavy metal dermatitides characteristically are persistent. British antilewisite (BAL; 2,3 dimercaptopropanol) developed during World War II may be employed in the treatment of arsenical drug eruptions. It has proved reasonably effective in treatment not only of arsenical, mercurial, and gold eruptions but also of some other heavy metal skin reactions. BAL is administered intramuscularly (in a repository vehicle) in a dosage of 3 mg. per kg. of body weight every four hours the first two days, every six hours the third day, and twice daily for the next 10 days. Local reactions, sometimes with abscess formation, are common after BAL injections. Other chelating agents may be employed for drug eruptions due to other agents, and penicillamine, although allergenic itself, may be useful in mercury poisoning.

A high chloride intake has been recommended in the treatment of bromodermas and iododermas. This should be employed with care. In the treatment of patients with high bromide or iodide serum levels, too vigorous sodium chloride therapy may produce severe toxic psychotic reactions.

Antihistaminics are useful for the relief of itching and for the suppression of urticarial lesions.

Local treatment for drug eruption follows the principles and procedures for topical therapy described elsewhere. Photosensitive patients should wear sun screens and avoid sunlight until their sensitivity subsides.

Supportive Treatment

Symptomatic treatment and good nursing are absolutely essential to the care of patients with severe and extensive drug eruptions, particularly if there is systemic involvement.

CORTICOSTEROIDS. These agents are of considerable value in reducing the inflammatory element in all drug eruptions. They are especially useful in widespread reactions. It should be remembered that corticotropin or prednisone may themselves be responsible for skin changes (acneiform and others).

Severe generalized drug eruptions should be treated initially with a high dosage; for example, 60 to 100 mg. prednisone (or its equivalent in prednisolone, triamcinolone, betamethasone, dexamethasone, or other corticosteroid). As the reaction comes under control, the dose may be decreased rather rapidly; for example, at a rate of 10 to 20 mg. per day. Usually a short course of 10 to 14 days of steroid therapy is sufficient, although at times longer treatment is necessary. The rate at which the offending drug is destroyed and eliminated by the body probably is the chief determinant of the duration of treatment. If the tapering of dosage is adjusted to the clinical response of the patient, there are rarely any rebound phenomena after cessation of treatment. Patients with diffuse exfoliative dermatitis may require a rather extended course of treatment, since in this overwhelming drug reaction recovery is often slow.

Prophylaxis

Drug eruptions will be reduced in number by more rigid legal control of the sale and distribution of certain sensitizing drugs, and by avoidance of indiscriminate use of drugs with a high potential for skin reaction. Drugs known to have a high allergenic potential should be given only for serious indications. The problem will never be completely resolved, however, since new drugs are constantly becoming available, and their reaction potentials are frequently not fully determined until they have been used widely for long periods of time. Patients should always be asked whether they have had previous reactions to drugs suggested for therapy, and certain patients (particularly asthmatics and atopics) should be considered as being especially prone to allergic reactions.

DRUGS MOST COMMONLY PRODUCTIVE OF CUTANEOUS REACTIONS

It is not possible to list here all the drugs used and all the cutaneous changes they have produced. For detailed listings, the reader is referred to the monographic account of Meyler (1964) and to the series on cutaneous side effects of systemic drugs in Dermatologica (1973 et seq.). Noteworthy among currently prescribed medications are the following drugs and their dermatologic reactions.

ALLOPURINOL (ZYLOPRIM). Allopurinol is used for control of hyperuricemia and is associated with skin disorders in 5 to 10 per cent of patients. Eruptions from this drug include a generalized erythematous, maculopapular dermatitis which in some instances progresses to a severe diffuse, exfoliative dermatitis. Usually there are no bullae. Marked systemic reactions have been described, including high fever, eosinophilia, renal insufficiency, and other signs of nephropathy (Mills, 1971). Alopecia and icthyosis secondary to administration of allopurinol (Auerbach and Orentrich, 1968) as well as toxic epidermal necrolysis (Kantor, 1970) have also been reported. Other organ involvement that may occur includes bone marrow depression, retinal (macular) lesions, and systemic allergic vasculitis.

ANALGESICS, ANTIPYRETICS. The salicylates, codeine, Demerol, and morphine may produce any of the common lesions (maculopapular, urticarial, bullous, pruritic; Fig. 7–4). Antipyrine, amino-

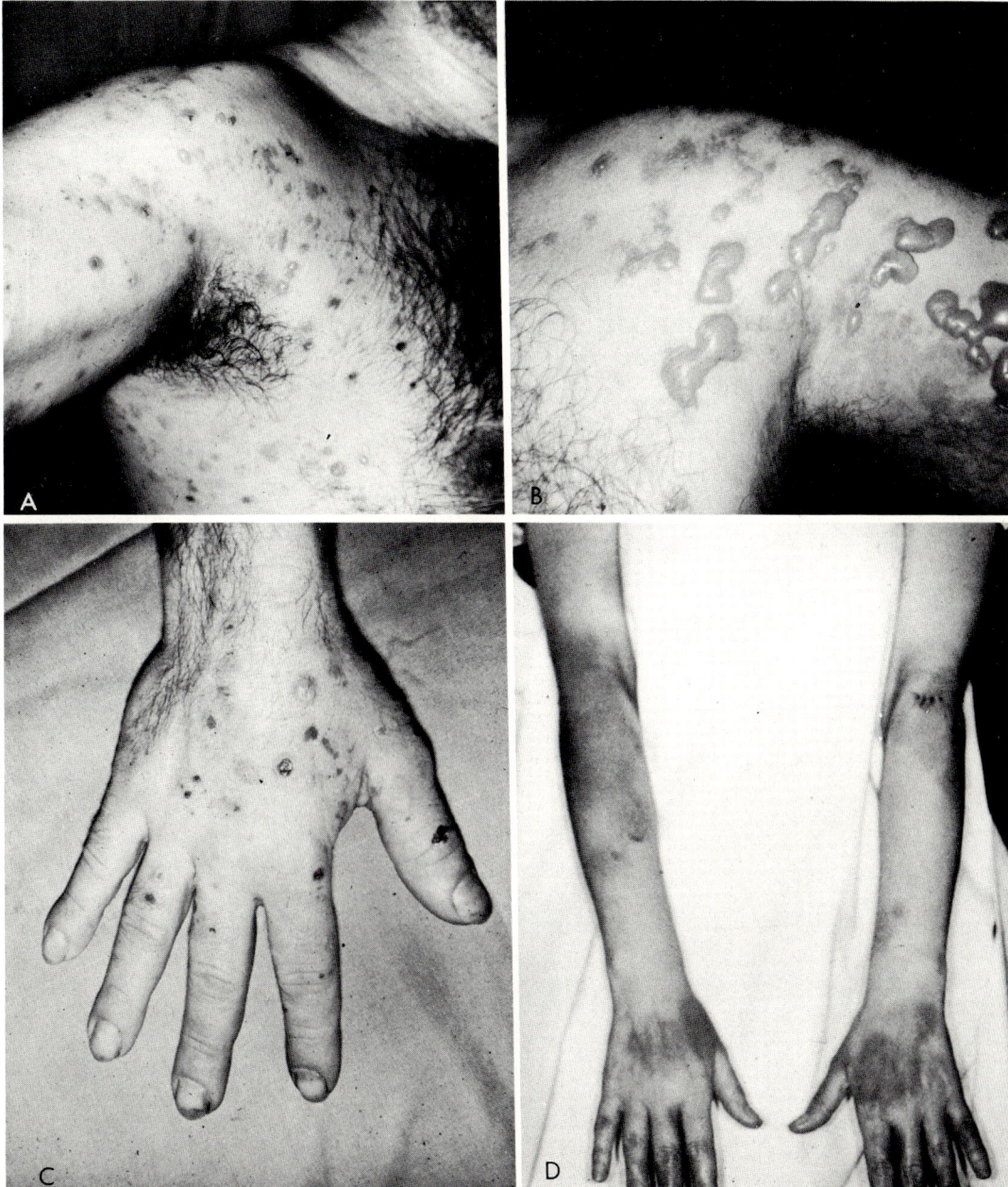

Figure 7–4 *A* and *B*, Bullous erythema multiforme due to aspirin. *C*, Erythema multiforme due to aspirin. *D*, Fixed drug eruption due to aspirin. (From Criep, L. H.: Dermatologic Allergy, Philadelphia, W. B. Saunders Co., 1967.)

pyrine, and phenacetin may show a similar pattern of cutaneous reaction. Antipyrine was the first drug to have been demonstrated as being responsible for the fixed drug eruption (Brocq, 1894). Acetaminophen rarely produces drug reactions but may on occasion cause methemoglobinemia, pruritic maculopapular eruptions, and urticaria; at least one instance of an apparent fixed drug eruption has been recorded (Henriques, 1970). While acetaminophen is probably the safest of the presently available substitutes for aspirin, it is by no means free of toxic and hypersensitivity reactions. A marked upsurge in its usage may be expected to increase the frequency of these reactions.

ANTIBIOTICS AND OTHER ANTIBACTERIAL COMPOUNDS. This group currently accounts for a major share of all dermatitis medicamentosa. Moreover, the penicillins, which are derived from 6-aminopenicillanic acid, are conspicuous among the antibiotics as a cause of drug eruptions. These include benzylpenicillin, methicillin, cloxacillin, flucloxacillin, ampicillin, and carbenicillin; all exhibit crosshypersensitivity (Levantine, 1972).

Prolonged therapy with a high total dose increases the incidence of hypersensitivity reactions. Parenteral administration is more apt to cause allergic reactions than oral ingestion. These reactions appear to be more frequent in patients with an active dermatophyte infection and trichophyton sensitivity, and atopic individuals are more susceptible to anaphylactic reactions. Patients may have unknowing contact with penicillin through contaminated food and syringes. Urticarial and morbilliform eruptions are the most common cutaneous manifestations of penicillin sensitivity (Figs. 7–5 and 7–6). The urticaria may be independent of or part of the anaphylactic reaction or serum sickness syndrome. Other clinical expressions seen are non-thrombocytopenic purpura, scarlatiniform, and fixed drug (which tend to be bullous) eruptions, pruritus ani, erythema nodosum, exfoliative dermatitis, erythema multiforme, systemic lupus erythematosus–like syndrome, polyarteritis nodosa, and toxic epidermal necrolysis.

Ampicillin. Levantine, 1972; Bronsert, 1971; Crow, 1970). Ampicillin is the most widely used of the synthetic penicillins.

Two main groups of eruptions occur. One is urticaria which may be associated with angioedema, serum sickness syndrome, and rarely anaphylaxis; the other group consists of dull red macular or maculopapular eruptions. The mucous membrane, particularly the palate, may be involved. A significantly high incidence of the latter type of eruptions occurs in patients with infectious mononucleosis. The eruptions are increased also in patients with cytomegalic virus infections, lymphatic leukemia, reticulosarcoma, and in patients with hyperuricemia who are being treated with allopurinol.

Cephalosporins. The cephalosporins are derivatives of 7-aminocephalosporanic acid and cross-react with penicillins. Cephalothin and cephapirin may produce remarkably uniform erythematous, maculopapular, pruritic eruptions primarily on the trunk. The lesions are initially discrete, but become confluent in some persons.

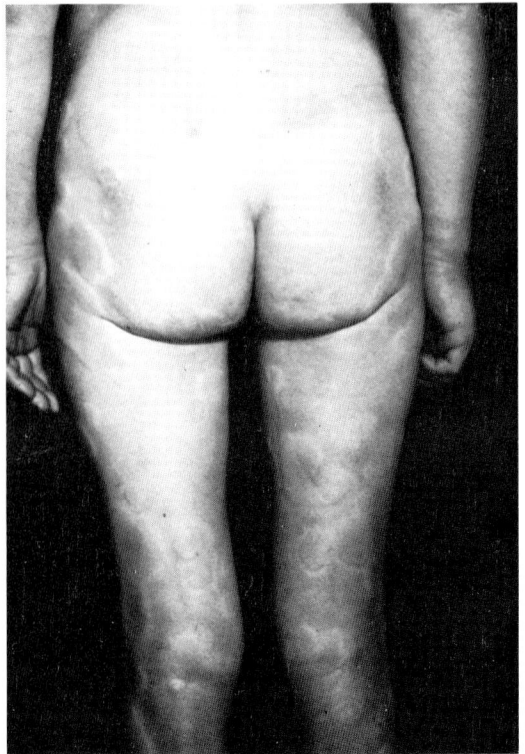

Figure 7–5 Urticaria due to penicillin. (From Criep, L. H.: Dermatologic Allergy. Philadelphia, W. B. Saunders Co., 1967.)

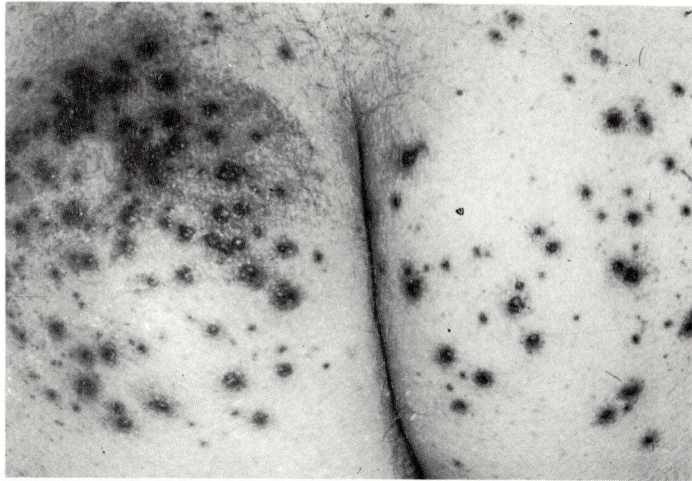

Figure 7–6 Severe allergic dermatitis in penicillin-sensitive patient. This patient had positive skin tests and positive passive transfer tests as well as hemagglutinating antibodies to penicillin. (From Criep, L. H.: Dermatologic Allergy. Philadelphia, W. B. Saunders Co., 1967.)

Although other antibiotics, such as streptomycin, show similar sensitizing potentials, the reactions are not seen as commonly. Stomatitis and pruritus ani and vulvae are concomitants of tetracycline and chloramphenicol therapy. Chloramphenicol (Chloromycetin) may also produce purpura, pellagrous dermatitis, or erythema multiforme. Other reactions may include: photosensitization (light sensitivity eruptions) due to tetracycline derivatives such as demethylchlortetracycline (Declomycin; Frost et al., 1971); discoloration of the teeth (Anthony, 1970) or lupus erythematosus–like syndrome, as well as fixed drug eruptions (Brown, 1974; Csonka et al., 1971); jaundice from novobiocin; black hairy tongue from penicillin; and Loeffler's syndrome, as well as various pruritic lesions, caused by dihydrostreptomycin, para-aminosalicylic acid, and isoniazid used in the therapy of tuberculosis. Photo-onycholysis due to tetracycline hydrochloride (Frank et al., 1971), demethylchlortetracycline, and doxycycline (Vibramycin) has been reported also.

Sulfonamides. The sulfonamides are notable causes of dermatitis medicamentosa (Fluker and Waugh, 1972; Kauppinen, 1972; Lehr, 1972; Fig. 7–7). The milder manifestations include pruritus or a morbilliform eruption. More severe reactions of all types may also be seen, and several unique features may be present. Photosensitization after sulfonamide treatment may occur as a polymorphic light eruption whose severity is determined by the degree of exposure to sunlight. Erythema nodosum may be seen at times during sulfonamide therapy. Sulfonamides are sometimes responsible for the appearance of generalized bullous (pemphigoid) and erythema multiforme–like eruptions, including Stevens-Johnson syndrome. These conditions may have a grave prognosis, and a number of instances of fatal outcome have been observed. Topical application of sulfonamide ointments may induce sensitivity which later becomes apparent on systemic administration. In addition, epidermolysis bullosa, fixed drug and other eruptions from sulfadiazine, photoallergic dermatitis due to the antidiabetic sulfonylureas (Harris, 1971), and other cutaneous reactions including urticaria, Stevens-Johnson syndrome, erythema multiforme, and fatal thrombocytopenic purpura from sulfamethoxypyridazine (Kynex) have been observed.

Cross-sensitization is so common as to make it imperative that patients with a cutaneous reaction to one sulfonamide do not receive another. This cross-sensitization extends further to include procaine (and other local anesthetics), para-aminobenzoic acid and para-aminosalicylic acid, all of which have a similar molecular structure.

ANTICHOLINERGIC AGENTS. Atropine, belladonna, and the synthetic anticholinergic agents (such as Banthine) may be responsible for a variety of cutaneous re-

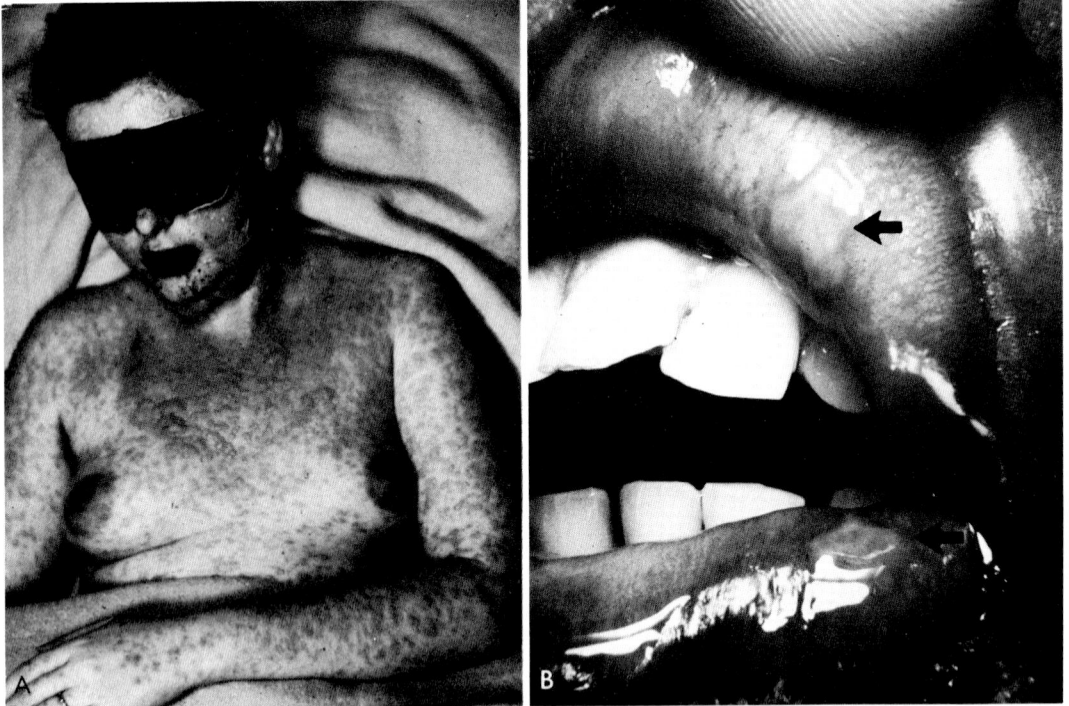

Figure 7–7   *A,* Extensive morbilliform and bullous eruption following sulfonamide therapy. *B,* Erosive lesions of erythema multiforme due to sulfonamide. (From Criep, L. H.: Dermatologic Allergy, Philadelphia, W. B. Saunders Co., 1967.)

actions, including morbilliform, eczematous, and urticarial eruptions.

ANTICOAGULANT DRUGS. Coumadin and Coumarin have produced extensive dermatitis, chiefly morbilliform, as well as local areas of necrosis (Nalbandian, 1970). *Heparin* and synthetic heparinoids cause alopecia of a diffuse type in a significant percentage of people. This is apparently a telogen effluvium and may affect hairs of the scalp, eyebrows, axillae, and pubic regions. It is reversible and requires no treatment other than discontinuance of the heparin. Heparin has also been known to produce morbilliform dermatitis and purpuric reactions. These may be due to impurities in the preparation. Phenindione, a short-acting synthetic anticoagulant similar in action to bishydroxycoumarin (but chemically unrelated) has been reported to cause jaundice, massive edema, and severe morbilliform dermatitis (along with agranulocytosis and other blood-cellular changes, hepatitis, and nephropathy).

ANTICONVULSANTS (Fig. 7–8). The newer antiepileptic drugs have been productive more of constitutional reactions than of cutaneous ones. The well-known diphenylhydantoin (Dilantin) hypertrophy of the gums and pigmentation from such drugs as mephenytoin (Mesantoin) constitute the most common mucocutaneous manifestations. However, more recently, visceral lupus erythematosus has been noted as a side effect of treatment with hydantoin derivatives. A syndrome simulating lymphosarcoma with exfoliative dermatitis has been induced by diphenylhydantoin sodium (Beerman and Wentzel, 1962). Tridione (trimethadione) and diphenylhydantoin occasionally produce a prominent acneiform eruption of the face (Jenkins and Ratner, 1972). An exanthem due to diphenylhydantoin therapy has also been reported (Robinson and Stone, 1970). Prolonged large doses of certain anticonvulsants, especially Dilantin, for mentally retarded patients with a severe seizure disorder may be responsible for a tissue proliferative syndrome characterized by coarsened facies, thickened calvaria, and hyperphosphatasia (Lefebure et al., 1972).

ANTIDIABETIC (ORAL) PREPARATIONS. Oral antidiabetic preparations, such as carbutamide, have been found to produce skin eruptions. These are sulfonamide derivatives having hypoglycemic effects. Carbutamide has yielded its place to tolbutamide (Orinase) which is considered a safer preparation. Tolbutamide is known to cause eczema and macular erythema in about 1 per cent of patients so treated, however, Chlorpropamide (Diabinese), another of the oral hypoglycemic agents, has been reported to be the causal agent of exfoliative dermatitis, eczema, photo-dermatitis, and erythema multiforme–like, erythema nodosum–like, purpuric, and papular eruptions. Photodermatitis and maculopapular eruptions have been reported from the use of phenformin and metformin (Almeyda and Baker, 1970; Harris, 1971).

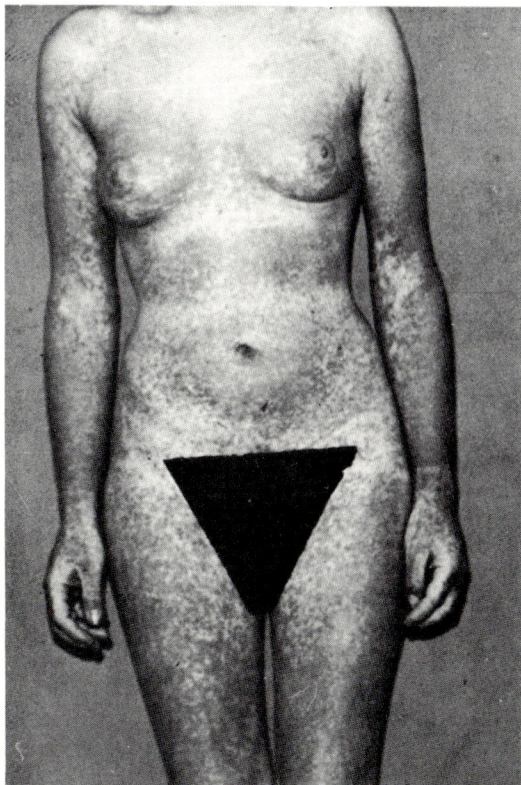

Figure 7–8 Acute dermatitis medicamentosa due to Dilantin. Such reactions to this drug are uncommon.

ANTIHISTAMINICS. Although commonly used in the treatment of drug eruptions, many antihistaminic compounds have themselves occasionally proved to be sensitizers and to produce drug eruptions. Fixed drug eruptions, eczematoid contact dermatitis, and urticaria have been reported to result from their administration.

ANTIMALARIALS. Antimalarials are important therapeutic agents in the management of lupus erythematosus and other conditions (Brown, 1972). A number of interesting sidelights have appeared in this connection (Huriez, 1969). Permanent anhidrotic asthenia, and psoriasis–like and prolonged lichen planus–like dermatitis have followed the development of quinacrine hydrochloride dermatitis. *Quinacrine* (Atabrine), which was administered to millions of persons during World War II, caused a distinctive drug eruption in some individuals, best described as an atypical lichen planus. The individuals affected showed violaceous and erythematous lichenoid plaques, at times associated with eczematous changes. The mucous membrane lesions were typical of lichen planus. Some patients developed generalized exfoliative dermatitis, and a significant number of instances of fatal hepatitis and aplastic anemia were also recorded. The cutaneous lesions may persist for many years after Atabrine ingestion has been terminated. Atrophic changes occur in the skin, and the sweat gland is commonly destroyed. If this latter change is widespread, anhidrosis and marked intolerance to heat results. Jaundice may also be simulated by the action of quinacrine. Malingering attributable to factitially produced "jaundice" by Atabrine ingestion can be uncovered by demonstrating fluorescence of the nails under Wood's light.

Chloroquine (Aralen), another of the expanding antimalarial family, also used in the treatment of photosensitivity and discoid lupus erythematosus, has shown a similar tendency to produce cutaneous reactions, although it does not destroy the sweat glands. Melanosis may be caused by camoquin hydrochloride. Exfoliative dermatitis, decrease in hair color, acute intermittent porphyria and other types of porphyria have also followed chloroquine ingestion. *Quinine* (also found in quinine water, vermouth, and cold tablets) has long been known to cause generalized pruritus as well as morbilliform, scarlatiniform, and vesicular eruptions. In addition, it may stimulate melanocytes, resulting in melanoderma. Soft drinks (for example, Bitter Lemon) containing even small amounts of quinine may also give rise to eruptions in sensitive individuals. Quinine and quinidine have caused hematopoietic as well as cutaneous problems, especially thrombocytopenic purpura. The cutaneous reactions, however, are not the most serious of those arising from the antimalarials, since ocular changes, aplastic anemia, leukopenia, and agranulocytosis have also been recorded. (see Fig. 7–9).

ANTITUBERCULOUS DRUGS. Levantine, 1972). Para-aminosalicylic acid, streptomycin, and isoniazid may produce macular, maculopapular, erythematous, acneiform eruptions, and exfoliative dermatitis. Patients may react to more than one drug of this group. Para-aminosalicyclic acid has been responsible for the development of urticaria and the lupus erythematosus–like syndrome.

APRESOLINE (HYDRALAZINE). Apresoline, an antihypertensive, apparently may sometimes induce systemic lupus erythematosus (L.E.) when used for pro-

longed periods. The skin manifestations are typical of those seen in lupus erythematosus and the diagnostic L.E. cell may even appear in the blood stream. The process may prove to be progressive even though the drug is discontinued. Systemic lupus erythematosus syndrome with its characteristic cutaneous manifestations can also be induced by diphenylhydantoin, isoniazid, procainamide, quinidine, and a number of other drugs (see earlier discussion in this chapter concerning the L. E. cell phenomenon).

ATARACTIC DRUGS. The medical literature is replete with reports of cutaneous reactions caused by the so-called tranquilizing drugs: phenothiazine derivatives such as chlorpromazine (Thorazine) and promazine hydrochloride (Sparine); Rauwolfia alkaloids (Reserpine); substituted propanediols or butanediols (meprobamate); and methaminodiazepoxide (Librium). The manifestations include desquamation of the skin over the fingers; contact dermatitis; lichenoid dermatitis; stomatitis and proctitis; purpuric, maculopapular, vesicular erythematosquamous, and pigmentary eruptions (chlorpromazine); photosensitization (phototoxicity, photo contact allergy, and photo cross-sensitivity); hemorrhage from multiple sites associated with chlorpromazine–induced

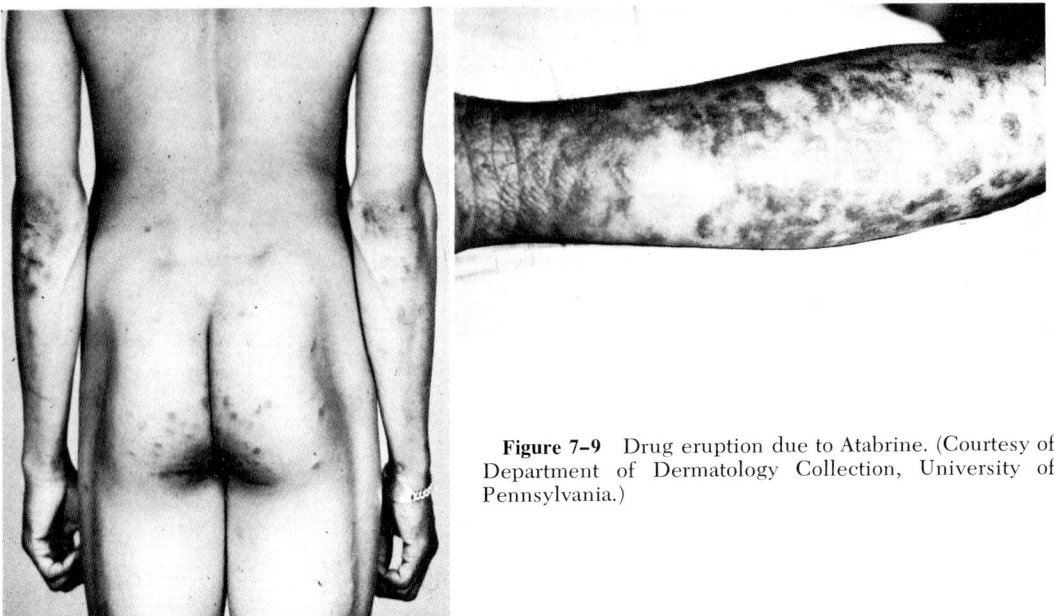

Figure 7–9 Drug eruption due to Atabrine. (Courtesy of Department of Dermatology Collection, University of Pennsylvania.)

jaundice; and nonthrombocytopenic purpura. Other distinctive signs of these reactions are agranulocytosis and abnormal lactation.

BIOLOGICALS. Serum sickness also has a cutaneous complement of morbilliform, scarlatiniform, urticarial, bullous, and purpuric lesions. Crude liver, insulin, estrogens, and heparin injections occasionally produce morbilliform and scarlatiniform eruptions, as well as urticaria and purpura.

BROMSULFOPHTHALEIN. Bromsulfophthalein can be responsible for a generalized severe coalescing morbilliform eruption, and for local necrosis of the skin if there is any escape into the tissue at the site of intravenous injection.

PHENYLBUTAZONE (BUTAZOLIDIN; Almeyda and Baker, 1970b). Phenylbutazone has been responsible for a number of cutaneous and mucocutaneous lesions, including exfoliative dermatitis. Both phenylbutazone and *oxyphenbutazone* have produced a reaction simulating Sjögren's syndrome with salivary gland enlargement, xerostomia, fever, and malaise. Phenylbutazone has also been reported to cause toxic epidermal necrolysis and fatal erythema multiforme, buccal ulceration, and allergic angiitis with ulcerated purpuric lesions. Other eruptions attributed to this drug include lichenoid lesions, erythroderma, acne necrotica, erythema nodosum, and blistering of the extremities, as well as sterile abscesses.

INDOMETHACIN. Indomethacin has been reported to cause pruritus, diffuse erythematous macular eruptions, alopecia, and urticaria. Mouth ulcers, erythema nodosum, thrombocytopenic purpura, allergic vasculitis, corneal deposits, retinal disturbances, periorbital edema, hepatitis and jaundice, ulcerations of the stomach, esophagus, and small bowel, and central nervous system reactions have been observed.

COLCHICINE DERIVATIVES. Alopecia totalis has been noted after diacetyl methylcolchicine therapy of acute gout. Vesicular dermatitis of the hands has also been seen in patients taking colchicine.

CENTRAL NERVOUS SYSTEM DEPRESSANTS. *Barbiturates* have produced nearly every possible skin reaction. Morbilliform, scarlatiniform, eczematous, urticarial, and bullous reactions may be encountered, and occasionally photosensitivity and fixed drug eruptions may be seen. However, the incidence of reactions is relatively low. Bullous skin lesions have been observed in barbiturate overdosage and carbon monoxide poisoning. The underlying pathology may be either edema and necrosis of epidermal cells surrounding the sweat pores or perhaps simply pressure necrosis (Groschel et al., 1970; Mandy and Ackerman, 1970). *Bromodiethylacetylcarbamine* (carbromal-Carbritol) produces a rather distinctive process which is different from bromism. The purpuric eruption appears first on the legs (ankles) and spreads slowly up the limbs to the buttocks and hips; later, if the drug is not withdrawn, it involves the forearms and trunk but the face is spared. Symmetric, reddish brown patches are seen, covered by fine scales on a background of tiny petechial spots and reticulate pigmentation. Itching may be severe on occasion. Resolution occurs slowly after withdrawal of the drug.

CHLORAL HYDRATE. The commonest types of eruptions produced by chloral hydrate are erythema, exanthemas, urticaria, eczematoid dermatitis, hemorrhagic lesions, erythema multiforme, fixed eruptions, ulcerative lesions, and pyoderma-like lesions. *Glutethimide* (Doriden), may cause a nonpurpuric, erythematous, morbilliform eruption.

CONTRACEPTIVES (ORAL) (A.M.A. Council on Drugs, 1970; Baker, 1969; Jelinek, 1970). The most frequent of the cutaneous reactions to oral contraceptives is chloasma (melasma). Irregular brown macules develop slowly on the face within one month to two years after starting therapy; the macules fade more slowly than melasma gravidarum and indeed may be permanent. Women who have had melasma during pregnancy are most susceptible to this reaction. All preparations cause the reaction, but the incidence depends on the total amount of estrogen and progestogen (dose and duration). Acne usually improves during use of the oral contraceptives because of the estrogenic component; however, it may worsen during the initial months, and also on discontinuance of the hormone. Moreover, some women previously free of acne may develop it. An irregular loss of hair can occur during or after the use of oral contraceptives, resembling postpartum telogen effluvium. Hirsutism has been reported occasionally in women who, for unknown reasons, are susceptible to the androgenic effects of some of these preparations. Other cutaneous manifestations possibly related to their use include erythema nodosum, erythema multiforme, hemorrhagic eruptions (purpura), pruritus, genital candidiasis, telangiectasia, and herpes gestationis. An uncommon side effect is the possible development of the lupus erythematosus syndrome. Photosensitization and phototoxicity as well as intermittent porphyria have also been reported with the use of oral contraceptives (Mathison and Haas, 1970).

CYTOSTATIC AGENTS. The cytostatic agents (Levantine and Almeyda, 1974) include: alkylating agents (for example, chlorambucil, cyclophosphamide, Endoxan, and nitrogen mustard), alkaloids (for example, vincristine), antimetabolites (for example, cytosine arabinoside, 5-fluorouracil, 6-mercaptopurine, and methotrexate), antibiotics (for example, bleomycin, daunorubicin, and actinomycin D), and others (for example, hydroxyurea, procarbazine, colchicine, and L-asparaginase). All of these drugs may produce some degree of alopecia of the anagen type interfering with hair growth in the proliferative phase. Microscopic examination of plucked or lost hairs will reveal the proximal arrow-shaped tips characteristic of these arrested anagen hairs. Regrowth of hair usually occurs if the drug is stopped and occasionally if the dose is reduced. A number of these drugs may also produce pigmentation and reactivation of radiation dermatitis (inducing an inflammatory reaction in previously irradiated skin). Any of the cytostatic agents may produce stomatitis, which may or may not be associated with agranulocytosis. Photosensitivity and erythema multiforme–like eruptions have also been reported with some of the cytostatic agents. Morbilliform eruptions and other miscellaneous dermatitides including acneiform eruptions have likewise been ascribed to several of the cytostatic agents. Gynecomastia and cutaneous carcinogenesis have also been noted.

Hyperpigmentation of the nails has been attributed to doxorubicin (adriamycin, an antitumor antibiotic).

DIGITALIS. Digitalis may but rarely induce any of the drug reaction patterns in the skin. Morbilliform, scarlatiniform, eczematous, and purpuric eruptions have been observed.

DIURETICS. *Diuril and HydroDiuril or Esidrix (Chlorothiazide and Hydrochlorothiazide).* Erythematous, papular, and papulovesicular pruritic lesions on the upper and lower extremities, associated with edema of the hands and feet, have been seen following Diuril therapy. Thrombocytopenic purpura, cutaneous allergic vasculitis, and photosensitivity eruptions have also occurred. *Acetazolamide* (Diamox), no longer used to any significant degree as a diuretic but currently used to treat glaucoma, has produced erythema multiforme and thrombocytopenic purpura. (See also the discussion under sulfonamides.)

ERGOTAMINE. Ergotamine, at times used systemically for the relief of pruritus and of migraine, may produce dermatitis, and, if administered in unusually large doses, may result in gangrene.

ESTROGENS. Estrogens administered orally to men being treated for carcinoma of the prostate has induced porphyria cutanea tarda. While the mechanism by which estrogens cause this reaction is not fully understood, it has been postulated that in certain individuals, estrogens activate a particular gene that controls the formation of specific liver enzymes. The resulting enzymatic changes may be responsible for the altered values of uroporphyrins and coproporphyrins in the urine and the symptoms of porphyria cutanea tarda (Stein et al., 1971).

GRISEOFULVIN. Urticarial, morbilliform, petechial, lupus erythematosus–like syndrome, and photosensitivity reactions have so far been observed (Fig. 7–10). There is no evidence to suggest the existence of a common antigenicity or cross-sensitivity in griseofulvin and penicillin, which are chemically dissimilar.

HALOGENS. Halogens still constitute an important source of cutaneous reactions because of their widespread use in many types of proprietary preparations, as well as their use in radiography or as a con-

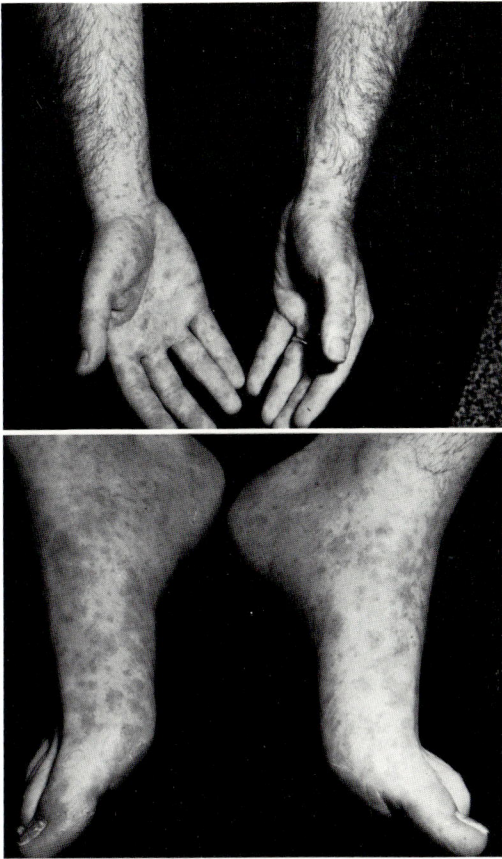

Figure 7-10 Drug eruption due to griseofulvin. (Courtesy of Department of Dermatology Collection, University of Pennsylvania.)

stituent of complex drugs (for example, Banthine). In addition, a certain number of patients with acne vulgaris may experience aggravation of their acne by the ingestion of certain vitamins with minerals, and of some iodine preparations. Iodides may affect infants via the transplacental route. Symptoms of iodism include mucous membrane ulceration, salivary gland swelling, metallic taste, and gastric distress, in addition to skin changes. Bromodermas and iododermas may resemble ordinary acne and are localized about sebaceous glands. The more severe forms may manifest themselves as granulomatous vegetating tumors (Fig. 7-11).

HEAVY METALS AND ARSENICALS. With the phasing out of the organic arsenicals for the treatment of syphilis, the problem of arsenical cutaneous reactions is limited largely to the inorganic arseni-

cals. An occasional patient may develop organic arsenical reaction from such products as vaginal suppositories containing acetarsol. Arsenic is still very rarely used in the form of potassium arsenite (Fowler's solution).

Arsenic and the arsenicals (organic and inorganic) have a notorious capacity to elicit a wide variety of serious skin lesions (Fig. 7-12). The former wide use of trivalent arsenical compounds as antisyphilitic agents produced numerous instances of cutaneous reactions, but these are now very rare. In addition to the morbilliform, eczematous, urticarial, bullous, erythema multiforme, exfoliative dermatitis, and purpuric eruptions, arsenic compounds (for example, Fowler's solution), when given over prolonged periods, may produce keratoses and cancer, both cutaneous and visceral. Toxic hepatitis and cirrhosis have also been reported. Obviously, such compounds should rarely if ever be dispensed.

Gold, currently employed in the treatment of rheumatoid arthritis and formerly used in discoid lupus erythematosus, has a very high sensitization index. In as many as 20 per cent of patients receiving gold therapy, some cutaneous reaction may be expected. The usual morbilliform, eczematous, urticarial, bullous, and purpuric lesions are found (Fig. 7-13). In addition, there may be nonspecific dermatitis and lichen planus–like and pityriasis-like eruptions (Penneys et al., 1974). The bone marrow, liver, and other tissues may also be shock sites.

Bismuth may duplicate these findings, but its sensitizing potential is much lower. Bismuth commonly produces a slate blue line at the gum margin, especially pronounced in patients with poor oral hygiene.

Mercurials have a similar capacity, but in addition have been shown to be responsible for the production of acrodynia or "pink disease." Ammoniated mercury ointment is a common offender in this regard. It is used on infants, who subsequently ingest small amounts of the ointment. Over prolonged periods, this intake of mercury leads to the development of acrodynia.

Thallium, at times unjustifiably used as a depilatory, may be accidentally ingested

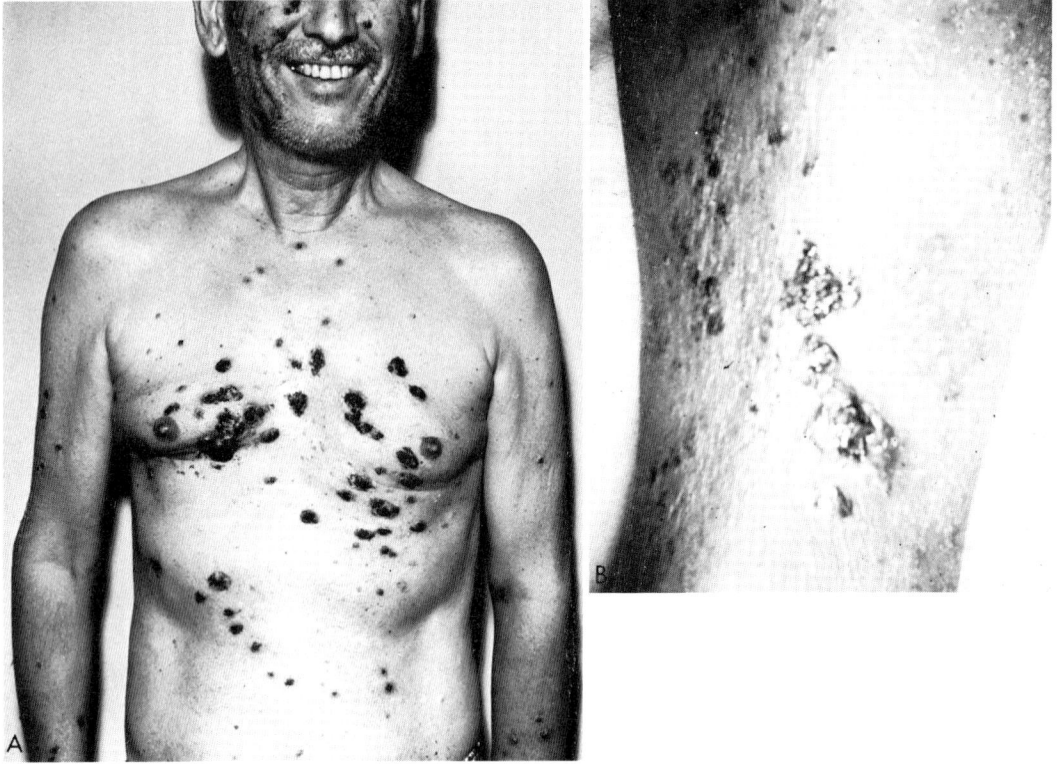

Figure 7–11   *A*, Drug eruption produced by iodides. (Courtesy of Department of Dermatology Collection, University of Pennsylvania.) *B*, Iododerma. (From Criep, L. H.: Dermatologic Allergy. Philadelphia, W. B. Saunders Co., 1967.)

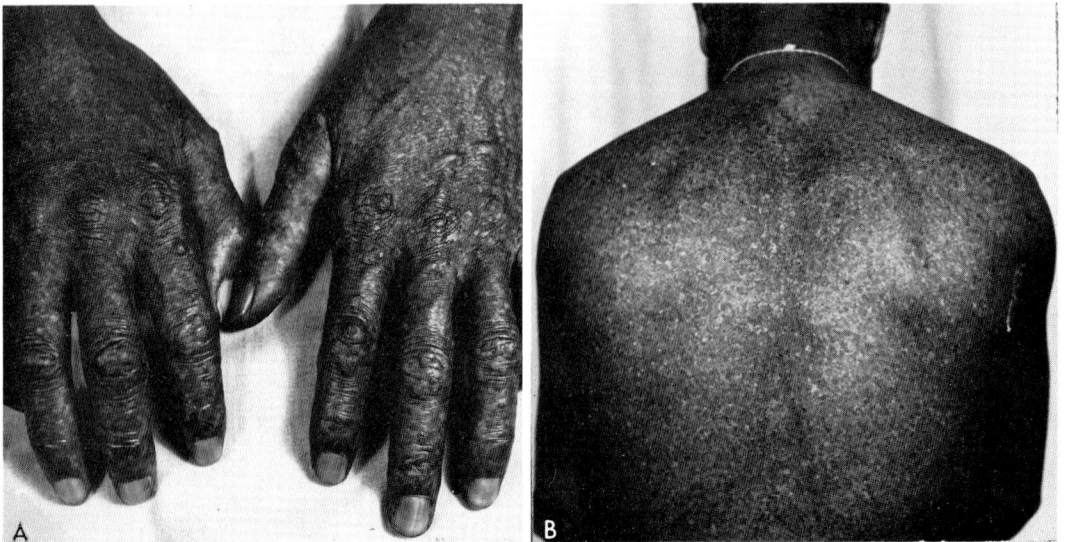

Figure 7–12   *A* and *B*, Keratoses (pre-malignant") and pigmentary changes following prolonged exposure to insecticide containing arsenic.

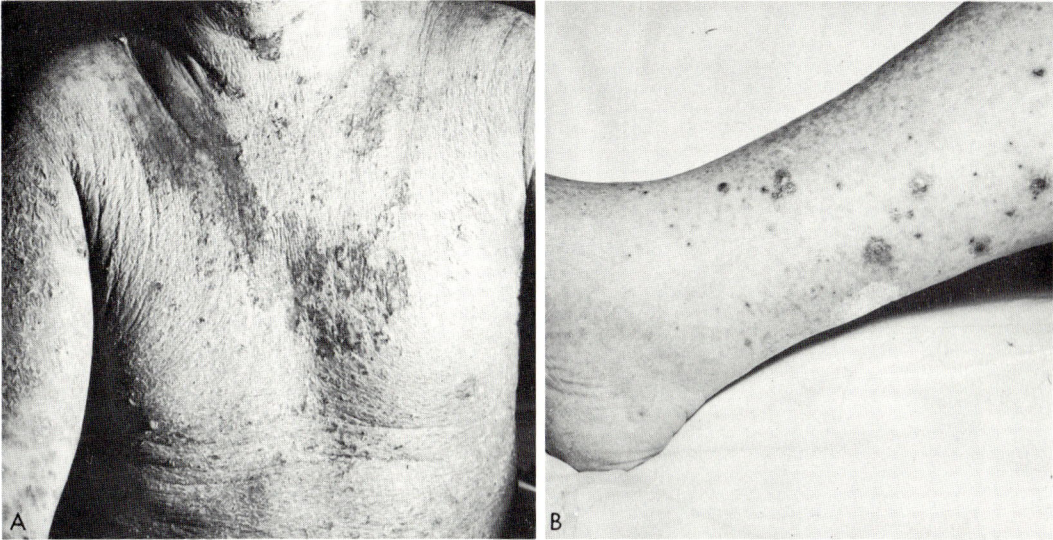

Figure 7–13 *A,* Exfoliative dermatitis due to gold. Prior to corticosteroid therapy, reactions of this severity were occasionally fatal, particularly after arsenical therapy. *B,* Proved sensitivity to "certified dye" in pimento cheese. Such "certification" implies lack of inherent toxicity, but some such compounds may induce sensitization on external use or internal administration.

by children, particularly when it is used as a rodenticide. Ingestion of thallium leads to alopecia and to severe neurologic and hepatic damage.

Silver, formerly a popular prescription in the form of silver nitrate and also silver proteinates (Argyrol), has left a now almost depleted group of patients with permanent, generalized, faintly violaceous, dusky hyperpigmentation (argyria; Fig. 7–14).

Topical silver nitrate, however, in stick form for localized application to suppress granulation tissue or as compresses on limited or extensive skin areas (for example, in the management of burns) apparently has not resulted in the development of argyria.

LAXATIVES. Phenolphthalein is the classic example here. It is present in over 100 proprietary preparations. Tons of it are actually ingested each year in the United States. Characteristically it causes a fixed drug eruption of multiple dusky red plaques. It also produces the usual morbilliform, scarlatiniform, bullous, or purpuric set of lesions. It may rarely cause granulomatous tumors. In view of the very broad use of phenolphthalein,

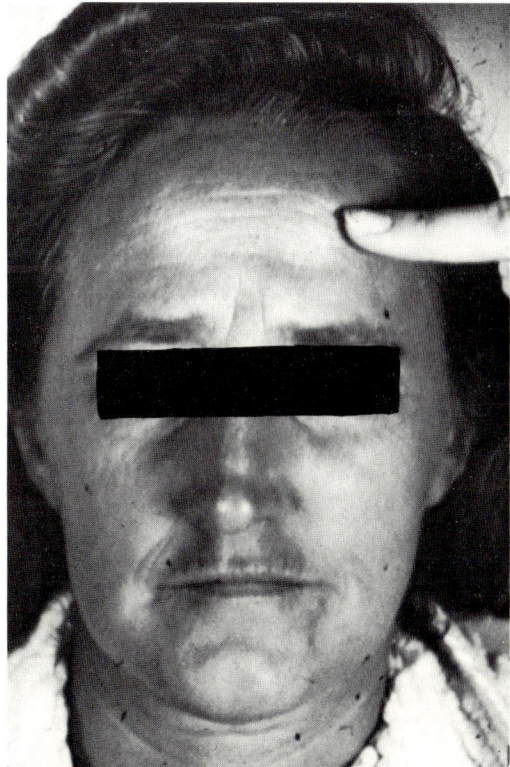

Figure 7–14 Generalized argyria from silver nitrate drops, given for "stomach trouble." (From Criep, L. H.: Dermatologic Allergy. Philadelphia, W. B. Saunders Co., 1967.)

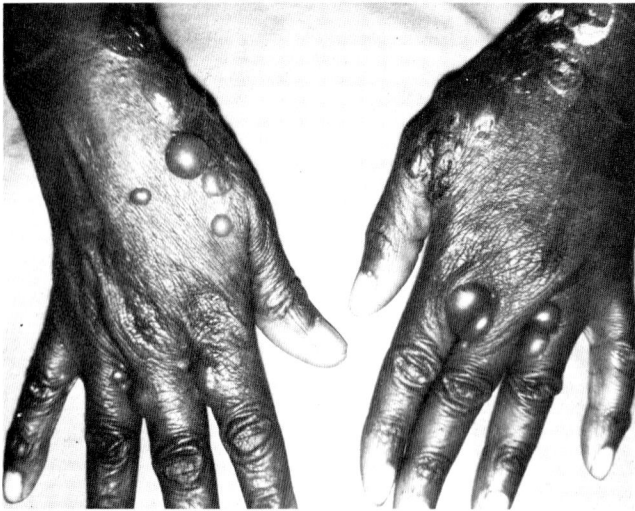

Figure 7-15 Bullous erythema multiforme due to phenolphthalein. (From Criep, L. H.: Dermatologic Allergy. Philadelphia, W. B. Saunders Co., 1967.)

the incidence of cutaneous sensitivity to it is relatively small (Fig. 7–15).

L-DOPA. L-dopa, which is used in the treatment of parkinsonism, may produce sweating, edema, hair loss, pallor, skin eruptions, and bad odor. (F.D.A., 1970). *Amantadine*, also used in the treatment of patients with parkinsonism, may produce livedo reticularis.

LITHIUM. Lithium carbonate, which is used for the treatment of manic-depressive patients, has produced maculopapular eruptions, alopecia, and flushed dry skin. These are reversible effects and the patients recover after the drug is discontinued. Effects in other organ systems are more grave.

METHOTREXATE. Methotrexate, an antimetabolite which has been of some value in the management of certain forms of psoriasis, must be used with extreme caution. Its more common toxic effects include nausea, diarrhea, malaise, fatigue, menstrual irregularities, and hematologic depression. Stomatitis, gingivitis, ulcers of the tongue and buccal mucosa, gastrointestinal ulceration, liver and kidney damage, as well as precipitation of diabetes, can also occur, but these entities are rare. Methotrexate has also been reported to have precipitated gout, pneumonitis, and possible chromosomal damage, if used in high dosages.

POLIOMYELITIS VACCINE. The incidence of cutaneous reactions to the Salk poliomyelitis vaccine is small. The cutaneous reactions include urticara and erythema multiforme among others. It is possible that the penicillin formerly found in the vaccine may play a prominent role in the production of the lesions.

SMALLPOX VACCINE (VACCINIA). Cutaneous eruptions may be caused by hypersensitivity to vaccine proteins. The eruptions may develop 9 to 12 days after vaccination and include roseola, vaccinia necrosum, erythema multiforme, and urticaria (Neff and Lane, 1970).

CORTICOSTEROIDS. Although corticosteroids are useful in the treatment of drug eruptions, they are not completely free from cutaneous ill effects. Cutaneous complications in patients treated with steroids include hyperpigmentation, acneiform eruptions, hirsutism, moonface, striae atrophicae, and delayed wound healing. These complications may be found with topical as well as systemically administered corticosteroids (Baer and Myrow, 1970).

TEMARIL. The oral antipruritic trimeprazine (Temaril) has caused urticarial lesions and nonspecific cutaneous eruptions. Like other phenothiazines, it may cause photosensitivity reactions and has also been associated with agranulocytosis.

THIOURACIL DERIVATIVES. Hair loss and pigmentation have been seen following the administration of thiouracil and its derivatives, including prophylthiouracil and other thioureas. These drugs may also induce a wide variety of non-distinctive eruptions.

MISCELLANEOUS DRUGS. *Antabuse* (tetraethylthiuram disulfide), used in treating alcoholism, has been reported to produce occasional skin reactions, primarily a fixed drug eruption.

A necrotizing angiitis indistinguishable from periarteritis nodosa has been found to occur in some drug addicts who have used *metamphetamine* alone or in combination with heroin or D-lysergic acid diethylamide.

Adverse cutaneous reactions to *insulin* have also been reported. Since insulin is a typical protein it may occasionally act as an antigen. Pruritus and urticaria have been reported most commonly. Spontaneous desensitization to local allergic reactions is frequent in diabetics using insulin and often no additional treatment is needed (Almeyda and Baker, 1970a).

REFERENCES

Ackroyd, J. F.: Thrombocytopenic purpura due to drug hypersensitivity. *In* Rosenheim, M. L., and Moulton, R., (eds.): Sensitivity Reactions to Drugs. Oxford, Blackwell, 1958.

Ackroyd, J. F., and Rook, A. J.: Gell, P. G. H., and Coombs, R. R. A., (eds.): *In* Clinical Aspects of Immunology. 2nd ed. Oxford, Blackwell, 1968.

Alarcon-Segovia, D.: Drug induced lupus syndromes. Mayo Clin. Proc. 44:664, 1969.

Alkalay, I., and Bullard, J. C.: Systemic lupus erythematosus following prolonged treatment with hydralazine. Ann. Allergy 29:35, 1971.

Almeyda, J., and Baker, H.: Adverse cutaneous reactions to hypoglycemic agents. Br. J. Dermatol. 82:634, 1970a.

Almeyda, J., and Baker, H.: Cutaneous reactions to anti-rheumatic drugs. Br. J. Dermatol. 83:707, 1970b.

A.M.A. Council on Drugs: Oral contraceptives. J.A.M.A. 214:2316, 1970.

Anthony, J. R.: Effect on deciduous and permanent teeth of tetracycline deposition in utero. Postgrad. Med. 48:165, 1970.

Arthritis Foundation: Bulletin on the Rheumatic Diseases 20:604, 1970.

Auerbach, R., and Orentrich, N.: Alopecia and ichthyosis secondary to allopurinol. Arch. Dermatol. 98:104, 1968.

Baer, R. L., and Harber, L. C.: Photosensitivity to drugs. Arch. Dermatol. 83:7, 1961.

Baer, R. L., and Myrow, R.: Complications of topical corticosteroid therapy. Arch. Bel. Derm. Syph. I XXVI:129, 1970.

Baker, H.: Adverse cutaneous reaction to oral contraceptives. Br. J. Dermatol. 81:946, 1969.

Bean, S. F.: Acneiform eruption from tetracycline. Br. J. Dermatol. 85:585, 1971.

Beerman, H.: Drug eruptions: A survey of recent literature. Am. J. Med. Sci. 218:446, 1949.

Beerman, H., Kirshbaum, B. A., and Criep, L. H.: Adverse drug reactions. *In* Criep, L. H.: Dermatologic Allergy, Philadelphia, W. B. Saunders Co., 1967.

Beerman, H., and Wentzel, H. E.: Exfoliative dermatitis due to Dilantin and lymphoma-like syndrome. Arch. Dermatol. 87:783, 1962.

Bleyer, W. A., Au, W. Y. W., Lange, W. A., Sr., et al.: Studies on the detection of adverse drug reactions in the newborn. J.A.M.A. 213:2046, 1970.

Brocq, L.: Eruption erythemato-pigmentée fixé due à l'Antipyrine. Ann. Dermatol. Syph. 5:308, 1894.

Bronsert, U.: Exantheme bei Ampicillin therapie. Med. Klin. 66:352, 1971.

Brown, R. K.: Discoid lupus erythematosus. Arch. Dermatol. 105:768, 1972.

Cohen, L. K.: Isoniazid-induced acne and pellagra. Arch. Dermatol. 109:377, 1974.

Coombs, R. R. A.: Fundamental concepts on allergic reactions to drugs. Br. J. Dermatol. 81:2, 1969.

Crow, K. D.: Ampicillin eruptions. Trans. St. John's Hosp. Dermatol. Soc. 56:35, 1970.

Delaney, T. J.: Tetracycline-induced fixed drug eruptions. Br. J. Dermatol. 83:357, 1970.

DeWeck, A. L.: Drug reactions. *In* Samter, M., (ed.): Immunological Diseases. Boston, Little Brown, 1972.

F.D.A.: Current Drug Information—Levodopa. Ann. Intern. Med. 73:445, 1970.

Fellner, M. J., and Baer, R. L.: Cutaneous reactions from drugs. Med. Clin. North Am. 49:711, 1965.

Fluker, J. L., and Waugh, M. A.: Fixed drug eruption due to sulphamethoxydiazine. Trans. St. Johns Hosp. Dermatol. Soc. 58:59, 1972.

Frank, S. B., Cohen, H. J., and Minkin, W.: Photo-onycholysis due to tetracycline hydrochloride and doxycycline. Arch. Dermatol. 103:520, 1971.

Frost, P., Weinstein, G. D., and Gomez, E. C.: Methacycline and demeclocycline in relation to sunlight. J.A.M.A. 216:326, 1971.

Gell, P. G. H., and Coombs, R. R. A.: Clinical Aspects of Immunology. Philadelphia, F. A. Davis Co., 1963.

Girard, J. P., Hildebrandt, F., and Favre, H.: Hypersensitivity to aspirin: Clinical and immunological studies. Helv. Med. Acta 35:86, 1969/70.

Grishman, E., and Churg, J.: Ultrastructure of dermal lesions in systemic lupus erythematosus. Lab. Invest. 22:189, 1970.

Groschel, D., Gerstein, A. R., and Rosenbaum, J. M.: Skin lesions as a diagnostic aid in barbiturate poisoning. N. Engl. J. Med. 283:409, 1970.

Guss, Stephen B.: Cutaneous manifestations of procainamide-lupus syndrome. Cutis 6:869, 1970.

Harber, L. C., and Bear, R. L.: Pathogenic mechanisms of drug induced photosensitivity. J. Invest. Dermatol. 58:327, 1972.

Harris, E. L.: Adverse reactions to oral antidiabetic agents. Br. Med. J. 3:29, 1971.

Henriques, C. C.: Acetaminophen sensitivity and fixed dermatitis. J.A.M.A. 214:2336, 1970.

Hicks, E. J., Long, K. R., Nordschow, C. D., et al.: Immunofluorescence studies in penicillin hypersensitivity. Int. Arch. Allergy Appl. Immunol. 37:495, 1970.

Huriez, C.: Conséquences sur la santé publique de l'évolution des affections vénériennes et cutanées durant le dernier quart de siède. Bull. Acad. Nat. Med. (Paris) *153*:396, 1969.

Hurley, H. J.: Personal communication, 1974.

Jelinek, J. E.: Cutaneous side effects of oral contraceptives. Arch. Dermatol. *101*:181, 1970.

Jenkins, R. B., and Ratner, A. C.: Diphenylhydantoin and acne. N. Engl. J. Med. *287*:148, 1972.

Kantor, G. L.: Toxic epidermal necrolysis azotemia, and death after allopurinol therapy. J.A.M.A. *212*:478, 1970.

Kirshbaum, B. A., and Beerman, H.: Photosensitization due to drugs. Am. J. Med. Sci. *248*:445, 1964.

Kirshbaum, B. A., Cohen, H. B., Beerman, H. et al.: The basophil degranulation test—A review of the literature. Am. J. Med. Sci. *253*:4, 1967.

Kirshbaum, B. A., Beerman, H., and Stahl, E. B.: Drug eruptions: A review of some of the literature. Am. J. Med. Sci. *240*:512, 1970.

Korbitz, B. D., Ramirez, G., Mackman, S., et al.: Coumarin induced skin necrosis in a sixteen year old girl. Am. J. Cardiol. *24*:420, 1969.

LaDu, B. N., Jr.: Pharmacogenetics: Defective enzymes in relation to reactions to drugs. Ann. Rev. Med. *23*:453, 1972.

Lefebure, E. B., Haining, R. G., and Labbe, R. F.: Coarse facies, calvarial thickening and hyperphosphatasia associated with long-term anticonvulsant therapy. N. Engl. J. Med. 286:1301, 1972.

Lehr, D.: Sulfonamide vasculitis. J. Clin. Pharmacol. *12*:5, 181, 1972.

Lentz, J. W., and Nicholas, L.: Penicilloyl-polylysine intradermal testing for penicillin hypersensitivity. Br. J. Vener. Dis. *46*:457, 1970.

Levantine, A.: Drug reactions: Adverse cutaneous reactions to the penicillins-ampicillin rashes. Br. J. Dermatol. *86*:293, 1972.

Levanthine, A., and Almeyda, J.: Cutaneous reactions to cytostatic agents. Br. J. Dermatol. *90*:239, 1974.

Lyell, A.: Toxic epidermal necrolysis: Eruption resembling scalding of skin. Br. J. Dermatol. *68*:355, 1956.

Mandy, S., and Ackerman, A. B.: Characteristic traumatic skin lesions in drug-induced coma. J.A.M.A. *213*:253, 1970.

Mathison, I. W., and Haas, K. L.: Light and photosensitivities observed during oral contraceptive therapy. Obstet. Gynecol. Survey *25*:389, 1970.

Meyler, L.: Side Effects of Drugs as Reported in the Medical Literature of the World. Fourth ed. Amsterdam, Excerpta Medica Foundation, 1964.

Mills, R. M.: Severe hypersensitivity reactions associated with allopurinol. J.A.M.A. *216*:799, 1971.

Nalbandian, R. M.: Skin necrosis induced by coumarin congeners. J.A.M.A. *211*:1169, 1970.

Neff, J. M., and Lane, J. M.: Vaccinia necrosum following smallpox vaccination for chronic herpetic ulcers. J.A.M.A. *213*:123, 1970.

Oates, R. K., and Tongue, R. E.: Phenytoin and the pseudolymphoma syndrome. Med. J. Austl. 2:371, 1971.

Penneys, N. S., Ackerman, A. B., and Gottlieb, N. L.: Gold dermatitis. Arch. Dermatol. *109*:372, 1974.

Pratt, C. B., and Shanks, E. C.: Hyperpigmentation of nails from Doxorubicin. Letter. J.A.M.A. *228*(4):460, 1974.

Robinson, A. M., and Stone, J. H.: Exanthem due to diphenylhydantoin therapy. Arch. Dermatol. *101*:462, 1970.

Rook, A., and Rowell, N. R.: Drug reactions. *In* Rook, A., Wilkinson, D. S., and Ebling, F. J. G., (eds.): Textbook of Dermatology. Oxford, Blackwell, 1968.

Sanders, W. E., Jr., Johnson, J. E., and Taggart, J. G.: Adverse reactions to cephalothin and cephapirin: Uniform occurrence on prolonged intravenous administration of high doses. N. Engl. J. Med. *290*:424, 1974.

Savin, J. A.: Current causes of fixed drug eruptions. Br. J. Dermatol. *83*:546, 1970.

Shelley, W. B.: Indirect basophil degranulation test for allergy to penicillin and other drugs. J.A.M.A. *184*:171, 1963.

Shelley, W. B., and Comaish, J. S.: New test for penicillin allergy—Fluorometric Assay of Histamine Release. J.A.M.A. *192*:36, 1965.

Stein, K. M., Raque, C. J., Zeigerman, J. H., et al.: Porphyria cutanea tarda induced by natural estrogens. A case report. Obstet. Gynecol. 38:755, 1971.

HYPERSENSITIVITY AND MISCELLANEOUS INFLAMMATORY DISORDERS

Samuel L. Moschella

Erythema is caused by the congestion of the small vessels of the dermal papillae and subpapillary plexus, may be localized, diffuse, or generalized, and is most frequently associated with a systemic disease or a drug reaction. It may be transient or persistent. The nature and duration of the lesion depend on the intensity, distribution, and the character of the perivascular inflammatory infiltrate. The responsible mechanisms for the vasodilatation may be intrinsic vessel changes, chemical mediators and drugs, neurogenic factors, and direct vascular injuries. Erythema is a frequent component of cutaneous reactions. Because of the inapparent cause of many of these erythemas, attempts to classify them on the basis of their clinical appearance have resulted in a large number of descriptive names. This confusion is best appreciated in the figurative erythemas which are characterized by fixed or migratory, circinate, arcuate, and polycyclical lesions and occur occasionally as a hypersensitivity reaction to infections, drugs, insect bites, and neoplasms. However, despite the failure to appreciate an underlying cause in many of these erythemas, some of these conditions have a natural history and a clinical appearance and behavior distinctive enough to warrant consideration as separate entities.

Localized erythema may be transient, as in blushing; may appear as flushing, as in the carcinoid syndrome or mastocytosis; may result from the physical insults of heat, cold, light, or trauma (for example, erythema ab igne); may be caused by such drugs as phenolphthalein, barbiturates, sulfonamides, and others which are responsible particularly for the fixed type; and may be toxic manifestations of the collagen diseases, dermatomyositis, lupus erythematosus, and rheumatoid arthritis.

385

Palmar erythema may occur as an isolated phenomenon in pregnancy, liver disease, and rheumatoid arthritis with or without spider telangiectasis and as part of psoriasis, pityriasis rubra pilaris and genodermatoses. Asymmetrical erythema of the feet associated with hyperhidrosis is seen. Occasionally, localized and diffuse erythema may antedate the appearance of lesions of other diseases such as bullous pemphigoid.

The generalized and diffuse erythematous eruptions are most frequently associated with viral and bacterial infections, drugs and the toxic states of moderate to severe constitutional illness. The exanthemic eruptions of infections are the scarlatiniform type caused by the exotoxin of the hemolytic streptococcus and seen rarely in infectious mononucleosis, the roseolar type of rubella, roseola infantum, secondary syphilis, and the morbilliform type of measles. Among the drugs that can cause similar exanthemic eruptions are allopurinol, anticonvulsants, barbiturates, chlorothiazides, chlorpromazine, meprobamates, novobiocin, para-aminosalicylic acid, penicillin, phenothiazines, phenylbutazone, quinine, streptomycin, sulfones, sulfonamides, tetracyclines, and thiouracil.

ERYTHEMA AB IGNE
(Erythema Caloricum)

Erythema ab igne (erythema caloricum – Finlayson et al., 1966) is an acquired in-flammatory condition produced by the exposure of the skin to moderately intense heat from open fireplaces, heating appliances (Fig. 8–1) or systems, or occupations (cooks, stokers, blacksmiths). On histopathologic examination the papillary blood vessels are dilated and have slight endothelial swelling, an intense perivascular infiltrate is noted, and melanin pigment is present throughout the epidermis in the macrophages and connective tissue. The disease occurs most frequently in women who expose their legs to heating systems for prolonged periods. The eruption, which is not preceded by an acute burn, is characterized by reticulated erythema, checkered pigmentation, and telangiectases (Fig. 8–1). Later, keratoses and even squamous cell carcinoma may develop (Peterkin, 1955). The erythema can fade, but the pigmentation can persist indefinitely.

SYMMETRIC ERYTHEMA OF SOLES (Symmetric Lividity of Soles of Feet)

Symmetric erythema of the soles (Hitch and Hansen, 1938; Hopkins et al., 1948) is a type of localized erythema most frequently seen in sneaker-wearing male athletes and military men of 20 to 30 years of age. They have hyperhidrosis. The onset is acute, and the condition tends to

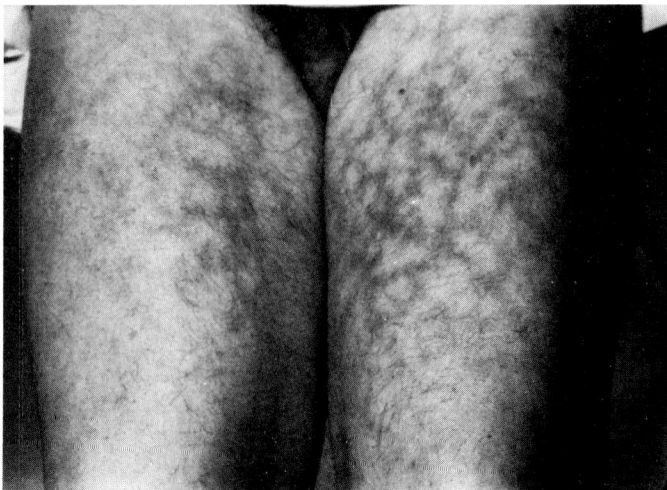

Figure 8–1 Erythema ab igne resulting from frequent prolonged application of a heating pad for chronic polymyalgia of unknown etiology.

be self-limited but recurrent. It involves the entire sole of the foot as well as the adjacent areas, creating a "moccasin" effect. The skin is erythematous with a well-defined border similar to that seen in psoriasis and *Trichophyton rubrum* infection of feet. The central area is soggy and cyanotic. The feet tend to be bromhidrotic, may be painful with or without fissures, and are prone to secondary fungal infection and contact dermatitis. Treatment is palliative and consists of local and systemic measures to reduce sweating which include wearing sandals and absorbent hosiery, the topical application of astringents, such as solutions of formaldehyde and glutaraldehyde, and sedation when necessary.

ERYTHEMA DYSCHROMICUM PERSTANS (Erythema Chromicum, Ashy Dermatosis of Ramirez, Dermatosis Cenicienta)

Erythema dyschromicum perstans is a chronic dermatosis of unknown origin that presents a characteristic localized ashen discoloration of the skin. The eruption was originally described by Ramirez in El Salvador in 1957 and has been reported almost exclusively in Central and North America (Knox et al., 1968; Ramirez). It has been classified as a member of the erythema perstans group (fixed erythemas) and described as a reaction pattern to intestinal parasitism, dermatophytosis, food, auto-immune disease, insect bites, acute rheumatic disease, and cancer (Convit et al., 1961; Stevenson and Miura, 1966). On histopathologic examination, vacuolization of the basal cell and lower prickle cell layers and a mixed infiltrate of mononuclear cells and melanophages about the blood vessels of the papillary dermis are seen. It affects both sexes between 7 and 63 years of age.

Although the lesions begin as erythematous macules that develop a slate-gray color, they are more frequently seen as localized variably hyperpigmented macules with an erythematous "active" border that may be raised slightly and

palpable. The lesions vary in size from millimeters to many centimeters, tend to coalesce and extend and cover large areas, involve the trunk, face, and limbs, are not symmetrical, and persist. Exacerbations are frequent in previously involved sites. Among the conditions to be considered in the differential diagnosis are local areas of melanosis, such as pinta, leprosy, lichen planus, fixed drug eruption, poikiloderma, and melasma. No effective or recommended therapy is known.

ERYTHEMA MULTIFORME (Herpes Iris, Dermatostomatitis, Erythema Polymorphe, Ectodermosis Pluriorificialis, Stevens-Johnson Syndrome)

Erythema multiforme is an acute and frequently recurrent inflammatory syndrome with skin and mucous membrane lesions and, in the more severe cases, with constitutional symptoms and visceral lesions (Fig. 8-2).

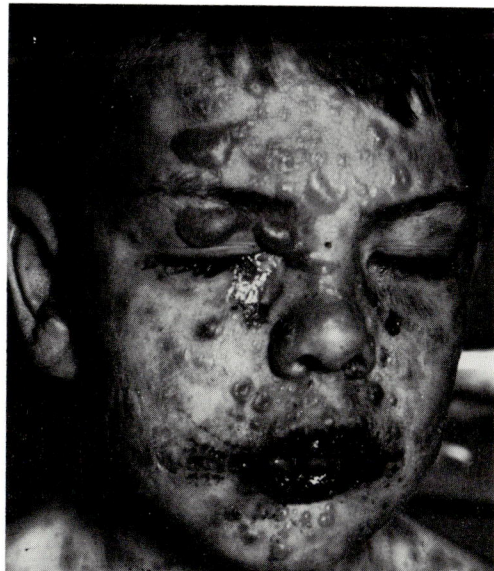

Figure 8–2 Severe case of erythema multiforme with not only cutaneous and mucous membrane lesions but also constitutional signs and symptoms (Stevens-Johnson syndrome).

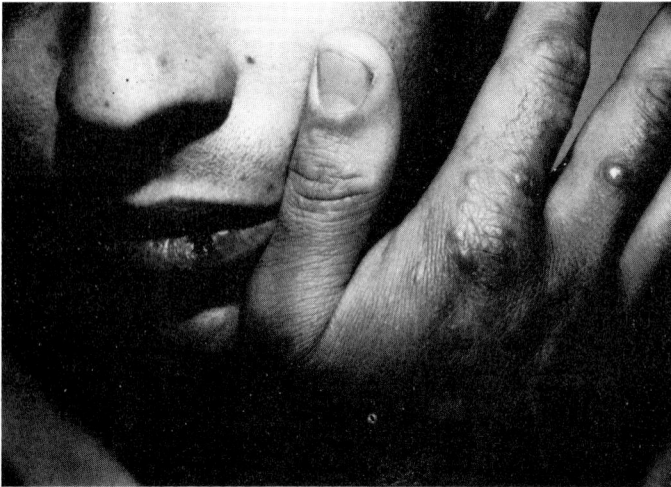

Figure 8–3 Herpes simplex associated with erythema multiforme bullosum.

The etiology is unknown. It appears to be a symptom complex secondary to many diseases and drugs causing the responsible toxic or hypersensitive phenomenon. The reported *causes* or *associated diseases* are as follows:

1. *Viral infections*—herpes simplex (Shelley, 1967, Fig. 8-3), Mycoplasma pneumonia (Eaton agent), vaccination with vaccinia and poliovirus vaccine, psittacosis, lymphogranuloma inguinale, milker's nodes, orf, mumps, Coxsackie B-5, influenza type A, ECHO viruses.

2. *Fungal infections*—histoplasmosis, coccidiomycosis.

3. *Bacterial infections*—typhoid fever, BCG vaccination, leprosy.

4. *Collagen disease*—lupus erythematosus, dermatomyositis, allergic vasculitis, periarteritis nodosa.

5. *Malignancy with or without radiation therapy*—carcinoma, lymphoma.

6. *Contact dermatitis*—poison ivy.

7. *Drug reactions*—penicillin, phenolphthalein, sulfonamides (Fig. 8-4) and related compounds, barbiturates, halogens, salicylates, and hydantoin.

In children and young adults, the eruptions are most frequently associated with infections; in older persons, they are associated with drugs and malignancies. As the techniques of viral isolation and identification, as well as the methods of detection of environmental toxins, are further developed, the number of idiopathic cases will be reduced.

Pathology

The microscopic picture is not diagnostic. The bulla is subepidermal, and a lymphocytic infiltrate is present about the capillaries and venules of the upper dermis. The roof of the blister usually consists of normal epidermis, but severe changes including necrosis may occur. No acantholysis is present. On electron microscopy, the basement membrane remains in the floor of the bulla. The lesion has to be differentiated histopathologically

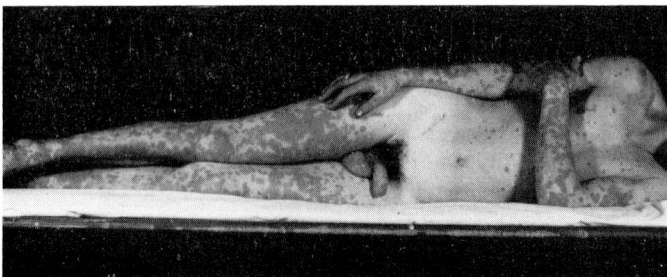

Figure 8–4 Patient with generalized erythema multiforme due to drug (sulfamethoxazole) for urinary infection.

from dermatitis herpetiformis and bullous pemphigoid. In dermatitis herpetiformis, microabscesses containing predominantly eosinophils are demonstrable at the tips of the papillae at the margins of the bullae. In bullous pemphigoid, direct homogeneous immunofluorescence of the basement membrane is seen.

Lesions of the gastrointestinal and respiratory tracts have been described at autopsy (Ashby and Lazar, 1951; Bloom and Lovel, 1964; Finland et al., 1948).

Clinical Manifestations

The clinical spectrum varies from a localized eruption of skin and mucous membranes to a severe fatal multisystem disorder (Keil, 1940). The disease occurs at any age, and the severe bullous forms are most frequently seen in boys and young adults. The disease is most frequently seen in the spring and fall and infrequently in the summer. Groups of cases have appeared during epidemics of atypical pneumonia, adenoviruses, and histoplasmosis. Two basic types of lesions are clinically appreciated: one is macular urticarial and the other is vesiculobullous. The eruption appears suddenly, is symmetrical, and has a predilection for the backs of the hands, palms, soles, extensor surfaces of limbs, and mucous membranes.

The trunk usually becomes involved only after severe involvement of the extremities. The lesions tend to appear in crops for two to three weeks. The individual lesions, which heal in about one week, may cause hypopigmentation or hyperpigmentation without scarring. The characteristic iris (target) lesion is urticarial with a dusky center that may blister and have successive bright red bordering rings (Fig. 8-5 A and B). Careful examination of the lesions may disclose fine petechiae. Fifteen per cent of the recurrent cases have been associated with and attributed to the accompanying herpes simplex.

The vesiculobullous lesions develop centrally in preexistent macules, papules, or wheals and may involve the mucous membranes more than the skin or only the mucous membranes in 25 per cent of the cases. In the plaque lesions, a marginal ring of vesicles may appear. A greater tendency exists for recurrences to occur in the vesiculobullous than in the papular type of eruption.

The Stevens-Johnson syndrome (Bukantz, 1968) is characterized by a sudden onset, a prodrome of 1 to 14 days, and severe mucous membrane as well as visceral involvement. The prodrome can consist of fever, malaise, coryza, cough, sore throat, chest pain, vomiting, diarrhea, myalgias,

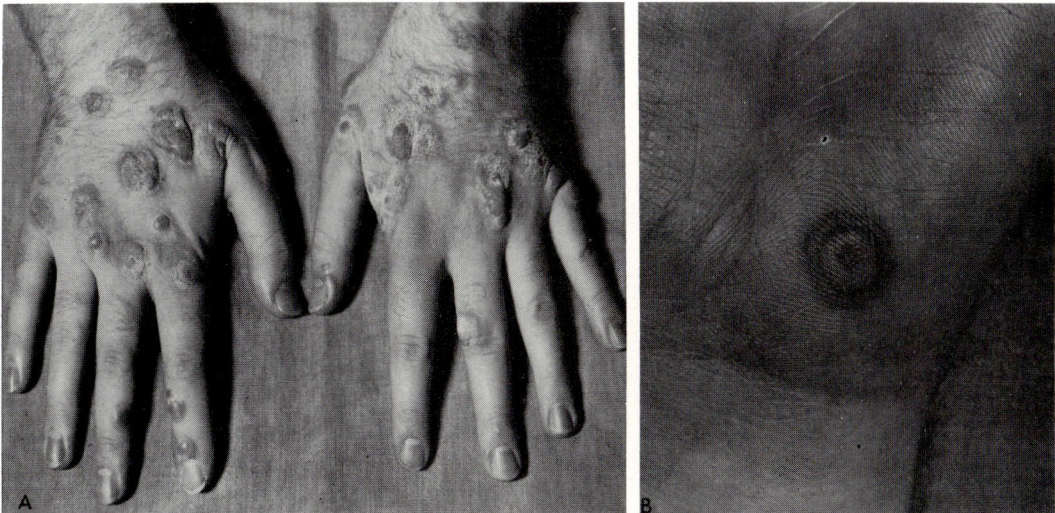

Figure 8-5 *A* and *B*, The classic and diagnostic "iris" lesions of erythema multiforme.

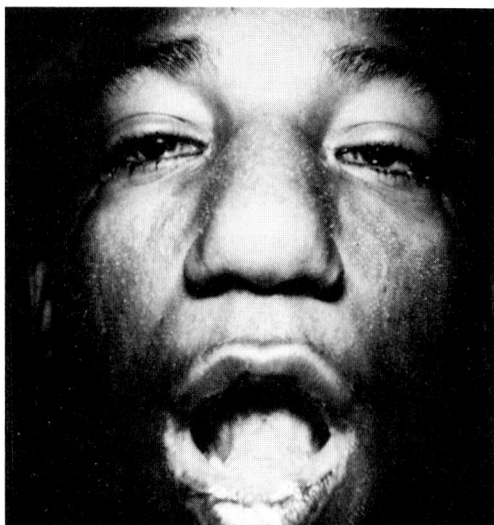

Figure 8–6 Severe mucocutaneous involvement (Stevens-Johnson syndrome) in a youth resulting from an anticonvulsant medication, mephenytoin.

and arthralgias of variable severity. The mucous membranes of the mouth, tongue, lips, eyes, nasal mucosa, genitalia, and rectum become involved (Fig. 8-6). The blisters in the skin rupture, forming erosions or ulcers, and in the mouth characteristically a gray or white pseudomembrane forms. The hemorrhagic crusting of the lips is impressive. The resultant balanitis and vulvovaginitis can lead to adherence of the prepuce to the glans and fibrotic bands or stenosis of the vagina. The eye changes are commonly a severe catarrhal or purulent conjunctivitis, bullae, corneal ulceration, anterior uveitis, and panophthalmitis; blindness or corneal opacities are sequelae. A paronychia and shedding of nails may result. The radiologic changes of the lungs when present are greater than the symptoms. Hematuria, renal tubular necrosis, and progressive renal failure have been reported (Comaish and Kerr, 1961).

Differential Diagnosis

Among the conditions to be considered in a differential diagnosis are the circinate or polycyclic urticarias; the toxic erythemas caused by infectious fevers or drugs; the blood-borne infections of meningococcemia, gonococcemia, and secondary syphilis; the blistering diseases of bullous pemphigoid, herpes gestationis, and pemphigus; the mucocutaneous disorders of Reiter's disease, Behçet's syndrome; the hand, foot, and mouth diseases (Coxsackie A-16, A-5, A-10); and the systemic vasculitides with cutaneous lesions, such as allergic vasculitis, lupus erythematosus, and periarteritis nodosa. Erythema multiforme has been seen in association with instances of toxic epidermal necrolysis and erythema nodosum. Whether herpes gestationis is part of the erythema multiforme syndrome remains to be established; recent immunofluorescent studies reveal basement membrane changes in herpes gestationis similar to those of bullous pemphigoid.

Treatment

The mild cases of erythema multiforme clear spontaneously in two to three weeks. The mortality is 5 to 15 per cent in severe untreated cases. The localized cases require only local and mild symptomatic treatment. The underlying precipitant causes, when appreciated, should be treated. In severe cases, large doses of systemic corticosteroids give symptomatic relief and questionably reduce mortality.

THE FIGURATIVE ERYTHEMAS

Although the figurative erythemas are generally very picturesque and sometimes striking, they are usually not sufficiently clinically distinctive to be considered as separate entities. These erythemas may be annular, arcuate, polycyclic (Fig. 8–7), migratory or fixed, and chronic or recurrent. Because, in all these conditions, a similar etiologic factor, namely, a hypersensitivity reaction to infections, insect bites, drugs, and neoplasms (Summerly, 1964) is occasionally demonstrable, the question is raised whether it is advisable to treat some of these conditions as separate clinical entities. Several figurative erythemas are known that have a clinical pattern, behavior, and etiology that merit the creation of an entity; they are erythema annulare centrifugum, erythema marginatum rheumaticum, erythema chronicum migrans, erythema gyratum perstans, and erythema perstans (Fig. 8–8).

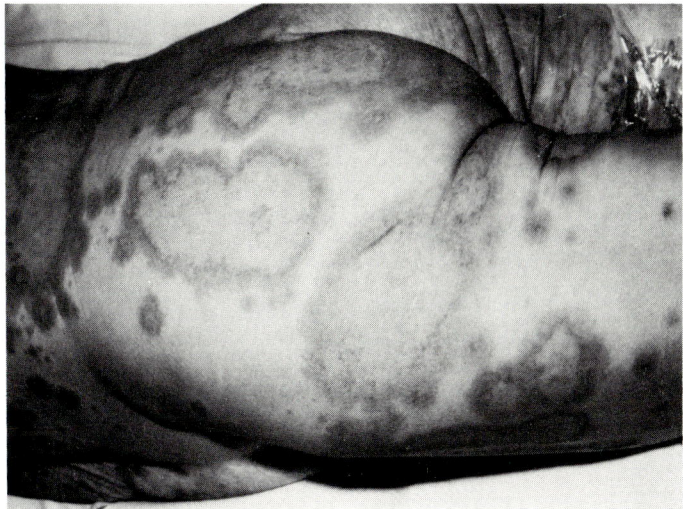

Figure 8–7 Generalized gyrate erythema, etiology undetermined.

ERYTHEMA ANNULARE CENTRIFUGUM (Fig. 8-9)

This title has been used to describe a chronic recurrent migratory erythema that has been reported as a hypersensitivity reaction (Lazar, 1963) to a fungal infection

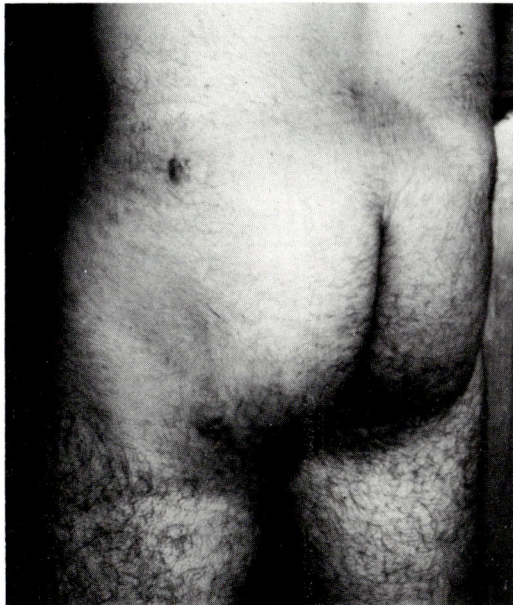

Figure 8–8 Erythema perstans. A persistent, slightly infiltrated erythema in a patient who had episodes of high fever, malaise, myalgia, and hyperhidrosis.

of feet (Fig. 8-10), moniliasis, fungus in blue cheese, blood dyscrasias, neoplasms, and other immunologic disturbances. The cause is rarely uncovered. A familial type (Beare et al., 1966) is to be suspected when it appears soon after birth, during infancy, or in other members of the family. The disorder usually affects young adults and middle-aged persons of either sex.

On histopathologic examination, a dense, coat-sleeve perivascular disposition of lymphocytes and a few eosinophils in the upper and middle dermis are seen; some parakeratosis and spongiosis of the epidermis may be seen.

The lesion presents as a small, pink, infiltrated papule that extends slowly peripherally, forming arcuate lesions with a palpable peripheral scaling border with some central hyperpigmentation; vesiculation rarely occurs. The lesions tend to be multiple but may be solitary and pruritic; they most commonly involve the buttocks, thighs, the upper arms, and, rarely, the face. The lesions usually last a few weeks, occasionally a few days or even months, and may recur for years.

The differential diagnoses are tinea corporis; annular granulomatous lesions such as granuloma annulare, sarcoid, syphilis, and leprosy; lupus erythematosus; lymphoma cutis; herald spot or atypical pityriasis rosea; and a petaloid cutaneous expression of seborrheic dermatitis.

Other migratory, annular, and configur-

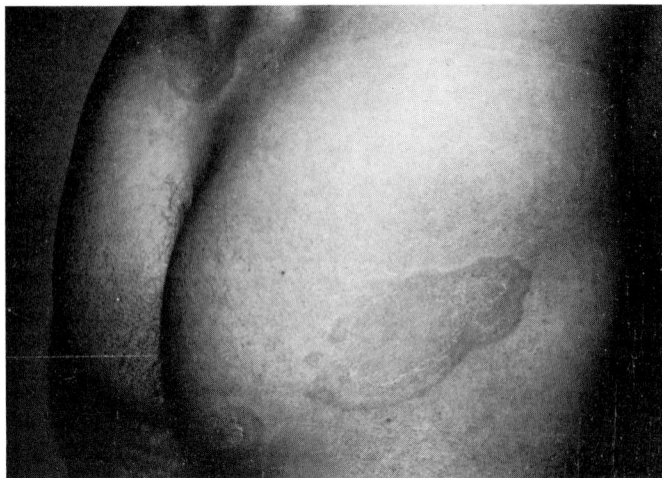

Figure 8–9 Erythema annulare centrifugum has a predilection for the bathing suit area and resembles a dermatophyte infection.

ate erythemas that have a more indurated border and histologically a deeper perivascular infiltration with less, if any, eosinophils have been included under this entity.

ERYTHEMA MARGINATUM RHEUMATICUM

Erythema marginatum rheumaticum (Keil, 1938; Perry, 1937) is a specific distinctive eruption occurring in about 10 per cent of patients with active rheumatic fever. It is usually associated with carditis, follows the onset of joint symptoms, and is seen more frequently in children than in adults. Two cutaneous lesions are seen: flat type (the so-called erythema circinatum or annulare) and a raised type (the so-called erythema marginatum). The lesions, which are ring or arcuate, may remain discrete or enlarge to form polycyclic or reticulate patterns ("chicken-wire"). They tend to appear on the trunk, especially the abdomen, less frequently on the limbs, and rarely on the face and hands. The lesions spread rapidly, are evanescent, fade in a few hours or at most several days, and may recur in crops in different areas for many weeks.

ERYTHEMA CHRONICUM MIGRANS

Erythema chronicum migrans (Flanagan, 1962) is an annular erythema that is caused

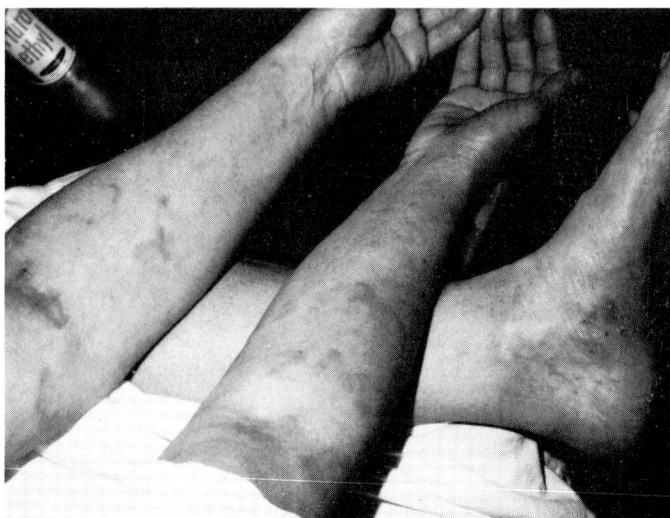

Figure 8–10 Erythema annulare centrifugum associated with recurrent attacks of tinea pedis.

by the bite of a tick and may be associated with regional lymphadenopathy and occasionally a lymphocytic meningitis. It occurs chiefly in northern Europe and rarely in America, affects most commonly children and young adults, and follows the bite of the tick of the family Ixodidae. The cause of the disease has been attributed to the tick bite, Spirochaeta, or more likely a rickettsial infection, since positive microagglutination tests against species of Rickettsia have been demonstrated (Degos et al., 1962). The meningitis is probably the result of a tick-borne virus infection. The eruption usually starts on the leg or an exposed area. The lesion originates about the site of the tick bite which leaves no clinical residua. It appears as an erythematous plaque within several weeks to many months after the initiating insult. The lesion extends peripherally, presents as an erythematous indurated ring of about 1 cm. in width, and can measure about 20 to 30 cm. or more in diameter. Unlike erythema annulare centrifugum, the lesion is solitary, but several lesions may be present as a result of multiple tick bites. The patient may complain of severe itching or burning. The ring fades completely in a few weeks to months. The lesion has to be differentiated from other erythematous annular lesions and erysipeloid of Rosenbach. The lesions usually clear in a few days with systemic penicillin therapy. Tetracycline has been reported as effective (Degos et al., 1962).

ERYTHEMA GYRATUM PERSTANS

This type of erythema (Purdy, 1959; Woerdeman, 1964) is a rare disorder that has been associated with malignant disease of the breast, lung (Fig. 8-11), and other areas. It is characterized by a generalized bizarre festooned pattern resembling the grain in wood and is created by irregular erythematous waves that spread progressively over the body. Removal of the malignancy may reverse the process.

ERYTHEMA PERSTANS

Erythema perstans has been used to describe a persistent erythema that does not develop an annular, circinate, or serpiginous pattern but is histologically similar to the figurative erythemas. The condition has to be differentiated from polymorphous light reaction, lymphocytoma cutis, lupus erythematosus, Jessner's lymphocytic infiltration of the skin, and leukemia cutis.

ERYTHEMA NODOSUM

Erythema nodosum (Blomgren, 1974; Gordon, 1961; Hannuksela, 1971; James, 1961; Michelson, 1958; Versey and Wil-

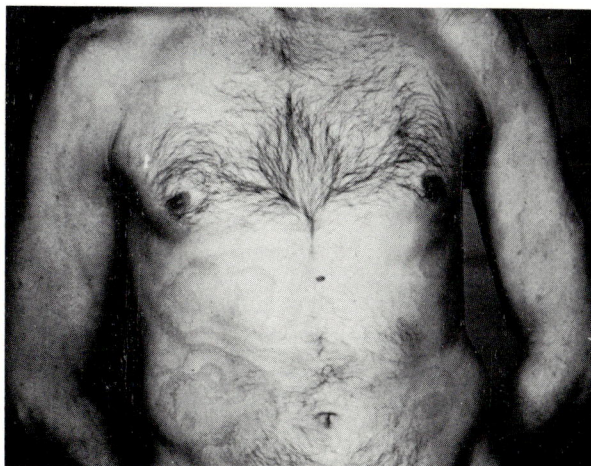

Figure 8–11 Erythema gyratum perstans in a patient with carcinoma of the lung.

kinson, 1959; Weinstein, 1969) is a syndrome that consists of an acute transitory eruption of tender erythematous nodules with special predilection for the lower extremities and prodromal symptoms.

Pathogenesis (Löfgren, 1946)

Erythema nodosum is not a specific entity but a syndrome caused by a delayed hypersensitivity reaction to infectious and noninfectious conditions. Although the etiologic causes are many, the most common are β-streptococcal and tuberculous infections and sarcoidosis (Fig. 8-12 *A* and *B*). Other responsible infections are the bacteria of Yersinia (Hannuksela and Avronen, 1969), the mycoses of coccidioidomycosis, histoplasmosis, North American blastomycosis, and kerion formation, and the viruses of psittacosis, lymphogranuloma venereum, ornithosis, cat-scratch fever, and possibly measles.

The onset of the eruption in the previously mentioned deep mycoses as well as in tuberculosis occurs at the time of the conversion of the coccidioidin, histoplasmin, and tuberculin skin tests respectively, to positivity. In coccidioidomycosis and histoplasmosis, erythema nodosum may be accompanied by erythema multiforme. The precipitating streptococcal infections are pharyngitis, tonsillitis, and scarlet fever; erythema nodosum is rarely, if ever, a manifestation of rheumatic fever. In tuberculosis, it occurs not only during the primary infection but also later during a massive bacillemia. Among the noninfectious states that may develop erythema nodosum are sarcoidosis, the enteropathies of ulcerative colitis and less frequently regional ileitis (Jacobs, 1959), drug therapy with sulfonamides, halogens, and recently contraceptives, Behçet's syndrome, the malignancies of Hodgkin's disease and leukemia, and the postradiated pelvic malignancies.

Histopathology

The histologic picture is not specific. The changes are predominantly in the

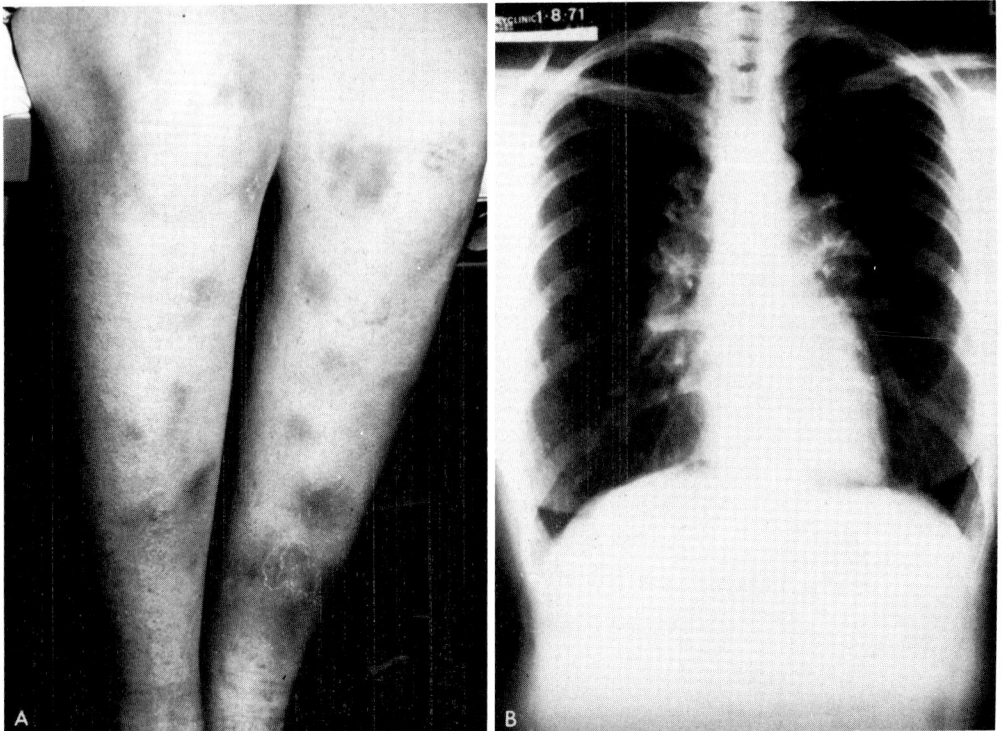

Figure 8-12 *A*, Erythema nodosum in a patient with hilar adenopathy. *B*, Liver biopsy revealed a granulomatous process consistent with sarcoidosis.

septal collagen of the lower dermis consisting of edema, inflammation of veins with some endothelial proliferation, and infiltration with mononuclear cells, neutrophils, and later giant cells. Fibrinoid changes and thrombosis of blood vessels are unusual, and necrotizing angiitis and fat necrosis are absent. The vessels in the upper dermis are dilated. The fat lobules adjacent to the upper septa may be involved secondarily. Small rosettes of histiocytes and lymphocytes radially surrounding tiny vascular slits in the connective tissue septa may be seen.

Clinical Picture

The incidence of this condition varies in different countries and has been lessened as a result of the advances in the treatment of infections. The decrease of erythema nodosum in children may be the result of the better control and treatment of tuberculosis. The disease has its greatest incidence in the spring and fall and is least common in the summer. Women experience this disorder three times more frequently than men; the peak incidence is between 20 and 35 years of age, and it is rare after 50 years of age.

The associated prodromal symptoms are fever, chills, malaise, and arthralgia. A prolonged prodrome including not only the previously mentioned symptoms but also fatigue, weight loss, cough, and depression suggests sarcoidosis as the underlying cause. The clinical manifestations of erythema nodosum are an eruption, episcleral nodules (Bluefarb, 1960), and hilar adenopathy. Discrete tender erythematous nodules, which tend to appear in areas where subcutaneous fat is present, as seen in the shins, knees, and ankles and occasionally in the thighs, lower arms, and face. The lesions measure 2 to 5 cm. or larger in size. They number from a few to several dozen and may appear in crops; they may coalesce to cover the entire shin and resemble erysipelas. They may evolve through a classic spectrum of color resembling a bruise (the so-called erythema contusiformis).

The eruption usually lasts three to six weeks but may continue for months. During the healing, a cigarette paper scale may appear on the surface. The lesions heal without suppuration, depression, or scar formation. Swelling of the feet and ankles may occur and persist, especially when the patient continues to be active. Arthralgias, which may precede, coincide, or follow the eruption, have been described in as many as 90 per cent of the cases and may be flitting and polyarthralgic (Truelove, 1960). Red superficial erythematous tender plaques may occur over the joints and result in a misdiagnosis of an acute arthritis. Episcleral nodules that histopathologically resemble Aschoff's bodies and the subcutaneous nodules of rheumatic fever develop in the palpebral fissure, are superficial and bilateral, and follow the course of the skin lesions.

Hilar adenopathy, which may be bilateral or unilateral, may occur as part of the symptom complex of erythema nodosum. Although it is seen in cases of erythema nodosum associated with tuberculosis, streptococcal disease, and coccidioidomycosis, one-half of the reported cases have been associated with sarcoidosis; it has not been described as resulting from drugs. The nodes, which are radiologically well delineated, tend to be symmetrical, reach their maximum size in one month, and regress in 12 to 18 months. Löfgren's syndrome is a classic expression of this disease and is characterized by fever, erythema nodosum skin lesions, and bilateral enlargement of the hilar nodes, as well as the right paratracheal node which may be palpable. It runs a benign course and has histologic evidence of sarcoidosis in the skin, liver, or lymph nodes, and very frequently a positive Kveim test.

Subacute nodular migratory panniculitis (Vilanova and Piñol Aguardé, 1959), described as a variant of erythema nodosum, is characterized by deep-seated nodular lesions which are seen almost exclusively in women, extend or coalesce to form large plaques especially over the knees and ankles, may persist for months, and may involute with orally administered potassium iodide therapy.

Differential Diagnosis

Differential diagnosis is usually that of red nodules on the lower extremities. The contusiform appearance of the lesion helps, although it may be seen in trauma, phlebitis, and localized infections. The conditions to be considered are:

INFECTIONS. Subsiding cellulitis, erysipeloid, septicemic nodules of staphylococcal, meningococcal, and gonococcal infections, borderline leprosy and lepromatous leprosy in reaction (erythema nodosum leprosum), Trichophyton granuloma, and nodular syphilids.

VASCULITIDES. Posttraumatic and migratory phlebitis, nodular vasculitis, and nodose lesions of the necrotizing vasculitides.

GRANULOMATOUS DISEASE. Sarcoidosis of the skin and the subcutaneous tissue, and insect bites.

PANNICULITIDES. Nodular migratory panniculitis, perniotic nodules, and nodular liquefying panniculitis.

NEOPLASMS. Lymphoma cutis and metastatic carcinoma.

Prognosis

Erythema nodosum is a benign process with a favorable prognosis. The lesions with "bruising" last longer. Early ambulation or excessive activity invites continued cropping of new lesions and persistent swelling and edema of feet and ankles. Arthralgias and stiffness may persist for months or years after the disappearance of the eruption. Recrudescences are infrequent; they have been reported in tuberculosis, coccidioidomycosis, sarcoidosis, and most frequently in streptococcal infections and drug reactions. Its presence in tuberculosis usually heralds a progressive pulmonary and generalized tuberculosis; in coccidioidomycosis, its presence is associated with a mild form of the disease; and in sarcoidosis, it has no prognostic significance.

Treatment

Treatment is primarily directed to the underlying disease. It has been recommended that erythema nodosum in the presence of a strong tuberculin skin test be treated with antituberculous drugs. Bed rest is indicated in all but the mild cases. In the resolving cases, firm supportive stockings are helpful. Salicylates are used for fever and joint and leg discomfort. Intralesional corticosteroid therapy may

be effective in those cases with only a few nodose lesions. Systemic corticosteroids may have an unfavorable effect on the underlying disease and do not shorten the course of erythema nodosum; recurrences after their withdrawal do occur. In severe cases they may be utilized for symptomatic relief, providing no evidence of tuberculosis is present. In cases of sarcoidosis, they are used to treat such indicated associated conditions as iritis.

ERYTHEMA TOXICUM NEONATORUM

Erythema toxicum neonatorum (toxic erythema of newborn, erythema neonatorum allergicum, urticaria neonatorum —Duperrat and Bret, 1961; Taylor and Boudurant, 1957) is a benign common macular erythematous eruption of brief duration found in the newborn. The nature of the eruption is unknown, an allergic cause cannot be established, and the presence of an irritant substance in the sebum has been advanced as being responsible. No infective agents have been demonstrated; newborn infants often react to nonspecific insults with an eosinophilic exudate. No racial, sexual, geographic, or seasonal variations are known.

Pathology

The early macular lesions have edema and perivascular and diffuse cellular infiltrate that consist predominantly of eosinophils in the upper dermis. Subcorneal and intra-epidermal sterile pustules appear later at the pilosebaceous orifice and around the eccrine pores; these lesions are associated with an eosinophilic leukocytosis (7 to 18 per cent) of the peripheral blood.

Clinical Picture

Erythema toxicum neonatorum is characterized by a macular erythematous eruption that may consist of several hundred macules and may be preceded by a diffuse transitory erythema. The lesions, which measure from a few millimeters to 2 cm. in diameter, appear mainly on the trunk and less frequently on the face and extremities, occur within 24 to 48 hours after birth, are rarely present at birth, and last four to six days. When the condition is more severe, the macules tend to become wheals or become associated with wheals and some of the lesions develop pustules that favor the pressure areas, the back, and buttocks. These eruptions may resemble flea bites, pustular miliaria, and impetigo. A presumptive diagnosis can be made from Leishman's stain of a pustule which reveals eosinophils. The eruption is asymptomatic and heals spontaneously.

TOXIC EPIDERMAL NECROLYSIS

Toxic epidermal necrolysis (Lyell's syndrome, epidermolysis necroticans combustiformis) is a toxic erythema of the skin that undergoes epidermal necrosis and peeling so that it appears to have been scalded (Koblenzer, 1967; Lyell, 1967; Melish and Glasgow, 1970; Samuels, 1967). There seem to be, two basic forms of toxic epidermal necrolysis, the child and adult types. In children, the cleavage of the epidermis that results from an acantholytic-dyskeratotic-cytolytic process is in the malpighian or granular layer and is usually induced by a staphylococcic toxin. In adults, it is characterized by a full-thickness cytolytic cleavage of skin above the basal layer and is usually precipitated by a drug.

The etiology (Lyell et al., 1969) of this syndrome is less obscure and is believed to be a reaction phenomenon to a toxin or allergen or both. Billingham and Streilin (1968) produced a similar disease in hamsters by the mechanism of homologous (runt) disease and suggested that the hypersensitivity mechanism may be important. This condition has been associated with drugs (Fig. 8-13); infections, especially staphylococcal phage-type 71 (Fig. 8-14 A and B); poisoning, especially carbon monoxide; lymphomas; and has followed measles, vaccination (Fig. 8-15), and radiotherapy. Among the drugs most frequently implicated are the sulfonamides, phenylbutazone, penicillin, aspirin, procaine, phenolphthalein, gold salts, and hydantoin. In drug-induced toxic epidermal necrolysis, direct immunofluorescence studies have shown intercellular fixation of immunoglobulins and complement globins in the basal cell layer which suggests that drugs bind to intercellular epidermal protein and that the basal cells are the site of damage (Stein et al., 1972). Where erythema multiforme and toxic epidermal necrolysis occur together, it is most likely caused by a common etiologic factor (Ohlenschlaeger, 1966). Cases described in the past as acute pemphigus, acquired epidermolysis bullosa, measles pemphigoid, and Ritter's disease (dermatitis exfoliativa neonatorum) were probably expressions of this disease.

Histopathology

The epidermis splits at the basal, malpighian, and granular levels, undergoes

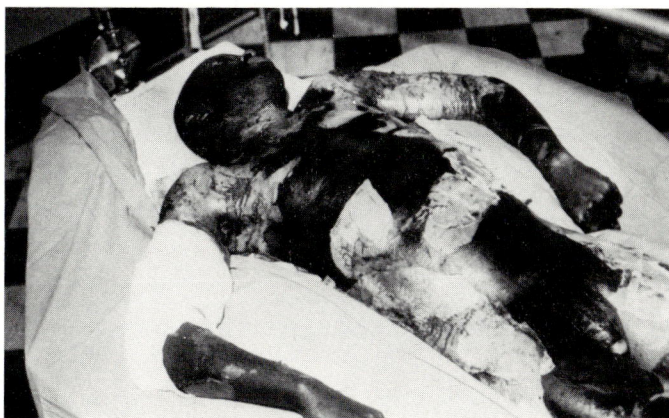

Figure 8–13 An almost fatal case of toxic epidermal necrolysis in an adult which was precipitated by oral penicillin.

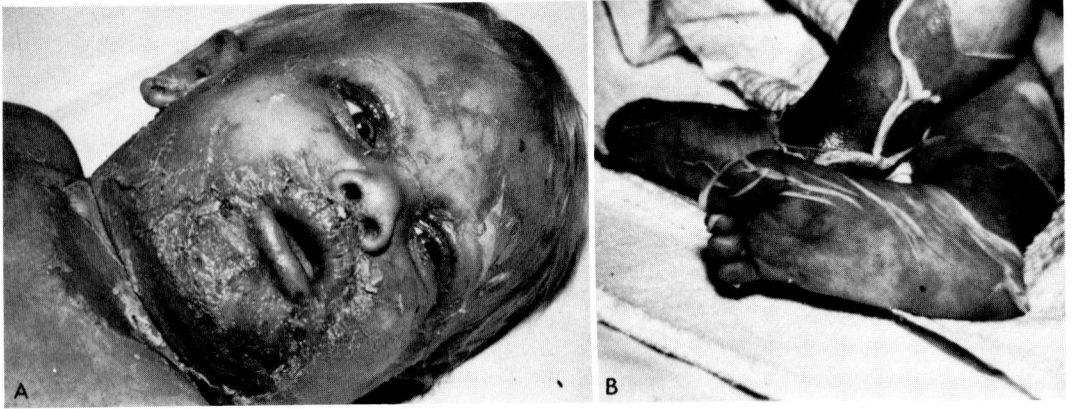

Figure 8–14   *A* and *B*, Toxic epidermal necrolysis caused by staphylococcal infection with phage Group II, type 71.

necrosis, and sloughs. Unlike erythema multiforme, no significant dermal infiltrate is present. At autopsy, no specific systemic lesions have been uncovered.

Clinical Picture

The disease affects persons of all ages, especially children, and races and sexes equally. It has the following clinical features: a prodrome, a toxic phase with the characteristic and diagnostic eruption, recovery in a few weeks, ability to recur, and possible death (25 to 30 per cent of cases). The prodrome consists usually of malaise, pyrexia, and marked tenderness and erythema of axillae and groins. A mild in-

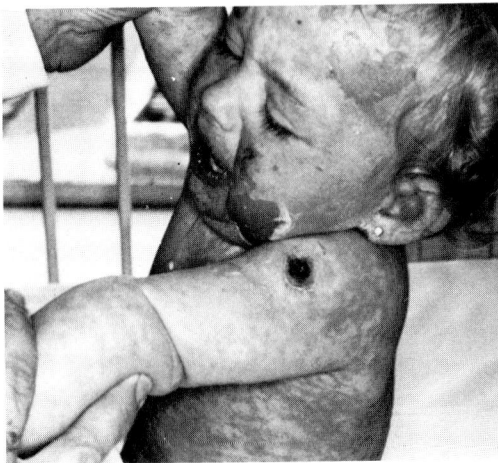

Figure 8–15   Vaccination complicated by toxic epidermal necrolysis.

flammation of the eyelids and mucous membranes of the eye, mouth, and genitalia may antedate all signs and symptoms for one to two weeks. From the sites of predilection, the intertriginous and periorificial areas and the trunk, the erythema and tenderness spread over the whole body but usually spare the hairy parts. Within 24 hours, the sodden necrotic skin begins to peel off in large sheets, leaving raw oozing areas resembling superficial scalds. Flaccid blisters sometimes occur and are passively and secondarily formed by the fluid filling the epidermal separations. Complete reepithelization occurs within 10 to 14 days without scarring. The infrequent permanent sequelae of corneal scarring, destruction of the eye, scarring alopecia, and nail destruction and scarring appear to be the result of an accompanying severe erythema multiforme (Stevens-Johnson syndrome).

Unlike the serum protein pattern in severe burns, the total protein, albumin, and IgG are not significantly affected in toxic epidermal necrolysis. Leukocytosis is usual, lymphocytosis occurs, and leukopenia can occur secondary to toxic bone marrow depression and thrombocytopenia secondary to disseminated intravascular coagulation.

The mortality rate is highest among children less than one year old, especially if more than 50 per cent of the skin is involved, and the elderly; it is relatively low in children from one to six years of age. Involvement of the mucous membranes is seen in more severe cases and tends to indicate a poor prognosis. Death usually results from fluid and electrolyte imbalance or sepsis or both.

Treatment

The treatment is in general similar to the treatment of burns, paying attention to electrolyte balance, demanding concentrated nursing service, and utilizing a turning frame. When systemic corticosteroids are given early, they may effectively and favorably influence the course of the disease and modify the recurrent attacks.

REITER'S SYNDROME

Reiter's syndrome (Fessinger-LeRoy-Reiter's syndrome, conjunctivourethrosynovial syndrome, postdysenteric arthritis, infective uroarthritis) is a symptom complex of unknown etiology and consists of the classic clinical triad of polyarthritis, nongonococcal urethritis, and conjunctivitis. Mucocutaneous lesions are present in 30 to 80 per cent of the cases (Ford, 1970; Kulka, 1962; Weinberger et al., 1962). The so-called enteric form of this syndrome presents with dysentery which is followed by one or all of the previously mentioned manifestations. The other form, the venereal type, which begins with a urethritis, is seen primarily in the United States, Great Britain, and western Europe; the enteric type predominates in eastern and southern Europe, North Africa, and Asia.

The disease affects young men of all races between 20 and 40 years of age, and rarely women and children. Women experience more frequently the dysenteric form of this condition. The syndrome has been associated with bacillary and nondysenteric diarrhea, venereally and nonvenereally acquired nongonococcal urethritis, and gonorrhea with or without an associated nonspecific urethritis. In the postdysenteric form, the dysentery bacilli seem to be related etiologically; however, in the venereal form, two classes of microorganisms — the Bedsonia agents and the Mycoplasmas — have been implicated but not substantiated. Because of an occasional report of a family incidence, the possibility of a genetic predisposition has been offered. Since psoriasis has eventually developed in patients with a classic Reiter's syndrome (Wright and Reed, 1964), a possible interrelationship between these diseases has been suggested (Perry and Mayne, 1965).

Histopathology

The skin shows hyperkeratosis, parakeratosis, acanthosis, and the classic spongiform pustule (unilocular polymorphonuclear pustule) in the upper malpighian layer. It differs from the other so-called pustular variants of psoriasis (pustular psoriasis, impetigo herpetiformis, and acrodermatitis continua) in the greater extent of the hyperkeratosis and parakeratosis and the failure of the spongiform pustule to be broken up during extrusion (Lapiere, 1961). No pathognomonic histologic changes of synovial tissue are present which, when the disease is chronic, resemble rheumatoid arthritis.

Clinical Picture

Before the onset of the disease, no prodromal symptoms occur. Sexual exposure or diarrhea antedates by days or three to four weeks the usual triad of organ involvement. Constitutional symptoms such as fever up to 102° F., malaise, anorexia, and weight loss usually accompany the onset of the disease and may last for several weeks. The conjunctivitis and urethritis commonly disappear in a few days or weeks, in contrast to the arthritis that continues. Although the initial attack is usually self-limited and clears spontaneously, exacerbations of ocular, urethral, and articular symptoms occur during the single course. Recurrences are seen up to five to eight times over a period of 6 to 12 years, involve one to all systems, and may produce sequelae.

The mucocutaneous lesions are frequent and rarely antedate the other classic manifestations. Skin lesions are more common in the venereal than in the enteric cases. The palms, soles (Fig. 8-16), penis, and the oral (Fig. 8-17) and urethral

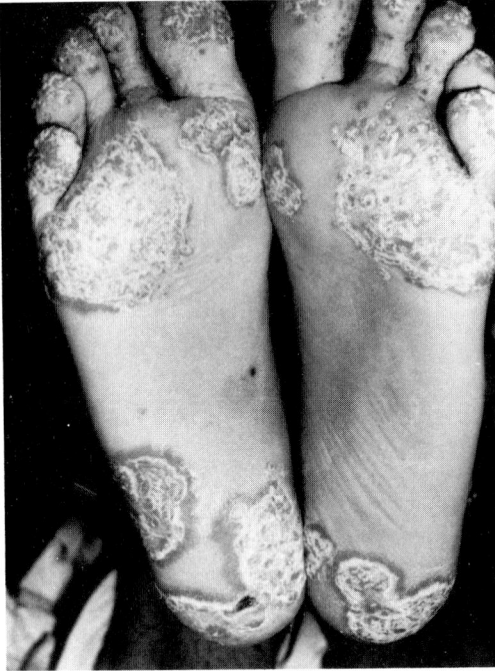

Figure 8-16 The classic keratoderma of the feet with geographic outline.

mucosa are the usual involved sites; a generalized exfoliative eruption rarely occurs. The keratoderma is appreciated especially on the soles but also on the hands, legs, and scalp; the lesions in the umbilical and buttock areas are more psoriasiform. The eruption usually appears about one month after the onset of the urethritis and follows the appearance of the arthritis. The initial lesion is an erythematous macule that vesiculates, becomes purulent, and develops a cone-shaped thick hyperkeratosis (keratosis blenorrhagicum, Fig. 8–18). The merging of the lesions creates the "mountain range" or "relief map" appearance. These lesions are self-limited and may last weeks to months. Scaling, erosive plaques may appear on the scrotum. Pustules occur beneath the nails near the lunula resulting in onycholysis and onychodystrophy. Thickening of the nails and subungual hyperkeratosis may occur. An exfoliative dermatitis may appear in severely ill patients who have fever, arthritis, and a protracted course, and may be fatal.

The mucosal lesions appear more frequently in the venereal form. The penis is most frequently involved. A circinate balanitis, which involves the corona and the glans and is best appreciated in the uncircumcised patient, is characterized by a coalescence of erosions in circumscribed erythema creating a circinate pattern (Fig. 8-19). In the uncircumcised patient, the eroded papules may become crusted and hyperkeratotic and resemble the lesions on the skin. In the oropharynx, diffuse erythema may be present that may vesiculate and erode. The palatal lesions may become purpuric. The superficial asymptomatic oral lesions last a few days. If the tongue is coated, confluence of the patches of denuded papillae simulates a geographic tongue. The oral lesions must be differentiated from erythema multiforme and aphthous and gonorrheic stomatitides.

The urethritis may be minimal, overlooked, or ignored by the patient. The urethral discharge is purulent and blood-stained, contains polymorphonuclear leukocytes and epithelial cells without bacteria, and is accompanied by dysuria. Hematuria results from an abacterial hemorrhagic cystitis. Urethral stricture and prostatovesiculitis are complications. In the enteric type, a urethritis, if present, tends to be mild and of short duration. Gonorrhea may antedate or coexist with the urethritis. In women, vaginitis, cervicitis, and cystitis occur.

The ocular lesions are conjunctivitis, iritis, and rarely keratitis. The conjunc-

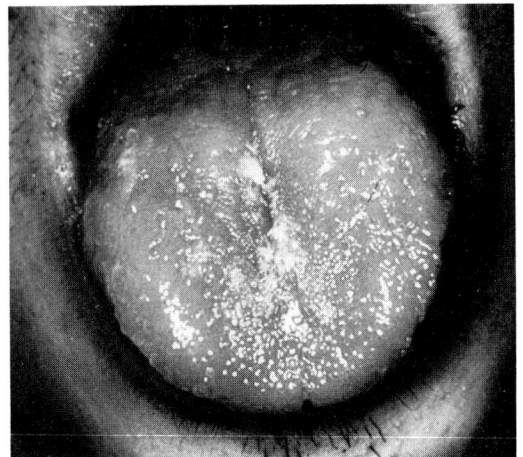

Figure 8-17 Mucous membrane lesion of glossitis.

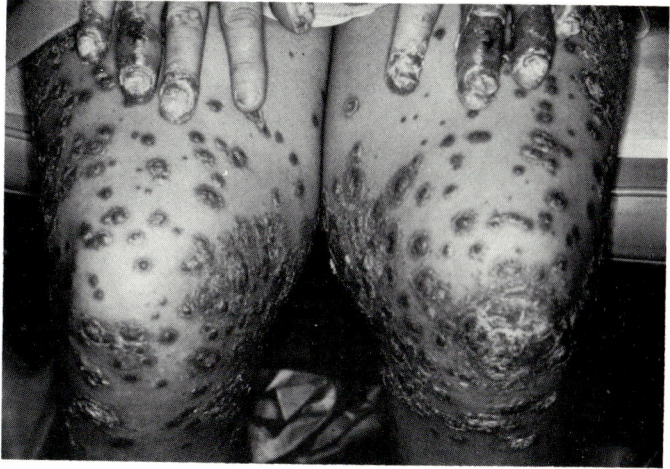

Figure 8–18 Rupioid skin changes with dystrophic nail changes.

tivitis may be so mild and evanescent as to be overlooked. It occurs in more than 50 per cent of the cases, tends to be bilateral and transient, lasts a few days, rarely has a purulent exudate or an associated lid edema, and resembles acute catarrhal conjunctivitis ("pink eye"). Keratitis or corneal ulcerations rarely occur. A nongranulomatous anterior uveitis occurs less frequently in the acute cases than in the severe protracted cases, especially those with sacro-iliitis with or without prostatitis.

Arthritis, which is the dominating feature of this syndrome, is almost always present. Initially, it may be polyarticular but finally, in a few days, it commonly affects symmetrically the large weight-bearing joints, the knees, and ankles, and less frequently and asymmetrically the joints of the upper extremities. The involved joints are usually hot, tender, and swollen with effusion, and have synovial thickening. The arthritis, which lasts two to four months and rarely more than a year, usually clears completely. When multiple attacks occur, residual joint damage is prone to develop. Low back pain results from sacro-iliitis which occurs early and in some cases exhibits clinically and radiologically ankylosing spondylitis similar to that seen in ulcerative colitis, regional ileitis, Whipple's disease, and psoriasis. Pain in the heel may be the result of periostitis of the calcaneal ligament and tendinitis of the plantar fascia and Achilles tendon.

Patients may have ST- and T-wave electrocardiographic changes presumably re-

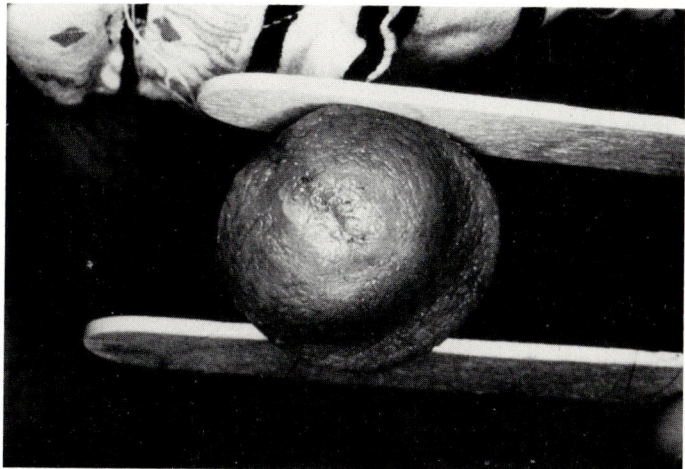

Figure 8–19 Circinate pattern of penile involvement, balanitis circinata.

sulting from pericarditis or myocarditis; aortic incompetence is rarely seen (Rodnan et al., 1964) and usually appears in patients who have had recurrent or prolonged disease with a high incidence of sacro-iliitis, iritis, and mucocutaneous manifestations (Paulus et al., 1972). Neuralgic amyopathy and pulmonary changes (pleurisy and infiltration) have been reported, but their specificity is questioned because of their rarity. Amyloidosis is rare.

Among the laboratory findings are a leukocytosis, an elevated sedimentation rate, a negative latex fixation test, and a normal serum uric acid. Cytologic and chemical changes of synovial fluid resemble those of rheumatoid arthritis and mild infection. The joint fluid has a high hemolytic complement activity and macrophages containing polymorphonuclear leukocytes (Pekin et al., 1967). Only two radiographic findings are suggestive of this disease; these are periostitis with periosteal new bone formation in the region of involved joints, especially in the inferior and posterior aspects of the os calcis producing calcanean spurs and subchondral sclerosis, and irregular outlines of one or both sacro-iliac joints (Sholkoff et al., 1970).

The diagnosis of Reiter's syndrome is easy when the classic triad with or without mucocutaneous lesions is present. Among the conditions to be considered in the differential diagnosis are psoriatic arthritis, severe erythema multiforme (Stevens-Johnson syndrome), and Behçet's syndrome. Pustular psoriasis can be distinguished by the family history of psoriasis, the greater amount of hand involvement than foot, the association of joint and skin exacerbations, and the absence of oral lesions, iritis, or genitourinary manifestations (except skin involvement of the penis). The arthritides from which it may be necessary to be differentiated are gonococcal and rheumatoid arthritis, and that of ulcerative colitis.

Treatment

In the acute febrile phase, the treatment consists of bed rest; antibiotics for urethritis; phenylbutazone, 100 mg. four times a day, for pain; and systemic corticosteroids, especially if the attack is severe. Salicylates are relatively ineffective. Intralesional steroids may be used when one or two joints are involved. The iritis requires local or systemic corticosteroids or both. Tetracycline, 250 mg. four times a day by mouth, seems to reduce the signs of urethritis but has no effect on the arthritis. Sexual promiscuity should be discouraged and, when the urethritis is recurrent, the conjugal partner should be treated with tetracycline. The arthropathy, when it persists, may be treated with antimalarials, indomethacin, gold and pyrotherapy. The skin lesions are treated the same as for psoriasis, with tar, topical steroids, sulfur precipitate, salicylic acid ointments, and systemic antimetabolites. Physiotherapy is advisable to prevent muscle wasting.

BEHÇET'S SYNDROME

Behçet's syndrome (Dowling, 1961; France et al., 1951; Mounsey, 1966) is a chronic and usually progressive multisystem disease clinically consisting of the triad of oral ulcerations, genital ulcerations, and inflammatory disease of the eyes. It was originally described in the middle East but is presently being reported worldwide. It usually appears in patients between the ages of 15 and 45 years; the classic expression favors the male. The causes advanced for this disease have been allergic owing to the presence of oral antimucosal antibodies in the patient's serum and the histologic evidence of inflammatory vasculitis, viral as a result of the reported isolation and the production of similar symptoms upon inoculation of rabbits, and vascular because of the high incidence of phlebitis or presence of a coagulation defect or both. The present state of our knowledge, however, fails to support these theories or to explain adequately the polymorphic and diverse clinical manifestations of this entity.

Histopathology

The mucocutaneous ulcerations show nonspecific inflammation with or without inflammatory infiltration of thrombosed arterioles. Widely disseminated, multifocal, small necrotic areas of the central nervous system, as well as a mild diffuse inflammatory meningoencephalitis, may be present.

Clinical Picture

Behçet's syndrome is characterized by frequent recurrences of variable duration and intensity, and various clinical expressions resulting from the multisystem involvement. In addition to the original triad, other described symptoms are pyoderma, polyarthritis and hydroarthrosis, erythema nodosum-like lesions, thrombophlebitis of small and large veins, central nervous system involvement, recurrent epididymitis and orchitis, abnormal skin responses to tests of delayed hypersensitivity, and pericardial, pulmonary, and gastrointestinal manifestations, including rectal and colonic ulcerations with even perforation. The syndrome may present as a spectrum of varying combinations of the previously mentioned symptoms. It has been suggested that incomplete forms of Behçet's disease presenting with less than the oral-genital-ocular syndrome exist (Curth, 1946). Until an etiologic agent is identified or a diagnostic test is available, in the absence of a cardinal symptom of the triad, one searches for the other associated signs and symptoms and anticipates the appearance of the lacking members of the triad to establish the diagnosis.

Constitutional symptoms, such as fever, malaise, and arthralgia, may be moderate or severe during the periods of activity. The oral and genital ulcerations are the initial symptoms followed within days, months, and even years by an iritis and the other elaborated manifestations. The thrombophlebitis and central nervous system involvement may dominate the clinical picture.

The oral ulcerations, which began as vesicles or pustules, are of two types: (1) a superficial erosive one similar to aphthae and (2) a deeply punched-out ulcer resembling periadenitis mucosae necroticans. The lips, gums, buccal mucosa, and tongue are usually involved, and in severe cases, the palate, pharynx, and esophagus are also affected. One or more ulcers may be present for years. The patient complains of pain, dysphagia, and fetor. The genital ulcers occur mainly on the scrotum, base of the penis, and labia and tend to be smaller than those of the mouth and pharynx. Perforation of the labia minora may occur. The mucocutaneous ulcers heal with scar formation.

The cutaneous lesions, which occur in 80 per cent of the cases, are follicular pustules, furunculosis, acneiform lesions, inflammatory dermal nodules, posttraumatic recurrent cellulitis, and the development of pustules at the sites of skin puncture. The dermal nodules resemble clinically erythema nodosum, appear mainly on the lower extremities, and exhibit histologically an angiitis of small vessels.

Conjunctivitis may be an early ocular lesion, but iritis or uveitis with hypopyon is most commonly seen. The ocular change may be unilateral but becomes bilateral. Keratitis, retinitis, choroiditis, and optic nerve atrophy have been described (Mamo and Baghdassarian, 1964). The eye involvement is the most frequent cause of disability.

The venous involvement (Haim et al., 1971) consists of the frequent superficial migratory thrombophlebitis, the occasional deep thrombophlebitis, and the rare phlebitis of retinal veins, dural sinus, and superior and inferior vena cava.

Any part of the neuroaxis except the lower motor neuron may be involved. Neurologic involvement (Pallis, 1966) appears in 15 to 20 per cent of cases, is of grave prognosis with 50 per cent mortality within one year, and presents as cranial nerve palsies, brain stem syndromes, meningoencephalitis, meningomyelitis, multiple sclerosis-like disorders, and organic confusional states.

The most frequent significant laboratory data are leukocytosis with an occasional striking eosinophilia, an elevated sedimentation rate, and a hypergammaglobulinemia with an increase in the α-2 component on electrophoresis.

The diseases to be considered in the differential diagnosis are erythema multiforme bullosum, systemic lupus erythematosus, sarcoidosis, syphilis, and ulcerative colitis.

The progress of the disease is slow, with spontaneous remissions and exacerbations. If the disease does not prove to be fatal, its activity diminishes and ceases after many years.

Treatment
(Haim and Sherf, 1966)

No specific treatment is known. Evaluation of therapeutic responses, especially with corticosteroids, is hampered by the clinical fluctuations in the natural course of the disease as well as by the lack of controlled studies. Improvement and continuous suppression of the ocular and central nervous system involvement with steroid therapy have sometimes been dramatic; unfortunately, the other involved systems have remained unaffected by this therapy. Because of the concept of auto-immunity and the presence of inflammatory vasculitis, immunosuppressive drugs, such as azathioprine, 2.0 to 2.5 mg. a day, and cyclophosphamide, 100 to 150 mg. a day, have been reported as effective and have resulted in smaller maintenance or suppressive doses of corticosteroids.

FAMILIAL MEDITERRANEAN FEVER

Familial Mediterranean fever (benign paroxysmal peritonitis, familial recurrent polyserositis, periodic disease—Ehrenfeld et al., 1961; Reimann et al., 1954; Siegal, 1964; Sohar et al., 1967) is an inherited disease with a peculiar ethnic predilection and is characterized by recurrent acute febrile attacks associated with polyserositis and insidious development of amyloidosis that rarely may be the first manifestation. It occurs almost exclusively in persons of Mediterranean stock, Jews especially, the Sephardic in Israel and the Ashkenazic in the United States, Arabs, Armenians, and Italians. Men are affected one and one-half times more frequently than women, and 90 per cent of the patients are affected by the end of the second decade although it may appear during the first year of life and rarely in the fourth decade or later. It is transmitted by an autosomal recessive gene. Its etiology and pathogenesis are unknown.

Histopathology

Histopathologic examination reveals an acute inflammation of the involved serosa; the remarkable reversibility of the process has been demonstrated by the normal histologic appearance of the previously involved organs on later examination. At necropsy, amyloidosis is usually the only finding of significance and is the cause of death. It is of the perireticulum type with characteristic parenchymal involvement. The renal glomeruli, adrenal gland, spleen (principally the red pulp), and pulmonary aveolar septa may be involved, and the hepatic sinusoids are spared.

Clinical Picture

Two phenotypes of familial Mediterranean fever are described, one characterized by self-limited recurrent acute febrile episodes of short duration with polyserositis, the other a rare variant presenting with amyloidosis as the initial manifestation of the disease.

Familial Mediterranean fever affects an individual in good health, begins with pain in the involved viscera, and is associated with fever that may be as high as 105° F. and lasts 12 to 36 hours. Although it has been described as a periodic disease, no periodicity or regular rhythm occurs; recurrences are irregular. The peritoneal "attack" is the most frequent type (95 per cent of cases) and the most common presenting sign (55 per cent of cases). Pleural involvement is seen in approximately 40 per cent of the patients. Synovitis is the second most common manifestation, occurs in about 75 per cent of cases, is usually monoarticular, involving the knee, ankle, hip, and shoulder, and lasts from one to seven days but may become protracted or chronic, lasting weeks and even a year. Despite prolonged involvement, spontaneous complete functional recovery occurs.

A cutaneous eruption has been described in 10 per cent of the cases. The most frequent and characteristic lesion is a painful tender, erythematous, sharply marginated, erysipelas-like patch that affects the skin of the calf, ankles, and dorsum of the foot. It may be the only sign during the febrile attack, may accompany the monoarthritis, and, like the arthritis, may be precipitated by trauma. Urticaria may accompany paroxysms of fever and abdominal complaints and may be recurrent. Schönlein-Henoch purpura has been associated with attacks, especially in children, and has recurred. Acute tender nodules, which histologically reveal a panniculitis or resemble periarteritis nodosa, have also been described.

Amyloidosis occurs in about 25 per cent of the cases and causes death in 90 per cent of the patients before the age of 40. No relationship is present between the age at onset, the type, frequency, and severity of the attacks, and the occurrence of amyloidosis. The course of amyloidosis consists of the preclinical phase appreciated by liver or rectal biopsy and the clinical phase marked by nephropathy (proteinuria, nephrotic syndrome, uremia, and death) and rarely gastrointestinal malabsorption syndrome.

Familial Mediterranean fever is a severe, chronic, incurable disease with an unpredictable and fatal course in a significant number of patients. Constant and complete remissions occur unexplainably during pregnancy. No effective therapy is known to prevent or shorten the attacks. A reduction in frequency of attacks has been reported in patients on a low fat diet (Mellinkoff et al., 1961).

RELAPSING POLYCHONDRITIS

(Polychondritis Chronica Atrophicans, Chondrolytic Perichondritis, Rheumatic Panchondritis, Generalized Chondromalacia of Von Meyenburg-Altherr, Familial Chronic Atrophic Polychondritis)

Relapsing polychondritis (Kaye and Sones, 1964; Self et al., 1967) is a distinctive but rare systemic disease of unknown cause. It is characterized by an inflammatory and degenerative process of both articular and nonarticular cartilage and has been classified as a connective or metabolic disease resulting in an enzymatic disruption of cartilage. The pathogenesis is currently attributed to the release or activation of lysosomal enzymes resulting in destruction of the connective tissue. The association of the disease with rheumatoid arthritis, lupus erythematosus, and Hashimoto's thyroiditis suggests that an auto-immune mechanism is responsible. Immunofluorescent studies (Dolan et al., 1966) demonstrated greater binding of conjugated test serum with normal collagen than controls and were advanced to support the immunologic pathogenic concept.

The majority of cases have appeared in Caucasians, but it has also been seen in Orientals and Negroes. Both sexes are almost equally affected, with a slight predominance in women. The disease favors persons between the third and fifth decade but has appeared in children as early as 2 years of age and adults in the late 60s.

Histopathology

The involved cartilage histologically reveals basophilic staining, fragmentation, replacement by fibrous tissue, and focal lymphocytic infiltrates. The cartilaginous changes have been attributed to the loss of chondroitin sulfate from the matrix.

Clinical Picture

The diagnosis is based upon the presence of recurrent inflammation of two or more cartilaginous sites (one of which is a sensory organ) and a compatible biopsy of an involved site. The course of the disease is extremely variable; it tends to be chronic with exacerbations and remissions over a period of months to years, each attack lasting days to months, but it may pursue a rapidly fulminant course. In general, the more severe and extensive the process, the more frequent and severe the relapses. Solitary sites of involvement usually occur without constitutional symptoms in contrast to the multisystem involvement that is associated with fever, malaise, anorexia, and weight loss. The inflammatory process that causes chondrolysis, dystrophy, and atrophy of cartilage typically affects the ears and the nasal septum as well as the peripheral joints, larynx, trachea, bronchi, epiglottis, thyroid, and the eustachian tube.

The external ear is involved in 85 per cent of cases; initially the pinnae are "beefy" red and tender (Fig. 8-20) and later become floppy, atrophic, and deformed with roentgenologically demonstrated calcification (Thurston and Curtis, 1966). Extensive swelling of the external auditory canal may cause a conductive deafness. Inflammation of the middle ear may occur with the appearance of eighth nerve deafness or labyrinthine symptoms of vertigo, tinnitus, and nausea. Nasal involvement occurs in 80 per cent of the cases and is characterized by septal tenderness and swelling with or without crusted erosions and an associated rhinorrhea and epistaxis; the late sequelae are a "saddle" deformity (Fig. 8-21) and calcification of the septum. Involvement of the intra-articular cartilages of the peripheral, sternocostal, intervertebral, and temporomandibular joints is clinically appreciated by erythema, heat, pain, and tenderness; a mild migratory arthralgia may affect all joints. Lesions of the respiratory tract, epiglottis, larynx, trachea, and bronchi can cause respiratory embarrassment and recurrent infection; fortunately, death from extensive involvement affects only a small percentage of the cases. The patients may present initially

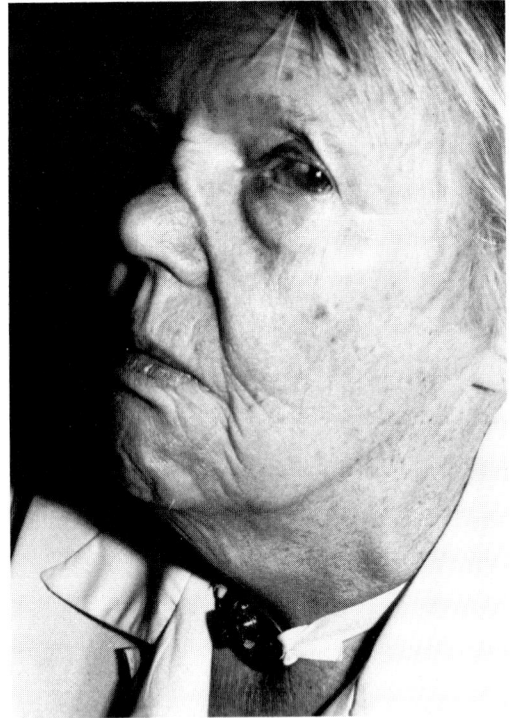

Figure 8–21   There is not only "saddle" deformity of the nose but also collapse of tracheal rings necessitating tracheostomy.

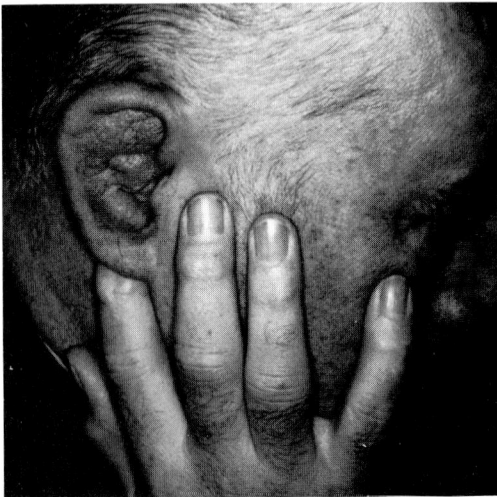

Figure 8–20   The "beefy" red ears with rheumatoid-like changes of the hands.

with hoarseness, dry nonproductive cough, progressive dyspnea, and dysphagia. With the collapse of the tracheal ring (Fig. 8-21) and bronchial wall, the patients may experience chronic bronchopulmonary infection, cardiorespiratory failure, and sudden complete obstruction with asphyxia; all may prove to be fatal. Over half of the patients experience eye problems; the common lesions are conjunctivitis, scleritis, and iritis, and the uncommon ones are keratoconjunctivitis sicca, iridocyclitis, chorioretinitis, optic neuritis, exophthalmos, ocular palsy, and cataracts. Medial aortopathy has recently been recognized as part of the syndrome (Hainer and Hamilton, 1969; Pearson et al., 1967). The most frequent lesion is aortic insufficiency but dissecting aortic aneurysm has been seen. The changes have been attributable to the disruption of the elastic fibers of the aorta typical of cystic medial necrosis.

The usual laboratory abnormalities, which are nonspecific, are an elevated sedimentation rate and anemia. Leuko-cytosis, eosinophilia, and the presence of the rheumatoid factor are occasionally seen and infrequently a positive L.E. test is noted. During the initial attack and exacerbations, an increase in urinary acid mucopolysaccharides occurs.

Among the diseases that may be enter-tained in the differential diagnosis are those diseases characterized by arthrop-athy, such as rheumatoid arthritis, rheu-matic fever, and Reiter's disease, those with auricular lesions, such as gout, chondrodermatitis nodularis chronica helicus, and external otitis with cellulitis, and those with respiratory tract involve-ment, such as midline lethal granuloma, Wegener's granulomatosis, lymphoma, syphilis, and tuberculosis.

The prognosis is uncertain; it may be-come inactive within a short time or may relapse for 20 years, and it may be fatal in a few cases.

Treatment

Therapy has been of a supportive na-ture. Systemic corticosteroids have their greatest efficacy in the laryngotracheo-bronchial manifestations where they are often lifesaving; they are suppressive in 30 to 60 mg. doses, usually cannot be with-drawn completely, and are continued on a maintenance of 5 to 20 mg.; they are least effective for scleral and arthritic symptoms. Long-term salicylate therapy may be help-ful. The effectiveness of immunosuppres-sive agents or antimetabolites in this syn-drome has not been reported. Once the cartilaginous rings of the respiratory tract have been destroyed, the maintenance of a patent airway with a permanent trache-ostomy is a lifesaving measure. Surgical replacement of the aortic valve with a prosthesis has been performed for aortic insufficiency.

REFERENCES

Ashby, D. W., and Lazar, T.: Erythema multiforme exudativum major (Stevens-Johnson syndrome). Lancet 1:1091-1095, 1951.

Bean, W. B.: Vascular Spiders and Related Lesions of the Skin. Springfield, Illinois, Charles C Thomas, 1958.

Beare, J. M., Froggatt, P., Jones, J. H., et al.: Familial annual erythema. An apparently new dominant mutation. Br. J. Dermatol. 78:59-68, 1966.

Billingham, R. E., and Streilein, J. W.: Toxic epider-mal necrolysis and homologous disease in ham-sters. Arch. Dermatol. 98:528-539, 1968.

Blomgren, S. E.: Erythema nodosum. Semin. Ar-thritis Rheum. 4:1, 1974.

Bloom, A., and Lovel, T. W.: Erythema multiforme with renal and myocardial injury. Proc. R. Soc. Med. 57:175-177, 1964.

Bluefarb, S. M.: Erythema nodosum with conjunc-tival nodules. Quart. Bull. Northwest. Univ. Med. Sch. 34:194-196, 1960.

Bukantz, S. C.: The Stevens-Johnson syndrome. D.M. 1-36, October, 1968.

Comaish, J. S., and Kerr, D. N.: Erythema multi-forme and nephritis. Br. Med. J. 2:84-88, 1961.

Convit, J., Kerdel-Vegas, F., and Rodriguez, G.: Erythema dyschromicum perstans: a hitherto un-described skin disease. J. Invest. Dermatol. 36:457-462, 1961.

Curth, H. O.: Recurrent genito-oral aphthosis and uveitis with hypopyon (Behçet's syndrome); re-port of 2 cases. Arch. Dermatol. 54:179-196, 1946.

Degos, R., Touraine, R., and Arouete, J.: [Chronic erythema migrans. (Discussion of a rickettsial origin.)] Ann. Dermatol. Syphiligr. 89:247-260, 1962.

Dolan, D. L., Lemmon, G. B., Jr., and Teitelbaum, S. L.: Relapsing polychondritis. Analytical litera-ture review and studies on pathogenesis. Am. J. Med. 41:285-299, 1966.

Dowling, G. B.: Behçet's disease. Proc. R. Soc. Med. 54:101-104, 1961.

Duperrat, B., and Bret, A. J.: Erythema neonatorum allergicum. Br. J. Dermatol. 73:300-302, 1961.

Ehrenfeld, E. N., Eliakim, M., and Rachmilewitz, M.: Recurrent polyserositis (familial Mediterranean fever; periodic disease). A report of fifty-five cases. Am. J. Med. 31:107-123, 1961.

Finland, M., Jolliffe, L. S., and Parker, F., Jr.: Pneu-monia and erythema multiforme exudativum; re-port of 4 cases and 3 autopsies. Am. J. Med. 4:473-492, 1948.

Finlayson, G. R., Sams, W. M., Jr., and Smith, J. G., Jr.: Erythema ab igne: a histopathological study. J. Invest. Dermatol. 46:104-108, 1966.

Flanagan, B. P.: Erythema chronicum migrans Afzelius in Americans. Arch. Dermatol. 86:410–411, 1962.

Ford, D. K.: Reiter's syndrome. Bull. Rheum. Dis. 20:588–591, 1970.

France, R., Buchanan, R. N., Wilson, M. W., et al.: Relapsing iritis with recurrent ulcers of mouth and genitalia (Behçet's syndrome); review: with report of additional case. Medicine 30:335-355, 1951.

Gordon, H.: Erythema nodosum. A review of one hundred fifteen cases. Br. J. Dermatol. 73:393-409, 1961.

Haim, S., and Sherf, K.: Behçet's disease. Presenta-tion of 11 cases and evaluation of treatment. Isr. J. Med. Sci. 2:69-74, 1966.

Haim, S., Barzilai, D., and Hazani, E.: Involvement of veins in Behçet's syndrome. Br. J. Dermatol. 84:238-241, 1971.

Hainer, J. W., and Hamilton, G. W.: Aortic abnor-malities in relapsing polychondritis. Report of a case with dissecting aortic aneurysm. N. Engl. J. Med. 280:1166-1168, 1969.

Hannuksela, M.: Erythema nodosum with special reference to sarcoidosis. A clinical study of 343 Finnish adult patients. Ann. Clin. Res. 3:1-64, (Suppl. 7) 1971.

Hannuksela, M., and Avronen, P.: Erythema nodosum due to yersinia enterocolitica. Scand. J. Infect. Dis. *1*:17-19, 1969.

Hitch, J. M., and Hansen, R. F.: Symmetric erythema of the soles. Arch. Dermatol. 38:881-892, 1938.

Hopkins, J. G., and others: Treatment of hyperhidrosis and symmetric lividities of feet. Arch. Dermatol. 57:850-857, 1948.

Jacobs, W. H.: Erythema nodosum in inflammatory diseases of the bowel. Gastroenterology 37:286-294, 1959.

James, D. G.: Erythema nodosum. Br. Med. J. *1*:853-857, 1961.

Kaye, R. L., and Sones, D. L.: Relapsing polychondritis. Clinical and pathologic features in fourteen cases. Ann. Intern. Med. 60:653-664, 1964.

Keil, H.: The rheumatic erythemas; a critical survey. Ann. Intern. Med. *11*:2223-2272, 1938.

Keil, H.: Erythema multiforme exsudativum (Hebra); a clinical entity associated with systemic features. Ann. Intern. Med. *14*:449-494, 1940.

Knox, J. M., Dodge, B. G., and Freeman, R. G.: Erythema dyschromicum perstans. Arch. Dermatol. 97:262-272, 1968.

Koblenzer, P. J.: Acute epidermal necrolysis (Ritter von Rittershain-Lyell). A clinicopathologic study. Arch. Dermatol. 95:608-617, 1967.

Kulka, J. P.: The lesions of Reiter's syndrome. Arthritis Rheum. 5:195-201, 1962.

Lapiere, S.: [Multilocular spongiform pustular dermatoses.] Ann. Dermatol. Syphiligr. 88:481-506, 1961.

Lazar, P.: Cancer, erythema annulare centrifugum, autoimmunity. Arch. Dermatol. 87:246-251, 1963.

Löfgren, S.: Erythema nodosum; studies on etiology and pathogenesis in 185 adult cases. Acta Med. Scand. [Suppl.] *174*:1-197, 1946.

Lyell, A.: A review of toxic epidermal necrolysis in Britain. Br. J. Dermatol. 79:662-671, 1967.

Lyell, A., Dick, H. M., and Alexander, J. O.: Outbreak of toxic epidermal necrolysis associated with staphylococci. Lancet *1*:787-789, 1969.

Mamo, J. G., and Baghdassarian, A.: Behçet's disease; a report of 28 cases. Arch. Ophthalmol. 71:4-14, 1964.

Melish, M. E., and Glasgow, L. A.: The staphylococcal scaled-skin syndrome. N. Engl. J. Med. 282:1114-1119, 1970.

Mellinkoff, S. M., Schwabe, A. D., and Lawrence, J. S.: A dietary treatment for familial Mediterranean fever. Arch. Intern. Med. *108*:80-85, 1961.

Michelson, H. E.: Erythema nodosum. Arch. Dermatol. 77:546-553, 1958.

Mounsey, J. P. D.: Behçet's syndrome — A spectrum. Trans. St. John's Hosp. Dermatol. Soc. 52:197-200, 1966.

Ohlenschlaeger, K.: Toxic epidermal necrolysis and Stevens-Johnson's disease. Acta Derm. Venereol. *46*:204-209, 1966.

Pallis, C. A.: Behçet's disease and the nervous system. Trans. St. John's Hosp. Dermatol. Soc. 52:201-206, 1966.

Paulus, H. E., Pearson, C. M., and Pitts, W., Jr.: Aortic insufficiency in five patients with Reiter's syndrome. Am. J. Med. 53:464-472, 1972.

Pearson, C. M., Kroening, R., Verity, M. A., et al.: Aortic insufficiency and aortic aneurysm in relapsing polychondritis. Trans. Assoc. Am. Physicians 80:71-90, 1967.

Pekin, T. J., Jr., Malinin, T. I., and Zvaifler, N. J.. Unusual synovial fluid findings in Reiter's syndrome. Ann. Intern. Med. 66:677-684, 1967.

Perry, C. B.: Erythema marginatum (rheumaticum). Arch. Dis. Child *12*:233-238, 1937.

Perry, H. O., and Mayne, J. G.: Psoriasis and Reiter's syndrome. Arch. Dermatol. 92:129-136, 1965.

Peterkin, G. A. G.: Malignant change in erythema ab igne. Br. Med. J. 2:1599-1602, 1955.

Purdy, M. J.: Erythema gyratum repens: report of a case. Arch. Dermatol. 80:590-591, 1959.

Ramirez, C. O.: Quoted by Knox, J. M., et al.

Reimann, H. A., Moadie, J., Semerdjian, S., et al.: Periodic peritonitis — heredity and pathology; report of 72 cases. J.A.M.A. *154*:1254-1259, 1954.

Rodnan, G. P., Benedek, T. G., Shaver, J. A., et al.: Reiter's syndrome and aortic insufficiency. J.A.M.A. *189*:889-894, 1964.

Samuels, M. J.: Toxic epidermal necrolysis. A report of 42 cases. Br. J. Dermatol. 79:672-677, 1967.

Self, J., Hammarsten, J. F., Lyne, B., et al.: Relapsing polychondritis. Arch. Intern. Med. *120*:109-112, 1967.

Shelley, W. B.: Herpes simplex virus as a cause of erythema multiforme. J.A.M.A. *201*:153-156, 1967.

Sholkoff, S. D., Glickman, M. G., and Steinbach, H. L.: Roentgenology of Reiter's syndrome. Radiology 97:497-503, 1970.

Siegal, S.: Familial paroxysmal polyserositis. Analysis of fifty cases. Am. J. Med. 36:893-918, 1964.

Sohar, E., Gafni, J., Pras, M., et al.: Familial Mediterranean fever. A survey of 470 cases and review of the literature. Am. J. Med. 43:227-253, 1967.

Stein, K. M., Schlappner, O. L., Heaton, C. L., et al.: Demonstration of basal cell immunofluorescence in drug-induced toxic epidermal necrolysis. Br. J. Dermatol. 86:246-252, 1972.

Stevenson, J. R., and Miura, M.: Erythema dyschromicum perstans. (Ashy dermatosis). Arch. Dermatol. 94:196-199, 1966.

Summerly, R.: The figurative erythemas and neoplasia. Br. J. Dermatol. 76:370-373, 1964.

Taylor, W. B., and Boudurant, C. P., Jr.: Erythema neonatorum allergicum; a study of the incidence in two hundred newborn infants and a review of the literature. Arch. Dermatol. 76:591-594, 1957.

Thurston, C. S., and Curtis, A. C.: Relapsing polychondritis. Report of a patient with "beefy" red ears and severe polyarthritis. Arch. Dermatol. 93:664-669, 1966.

Truelove, L. H.: Articular manifestations of erythema nodosum. Ann. Rheum. Dis. *19*:174-180, 1960.

Versey, C., and Wilkinson, D. S.: Erythema nodosum; a study of seventy cases. Br. J. Dermatol. 71:139-155, 1959.

Vilanova, X., and Piñol Aguadé, J.: Subacute nodular migratory panniculitis. Br. J. Dermatol. 71:45-50, 1959.

Weinberger, H. W., Ropes, M. W., Kulka, J. P., et al.: Reiter's syndrome, clinical and pathologic observations. A long term study of 16 cases. Medicine *41*:35-91, 1962.

Weinstein, L.: Erythema nodosum. D. M. pp. 1-30, June, 1969.

Woerdeman, M. J.: Erythema gyratum repens. Dermatologica *128*:391-392, 1964.

Wright, V., and Reed, W. B.: The link between Reiter's syndrome and psoriatic arthritis. Ann. Rheum. Dis. 23:12-21, 1964.

CHAPTER

9

PAPULOSQUAMOUS ERUPTIONS AND EXFOLIATIVE DERMATITIS

Harry J. Hurley

The natural consequences of epidermal proliferation are the formation and shedding of keratin scales. The loss of the dead corneum normally occurs imperceptibly and undramatically as the outermost cells or their aggregates are progressively dehydrated, fragmented, loosened, and lost. In any disease state in which epidermal cell growth and maturation are disturbed, this normally inapparent sequence becomes apparant. Keratinous scales accumulate on the skin and their loss is recorded on clothing or other articles of contact. The scales produced by these diseases show great variation morphologically, reflecting their disparate pathogenesis. Some are distinctive enough in appearance to be useful in clinical diagnosis. Moreover, there is a degree of erythema in many of these disorders marking macular or more often papular change. The distinctive composite scale and papule of these diseases has prompted their didactic grouping as papulosquamous eruptions. Although this organizational plan has been discarded in some of the other current major textbooks of dermatology, the authors of this book have elected to retain it since it serves to direct the examiner quickly from what is seen on the patient to a systematic mental and laboratory analysis of the dermatosis and when necessary to the appropriate section in a reference source. In addition, there is no better primer for the acquisition of skill in dermatologic diagnosis than the papulosquamous eruptions. Proficiency in their diagnosis prepares the student well for the identification of other skin diseases.

All of the papulosquamous eruptions can be compared to psoriasis, which is perhaps the most troublesome and most studied disease of the group. In addition to psoriasis, the papulosquamous eruptions include seborrheic dermatitis, which is discussed in detail in Chapter 3, pityriasis rosea, pityriasis rubra pilaris, lichen planus, lichen nitidus, lichen striatus, and a group of conditions considered under the heading parapsoriasis. Tinea corporis, a superficial fungal infection, and tinea versicolor, an infection due to *Pityrosporon orbiculare*, may be maculosquamous or papulosquamous eruptions; they are described in Chapter 13. It should be stressed also that drug eruptions, the modern day mimic of disease, and secondary syphilis, the great imitator of days past, are commonly papulosquamous in character and must always be included in the differential diagnosis of the condition of any patient with scaly macular or papular lesions. In fact, in terms of frequency alone, drug eruptions are probably the most important of the group. They are discussed in Chapter 7.

The final section of this chapter is devoted to exfoliative dermatitis. Among the cutaneous and systemic conditions that may give rise to an exfoliative dermatitis are several of the papulosquamous eruptions, notably psoriasis, seborrheic dermatitis, pityriasis rubra pilaris, lichen planus, and pityriasis rosea.

PSORIASIS

Psoriasis is a common scaly erythematous disease of unknown etiology showing wide variation in severity and distribution of skin lesions. It usually follows an irregular chronic course which is marked by remissions and exacerbations of unpredictable onset and duration. A genetic influence in the pathogenesis of psoriasis is now unquestioned but despite intensive investigation over the past 20 years, resulting in the accumulation of much new data and many concepts relating to the altered morphology and function of psoriatic skin, the cause of the disease remains obscure. The only significant systemic association is arthritis, which is seen in a minority of the patients and which should now be regarded as a spectrum of clinical joint disease, ranging from a special predominantly acral form to rheumatoid arthritis or arthritis mutilans. The designation "psoriasis" has been preferred for many years and there are no synonyms of importance.

Historical Features

Psoriasis is one of the oldest of all recorded skin diseases. Celsus probably described it originally in 35 to 40 A.D. During biblical times and thereafter, it and certain other skin disorders were regarded as forms of leprosy. The term "lepra" was used even in Willan's classic description of psoriasis in 1808. The voluminous literature of recent years has focused on the ultrastructural, functional, and biochemical alterations of the epidermis in psoriasis, the importance of inheritance in its pathogenesis, and the treatment of the disease with antifolic and other cytotoxic medications.

Epidemiology

Psoriasis is found all over the world but its recorded prevalence in different areas varies from less than 1 per cent to perhaps as high as 6 per cent of the population. The higher figures, however, are from closed patient groups, in hospitals or institutions, and are possibly not representative. In the United States, its frequency is in the range of 1 to 2 per cent, although as yet there are no comprehensive studies of the prevalence of psoriasis in North America. The current Health and Nutrition survey should provide more precise figures on the prevalence of psoriasis in the United States. The incidence of the disease is particularly low in the Japanese (Shima and Havin, 1962), and in American Indians and Negroes (Simons, 1949), especially those of West African origin (Verhagen and Koten, 1967), who comprise the bulk of the American Negro population and in whom the disease is also uncommon. Males and females are equally predisposed and all age groups are affected, although the onset of the disease is less common in the very young and the elderly. However, true congenital psoriasis, with active lesions present at birth, has been reported (Lerner and Lerner, 1972). Familial occurrence has been described often and reflects a genetic predisposition, as discussed below. There is no epidemiologic evidence to support the theory that psoriasis is an infectious disease. Psoriasis is usually less severe in summer than in winter, but its onset in summer months is strikingly high (Hellgren, 1964).

Etiology and Pathogenesis

The riddle of psoriasis remains unsolved, despite intensive basic and clinical investigation. At one time or another almost every conceivable causative influence, including microbiologic, metabolic, and immunologic causes, "liver disease," and food intolerance, has been indicted, but conclusive evidence is lacking for any and all of these. It is convenient to consider the pathogenesis of psoriasis under three sections: genetic predisposition, precipitating factors, and structural and biochemical alterations.

GENETIC PREDISPOSITION. There is no longer any doubt that the tendency to develop psoriasis is genetically determined, although development of the disease is also influenced by environmental factors. The familial concentration of the disease and the higher concordance rates for psoriasis in monozygotic over dizygotic twin pairs (Farber et al., 1974) emphasize the role of heredity in the pathogenesis of the disease. Early studies suggested autosomal dominant transmission with incomplete penetrance (Romanus, 1945), and studies of large families support this (Abele et al., 1963). Lomholt (1963), however, in his exhaustive Faroe Island survey, concluded that either dominant inheritance with incomplete penetrance or double recessive inheritance was operative. A mechanism involving two recessive genes was suggested by Sternberg et al. (1951). Burch and Rowell (1965) proposed two distinct subpopulations, both autosomal and sex-linked, to explain a number of discrepancies unaccountable on the basis of previously suggested modes of transmission. It is apparent that the genetic transmission of a psoriatic tendency is more complicated than was previously suspected, and probably reflects the presence of subpopulations involving different genetic loci. Of interest in this regard are recent studies relating two HL-A antigens and psoriasis (Krain, 1974). One of the HL-A antigens, W-17, was found useful as a genetic marker for the detection of a subgroup of psoriatic patients characterized by a high rate of affected relatives and a mean age of onset of 18.2 years. Patients of the subgroup showing antigen HL-A$_{13}$, however, display little or no heritable psoriatic tendency, have milder, more reversible disease than the W-17 subgroup, and often give a history of antecedent streptococcal infections. Interestingly, the HL-A$_{13}$ antigen cross-reacts with a type M protein of group A beta-hemolytic streptococci, a finding which may explain the association of the HL-A$_{13}$ antigen and this particular subgroup of psoriatic patients.

In conclusion, the concept of multifactorial inheritance, which dictates that multiple heritable (that is, polygenic) and environmental factors are necessary for manifestation of the trait, perhaps best explains the predisposition to psoriasis (Watson et al., 1972). Most important of the environmental factors is local trauma, which will be discussed below.

PRECIPITATING FACTORS. Although the majority of patients with psoriasis may give no history of an antecedent precipitating or provocative influence, there is a significant number who do. Trauma, infection, endocrine factors, climate, and emotional stress have all been cited. Psoriasis may first appear at sites of local injury, scars, and vaccinations (Reiss, 1949), presumably as part of the Koebner phenomenon mechanism, the dynamics of which are still unexplained. Infection, especially with hemolytic streptococci, is a not uncommon inciting influence in children, frequently productive of a guttate form of psoriasis (Norrlind, 1955; Whyte and Baughmann, 1964). Psoriasis has appeared after other bacterial and certain viral infections, also, and has cleared with resolution of the infection, although the association and the sequence are not that regular. Pregnancy, possibly as a result of increased corticosteroid secretion, may exert a salutary influence on psoriasis. The effect is less often reproduced by the oral contraceptives, however. Variations in psoriasis with climatic or seasonal change were mentioned earlier. The onset or exacerbation of psoriasis is commonly attributed to emotional stress, but the association is by no means constant or predictable. An occasional patient may actually clear after psychic stress. However, few physicians who have followed large numbers of patients suffering the "heartbreak of psoriasis" would deny the provocative influence of emotional stress in this disease. Personality studies of psoriatic patients have not been revealing.

STRUCTURAL AND BIOCHEMICAL AL-TERATIONS. The two most conspicious alterations in psoriatic skin are the epidermal hyperplasia and the dermal capillary derangements. Which comes first is still debatable, based on the assembled evidence; moreover, a host of biochemical abnormalities, all or most of which reflect the accelerated epidermopoiesis of the disease, have been recorded. The earliest inciting influence, from which the dermal and epidermal alterations would derive, may indeed be chemical in nature. The precise role of focal collections of leukocytes in the early stages of the pathologic process is still unclear.

A geometric analysis of the proliferative epidermis in psoriasis reveals a several-fold increase in the number of germinative basal cells per unit surface area (Soltani and Van Scott, 1972; Van Scott and Ekel, 1963), which is brought about by enlargement and upward proliferation of the dermal papillae and consequent lengthening of the rete ridges. There is also an increase in the mitotic cycle (Weinstein and Frost, 1968). As demonstrated by autoradiographic techniques, the turnover time is dramatically shortened from 28 days to 3 or 4 days (Weinstein and Van Scott, 1965). The rapid transit time for epidermal basal cells results in signs of disturbed keratinization microscopically and clinically. There is a reduction in tonofilament formation and in keratohyaline granules in the precociously developing epidermis. Many chemical abnormalities, including high concentrations of lipids and phospholipids, an increase in acid mucopolysaccharides, alpha amino acids and sulfhydryl groups, and the retention of taurine, are also seen. The increased urinary excretion of uric acid reflects the accelerated formation and degradation of nucleoproteins and correlates with the extent of cutaneous involvement. It should not be regarded as a sign of concurrent gout, although there have been reports of the occasional association of this disease and psoriasis.

The dermal capillary loops of both involved and uninvolved skin of psoriatics are dilated and abnormally tortuous (Holti, 1964). Neutrophils and enzymes may be "squirted" into the epidermis from these distorted vessels (Pinkus and Mehregan, 1966) and stimulate some of the earliest dermo-epidermal changes. Electron microscopic studies have recently revealed markedly attenuated vessel walls and gaps between the endothelial cells, primarily in the arterial capillary and less frequently in the venous capillary and in the postcapillary venule (Braverman et al., 1972). The loss of white and red blood cells and albumin, as well as enzymes and other substances, through these gaps into the dermis and chemotactically into the epidermis is readily appreciated.

Among the possible chemical regulators of epidermal mitotic activity is cyclic-AMP (adenosine-3′,5′-monophosphate), which has been found to be reduced in psoriatic skin (Voorhees et al., 1972). Cyclic-AMP also promotes cellular differentiation and regulates glycogen metabolism, both of which are abnormal in the unstable psoriatic epidermis. If validated, this finding could offer other possible therapeutic approaches to this disease in addition to clarifying its pathogenesis.

The pathogenesis of pustular psoriasis is similar to that of classic psoriasis except that the microabscesses of the latter become visible macroabscesses in pustular psoriasis. Identical vascular changes are found in both diseases (Braverman et al., 1972) and autoradiographic studies reveal an even more rapid proliferation in pustular psoriasis than in ordinary psoriasis (De La Brassine and Couteaux-Dumont, 1972). Hypoalbuminemia, hypocalcemia, hyperuricemia, and other systemic abnormalities may be found in generalized pustular psoriasis, and several strange precipitating influences, such as iodide, progesterone, salicylate, and mycostatin hypersensitivity, have been recorded for this variant.

Clinical Manifestations

Psoriasis presents many faces to the clinician. Although its ravages are limited essentially to the skin and joints, it is a remarkably protean disorder, producing a surprising variety of clinical patterns. The threads of recognizable clinical and histopathologic features bind all of these expressions to a common pathogenetic process, however. It is essential, therefore, for the observer to have a full appreciation of the diagnostic elements of classic psoriatic skin lesions, which must be studiously searched for in some patients. Subtle or obvious distortions of the nails are also frequent findings in the psoriatic, many times clinching the clinical diagnosis. Mysteriously, for a disease which so markedly alters keratinization, alopecia or even minor disturbances in the quality of hair or its rate of growth have never been described. Rare also are true mucosal changes, although involvement of the glans penis is quite common. Pruritus is a variable feature of psoriasis and may bear little relationship to the severity of the disease. The clinical discussion here begins with a description of the vital quali-

ties of the psoriatic skin lesion, and continues with a consideration of the sites of predilection, the Koebner phenomenon, the bacteriology of psoriatic skin, psoriatic nail disease, the various clinical forms of psoriasis, psoriatic arthritis and the systemic associations of psoriasis.

MORPHOLOGY OF THE PSORIATIC LESION. A sharp, definable border, a bright red color, and a silvery white scale delineate the lesions of psoriasis (Fig. 9–1) and reflect the pathologic dynamics of the disease. The sharp border, which can usually be felt as well as seen, abruptly demarcates the epidermal hyperplasia and dermal changes of psoriasis. Interestingly, the skin immediately surrounding the psoriatic patch may appear somewhat paler than

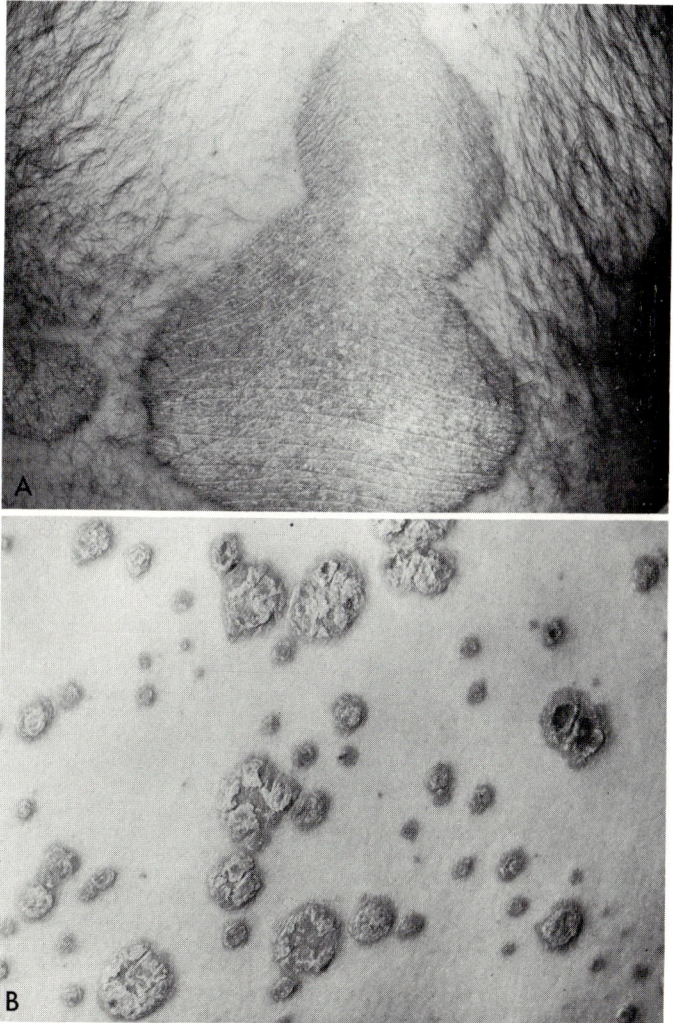

Figure 9–1 Morphology of psoriatic skin lesions. Sharply marginated border and white scales are apparent in close-up views of large plaques (*A*) and smaller guttate lesions (*B*) of psoriasis.

normal skin, and is apparently less reactive to certain therapeutic and pharmacologic stimuli, possibly because of impending or resolving involvement by the inflammatory process. The bright red color, which on dependent areas may have a violaceous hue, is indicative of the dilated superficial vasculature, particularly of the dermal papillae, of psoriasis. These capillaries so closely approach the skin surface at the apex of the elongated dermal papillae that the removal of psoriatic scales frequently produces fine bleeding points (Auspitz sign).

The scale of psoriasis is an almost constant feature, except possibly after effective topical or systemic therapy. Characteristically silvery white, it may assume a duller, less reflective white appearance as the scales become thicker. These scales are normally rather loosely adherent and are the result of the greatly accelerated and incomplete keratinization process. They may be very thin, usually curling slightly as they detach, or may be piled up

and thickened to produce a keratin plate or mound over the erythematous skin lesions.

Pustules are not a regular feature of most clinical types of psoriasis, although on close inspection and with the aid of magnification they can sometimes be seen, especially during acute episodes. Like the lesions of pustular psoriasis, to be discussed later, they apparently represent occasional enlargement, to a grossly visible size, of the microabscesses which are a cardinal microscopic component of the disease.

Bullae have been seen during acute phases of psoriasis, but they are exceptionally rare developments of the pathologic process. Psoriasis does not produce scarring.

SITES OF PREDILECTION. Although no region is exempt from involvement, the areas most commonly affected by psoriasis are the elbows and knees, the scalp, and the lumbosacral skin (Fig. 9–2). If one accepts hat band pressure, hair brushing, or simply rubbing or scratching as sources of

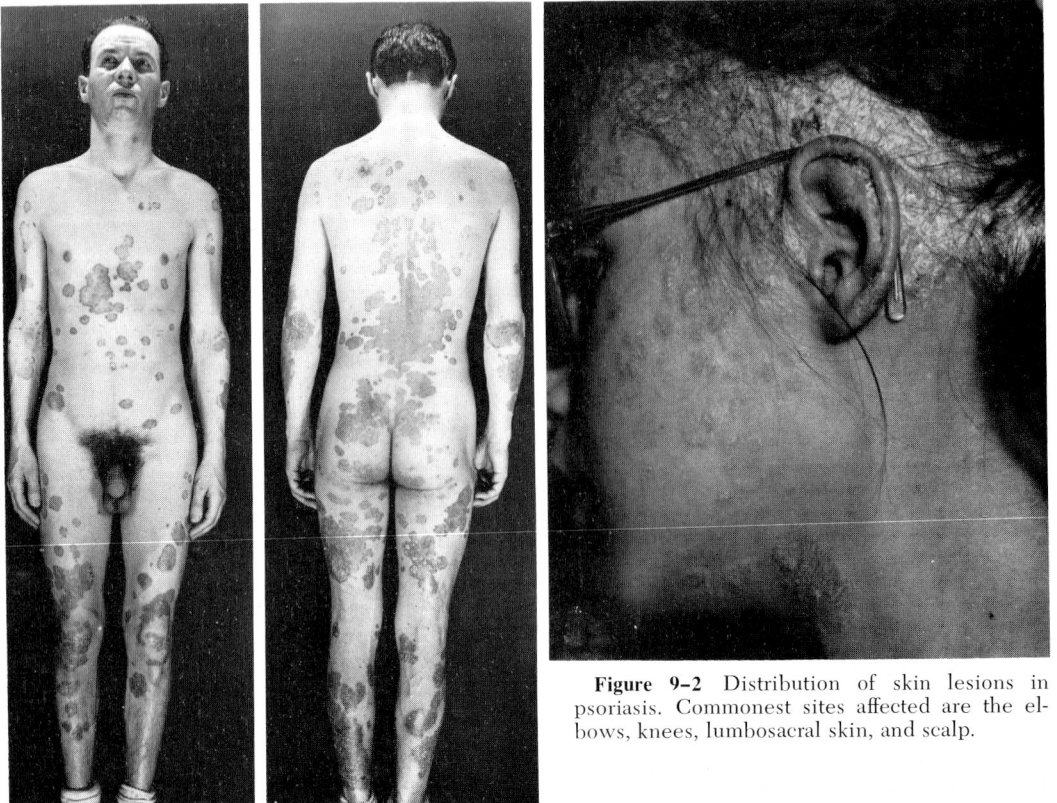

Figure 9–2 Distribution of skin lesions in psoriasis. Commonest sites affected are the elbows, knees, lumbosacral skin, and scalp.

injury for the scalp skin, all of these sites have in common a tendency to fairly regular local trauma. These common localizations have been attributed to Koebner or isomorphic reactions. The predisposition of scalp skin may have another explanation, of course, for local injury may not be a factor in the majority of patients. Flexural or inverse psoriasis, in which the intertriginous areas are involved, is a less common distribution pattern, although it can be combined with "extensor surface" psoriasis. If severe and uncontrolled, psoriasis can produce a generalized exfoliative erythroderma.

It has been postulated (Van Scott and Ekel, 1963) that involvement of most mucosal surfaces (mouth and vagina) is absent because these epithelial surfaces are normally as rapidly proliferative as is psoriatic skin, with turnover times as short as the skin lesions of psoriasis. Parakeratotic stratum corneum normally formed on these moist mucosal surfaces is presumably shed quickly and not seen. Mucosal surfaces with slower, "orthokeratotic" maturation of epidermis, such as the glans penis, may show psoriatic lesions.

PSORIATIC NAIL DISEASE. Nail involvement is common in psoriasis, and is seen in at least 30 per cent of cases, especially those of long standing (Fig. 9–3). Fingernails show changes more often than do toenails. Pitting or punctate dimpling of the nail plate is the most common finding and results from focal psoriasis in that part of the nail matrix that gives rise to the superficial nail plate (Zaias, 1969). The resultant punctate parakeratotic psoriatic horn falls out of the newly emergent nail, leaving a small pitlike deformity. Yellowish discoloration and onycholysis of the nail at the free or lateral edges may also be seen along with subungual hyperkeratosis, thickening and crumbling, and splitting or grooving of the nail. These findings reflect psoriasis of the hyponychium and distal nail bed.

It is important to realize that psoriasis does not produce the destructive cicatricial change of lichen planus which may result in a bandlike pterygium or loss of the nail. Acute fulminant psoriasis or pustular psoriasis affecting the paronychial and proximal nail fold skin may also result in nail dystrophy. Classic psoriatic arthritis, affecting the distal interphalangeal joints, is usually associated with nail dystrophy (Baker et al., 1964). Nail involvement in the absence of psoriatic skin lesions is rare and would be difficult to prove. It is sometimes seen in young children. Careful examination of the psoriatic patient usually reveals some psoriatic skin change, or will in time.

The thickened or onycholytic psoriatic nail or subungual tissue frequently contains *Candida albicans* and Pseudomonas organisms. The latter may at times produce a greenish discoloration of the nails.

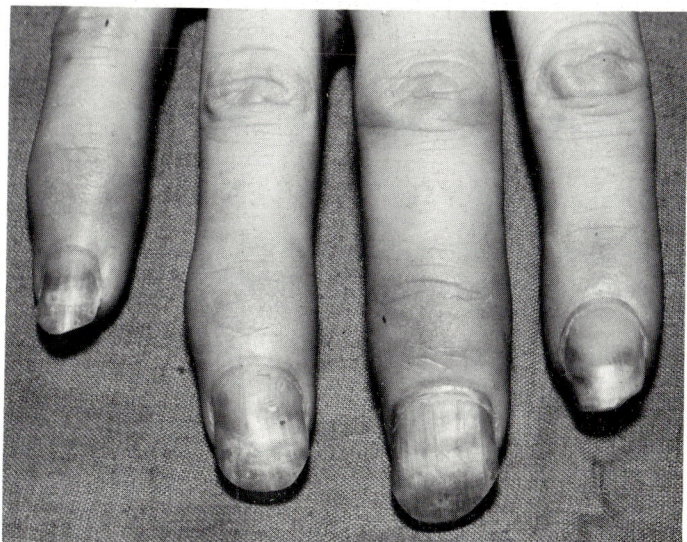

Figure 9–3 Nail changes in psoriasis. Note characteristic pitting or dimpling of the nail plate and onycholysis of the distal nail. Thickening and yellowish discoloration of the nail and subungual hyperkeratosis are also commonly seen.

The psoriatic nail is apparently peculiarly resistant to invasion by superficial (ringworm) fungi, however (White and Laipply, 1952).

THE KOEBNER OR ISOMORPHIC PHENOMENON. Among the special features of psoriasis is the capacity to reproduce skin lesions at sites of local injury (Eddy et al., 1964; Farber et al., 1965; Hellgren, 1964; Hurley and Shelley, 1955). Originally described by Koebner in 1877, this reactive phenomenon has intrigued many investigators searching for basic clues to the cause of psoriasis. Although best-known in psoriasis, the Koebner phenomenon may occur also in certain other skin diseases, notably lichen planus, lichen nitidus, pityriasis rubra pilaris, and Darier's disease. Moreover, a pathogenetic role for the Koebner phenomenon in psoriatic arthritis has also been suggested (Moll and Wright, 1973). While the precise mechanism is unknown, the important features of the Koebner or isomorphic phenomenon in psoriasis can be summarized as follows:

1. The reaction may follow simple irritation, physical injury, wounds, sunburn (Fig. 9–4), x-radiation, vaccination, or may occur in preexisting disease, such as an eczematous dermatitis or an old scar.

2. The trauma must reach or act on the papillary layer of the dermis, but epidermal injury is also necessary. Simple vasodilatation, vasoconstriction, or suction injury which spares the epidermis will not evoke the reaction.

3. It occurs in almost half but apparently not in all psoriatics at some time during their disease.

4. The Koebner reaction can be enhanced or inhibited by certain chemicals and cytotoxic agents.

5. An interval of 8 to 10 days after the injury usually precedes the development of the psoriatic skin lesion but it may appear within 3 days or be delayed as long as 18 days. Capillary alterations precede the skin changes.

6. When it follows an accident, industrial injury, or medical therapy, the Koebner phenomenon may have medicolegal importance.

7. The practical significance of the Koebner phenomenon as a precipitating cause of psoriatic skin lesions should be emphasized to all patients with the disease.

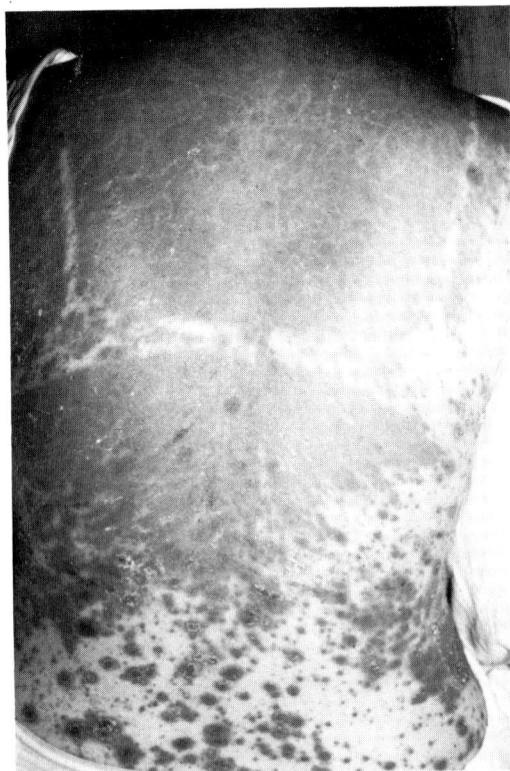

Figure 9–4 Sunburn-induced Koebner phenomenon in psoriasis.

Avoidance of local skin injury may significantly decrease the cutaneous involvement in some patients.

BACTERIOLOGY OF PSORIASIS. The colonization of dermatitic skin by bacteria not only may result in secondary infection and aggravation of the skin lesions but also may provide a significant source of infection to other individuals, particularly those in the hospital. Microbiologic studies have revealed increased numbers of *Staphylococcus aureus* and resident cocci on involved as opposed to the uninvolved skin of psoriatics (Marples et al., 1973), although the number of organisms found was not remarkably high. Moreover, occlusion of the skin lesions with a vapor-impermeable plastic film led to a dramatic increase of all organisms, especially *S. aureus*, which apparently increases disproportionately to the remainder of the flora. Frank pustule formation or impetiginous crusting was not seen with this increased staphylococcal growth, but an intensification of the inflammatory process was evident along with a relative resistance of the lesions to otherwise effective topical medicaments, such as corticosteroids. This refractoriness could be reversed by local treatment with broad-spectrum antibiotics. It is possible that the improvement in psoriatic skin lesions sometimes seen after systemic and local antibiotics may be directly attributable to the reduction of the microflora.

Although nosocomial infection from psoriatic skin lesions has in fact been reported quite infrequently, exfoliation of psoriasis scales is a definite hazard as a source of hospital cross-infection (Payne, 1967). It is to be emphasized that the lesions of pustular psoriasis, both the localized and generalized varieties, are sterile, at least until ruptured.

CLINICAL FORMS OF PSORIASIS. *Common Plaque or Nummular Psoriasis.* The commonest form of the disease is the plaque or nummular variety in which round or oval lesions of one to many centimeters are found on the elbows or knees, scalp and trunk (Fig. 9–2). After an insidious onset, this type of psoriasis may remain stationary for long periods of time. Exacerbations may bring small guttate lesions along with the large plaques (Fig. 9–5). Serpiginous, annular, gyrate, and zonal arrangement of lesions may be seen along with Koebner-induced linear papules produced by scratching. Thick, inveterate, or rupial plaques may occur in patients with very chronic involvement of the elbows, knees, or hips.

Inverse or Flexural Psoriasis. Psoriasis can involve the intertriginous folds of the axillae and of inguinal, inframammary, intergluteal, and perianal skin either as the dominant clinical expression or in association with lesions of other sites (Fig. 9–3). At times, flexural psoriasis can be difficult to distinguish from seborrheic dermatitis, especially early in its development, and the terms "seborrheic psoriasis" or "seborrhiasis" have been applied to this condition. Because of the maceration produced by wetness and rubbing, flexural psoriasis may often be a stubborn therapeutic problem. Bacteria are often quite numerous in the lesions.

Guttate Psoriasis. The abrupt appearance of a shower of small, droplike psoriasis lesions with a less prominent scale than usual over much of the skin surface, but especially on the trunk and proximal extremities, should suggest this special syndrome. It is seen primarily in children

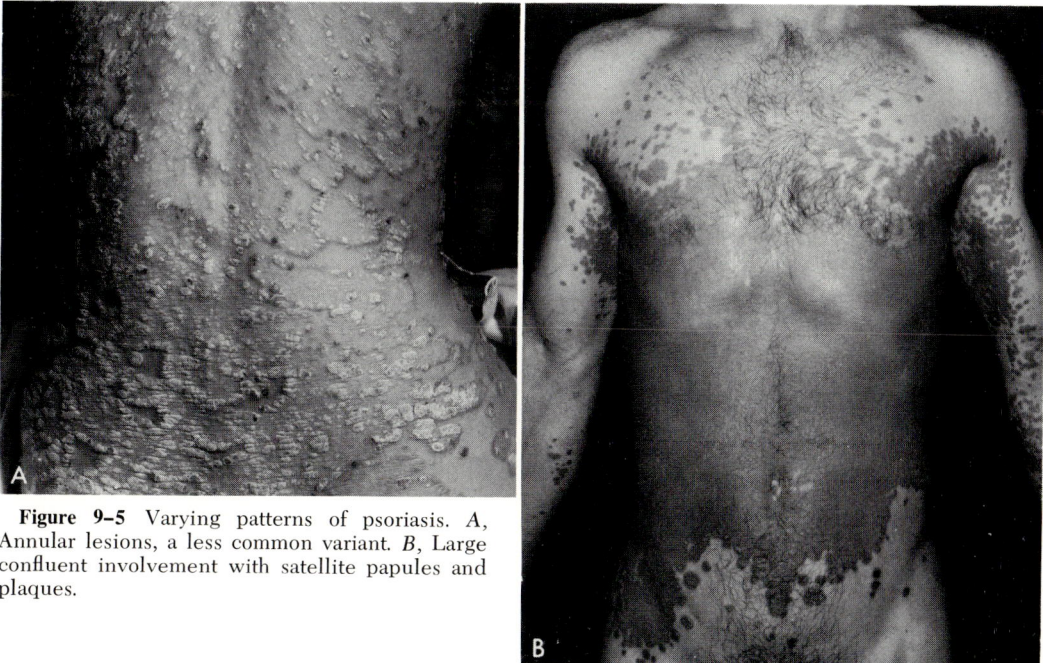

Figure 9–5 Varying patterns of psoriasis. *A,* Annular lesions, a less common variant. *B,* Large confluent involvement with satellite papules and plaques.

and young adults and commonly occurs a few weeks after streptococcal infections (Whyte and Baughmann, 1964). Elevated ASO titers are usually found. The lesions often gradually disappear after resolution of the infection.

Palmar Psoriasis. A distinctive, patchy, hyperkeratotic type of psoriasis affecting principally contact points of the volar surface of the fingers and palms, this form of the disease may exist alone or in combination with mild psoriasis, usually of the elbows, knees, and scalp. The lesions are thought to be related to local physical or chemical injury and are thus volar Koebner phenomena. It may involve one palm more than the other, as in tennis players, golfers, or industrial workers. Strangely, the same changes are less common on the soles. Palmar psoriasis is often confused with chronic contact dermatitis. It runs a protracted course of a few to several years, but may persist indefinitely. Palmar psoriasis is to be distinguished from pustular psoriasis of the palms and soles.

Psoriasiform Neurodermatitis. Chronic psoriatic plaques may itch intensely, provoking considerable scratching and a lichenoid appearance. A rather common syndrome, however, is the lichenoid neurodermatitis of the occipital scalp and nape of the neck which develops a psoriasiform appearance (Fig. 9–6). The majority of patients with this condition, usually women, have no psoriasis elsewhere, and would best be regarded as having a primary neurodermatitis rather than psoriasis. A minority do show evidence of some psoriasis at other sites, however.

Pustular Psoriasis. There are two clinically dissimilar conditions to which the name pustular psoriasis has been applied, namely, localized pustular psoriasis (Barber) and generalized pustular psoriasis (Von Zumbusch).

Localized Pustular Psoriasis. Also known as pustular psoriasis of the palms and soles, this sterile pustular eruption affects the digits and volar skin of the hands or feet, or both, usually in the presence of papulosquamous psoriasis elsewhere. The paronychial skin may be involved, with swelling, erythema, and considerable local discomfort (Fig. 9–7). Upon remission, the areas may remain scaly and red, with a ten-

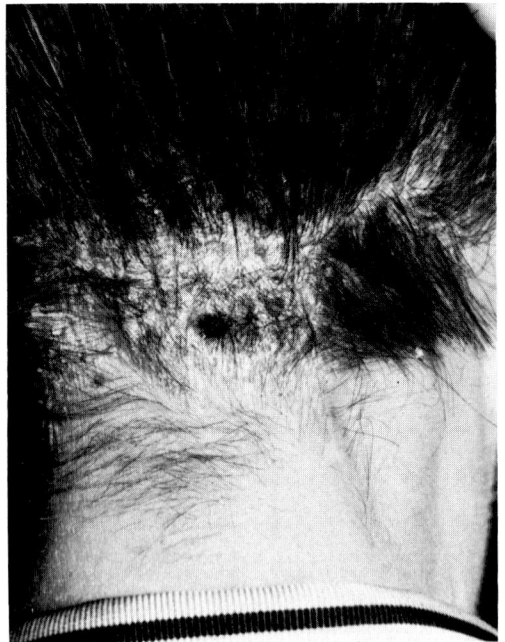

Figure 9–6 Characteristic site for psoriasiform neurodermatitis.

dency to fissure, but will show only an occasional pustule. These pustules may be hemorrhagic. Histologically the lesions infrequently show the epidermal and dermal features of psoriasis but regularly exhibit unilocular intra-epidermal pustules which are filled with neutrophils and are free of bacteria. There is also some inflammatory exudate in the dermis. Patients with this condition are otherwise well with no clinical or laboratory evidence of other organ system involvement. The process runs a chronic course with only a slim chance of significant remission. Localized pustular psoriasis is difficult to distinguish from pustular bacterid, which allegedly is a reaction to a focus of infection elsewhere in the body, and from acrodermatitis continua and dermatitis repens, which are of unknown etiology and are purportedly different histologically because of the presence of the spongiform pustules of Kogoj.

Generalized Pustular Psoriasis (Von Zumbusch). Generalized pustular psoriasis is a rare, at times fatal, pustular eruption developing suddenly in psoriatic patients with mild to moderate involvement, or in those with psoriatic arthritis or exfoliative psoriasis. The attacks are preceded by high fever, leukocytosis, arthralgia, malaise, and other constitutional signs. An aura of burning may occur prior to the appearance of the erythema and pustules which are seen in groups de novo or in and around old lesions of psoriasis, especially in the inguinal, axillary, and other flexural areas. The pustules may coalesce, thereby forming large lakes or sheets of pus. Around the nails the changes may be especially annoying, and subungual collections of pus are not uncommon with the thickened dystrophic nails. The tongue and buccal mucosa may also be involved. The attacks subside gradually within several days to weeks; the skin desquamates and gradually returns to its normal state. Hypocalcemia, possibly related to hypoalbuminemia (Braverman et al., 1972), is often seen, as in impetigo herpetiformis. Generalized pustular psoriasis may occur in children, often without antecedent papular psoriasis. It has a better prognosis than the adult disease and is more likely to resolve spontaneously after a few weeks of bland topical therapy (Khan et al., 1972).

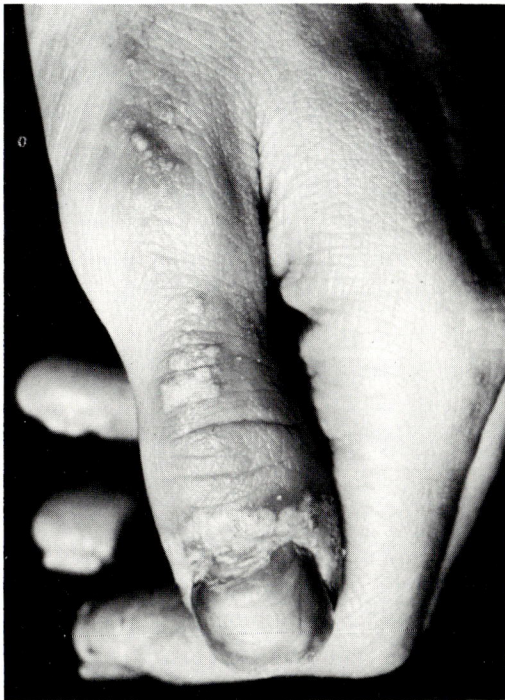

Figure 9-7 Localized pustular psoriasis. Note intense paronychial inflammation with pustules and nail dystrophy.

Pustular psoriasis has been precipitated by systemic steroids (Braverman et al., 1972; Champion, 1959), iodide, salicylates, and progesterone (Shelley, 1972), penicillin (Privat et al., 1969), and nystatin (Petrozzi and Witkowski, 1971), the latter in a patient sensitive to Candida antigens, which were apparently released and absorbed after administration of the nystatin. The course of generalized pustular psoriasis is little influenced by any therapy, including high dosage corticosteroids and methotrexate. The successful treatment of several patients with high doses of cloxacillin and cephaloridine (Malkinson and Pearson, 1972) awaits confirmation.

Recurrent attacks are usually progressively more severe and death from infection or electrolyte imbalance is eventually seen in many of the patients.

Exfoliative Psoriasis. Exfoliative or erythrodermic psoriasis may develop from chronic psoriasis or rarely may occur as the initial manifestation of the disease. It may appear as a reaction to topical therapy or as a result of too vigorous light therapy, which provokes extension of the psoriasis to a more generalized erythrodermic condition. Patients with exfoliative psoriasis generally are responsive to other therapy, thoughtfully employed, and will usually remit to their original psoriatic state. Some, however, behave as if they have a serious systemic illness, showing constitutional signs and resistance to treatment. The latter group often have psoriatic arthritis, or less commonly, generalized pustular psoriasis. These patients have a grave prognosis, show little tendency to remit appreciably, demonstrate increasing toxicity, and may die.

Psoriatic Arthritis. Although the association between psoriasis and an inflammatory arthritis has been known for over 150 years (Alibert, 1818), the recognition of psoriatic arthritis as a distinct clinical entity awaited the accumulation of epidemiologic, genetic, clinical, radiologic, and laboratory evidence over the past three decades (Moll and Wright, 1973; Reed, 1961; Wright and Moll, 1971).

Psoriasis has been shown to be more common among arthritics, and arthritis more common in psoriatics, than either disease is in the normal population (Baker, 1966). More precisely, Leczinsky (1948) in a 10-year survey, found the prevalence of arthritis in psoriatic patients to be 6.8 percent, which is well above that of arthritis in the non-psoriatic population. Although females show a greater tendency to develop psoriatic arthritis than do males, this preponderance may be attributable to the decided female predilection for one type of psoriatic arthritis, namely, that which is indistinguishable from rheumatoid arthritis.

Genetic factors are of demonstrable importance in the pathogenesis of psoriatic arthritis (Moll and Wright, 1973) just as they are in psoriasis. Moreover, the findings favor a multifactorial form of inheritance as has been suggested in studies of psoriasis also. Among the environmental influences, trauma has been deemed important in precipitating psoriatic arthritis in genetically predisposed individuals. Thus, joint injury may be viewed as a Koebner phenomenon similar, in concept at least, to the Koebner phenomenon-induced lesions of cutaneous psoriasis. As to the possible mechanism of this trauma-inducing effect, an enzyme deficiency resulting in lower joint levels of hyaluronic acid, which purportedly makes the joint tissue more vulnerable (Cotton and Muir, 1964), and a neurotrophic effect, analogous to that seen in leprosy, diabetes, and syphilis, have been proposed.

A more distinct clinical image of psoriatic arthritis has also emerged in recent years. It now appears clear that three major clinical types of psoriatic arthritis may be defined:

1. Patients with distal interphalangeal arthritis as the exclusive or predominant clinical expression (Fig. 9–6). This was the group of patients who for years were accepted as having "classic psoriatic arthritis" since they clearly did not fit the usual pattern of digital involvement in rheumatoid arthritis which preferentially affects the proximal interphalangeal and metacarpophalangeal joints.

2. Patients with clinical arthritis mutilans often complicated by digital "telescoping" and those showing involvement of the sacroiliac joints. Increasing attention has been paid to what has been called psoriatic spondylitis, which some regard as a very special variant of psoriatic arthritis. It is not yet clear whether psoriatic spondylitis is the equivalent of idiopathic ankylosing spondylitis; this is the view of many observers, however. Although a peripheral psoriatic arthritis overshadows the sa-

croiliitis in many of these patients, the reverse clinical picture with negligible digital involvement may also be seen. Reed (1961) has emphasized the possible development of a special form of spondylitic heart disease, characterized by aortic insufficiency, persistent conduction defects, and otherwise inexplicable cardiomegaly, in patients with psoriatic spondylitis. A pustular or exudative form of psoriasis appears to be more common in these patients.

3. Patients demonstrating an arthritic pattern indistinguishable from that of rheumatoid arthritis. These patients would show the usual clinical elements of rheumatoid arthritis, such as early morning stiffness, symmetric involvement, fusiform swelling of the proximal finger joints, ultimately ulnar deviation, rheumatoid nodules, and, commonly, rheumatoid factor in the serum.

The onset of psoriatic arthritis is usually insidious, but an acute, goutlike beginning is seen occasionally. The age of onset is similar for psoriatic arthritis and rheumatoid arthritis. The traditional view that the onset of arthritis coincides with that of skin lesions is apparently no longer valid (Baker et al., 1963). Actually a closer temporal relationship has been demonstrated for nail and joint involvement (Wright, 1956). Over 80 per cent of patients with psoriatic arthritis have nail involvement, and a correlation between involvement of distal joints and the associated nails has been observed.

Other clinical findings that have been found at times in psoriatic arthritis include high fever, sclerodactyly, minimal adenopathy, absence of subcutaneous nodules, little muscle wasting, occasional tendon sheath effusions, ocular inflammation, and gastrointestinal amyloidosis (Wright and Moll, 1971).

It must be recognized that other seronegative arthritides such as Reiter's disease, Behçet's syndrome, the intestinal arthritides, and idiopathic ankylosing spondylitis may show many of the clinical features of psoriatic arthritis and at times are difficult if not impossible to distinguish from it.

X-ray examination of affected joints reveals a number of changes which are characteristic of, if not entirely specific for, psoriatic arthritis (Avila et al., 1960; Baker, 1965). These include:

1. Predilection for distal interphalangeal joints with relative sparing of metacarpo-

phalangeal, metatarsophalangeal, and proximal interphalangeal joints.

2. "Whittling" of terminal phalanges.

3. "Pencil in cup" changes

4. Peripheral arthritis mutilans showing marked osteolysis and ankylosis.

5. Gross destruction of isolated small joints.

6. "Fluffy" periostitis.

7. Atypical spondylitis. Paravertebral ossification has also been described in psoriatic spondylitis but apparently is a rare finding (Wright and Moll, 1971).

Histologic study of synovial fluid and joint tissue specimens has not revealed any significant microscopic distinction between psoriatic arthritis and rheumatoid arthritis (Bauer et al., 1941; Delbarre, 1967), although an excessive fibrous reaction has been empahsized in psoriatic arthritis (Costa and Solnica, 1966).

The regular absence of rheumatoid factor in the serum is the most important laboratory finding in psoriatic arthritis. Serologic tests for L.E. cells, antinuclear factor, and other auto-antibodies are also negative. Hyperuricemia is found in 10 to 20 per cent of patients but it is usually only a mild elevation over the normal. Other nonspecific findings that may be found include anemia and increased sedimentation rate, both of which are more pronounced during more severe attacks, and elevated gamma and alpha-2 globulins (Baker et al., 1963).

The course of psoriatic arthritis can be expected to be chronic, with remissions and exacerbations, as in cutaneous psoriasis. Resolution of skin lesions may be followed by improvement of psoriatic arthritis but this is not a constant relationship. Psoriatic arthritis tends to be less painful and disabling than rheumatoid arthritis except for the rare cases of arthritis mutilans, which are incapacitating. In severe cases, death is possible and not uncommonly results from complications of corticosteroid therapy (Reed and Wright, 1966).

The treatment of psoriatic arthritis is the responsibility of the rheumatologist and will not be considered here. It is worth emphasizing, nevertheless, that antimalarial drugs are contraindicated because of the significant danger of exfoliative dermatitis in these patients. Gold carries no such high risk of an untoward reaction, however; it is no more likely to produce signs of

toxicity in psoriatic arthritis than in rheumatoid arthritis.

SYSTEMIC ASSOCIATIONS. The major concomitant organ system involvement in psoriasis is inflammatory arthritis, as discussed above. Indeed, other systemic associations are unusual in psoriasis, although two are worthy of mention. A psoriatic myopathy has been described (Mom et al., 1970); in addition, a dermatogenic enteropathy, the frequency and severity of which are directly proportional to the extent of the skin involvement, may also develop in exfoliative psoriasis (Shuster, 1968). A similar enteropathy can apparently be seen in other extensive dermatoses. It is to be distinguished from the enteropathy of dermatitis herpetiformis, however, from which it differs in several respects. Certain patients with psoriatic arthritis may also show the rare complications of spondylitic heart disease, ocular inflammation, and gastrointestinal amyloidosis, as discussed above.

Histopathology

The microscopic features of psoriasis reflect the increased cellular activity of the epidermis and the dermal alterations which were outlined earlier under the heading Etiology and Pathogenesis. They show some variation, however, depending on the age and clinical form of the lesions, their location, and the influence of treatment.

The salient histopathologic findings of psoriasis include:

1. Acanthosis, with elongation of the rete ridges.

2. Elongation and clubbing of the dermal papillae.

3. Parakeratosis, usually dominating an associated hyperkeratosis.

4. Thinning or absence of the granular layer, a consequence of the epidermal proliferation.

5. Increased mitoses primarily in the multiple layers of basal cells of the psoriatic lesions and possibly in the lower malpighian layer. This is to be contrasted with the presence of mitoses only in the single basal cell layer of normal skin.

6. Edema and a mild to moderate dermal infiltrate consisting primarily of lymphocytes and monocytes.

7. Epidermal microabscesses composed of focal collections of neutrophils in the stratum corneum or immediately below it. These ab-

scesses are to be differentiated from the mononuclear microabscesses of mycosis fungoides. Microabscesses indistinguishable from those of psoriasis can be seen also in some lesions of seborrheic dermatitis, acrodermatitis continua, and keratosis blenorrhagica.

8. Under the electron microscope, changes reflecting the increased epidermopoiesis are seen, including reduction in tonofilament formation, decreased desmosomes, increased mitoses, and the abnormal retention of nuclei, endoplasmic reticulum, and mitochondria in the outer layers.

The constellation of changes described above should prompt a histologic diagnosis of psoriasis but other conditions, especially localized neurodermatitis and seborrheic dermatitis, may resemble psoriasis and at times may be difficult or impossible to differentiate.

Diagnosis

In patients with well-developed skin lesions in the usual areas, the diagnosis of psoriasis should pose no problem. While suggestive of or consistent with psoriasis, the histopathologic findings are not specific and thus will not establish the diagnosis with certainty. Other papulosquamous eruptions may be difficult to distinguish in certain patients, although continued observation should permit the development and recognition of distinctive clinical features of the disease and allow an unequivocal diagnosis. Lichen planus, seborrheic dermatitis, parapsoriasis, pityriasis rubra pilaris, and pityriasis rosea are representative of this group of eruptions. Seborrheic dermatitis may easily be confused or may coexist with flexural psoriasis, virtually preventing meaningful separation of the disorders. Drug eruptions may also mimic psoriasis, just as they can simulate almost every other skin eruption. Some of the special or atypical expressions of psoriasis may be imitated by Reiter's syndrome, mycosis fungoides, psoriasiform tertiary syphilis, localized neurodermatitis, certain superficial fungal infections, and congenital ichthyosiform erythroderma. In all of these disorders, the diagnosis is usually possible by a careful study of the clinical features, biopsy examination, and appropriate laboratory studies. Cytologic study of psoriatic scales using a special adhesive slide technique may be helpful in differentiating psoriasis from many other dermatoses, although not from seborrheic dermatitis or mycosis fungoides (Goldschmidt and Thew, 1973).

There are no laboratory tests which will identify psoriasis. The blood count, urinalysis, sedimentation rate, and other hematologic, chemical, and serologic studies should be within normal limits in most cases of psoriasis. An elevated blood uric acid may be found in 10 to 20 per cent of patients with psoriasis, especially those with widespread involvement. Moreover, there are certain nonspecific laboratory findings in some patients with psoriatic arthritis which are discussed earlier in this chapter (p. 421).

Treatment

Although the etiology of psoriasis remains obscure, enough is known of its pathogenesis to explain the efficacy of modern day therapy and that of much of the older treatment that has been employed. Most if not all of the predictably effective modes of therapy, old and new, apparently clear the skin of lesions by inhibiting the accelerated epidermal proliferation characteristic of psoriasis. What is uncertain, however, is whether or not a remission of significant duration, at least several months, can be achieved in any given patient by therapy, even that which predictably resolves the skin lesions within days. In general, it can be said that the more dramatically effective remedies, notably the systemic cytotoxic medications and the corticosteroids, are less likely to produce a lasting remission. Such drugs are used in the more severe psoriatic who is less likely to remit, but even when used in patients with milder psoriasis, long remissions are not the rule. Indeed, when these medications are discontinued or the dosage is lowered, the psoriasis often flares. This is especially true of the corticosteroids.

Before initiating therapy, the physician should explain to the patient that treatment is not expected to permanently cure his disease but that a remission of months to years is possible and is the desired objective. It should be explained further that psoriasis is not a contagious disease, that there is very little likelihood that the patient's general health will be affected nor will other organs be involved, although the slight risk of an inflammatory arthritis must be acknowledged. Finally, while total clearing of the skin lesions is desirable, a few small, insignificant, and essentially asymptomatic, scaly papules may be best ignored unless they are cosmetically compromising. There is a good chance that some or all of these lesions will in time clear spontaneously or with the summer sun.

GENERAL MEASURES. A weight reduction program is sometimes helpful in the management of the psoriatic and should be instituted in all overweight individuals. The beneficial effect is probably related principally to a reduction in the supply of protein. It has been demonstrated that a starvation diet will frequently result in resolution of psoriatic skin lesions (Lerner and Lerner, 1964, Simons, 1949). Patients who are not overweight are not likely to clear from any diet short of a starvation diet, whether it be of a weight reduction type or one which eliminates a specific amino acid, protein, lipid, vitamin, mineral, or any other dietary constituent (Zackheim and Farber, 1969). In short, patients should be advised to eat as balanced a diet as possible, to avoid excessive weight gain, and to ignore the suggestions of overzealous relatives and friends who "prescribe" the elimination from or addition to the diet of any food or dietary element.

During an acute episode, the possibility of minimizing or relieving emotional stress should be explored, although psychotherapy is certainly not recommended as a routine approach. Vacations are surprisingly beneficial in some patients, not unlike the effect of hospitalization without a change in therapy. If sleeping is a problem, nighttime sedation, at least until the acute phase has subsided, is desirable. Ataractics or antihistamines may be used to minimize pruritus but none of these drugs regularly produces a marked antipruritic effect.

Inquiry and study of the patient regarding a preceding acute or chronic focus of infection may prove very rewarding. The most dramatic cases are those with guttate psoriasis following streptococcal pharyngitis, but other less well-documented examples of infection-induced psoriasis are known also and eradication of an existing infection is an avenue which should never be overlooked.

The importance of the Koebner phenomenon in precipitating new lesions is worth stressing, especially in certain forms of psoriasis. Excessive scratching should be avoided, therefore, and sun or ultraviolet light exposure, which in moderate doses is usually helpful in most patients, should never be excessive in order to prevent a sunburn-induced Koebner reaction. In palmar psoriasis, the occupation and hobbies of the individual may have to be investigated to expose a source of local trauma to the volar skin.

SPECIFIC THERAPY. Few maladies have been exposed to more empiric therapeutic measures than has psoriasis. Most have been discarded because of toxicity or lack of efficacy. Vitamin B_{12} injections and B complex therapy have no consistently beneficial effect. Indomethacin has not been helpful (Kern, 1966), nor has penicillamine or other chelating agents. Although their value in light-induced psoriasis has been stressed (O'Quinn, 1964), chloroquine and other antimalarials are probably contraindicated in psoriasis because of their tendency to induce exfoliative dermatitis (Baker, 1966). Calciferol and vitamin D have no place in the treatment of the psoriatic, nor has autohemotherapy, liver injections, systemic vitamin A, or arsenic. Topical ammoniated mercury is also of limited value and with the advent of safer, more effective therapy, has all but been abandoned. Griseofulvin and levodopa (Barbeau and Giroux, 1972) are other remedies of purported efficacy which deserve further study.

A number of rational, predictable forms of therapy are currently available. Properly employed they provide an effective approach to the care of most patients with psoriasis. During the acute eruptive phase, therapy should be more conservative, with bland topical preparations predominating. In general, psoriatics prefer occlusive ointment bases such as petrolatum or a hydrophobic cream which produce a greater lubricating or softening effect and with which there is less curling and movement of the scales than with a hydrophilic cream or lotion. In hairy flexural areas such as the axilla and inguinal skin, the hydrophilic vehicles are better tolerated. Wet dressings with aqueous solutions, dispersible oil or tar oil suspensions, or propylene glycol–water mixtures (40/60) facilitate removal of scales and provide symptomatic relief of pruritus. Scalp lesions may be treated with lotions or creams. Removal of scales is facilitated by shampooing with or without preliminary compresses with warm mineral oil.

Topical Corticosteroids. Depending on their concentration, frequency and technique of application, and the type and severity of the psoriasis, almost all of the topical corticosteroid preparations are more or less effective in suppressing the skin lesions. They act primarily as antiinflammatory agents and secondarily retard the excessive epidermal proliferation. Hydrocortisone in 1 per cent concentration and above, betamethasone valerate (0.1 per cent), triamcinolone acetonide (0.1 per cent), fluocinolone acetonide (0.025 per cent), and fluocinonide (0.05 per cent) are among the most effective topical corticosteroids. High potency topical corticosteroids, such as fluocinolone acetonide (0.2 per cent) and triamcinolone acetonide (0.5 per cent), are also available for short-term use on small skin areas which are especially recalcitrant. In general, petrolatum or other hydrophobic bases are preferred by psoriatics but hydrophilic creams or lotions are comfortable in many patients and are especially suitable for flexural and hairy areas.

The effects of topical corticosteroids can be enhanced considerably by occlusion of the skin surface with polyvinylidine or polyethylene plastic films, which markedly increase the percutaneous absorption of the medication. These are available as gloves, boots, bags, and suits (the plastic "jogging suit" is a suitable general body occlusive cover). Moreover, the incorporation of corticosteroid into a polyethylene adhesive tape has facilitated the treatment of certain limited areas with the occlusive method. Local atrophy and striae are complications of long-term use of topical steroids, especially under occlusion. With widespread application, there is measurable systemic absorption of the corticosteroid (Champion, 1966).

Tars. Tars of various types have long been used in psoriasis and are still popular today in wet dressings, shampoos, and other topical preparations. Their action is still unclarified, although an anti-inflammatory effect is acknowledged as at least one effect. A common practice in the management of extensive psoriasis is the use of tar baths daily prior to the application of topical corticosteroids or in conjunction with ultraviolet light (U.V.L.) treatments as part of the *Goeckerman technique.* There are many modifications of the latter treatment method which consists essentially of a series of progressively stronger U.V.L. treatments along with the local use of tars to sensitize the psoriatic skin to the ultraviolet radiation. Crude coal tar in petrolatum (4 to 10 per cent) is perhaps the most effective tar for the technique but it is messy and unpleasant to use. Liquor carbonis detergens solution or in 5 to 10 per cent concentration in a hydrophilic cream, with or without salicylic acid (3 to 5 per cent), is more palatable. The patient should bathe or wash off the scales and residual topical medication prior to the light therapy, which should be given daily or every other day and should be pushed to the erythema level but not beyond. The Goeckerman regimen may be performed on an outpatient basis but in severe cases is best used in the hospital where the added advantages of rest, sedation, and simply change of environment enhance the therapeutic effect. The new Psoriasis Day Care Center concept, which permits ambulatory full or partial day treatment programs usually over periods of two to three weeks, utilizes the Goeckerman regimen as well as other treatment methods such as the Ingram technique (Farber, 1974). Properly used, the Goeckerman regimen is one of the safest and most effective treatments available for psoriasis, and is among the best ways to induce a lasting remission. Complications include folliculitis and occasionally aggravation of the disease, if the light therapy is too aggressive or if the patient is in an acute eruptive stage or is sensitive to tar.

Ingram Technique. An effective treatment developed in England consists of daily tar baths and gentle scrubbing to remove excessive scales, followed by ultraviolet light therapy and subsequent application of anthralin in 0.1 to 0.8 per cent concentration in a stiff Lassar's paste (Bowers et al., 1966; Ingram, 1953). An anthralin pomade can be used on the scalp. The weaker strengths should be employed initially, and it is usually not necessary to proceed beyond 0.5 per cent. Cotton stockinette dressings or pajamas are worn while the paste is on the skin overnight. Care should be taken to avoid contacting the eyes with the anthralin. Local yellow-brown staining of the skin is a transient aftereffect of the anthralin but should not discourage its use. Anthralin apparently has a low order of systemic toxicity even when used over wide areas of the body (Gay et al., 1972). The ultraviolet therapy can be omitted from the above routine with little loss of efficacy in many patients.

Intralesional Corticosteroids. Prompt resolution of small areas of psoriasis can be accomplished through intralesional injection of corticosteroid suspension either through a small (26 gauge) needle or pressure jet injection apparatus. The most commonly used steroid is triamcinolone acetonide in a 0.1 to 2 per cent concentration. The steroid must be in suspension so that the injected particles will remain localized to the inflamed skin to exert their effect over weeks to several months. It may be diluted to any desired concentration with saline or a local anesthetic which minimizes the injection pain. Local atrophy may follow the injection of too concentrated a suspension of triamcinolone, but this usually disappears within 6 to 9 months. Repeated or excessive use of this technique can also lead to systemic effects of the injected corticosteroid.

Systemic Corticosteroids. Oral or parenteral corticosteroid treatment of psoriasis is indicated only for the severe or life-threatening forms of the disease, such as exfoliative psoriasis, certain cases of generalized pustular psoriasis, and psoriatic arthritis. A "rebound" effect upon cessation of therapy is the rule with these drugs, and their prolonged use leads inevitably to one or more signs of toxicity. Triamcinolone seems to be the most dramatically effective of the steroids but also may be productive of certain distinctive side effects, particularly myopathy. Intramuscular injection of triamcinolone is preferable in some patients and the rebound effect may be less pronounced than after oral administration.

Methotrexate. Cellular poisons which inhibit the rapid mitoses of the epidermal cells in psoriasis have long been known to cause involution of the skin lesions. Arsenic was administered in years past and more recently the folic acid antagonists, aminopterin (Rees, 1964) and its less toxic analog, amethopterin or methotrexate, have been used. The initial surge of enthusiasm for the latter compounds has been replaced by a more sober judgment that they should be used only in patients with extensive or resistant psoriasis. Guidelines for the use of methotrexate have been prepared by the Psoriasis Task Force of the National Program for Dermatology (Roenigk et al., 1972) and revised (Roenigk et al., 1973). Physicians planning to use methotrexate should be thoroughly familiar with the indications, contraindications, dosage schedules, methods of administration, and necessary laboratory studies to be performed before administering it to any patients. In particular, the diagnosis and need for methotrexate therapy should be established by dermatologic consultation (see also page 1630).

Other Systemic Antimitotic Agents. The exhaustive survey of cytotoxic compounds for use in cancer chemotherapy has provided several additional drugs for therapeutic trial in psoriasis. To date none have been found which are remarkably superior in safety or efficacy to methotrexate. Two such compounds which have received considerable attention are hydroxyurea (Leavell et al., 1973; Moschella and Greenwald, 1973) and triacetyl azauridine (Turner and Calabres, 1964). Like methotrexate, these compounds are potent antimetabolites which carry a high risk of acute and chronic toxicity. They appear to offer little or no advantage over methotrexate except possibly as alternatives in severe and resistant psoriasis or in patients with methotrexate sensitivity. The same special care should be given in the selection and treatment of patients as is used with methotrexate. Continued study of these and other similar compounds may one day provide an effective and relatively safe antimitotic approach to the management of psoriasis. Of interest is the apparent successful use of a combined methotrexate-hydroxyurea regimen in a small series of patients with intolerance to one or both of these medications used separately (Sauer, 1973). Allopurinol, a xanthine oxidase inhibitor used in gout, is of doubtful benefit in psoriasis. Claims of its remarkable efficacy without rebound effect (Viglioglia et al., 1970) have been countered by studies indicating that it is useless (Feuerman and Nir, 1973).

Topical Vitamin A and Antimitotic Agents. Topical vitamin A acid apparently does not produce a dramatically effective response in psoriasis (Frost and Weinstein, 1969, Peck et al., 1973). Indeed, appreciable clearing was seen only with occlusion and then in less than half of the patients studied. Moreover, prompt recurrence of the lesions is likely upon cessation of treatment.

The use of topical antimitotic agents, such as methotrexate, mechlorethamine and 5-fluorouracil, among others, was a natural sequela to the demonstration of the efficacy of systemic administration of such chemicals in psoriasis. Although these compounds may produce some resolution of lesions of psoriasis after topical application, they have not proved satisfactory with or without occlusion because of local irritancy, allergic sensitization, or poor clinical response (Tsuji and Sugai, 1972; Van Scott and Reinertson, 1969; Zackheim et al., 1972).

Ultraviolet Light Therapy. Even without adjuvant light-sensitizing therapy, a series of sun exposures or artificial ultraviolet light treatments may be remarkably effective in many psoriatic patients. Excessive light exposure which would be productive of a burn is to be avoided, however, since Koebner-induced lesions of psoriasis may ensue. Moreover, certain patients are light sensitive and may experience exacerbations in the summer or on exposure to ultraviolet light. It is well to remember also that the skin is more light sensitive after occlusion with plastic films so that if occlusive therapy using topical corticosteroids is combined with light therapy, the light exposures must be more limited. The classic use of ultraviolet light therapy in psoriasis is in the Goeckerman regimen described previously.

The mechanisms responsible for the beneficial effect of ultraviolet radiation in psoriasis have not been elucidated (Hodgen and Hill, 1972). An antimitotic effect of the ultraviolet light on epidermal cells may be operative, similar to the mitotic inhibition of ultraviolet light on mammalian cells in tissue culture (Epstein et al., 1970). The precise wavelengths of ultraviolet radiation which are of therapeutic value in psoriasis are imperfectly known. The erythema-producing wavelengths (290 to 320 nm.) appear to be effective generally, but more restricted bands of ultraviolet radiation, such as 360 nm. and longer wavelengths, may be of value. Topical psoralen therapy to sensitize the skin to long wave ultraviolet radiation is apparently beneficial in some psoriatics also (Walter et al., 1973). The latter approach has been combined with a low strength anthralin paste regimen to successfully treat resistant psoriasis (Willis and Harris, 1973).

Worthy of mention are two special ultraviolet light cabinets utilizing tubular sunlamps or black light lamps which facilitate the administration of light therapy. The Zimmerman (1958) box permits head-to-toe irradiation in a single exposure and can fit neatly into a small area in an office, hospital, or home. Witten (1973) has also devised a folding ultraviolet light box with similar treatment capabilities which takes up even less space. (See also p. 1635.)

X-ray and Grenz Ray Therapy. Conventional x-ray treatment of psoriasis is rarely used today. Grenz rays are often helpful in selected patients with localized psoriasis which is resistant to other therapy. The response is generally short lived, however.

Course and Prognosis

The capricious and unpredictable course of psoriasis is perhaps its most exasperating feature. Remissions and exacerbations are the rule in most cases, but some patients remain relatively unchanged for years after the onset of the disease. With one or another form of therapy, satisfactory control of the disease is possible in the majority of patients. The special severe forms of psoriasis, such as generalized pustular psoriasis and exfoliative psoriasis, are disabling and may be fatal. Psoriatic arthritis is usually simply chronic and annoying but some forms, such as psoriatic spondylitis and arthritis mutilans, are incapacitating. Secondary infection in psoriasis is unusual, except in the intertriginous varieties or after occlusive therapy. Despite the widespread use of tars and ultraviolet radiation, the development of basal or squamous cell cancer in psoriatic plaques is a rare complication (Franks and Barner, 1947; Vickers and Ghadially, 1961).

PITYRIASIS ROSEA

Pityriasis rosea is an acute or subacute, clinically distinctive, and self-limiting exanthematous disease of unknown etiology. Except for some constitutional symptoms, which are usually mild and may be seen prodromally or during the early active phase of the disease, there is no indication of any other organ system involvement and there are no complications or sequelae. All of the old synonyms reflected the morphologic features of the eruption and were discarded long ago in favor of the above designation.

Historical Features

The original description of this disease can be traced to the 1860 report of Gibert, who applied the name "pityriasis rosea." The early writing is concerned chiefly with the clinical aspects of the disease and its unusual expressions (Klauder, 1924; Niles and Klumpp, 1940; Percival, 1932). More recently the literature has emphasized etiologic agents of possible importance (Bunch and Tilly, 1961; Garcia e Silva and Gardner, 1968; Nurse, 1969; Raskin, 1968), although clinical features of the disease continue to be emphasized or summarized (Bjornberg and Hellgren, 1962; Hellgren, 1972; Hurley and English, 1961; Kestel, 1968; Lipman Cohen, 1967; Silvers and Glickman, 1964).

Epidemiology

The disease is common, has a worldwide distribution, and affects all races. Females are affected slightly more often than males. Adolescents and young adults comprise the bulk of patients with pityriasis rosea, but it has been seen in individuals 90 years old (Bjornberg and Hellgren, 1962) and in infants as young as 3 months of age (Hyatt, 1960). Seasonal incidences have been stressed over the years and may be the result of minor epidemic clustering of cases. The fall and spring were formerly believed to be the seasons of highest frequency, but an increase in cases in winter months has been mentioned more recently. There is no apparent variation in incidence from year to year and no predisposition in relation to inheritance, occupation, habitat, personality type, blood group antigens, or any other physical or chemical parameter. Curiously, the concurrent development of the disease in families is uncommon, although it has been described (Bjornberg and Hellgren, 1962; Shelton, 1949; White, 1973). Host resistance may play a major role in individual susceptibility, thus preventing major epidemics of the disease. If this is an infectious disease, the precise mode of transmission is unknown.

Etiology and Pathogenesis

The clinical features and course of pityriasis rosea strongly suggest an infectious cause, possibly viral in nature. The prodromal symptoms, the "primary" lesion which may represent the inoculation site of an infectious organism, the efflorescent exanthem and rarely enanthem, the constitutional reaction which, though present in the minority of patients, can be fairly severe, and the spontaneous resolution after several weeks, all point to a disease of microbial origin. Moreover, second attacks are quite rare suggesting that a lifelong immunity is conferred on anyone afflicted. Salin and colleagues' report (1957) of much shortened courses of pityriasis rosea in patients given injections of disease-specific convalescent sera also supports the hypothesis that the disease is caused by an infectious agent which stimulates a protective antibody response. Nonetheless, claims of the pathogenic role of fungi, bacteria, spirochetes (Marshall, 1956), and more recently a virus (Raskin, 1968) have not been substantiated, and transmission of the disease through skin samples has been so irregular as to be of doubtful significance (Marshall, 1956; Rantuccio and Mancosu, 1964). The old and frequent observation relating the onset of pityriasis rosea to the wearing of a new or recently cleaned garment (Epstein, 1943) continues to be made but no etiologic relationship has been established and it is impossible to assess its importance. Certainly no mite, louse, or other insect has been regularly found on these patients or their clothing, nor have bites from these organisms been identified. Finally, microscopic and laboratory findings are nonspecific in nature and do not suggest a viral or other microbial etiology. The latest etiologic probe portrays pityriasis rosea as an auto-immune disease (Burch and Rowell, 1970).

Clinical Manifestations

Mild prodromal symptoms, such as malaise, fatigue, headache, and sore throat, are seen only occasionally, a few days preceding the skin involvement. In most patients, a "herald plaque" is the earliest change and is usually a solitary, oval to circular, annular lesion 2 to 6 cm. in diameter, although a plaque of larger dimension, up to 10 to 12 cm. and rarely two herald plaques, have been described. Herald plaques occur most often on the trunk or proximal arms or thighs but have been seen rarely on the penis, face, and scalp. This primary lesion is often mistaken by patient and physician for a ringworm infection since it shows a raised border and is usually covered by fine branny scales (Fig. 9–8). The appearance of the other skin lesions, the exanthem of pityriasis rosea, which follows after an interval usually measuring 3 to 14 days but at times may be as short as a few hours or as long as 6 to 8 weeks, should dispel that impression. These secondary eruptive lesions are clinically distinctive and when well-developed are quickly recognized by the trained eye. They are characteristically oval in shape with a long axis in the lines of cleavage (Figs. 9–8 and 9–9). On the trunk this feature is quite conspicuous, especially on the lateral or posterior thorax, the axillary lines, and the abdomen. These lesions, normally flat, erythematous, or fawn-colored plaques measuring 0.5 to 1.5 cm. in diameter, are essen-

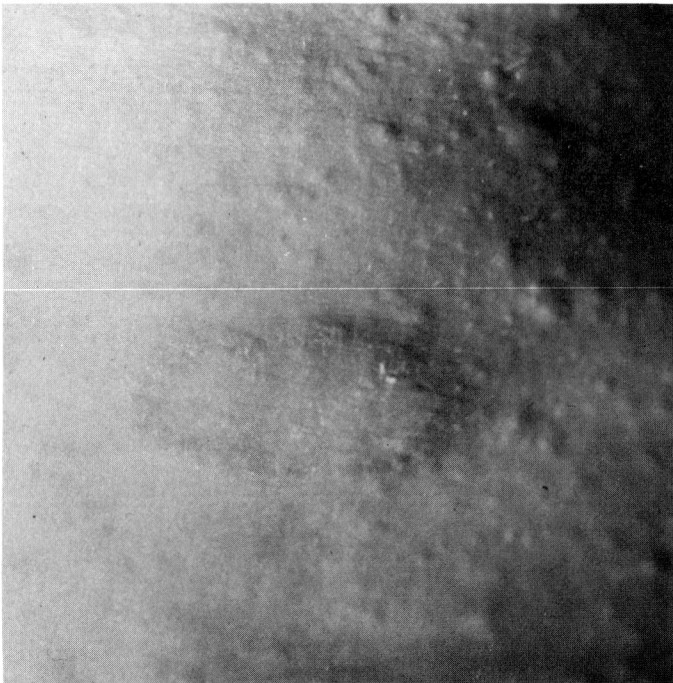

Figure 9–8 Annular herald plaque of the trunk in pityriasis rosea. Resemblance to tinea corporis (ringworm infection) is apparent. Note papular exanthematous lesions nearby.

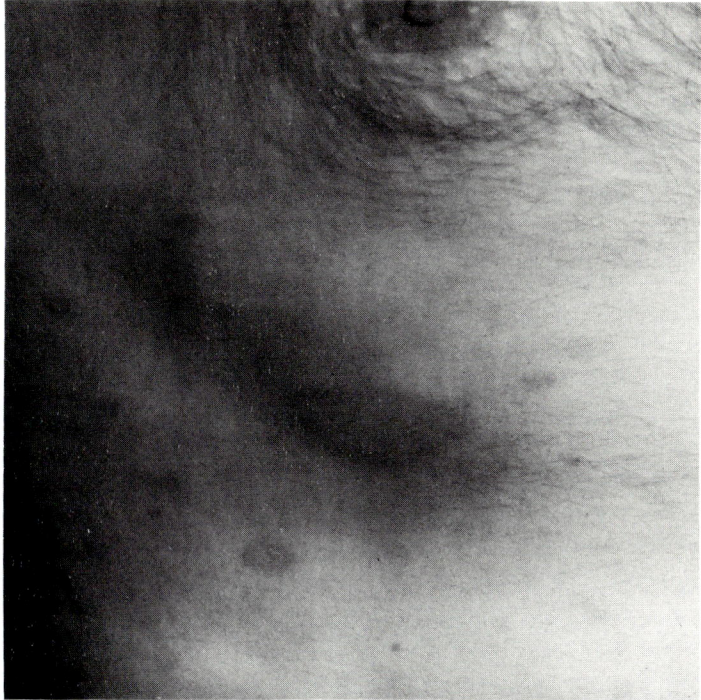

Figure 9–9 Herald plaque and characteristic oval lesions of pityriasis rosea. Observe arrangement of lesions in lines of cleavage.

tially miniatures of the herald plaque. Their annularity is produced by a raised, edematous, and at times finely vesicular border and a unique fine scale which tends to peel peripherally, producing a special collarette. Smaller papular lesions, only a few millimeters in length, are often seen in extensive eruptions and may not develop the characteristic clinical features of the better-developed lesions described above. New lesions continue to appear during the first weeks of the eruption.

Although a papulosquamous eruption usually accompanies the disease, unusual lichenoid, vesicular, pustular, urticarial, and even purpuric forms may be seen, more often in children than in adults. Negro children, especially, both in America and in Africa (Marshall, 1956), may show the papular or lichenoid lesions. In all of these patients, however, the diagnosis can be suspected on clinical examination since some of the typical features described above remain or evolve in many of the lesions. The more florid nature of the eruption, the regular peripheral distribution of lesions, and the constancy of generalized lymphadenopathy have been

emphasized recently in African patients with pityriasis rosea (Vollum, 1973).

The major distribution of lesions is usually on the trunk, neck, and proximal extremities; involvement of the face and scalp is unusual. Less commonly, patients may show an inverse distribution of lesions on the face and extremities as opposed to the trunk. Children apparently develop this atypical distribution more often. Even "localized" forms (Vidal) of pityriasis rosea essentially restricted to one axilla or inguinal region (Hurley and English, 1961; Klauder, 1924) but sooner or later usually demonstrating at least a few scattered lesions of the trunk, are well known and are seen usually in adults. Involvement of the volar skin in pityriasis rosea is almost invariably vesicular in type, a feature which distinguishes it from secondary syphilis. In severe cases of the disease, the lesions are so numerous as to be confluent (Fig. 9–10) and may be accompanied by more prominent constitutional signs, such as fever (100 to 102°F.), malaise, loss of appetite, and definite if not marked lymphadenopathy, principally of the anterior cervical nodes.

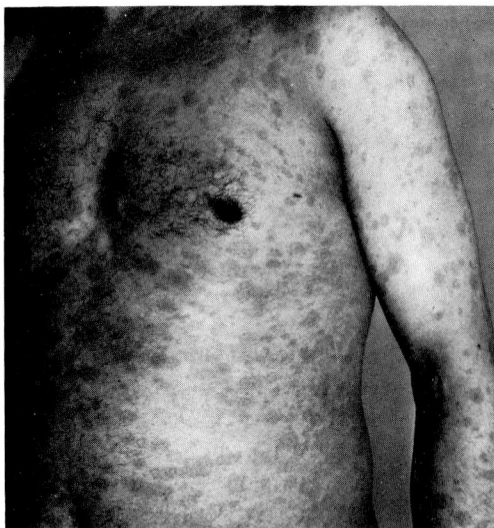

Figure 9–10 Extensive pityriasis rosea with numerous lesions in typical arrangement and distribution.

Pruritus is usually present in pityriasis rosea but may be surprisingly mild, even in extensive cases. Post-inflammatory hypopigmentation or hyperpigmentation after pityriasis rosea is uncommon and occurs primarily in Negroes. Mucous membrane involvement, though unusual, may be seen, usually in the form of red patches which are sometimes hemorrhagic, erosive, or bullous. Pitting of the fingernails has been reported after pityriasis rosea (Silvers and Glickman, 1964), but this or any other alterations of the nails are extraordinary features of the disease. Second attacks of pityriasis rosea are rare, but have been described (Bjornberg and Hellgren, 1962). Relapse or recrudescence of lesions is exceptional; it may be observed in patients in whom systemic corticosteroid therapy is discontinued prematurely, however. Involvement of internal organs has never been documented in pityriasis rosea.

Pathology

The histopathologic picture is nonspecific. There are edema and a chronic inflammatory infiltrate in the dermis which is chiefly lymphocytic with a few neutrophils. The epidermis shows spongiosis and occasionally superficial vesicle formation in the upper malpighian layer or sub-

corneally. A parakeratotic scale is found irregularly along the epidermal surface. Viral inclusions or other cytoplasmic alterations suggestive of viral infection have not been identified. Electron microscopic study has failed to add any distinctive ultrastructural elements of fundamental importance.

Diagnosis

Pityriasis rosea is diagnosable on the clinical grounds mentioned previously, with requisite exclusion of secondary syphilis and a drug reaction in certain cases. Serologic test for syphilis (STS) is indicated in the majority if not all patients with a pityriasis rosea type of eruption. The classic sequence of a primary herald plaque, when it is present, and the distinctive secondary lesions, so readily recognized by those familiar with the disease, is not duplicated by other conditions. Medallion-type seborrheic dermatitis may pose a diagnostic problem at times, but the absence of a herald plaque, the scalp involvement, and the greasy seborrheiform scales serve to distinguish this disorder. Moreover, the chronic course of seborrheic dermatitis contrasts sharply with the subacute and self-limiting course of pityriasis rosea. Other papulosquamous eruptions, especially psoriasis and parapsoriasis en plaque, may deserve consideration in certain patients, but careful clinical study of the skin lesions will usually permit differentiation. The smaller and more widespread lesions of tinea versicolor may resemble pityriasis rosea but this fungal infection can be quickly identified by a microscopic examination of a KOH preparation of skin scrapings. Tinea corporis may be confused with the herald plaque or with lesions of localized pityriasis rosea and may justify mycologic study of the marginal scales or vesicular element of the lesions. There are no laboratory studies of diagnostic importance. Indeed, the blood count, urinalysis, and other tests are within normal limits.

Treatment

Reassurance and symptomatic therapy are all that is required in most cases. Topical management should be as bland as possible in order to minimize excessive irritation or drying. A topical steroid in a hydrophilic cream base is usually preferred along with colloidal starch or oatmeal-oil baths. Antihistamines or ataractics may allay pruritus. In severe cases the administration of systemic corticosteroids, in an initial daily dose of 30 to 40 mg. of prednisone or its equivalent, is suppressive but probably does not shorten the course of the disease. A low maintenance dose is therefore required for the anticipated duration of the process. This author has seen no complications from corticosteroid therapy but the usual precautionary and adjunctive measures for such medication should apply. Ultraviolet light treatment is said to hasten involution of more chronic cases but is certainly not dramatically effective. The possible efficacy of sulfone therapy used empirically (Anderson, 1971) requires confirmation.

Course and Prognosis

Most cases of pityriasis rosea clear in six to eight weeks; shorter (three to four weeks) or longer (10 to 14 weeks) courses are possible, however. If an eruption persists beyond 14 weeks, another diagnosis should be entertained. There are no known systemic or local complications or sequelae of pityriasis rosea. The prognosis for return of the skin to normal is excellent and the patient's general health should be unaffected. If acquired during pregnancy, no fetal abnormalities are to be anticipated.

PITYRIASIS RUBRA PILARIS

Pityriasis rubra pilaris is a rare, scaly, erythematous, cutaneous disease of unknown etiology. Although it shares certain features with psoriasis and seborrheic dermatitis, pityriasis rubra pilaris shows a preference for the follicular apparatus as reflected in distinctive focal changes histologically and clinically. Current knowledge requires the delineation of a familial, genetically influenced form of pityriasis rubra pilaris as well as an acquired form, in

which a heritable tendency has not yet been demonstrated. No systemic diseases have been regularly found in patients with pityriasis rubra pilaris, although several cases of associated muscle or joint disease (Aguilar et al., 1973; Kierland and Kulwin, 1961; Orbaneja et al., 1962; Waldorf and Hambrick, 1965) have been described. Synonyms include *pityriasis pilaris, lichen rubra acuminatus, lichen psoriasis and Devergie's disease.*

Historical Features

Devergie's careful clinical description in 1857 deserves recognition as the initial treatise on pityriasis rubra pilaris. Attempts to correlate the disease with vitamin A deficiency, along with reports of the therapeutic efficacy of systemic and topical vitamin A (Gross et al., 1969), highlight the more recent literature.

Epidemiology

There are no conclusive data on the incidence of pityriasis rubra pilaris but it is clearly a rare disorder. While best known in Europe and North America, it is apparently not restricted to these geographic regions. There is no known racial variation but this author's experience suggests a higher frequency of the disease in Caucasians. Both sexes are affected equally and there is no other predilectional factor, such as habitat, occupation, ethnic origin, and body or personality type, that is of importance.

Etiology and Pathogenesis

The causal factors involved in this disease remain obscure. In the familial cases, there is evidence of genetic transmission of the simple autosomal dominant type (Leitner and Ford, 1947). Moreover, many believe that patients with the acquired form of the disease, which usually develops later in life but may show mild, easily overlooked features at an early stage, may simply represent delayed expression of a heritable disorder. The disease appears to represent a special disturbance of keratinization but the precise defect remains a mystery. Accelerated epidermal proliferation in pityriasis rubra pilaris is evident by the decreased transit time of radioactive-labeled amino acids through the skin (Porter and Shuster, 1968) and by the salutary clinical effect of inhibitors of epidermal maturation such as the antifolic drugs (Brown and Perry, 1966).

Since the studies of Frazier and Hu in 1931, in which skin lesions suggestive of pityriasis rubra pilaris were described in vitamin A–deficient individuals, interest has centered on the pathogenetic importance of hypovitaminosis A in pityriasis rubra pilaris (Logan, 1972). Despite nagging suggestive evidence implicating vitamin A deficiency, however, there has been no conclusive demonstration of its relationship to pityriasis rubra pilaris. To begin with, the cutaneous lesions of the vitamin A depletion syndrome are not exact replicas of pityriasis rubra pilaris and can be differentiated clinically (Lowenthal, 1933). Low plasma vitamin A levels are also not regularly found in pityriasis rubra pilaris and do not correlate well with the clinical severity of the disease. In humans, deprivation of vitamin A and carotene for as long as 22 months has not resulted in development of pityriasis rubra pilaris, and studies in rats and humans have emphasized the role of the B group of vitamins vis-á-vis vitamin A in the reversal of phrynoderma (Moult, 1943; Shrank, 1966; Sullivan and Evans, 1945). Further clarification of the complex facets of vitamin A

metabolism and absorption, including the genetic variations, may one day resolve the presently muddled picture.

Clinical Manifestations

The earliest sign of the disease is usually a scaling seborrheiform change of the scalp which at times can be quite severe. The follicular involvement of the inflammatory process is curiously absent on the scalp, however. This is soon followed by involvement of the face and ears and at this point the picture suggests seborrheic dermatitis. Later, however, the palms and soles develop scaly, red patches and ultimately a diffuse, thick hyperkeratotic appearance which may be fissured and painful. On the soles this has been aptly described as a "keratodermic sandal." Keratotic, acuminate, reddish papules then appear in turn on the dorsal aspects of the hands and fingers, the extensor surfaces of the wrists and forearms, and eventually on wide areas of the trunk, neck, and extremities (Fig. 9–11). In all of these areas except the dorsal fingers, the lesions evolve from the discrete, follicularly oriented papules to confluent and larger plaques in which the rough nutmeg grater-like surface is replaced by a thickened, more diffusely scaly erythematous alteration (Fig. 9–12). On the dorsal fingers, however, the papules remain discretely

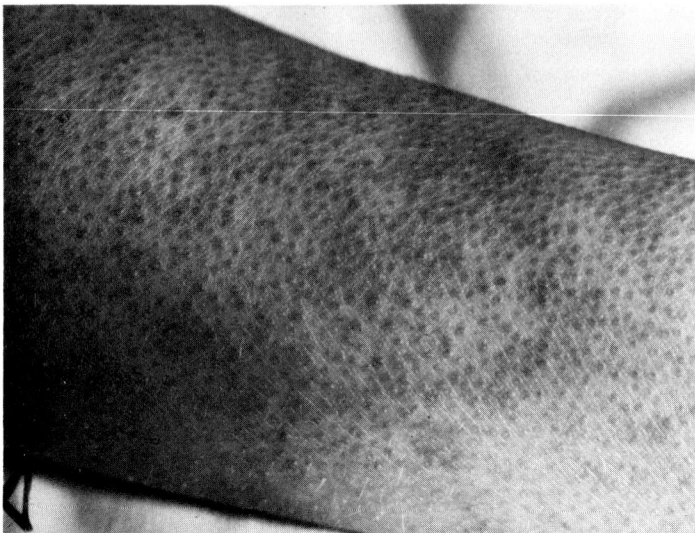

Figure 9–11 Characteristic follicular papules of pityriasis rubra pilaris. These early lesions may later be replaced by confluent scaly plaques (see Figure 9–12).

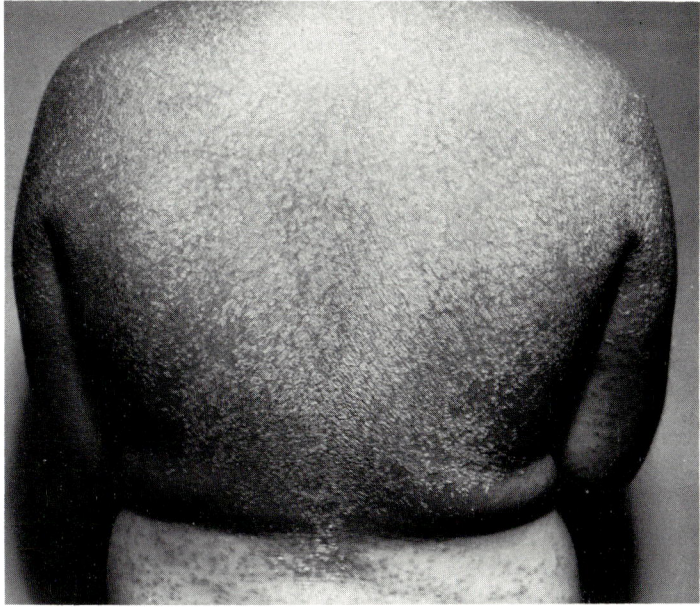

Figure 9-12 Diffuse scaly erythematous lesions of the trunk in pityriasis rubra pilaris. Follicular orientation of the lesions may be inapparent in such confluent involvement except on the dorsal fingers, where it remains as a special diagnostic feature of this disease.

follicular, a sign of diagnostic importance. Additional noteworthy clinical features of the lesions of the trunk are the salmon color of the scaly plaques and the presence of small islands of normal skin within large coalescent areas of the eruption. At times the disease can eventuate in an exfoliative dermatitis, and on the face thick, heavy scaling and ectropion of the eyelids may develop. On other areas, aside from the follicular localization, the scaling of the eruption is classically fine and pityriasiform, as its designation implies, but may at times be psoriasiform or similar to the large, thick scales of lamellar ichthyosis.

As in psoriasis, hair growth is essentially undisturbed but the nails are often dull, thickened, and may show transverse striations. The characteristic psoriatic pitting of the nails is not seen in pityriasis rubra pilaris, however. The mucous membranes are not affected often, but whitish papules resembling oral lichen planus have been reported (Baden and Roth, 1968), and in one unusual patient a diffusely rough, gray-white alteration of the entire buccal mucosa resembling frosted glass was described (Marshall, 1952). The disease may also rarely present as a scarring erythematous plaque dermatosis involving primarily the face, mouth, and scalp and clinically resembling discoid lupus erythematosus but with characteristic follicular lesions elsewhere. The familial form of pityriasis rubra pilaris usually begins in childhood and is milder than the acquired form, which usually develops in middle age.

Pruritus is usually not a prominent feature of pityriasis rubra pilaris and is often completely absent. The reported association of certain muscle or connective tissue diseases, such as myasthenia gravis, polymyositis, and muscular dystrophy, may well be coincidental but deserves further study.

Pathology

Although not always diagnostic, the histopathologic features are at least strongly suggestive of the disease. The essential follicular involvement, as manifested by focal hyperkeratosis, parakeratosis, and adjacent mild irregular acanthosis and a perifollicular inflammatory infiltrate, is characteristic. Liquefaction degeneration of the basal layer is often present and extends along the hair follicle. The interfollicular skin may show some of the epithelial changes described previously, but they are less prominent. At times, especially in old or resolving lesions, psoriasis or lichenoid neurodermatitis may resemble pityriasis rubra pilaris. Monro abscesses are not seen in pityriasis rubra pilaris.

Diagnosis

The diagnosis of pityriasis rubra pilaris is established by the clinical and histopathologic features described previously. Psoriasis and seborrheic dermatitis may be difficult to distinguish in certain cases but the diagnosis eventually becomes evident as the more characteristic features of pityriasis rubra pilaris develop and as signs of the other disorders fail to appear. Avitaminotic patients with skin changes resembling pityriasis rubra pilaris usually have other signs of vitamin deficiency as well, and a diagnostic problem rarely exists. Keratosis pilaris is more limited in distribution and does not show the digital, scalp, or extensive trunk involvement of pityriasis rubra pilaris.

Treatment

Oral vitamin A, in daily doses of 200,000 to 600,000 units, will result in clearing of many cases of pityriasis rubra pilaris within two to three months. As little as 100,000 units daily may be effective in children (Huntly, 1971). This response is not regularly predictable, however, even in patients with low plasma levels of vitamin A (Cornbleet, 1954). Discontinuance of therapy often results in relapse, but prolonged remissions have apparently been produced in some patients. After several months of continuous therapy the vitamin A must be discontinued for a rest period of at least two to three months in order to avoid development of vitamin A toxicity, which is marked by anorexia, pruritus, dry skin, loss of hair, hyperostoses, and subcutaneous swellings.

Pityriasis rubra pilaris has responded also to azathioprine (Hunter and Forbes, 1972), systemic methotrexate (Brown and Perry, 1966), and corticosteroids, but the risk of attendant side effects is always present. These drugs are indicated particularly in patients with exfoliative dermatitis. Appropriate precautionary measures, monitoring, and adjuvant medica-

tions should be used in these patients. Topical vitamin A acid has shown promise, especially under occlusion, in some patients (Gunther, 1972).

Course and Prognosis

The disease is usually quite chronic, persisting for an indefinite period. Remissions and exacerbations are not as common as in psoriasis. Some patients may clear completely, however, at times fairly abruptly (Davidson et al., 1969). This latter course is more common in the acquired form of pityriasis rubra pilaris, which is usually more severe. Devergie and the earlier writers emphasized the possible fatal outcome of a high percentage of their cases but the outlook is rarely that grave today, even without the medications currently available.

LICHEN PLANUS

Lichen planus is a relatively common, clinically and histologically distinctive, inflammatory cutaneous disease of unknown etiology. Classically a papulosquamous disorder, it may present as vesicular or bullous, hypertrophic, atrophic, annular, follicular, erosive, actinic, or erythematous variants. Eruptions similar to lichen planus have been induced by certain drugs, heavy metals, photographic chemicals, and apparently by a few systemic diseases. One synonym, *lichen ruber planus*, is still commonly used today, especially in the European literature.

Historical Features

Erasmus Wilson's description of 50 cases in 1869 is recognized as the first account of the disease. In the century that has followed, the knowledge of this disease has increased principally in an improved understanding of its clinical variations and the microscopic and ultrastructural features; however, there has been some increased insight into the pathogenetic mechanisms involved in some cases.

Epidemiology

The incidence of lichen planus has been placed at between 0.1 and 1.2 per cent, depending on the region of the world under study (Calnan and Meara, 1957; Depaoli, 1964; Schmidt, 1961). In the United States, it is certainly not increasing in frequency; indeed, there may be fewer cases than in the past. Men and women are equally prone to this disorder, and it has been seen in all racial groups. Although it has been reported in infants, it is rare in the very young and elderly; the usual group affected is that between 30 and 60 years of age. Lichen planus has been described in all geographic regions of the world, but in the tropical climates it affects the young more commonly and may show special clinical expressions.

Etiology and Pathogenesis

Lichen planus remains a dark etiologic mystery, although some light has been focused on the disease fairly recently. Three pathogenetic theories seem worthy of mention, despite limited supportive evidence. A viral cause has long been suspected and is based on both histologic and electronmicroscopic findings (Aplas, 1957; Swanbach and Thyressen, 1964; Thyresson and Moburger, 1957). Psychogenic influences appear to be of striking importance in many patients and have been frequently related to the onset of the disease, the precipitation of additional attacks, and their resolution as the stressful factors have been removed.

The accumulated cases of lichen planus related to drugs, heavy metals, and the photographic industry have prompted the hypothesis that susceptible enzyme-deficient individuals may selectively respond with a lichen planus–like eruption on exposure to these chemicals. The interesting finding of a deficiency of glucose-6-phosphodehydrogenase in lichen planus skin (Cotton et al., 1972) is consonant with this theory. Moreover, it seems particularly applicable to Atabrine, a drug known to induce a hemolytic anemia in individuals with an erythrocyte glucose-6-phosphodehydrogenase deficiency. Reconciliation of alternative theories is possible if one assumes that lichen planus is a reaction pattern of genetically predisposed individuals, which is triggered by exposure to chemicals of microbiologic, pharmacologic, or industrial origin. There is little evidence that the disease is genetically determined, however, although its rare familial appearance has been reported (Depaoli, 1970; DuPont, 1972). The recent localization of immunoglobulins in lichen planus lesions (Waisman et al., 1973) has not yet been fully assessed but may reflect nonspecific binding by damaged epidermal cells and not the presence of true auto-antibodies. There is no other evidence suggesting an auto-immune pathogenesis for lichen planus.

Clinical Manifestations

The lesions of lichen planus are characteristically polygonal, flat papules of violaceous hue, showing a fine but often inconspicuous scale (Fig. 9–13). Close study of the lesions may reveal whitish lines or spots which have been called Wickham's striae. These have been attributed to focal epidermal thickening which was correlated histologically (Summerly and Wilson-Jones, 1964). The papules are usually of fairly uniform diameter, about 2 to 4 cm., but may be of pinhead size. They are commonly discrete but may coalesce to form plaques or annular lesions, or may show a linear configuration, probably as part of a Koebner phenomenon induced by scratching.

Any part of the skin can be affected by lichen planus but the most commonly involved sites are the lumbar region, genitalia, ankles and anterior lower legs, where the lesions may commonly persist and become hypertrophic, and the flexor aspects of the wrists. The latter are loci which are rarely spared. When the palms and soles are affected, the lesions are often yellow-brown in color with a more prominent scale or appear as punctate keratoses. A very rare form of lichen planus in which erosive or ulcerative changes are seen on the soles of the feet has been described in association with toenail and scalp involvement, resulting in anonychia and alopecia (Cram et al., 1966). Mucous membrane involvement is seen in over 50 per cent of patients with lichen planus, occasionally with concomitant skin lesions. Such lesions appear most often on the buccal mu-

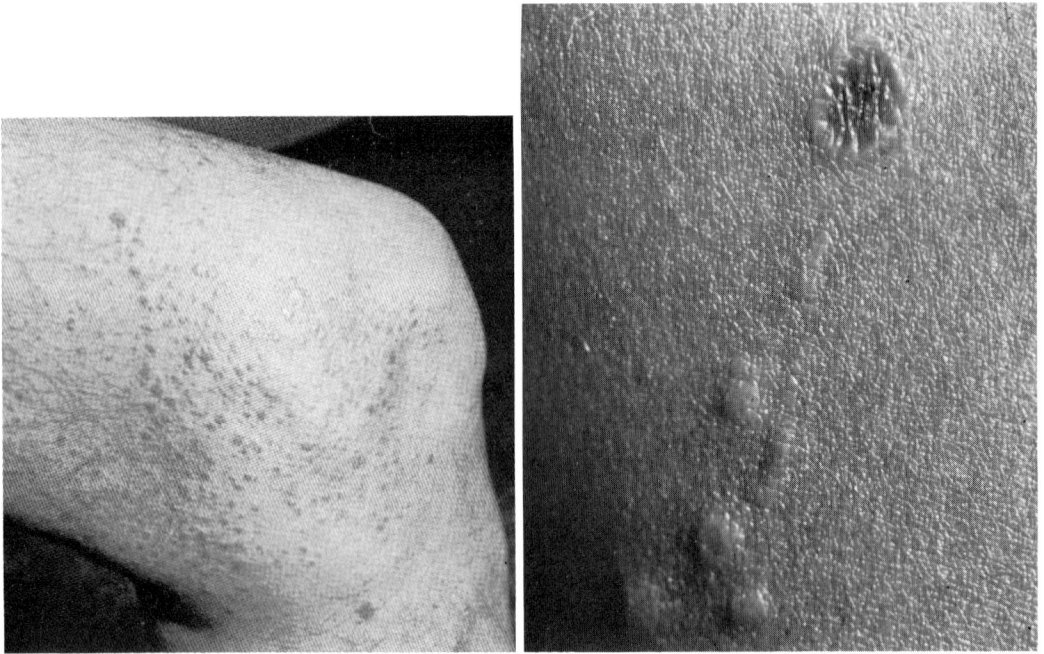

Figure 9–13 Lichen planus papules. Oval or angular character of these small papules is apparent and there is a suggestion of a linear Koebner reaction. There is little or no scaling evident in some of these lesions, and prominent fine scaling in others.

cosa, as a lacy white network or as white papules or plaques (Fig. 9–14), and on the tongue in the form of slightly depressed white plaques (Shklar, 1972). Conjuncti- val, anal, rectal, penile, vulvovaginal, laryngeal esophageal, gastric, colonic, urinary bladder and eardrum involvement has also been seen.

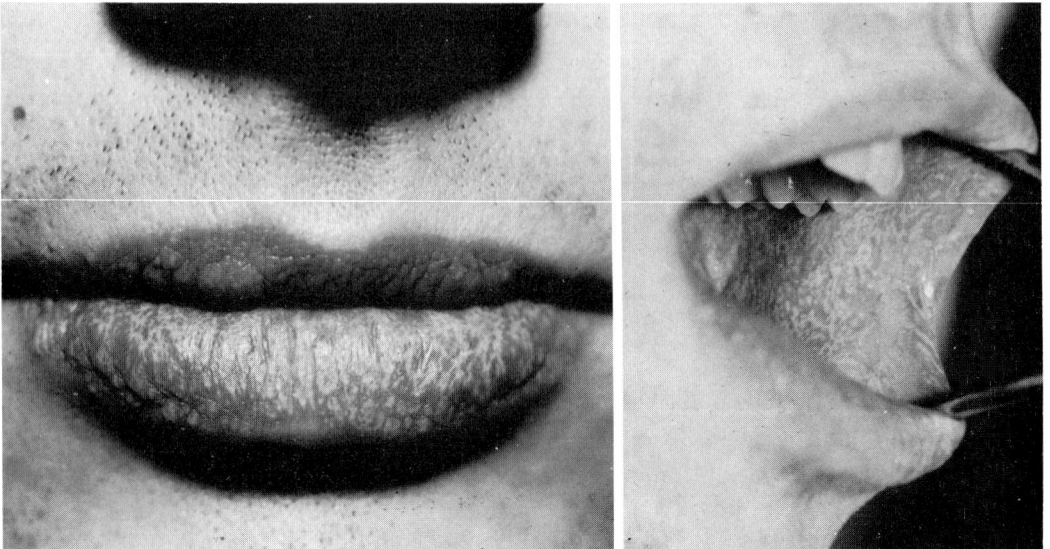

Figure 9–14 Typical papular lesions of the lips and buccal mucosa in lichen planus. The lacy, white appearance of the lesions of the mucosal surface is characteristic.

Pruritus is usually a prominent symptom in patients with lichen planus, although there are some patients who deny any itching, despite widespread involvement. Moreover, there are special clinical forms of lichen planus, to be discussed later, which show little or no pruritus.

Perhaps 10 per cent of patients with lichen planus show some alteration of the nails, reflecting mild or marked focal or diffuse inflammation of the nail matrix and at times the posterior nail fold. Thus, the nail plate may show transient simple thinning, longitudinal striations or grooves, splitting and other distortions, as well as atrophy and permanent loss of the nail (Zaias, 1970). A particularly distinctive change is the formation of a pterygium, a wing-shaped scar extending from just beyond the nail matrix to the edge of the nail. It results from inflammatory fusion of the posterior nail fold and nail plate and may be duplicated only by local trauma, infection, or peripheral vascular disease.

Hair loss occurs in lichen planus when there is destruction of the follicles by the inflammatory process. This results in patches of atrophic alopecia resembling that seen in pseudopelade. It is to be emphasized that the classic angular violaceous papules of lichen planus are not seen on the scalp in these patients but may be found elsewhere in the usual cutaneous or mucosal sites. Moreover, non-cicatricial alopecia, as seen in systemic lupus erythematosus or secondary syphilis, is apparently not a feature of lichen planus, even the acute explosive form.

Lichen planus may develop suddenly or slowly. In the acute form, widespread skin involvement with discrete lesions which tend to become confluent is the rule. These cases may abate completely within a few months, may remit partially and at irregular intervals over months to years, or may progress into chronic lichen planus. In the latter instance, hypertrophic, deeply violaceous lesions are likely, especially on the ankles and lower third of the legs, but may also be seen on the wrists and other areas (Fig. 9–15). These lesions are usually markedly pruritic.

A special feature of lichen planus, in contradistinction to the other papulosquamous disorders, is its capacity to produce very restricted clinical expressions or localizations of the inflammatory process. The disease may affect only some or all of the nails, often resulting in a characteristic scarring anonychia, as described previously. The oral or genital mucosa (the latter more often in males), the soles of the feet, or the scalp may be similarly selected. In each instance a biopsy specimen should confirm the clinical suspicion.

A number of special clinical forms of lichen planus, based on a predominance of nonpapular skin lesions, or an unusual configuration or distribution of the skin lesions, are worthy of mention. (Cram and Muller, 1966). Although papular lesions are by far the commonest expression of lichen planus, small vesicles and bullae may be seen as part of the general papular eruption. An even rarer clinical form, which has been called *lichen planus pemphigoides*, shows large bullae arising from

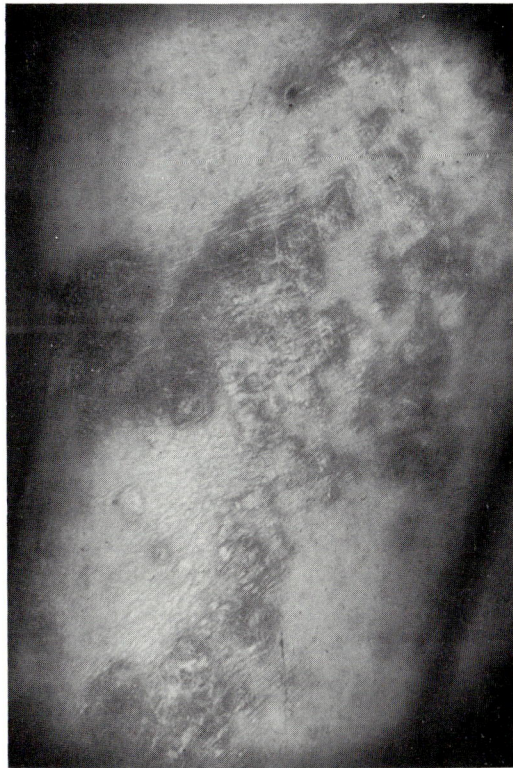

Figure 9–15 Thickened papular lesions of hypertrophic lichen planus of the legs. These lesions tend to be intensely pruritic. Note the linear Koebner reaction papules (lower part of the photograph) which were probably induced by scratching.

normal or involved skin, and is easily confused with other bullous disorders. Moreover, at a later stage when there has been some attempt at healing of affected areas, it may resemble acrodermatitis chronica atrophicans, lichen sclerosus et atrophicus, or morphea, especially on the legs. *Annular lichen planus,* another variant evolving commonly from more chronic forms of the disease, results from the ring-like grouping of papules. It is common on the penis and lower trunk but may develop anywhere. *Follicular lichen planus,* also called lichen planopilaris, is characterized by the presence of acuminate, keratotic follicular lesions of the scalp, often leading to local atrophy or alopecia. Typical cutaneous or mucosal lesions may be missing in some of the patients with this condition. Linear lichen planus, in a dermatomal or zosteriform pattern, is also seen occasionally.

A distinctive variant known as *lichen planus actinicus* occurs in tropical or subtropical areas principally in children and young adults of Oriental extraction. The lesions develop on exposed skin areas and are presumably light-induced, although there has been no delineation of the responsible wavelengths. The lesions may be pigmented, dyschromic, or granuloma annulare–like and may be confused with discoid lupus erythematosus. Pruritus is commonly minimal or absent (Almeyda, 1970; Dostrovsky and Sagher, 1949; Katzenellenbogen, 1962).

The designation *lichen planus erythematosus* has been applied to an unusual form of the disease occurring primarily in elderly patients. Soft, nonpruritic, slightly erythematous or purpuric papules with or without mucosal and nail involvement are seen, usually on the forearms. Some areas are poikiloderma-like and exhibit histologically a marked vascular element, degeneration of collagen, and the characteristic features of lichen planus.

Malignant change has been described in some chronic hypertrophic forms of lichen planus (Kronenberg et al., 1971) and notably in ulcerative lesions of the tongue or oral mucosa.

LICHEN PLANUS-LIKE ERUPTIONS OF CHEMICAL ORIGIN. *Drugs.* A number of medications, such as streptomycin, para-aminosalicylic acid, methyldopa, quinidine, gold, bismuth, phenothiazine, thiazides, chloroquine, and Atabrine, are known to cause lichen planus-like eruptions (Almeyda and Levantine, 1971; Pillsbury and Livingood, 1968; Sulzberger et al., 1947). At times these may be difficult if not impossible to distinguish from idiopathic lichen planus. The Atabrine-induced disorder is of particular interest and shows features both common to and missing from ordinary lichen planus. Mucous membrane involvement may be indistinguishable clinically and histologically, although an eosinophilic infiltrate has been emphasized with Atabrine. Scaling and atrophy of skin is often more prominent in the Atabrine disorder. Thick hypertrophic plaques also have been described. Destruction of the appendages, resulting in hair loss and anhidrosis, is not uncommon. Examination of suspicious lesions under ultraviolet light (360 nm.) often reveals fluorescence at Atabrine-impregnated sweat pores.

Other Chemical Exposures. The fascinating reports of Buckley (1958) and de Graciansky (1966) describe the special features of lichen planus-like eruptions developing after exposure to color film developers. The responsible chemicals are substituted paraphenylenediamine salts but include 2-amino-5-diethylamino toluene monochloride (CD_2, 4-amino-N-diethylaniline sulfate (TTS), and antimony trioxide. Contact with these substances may provoke an eczematous reaction initially which may become lichenoid. There may also be a blend of eczematous and lichenoid changes or simply the lichenoid eruption. External contact is the primary exposure route but the possibility that inhalation or ingestion may be an avenue of entry has not been excluded. The eruption can be quite widespread, but mucosal surfaces are usually uninvolved. Patch test responses to the offending chemicals are eczematous initially but may become lichenoid. Histologically the picture is often nonspecific but may resemble the changes of lichen planus quite closely. Resolution is slow, with residual hyperpigmentation a common finding. Similar reactions have been described after exposure to dust from blueprints containing diazodiethylaniline (Scarpa and Ferrea, 1968).

LICHEN PLANUS AND SYSTEMIC DISEASE. Eruptions resembling lichen planus, at least clinically, have been described in association with polymyositis and malignant lymphoma, as well as with the malabsorption syndrome (Feuerman and Sandbark, 1971). Bullous lichen planus has been described in several patients in association with adrenal or perirenal tumors (Magnusson, 1967). In some of these patients the eruption apparently cleared following removal of the tumor. The great majority of patients with lichen planus, however, have no related systemic disorders. The observation that older patients with lichen planus are likely to be hypertensive (Allende, 1950) has not been confirmed, nor has the reported frequent association of oral lichen planus and diabetes mellitus (Jolly, 1972).

Pathology

The histopathologic features of lichen planus are diagnostic in the great majority of cases. The epidermis shows hyperkeratosis, a thickened, granular layer, patchy acanthosis, and liquefaction of the basal cell layer, which some regard as the primary event in the disease (Sarkany and Gaylarde, 1971). Eosinophilic colloidal bodies, apparently degenerated epidermal cells and not viral structures, are also commonly found in the lower epidermal layer. The most striking element is a dense band-like lymphocytic and histiocytic infiltrate which hugs the epidermis and is sharply defined inferiorly. Bullous forms of the disease show dermoepithelial separation, and in follicular lichen planus the infiltrate surrounds the hair follicle and may eventually destroy it. The lichen planus papule has shown a proliferative microvasculature, especially peripherally (Glickman et al., 1964). Ultrastructural changes include tonofibril damage and aggregation, and breakdown and decrease in desmosomes and intranuclear particles which apparently are not viral in origin (Goltz and Hult, 1963; Johnson and Fry, 1967). Immunofluorescent studies have revealed globular deposits of immunoglobulin at the dermo-epidermal junction in over 95 per cent of lichen planus lesions, including those which are Koebner-induced (Waisman et al., 1973). This finding is not specific for lichen planus, although it helps distinguish it from many other disorders.

Diagnosis

Exclusion of causative drugs or chemicals is essential in all patients with lichen planus. Among the other disorders which may at times be confused with certain forms of lichen planus are psoriasis, secondary syphilis, localized neurodermatitis, pityriasis rosea, discoid lupus erythematosus, disseminated granuloma annulare, flat warts, leukoplakia, lichen sclerosus et atrophicus, Kaposi's sarcoma, primary localized amyloidosis, pseudopelade, and folliculitis decalvans. Analysis of the complete clinical picture, however, along with study of biopsy specimens, other appropriate laboratory tests, and further observation should permit unequivocal diagnosis of the given condition.

Treatment

Lichen planus can be a most distressing disorder therapeutically. Removal of offending drugs or chemical exposures is indicated whenever necessary. Local symptomatic treatment with corticosteroid creams or sprays, along with soothing colloidal baths, may be helpful in widespread involvement. Intralesional corticosteroid injections produce prompt involution of lesions and are useful for a limited number of lesions. Occlusive dressings over topical corticosteroids are also helpful. Hyperkeratotic lesions have apparently responded to topical retinoic acid, 0.1 per cent in an ointment base (Gunther, 1971). A two to three week course of systemic corticosteroids, such as prednisone, in 25 to 35 mg. daily doses, may be curative but usually produces at best only a temporary interruption of the disease. Ataractics and sedatives are sometimes helpful, especially in those patients in whom emotional stress is felt to be responsible for the condition. Rest, vacations, resolution of pressing problems, and psychotherapy have been helpful occasionally in special patients. The empiric use of bismuth and other heavy metals with their attendant risks is no longer advocated, and neither these metals nor other unfounded remedies such as penicillin, vaccines, vitamins, antimalarials, calcium gluconate, grenz ray, ultra-violet light, and physical therapy have any predictable effect on the course of this disease (Altman and Perry, 1961; Samman, 1961). Of some interest, however, is the report of the beneficial effect of griseofulvin in a double-blind study (Sehgal et al., 1972). Oral lichen planus may require surgical management, possibly by excision (Emslie and Hardman, 1970), because of the danger of squamous cell cancer. Oral lesions of lichen planus have apparently cleared after removal of copper inlays used in dental reconstruction (Fryholm et al., 1969).

Course and Prognosis

In acute lichen planus the outlook is more favorable and resolution can be expected in 6 to 18 months. Relapse or recurrence is possible, but the eruption usually clears again within several months. Chronic lichen planus may last for more than 10 to 15 years. This is particularly true for the hypertrophic form, oral lichen planus, and lichen planopilaris. It is unlikely that any form of treatment, although temporarily suppressive or symptomatically helpful, significantly shortens the course of the disease. There are no complications of lichen planus aside from the local pigmentary and atrophic sequelae and the danger of the development of squamous cell cancer in mouth lesions, which is slight.

LICHEN NITIDUS

Lichen nitidus is a chronic, generally asymptomatic micropapular dermatosis usually affecting the penis, forearms, breast, and other portions of the trunk. Once thought to be a tuberculid, it is now regarded as a disease of unknown etiology. A distinctive granulomatous pattern characterizes lichen nitidus histologically. There are no synonyms of importance.

Historical Features

The credit for the initial description of the disease belongs to Felix Pinkus (1907).

Subsequent reports have been clinically oriented, often dealing with the possible relationship of lichen nitidus to tuberculosis and in later years to lichen planus. The literature of recent times has been strikingly barren, however, in reference to the etiology or treatment of the disease.

Epidemiology

Lichen nitidus is not a common disease. Its prevalence has never been established and indeed might be difficult to determine accurately since lesions similar or identical to lichen nitidus are apparently seen in up to 30 per cent of patients with lichen planus. There has been no comprehensive epidemiologic study of the disease but it appears to be more common in young adults and children, in males, and, in the United States at least, in Negroes. There are no predisposing genetic or occupational influences, nor is there an association with any systemic or cutaneous disease other than lichen planus (see below).

Etiology and Pathogenesis

It is easy to understand the early attempts to link lichen nitidus to tuberculosis, a condition with which many diseases of questioned etiology, especially those of granulomatous character, were coupled in the early twentieth century. Its clinical resemblance to lichen scrofulosorum and its granulomatous histology quickly suggested the association. Subsequent careful histologic, microbiologic, and clinical study of patients with lichen nitidus have extinguished the tuberculosis theory. A second plausible hypothesis is that lichen nitidus represents a granulomatous response to an as yet undiscovered agent, possibly infectious in nature. If so, the process must be limited to the skin since no other organ system involvement, including the lymphatics, has been demonstrated. There is also no evidence of a relationship to sarcoidosis.

In some patients at least it seems plausible to relate lichen nitidus to lichen planus (Stankler, 1967). Coexistence of the two diseases is an ordinary occurrence, signaling either a common etiology of the disorders or a common vulnerability of certain patients to two disparate disorders. The former possibility may be the more popular Ellis, 1957; Ellis and Hill, 1938; Wilson and Bett, 1961) but has little significance at this time, since lichen planus is also of unknown etiology. Those in favor of a separate etiology, however, emphasize that the majority of patients with lichen nitidus have no signs of lichen planus and there are discernible differences, clinically and histologically, between the two diseases (Pinkus, 1973). Moreover, immunoglobulin deposits, which are localized to the dermo-epidermal interface in over 95 per cent of lichen planus lesions, are absent in lesions of lichen nitidus (Waisman et al., 1973).

Clinical Manifestations

The lesions of lichen nitidus are characteristically discrete, smooth, flat minipapules which are roughly circular in outline but at times may show a suggestion of angularity. They are uniformly pinpoint to pinhead in size (Fig. 9–16). A tendency to grouping of lesions is common, and they may be pink or flesh-colored and present a glistening appearance. A central dell or aperture is evident in some of the lesions, but there is no spiny trichotic or hyperkeratotic apex. Scales are classically absent or insignificant except in confluent lesions when a fine pityriasiform scale or, more rarely, a psoriasiform scale has been described. Itching is not a common feature of lichen nitidus, unlike lichen planus. Lesions may occur almost anywhere on the skin surface but the favorite sites are the shaft and glans of the penis, the flexural aspects of the forearms and wrists, the breasts, the abdomen, and the buttocks. The palms may also be involved, presenting a strange, roughened appearance which may be confounding to the uninitiated. Koebner-induced lesions, from rubbing or scratching and those in scars, resulting in a linear arrangement, have been described (Pinkus and Shair, 1952). Oral lesions are seen occasionally, possibly only in those patients with associated lichen planus. Widespread involvement may produce confluence of lesions in which the individual papules are seen only as satellites or at the periphery of a plaque.

The concurrence of lichen nitidus and

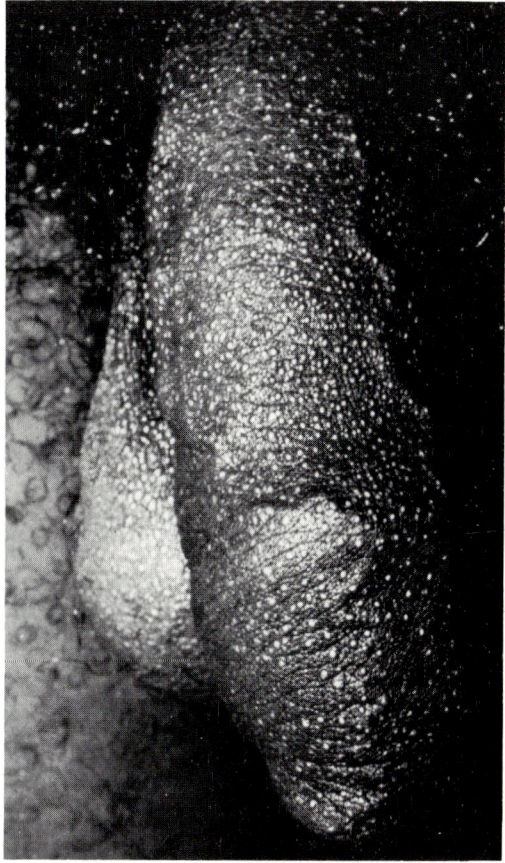

Figure 9–16 Typical flat, minipapules of lichen nitidus. Uniformly pinpoint to pinhead in size, these papules are usually flesh colored and glistening in appearance.

lichen planus is common and all patients with lichen nitidus should be scrutinized for evidence of the other disease. While a 25 to 30 per cent incidence of lichen nitidus lesions has been recorded in lichen planus patients, the frequency of the development of lichen planus in patients with primary lichen nitidus has not been established.

There are no constitutional complaints in lichen nitidus nor any signs of other organ systemic involvement.

Pathology

The histologic picture is pathognomonic, consisting of a circumscribed granulomatous change placed superficially in the papillary dermis, compressing and at times invading the overlying epidermis.

Elongation of marginal rete pegs is common, producing an encircling of the granuloma. A hyperkeratotic or parakeratotic scale is commonly seen capping the affected epidermis. Pinkus (1973) has stressed the diagnostic importance of a central focus of parakeratosis in the lesions. On volar skin, this may be in the form of a dense parakeratotic plug in the center of the papule, a distinctive change never seen in lichen planus. There is no central caseation in the granulomatous infiltrate which consists of a collection of lymphocytes, histiocytes, some epithelioid cells, and a few Langhans' giant cells. A true tuberculoid or sarcoidal patterning of these mini-granulomas has not been seen. Microorganisms are not identifiable with acid-fast, Gram, or PAS techniques.

Diagnosis

Lichen nitidus should present little problem in clinical diagnosis except in special instances. A biopsy specimen will establish the diagnosis in disputed cases. Lichen planus has a distribution similar to lichen nitidus and may coexist with it. The special features of lichen planus, such as the violaceous color and Wickham's striae of the lesions, the characteristic mucosal change, and the presence of itching, serve to distinguish the two diseases. Confluent plaques of lichen nitidus may resemble psoriasis or localized neurodermatitis. Sarcoidosis might be a consideration in certain cases of lichen nitidus. Flat warts should be recognizable on close inspection. Keratosis pilaris shows acuminate papules unlike the small smooth lesions of lichen nitidus. The indolent, flat lesions of lichen scrofulosorum may closely resemble those of lichen nitidus, but are perifollicular, may be scaly and inflammatory, and occasionally are surmounted by a small pustule. Lichen scrofulosorum occurs principally in children and is a tuberculid, developing hematogenously from glandular, bone, or joint tuberculosis. A strongly positive tuberculin skin test is characteristic. Lichen spinulosus lesions show an acuminate, spiny apex which may be felt as well as seen, distinguishing it from the smooth, flat lesions of lichen nitidus.

The hematologic, urinologic, and chemi-cal profiles of patients with lichen nitidus are within normal limits.

Treatment

There is no effective empiric or rational therapy for lichen nitidus. Symptomatic treatment is usually unnecessary since it is generally symptomless. Topical or intralesional corticosteroids may be used on confluent plaques.

Course and Prognosis

Lichen nitidus may resolve within a few weeks but this is an exceptional occurrence. A chronic course of a few to several years is to be anticipated in most cases and some patients apparently show activity almost indefinitely. When healing occurs, the skin shows no residual atrophy or hypo- or hyperpigmentation.

LICHEN STRIATUS

Lichen striatus is a clinically distinctive, self-limiting linear eruption of unknown etiology. The prevalence of this disease is unknown but it is certainly not a rarity. Children between the ages of 5 and 12 years represent the usual group affected although the disease has been seen in infancy and old age. Girls are affected at least twice as often as boys. There is no known racial variation in incidence nor any predisposition based on heredity, habitat, occupation, diet, or other factors. The condition has been described almost exclusively in the United States and Europe but there is little reason to doubt its occurrence in most of the rest of the world. Although the disease had been described and named earlier by European authors (Fantl, 1914), Senear and Caro in 1941 were probably the first to distinguish lichen striatus from other linear or zonal dermatoses.

Etiology and Pathogenesis

The zonal or dermatomal distribution of the eruption has long suggested pathogenetic mechanisms involving nerves, blood vessels, lymphatics or unclarified embryologic alterations of delayed emergence. There is no support for any of these hypotheses, however, and no evidence indicating an infectious origin.

Clinical Manifestations

Of rather abrupt onset, this eruption consists initially of discrete, pink papules, 2 to 4 cm. in width, which soon coalesce, some to form small plaques. The lesions extend linearly over the affected part, reaching a length of several centimeters or running the entire length of an extremity. They may be interrupted or may form a continuous, long, eruptive change and are at times matched by parallel linear bands of lesions. One arm or leg is usually affected, although the buttocks, neck, and trunk may be involved. The involvement of more than one extremity is seen rarely (Johnson, 1946). Classically, the lesions are papular or lichenoid, with an inconspicuous scale. Verruciform and vesiculobullous lesions have been described (Staricco, 1959) although they are rare. Pruritus is not usually a prominent feature but can be marked, especially if there is secondary irritation.

Pathology

The histopathologic picture is that of a chronic dermatitis with certain special features (Lee, 1951; Staricco, 1959). Dermal and epidermal changes correlate well, although the degree and character of the alterations vary along the length of most specimens. A dense perivascular lymphocytic and histiocytic infiltrate is characteristic but periappendageal collections, even to the point of disruption of the follicles or glands, may be seen. The infiltrate may invade the epidermis but is not bandlike as in lichen planus. The epidermis shows hyperkeratosis, parakeratosis, acanthosis, spongiosis, and not uncommonly dyskeratotic cells. A thickened, granular layer may also be present.

Diagnosis

The condition is most often confused with linear nevi, which persist indefinitely. Lichen striatus should be distinguishable histopathologically, however. A linear arrangement of viral verrucae is not uncommon but is usually of much shorter length than the evolving lesions of lichen striatus and is often associated with warts on other skin areas. Lichen planus and psoriasis may also show a linear distribution but only as part of the usual clinical picture and should not be a diagnostic problem.

Treatment and Course

Topical corticosteroids or a simple bland emollient cream to minimize dryness are all that are required since the disorder disappears spontaneously, usually within 12 weeks. Longer courses have been seen but very rarely extend beyond six to nine months. There is no internal involvement, and no local complications or sequelae are to be anticipated.

PARAPSORIASIS

To trace the history of the disorders grouped under the heading "parapsoriasis" would serve only to confound students and tire the cognoscenti. It is a tale which, from a well-intentioned beginning (Brocq, 1903), grew over the years into a taxonomic maze. Parapsoriasis is today accepted as a designation applicable to perhaps three disorders of distinctly different pathogenesis and natural history. Only tradition and a lack of clarifying information justify the continued nosologic grouping of these disorders. Except for an occasional clinical morphologic similarity, none of these conditions bears any relationship to psoriasis, despite the nominal implication to the contrary. Based on incidence alone, the parapsoriasis disorders are relatively unimportant conditions. Taken together, they constitute well under 0.1 per cent of skin diseases encountered in any clinical setting.

Although any classification of parapsoriasis is imperfect, the one used below, modified from that of Pillsbury et al. (1956), is as simple and accurate as can be made, based on present knowledge. The single appellation chosen for each disorder will be used throughout the discussion that follows. At the beginning of the discussion of each disorder the major synonyms will be cited once, to orient the reader, along with any requisite commentary. The following entities are considered under the heading parapsoriasis:

Acute vasculitic parapsoriasis
Chronic parapsoriasis
  Guttate parapsoriasis
  Parapsoriasis en plaques, including the poikilodermatous and retiform variants

ACUTE VASCULITIC PARAPSORIASIS

This condition, which is also known as Mucha-Habermann disease and pityriasis lichenoides et varioliformis acuta, is an acute or subacute and at times relapsing papulovesicular disorder of unknown etiology. It is histologically a lymphocytic vasculitis, which clearly separates it pathogenetically from the other parapsoriatic disorders.

Epidemiology

The precise incidence of acute vasculitic parapsoriasis is unknown but it is not a rare disorder. There seems to be no sexual or racial predisposition, and while both the very young and elderly have been affected, most cases occur in young adults. The disease has been reported principally in North America and Europe but has also appeared in Japan, South Africa, and Australia.

Etiology and Pathogenesis

Although no causative agent has been identified, the clinical picture suggests that an infectious agent, possibly a virus, is responsible. Efforts to isolate an organism have failed, however, (Nazarro, 1953). Angiitis secondary to allergic hypersensitivity has also been considered but there is no immunologic support for this hypothesis.

Clinical Manifestations

The eruption usually has a fairly abrupt onset, involving much of the skin surface within a few days. Small erythematous and edematous papules, 1 to 3 mm. in diameter, represent the initial change, and they are soon surmounted by a vesicle which in the more severe cases may be hemorrhagic and at times pustular. The lesions eventually rupture, leaving crusted erosions or punched-out ulcers, consistent with the infarction-like effect of the underlying vasculitis (Fig. 9–17). Some of the papular lesions fail to ulcerate and may develop a nondescript scale and ultimately some degree of post-inflammatory hyperpigmentation. The deeper lesions leave small depressed scars as in variola or papulonecrotic tuberculid (Fig. 9–17). Lesions in all stages of development are commonly seen, and a fresh wave of papules may appear as old ones are healing. The trunk is usually the site of heaviest involvement, with the axillae and extremities, especially the flexor surfaces, also commonly showing lesions. Limitation to sun-exposed areas has been observed but is not a regular feature. Lesions of the palms and soles are less common and oral or genital mucosal involvement is exceptional. The face is usually spared. Symptoms are often absent, although low-grade itching or burning may be noted early in the evolution of new lesions. Constitutional signs, including fever, malaise, headache, and rarely arthralgia, may occasionally precede or accompany the earliest evidence of acute vasculitic parapsoriasis. There are no regularly observed abnormal laboratory findings in this disease.

Pathology

The histopathologic picture is distinctive and is highlighted by a lymphocytic perivasculitis and vasculitis of the small dermal blood vessels (Szymanski, 1959). Dilation and engorgement of these blood vessels is seen early, with subsequent thickening of the vessel walls, occlusion, and consequent infarction necrosis of the adjacent dermis and epidermis. At the appropriate stage, the vesicular lesions, some hemorrhagic or pustular, can be seen. Earlier, edema and inflammatory infiltration of the dermis, close to or invading the epidermis are present.

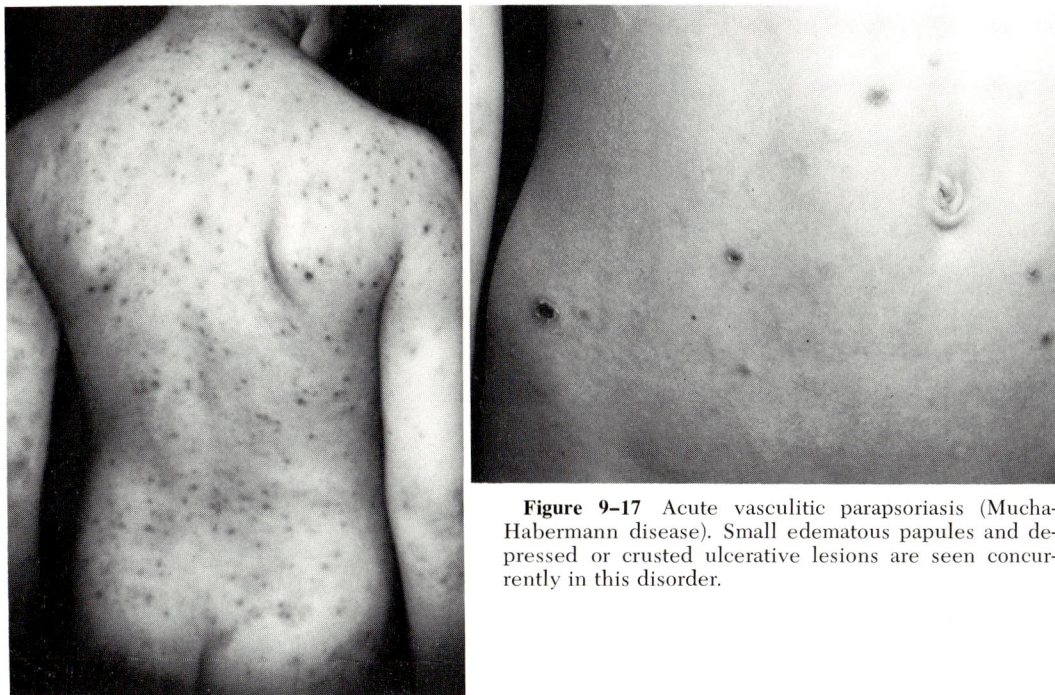

Figure 9-17 Acute vasculitic parapsoriasis (Mucha-Habermann disease). Small edematous papules and depressed or crusted ulcerative lesions are seen concurrently in this disorder.

Diagnosis

Acute vasculitic parapsoriasis is most often confused with varicella, but variola, leukocytoclastic angiitis, insect bites, lymphomatoid papulosis, and papuloneurotic tuberculid should also be considered in the differential diagnosis. Cytologic smears, culture, and serologic studies will distinguish the viral diseases, and the other conditions can be excluded histologically if not by careful analysis of the clinical features. Leukocytoclastic angiitis, it should be emphasized, is a neutrophilic vasculitis in contrast to the lymphocytic vasculitis of vasculitic parapsoriasis.

Treatment

There is no specific therapy for vasculitic parapsoriasis. Systemic corticosteroids in moderate dosage over a two to three week period may be beneficial at times. The course of therapy may be reinstituted if advisable when relapse occurs. ACTH is also effective (Winkelmann and Lorenc, 1959), and improvement has been described after antimalarials (Nagy and Balagh, 1959) and calciferol (Canizares,

1952). Tetracycline in high doses is apparently helpful in certain patients (Shelley and Griffith, 1969). Finally, methotrexate, through an as yet unexplained mechanism, may clear acute vasculitic parapsoriasis, often after the comparatively small dose of 7.5 mg. to 20 mg. weekly by mouth. Relapse usually follows discontinuance of therapy, however, and the drug should not be employed regularly for this disease. It is reserved for special troublesome patients in whom other therapy is ineffective or contraindicated.

Course and Prognosis

The disease may fade within a few weeks or last for several months and less commonly for a few years. In the longer cases there is a tendency toward short remissions followed by new outbreaks. Recovery is the rule in vasculitic parapsoriasis, however, and there is no progression to lymphoma. Attempts have been made to relate acute vasculitic parapsoriasis to chronic guttate parapsoriasis, based on the rare alleged concurrence of the two conditions. In such patients the term *pityriasis lichenoides chronica* has usually been used as a synonym for chronic guttate parapsoriasis. The problem remains unclarified. Although time and further study may dictate otherwise, this author believes the association should be regarded as fortuitous and pathogenetically insignificant.

CHRONIC PARAPSORIASIS

Guttate Parapsoriasis

Guttate parapsoriasis is a virtually asymptomatic papulosquamous disease of unknown etiology which is not to be regarded as a prelymphoma. It is a rare disease, occurring most commonly in young adults. Approximately two-thirds of the patients are males. There are no known racial, occupational, or other predisposing factors. The French (parapsoriasis en gouttes) and Latin (parapsoriasis guttata) equivalents are used regularly as synonyms for guttate parapsoriasis. The term *pityriasis lichenoides chronica* has also been used synonymously, often in a special etiologic context (see below).

Etiology and Pathogenesis

No studies or even any meaningful clues suggesting the cause of this disease are available. It is apparently without any genetic influence and bears no relationship to a cutaneous or systemic lymphoma. Some observers describe as a type of guttate parapsoriasis, pityriasis lichenoides chronica, which they consider to be a chronic form of vasculitic parapsoriasis.

Clinical Manifestations

The disease usually has a gradual and undramatic onset without any constitutional signs. Small to moderate-sized papules, 1 to about 10 mm. in diameter, are seen developing primarily on the trunk and proximal extremities. The lesions are reddish brown in color and are slightly infiltrated. The hands and feet, usually the dorsal aspect but rarely the volar, may also be involved occasionally, along with the face. A thin, adherent scale is commonly found and when removed reveals a shiny

brown surface devoid of bleeding points. No lesions are found on the mucous membranes. Itching is almost invariably absent but when present is quite mild.

Pathology

A nonspecific dermatitis characterizes this disease histopathologically. There are a mild to moderate acanthosis and spongiosis of the epidermis. A few lymphocytes may invade the epidermis, and there is a prominent perivascular lymphocytic and histiocytic infiltration of the dermis. The vessels are not invaded by round cells as they are in acute vasculitic parapsoriasis. Plasma cells and neutrophils are also insignificant components of the inflammatory infiltrate.

Diagnosis

The diagnosis is made purely on clinical grounds and largely by exclusion. Among the alternative conditions to be considered are a drug eruption, pityriasis rosea, secondary syphilis, lichen planus, psoriasis, and parapsoriasis en plaques. A careful drug history, appropriate laboratory tests for syphilis, and often a biopsy specimen are required to distinguish these disorders after a critical analysis of the clinical features of the eruptive process.

Treatment

No effective therapy is available. Local application of emollient creams and steroid preparations may be used but do not influence the course of the disease.

Course and Prognosis

A chronic course lasting from several months to 5 or 10 years is to be expected, but remissions of variable duration are common. Eventual permanent resolution is the rule, however, without any local or systemic complications or sequelae.

Parapsoriasis en Plaques

Present day knowledge dictates that parapsoriasis en plaques should be subdivided into benign and premalignant (pre-lymphoma) forms. Between 5 and 25 per cent of patients with this condition belong in the latter category and most can be identified clinically with the development of atrophy, poikiloderma, or the reticulate pattern of the eruption. Some of the synonyms that have been used for parapsoriasis en plaques include, for the benign type, xanthoerythrodermia perstans, parapsoriasis en plaques disseminées, and chronic superficial dermatitis, and for the premalignant type, poikiloderma vasculare atrophicans, parapsoriasis lichenoides, and parakeratosis variegata.

Epidemiology

Both benign and premalignant forms are diseases primarily of middle age. Careful epidemiologic surveys are unavailable. Caucasians seem to be predisposed but there is no sexual or genetic predilection.

Etiology and Pathogenesis

The cause of both the benign and premalignant forms of parapsoriasis en plaques is unknown. No precipitating factors have been identified with the transformation to malignancy.

Clinical Manifestations

The benign type of parapsoriasis en plaques is characterized by round to oval, poorly defined, flat dermatitic plaques usually 2 to 4 cm in diameter. The color of the lesions varies from yellow (xantho-erythrodermia) to red and there is no vesiculation or crusting as in the usual eczematous dermatoses, nor is there prominent infiltration. Fine, superficial scaling of the lesions is characteristic. The trunk and extremities are involved preferentially; the face, scalp, hands, and feet are rarely affected. The eruption commonly involves both sides of the body but tends to be less symmetric than the premalignant forms. Mucous membrane lesions have never been described nor is there any alteration of hair or nail growth or change in the general health of the individual. Pruritus is usually absent or is a minor complaint.

Patients with premalignant parapsoriasis en plaques are placed in one of three clinical categories, all of which are simply different manifestations of the same basic pathologic process. The first group consists of those patients with an eruption suggestive of the benign form of parapsoriasis en plaques, as described above, but showing changes in some of the lesions toward atrophy or poikiloderma. A red-blue color of the plaque is noted, there may be some telangiectasia, patchy hyperpigmentation, and a cigarette paper-like wrinkling of the lesions. Involvement of the flexural creases, the buttocks, and the breasts, often symmetrically, is common. A second class includes those patients with poikiloderma which completely overshadows or is present in the absence of scaly parapsoriatic plaques. The process may be localized to portions of the trunk, the buttocks, the axillae, the flexural areas, or the extremities, and rarely may be generalized; individuals so affected have been labeled as having the so-called idiopathic poikiloderma vasculare atrophicans. Mucous membrane involvement is seen exceptionally. Drying of the lesions, especially during cold weather or with excessive bathing, may lead to irritation and a slight burning reaction, but there is usually little or no itching until the lesions change toward a lymphoma, becoming infiltrated and assuming a specific histologic picture.

The third group of patients represent an unusual clinical variant known as the retiform variant of parapsoriasis en plaques. These patients usually maintain a picture suggestive of parapsoriasis en plaques with a dramatic striped pattern or network of lesions over much of the skin surface affecting preferentially the intertriginous areas, lower trunk, buttocks, and thighs. Intermixed with the above retiform eruption and poikilodermatous changes are deeply erythematous plaques which may show small lichenoid papules. This rare eruption progresses rather regularly to a lymphoma.

Pathology

A nonspecific dermatitis characterizes the early phase and in many cases there may be histologic signs of poikiloderma; namely, dilatation of superficial capillaries, an abundance of melanophores, a predominantly lymphocytic infiltrate in the upper dermis and at times invading the epidermis (which is generally thinner overall), and a few intra-epidermal mononuclear microabscesses. With transformation to a lymphoreticulosis, abnormal cells are present and are eventually identified.

Diagnosis

Parapsoriasis en plaques, both the chronic benign type and the prereticulotic variety (before poikilodermatous changes are evident), may resemble nummular atopic dermatitis, the medallion type of seborrheic dermatitis, Sulzberger-Garbe syndrome, and certain drug eruptions, including fixed drug eruptions. Careful analysis of the clinical features and history, the histologic findings, and the response to treatment permit an unequivocal diagnosis.

Radiodermatitis and the other poikilodermas are to be distinguished from poikilodermatous parapsoriasis on the basis of the clinical signs and the histologic findings. Retiform parapsoriasis is so distinctive a clinical picture as to rarely present a diagnostic problem.

Treatment

No curative treatment is available for any of these forms of parapsoriasis. Emollient or corticosteroid creams, which are rather ineffective in suppressing the inflammatory element, are helpful in minimizing the dryness many patients exhibit, particularly in cold weather. Superficial x-ray or grenz ray therapy may produce temporary regression of isolated infiltrated plaques, and teleroentgentherapy may be useful in certain prelymphomatous forms. Later, when the change to lymphoma is apparent, the treatment is that of the lymphoma as outlined elsewhere (see Chap. 29).

Course and Prognosis

A chronic course of years is to be expected for parapsoriasis en plaques and it is virtually unremitting during its course. The great majority of patients, at least 75 per cent and perhaps 95 per cent of them (Lapiere, 1949; Shelley, 1974), never develop lymphoma, although they may die having had parapsoriasis for 20 or more years. The telltale clue to the identity of those patients who will develop lymphoma is the poikilodermatous alteration of the eruption which may appear quite early in the course of the disease (Samman, 1964). Mycosis fungoides is the usual clinical type of lymphoma which ultimately develops in these patients, although other lymphomas or reticuloses have been described.

EXFOLIATIVE DERMATITIS

The designation exfoliative dermatitis refers to the involvement of all or most of the skin surface by a scaly erythematous dermatitis. Erythroderma is favored as a synonym by the British. The widespread inflammatory and exfoliative eruption produces secondary effects on other organ systems and on the body as a whole, some of which can be quite debilitating.

The epidemiologic features of exfoliative dermatitis reflect the composite epidemiology of all of the diseases which cause this disorder. As a set of separate characteristics they are of little value. Some statistics on incidence are worthy of mention, however. Approximately 1 per cent of patients hospitalized for skin disease show exfoliative dermatitis (Gentele et al., 1958). Males are victims of the condition at least twice as often as are females and over three-quarters of the patients are over the age of 40. The available surveys generally exclude the very young, however, who may have atopic dermatitis and certain inherited dermatoses which can result in exfoliative dermatitis.

Etiology and Pathogenesis

The modern interpretation of exfoliative dermatitis no longer includes the old etiologic classification of the disorder into primary and secondary types. Exfoliative dermatitis is always a secondary or reactive process to an underlying cutaneous or systemic disease. As knowledge and diagnostic methods improve, the number of cases of exfoliative dermatitis with an unidentifiable cause should decrease.

The mechanisms responsible for the development of exfoliative dermatitis secondary to a systemic disease are unknown. Auto-allergic mechanisms have not been demonstrated. Speculation that the underlying disorder may release chemicals which act as cutaneous toxins or may suppress the normal immunologic protective mechanisms is unsupported by experimental or clinical evidence. Extension of a preexisting skin disease to produce an exfoliative dermatitis is readily understood, as is the universal involvement of the skin by an exogenous agent.

An etiologic classification showing the relative incidence of the underlying causes of exfoliative dermatitis is shown in Table 9–1.

Clinical Manifestations

The onset of exfoliative dermatitis may be acute, particularly when a reticulosis, drug reaction, or contact allergy with universal exposure is responsible. Most of the cutaneous diseases which can eventuate in an exfoliative dermatitis do so more gradually, however. In the untreated individual,

TABLE 9–1 CAUSES OF EXFOLIATIVE DERMATITIS*

Disease	Incidence (Per Cent)
Preexisting cutaneous disease	40
Psoriasis	
Atopic dermatitis	
Seborrheic dermatitis	
Eczema of unknown origin	
Stasis dermatitis	
Pityriasis rubra pilaris	
Ichthyosiform dermatoses	
Pityriasis rosea	
Pemphigus foliaceus	
Lichen planus	
Scabies	
Toxic epidermal necrolysis	
Contact dermatitis	10
Drugs	10
Lymphoma and leukemia	15
Idiopathic	25

*Based on analysis of our own cases and the reports of Rook et al. (1968), Wilson (1954), Gentele et al. (1958), and Abrahams et al. (1963).

the extensive involvement, once stabilized, tends to change little, and waxing and waning between a widespread and limited eruption are not to be expected.

There is a general tendency to view exfoliative dermatitis, regardless of cause, as an end-stage process in which identifiable features of the underlying disorder are lost. This is true in many cases, but in others, careful and continued clinical observation may reveal local changes which are characteristic of the primary disease. There are also certain clinical signs of diagnostic importance which are associated with some underlying disorders and not with others. It is appropriate, therefore, to cite the distinctive clinical features of the disorders that may give rise to exfoliative dermatitis.

PSORIASIS. As it is developing, exfoliative psoriasis may show heavier involvement in the areas where psoriasis is most common, namely, the elbows, knees, scalp, and lumbosacral skin. In addition, the characteristic silvery-white scale and sharp margin on the lesions may persist. Once generalized involvement has occurred these special features will be lost or difficult to discern. Psoriatic pustules may develop in some areas during acute attacks and generalized pustular psoriasis can be an unfortunate complication at times (p. 419). A characteristic nail dystrophy can be seen in many patients with psoriatic erythroderma.

ATOPIC DERMATITIS. Generalization of atopic dermatitis usually follows exacerbation of chronic localized eczema of the antecubital-popliteal and face-neck areas. The "white line" response may be especially prominent in these patients and pruritus is often severe. In youngsters, regional adenopathy, at times quite marked, is often present. Among the atopic stigmata, the atopic epicanthal fold of the lower eyelid should be looked for. Eosinophilia is common. The complications of significance in atopic exfoliative dermatitis include secondary bacterial infection and atopic cataracts which are apparently more common in the patient with severe or chronic atopic dermatitis.

STASIS DERMATITIS. Signs of venous insufficiency, such as varicosities, edema, patchy post-inflammatory hyperpigmentation from previous dermatitic episodes, and active ulcers or healed scars usually at the ankle along the course of the greater or lesser saphenous veins, may be present. Exfoliative dermatitis from stasis dermatitis may result from "autosensitization" (Parish et al., 1965) or from contact allergy to an applied topical medicament.

PITYRIASIS RUBRA PILARIS. The clinical clues to an exfoliative dermatitis arising from pityriasis rubra pilaris include follicular papules on the dorsal aspects of the fingers, toes, knees, and elbows, the thick scaling of the palms and soles, and the persistence of islands of normal skin within diffusely erythrodermic areas.

Facial scaling may be particularly heavy, and ectropion is seen occasionally. The nails may be thickened and transversely striated but do not show the pitting typical of psoriasis.

PEMPHIGUS FOLIACEUS. Rupture of bullae may leave moist erosive or crusted areas. Although the bullae usually rupture quickly, they may remain intact in places and can be detected on close examination of the patient. An arcuate or gyrate pattern of the lesions is common on the trunk, especially the anterior thorax. Old lesions may develop a vegetative or keratotic appearance.

LICHEN PLANUS. The violaceous color, fine reticulate scale, and angulation of the papules may be perceived as lichen planus progresses to exfoliative dermatitis and as the generalized process recedes. Oral, penile, vaginal, and other mucosal surfaces may reveal the characteristic lacy white lesional network seen in this disease. Involvement of the nails, if present, may be suggestive, especially if anonychia or pterygium formation are present. Lichen planus is an uncommon cause of exfoliative dermatitis, although drug-induced lichen planus or lichenoid eruptions more readily become generalized.

NORWEGIAN SCABIES. Chronic infestation by the scabetic mite may result in widespread scaly erythema, with thick crusted lesions of the hands and feet and nail involvement. The mites may be found on microscopic examination of the scales or crusts under potassium hydroxide.

CONTACT AND PHOTOCONTACT DERMATITIS. Vesicles, the primary lesions of allergic and primary irritancy contact dermatitis, may be visible early in the course of the process or during an acute exacerbation. They are absent in the very chronic cases, however. The characteristic exposure patterns of the given contactant are also missing, but more pronounced inflammation at the primary contact sites and the relative sparing of other areas may suggest the type of contactant responsible. Thus, airborne contact allergens affect the eyelids preferentially, and relative sparing of the submental skin and covered areas is common in severe photocontact dermatitis. Photocontact and straight contact allergy may coexist in some chronic cases.

DRUGS. There are no special clinical signs to indicate that drugs are the cause of exfoliative dermatitis. However, the reactions are classically rather acute in onset and symmetric in distribution, with erythema a prominent feature generally accompanied by a purpuric element in dependent skin areas. Penicillin, sulfonamides, barbiturates, gold, isoniazid, and phenothiazines are among the most important of the commonly used medications which may induce exfoliative dermatitis.

TOXIC EPIDERMAL NECROLYSIS. This condition, which has also been called the "scalded skin syndrome" and Ritter's disease (in infants), may develop following bacterial infection, especially the group II phage type 71 of *Staphylococcus aureus*, as a reaction to drugs, and possibly after certain viral infections such as measles (Koblenzer, 1967; Lyell, 1967). Apparently a unique, as yet unclarified hypersensitivity reaction restricted to the skin, toxic epidermal necrolysis produces a striking clinical picture. An intense erythema of portions of the face, especially the perioral and medial cheek skin, is an early feature. Exquisitely tender skin, reminiscent of burned skin, is also present, producing restlessness and marked irritability. The process extends quickly to affect most of the skin surface but generally sparing the scalp. Superficial fine vesicles or bullae form and rupture easily. Large sheets of epidermis are lost, leaving erosive red areas. The conjunctivae and the oral, nasal, genital, and anal mucosa may also be affected. Some cases may appear to have concurrent Stevens-Johnson syndrome or at least be difficult to distinguish from that disorder.

SEBORRHEIC DERMATITIS (LEINER'S

DISEASE). An infrequent cause of exfoliative dermatitis in the adult, seborrheic dermatitis may also rarely produce a distinctive exfoliative dermatitis in infants, usually in those under three or four months of age. The pediatric form has been called Leiner's disease and among its clinical features are generalized lymphadenopathy and a severe recalcitrant diarrhea. In many patients the process begins with an almost universal erythroderma while in others it is initiated by an erythematous or seborrheic eruption of the diaper areas, face, or scalp. Certain familial cases of Leiner's disease, which are especially severe and frequently fatal, have a functional defect in the fifth component of complement (C5) which is detectable only by functional assay and not by simple immunochemical quantitative determination (Jacobs and Miller, 1972). These infants may be saved by administration of fresh plasma. Leiner's disease is most often confused with toxic epidermal necrolysis (Ritter's disease) and with atopic dermatitis.

LYMPHOMA AND LEUKEMIA. The exfoliative dermatitis produced by lymphomas and leukemia may defy elucidation for months or years. Pruritus is often quite severe so that excoriations are common. The skin eventually becomes infiltrated, and distortion of facial features may occur, resulting in a leonine facies. Lymphadenopathy, showing specific or nonspecific histologic changes, is common. Among the lymphomas, mycosis fungoides, reticulum cell sarcoma, and Hodgkin's disease are common causes of an exfoliative dermatitis. The Sézary syndrome, an erythroderma with a leukocytosis and atypical lymphocytes in the skin and blood, has received considerable attention in recent years. Its nosologic status is still unclarified and many regard it simply as a modified clinical expression of one of the lymphomas or leukemia, into which it almost invariably eventuates in time. Of interest is the recent demonstration of small and large T-cell variants among the Sézary lymphocytes (Lutzner et al., 1973). Winkelmann (1973) has emphasized that the Sézary syndrome is not a lymphoma, although it may develop into one, and that it may be brought into remission with a low-dose alkylating agent and prednisone therapy.

IDIOPATHIC. The cause of exfoliative dermatitis will remain undiscovered in a significant number of patients, ranging from about 10 per cent in some series (Gentele et al., 1958; Rook et al., 1972) to almost 50 per cent in others (Abrahams et al., 1963).

Continued, careful observation and study will in time expose the causative influences in some of these patients. Interestingly an occasional unexplained temporary remission may be seen in these patients, but spontaneous, complete clearing is rare.

OTHER CLINICAL AND METABOLIC EFFECTS OF EXFOLIATIVE DERMATITIS. Fever, usually low grade, and chilly sensations are common as exfoliative dermatitis develops. These signs come and go as the acuteness of the inflammatory reaction, manifested principally by erythema, waxes and wanes. Malaise and some weakness are noted in some patients but a marked constitutional reaction is not usually seen except perhaps in those patients with an acute leukemia. Because of the erythema the skin of the patient with exfoliative dermatitis feels warm or even hot to the touch. In addition to a feeling of being cold, the more outstanding subjective complaints include tightness of the skin, especially during the acute phase. In chronic cases the skin may hang loosely in certain areas and appear stretched after resolution of edematous inflammation of long standing. Loss of hair on the scalp and body occurs after several weeks, and dystrophic nail changes are common. In dark-skinned individuals, post-inflammatory hyperpigmentation and less often hypopigmentation are seen in a patchy or diffuse pattern.

Gynecomastia is a common finding in almost all patients with exfoliative dermatitis of at least several weeks duration. It is apparently a hormonally mediated change, although the precise mechanism is still unknown. Hyperestrogenism is present, marked by increased urinary excretion of estrogens (Shuster and Brown, 1962).

Nonspecific lymphadenopathy, at times of surprising dimensions, is not unexpected in view of the persistent or recurring extensive inflammatory reaction in the skin of patients with exfoliative dermatitis. The nodes are nontender and discretely enlarged and have a firm, rubbery consistency. Usually the most prominent nodes are those of the cervical and axillary chains. The terms *dermatopathic lymphadenitis* and *lipomelanotic reticulosis* have been applied to this nonspecific lymphadenopathy. Biopsy study of enlarged nodes should be performed in all patients in whom the etiology of the exfoliative dermatitis has been difficult to establish. Cytologic examination of aspirates of enlarged nodes has also been recommended to establish the diagnosis of lymphoma but has proved a disappointing technique for this author.

The extensive erythema and scaling of exfoliative dermatitis are productive of significant and at times profound physiologic changes. A markedly augmented blood flow through the skin (Fox et al., 1965) and consequent increased heat loss from the body are seen in these patients (Zoon and Mali, 1957). Temperature regulation may be disturbed, and the danger of hyothermia exists (Krook, 1960). A compensatory increase in the metabolic rate ensues which has been shown to be unrelated to a primary increase in thyroid function (Krook, 1961).

Transepidermal water loss, largely a measure of water loss through keratinization, is greatly increased, and the loss of protein through scaling may reach substantial levels. Exfoliation may produce a protein loss of 9.0 gm. per m.² of skin surface per day and still not result in clinical or laboratory signs of negative nitrogen balance (Freedberg and Baden, 1962). With more severe scaling, however, protein losses as high as 17 gm. per m.² of skin surface per day may occur, resulting in negative nitrogen balance. The serum protein falls owing to a lowered serum albumin resulting from (1) increased loss of protein from both the exfoliative skin and the gastrointestinal tract and (2) plasma dilution secondary to cardiovascular alterations (Shuster and Wilkinson, 1963, Teckner and Baset, 1960). There is a relative increase in the globulin fraction of the serum. Folate loss may also occur through the "sloughing skin" of exfoliative dermatitis, resulting in a decreased serum folate (Held, 1969). Anemia has not yet been described as a result of this change, however. The hemodynamic alterations that occur in exfoliative dermatitis may produce a high-output cardiac failure (Shuster, 1963). During the active erythrodermic phase, the cardiac output is increased and returns to normal as the skin improves (Voigt et al., 1966).

The widespread cutaneous inflammation and defoliation may also result in an enteropathy, as manifested principally by steatorrhea, which tends to resolve with clearing of the exfoliative dermatitis (Shuster, 1968). Among other clinical findings in these patients are hepatomegaly, which is found in a minority of patients and has no known etiologic significance (Abrahams et al., 1963), and splenomegaly, which has been seen only in patients with lymphoma or leukemia. In many patients congestive failure may account for the hepatomegaly (Frost and Weinstein, 1972). Such individuals may also exhibit other signs of cardiac failure such as dyspnea and edema.

Pathology

Unless the primary diagnosis is otherwise apparent, a biopsy specimen should always be secured in these patients. Moreover, additional biopsies are necessary in many patients, especially those in whom a lymphoma is suspected. If obtained from a site showing residual clinical signs of the primary disease, the biopsy may reveal histologic changes which will confirm the clinical impression. Thus, care should be taken to obtain a specimen from an early representative lesion so that the specific or suggestive microscopic elements of pityriasis rubra pilaris, lichen planus, or pemphigus foliaceus may be found. Some of the other conditions, namely, psoriasis, seborrheic dermatitis, and atopic dermatitis, which normally exhibit rather nonspecific changes histologically are often difficult if not impossible to identify as the underlying cause of exfoliative dermatitis. In patients with a lymphoma, the specific cytologic features will ultimately be evident. During the full-blown exfoliative erythrodermic phase with generalized involvement, a number of nonspecific microscopic features may be seen in the skin, including hyperkeratosis, parakeratosis, and acanthosis in the epidermis, plus edema, vasodilation, and a perivascular infiltrate consisting of lymphocytes, histiocytes, and some eosinophils in the dermis.

Laboratory Findings

Any and all laboratory studies which might establish the primary cause of the exfoliative dermatitis should be performed. Unfortunately, there are few studies which are helpful in the majority of cases. Leukemia can be detected from a blood count and marrow study. A greater number of eosinophils may be present in the skin of the atopic with exfoliative dermatitis. Other nonspecific findings which will not elucidate the causes of an exfoliative dermatitis are an elevated sedimentation rate, decreased serum albumin and a relative increase in serum globulin, and signs of cardiac failure and intestinal dysfunction (described above).

Diagnosis

The distinction between a dermatitis which is simply extensive and acute and a true exfoliative dermatitis or erythroderma may at times be arbitrary. An extensive eczematous dermatitis due to contact allergy or a drug eruption may resolve fairly quickly with treatment and elimination of the exposure, and the classic clinical elements of exfoliative dermatitis, namely, the erythroderma and recurring desquamation, will not be evident. Once the process has become more chronic or stable as an extensive exfoliative dermatitis, however, there should be little difficulty in labeling it. Identification of the specific cause of exfoliative dermatitis in a given patient has been discussed previously. It requires a careful analysis of the clinical features; laboratory findings; biopsy study of skin, marrow, and lymph nodes; chest x-ray; and any other studies that could uncover the etiologic process. Since the ultimate picture of exfoliative dermatitis may be amorphous and lack suggestive clinical clues, the examiner should be cognizant of all of the etiologic possibilities and study the patient appropriately. Unfortunately, between 10 and 50 per cent of patients with exfoliative dermatitis may have to be regarded as idiopathic, with no identifiable cause after extensive study.

Treatment

Hospitalization, where appropriate dermatologic nursing care, supportive measures, and laboratory studies are available, is generally indicated for the patient with exfoliative dermatitis. Systemic corticosteroids are necessary in the majority of patients. The precise initial daily dosage will vary from patient to patient but is usually in the range of 30 to 40 mg. of prednisone. It should be increased by 20 mg. if there is no improvement in three or four days. Further increases to a level which will produce clearing of the eruptions may be necessary. The ordinary adjuvant measures used in patients given systemic corticosteroids should be instituted. In many patients in whom there is no primary diagnosis and thus no specific treatment, long-term administration of corticosteroids may be required. An effort should be made to keep the maintenance dose as low as possible. Systemic antibiotics are advisable in many patients, since bacterial infection of moist exfoliative skin is common and represents a significant hazard. Topical approaches include lukewarm or tepid colloidal baths with cornstarch or oatmeal powder suspensions followed by the application of bland, non-irritating lotions such as a simple wetting lotion with 15 per cent olive oil, or an oil-lime water lotion. Corticosteroids in lotions or creams are not dramatically beneficial but may allay the inflammation and pruritus somewhat. Because of the extensive surface area involved, there may be significant systemic absorption of topically applied corticosteroids. There would be an even more pronounced effect with occlusion. In addition, the risk of secondary bacterial infection of the skin areas is substantially increased with the occlusive technique.

Exfoliative psoriasis or pityriasis rubra pilaris may require the administration of methotrexate, in accordance with the guidelines recommended for its use in these diseases (Brown and Penny, 1966; Roenigk et al., 1972). The management of patients with leukemia or lymphoma requires the collaboration of the hematologist or radiologist.

Course and Prognosis

The course of exfoliative dermatitis is dependent on the nature and response to treatment of the underlying disorder. An identified contactant or drug can be eliminated. Some of the skin diseases that give rise to exfoliative dermatitis may resolve spontaneously or remit temporarily. The prognosis in many patients, however, especially those in the idiopathic group, is generally poor since many will persist almost indefinitely in this state and fatal complications such as infection with septicemia, pneumonia, or heart failure are possible. The outlook for patients with lymphoma or leukemia will reflect the anticipated course of this specific type of reticulosis.

REFERENCES

Psoriasis

Abele, D. C., Dobson, R. L., and Graham, J. B.: Heredity and psoriasis. Arch. Dermatol. 88:38, 1963.

Alibert, J. L.: Précis Théorique et Pratique sur les Maladies de la Peau. Vol. 1. 1st ed. Paris, Caille and Ravier, 1918, p. 21.

Avila, R., Pugh, D. G., Slocumb, C. H., et al.: Psoriatic arthritis: A roentgenologic study. Radiology 75:69, 1960.

Baker, H.: The Relationship between Psoriasis, Psoriatic Arthritis and Rheumatoid Arthritis. An Epidemiologic, Clinical and Serological Study. M. D. Thesis. University of Leeds, 1965.

Baker, H.: The influence of chloroquine and related drugs on psoriasis and keratoderma blenorrhagicum. Br. J. Dermatol. 78:161, 1966.

Baker, H., Goldring, D. N., and Thompson, M.: Psoriasis and arthritis. Ann. Intern. Med. 58:909, 1963.

Baker, H., Goldring, D. N., and Thompson, M.: The nails in psoriatic arthritis. Br. J. Dermatol. 76:549, 1964.

Barbeau, A., and Giroux, J. M.: Levodopa and psoriasis. Lancet 1:204, 1972.

Bauer, M., Bennett, G. A., and Zeller, J. W.: Pathology of joint lesions in patients with psoriasis and arthritis. Trans. Assoc. Am. Physicians 56:349, 1941.

Bowers, R. E., Dalton, D., Furdson, D., et al.: The treatment of psoriasis with UVR, dithranol paste and tar baths. Br. J. Dermatol. 78:273, 1966.

Braverman, J. M., Cohen, I., and O'Keefe, E.: Metabolic and ultrastructural studies in a patient with pustular psoriasis. Arch. Dermatol. 105:189, 1972.

Burch, P. R. J., and Rowell, M. R.: Psoriasis: Aetiological aspects. Acta Derm. Venereol. 45:366, 1965.

Champion, R. H.: Generalized pustular psoriasis. Br. J. Dermatol. 71:384, 1959.

Champion, R. H.: Treatment of psoriasis. Br. Med. J. 2:993, 1966.

Costa, F., and Solnica, J.: Lu Polyarthritis psoriasique. Rev. Fr. Etud. Clin. Biol. 11:578, 1966.

Cotton, D. K., and Muir, P. D.: An hypothesis on the aetiology of psoriasis. Br. J. Dermatol. 76:519, 1964.

De La Brassine, M. F., and Couteaux-Dumont, E. M.: Tritiated thymidine labelling of epidermis in pustular psoriasis. Arch. Dermatol. 106:768, 1972.

Delbarre, F.: Interest in the study of intraleucocytic "inclusions" in the diagnosis of sero-negative polyarthritis. 6th European Congress of Rheumatology. London, 1967, p. 65.

Eddy, D. D., Ascheim, E., and Farber, E. M.: Experimental analysis of isomorphic (Koebner) response in psoriasis. Arch. Dermatol. 89:579, 1964.

Epstein, I. H., Fukuyma, K., Fye, K.: Effects of ultraviolet reduction on the mitotic cycle and DNA, RNA and protein synthesis in mammalial epidermis in vivo. Photochem. Photobiol. 12:57, 1970.

Farber, E. M.: Psoriasis Center. Int. Psoriasis Bulletin 1:1, 1974.

Farber, E. M., Nall, L. M., and Watson, W.: Natural history of psoriasis in 61 twin pairs. Arch. Dermatol. 109:207, 1974.

Farber, E. M., Roth, R. J., Ackermin, E., et al.: Role of trauma in isomorphic response in psoriasis. Arch. Dermatol. 91:246, 1965.

Feuerman, E. J., and Nir, M. A.: Allopurinol in psoriasis. Br. J. Dermatol. 89:83, 1973.

Franks, A. G., and Barner, J. L.: Basal cell epithelioma in psoriatic patch. Arch. Derm. Syph. 55:375, 1947.

Frost, P., and Weinstein, G.: Topical administration of vitmain A acid for ichthyosiform dermatoses and psoriasis. J.A.M.A. 207:1863, 1969.

Gay, M. W., Moore, W. J., Morgan, J. M., et al.: Anthralin Toxicity. Arch. Dermatol. 105:213, 1972.

Goldschmidt, H., and Thew, M.: Exfoliative cytology of psoriasis and other common dermatoses. Arch. Dermatol. 106:476, 1973.

Hellgren, L.: Psoriasis: The Prevalence in Sex, Age and Occupational Groups in Total Populations in Sweden: Morphology, Inheritance and Association With Other Skin and Rheumative Diseases.

Hellgren, L.: Psoriasis: Statistical, clinical and laboratory investigation of 255 psoriasis patients and matched healthy controls. Acta Derm. Venereol. 44:191, 1964.

Hodgen, C., and Hill, E.: Ultraviolet reduction and psoriasis. Arch. Dermatol. 106:498, 1972.

Holti, G.: Vascular phenomena diagnostic of latent psoriasis. Br. J. Dermatol. 76:503, 1964.

Hurley, H. J., and Shelley, W. B.: The induction of Koebner's phenomenon in psoriasis with roentgen irradiation. Am. J. Radiol. 73:984, 1955.

Ingram, I. T.: The approach to psoriasis. Br. Med. J. 2:591, 1953.

Kern, A. B.: Indomethacin for psoriasis. Arch. Dermatol. 93:239, 1966.

Khan, S. A., Peterkin, G. A., and Mitchell, P. C.: Juvenile generalized pustular psoriasis. Arch. Dermatol. 105:67, 1972.

Koebner, H.: Zur Aetiologie Der Psoriasis. Vgscha. Derm. Syph. 4:203, 1877.

Krain, L. S.: Histocompatibility antigens. A laboratory and epidemiologic tool. J. Invest. Dermatol. 62:67, 1974.

Leavell, U. W., Jr., and Yarbro, J. W.: Hydroxyuria: A new treatment for psoriasis. Arch. Dermatol. 102:144, 1970.

Leavell, U. W., Merpack, I. P., and Smith, C.: Survey of the treatment of psoriasis with hydroxyuria. Arch. Dermatol. 107:467, 1973.

Leczinsky, C. G.: The incidence of arthropathy in a ten year series of posoriasis cases. Acta Derm. Venereol. 28:483, 1948.

Lerner, M. R., and Lerner, A. B.: Psoriasis and protein intake. Arch. Dermatol. 90:217, 1964.

Lerner, M. R., and Lerner, A. B.: Congenital psoriasis. Arch. Dermatol. 105:598, 1972.

Lomholt, G.: Psoriasis: Prevalence, Spontaneous Course and Genetics. Copenhagen, GAD, 1963.

Malkinson, F. D., and Pearson, R. W.: Successful treatment of generalized pustular psoriasis (Zumbach) by systemic antibiotics controlled by blood culture. *In* Malkinson, F. D., and Pearson, R. W., (eds.): Year Book of Dermatology. Chicago, Year Book Medical Publishers, Inc., 1972.

Merples, R. R., Heston, C. L., and Kligman, A. M.: Staphylococcus aureus in psoriasis. Arch. Dermatol. 107:568, 1973.

Moll, J. M. H., and Wright, V.: Familial occurrence of psoriatic arthritis. Ann. Rheum. Dis. 32:181, 1973.

Mom, A. M., Polak, M., Fabeiro, J. A., et al.: The psoriatic myopathy. Dermatologica 140:214, 1970.

Moschella, S. L., and Greenwald, M. A.: Psoriasis with hydroxyurea. Arch. Dermatol. 107:363, 1973.

Norrlind, R.: The significance of infection in the organization of psoriasis. Acta Rheum. Scand. 1:135, 1955.

O'Quinn, S. E.: Psoriasis, Ultraviolet light and chloroquin. Arch. Dermatol. 90:211, 1964.

Payne, R. W.: Severe outbreak of surgical sepsis due to staphylococcus aureus of unusual type and origin. Br. Med. J. 4:17, 1967.

Peck, G. L., Key, D. J., and Guss, S.: Topical vitamin A acid in the treatment of psoriasis. Arch. Dermatol. 107:245, 1973.

Petrozzi, J. W., and Witkowski, J.: Acrodermatitis perstans. Generalization following therapy with nystatin. Arch. Dermatol. 103:442, 1971.

Pinkus, H., and Mehregen, A. H.: The primary histologic lesion of seborrheic dermatitis and psoriasis. J. Invest. Dermatol. 46:109, 1966.

Privat, Y., Faye, I., and Allain, G.: Psoriasis pustuleux de haute gravité probablement induits par la pénicilline. Bull. Soc. Fr. Dermatol. Syphiligr. 76:505, 1969.

Reed, W. B.: Psoriasis and arthritis. Acta Derm. Venereol. 41:396, 1961.

Reed, W. B., and Wright, V.: *In* Hill, A. G. D., (ed.): Modern Trends in Rheumatology. London, Butterworth and Co., 1966, pp. 375–383.

Rees, R. B.: Aminopterin for psoriasis. Arch. Dermatol. 90:544, 1964.

Reiss, F.: Psoriasis and adrenocortical function. Arch. Dermatol. Syph. 59:78, 1949.

Roenigk, H. H., Maibach, H. I., and Weinstein, G. D.: Guidelines: Methotrexate therapy for psoriasis vulgaris. Arch. Dermatol. 105:363, 1972.

Roenigk, H., Maibach, H., and Weinstein, G.: Methotrexate therapy for psoriasis. Arch. Dermatol. 108:35, 1973.

Sauer, G. C.: Combined methotrexate and hydroxyurea therapy for psoriasis. Arch. Dermatol. 107:369, 1973.

Shelley, W. B.: Generalized pustular psoriasis. *In* Consultations in Dermatology. Philadelphia, W. B. Saunders Co., 1972, pp. 210–215.

Shima, T., and Havin, K.: Incidence of psoriasis in Japan. Derm. Urol. 24:506, 1962.

Shuster, S.: Dermatogenic enteropathy. N. Y. State Med. J. 68:3160, 1968.

Simons, R. D.: Additional studies in psoriasis in the tropics and in starvation camps. J. Invest. Dermatol. 12:285, 1949.

Soltani, K., and Van Scott, C. J.: Patterns and sequence of tissue changes in incipient and evolving lesions of psoriasis. Arch. Dermatol. 106:484, 1972.

Sternberg, A. G., Becker, S. W., Jr., Fitzpatrick, J. B., et al.: A genetic and statistical study of psoriasis. Am. J. Hum. Genet. 3:267, 1951.

Tsuji, T., and Sugai, T.: Topically administered fluorouracil in psoriasis. Arch. Dermatol. 105:208, 1972.

Turner, R. W., and Calabres, P.: The effect of triacetyl azauridine on psoriasis. J. Invest. Dermatol. 43:551, 1964.

Van Scott, E. J., and Ekel, T.: Kinetics of hyperplasia in psoriasis. Arch. Dermatol. 88:373, 1963.

Van Scott, E. J., and Reinertson, R. P.: Morphologic and physiologic effects of chemotherapeutic agents in psoriasis. J. Invest. Dermatol. 33:357, 1959.

Verhagen, A. R. H. B., and Koten, J. W.: Psoriasis in Kenva. Arch. Dermatol. 96:39, 1967.

Vickers, C. F. D., and Ghadially, F. N.: Keratoacanthomata associated with psoriasis. Br. J. Dermatol. 73:120, 1961.

Viglioglia, P. A., Plante, G. E., Viglioglia, J., et al.: Allopurinol in psoriasis. Dermatologica 141:203, 1970.

Voorhees, J. J., Duell, E. A., Bass, L. J., et al.: Decreased cyclic AMP in the epidermis of lesions of psoriasis. Arch. Dermatol. 105:695, 1972.

Walter, J. F., Voorhees, J. J., Kelsey, W. A., et al.: Psoralens plus black light inhibits epidermal DNA synthesis. Arch. Dermatol. 107:861, 1973.

Watson, W., Cann, H. M., Farber, E. M., et al.: The genetics of psoriasis. Arch. Dermatol. 105:197, 1972.

Weinstein, G. D., and Frost, P.: Abnormal cell proliferation in psoriasis. J. Invest. Dermatol. 50:254, 1968.

Weinstein, G. D., and Van Scott, E. J.: Autoradiographic analysis of turnover times of normal and psoriatic epidermis. J. Invest. Dermatol. 45:257, 1965.

White, C. J., and Laipply, T. C.: Histopathology of nail diseases. J. Invest. Dermatol. 19:121, 1952.

Whyte, H. J., and Baughmann, R. D.: Acute guttate psoriasis and streptococcal infection. Arch. Dermatol. 89:350, 1964.

Willan, R.: On Cutaneous Diseases. P 105, London, 1808.

Willis, I., and Harris, D. R.: Resistant psoriasis. Arch. Dermatol. 107:358, 1973.

Witten, V.: A folding ultraviolet light box. Arch. Dermatol. 107:716, 1973.

Wright, V.: Psoriasis and arthritis. Ann. Rheum. Dis. 15:348, 1956.

Wright, V.: Psoriatic arthritis. A comparative study of rheumatoid arthritis and arthritis associated with psoriasis. Ann. Rheum. Dis. 20:123, 1961.

Wright, V., and Moll, J. M. N.: Psoriatic arthritis. Bull. Rheum. Dis. 21:627, 1971.

Zackheim, H. S., and Farber, E. M.: Low protein diet and psoriasis. Arch. Dermatol. 99:580, 1969.

Zackheim, H. S., Arnold, J. G., Farber, E. M., et al.:

Topical therapy of psoriasis with mechloretha-mine. Arch. Dermatol. 105:702, 1972.

Zaias, N.: Psoriasis of the nail. A clinico-pathologic study. Arch. Dermatol. 99:567, 1969.

Zimmerman, M. C.: Ultraviolet light therapy. Arch. Dermatol. 78:646, 1958.

Pityriasis Rosea

Anderson, C. R.: Dapsone treatment in a case of vesi-cular pityriasis rosea. Lancet 2:493, 1971.

Bjornberg, A., and Hellgren, L.: Pityriasis rosea. A statistical, clinical and laboratory investigation of 826 patients and matched healthy controls. Acta Derm. Venereol. 42 (Suppl. 50):1, 1962.

Bunch, L. W., and Tilley, J. C.: Pityriasis rosea. A histologic and serologic study. Arch. Dermatol. 84:79, 1961.

Burch, P. R. J., and Rowell, N. R.: Pityriasis rosea—an autoaggressive disease. Br. J. Dermatol. 82:549, 1970.

Epstein, S.: Etiology of pityriasis rosea. Urol. Cutan. Rev. 47:641, 1943.

Garcia e Silva, L., and Gardner, P. S.: Pityriasis rosea—a virological study. Br. J. Dermatol. 80:514, 1968.

Gilbert, C.: Traite Pratique des Maladies de la Peau. 5th ed. Paris, 1860, p. 402.

Hellgren, L.: Pityriasis Rosea. Die Prevalenz in Geschlechts—Alters- und Beruffsgruppen in den ganze Beval Kerungsgruppen. Hautarzt 23:492, 1972.

Hurley, H. J., and English, R.: Localized pityriasis rosea. J.A.M.A. 178:766, 1961.

Hyatt, H. W.: Pityriasis rosea in a three month old in-fant. Arch. Pediatr. 77:364, 1960.

Kestel, J.: Oral lesions in pityriasis rosea. J.A.M.A. 205:597, 1968.

Klauder, J.: Pityriasis rosea. J.A.M.A. 82:178, 1924.

Lipman Cohen, E.: Pityriasis rosea. Br. J. Dermatol. 79:533, 1967.

Marshall, J.: Pityriasis rosea. S. Afr. Med. J. 30:210, 1956.

Niles, H. D., and Klumpp, M. M.: Pityriasis rosea. Review of literature and report of two hundred and nineteen cases, in thirty-eight of which convales-cent serum was used. Arch. Dermatol. Syph. 41:265, 1940.

Nurse, D.: Pityriasis rosea. Aust. J. Dermatol. 10:38, 1969.

Percival, G. H.: Pityriasis rosea. Br. J. Dermatol. 44:241, 1932.

Rantuccio, F., and Mancosu, A.: Osbervazione Etio-logiche, Patogenetiche E Cliniche in Tema Di Pi-tiriasi Rosea Di Gibert. G. Ital. Dermatol. Sif. 105:513, 1964.

Raskin, J.: Possible dermatropic virus associated with pityriasis rosea. Acta Derm. Venereol. 48:474, 1968.

Salin, R. W., Curtis, A. C., and Wheeler, A.: Treat-ment of pityriasis rosea with convalescent plasma, gamma globulin and pooled plasma. Arch. Derma-tol. 76:659, 1957.

Shelton, J. M.: Pityriasis rosea. Report of three cases within one household. Arch. Dermatol. Syph. 59:115, 1949.

Silvers, S. H., and Glickman, F. S.: Pityriasis rosea followed by nail dystrophy. Arch. Dermatol. 90:31, 1964.

Vollum, D.: Pityriasis rosea in the African. Trans. St. John's Hosp. Dermatol. Soc. 59:269, 1973.

White, W.: Pityriasis rosea in sisters. Br. Med. J. 2:245, 1973.

Pityriasis Rubra Pilaris

Aguilar, A. R., Gomez, F., Beles, F. T., et al.: Pityriasis rubra pilaris with muscle and joint involvement. Dermatologica 146:361, 1973.

Brown, J., and Perry, H. O.: Pityriasis rubra pilaris. Arch. Dermatol. 94:636, 1966.

Cornbleet, T.: Liver vitamin A in Darier's and De-vergie's diseases. J. Invest. Dermatol. 23:71, 1954.

Davidson, C. L., Winkelman, R. K., and Kurland, R. R.: Pityriasis rubra pilaris: A follow-up study of fifty-seven patients. Arch. Dermatol. 100:175, 1969.

Devergie, A. M. G.: Pityriasis pilaris. In Martinet, L.: Traite Pratique des Maladies de la Peau. 2nd ed. Paris, 1857, pp. 454–464.

Frazier, C. N., and Hu, C. K.: Cutaneous lesions as-sociated with a deficiency of vitamin A in man. Arch. Intern. Med. 48:507, 1931.

Gross, D. A., Landau, J. W., and Newcomer, V. D.: Pi-tyriasis rubra pilaris. Report of a case and analysis of the literature. Arch. Dermatol. 99:710, 1969.

Gunther, S.: Topical administration of vitamin A acid (Retinoic acid) in enzyme, hypertrophic lichen planus and pityriasis rubra pilaris. Dermatologica 145:344, 1972.

Hunter, G. A., and Forbes, I. J.: Treatment of pi-tyriasis rubra pilaris with azathioprine. Br. J. Der-matol. 87:42, 1972.

Huntly, C. E.: Pityriasis rubra pilaris. Am. J. Dis. Child. 122:22, 1971.

Kierland, R. R., and Kulwin, M. H.: Pityriasis rubra pilaris. A clinical study. Arch. Dermatol. Syph. 61:925, 1950.

Leitner, Z. A., and Ford, E. B.: Vitamin A and pi-tyriasis rubra pilaris. Br. J. Dermatol. 59:407, 1947.

Logan, W. S.: Vitamin A and keratinization. Arch. Dermatol. 105:748, 1972.

Lowenthal, L. J.: A new cutaneous manifestation in the syndrome of vitamin A deficiency. Arch. Der-matol. Syph. 28:700, 1933.

Marshall, J.: Case of pityriasis rubra with lesions of buccal mucosa. Arch. Dermatol. Syph. 66:626, 1952.

Moult, F. H.: Histopathology of rat skin in avitamin-osis A. Arch. Dermatol. 47:768, 1943.

Orbaneja, J., Torres, M., Garein-Perez, A., et al.: Dis-trofia muscular progressiva y PRP. Actas Dermosi-filiogr. 50:179, 1959.

Porter, D., and Shuster, S.: Epidermal renewal and amino acids in psoriasis and pityriasis rubra pilaris. Arch. Dermatol. 98:339, 1968.

Shrank, A.: Phyrmoderma. Br. Med. J. 1:29, 1966.

Sullivan, M., and Evans, V. J.: Nutritional dermatoses in the rat. XI. Vitamin A deficiency superimposed on vitamin B complex deficiency. Arch. Dermatol. Syph. 51:17, 1945.

Waldorf, D. S., and Hambrick, G. W.: Vitamin A–responsive pityriasis rubra pilaris with myasthenia gravis. Arch. Dermatol. 92:424, 1965.

Lichen Planus

Allende, M. F.: Lichen planus and its possible associ-ation with vascular hypertension. J. Invest. Derma-tol. 15:7, 1950.

Almeyda, J.: Lichen planus actinicus. Br. J. Dermatol. *82*:426, 1970.

Almeyda, J. and Levantine, A.: Lichenoid dry eruptions. Br. J. Dermatol. *85*:604, 1971.

Altman, J., and Perry, H. O.: The variation and course of lichen planus. Arch. Dermatol. *84*:179, 1961.

Aplas, V.: Untersuchungen zur Histo- und Pathogenese des Lichen Ruber Planus. Arch. Klin. Exp. Derm. *204*:297, 1957.

Buckley, W. R.: Lichenoid eruptions: Following contact dermatitis. Arch. Dermatol. *78*:454, 1958.

Calnan, C., and Meara, R. H.: St. John's Hospital Diagnostic Index. Trans. St. John's Hosp. Dermatol. Soc. *39*:56, 1957.

Copeman, P. W. M., Schrocter, A. L., and Kurland, R. R.: An unusual variant of lupus erythematosus or lichen planus. Br. J. Dermatol. *83*:269, 1970.

Cotton, D. W. K., van den Hurk, J. J. M. A., and van den Staak, W. B. J. M.: Lichen planus, an inform error of metabolism. Br. J. Dermatol. *87*:341, 1972.

Cram, D. L., and Muller, S. A.: Unusual variations of lichen planus. Mayo Clin. Proc. *41*:677, 1966.

Cram, D. L., Kierland, R. R., and Winkelmann, R. K.: Ulcerative lichen planus of the feet. Arch. Dermatol. *93*:692, 1966.

de Graciansky, P., and Boulle, S.: Skin disease from color developers. Br. J. Dermatol. *78*:297, 1966.

Depaoli, M.: Lichen ruber planus familiaria. G. Ital. Dermatol. *45*:11, 1970.

Depaoli, M.: Rilievi clinico-statistici sul lichen ruber planus (noted 26 per cent of cases emotional stress). Minerva Dermatol. *39*:166, 1964.

Dostrovsky, A., and Sagher, F.: Lichen planus in subtropical countries. Arch. Dermatol. Syph. *59*:308, 1949.

DuPont, A.: Familial lichen planus. Arch. Belg. Dermatol. Syph. *28*:171, 1972.

Emslie, E. S., and Hardman, F. G.: The surgical treatment of oral lichen planus. Trans. St. John's Hosp. Dermatol. Soc. *56*:43, 1970.

Feuerman, E. J., and Sandbark, M.: Lichen planus pemphigoides with extreme melanosis in a patient with malignant lymphoma. Arch. Dermatol. *114*:61, 1971.

Fryholm, K. O., Frithiof, L., Fernstrom, A. B., et al: Allergy to copper derived from dental alloys as a possible cause of oral lesions of lichen planus. Acta. Derm. Venereol. *49*:268, 1969.

Glickman, F., Rapp, Y. and Funk, L.: Capillary microscopy. Inflammatory dermatosis. Arch. Dermatol. *89*:500, 1964.

Goltz, R. W., and Hult, A. M.: Zur histochemischen Natur der Kolloidkorper beim Lichen Ruber Planus. Hautarzt *96*:355, 1963.

Gunther, S.: Retinoic acid in the treatment of lichen planus. Dermatologica *143*:315, 1971.

Johnson, F. R., and Fry, L.: Ultrastructural observations in lichen planus. Arch. Dermatol. *95*:596, 1967.

Jolly, M.: Lichen planus and its association with diabetes mellitus. Med. J. Aust. *1*:990, 1972.

Katzenellenbogen, I.: Lichen planus actinicus (lichen planus in subtropical countries). Dermatologica *124*:10, 1962.

Kronenberg, K., Fretzin, D., and Potter, B.: Malignant degeneration of lichen planus. Arch. Dermatol. *104*:304, 1971.

Magnusson, B.: Lichen ruber bullosus and tumors in internal organs. Dermatologica *134*:166, 1967.

Pillsbury, D. M., and Livingood, C. S.: Dermatology. *In* Anderson, R. S., (ed.): Internal Medicine in World War II. Washington, D. C., Department of the Army, 1968, pp. 543–675.

Samman, P. D.: Lichen planus. An analysis of 300 cases. Trans. St. John's Hosp. Dermatol. Soc. *46*:36, 1961.

Sarkany, I., and Gaylarde, P. M.: Ultrastructural and light microscopic changes of the epidermo-dermal junction. Trans. St. John's Hosp. Dermatol. Soc. *57*:139, 1971.

Scarpa, C., and Ferrea, E.: Allergological researches with cadmium, beryllium and arsenic and a case of lichen planus from diazodiethylaniline. Panminerva Med. *10*:93, 1968.

Schmidt, H.: Frequency, duration and localization of lichen planus. Acta. Derm. Venereol. *41*:164, 1961.

Sehgal, V. N., Abraham, G. J. S., and Malik, G. B.: Griseofulvin therapy in lichen planus. A double blind controlled trial. Br. J. Dermatol. *87*:383, 1972.

Shklar, G.: Lichen planus as an oral ulcerative disease. Oral Surg. *33*:376, 1972.

Sulzberger, M. B., Hermann, F., and Zak, F. G.: Studies of sweating. I. Preliminary report with particular emphasis on a sweat retention syndrome. J. Invest. Dermatol. *9*:221, 1947.

Summerly, R., and Wilson-Jones, E.: The microarchitecture of Wickhan's striae. Trans. St. John's Hosp. Dermatol. Soc. *50*:157, 1964.

Swanbach, G., and Thyresson, N.: Electron microscopy of intravascular particles in lichen ruber planus. Acta. Derm. Venereol. *44*:105, 1964.

Thyresson, N., and Moburger, G.: Cytologic studies in lichen ruber planus. Acta. Derm. Venereol. *37*:191, 1957.

Waisman, M., Dundon, B. C., and Michel, B.: Immunofluorescent studies in lichen nitidus. Arch. Dermatol. *107*:200, 1973.

Wilson, E.: On lichen planus. J. Cutan. Med. *8*:117, 1869.

Zaias, N.: The nail in lichen planus. Arch. Dermatol. *101*:264, 1970.

Lichen Nitidus

Ellis, F. A.: Histopathology of lichen planus based on analysis of one hundred biopsy specimens. J. Invest. Dermatol. *48*:143, 1967.

Ellis, F. A., and Hill, W. F.: Is lichen nitidus a variety of lichen planus? Arch. Dermatol. Syph. *38*:569, 1938.

Pinkus, F.: Ueber eine Neue Knoetchen foermige Haut-Eruption: Lichen Nitidus. Arch. Dermatol. Syph. *85*:11, 1907.

Pinkus, H.: Lichenoid tissue reactions. Arch. Dermatol. *107*:840, 1973.

Pinkus, H., and Shair, H. M.: Koebner phenomenon in lichen nitidus: report of two cases. Arch. Dermatol. Syph. *65*:82, 1952.

Stankler, L.: The identity of lichen planus and lichen nitidus. Br. J. Dermatol. *79*:125, 1967.

Waisman, M., Dundan, B. C., and Michel, B.: Immunofluorescent studies in lichen nitidus. Arch. Dermatol. *107*:200, 1973.

Wilson, H. T. H., and Bett, D. C. G.: Miliary lesions in lichen planus. Arch. Dermatol. *83*:920, 1961.

Lichen Striatus

Fantl, G.: Lichen striatus: Beitrag zur Kenntnis der Strichtormigen Hauter Krankeingen. Dermatol. Monatsschr. 58:593, 1914.

Johnson, H. M.: Lichen striatus. Arch. Dermatol. Syph. 53:51, 1946.

Lee, H.: Lichen striatus. Lancet 1:615, 1951.

Senear, F. E., and Caro, M. R.: Lichen striatus. Arch. Dermatol. Syph. 43:116, 1941.

Staricco, R. G.: Lichen striatus. A study of fifteen new cases with special emphasis on the histopathological changes and a review of the literature. Arch. Dermatol. 79:311, 1959.

Parapsoriasis

Brocq, L.: Parapsoriasis. J. Cutan. Derm. 21:315, 1903.

Burke, O. P., Adams, R. M., and Arundell, F. O.: Febrile ulceronecrotic Mucha-Habermann's disease. Arch. Dermatol. 100:200, 1969.

Canizares, O.: Parapsoriasis. Its treatment with calciferol. Arch. Dermatol. Syph. 65:685, 1952.

Cornielson, R. L., Knox, J. M., and Everett, M. A.: Methotrexate for the treatment of Mucha-Habermann disease. Arch. Dermatol. 106:507, 1972.

Ingram, J. T.: Pityriasis, lichenoides, and parapsoriasis. Br. J. Dermatol. 65:293, 1953.

Lapiere, M. S.: Evolution et prognostique du parapsoriasis en plaques. Ann. Dermatol. Syph. 9:609, 1949.

Nagy, E., and Balagh, E. E.: Clinical findings in treatment of Mucha-Habermann's disease with acridine and quinoline derivatives. Dermatologica 118:391, 1959.

Nazarro, P.: Ricerche etiologiche in due casi di malattia di Mucha. Minerva Dermatol. 28:310, 1953.

Pillsbury, D. M., Shelley, W. B., and Kligman, A. M.: Dermatology. Philadelphia, W. B. Saunders Co., 1956.

Samman, P. D.: Survey of reticuloses and premycotic eruptions. Br. J. Dermatol. 76:1, 1964.

Shelley, W. B.: Poikiloderma vasculare atrophicans. In Consultations in Dermatology II. Philadelphia, W. B. Saunders Co., 1974.

Shelley, W. B., and Griffith, R. F.: Pityriasis lichenoides et varioliformis acuta. Arch. Dermatol. 100:596, 1969.

Szymanski, F.: Pityriasis lichenoides et varioliformis acuta. Arch. Dermatol. 79:7, 1959.

Winkelmann, N. R. K., and Lorenc, F.: Treatment of acute parapsoriasis with corticotropin (ACTH) Arch. Dermatol. 79:512, 1959.

Exfoliative Dermatitis

Abrahams, I., McCarthy, J. T., and Sanders, S. L.: One hundred and one cases of exfoliative dermatitis. Arch. Dermatol. 87:96, 1963.

Fox, R. H., Shuster, S., Williams, R., et al.: Cardiovascular, metabolic and thermoregulatory disturbances in patients with erythrodermic skin diseases. Br. Med. J. 1:619, 1965.

Freedberg, I. M., and Baden, H. R.: The metabolic response to exfoliation. J. Invest. Dermatol. 38:277, 1962.

Frost, P., and Weinstein, G.: Exfoliative dermatitis. In Demis, J., et al. (eds.): Clinical Dermatology I. Unit 1–15: 1–7, 1972. Hagerstown, Maryland, Harper and Row, 1972.

Gentele, H., Lodi, A., and Skop E.: Dermatitis exfoliative. Acta Derm. Venereol. 38:269, 1958.

Held, D. H.: Folate losses from the skin in exfoliative dermatitis. Arch. Intern. Med. 123:51, 1969.

Jacobs, J. C., and Miller, M. E.: Fatal familial Leiner's disease: A deficiency of the opsonic activity of serum complement. Pediatrics 49:225, 1972.

Koblenzer, P. J.: Acute epidermal necrolysis (Ritter Von Rittershain-Lyell). Arch. Dermatol. 95:608, 1967.

Krook, G.: Hypothermia in patients with exfoliative dermatitis. Acta Derm. Venereol. 40:142, 1960.

Krook, G.: The functioning of the thyroid in exfoliative dermatitis. Acta Derm. Venereol. 41:443, 1961.

Lutzner, M. A., Edelman, R. L., Smith, R. W., et al.: Two varieties of Sézary syndrome, both bearing T-cell markers. Lancet 2:207, 1973.

Lyell, A.: A review of toxic epidermal necrolysis in Britain. Br. J. Dermatol. 79:662, 1967.

Parish, W. E., Rook, A. J., and Champion, R. H.: A study of autoallergy in generalized eczema. Br. J. Dermatol. 77:479, 1965.

Rook, A. J., and Wilkinson, D. S.: Textbook of Dermatology. 2nd ed. Philadelphia, F. A. Davis Company, 1972.

Shuster, S.: High-output cardiac failure from skin disease. Lancet 1:1338, 1963.

Shuster, S.: Dermatogenic enteropathy. N. Y. State Med. J. 68:3160, 1968.

Shuster, S., and Brown, J. B.: Gynecomastia and urinary estrogens in patients with generalized skin disease. Lancet 2:1358, 1962.

Shuster, S., and Wilkinson, P.: Protein metabolism in exfoliative dermatitis and erythroderma. Br. J. Dermatol. 75:344, 1963.

Teckner, A., and Baset, A.: Serum proteins and liver function in exfoliative dermatitis. Br. J. Dermatol. 72:138, 1960.

Voigt, C. C., Knonthal, H. L., and Crouse, R. G.: Cardiac output in erythrodermic skin disease. Am. Heart J. 72:615, 1966.

Wilson, H. T. H.: Exfoliative dermatitis. Arch. Dermatol. 69:577, 1954.

Winkelmann, R. K.: T-cell erythroderma (Sézary syndrome). Arch. Dermatol. 108:205, 1973.

Zoon, J. J., and Mali, J. W. H.: The influences of erythroderma on the body. Arch. Dermatol. 75:573, 1957.

CHAPTER

10

BULLOUS DISEASES

Samuel L. Moschella

Blisters or bullae (Falco-Braun, 1969; Stoughton, 1964) result from the accumulation of fluid between the cells of epidermis or between the cells of epidermis and corium. Some form of cell damage is necessary to cause the fluid, whose composition is similar to serum, to enter the spaces of these previously damaged sites. Knowledge of the cause and pathogenesis of blister formation is limited. With the current, improved, investigative techniques utilizing electron microscopy, and with the advances in histochemistry and immunology, an understanding of the pathodynamics has increased, but knowledge of responsible biochemical changes is still wanting.

The classification of these blister diseases is presently based on histologic-morphologic criteria that have been refined further by electron microscopy. The histologic findings used to classify blister formation are primary cell damage, spongiosis, acantholysis, subcorneal blistering, and dermo-epidermal loss of continuity. Since the blisters may form at the same site in several skin diseases with different causes, the histologic appearance alone is sometimes inadequate for diagnosis. Among the conditions that may cause primary cell injury are certain virus infections, such as herpes simplex, herpes zoster, varicella, variola, and vaccinia, and congenital bullous ichthyosiform erythroderma. Spongiosis is seen in eczematous diseases; acantholysis is appreciated in the pemphigus group, subcorneal pustular dermatosis, thermal injury, topical chemical application, and ultraviolet burn; subcorneal blister is found with impetigo; and the dermo-epidermal separation appears with pemphigoid, dermatitis herpetiformis, and erythema multiforme. Acantholysis (Falco-Braun, 1969) depends on the separation of the intercellular contacts between the malpighian cells; it is not a lytic process but is the result of the inability of epidermal cells to establish intercellular contact because of the impairment of the three main structures, desmosomes, simple desmosomes, and nexus (zona occludens), and intercellular muco-polysaccharide-protein complexes.

Patients with pemphigus vulgaris have a

459

serum antibody that is directed against the intercellular substance of epidermal prickle cells which can be demonstrated immunohistologically and appears to inhibit the formation of intercellular contacts (desmosomes and synthesis of epidermal intercellular substances). The mechanism of the dermo-epidermal separation (Falco-Braun, 1969) is dermo-epidermal disjunction by disintegration of basal cells (hereditary epidermolysis simplex of autosomal-dominant type), cleft formation in the intermembranous space (autosomal-dominant epidermolysis bullosa hereditaria lethalis, erythema multiforme bullosum, bullous pemphigoid, bullous lichen planus, and suction blister), disintegration of the connective tissue of subjacent corium (recessive epidermolysis bullosa dystrophica and porphyria cutanea tarda), and destruction of the dermo-epidermal junction after dermal injury (erythema multiforme bullosum and dermatitis herpetiformis). Among the diseases with subepidermal blister formation are erythema multiforme, bullous pemphigoid, dermatitis herpetiformis, benign mucous membrane pemphigus, epidermolysis bullosa dystrophica, prophyria cutanea tarda, urticaria pigmentosa bullosa, lichen ruber pemphigoides, bullous lichen sclerosis et atrophicans, pityriasis lichenoides et varioliformis acuta, lupus erythematosus pemphigoides, and thermal burns.

The mechanism by which blisters of skin disease arise is as yet an unsolved problem. The present state of our knowledge makes it impossible to classify and discuss the bullous diseases on an etiologic basis. A number of conditions are of genetic origin and, on this basis alone, can be differentiated; the remainder are described only as separate clinical entities. The nomenclature and classification of the chronic bullous diseases used in this chapter follow the views of Lever (1965) and are based not only on the clinical features but also on the histologic findings.

PEMPHIGUS

Pemphigus (Lever and Hashimoto, 1969; Newcomer and Landau, 1971) describes a group of chronic blistering diseases of un-known etiology and is characterized clinically by the involvement usually of healthy appearing skin and mucous membrane, histologically by the presence of the diagnostic acantholysis with resultant intradermal bullae, and immunologically by the presence of circulating auto-antibodies to an intercellular epidermal antigen.

The disease is worldwide and has an unexplainably higher incidence in the Jewish race. It is a disease of middle-aged persons but has occurred in children and even in families as fogo selvagem (Brazilian pemphigus foliaceus). The basic cause for the formation of bullae in pemphigus is obscure. There is no proof of a virus or the circulating auto-antibodies being responsible for the formation of blisters. The question still being asked is: "Are these antibodies primary or secondary?" These circulating antibodies occur in the serum without cutaneous lesions and in burned patients. Injection of sera containing anti-epithelial antibodies does not produce bullae in animals or man. In animals, fixation of the anti-epithelial humoral antibody to the epithelium with the production of acantholytic cells occurs only after the skin has been induced by local treatment which permits permeation of plasma containing the antibody (Grob and Inderbitzin, 1968). The clinical and serologic overlap between pemphigus vulgaris, myasthenia gravis, systemic lupus erythematosus, and thymic disease encourages further immunologic interpretations. The mechanism of bulla formation is presumed to be the result of enzyme activity affecting the desmosomes.

The pemphigus complex consists of pemphigus vulgaris, vegetans, and foliaceus. It has been divided into two types based on the level of the intra-epidermal blister formation: one is, suprabasally, pemphigus vulgaris, and the other, subcorneally, pemphigus foliaceus. Pemphigus vulgaris includes pemphigus vegetans, the malignant Neumann type, and the benign Hallopeau type. Pemphigus foliaceus includes two variants, the more benign and localized form, pemphigus erythematosus, and the endemic and possibly infectious type, fogo selvagem. It has been suggested that pemphigus vulgaris and pemphigus foliaceus are different diseases because of genetic factors, clinical and histologic presentations, some ultrastructural alterations seen on electron microscopy, and the relatively infrequent clinical transition of pemphigus foliaceus to pemphigus vulgaris and the failure to substantiate this change.

PEMPHIGUS VULGARIS

Pemphigus vulgaris (Asboe-Hansen, 1970; Hurst, 1970) has a characteristic clinical and predictable course. The disease appears most frequently in Mediterranean people, especially in Jews, who tend to have a more rapidly progressive course. It often affects persons who are debilitated.

The earliest change histopathologically is intercellular edema with loss of intercellular bridges in the lower epidermis and the development of suprabasal clefts and bullae. The bullae contain single or clusters of acantholytic cells. The Tzank test is a rapid cytologic examination that demonstrates the acantholytic cells in the bullae of pemphigus vulgaris and is performed by opening a blister, scraping its base, making a smear, and finally staining the smear with Giemsa's stain to demonstrate these supportive diagnostic cells. Acantholytic cells are also seen in non-acantholytic vesiculobullous (herpes simplex, herpes zoster, and varicella) and pustular (impetigo, halodermas, and subcorneal pustular dermatosis) dermatoses.

The course of the disease (Sanders and Nelson, 1965) varies from acute with a fulminating malignant course to chronic. The disease may remain localized for months with a few lesions, especially in the mouth or scalp and in the axillae and inguinal regions. A generalized bullous phase usually appears within one year. In more than 50 per cent of patients, the oral mucosa is involved initially and portends a more serious prognosis. In patients with active disease, involved and uninvolved skin may be dislodged by sliding pressure with a finger, the so-called Nikolsky sign which is seen in other acantholytic and non-acantholytic diseases. Because of constant trauma, the bullae are frequently seen in the mouth (Fig. 10–1); the vermilion border of the lips is frequently involved. Other mucosal surfaces similarly affected are those of the anogenital area, the conjunctiva, and the pharynx and larynx, the latter with a resultant hoarseness. The painful oral and pharyngeal lesions make ingestion of food difficult, resulting in further debilitation of the patient. Like the cutaneous lesions, the superficial mucosal ulcerations and denudation show little tendency to heal spontaneously, extend peripherally with shedding of the epithelium, and heal without scarring.

The eruption favors the seborrheic areas such as the scalp, midface about the eyes, nostrils, and mouth, sternum, mid-back, umbilicus, and groin. Since pressure may cause denudation of the skin, the pressure areas (back, flexures, and feet) are often in-

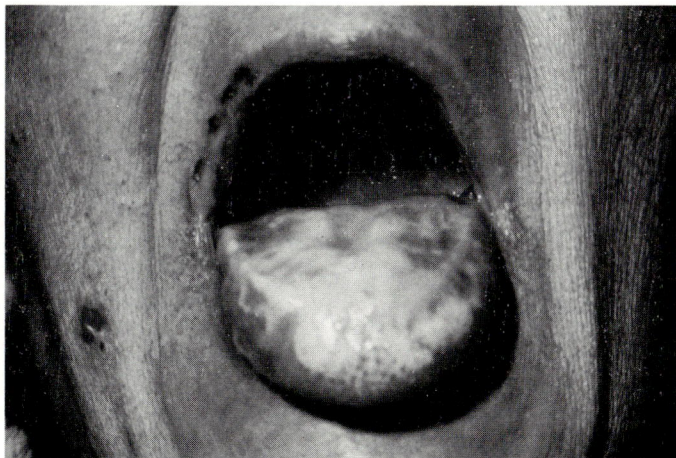

Figure 10–1 Characteristic erosive lesions of pemphigus vulgaris on the tongue; the oral lesions antedated the cutaneous and other mucous membrane lesions by six months.

volved. The blisters are small but can be large, are flaccid (Fig. 10-2), arise in normal skin, may be clear, hemorrhagic, or pustular, and rupture easily. Vertical pressure on the bulla may move it into the surrounding normal appearing skin. The detached skin may form peripheral epidermal collarettes and can cover large areas. The denuded intertriginous lesions tend to become vegetative (Figs. 10–3 and 10-4). The erosions may bleed, are occasionally pruritic, and heal with hyperpigmentation. An associated increased susceptibility to oral, intertriginous, and paronychial bacterial and monilial infections is even greater during the administration of corticosteroid and immunosuppressive therapy.

Systemic involvement has not been appreciated in patients with pemphigus. The nonspecific autopsy findings found in the viscera such as the central nervous system are presumed to be the result of metabolic rather than organic changes.

Among the differential diagnosis of the oral involvement are aphthosis, lichen planus, and benign mucous membrane pemphigus, and of the cutaneous lesions are erythema multiforme, bullous pemphigoid, and toxic epidermal necrolysis.

The laboratory findings in pemphigus are hypoalbuminemia, probably secondary to protein loss through denudation and starvation, and an elevation in the α-2 globulins. Eosinophilia is seen and becomes reduced in severely ill patients.

In the days before steroid therapy, the mortality rate was 95 per cent, death occurring usually within 14 months. The cause of death was the results of secondary infection, starvation, and a toxic state. Corticosteroid therapy has reduced the mortality rate to 40 per cent with the causes of death being uncontrolled pemphigus and the complications of corticosteroid therapy, namely, hypercorticoidism, septicemia, and thromboembolism.

Treatment

Corticosteroid therapy is the treatment of choice in pemphigus vulgaris; immuno-

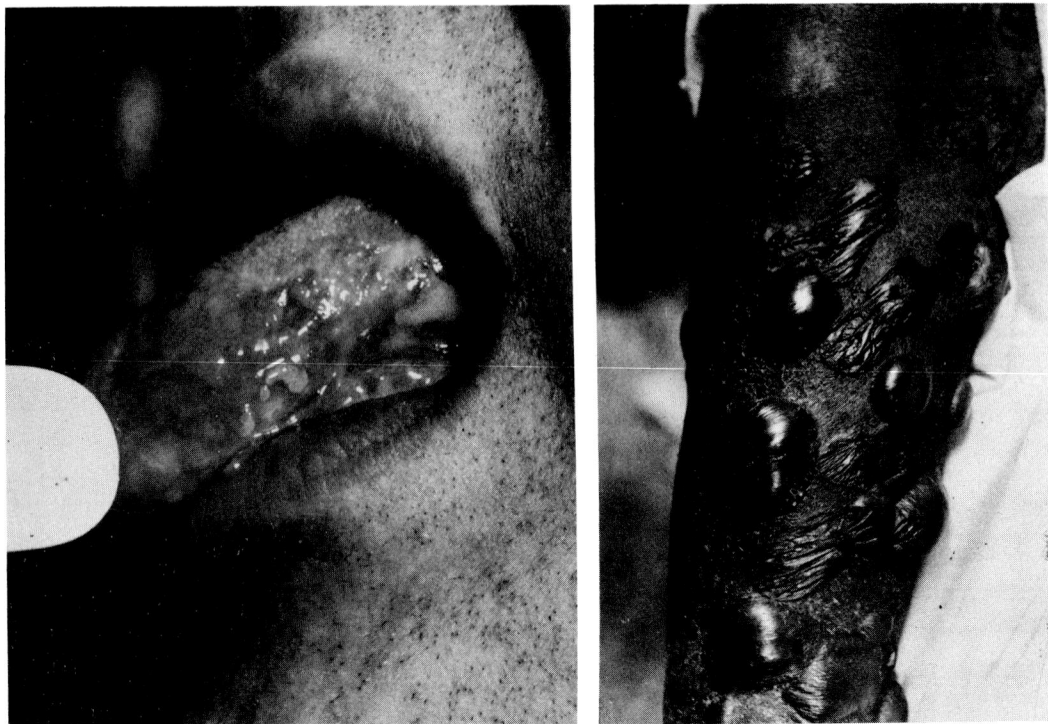

Figure 10-2 Extensive cutaneous involvement of pemphigus vulgaris with large flaccid bullae; these lesions developed in normal-appearing skin.

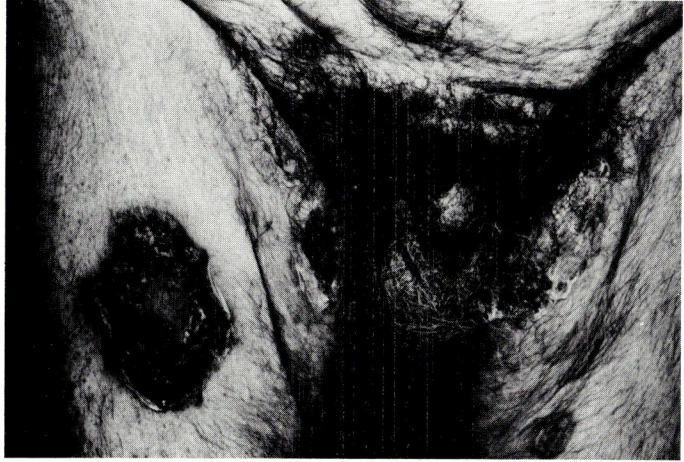

Figure 10–3 The inguinal lesions with the detached skin forming peripheral epidermal collarettes of pemphigus vulgaris.

suppressants are a useful adjunct to corticosteroids and, in some cases, are an effective substitute. Corticosteroids should be initiated promptly and in a large enough dose over a sufficient period of time to suppress the appearance of new lesions; this initial dose varies from 80 to 300 mg. a day of prednisone, depending on the severity and rapidity of progression of the disease. Once the disease is controlled, the dose is rapidly reduced to an effective maintenance level that is then cut further and more gradually in logarithmic manner. Alternate-day maintenance therapy is desirable, if possible, to minimize the side effects of long-term steroid therapy. Im-

munosuppressants may be added in an attempt to reduce the maintenance dose of corticosteroid therapy or to replace it as a result of the potential complications or the patient's intolerance to the latter.

Because pemphigus is thought by some to be an auto-immune phenomenon and because the level of auto-antibodies correlates with the severity of the disease, immunosuppressant therapy is being used and evaluated (Jablonska et al., 1970). Whether chemotherapy is effective by suppressing antibody formation or inflammation or both is not understood. The hesitancy for therapeutic use of these drugs is not only because of their potential toxicity but also because of their carcinogenic effect. Among the drugs being used and evaluated are methotrexate, azathioprine, and cyclophosphamide. Methotrexate has been useful mainly in conjunction with systemic corticosteroid therapy but has also been of value when used alone, especially in early localized lesions. Whether methotrexate given over a prolonged period of time is safer than prednisone so administered is uncertain. The dose of methotrexate (amethopterin) is 25 mg. to 100 mg. orally, intravenously, or intramuscularly at weekly intervals. Azathioprine (imidazole derivative of 6-mercaptopurine) seems to be effective when combined with corticosteroids. Since it takes several months for the therapeutic impact of azathioprine to be appreciated clinically, the corticosteroid dose should be reduced gradually and replaced later if possible by azathioprine.

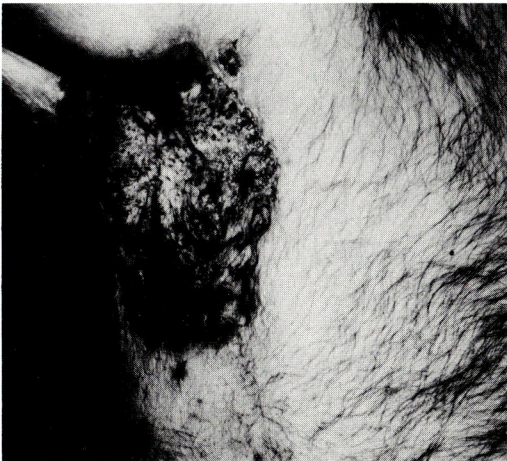

Figure 10–4 The chronic lesions of pemphigus vulgaris on the axillae have become vegetative.

The dose of azathioprine is 100 mg. to 200 mg. orally a day. Cyclophosphamide, 100 mg. to 200 mg. orally a day, has been used infrequently but successfully alone or with prednisone.

Pemphigus Vegetans

Pemphigus vegetans (Lever, 1965), which is a variant of pemphigus vulgaris, can present as two types—the Neumann or the Hallopeau; the rare latter form has a more favorable prognosis.

Pemphigus vegetans, the Neumann type, usually behaves like pemphigus vulgaris except that it appears at an earlier age. Most of the denuded areas, especially of the face, axillae, genitals, and other intertriginous areas develop vegetations that are pustular and later become verrucoid. Oral lesions are almost always present. On histologic examination the initial lesion has the same appearance as pemphigus vulgaris but later develops upward proliferation of papillae, downward growth of epidermis, and intra-epidermal abscesses consisting almost entirely of eosinophils. The clinical course is more prolonged than pemphigus vulgaris and may even undergo spontaneous remission with complete clearing of the skin. However, when the disease becomes more acute, the clinical picture of pemphigus vulgaris may predominate and the disease may even end fatally. Treatment is similar to that of pemphigus vulgaris.

Pemphigus vegetans (Hallopeau type, pyodermite vegetante) is also a relatively benign form of pemphigus that has a chronic, prolonged course but can behave like pemphigus vulgaris and terminate fatally. The primary lesions are pustules that coalesce, extend peripherally, become vegetative, and cover large areas of the axillae and perineum. In the mouth, the characteristic velvety granulomatosis may be seen. The early lesions, which are histologically similar to the Neumann type, show suprabasal acantholysis, numerous eosinophils, and epidermal hyperplasia with eosinophilic abscess formation in the vegetative lesions. Later in the disease, papillomatosis and hyperkeratosis without abscess formation appear.

Pemphigus Foliaceus

Pemphigus foliaceus (Perry and Brunsting, 1965) has been used to describe a generalized condition that is presumed to be related, because of histologic evidence, to pemphigus erythematosus, considered to be a localized variant, and to Brazilian pemphigus foliaceus (fogo selvagem), thought to be an endemic viral-induced type. The histologic change is acantholysis in the subcorneal and granular layers of the epidermis with the appearance of acantholytic cells, clefts, and bullae; in the older lesions, the acantholytic process may appear in any part of the epidermis. Pemphigus foliaceus is a benign disease that mainly affects elderly persons but occurs also in children. Although it may have an acute onset with a rapid spreading, it frequently begins with a few lesions scattered about the head and upper trunk in a seborrheic distribution (Fig. 10-5 *A* and *B*) and spreads slowly. During the early stage of the disease, the bullae are small and flaccid, and, when they are grouped, the eruption may initially resemble dermatitis herpetiformis. The subcorneal vesicles and bullae rupture easily and leave shallow and painful erosions. Oral lesions are usually absent, but, in the rare fulminating case, diffuse superficial exfoliation of the oral mucosa occurs. Characteristic superficial denudation may occur in erythematous areas of the skin and spread with the formation of sharp serpiginous borders and large loose scales.

When the process becomes widespread (Fig. 10-6), a generalized erythroderma that, unlike an exfoliative erythroderma, has moist scaling and crusting, gives off an unpleasant odor, and may have a few blisters, especially of the palms and soles. The more localized type may become generalized and vice versa. Extension of the disease may result from emotional stress or exposure to heat and sunlight. Although the disease may be widespread, the patients appear to be in good health and experience a relatively more benign course for ten or more years. The disease may be fatal, especially in persons more than 50 years of age. Periods of spontaneous partial remission are seen.

Prior to the availability of effective systemic therapy, the mortality rate was about

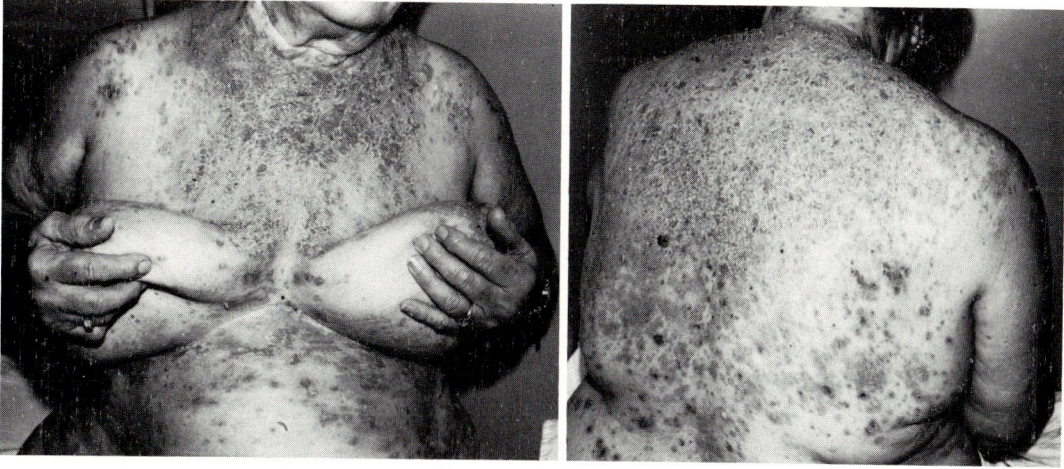

Figure 10–5 Rapid spreading pemphigus foliaceus involves the anterior and posterior seborrheic areas.

60 per cent. When the disease is mild, no treatment is necessary; if it is extensive, sufficient corticosteroid to control but not to suppress blister formation is the goal of therapy. Immunosuppressants, such as methotrexate and azathioprine, have been effective, and the former had been used most frequently.

Pemphigus Erythematosus

Pemphigus erythematosus—Senear-Usher syndrome (Lever, 1965)—is an abortive localized variant of pemphigus foliaceus that may become generalized. It is considered a form of pemphigus folia-

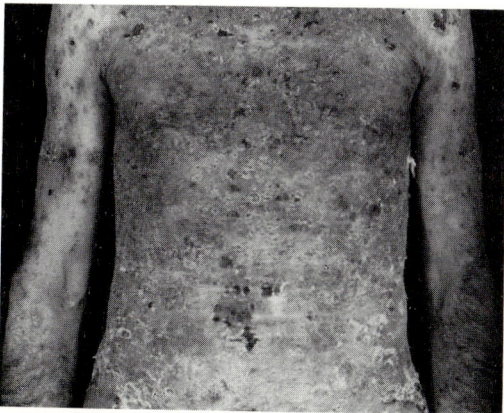

Figure 10–6 A generalized erythroderma that, unlike exfoliative erythroderma, has a moist scaling and crusting which causes an unpleasant odor.

ceus because of the similar histologic appearance, the frequent presence of few lesions for months in both, the absence of oral lesions, the good health of patients, and the better prognosis than in other types of pemphigus. The distribution of the cutaneous lesions favoring the seborrheic areas of the head and upper trunk is similar to pemphigus foliaceus. The classic lesion frequently seen is sharply demarcated heavy crusting in the "butterfly" area with follicular plugging (carpet tacks). The condition (Fig. 10-7 *A* and *B*) can clinically resemble lupus erythematosus and seborrheic dermatitis. It may remain localized for a long period, require no treatment, and even clear spontaneously. Topical, occlusive, concentrated or intralesional corticosteroids may be useful; in the more severe cases, systemic corticosteroids or immunosuppressants are effective.

Fogo selvagem, the Brazilian variant of pemphigus foliaceus (Brown, 1954), occurs endemically in children and young adults, especially women, and affects Brazilians and their families as well as immigrants. Histologic examination of the involved skin reveals not only the acantholysis and cleavage of the subcorneal and granular layers but also papillomatosis. At the onset, a bullous eruption appears mainly localized to the seborrheic areas. As the disease progresses, the bullae become more widespread. The rupturing of the bullae produces a crusting exfoliative

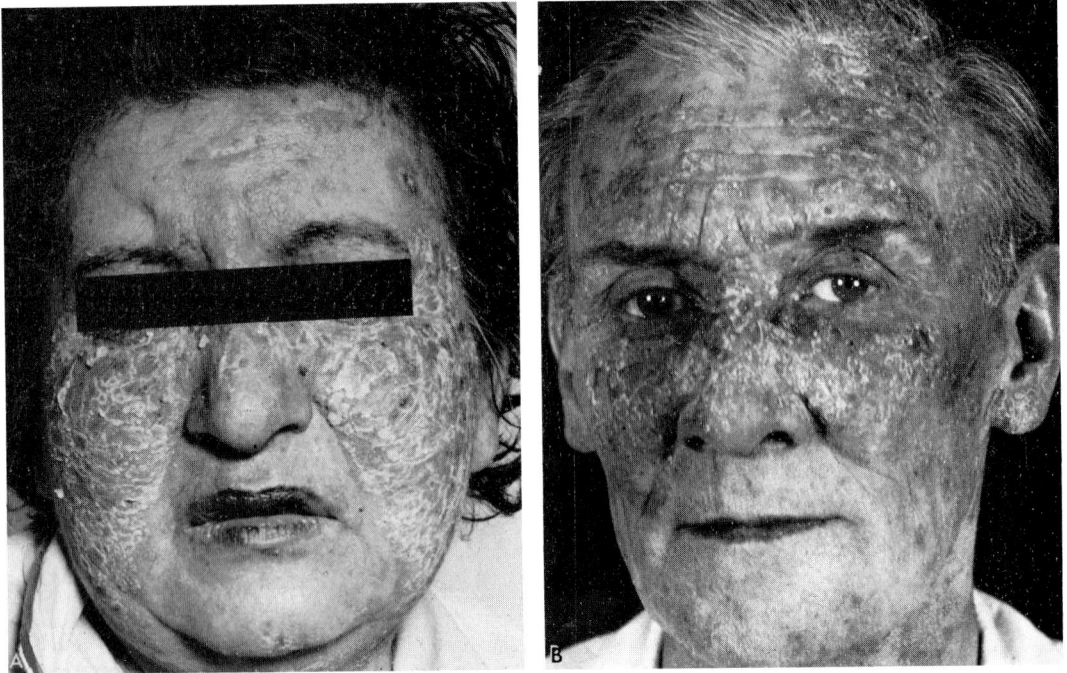

Figure 10–7 *A* and *B*, Facial lesions of pemphigus erythematosus that resemble superficially lupus erythematosus and seborrheic dermatitis.

erythroderma with circinate patterns, and the patient becomes cachectic. At this stage of the disease, alopecia of the scalp, eyebrows, eyelids, and axillae occurs. Nikolsky's sign is present only at the site of lesions. Oral lesions are absent. Papillomatosis of skin produces gyrate rugae. Hyperkeratosis and hyperpigmentation are seen. The musculoskeletal changes are serous effusions in large joints, osteoporosis, and muscular atrophy. The mammae and testes may become atrophic. Twenty-five per cent of the patients now experience recovery within two years in contrast to 40 per cent of patients who died prior to the advent of corticosteroid therapy. Systemic antimalarials and a local tar preparation, Jamarsan, as well as local corticosteroids, are useful therapeutic adjuncts.

BENIGN MUCOSAL PEMPHIGOID

Benign mucosal pemphigoid – cicatrizing pemphigoid, ocular pemphigus (Lever, 1965; McCarthy and Shklar, 1958) – is a chronic blistering disease of unknown origin with predilection for mucous membranes and less frequently the skin, and with a tendency to scarring. The disease mainly affects persons more than 60 years of age but can appear during the second through the sixth decade of life. Women are afflicted twice as often as men. No racial predilection is found. On histopathologic examination of the bullae, a subepidermal blister without acantholysis and with a severe inflammatory infiltrate and subsequent fibrosis is noted. On periodic acid-Schiff staining, the basement membrane appears to separate with the epithelium from the underlying corium. Immunofluorescence studies have revealed deposits of immunoglobulins (IgG) at the dermo-epidermal junction of involved skin and mucous membranes of patients with benign mucosal pemphigoid; no circulating antibasement membrane antibodies have been detected (Bean et al., 1972; Holubar et al., 1973).

The mucous membranes are almost always affected, and the skin is affected in about one-third of cases. The mucous membranes of the oral cavity, conjunctivae, and pharynx, larynx, esophagus, genitalia, and anus are involved.

The mouth is usually involved for months or even years before other manifestations are seen. Two types of lesions are seen in the mouth—the characteristic desquamative gingivitis (Shklar and McCarthy, 1971) and a vesiculobullous eruption. The gingivitis is diffuse or patchy, appears only when teeth are present, heals slowly, and may persist for years without significant change. When the vesicles and bullae develop, they appear rapidly, are intact for two to three days, and heal within one and one-half to four weeks. Coalescence of lesions creates large areas of denudation. Unlike pemphigus, the lesions do not have threads of epithelium, are usually not painful, do not interfere with eating, and are not associated with excessive salivation. Scarring, when present, can resemble the delicate, white, lacy lesions of lichen planus. Cicatrization occurs most frequently in the area of the soft palate, tonsillar pillars, and uvula, and adhesions may form between the buccal mucosa and alveolar processes and in the pharyngeal area. Laryngeal involvement results in recurrent soreness and hoarseness and may reveal adhesive bands on laryngoscopy. Esophageal stricture with accompanying dysphagia may develop. Nasal mucosal involvement causes symptoms of chronic rhinitis. The anogenital orifices may become stenosed and symptomatic from the resultant adhesions.

Involvement of the ocular mucous membranes is seen in about 75 per cent of the patients, is occasionally the initial manifestation for years, and is the most conspicuous and distressful symptom. The initial simple catarrhal conjunctivitis causes ocular burning and smarting and photophobia. As the process continues, scarring and shrinking of conjunctivae result in symblepharon and narrowing of the palpebral fissure (Fig. 10–8). Corneal damage may result from the conjunctival inflammation that leads to vascularization and opacity, from extension of pannus from the conjunctiva, from conjunctival scarring leading to entropion and trichiasis that cause corneal ulceration and opacity, and from obstruction of the lacrimal duct and destruction of the lacrimal gland that lead to xerosis and degeneration of the cornea.

Two types of skin lesions are seen—a recurrent vesiculobullous nonscarring eruption usually involving the inguinal area and extremities and becoming occasionally generalized, and a localized erythematous plaque with recurrent vesicles and bullae that appear on the scalp and face near the affected mucous membranes and heal with smooth atrophic scars and permanent alopecia.

In patients with benign mucosal pemphigoid, the differential diagnoses of the oral lesions are desquamative gingivitis, bullous pemphigoid, bullous lichen planus, pemphigus, and erythema multiforme; of the conjunctivae are severe erythema multiforme, epidermolysis bullosa, and burn; of the generalized skin eruption are bullous pemphigoid and erythema multiforme; and of the localized cutaneous form are localized pemphigus foliaceus and the so-called localized dermatitis herpetiformis.

The disease does not affect the general health. Blindness occurs in less than 20 per cent and generally useful vision remains in at least one eye. The course of the disease is punctuated by periods of activity and remission every few months continuing for many years.

There is no specific therapy, and the aim of therapy is to control the disease process as much as possible for an indefinite period in order to reduce symptoms and undesirable sequelae. Local and systemic

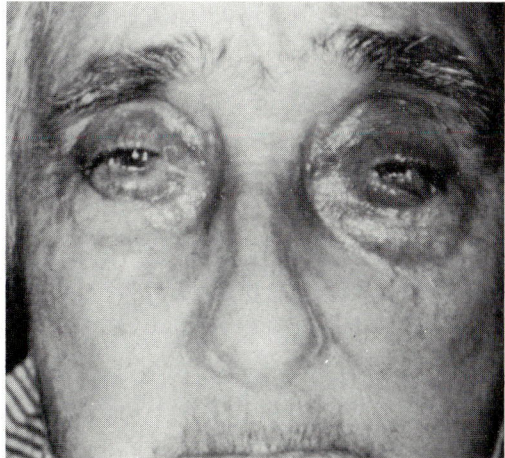

Figure 10–8 Benign mucosal pemphigoid. Chronic eye involvement with scarring and shrinking of the conjunctivae resulting in symblepharon and narrowing of the palpebral fissure.

measures are utilized. The oral and perio- dontal lesions require good dental care with elimination of irritation from trauma- tic, chemical, or bacterial factors. Dentures may be necessary to minimize tissue trauma. Topical anesthetic agents may be applied to render eating less painful; usu- ally oral lesions are not sufficiently in- capacitating or uncomfortable to warrant courses of systemic corticosteroid therapy; topical steroid therapy has been disap- pointing. For the ocular lesions, subcon- junctival injections of corticosteroids are given at weekly intervals and are of ques- tionable value. Unfortunately, large doses of systemic steroids are usually required to control this disease and are not practical for indefinite administration because of the potential and serious side effects. The eyelashes should be removed in cases of entropion. The ocular adhesions may be lysed and contact lenses may temporarily inhibit further visual damage. Systemic steroids are best used for limited periods to inhibit or reduce further esophageal and laryngeal structure formation and to con- trol the generalized bullous eruption. The early adhesions can be dislodged by re- peated esophageal bougienage.

BENIGN FAMILIAL CHRONIC PEMPHIGUS (Hailey-Hailey Disease)

Benign familial chronic pemphigus (Hailey-Hailey disease) is an incomplete autosomal dominant genodermatosis. It has been postulated that the pathologic genetic defect is the failure of tonofila- ments to connect properly with their desmosomes and the epidermal cells. Be- cause of this defect in the tonofilament- desmosome complex, the skin can experi- ence acantholysis with blister formation when exposed to traumatic or infectious stimuli or other cutaneous disorders (Wil- gram and Winstock, 1966).

Histopathology (Lever, 1967)

Like pemphigus vulgaris, suprabasal acantholysis with blister formation is present; however, it differs from pemphi- gus vulgaris by the presence of more acan- tholysis, greater loss of intercellular bridges, and evidence of dyskeratosis. The retention of some of the intercellular bridges holds the cells loosely together and is responsible for the so-called di- lapidated brick-wall appearance. There is an upward proliferation of papillae into the lacunae. Unlike Darier's disease, the suprabasal separation and acantholysis are greater but the dyskeratosis consisting of corps ronds and grains is less.

On electron microscopic examination, the number of desmosomes is reduced, and the tonofilaments, which are greatly increased and unattached to the desmo- somes, lie within the cytoplasm, often sur- round the nucleus, and appear in large whorls.

Clinical Manifestations (Lever, 1965)

Benign familial pemphigus affects both sexes equally. It occurs most frequently in Caucasians, less in Negroes and Orientals, and during the second and third decades. About two-thirds of the patients have a family history of the disease. The eruption is adversely affected by a hot, humid climate.

The eruption is characterized clinically by the appearance of groups of flaccid vesicles in normal or erythematous skin. They become turbid, rupture, and crust. The lesions may simultaneously heal cen- trally with residual hyperpigmentation and extend peripherally with the develop- ment of new lesions. The central area may persist and have a relatively flat, moist, verrucoid appearance. The lesions tend to heal spontaneously within several months and recur in the same locations. The sites of predilection are the intertriginous areas and the sides (Fig. 10-9) and nape of the neck. The disease rarely becomes wide- spread (Fig. 10-10) and can involve the oral mucosa. The pruritic eruption may be malodorous. Burning of the skin or pain from intertriginous fissures occurs.

The eruption must be differentiated from impetigo, monilial infection, pemphi- gus vegetans, and atypical Bowen's dis- ease and extramammary Paget's disease. Whenever a patient has a persistent, re- sistant, chronic intertriginous dermatitis, one should suspect the possible presence

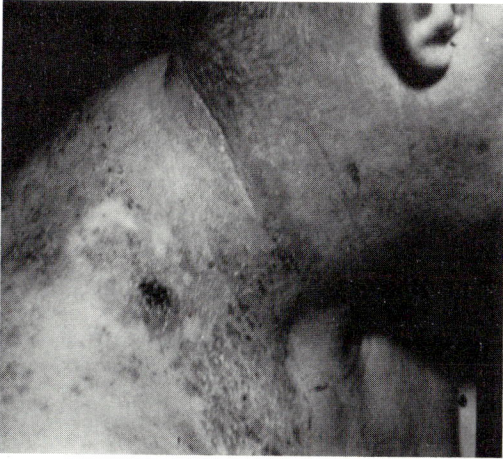

Figure 10–9 Benign familial chronic pemphigus (Hailey-Hailey disease) involving the side of the neck, a favorite site, and exhibiting peripherally small flaccid vesicles with central clearing.

of benign familial pemphigus (Lyles et al., 1958).

The relationship between Darier's disease and benign familial pemphigus is unsettled; some believe that benign familial pemphigus is a vesicular variant of Darier's disease. It appears that Darier's disease can have a vesicular component and benign familial pemphigus can have corps ronds; however, until more information is available, it is probably best to maintain these conditions as distinct entities.

The disease can remit spontaneously for long periods but rarely permanently and is less severe after the fifth decade.

Treatment

Although antibiotics may be effective locally, they are more effective when given systemically. Bacterial cultures and sensitivity tests are advocated for the selection of the appropriate antibiotic. The antibiotic has to be used continuously unless the disease is going into a remission. Sulfonamides, and particularly the related sulfones, may be effective. Topical and intralesional corticosteroids have been helpful. Systemic corticosteroids can suppress the disease, but the problems of induced hypercorticoidism and rebound phenomenon are inherent. Grenz ray therapy may induce a remission for several months. Severe medically resistant areas of involvement can be treated effectively by wide excision followed by split-thickness skin grafting (Thorne et al., 1968).

BULLOUS PEMPHIGOID

Bullous pemphigoid is a chronic and relatively benign subepidermal blistering disease usually of the elderly and without histopathologic acantholysis.

Etiology

The etiology of this disease is unknown. The finding of a serum antibody to the

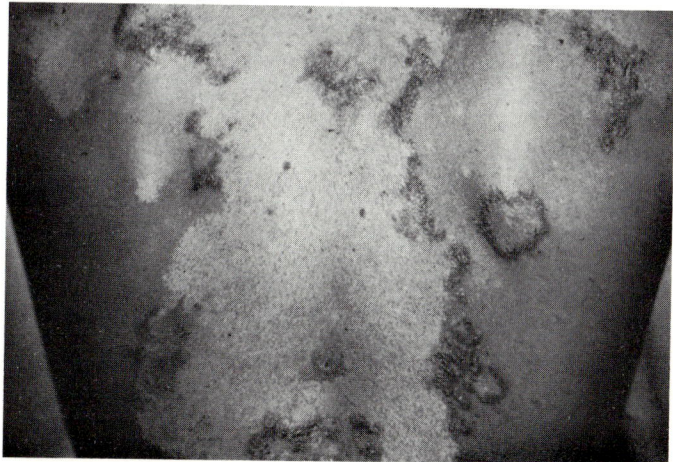

Figure 10–10 Unusual extensive involvement by benign familial chronic pemphigus (Hailey-Hailey disease).

basement membrane of skin has stimulated speculation that this distinct entity
results from an auto-immune process. The
evidences (Sams, 1970) advanced to favor
this concept are the demonstration of a
serum IgG antibody to the patient's basement membrane, the ability of the antibody to fix complement, the presence of
antibody and complement at the exact site
of pathologic change, and the predominance of polymorphonuclear leukocytes in
inflammatory infiltrate. The evidences offered against this idea are the inability to
transfer the disease passively and the failure to measure consistently the activity of
the disease with the serum antibody levels.

The disease occurs predominantly in
patients more than 60 years of age but appears infrequently before the age of 40 and
in children. No racial predilection is found,
and it affects women more frequently
under the age of 60 and men after the age
of 70. Currently, no firm evidence is present that pemphigoid is causally related to
malignancy. A pemphigoid eruption, especially with involvement of mucous membranes, has been described (Rook, 1968) as
being associated with malignant disease,
but without immunologic and electron
microscopic studies of the bullae one cannot speculate about the relationship of
malignancy to bullous pemphigoid.

Pathology

The earliest histopathologic changes
seen are numerous subepidermal micro-
vacuoles that coalesce to form bullae. In
the peribullous area, not only microva-
cuoles can be seen but also rarely an intra-
papillary accumulation of neutrophils and
eosinophils (microabscesses). In the
erythematous areas of the skin, a vasculitis
with endothelial swelling and degeneration, an infiltrate of neutrophils and
eosinophils, and nuclear dust may be seen.
Ultramicroscopy reveals that the basement membrane is free of interruption or
local destruction and a bulla which lies
above it (Jakubowicz and Dabrowski,
1970). On immunofluorescent studies, a
linear staining for IgG is usually seen
along the dermal papillae which form the
floor of the bulla (Chorzelski et al., 1971).

Clinical Manifestations

Bullous pemphigoid is a chronic disease that may last for a few months to several years and may be punctuated by exacerbations and remissions. A generalized
pruritus or a prodromal urticarial or eczematous eruption or both may be present
before the onset of the classic eruption.
Some patients may experience only a
localized eruption for several months
before generalization develops. Large,
tense, irregular bullae are characteristic;
they do not break as easily as those of
pemphigus vulgaris, tend to heal, may be
hemorrhagic, and arise usually on erythematous skin but may arise in normal
appearing skin. The erythematous areas
may have central clearing with a resultant
figurative pattern, and the subsequent
bullae appear in the serpiginous borders;
this type of eruption may clinically resemble erythema multiforme. The occasional clinical presentation of grouped
vesicles may suggest the diagnosis of
dermatitis herpetiformis. Although the
entire skin may be involved without any
pattern of distribution, there is a predilection for the lower abdomen, groin, inner
aspects of thighs, and the flexor areas of
forearms (Fig. 10-11). Mucosal lesions
confined to the mouth are seen and consist
of small tense bullae that rupture and heal
quickly and do not interfere too much with
mastication and swallowing. The disease
is not usually accompanied by constitutional symptoms; fever is uncommon; the
general health of the patient is unimpaired,
but the patient experiences great discomfort. Pruritus is generally present and can
be very severe. A leukocytosis is usually
present.

The primary or localized type of bullous
pemphigoid appears most frequently in
the lower limbs, especially the shins, and
rarely the umbilicus, and is seen usually in
the elderly. The bullae often occur in a
preexisting inflammatory skin condition,
such as stasis ulcer. They heal slowly
and recur intermittently for several
months.

The diseases that may be considered in
the differential diagnosis are pemphigus
vulgaris, erythema multiforme, and the
generalized eruption of benign mucosal
pemphigoid.

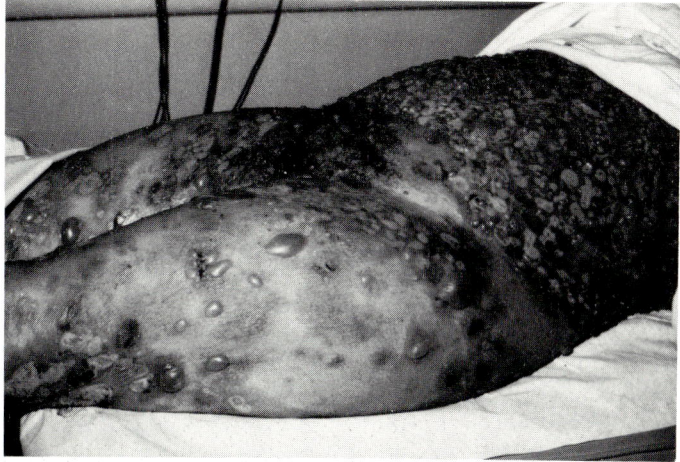

Figure 10-11 Bullous pemphigoid. The patient had a generalized pruritic eruption consisting of small and large tense bullae with a predilection for the lower abdomen and groin; the eruption responded to oral corticosteroids and was subsequently controlled by immunosuppressants.

Treatment

Bullous pemphigoid, which may remit spontaneously, was occasionally fatal prior to the onset of effective therapy because of debility and complicating infection, such as bronchopneumonia. Systemic corticosteroids are indicated in moderate to severe cases, and the dosage is not as high as that required for the treatment of pemphigus vulgaris. Intralesional steroids and topical fluorinated steroids under plastic occlusion should be attempted in the localized or mild cases respectively. In an attempt to avoid or lessen the side effects of prolonged systemic corticosteroid therapy, especially in the elderly, antimetabolites, such as methotrexate and azathioprine, may be added to reduce or replace the required amount of systemic corticosteroid.

LOCALIZED CHRONIC PEMPHIGOID

Localized chronic pemphigoid (MacVicar and Graham, 1966) is a localized chronic blistering disease that results in scarring of affected sites and is of unknown etiology. This condition was so named because it describes the clinical nature and classifies it as a subepidermal bullous dermatosis. Unlike bullous pemphigoid, direct and indirect immunofluorescent studies of the basement membrane of involved and uninvolved skin were normal (Trepanier, 1970). Immunologic studies to establish a relationship of this disorder with dermatitis herpetiformis have not been reported.

On histopathologic examination, a subepidermal blister is seen and, with histochemical stains, the basement membrane is shown to line the floor of the bulla. The base of the bulla shows festooning, which is characterized by the projection of intact dermal papillae into the bulla. Collections of eosinophils and neutrophils at the top of the dermal papillae are found. An inflammatory infiltrate, often diffuse and at times perivascular, is seen in the upper corium.

Clinical Manifestations

The disease has a predilection for the middle-aged and older, particularly Caucasian, men. The age range has been reported from 25 to 73 years. The pruritic eruption is characterized by vesicles and bullae that appear a few at a time in one or more circumscribed plaques on the head, scalp, face, and neck. Successive flares appear over a period of 1 to 15 years; the disease spontaneously clears in about four years with atrophic scarring of the affected sites. Brief episodes of a generalized eruption resembling dermatitis herpetiformis were reported to develop in two patients, and another patient was described as having intermittent lesions of the mouth, pharynx, and conjunctiva (Brunsting and

Perry, 1957); it is questionable whether these three incidences represented localized chronic pemphigoid.

The differential diagnosis of the lesions free of blisters includes discoid lupus erythematosus, neurotic excoriations, lupus vulgaris, and fixed drug eruptions; in the presence of bullae, the differential diagnoses are recurrent herpes simplex, bullous lupus erythematosus, benign mucous membrane pemphigus, dermatitis herpetiformis, bullous lichen planus, and porphyria cutanea tarda.

Treatment

The lesions may be improved and occasionally healed with sulfones or sulfapyridine. Topical corticosteroids, with or without occlusion, and intralesional corticosteroids are helpful adjunctive measures. Systemic corticosteroids will clear up the eruption which recurs upon the discontinuance of this therapy.

HERPES GESTATIONIS

Herpes gestationis is a very pruritic, polymorphous, vesiculobullous eruption that occurs during pregnancy and puerperium and tends to recur in subsequent pregnancies.

Etiology

In view of its clinical and histological resemblance to erythema multiforme, the concept that this may represent a hypersensitivity or toxic reaction to fetal or placental products or hormones or their metabolites has been entertained. The presence of Rh isosensitization (Cawley et al., 1952), the reported increased incidence of fetal anomalies and spontaneous abortions, and the precipitation of the disease in previously affected women by anovulatory medication have been offered as supportive of the above concept. High doses of pyridoxine have been described as effective therapy, and its success was attributable to replacement (Fosnaugh et al., 1961); unfortunately, in three personal cases so treated, it was ineffective.

Histopathology

The histopathologic picture is a subepidermal bulla with polymorphonuclear, especially eosinophilic, leukocytes in the blister fluid and dermis and is indistinguishable from that of erythema multiforme, bullous pemphigoid, and the later lesions of dermatitis herpetiformis.

Clinical Manifestations (Osmundsen, 1966; Russel and Thorne, 1957)

The disease affects pregnant women from two weeks after conception into the puerperal stage, but most frequently during the second trimester. The incidence of the disease is roughly 1 in 4000 pregnancies.

The onset and relapses may be accompanied by the constitutional symptoms of fever, malaise, nausea, and headaches. The lesions heal with residual hyperpigmentation but with no scarring unless deep excoriations or secondary infection is present. The disease is characterized by a pruritic, tense, vesiculobullous eruption that appears on an erythematous, diffusely edematous, or urticarial base (Fig. 10-12 A and B and Figure 10-13). The pruritus may antedate the eruption by days. The lesions tend to appear in crops and may coalesce and spread, creating circinate and arcuate patterns. Initially the eruption is localized but becomes generalized, favoring the extremities, including the hands and feet; the trunk, especially the buttocks and the lower abdomen and particularly the umbilical areas, is usually involved. Bilateral symmetry of lesions is not seen. Mucous membrane lesions occur.

A transient herpetiform eruption characterized by vesicles, papules, and pustules may occur in the fetus, clears spontaneously after a few weeks, and has no effect on the development of the infant.

The laboratory studies may reveal a leukocytosis, and an eosinophilia of 10 per cent and greater is usually seen. The IgA may be increased, and the albumin in the serum may be normal or slightly lowered (Kjartansson et al., 1966).

Herpes gestationis resembles most closely bullous pemphigoid and in less severe cases erythema multiforme. It is

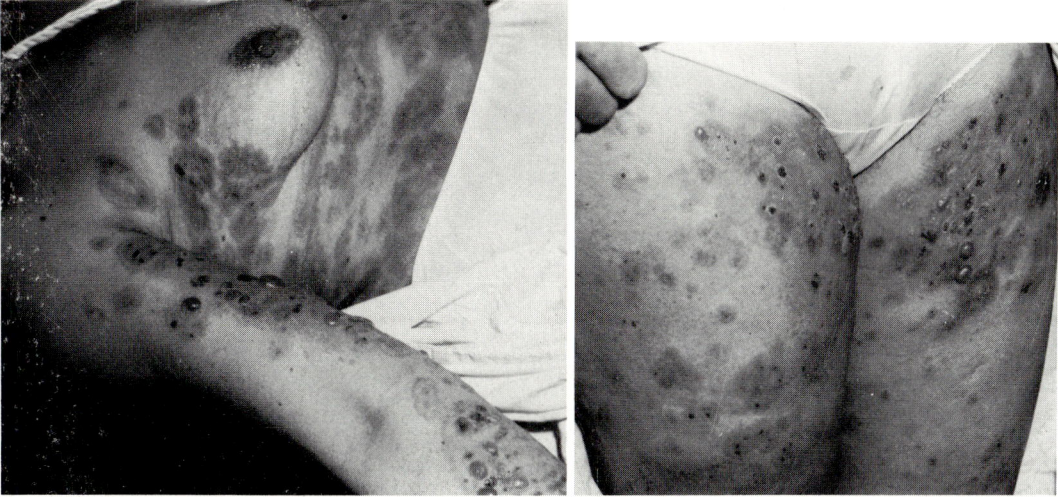

Figure 10–12 Second successive attack of herpes gestationis in two pregnancies; onset in first pregnancy at three months and in second pregnancy at one month. In both pregnancies, the disease was successfully controlled by prednisone; the deliveries and fetuses were normal.

distinct from dermatitis herpetiformis because it is a self-limited condition associated with pregnancy and similar hormonal states; it lacks the symmetry, the degree of pigmentation, and the scarring of dermatitis herpetiformis; it is predominantly a bullous disease and has oral lesions; and it responds best to steroid therapy and lacks, if any, the dramatic response to sulfapyridine and sulfones seen in dermatitis herpetiformis (Tolman et al., 1959).

The course of the disease is characterized by alternating exacerbations and remissions. The earlier in pregnancy its onset, the less likely it is to persist for any length of time into the postpartum period; however, the later its onset, especially just before delivery, the more likely it is to continue into the postpartum period. After its usual temporal onset, it extends at most for a few weeks after delivery; however, it may have minor recurrences at menses for 6 to 18 months after delivery.

The disease has no effect on the mother but can result in a high incidence of fetal anomalies, death, and abortions. Whether this is due to the disease or the drugs used in the past is not known; however, with the use of corticosteroids, the author's experience in three cases showed no fetal or delivery problems.

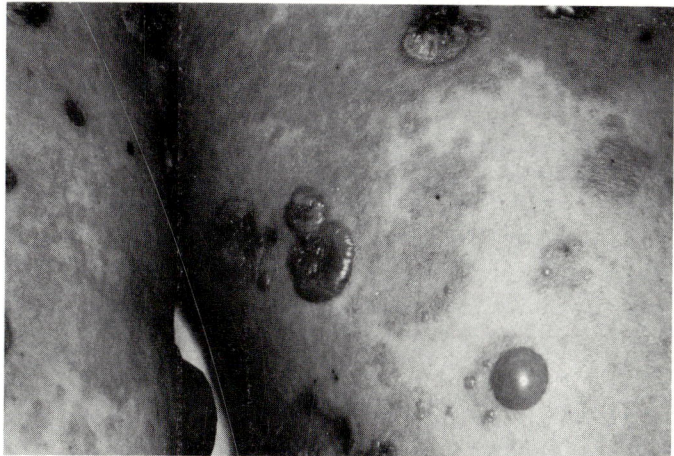

Figure 10–13 Close-up of tense bullae of herpes gestationis on erythematous base and in other parts of the body in the borders of figurative and circinate erythematosus urticarial lesions; patient was successfully treated by prednisone.

Treatment

Symptomatic treatment, such as baths and topical and systemic antipruritics, may be used as adjunctive measures. The most effective and usually the only successful therapy is systemic corticosteroids daily, 15 to 40 mg. of prednisone or its equivalent.

DERMATITIS HERPETIFORMIS
(Duhring's Disease)

Dermatitis herpetiformis is a rare, unknown, chronic, recurrent eruption characterized by erythematous papules, vesicles, and, infrequently, blisters.

The etiology of this disease is unknown, and it is believed that it may represent a reaction pattern. Although the causative factors are not appreciated, it has been associated with disturbances in mental health, hormonal changes, and vaccination. No familial incidence or genetic transmission is known. Dermatitis herpetiformis may coexist with carcinoma which, when the carcinoma is successfully treated, is followed sometimes by its regression. Despite a recent report in the literature (Mansson, 1971), the risk of development of malignancy does not appear to be increased in patients with dermatitis herpetiformis. For some unexplained reason, some patients show a positive patch test to halogens and an exacerbation of their eruption upon the ingestion of halogens.

In over two-thirds of the patients with dermatitis herpetiformis, an enteropathy is present similar to, but less pronounced than, that seen in the celiac syndrome (Shuster et al., 1968). The disaccharidase activity varies with the histologic changes in the small intestine in dermatitis herpetiformis. Shuster et al. found that the gluten-free diet did not affect the eruption and did not reduce the dose of sulfones necessary to control the disease; however, others have described improvement of the dermatitis herpetiformis with a gluten-free diet.

Direct immunofluorescent staining (IF) of adjacent uninvolved perilesional skin at the dermo-epidermal junction is seen (Chorzelski et al., 1971). The IF pattern may be microgranular, fibrillar, and linear continuous along the basement membrane. Although IgA is the predominant demonstrable immunoglobulin, IgG and IgM may be deposited; complement is also deposited in the tips of the dermal papillae. IF studies can aid in the differential diagnosis of the unusual clinical blister variants of dermatitis herpetiformis and bullous pemphigoid. No significant serum complement and circulating immunoglobulin levels have been demonstrated (Fraser et al., 1971). Similar immunofluorescent patterns in the upper gastrointestinal tract of patients have been reported but not confirmed.

Histopathology (Clark et al., 1965; MacVicar et al., 1963)

The earliest histologic change appreciated is a papillary crescentic or globular deposition of fibrin which appears before the development of the characteristic papillary microabscesses (Mustakallio et al., 1970). These abscesses are best seen not only in the erythematous lesions but also in the vicinity of the early blisters. They are composed of masses of neutrophils that enlarge and coalesce and result in a dermo-epidermal separation and multilocular vesiculation that later becomes unilocular (Piérard, 1963). The vesicles and bullae can rarely be subcorneal. Eosinophils are unusual during the initial evolution of the lesion. A vasculitis of the superficial dermal vessels is seen infrequently. The most characteristic ultrastructural change in dermatitis herpetiformis is widespread destruction of the basement membrane of the skin.

Clinical Manifestations (Smith, 1966; Tolman et al., 1959; Unger, 1969)

The disease most frequently appears between the second decade and the fifth decade, although it may occur in children, usually after five years of age. Men are affected two times more frequently than women. The disease is seen in all races.

The onset may be sudden, and no associated or prodromal constitutional symptoms are seen. Pruritus and occasionally a burning sensation are usually the initial prodromal symptoms. The early lesions are erythematous macules or papules that have superimposed small tight vesicles. Bullae are rare and best appreciated in subsequential exacerbations or relapses due to a lapse of therapy. One is impressed by the bilateral symmetry of the grouped lesions classically presenting the mirror image. The vesicles are difficult to find because of their early excoriation. The occasional annular or gyrate pattern may result from the appearance of vesicles in the border of erythematous plaques or in the central clearing of grouped vesicles. Temporary postinflammatory pigmentation occurs; secondary superficial scars are seen infrequently. An eosinophilia of 10 per cent or greater may be present.

The eruption (Figs. 10-14 and 10-15) classically involves the extensor surfaces of the elbows and knees, buttocks, sacral and scapular areas, and the scalp; other involved sites are the axillary folds, shoulders, trunk, face, malar areas, and ears. Mucous membrane lesions are rare and heal rapidly.

The diseases to be differentiated are ectoparasitic infestation, such as scabies, lichen urticatus, bullous urticaria, neurotic excoriations, pityriasis lichenoides et varioliformis acuta, folliculitis, disseminated neurodermatitis, stasis eczema with "ide" reaction, nickel dermatitis, tinea corporis (especially of the sacral area,

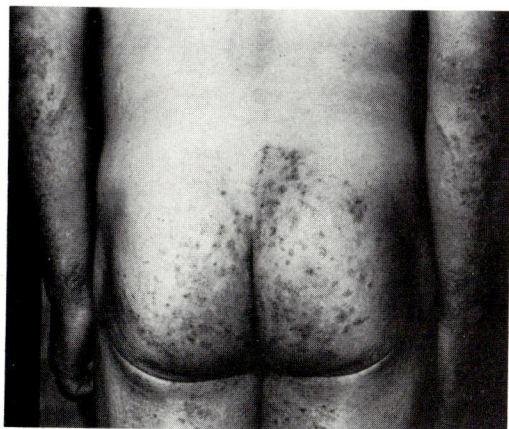

Figure 10–15 Patient had not only dermatitis herpetiformis but also rheumatoid arthritis and Sjögren's syndrome.

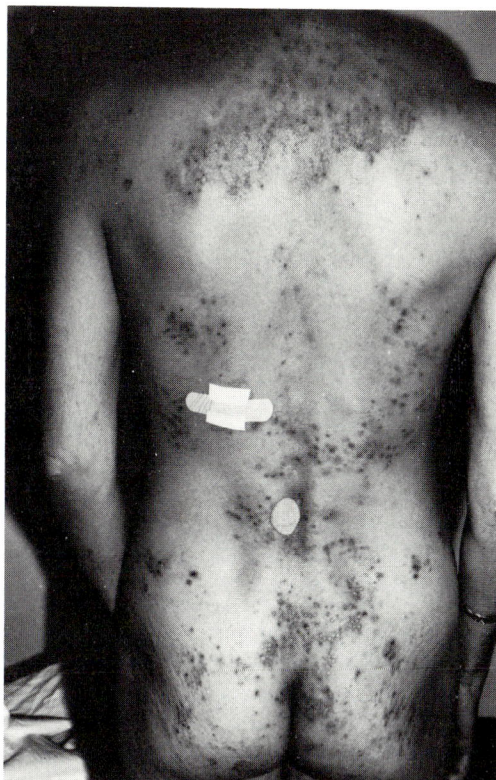

Figure 10–14 Classic distribution of dermatitis herpetiformis—elbows, buttocks, also knees; unfortunately, the patient was allergic to sulfapyridine and sulfones and many of the problems of continued systemic corticosteroid therapy also developed.

Fig. 10-16), bullous lichen planus, and bullous pemphigoid.

A syndrome consisting of a vesicular eruption resembling dermatitis herpetiformis associated with pyoderma gangrenosum and rheumatoid arthritis has been described (Ayres and Ayres, 1958).

Dermatitis herpetiformis usually has a chronic course punctuated by periods of remissions and exacerbations, and lasts about 5 to 10 years but may continue for 20 years or more. The reports stating that the intensity of the disease diminishes over the years have been disputed. Prolonged and permanent remissions are unusual and occur only after years.

Treatment

Fortunately, we have two drugs, sulfapyridine (Tolman et al., 1959) and diaminodiphenylsulfone (DDS, dapsone, Avlosulfon; Lorincz and Pearson, 1962),

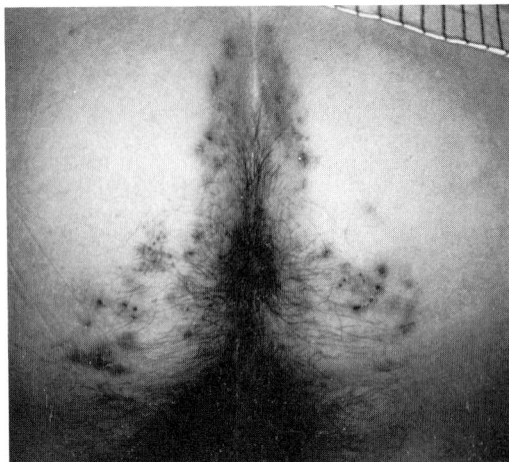

Figure 10-16 An unusual presentation of dermatitis herpetiformis that had been treated for 18 months as a tinea corporis.

that effectively control the symptoms and suppress the disease. Sulfapyridine, 2 gm. a day, is given initially, and the dose is tapered with improvement to 0.5 gm. to 1.0 gm. a day as the controlling and maintenance dose. The side effects of sulfapyridine are fever, headache, gastrointestinal symptoms (anorexia, nausea, vomiting), hematologic disturbances (leukopenia, hemolytic anemia, methemoglobulinemia), hepatitis, renal damage, psychosis, and dermatitis. The initial treatment with DDS is 200 mg. a day and may have to be increased to 300 mg. a day; the maintenance dose is 50 mg. to 100 mg. a day. The side effects of DDS are morning headache, methemoglobulinemia, anemia resulting from delayed red cell survival and hemolysis, toxic epidermolysis, and a syndrome characterized by fever, exfoliative dermatitis, liver necrosis, and lymphadenitis. Patients intolerant of the above drugs may require systemic corticosteroids because of the severity of the disease. These drugs, unfortunately, have to be administered for prolonged periods and in such doses as to produce iatrogenically a hypercorticoid state with its incumbent problems. The local application of steroids with or without occlusion and the use of oral antipruritic agents may be helpful adjunctive measures that may permit lowering of the effective dose of the systemically administered drug.

CHRONIC NONHEREDITARY VESICULOBULLOUS DISEASES IN CHILDHOOD

Originally, the chronic nonhereditary vesiculobullous diseases in children were called juvenile dermatitis herpetiformis. Kim and Winkelmann (1961) divided these diseases into the papular type similar to dermatitis herpetiformis and the bullous type which they called bullous pemphigoid of children because of its similarity to bullous pemphigoid of the elderly. Since they could not find immunologic changes in the skin and sera of children with the bullous type of eruption, Jordan et al. (1970) suggested that this entity be named benign chronic bullous dermatosis of childhood. Bean et al. (1970) have reported a case of bullous pemphigoid in a child with circulating antibodies to the basement membrane of skin; Jablonska et al. (1971) described cases in children each of whom had a clinical course and immunologic picture characteristic of adult dermatitis herpetiformis.

In summary, juvenile dermatitis herpetiformis appears to be a syndrome of multiple etiology and includes cases corresponding fully to bullous pemphigoid and dermatitis herpetiformis in adults as well as cases that resemble clinically bullous pemphigoid without any immunologic changes.

JUVENILE PEMPHIGOID

Juvenile pemphigoid is a chronic recurrent bullous eruption of unknown etiology that occurs in children; it resembles the bullous pemphigoid of adults and is unlike dermatitis herpetiformis of adults. Most reported cases failed to exhibit the immunologic phenomena of the bullous pemphigoid of the elderly; however, cases are described with circulating antibodies to the basement membrane zone of skin and in vivo bound IgG in this location. Biopsy results have shown inflammatory infiltrates in the intestinal villi in cases of the bullous pemphigoid and dermatitis herpetiformis types of eruption in children. The majority of the cases are seen in boys less than five years of age (Fig. 10-17); it has been seen in infants in the first weeks of life. On histopathologic examination, the bullae, which have an intact epidermis, are subepidermal and contain leukocytes. An eosinophilia of 5 to 10 per cent is present.

The onset of the disease is acute, usually with little, if any, constitutional symptoms. The growth and development of the afflicted child are unaffected. The mild pruritic eruption consists mainly of tense bullae that range from 0.25 to 2 cm. in diameter, appear often in normal skin but also on an erythematous base, may become hemorrhagic, and frequently form at the periphery of annular and polycyclic plaques formed by coalescence or extension of lesions. The denuded areas tend to heal rapidly, may become impetiginized and less frequently eczematized, and may heal with pigmentation and, rarely, scar-

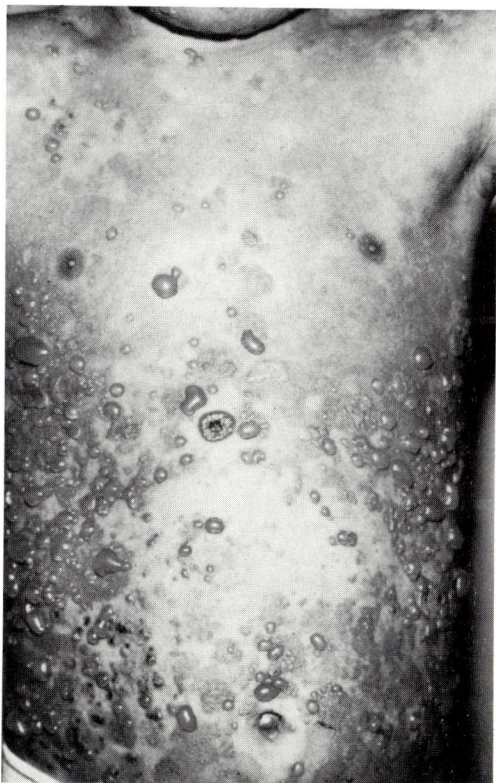

Figure 10-17 A three-year-old boy with generalized blister disease that was improved by sulfapyridine; unfortunately, immunologic basement membrane studies were not performed.

ring. The eruption becomes usually generalized. It has a predilection for the genitalia, bathing suit area, and face, and tends to concentrate in these areas. Few and scattered lesions of extremities may be present. The mucous membranes are rarely involved.

Among the conditions that may be considered in the differential diagnosis are impetigo contagiosa, epidermolysis bullosa, incontinentia pigmenti, urticaria pigmentosa, and acrodermatitis enteropathica. The course of the disease is usually chronic with remissions and recurrences over a period of three to four years; spontaneous remissions occur and may be complete within a few weeks.

No consistent or significantly effective treatment is known, although the sulfones and sulfapyridine may sometimes be effective. Systemic corticosteroids in relatively large doses may suppress the eruption which recurs upon the reduction of the dose. In severe and resistant cases, a combination of sulfones or sulfapyridine and corticosteroids may be helpful. Other adjunctive measures, such as baths, topical corticosteroids, and antipruritics, may be helpful.

SUBCORNEAL PUSTULAR DERMATOSIS (Sneddon-Wilkinson Disease)

Subcorneal pustular dermatosis is a benign but chronic relapsing pustular disease with a characteristic histologic picture of a subcorneal bulla filled with polymorphonuclear leukocytes.

Etiology

The etiology and pathogenesis of this disease are unknown. The pustules are primary and sterile; no associated local or systemic infections are present. No qualitative or quantitative changes in the serologic proteins have been described. The in vitro demonstration of antigen-antibody complement complexes in the stratum corneum suggests that part of the tissue damage may be mediated immunologically by a chemotactic trimolecular complex (C5, 6, 7) of the complement system that initiates the transepidermal migration of neutrophils and the development of blisters (Krogh and Toüder, 1970).

Pathology

The contents of the subcorneal bulla are almost completely neutrophils, occasionally eosinophils, and a few acantholytic cells that are probably secondary to the effect of proteolytic enzymes of the polymorphonuclear leukocytes. The underlying epidermis exhibits some spongiosis but no spongiosiform pustules. A mild perivascular infiltrate of polymorphonuclear cells is seen in the upper dermis. The histopathologic differential diagnosis with impetigo and pemphigus foliaceus may be quite difficult and at times even impossible.

Clinical Manifestations (Burns and Fine, 1959; Ellis, 1958; Sneddon and Wilkinson, 1956)

This uncommon disease appears four times more frequently in women than men and occurs in the fourth and fifth decades of life. Constitutional signs or symptoms are rarely present. The primary lesion is a small pustule on an erythematous base or a transient vesicle that quickly becomes a pustule. The pustules tend to appear in crops and waves and to form annular or gyrate spreading patches of dermatitis that may coalesce, creating serpiginous patterns. The lesions scale and crust and clear with a residual brownish hyperpigmentation; they tend to recur in the same sites over a number of years. The eruption favors the trunk and the intertriginous areas of the groin (Fig. 10–18 A), axillae (Fig. 10-18 B), breasts, and limbs, but no mucous membrane lesions are

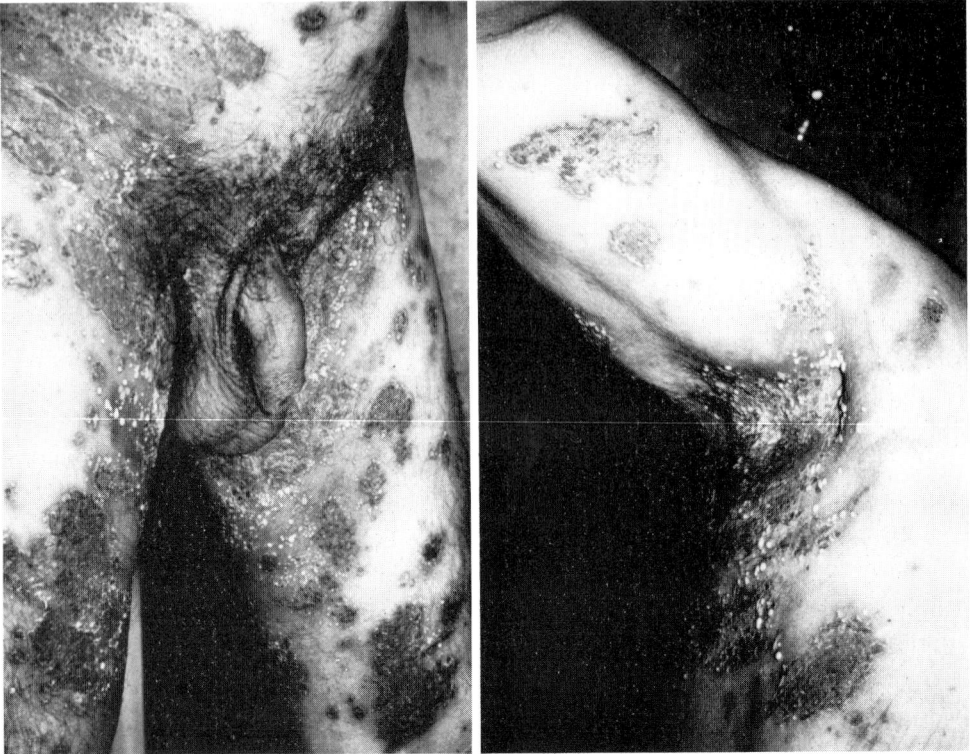

Figure 10–18 Chronic, generalized, predominantly intertriginous, subcorneal, pustular dermatosis of three years' duration characterized by primary pustules, a resistance to all forms of therapy, and frequent flares with moderately severe constitutional symptoms.

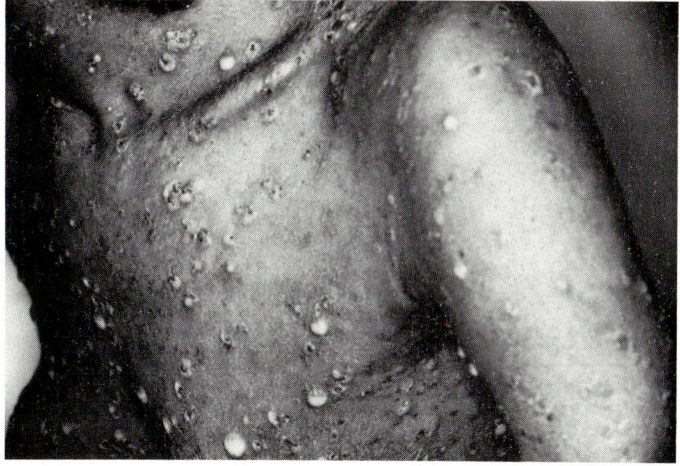

Figure 10–19 Discrete, flaccid, turbid bullae and pustules are the lesions of this rare type of subcorneal pustular dermatosis.

found. The face is not usually involved, but a follicular variant with subcorneal pustules in the upper part of the hair follicle has been reported as involving the

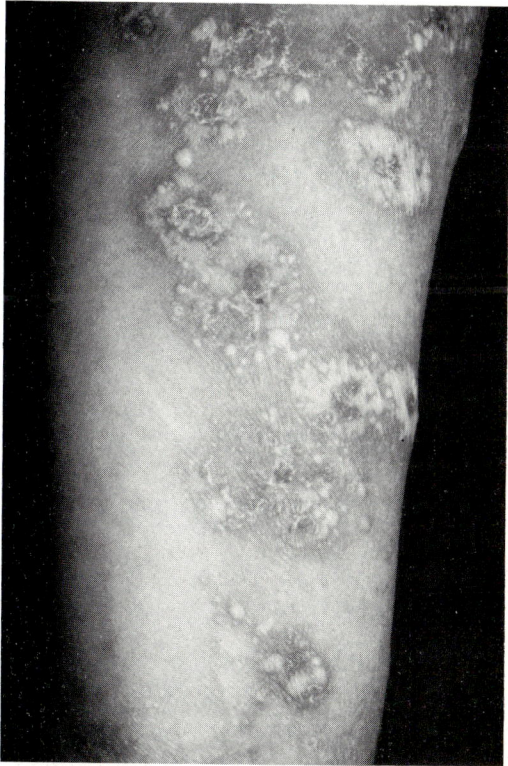

Figure 10–20 This patient had a sudden onset of generalized patchy dermatitis with many scattered pustules and "lakes" of pus resembling pustular psoriasis of Von Zumbusch.

face (Ise and Ofuji, 1965). The eruption may be moderately pruritic and is non-scarring. A few scattered or many bullae that rapidly become purulent with an appreciable purulent fluid level and favor the trunk may occur during the course of the disease and are rarely the initial or only expression of this disease (Fig. 10-19).

The disease is chronic with intermittent flare-ups and lasts five to eight years. The clinical differential diagnoses are bullous impetigo, pustular psoriasis of Von Zumbusch (Fig. 10-20), and pemphigus foliaceus.

Treatment

The sulfas (especially sulfapyridine) or the sulfones (especially DDS, diaminodiphenylsulfone) or both usually give partial and occasionally complete relief (Lorincz and Pearson, 1962). Corticosteroids, even in large doses, are not very effective. Antibiotics are useless. Antimetabolites, methotrexate, hydroxyurea, and azathioprine have proved to be ineffective in two patients treated by the author. The Goeckermann treatment may be a useful adjunctive measure.

The dose of DDS is 200 mg. a day initially and, when possible, 50 mg. to 100 mg. as a maintenance dose. When sulfapyridine is used, 2 gm. to 3 gm. is given initially to control the disease process and later 0.5 gm. to 1.0 gm. is given daily for maintenance therapy.

REFERENCES

Asboe-Hansen, G.: Diagnosis of pemphigus. Br. J. Dermatol. 83:81, 1970.

Ayres, S., Jr., and Ayres, S., III: Pyoderma gangrenosum with an unusual syndrome of ulcers, vesicles, and arthritis. Arch. Dermatol. 77:269, 1958.

Bean, S. F., Good, R. A., and Windhorst, D. B.: Bullous pemphigoid in an 11-year-old boy. Arch. Dermatol. 102:205, 1970.

Bean, S. F., Waisman, M., Michel, B., et al.: Cicatricial pemphigoid. Immunofluorescent studies. Arch. Dermatol. 106:195, 1972.

Brown, M. V.: Fogo selvagem (pemphigus foliaceus). Arch. Dermatol. 9:589, 1954.

Brunsting, L. A., and Perry, H. O.: Benign pemphigoid. A report of seven cases with chronic scarring, herpetiform plaques about the head and neck. Arch. Dermatol. 75:489, 1957.

Burns, R. E., and Fine, G.: Subcorneal pustular dermatoses. Arch. Dermatol. 80:72, 1959.

Cawley, E. P., Wheeler, C. E., and Wilhite, P. A.: Herpes gestationis and Rh factor. South Med. J. 45:827, 1952.

Chorzelski, T. P., Beutner, E. H., Jablonska, S., et al.: Immunofluorescence studies in diagnosis of dermatitis herpetiformis and its differentiation from bullous pemphigoid. J. Invest. Dermatol. 56:373, 1971.

Clark, W. H., Jr., Yip, S. Y., and Tolman, M. M.: Abstract. The histogenesis of dermo-epidermal separation in dermatitis herpetiformis. Fed. Proc. 24:433, 1965.

Ellis, F. A.: Subcorneal pustular dermatoses. Arch. Dermatol. 78:580, 1958.

Falco-Braun, O.: The pathology of blister formation. *In* Kopf, A. W., and Andrade, R.: The Year Book of Dermatology. Chicago, Year Book Medical Publishers, Inc., 1969, pp. 6-42.

Fosnaugh, R. P., Bryan, H. G., and Orders, R. L.: Pyridoxine in the treatment of herpes gestationis. Arch. Dermatol. 84:90, 1961.

Fraser, N. G., Beck, J. S., and Albert-Recht, F.: Serum complement (C'3) and immunoglobulin levels in dermatitis herpetiformis. Br. J. Dermatol. 85:314, 1971.

Grob, P. J., and Inderbitzin, Th.M.: Experimental studies on the pathogenesis of acantholysis in pemphigus. Internat. Cong. Dermatologicae 2:1158, 1968.

Holubar, K., Hönigsmann, H., and Wolff, K.: Cicatricial pemphigoid. Immunofluorescent investigations. Arch. Dermatol. 108:50, 1973.

Hurst, H. G.: Pemphigus and pemphigoid: Some current concepts. Can. Med. Assoc. J. 103:1279, 1970.

Ise, S., and Ofuji, S.: Subcorneal pustular dermatoses. A follicular variant? Arch. Dermatol. 92:169, 1965.

Jablonska, S., Chorzelski, T., and Blaszczyk, M.: Immunosuppressants in the treatment of pemphigus. Br. J. Dermatol. 83:315, 1970.

Jablonska, S., Chorzelski, T., Beautner, E. H., et al.: Juvenile dermatitis herpetiformis in the light of immunofluorescence studies. Br. J. Dermatol. 85:307, 1971.

Jakubowicz, K., and Dabrowski, J.: The ultrastructure of bullous changes in pemphigoid. Przegl. Dermatol. 57:291, 1970.

Jordan, R. E., Bean, S. F., Triftshauser, C. T., et al.: Childhood bullous dermatitis herpetiformis: Negative immunofluorescent tests. Arch. Dermatol. 101:629, 1970.

Kim, R., and Winkelmann, R. K.: Dermatitis herpetiformis in children: Relationship to bullous pemphigoid. Arch. Dermatol. 83:895, 1961.

Kjartansson, S., Fusaro, R. M., and Peterson, W. C., Jr.: Dermatitis herpetiformis and herpes gestationis. Analysis of gamma-A and gamma-M serum proteins by immunoelectrophoresis. J. Invest. Dermatol. 46:480, 1966.

Krogh, H. K., and Toüder, I. O.: Subcorneal pustular dermatoses pathogenetic aspects. Br. J. Dermatol. 83:429, 1970.

Lever, W.: Benign Mucosal Pemphigoid, Pemphigus and Pemphigoid. Springfield, Illinois, Charles C Thomas, 1965, pp. 40–72 and 103–118.

Lever, W. F.: Histopathology of the Skin. Ed. 4. Philadelphia, J. B. Lippincott Company, 1967, pp. 72–74.

Lever, W. F., and Hashimoto, K.: The etiology and treatment of pemphigus and pemphigoid. J. Invest. Dermatol. 53:373, 1969.

Lorincz, A. L., and Pearson, R. W.: Sulfapyridine and sulfone type drugs in dermatology. Arch. Dermatol. 85:2, 1962.

Lyles, T. W., Knox, J. M., and Richardson, J. B.: Atypical features in familial benign chronic pemphigus. Arch. Dermatol. 78:446, 1958.

MacVicar, D. N., and Graham, J. H.: Abstract. Localized chronic pemphigoid: A clinicopathologic and histochemical study. Am. J. Pathol. 48:52a, 1966.

MacVicar, D. N., Graham, J. H., and Burgon, C. F., Jr.: Dermatitis herpetiformis, erythema multiforme, and bullous pemphigoid: A comparative histopathological and histochemical study. J. Invest. Dermatol. 41:289, 1963.

Mansson, T.: Malignant disease in dermatitis herpetiformis. Acta Derm. Venereol. 51:379, 1971.

McCarthy, P. L., and Shklar, G.: Benign mucousmembrane pemphigus. N. Engl. J. Med. 258:726, 1958.

Mustakallio, K. K., Blomquist, K., and Laiho, K.: Papillary deposit of fibrin, a characteristic of initial lesions of dermatitis herpetiformis. Ann. Clin. Res. 2:13, 1970.

Newcomer, V. D., and Landau, J. W.: Recent advances in the diagnosis and treatment of pemphigus. Calif. Med. 114:1, 1971.

Osmundsen, P. E.: Herpes gestationis. Report on five cases. Dermatologica 132:393, 1966.

Perry, H. O., and Brunsting, L. A.: Pemphigus foliaceus. Arch. Dermatol. 91:10, 1965.

Piérard, J.: De l'aspect histologique des plaques érythémateuses de la dermatite herpétiforme de Duhring. Ann. Dermatol. Syphiligr. 90:121, 1963.

Rook, A. J.: A pemphigoid eruption associated with carcinoma of the bronchus. Trans. St. Johns Hosp. Dermatol. Soc. 54:152, 1968.

Russell, B., and Thorne, N.: Herpes gestationis. Br. J. Dermatol. 89:339, 1957.

Sams, W. M., Jr.: Bullous pemphigoid. Is it an immunologic disease? Arch. Dermatol. 102:485, 1970.

Sanders, S. L., and Nelson, C. T.: Pemphigus and pemphigoid. Med. Clin. North Am. 49:681, 1965.

Shklar, G., and McCarthy, P. L.: Oral lesions of mucous membrane pemphigoid. Arch. Otolaryngol. 93:354, 1971.

Shuster, S., Watson, A. J., and Marks, J.: Coeliac syndrome in dermatitis herpetiformis. Lancet 1:1101, 1968.

Smith, E. L.: The diagnosis of dermatitis herpetiformis. Trans. St. Johns Hosp. Derm. Soc. 52:176, 1966.

Sneddon, T. B., and Wilkinson, D. S.: Subcorneal pustular dermatoses. Br. J. Dermatol. 68:385, 1956.

Stoughton, R. B.: The pathophysiology of blister formation. *In* Rook, A., and Champion, R. H.: Progress in the Biological Sciences in Relation to Dermatology. Cambridge, Cambridge University Press, 1964, pp. 431–441.

Thorne, F. L., Hall, J. H., and Mladick, R. A.: Surgical treatment of familial chronic pemphigus (Hailey-Hailey disease). Arch. Dermatol. 98:522, 1968.

Tolman, M., Moschella, S. L., and Schneiderman, R. N.: Dermatitis herpetiformis: Specific entity or clinical complex? J. Invest. Dermatol. 32:557, 1959.

Trepanier, Y.: Localized bullous dermatitis herpetiformis. Arch. Dermatol. 101:98, 1970.

Unger, W. P., and MacVicar, D. M.: Dermatitis herpetiformis. Cutis 5:807, 1969.

Wilgram, G. F., and Weinstock, A.: Advances in genetic dermatology. Dyskeratosis, acantholysis, and hyperkeratosis, with a note on the specific role of desmosomes and keratinosomes in the formation of the horny layer. Arch. Dermatol. 94:456, 1966.

CHAPTER

11

BACTERIAL INFECTIONS

Section I

FUNDAMENTAL CUTANEOUS MICROBIOLOGY

Richard R. Marples

The normal skin of healthy subjects is very resistant to invasion by most bacteria. Although some bacterial diseases such as impetigo or furunculosis are common, exposure to the organisms responsible is far more frequent than the diseases they cause. Disease is not inevitable just because pathogenic bacteria are present. The host itself must be susceptible. Infection develops when the right combination of causative factors exists; a particular bacterium usually represents only one of the etiologic agents. There are almost always a number of interacting causes for infection of any body tissue, some direct, some indirect, which create circumstances leading to infection and aid in its persistence.

In understanding the causes and the quixotic and changeable course of various bacterial infections in different patients, it is helpful to have some knowledge of the bacteriology of the normal skin, what reciprocal relationships exist between the skin and its microflora, what forces keep the bacterial flora "normal," and what forces produce definite abnormality. Such an approach yields some insight into the pathogenesis of bacterial infections of the skin, though the host-parasite relationships between human skin and the millions of bacteria which reside in and on it are by no means fully understood.

FLORA OF NORMAL SKIN

The skin's surface provides many nutrients for the growth of organisms. It contains fats, proteins, nitrogenous substances, minerals, and so forth which are produced as by-products of keratinization or by the cutaneous appendages. The nutrient that is in shortest supply over much of the skin is water. Simple carbohydrates such as glucose are present in very small quantities but amino acids and the glycerol in triglycerides are abundant substitutes. Much of the surface of the skin is thus inhospitable to bacteria, but dense populations of microorganisms are resident in moist intertriginous regions.

The scalp and face, where sebaceous secretions may hinder the evaporation of water, and the stratum corneum, more permeable than abdominal or forearm skin, also carry large numbers of organisms. The microbial flora of each region of the skin seems to differ in detail from other regions. Climatic conditions, sweating, body hygiene, and, of course, skin disease and a host of other factors influence the composition of the microflora. Differences in the numbers and kinds of microorganisms may also be detected in normal individuals living under the same conditions which, in turn, are often resistant to changing conditions affecting the skin flora.

Since the skin is exposed, microorganisms from the nasopharynx, the gut, and the external sources are continuously being deposited on it. It is exceedingly useful to distinguish between the resident and the transient microflora. The resident flora includes organisms which are found more or less regularly in appreciable numbers on the skin of most normal individuals. These organisms form stable communities on the skin's surface and are not easily dislodged. Pathogenic bacteria are not ordinarily a regular part of this flora; the resident population is able to maintain itself against the constant pressure of competitive organisms which are continuously contaminating the skin's surface.

The number of species comprising the resident flora is surprisingly small considering the chances of potential colonists reaching the skin. Most of the bacterial isolates can be placed in two families, the Micrococcaceae and the Corynebacteriaceae, with a few isolates classified in the Enterobacteriaceae and other families. Among the fungi, Pityrosporum and perhaps Candida species are resident.

The transient flora includes a multiplicity of organisms, but these do not maintain themselves indefinitely on the normal skin. They are more readily removed from the normal skin by scrubbing and by disinfectants, though they are exceedingly difficult to dislodge from diseased skin. Pathogens as well as nonpathogens make up the transient flora, and the list of them is very long. Almost any organism may survive temporarily on the cutaneous surface under appropriate conditions, and a complete roll call of transient organisms would include essentially all the microorganisms found in the environment of man. Species of Candida and Cryptococcus are among the more common fungus transients. Although certain weed molds, such as Aspergillus and Penicillium, can be cultured from the skin's surface, it is doubtful whether these can grow and reproduce on the normal surface, even temporarily.

Sources within and without the body furnish the supply of transient organisms. Organisms from the nasopharynx and the gastrointestinal tract shower the skin repeatedly, particularly in mucocutaneous regions. Obviously, the hands have a great opportunity to acquire transient organisms. Surgeons who are in daily attendance on patients with infected wounds readily acquire a pathogenic transient flora. Nonetheless, transient organisms persist appreciably on the skin only if there is continuous replenishment from some external or internal source, or if the integrity of the skin is disturbed by disease or by injury.

CLASSIFICATION OF ORGANISMS IN NORMAL FLORA

The effect of improved classifications of the organisms present on the skin has been to increase the differences detectable between various regions and between health and disease. It is likely that a greater understanding of the ecologic factors which control the skin flora and prevent colonization by potentially pathogenic species will follow the application of these classifications and eventually lead to changes in therapy.

Micrococcaceae

The gram-positive, catalase-positive cocci are a major part of the microflora of the skin in health and disease. The most widely used system for subdivision of these organisms depends on a few relatively simple biochemical tests and divides the family into two genera, Staphylococcus and Micrococcus, on the basis of the production of acid from glucose under anaerobic conditions (Baird-Parker, 1963, 1965). Each genus is then divided into biochemical types SI to SVI and M1 to M8. Some of the Micrococcus types may truly be staphylococci but the scheme is useful as it stands.

Staphylococcus aureus is classified as SI in this system, based on the characters of coagulase production and anaerobic fermentation of mannitol. This organism is only rarely found in large numbers of the normal skin of adults but frequently contaminates the skin from its headquarters in the nose and perineum. Dermatitic skin is frequently colonized by *S. aureus,* which is the most frequent cause of secondary infection of wounds and also produces the primary infections typical of the species.

The organisms classified as SII and SV can be called *S. epidermidis.* A strain of this group can be isolated from nearly every sample of normal skin. The organisms may be isolated in increased numbers from acne lesions and from areas of dermatitis, as well as from surgical implants and minor skin septic lesions, and must be considered as having some pathogenicity, though less than *S. aureus.* The other biochemical types are less frequently found but note should be taken that SVI strains produce acid from mannitol aerobically but not anaerobically. There is no place for the old name. *S. albus.*

Among the Micrococcus types, M1 and M2 are frequently found in intertriginous areas and M3 is usually dominant on the scalp in normal adults. The coccus, often named *Sarcina lutea,* which forms large yellow colonies, is classified as M7. These organisms are recovered less frequently from dermatitic skin than from normal skin and probably have even lower pathogenicity than *S. epidermidis.*

Aerobic Diphtheroids

There is still need of an adequate classification of this large group of organisms which are particularly prominent in moist intertriginous regions but are also found in samples from all normal skin areas. Several important groups have been established, but even the genera to which isolates should be assigned are at present contentious. An important finding is that many strains on the skin require lipid supplements in artificial media. These lipophilic diphtheroids are very common in the axilla, where they appear to play an important role in the regulation of the flora; a similar role is likely in other intertriginous regions. Various subgroups can be defined.

The strains grouped as *Corynebacterium minutissimum* are characteristically fluorescent on special media; the same porphyrin fluorescence is seen in erythrasma or on normal skin when these organisms are present. They are frequently found, in the absence of symptoms, in the toe webs. The reason why the lesions of erythrasma are produced occasionally by this normal resident is obscure.

Other strains of aerobic diphtheroid have a powerful urease and may be of significance in some cases of diaper rash; they may be recovered from the diaper area and also from the nose in infants. Similar strains are present in the adult axilla. Organisms similar to those of Nocardia are found in association with *C. minutissimum* and lipophilic diphtheroids in the axilla of some subjects. Occasionally, the growth of these organisms may become visible (trichomycosis axillaris). Many other strains can be found in the toe webs but their association with disease is less certain. Pitted keratolysis of the sole may sometimes be due to a coryneform bacterium. *C. diphtheriae* may be a relatively benign secondary colonist of lesions in tropical countries, though severe disease may occur in the non-immune.

Attempts at classification based on a variety of primary criteria have been made but show little agreement, often because the lipophilic nature of many isolates has not been recognized. Others base many subdivisions on the production of acid from carbohydrates, a type of test suscepti-ble to difficulty in this group.

Anaerobic Diphtheroids

Anaerobic diphtheroids may be re-covered from many normal skin sites, but high numbers are also found in areas rich in sebaceous glands. They are almost universally present in lesions of acne vulgaris and have been implicated caus-ally in this disease. It is now possible to divide this group of skin residents into three species—*Corynebacterium acnes, C. granulosum,* and *C. avidum*—on the basis of phage susceptibility, colonial morphol-ogy, and a small number of biochemical tests. Some workers prefer, with some rea-son, to include these species in the genus Propionibacterium, while others continue to place them in Corynebacterium until a definitive classification of the non-sporing, gram-positive rods is available.

C. acnes is the most numerous and most frequent anaerobic diphtheroid on the skin of the scalp and face. *C. granulosum* is found with *C. acnes* in acne lesions, in the nose, and occasionally on the skin. *C. avidum* has been recovered most fre-quently from the axilla. The importance of *C. acnes* and *C. granulosum* in acne is debatable, though anaerobic diphtheroids as a group seem to play a role in the hy-drolysis of lipids.

Gram-Negative Organisms

Some members of the family Entero-bacteriaceae—*Klebsiella, Enterobacter,* and *Proteus*—appear as resident skin or-ganisms in the axilla, toe webs, or nose of some individuals. Another genus of more uncertain classification is Acinetobacter, which includes organisms formerly re-ferred to as Mima and Herellea.

Pseudomonas may colonize the skin under abnormal circumstances but it is rare on normal skin. Treatment with topi-cal or systemic antibacterial agents may encourage colonization of the skin by gram-negative organisms.

Other Bacteria

Some strains of beta-hemolytic strep-tococci appear to be able to colonize the skin before causing lesions of impetigo to appear and before carriage in the nose or throat can be detected. Other streptococci have been found on the skin of children in the absence of disease but these organisms are rare on adult skin. Bacillus and Clos-tridium spores are deposited on the skin but it is doubtful that these organisms are resident. Any organism present in the en-vironment or seeded from the oropharynx or gut may be transiently present.

Fungi

Pityrosporum ovale and *P. orbiculare* are regularly resident on the skin. *P. ovale,* the so-called bottle bacillus, is abundant on the scalp and may also be seen in smears of comedones. Since it is a lipid-dependent yeast, its existence in areas richly supplied with sebaceous glands is explicable. There is no convincing evi-dence that this organism causes dandruff or seborrheic dermatitis. The yeast does become more abundant in these condi-tions but an etiologic relationship has not been proved.

P. orbiculare appears to be a phase of *Malassezia furfur,* the pathogenic agent of tinea versicolor, but it is also found on normal skin. An interesting feature is the possibility of determining the factors which cause this organism to produce dis-ease in a susceptible host, though it ordinarily persists without giving rise to gross evidences of its presence.

Candida parapsilosis and other yeasts may be resident in small numbers.

LOCATION OF SKIN FLORA

The organisms resident on the skin are not distributed at random over its surface and through its thickness. They do not occur in or between the living cells of the epidermis or its appendages but appear in the outer desquamating portion of the stratum corneum only. The microbes are aggregated into microcolonies which can be visualized by electron microscopy. The greatest number are found in the infundi-bulum of the hair follicle, with a few scattered small microcolonies on the general skin surface. The sweat duct is not colonized. Evidence from a variety of technical methods indicates that the deeper layers of the stratum corneum are not invaded by the normal flora but that sebaceous follicles, folds, and creases are often densely colonized. The depth that some infoldings have is quite sufficient to account for the difficulty in killing or removing all organisms from an area of skin, even if the protective effects of sebaceous secretions are discounted.

In disease states, invasion of the stratum corneum by dermatophyte fungi or *C. minutissimum* may permit deeper ingress by normal flora organisms; these organisms may also be included purely by chance in developing lesions such as follicular pustules. Survival of different species may be selective and account, for example, for the preponderance of SII isolates in acne lesions or for the recovery of *C. acnes* from chemically induced pustules. Direct invasion by pathogenic organisms is more properly treated elsewhere, but enzymes, products of metabolism, and other toxins may diffuse across the horny layer and cause changes in the skin without the organism invading any more deeply than the normal flora living space.

Quantitative Aspects

There are great technical difficulties in estimating the quantities of organisms that a given surface of skin supports. Two main approaches have been tried: in one, the microcolonies are enumerated either by pressing a velvet pad or agar surface to the skin or by removing layers of skin with cellophane tape or adhesives; in the other, the organisms are washed from the skin and dispersed in some fluid, often saline or broth, but, more efficiently, in a buffered non-ionic detergent solution. Biopsy followed by homogenization of whole skin, although the most accurate method, is impracticable except in surgical studies or experiments. The contact methods are capable only of sampling the very outermost layer of the skin and perhaps of detecting only easily detached microcolonies. They have the disadvantage that dispersion of microcolonies by treatment leads to a false increase in count. The wash

methods remove more layers of skin and penetrate some of the crevices but removal of all the organisms from deep sites such as the sebaceous follicle is not usually attained. Samples, however, are quite repeatable and useful, since buffering eliminates charge effects and the detergent keeps the organisms dispersed. The counts obtained show a log-normal distribution and differ markedly from region to region. Aerobic counts of 1×10^6 organisms per square centimeter have been found on the scalp, 1.5×10^6 in the apex of the axilla, 4×10^4 on the forehead, and 10^2 to 10^3 on unspecialized skin of the arm or trunk. Counts of anaerobic diphtheroids are of the order of 10^6 on the scalp and forehead but only about 10^4 in the axilla and 10^2 on the skin of the arm or abdomen.

Certain persons may unquestionably be characterized as having consistently high counts, while others show relatively constant low counts. Thus, the average figure for the population as a whole cannot be used to characterize a particular individual. The number of organisms on the hands and forearms may be estimated by the technique of Price, which involves a series of successive one-minute scrubs in 15 wash basins. The number of organisms in each basin yields a curve which reflects the rate of removal of organisms from the surface. Individuals have characteristic Price curves. Thus, not only is each individual typified by the total level of skin bacteria but also the form of the Price curve tends to be individually peculiar. About 90 per cent of the bacteria recovered by this method derive from the hands; the forearms account for the remainder. The range of total bacteria recovered is 2,500,000 to 60,000,000 for different individuals. The total population that can develop on an individual's skin is controlled by ecologic factors which are not yet understood, but it is clear that the skin of some persons supports more organisms than the skin of others.

FORCES WHICH INFLUENCE THE TYPE AND DISTRIBUTION OF MICROORGANISMS ON THE SKIN

The factors which determine the survival and population size of resident bacteria are the same as those considered important in the "self-degerming capacity" of the skin. As has been stated, water is in short supply over much of the skin's area and appears to limit the size of populations, both of resident and nonresident organisms. Moist intertriginous regions have characteristically high aerobic counts, while the areas with marked sebaceous development, such as the face, scalp, and upper trunk, bear large numbers of anaerobic diphtheroids as well. Oily secretions may reduce evaporation of water. If water loss from an area of dry skin, such as the forearm, is prevented by an occlusive plastic film dressing, the bacterial count increases from about 10^3 organisms to 10^7 organisms per square centimeter within two days. Adding water to such a dressing is followed by a further increase in count. Dermatitic skin is more permeable to water than normal skin and, correspondingly, a higher bacterial count is found.

Decreased hydration of the skin's surface during the winter months probably accounts for the slightly lower bacterial counts found at this time. Certain organisms, such as gram-negatives from the gastrointestinal tract, ordinarily do not survive on the skin's surface because they are easily killed by desiccation, but they are able, at least temporarily, to gain a foothold and persist on the skin under conditions of high humidity.

Gram-negative organisms die just about as rapidly in inanimate surfaces, such as glass, as they do on the skin. In other words, the skin has no specific way of destroying these organisms. If the skin's surface is kept wet following the deposition of the bacteria, they fail to die, and may even multiply. *Escherichia coli* may persist for weeks on the skin of individuals who are kept in an artificially humid climate. The presence of serum also prevents rapid dehydration and enables gram-negative organisms to survive.

Other factors clearly are involved in the disappearance of some inoculated bacteria even when the inoculum is protected from desiccation. Pseudomonas organisms forced to compete with a large number of cocci under an occlusive dressing survived better than when made to compete with diphtheroids but less well than when the skin was "degermed" with ethanol. Streptococci disappear even under occlusive dressings.

One possible contributing factor would seem to be the acidity of the skin. Proponents of the "acid mantle" theory note that exposed skin has a pH of between 5 and 6, while intertriginous areas are neutral or even slightly alkaline, and that this corresponds to the presence of few and many bacteria. These theorists hold that it is the acidity which prevents growth of resident organisms and of colonists reaching the skin. Several facts indicate that this attractive hypothesis is largely incorrect. Occlusion of the acidic skin of the forearm is followed by growth of resident organisms and a rise in pH, suggesting that the alkali is microbially produced. Organisms from the skin are no more tolerant of acidity than *Staphylococcus aureus* and streptococci which, nonetheless, do not readily become established among the cutaneous flora.

Antibacterial substances in the surface lipid do seem to play a role. Inocula of *Streptococcus pyogenes*, *Staphylococcus aureus*, and *Candida albicans* die less quickly when the sites are washed with acetone and other lipid solvents than when in the presence of the skin lipid only, even under circumstances which prevent desiccation. *E. coli* and *Pseudomonas aeruginosa* are unaffected. *S. pyogenes* seems particularly susceptible to free fatty acids, which form about one-fifth of the surface lipid. Whether this should be regarded as a skin product or a product of microbial action depends on the viewpoint of the reader. The secretion of sebaceous glands initially contains very little unesterified fatty acid but, during the secretion's delivery to the surfaces, microbial lipases from anaerobic diphtheroids and, to a lesser extent from Pityrosporum, partially hydrolyse the triglyceride, liberating the fatty acids. These chemical antibacterial agents may thus be considered to be mutual products of the human and his flora, and are of value to both.

Other products of the resident flora may also be important in determining the population composition of a region as well as in preventing successful colonization from outside. Several antibiotics have been demonstrated to be produced by coagulase-negative staphylococci, and the production of similar substances has been ascribed to lipophilic diphtheroids. These antibiotics, of varied composition though some are polypeptides, are most active against gram-positive organisms and may limit the growth of resident competitors. Agents inimical to Pseudomonas are suspected of being produced by resident bacteria. In one study, these organisms did not colonize the skin until the normal flora had been eliminated by antibacterial soaps. In another study in which one foot was protected by silicone grease and both feet were immersed in water, colonization was seen only on the unprotected foot. Lixiviation of an inhibitor was suggested.

Even within a species in the normal flora, significant interactions seem to occur. The phenonemon of bacterial interference, in which a resident strain prevents colonization by another strain of the same species by a mechanism that is completely unknown, has been applied clinically in controlling nursery epidemics due to *S. aureus*. A less virulent strain of the species was inoculated onto the umbilicus of the newborn infant at birth, thus reducing the chance of acquisition of the epidemic phage 80/81 strain prevalent in the nursery. Similar inoculations of the nose have been effective in some cases of recurrent furunculosis. A mechanism of this sort may be the method by which the flora of each person retains its individuality over long periods of time.

Exposure to potential colonists has an effect on the flora of the skin. Recovery of transient *S. aureus*, for example, from normal skin is enhanced if a heavily colonized lesion is nearby; these organisms may also be recovered from the normal skin of the attendants of a patient who is thus infected. The more diverse flora found on children's skin may be due in part to great exposure to environmental sources, as well as to the reduced level of free fatty acids. If given increased opportunities in these circumstances, colonization of the skin by rarer members of the normal flora is likely to occur.

In summary, therefore, it may be stated that the primary factor determining the numbers and kinds of organisms found on the skin is the availability of water. Gram-negative organisms are particularly susceptible to desiccation. A second factor is the presence of lipid antibacterial agents, probably fatty acids. Streptococci are inhibited by these agents. A third and probably highly significant factor is the presence of a normal flora resident on the skin which, by ecologic forces, controls its own composition and prevents colonization.

MICROBIOLOGIC PRINCIPLES OF SKIN INFECTIONS

Many diagnostic sins are concealed under the term "skin infection"; there is a need for more strict criteria. It is too often not appreciated that the presence of a pathogenic bacterium in a lesion does not necessarily indicate a bacterial disease. The first problem is to separate clearly primary from secondary infections. The distinction is important; however, the criteria needed to make this distinction are not altogether rigid.

Primary bacterial infections are those which originate in skin that grossly appears to be healthy, usually are incited by a single organism, and have characteristic morphologic features. The etiologic role of the organism as the inciting pathogenic agent is usually very clear in primary infections. Adequate antibacterial therapy usually produces prompt and complete cure. Commonplace examples of such infections are impetigo, ecthyma, and furuncles. In secondary infections, on the other hand, the organisms do not play a prominent role in initiating the disease but may be important in protracting or intensifying it. Secondary infections develop in a variety of preexisting skin disturbances such as cuts, burns, abrasions, contact dermatitis, fungal and viral infections, insect bites, drug eruptions, and so forth.

Any change in the integrity of the skin paves the way for establishment of potentially pathogenic organisms and the possibility of a secondary infection. A variety of different organisms may be implicated and the morphologic features of the lesion are variable, depending on the primary disease. Unlike the more or less characteristic course of primary infections, the course and outcome of secondary infections are unpredictable.

Recognizing a secondary infected lesion is not always easy. Transitions between primary and secondary infections occur; thus, diphtheria of the skin frequently originates in a previous lesion, such as a cut, scratch, or patch of dermatitis, but because the morphologic changes and course of the disease are characteristic and attributable to a single organism, cutaneous diphtheria is regarded as a primary infection. Nonresident organisms regularly contaminate all types of skin lesions; a new and very divergent microflora is characteristic of dermatitic skin. In particular, transient bacteria become established, and of these, pathogenic staphylococci are predominant and constant. Hemolytic streptococci are also common colonists. Since both of these organisms are potential pathogens, the pathologic significance of their presence must be assessed. The mere association of these organisms, even in large quantities, with a skin lesion does not necessarily mean that there is a true secondary infection. The problem is to separate secondary colonization from secondary infection.

By colonization is meant that a potential pathogen is now living on the skin or on the lesion but its presence is causing no reaction in the host. Colonization in this sense is exemplified by the carriage of *S. aureus* in psoriatic lesions. The numbers are not large and destruction of the organism by antibiotics is not associated with clinical improvement. The first level of secondary infection occurs when the numbers of *S. aureus* are larger and treatment ameliorates the apparent severity of the underlying disease. In this form, toxins from the organisms penetrate the skin, eliciting the inflammatory response or even causing cell death in the epidermis; however, a leukocytic exudate is not present. An example of this type of toxic secondary infection may be seen in chronic eczema, especially atopic dermatitis in children. Occlusive therapy of psoriasis and other diseases may transform colonization by *S. aureus* into toxic secondary infection or into more severe forms. Recognition of this degree of infection is difficult. The responses of the host are the manifestations of disease; if

nothing happens to the host there is no disease. Immunologic responses may reveal the presence of true infection, but in the case of streptococcal disease the response to skin infections is not always as distinct as is that to pharyngeal infection. Colonization of varicose ulcers and other exudative lesions may lead to large numbers of potential pathogens but there is little evidence that these cause any damage to the host.

A smear made by swabbing the lesion may be helpful in determining whether or not secondary infection is actually present, since the finding of polymorphonuclear leukocytes yields direct evidence that the defenses of the host have swung into operation. These cells are quickly mobilized in response to injury created by the invading pathogenic streptococci and staphylococci. Leukocytes are usually absent in lesions in which the pathogenic organisms are simply colonists. At the same time, the smear technique demonstrates the kinds and relative abundance of the bacteria present. Streptococci and staphylococci are easily visualized, although, of course, specific recognition of species is impossible. The presence of appreciable numbers of bacteria in combination with a recognizable leukocyte response is strongly indicative of secondary infection. While phagocytes are not uniquely an expression of bacterial infection, and many nonbacterial stresses will elicit polymorphonuclear leukocytes, the absence of bacteria in smears from such lesions makes it clear that their origin is nonbacterial.

The presence of leukocytes which are actively engulfing bacteria is further evidence of secondary infection, though the significance of this test is certainly not absolute, and the findings must be correlated with the clinical data. In particular, the value of this test in the case of infections with gram-negative organisms will require further evaluation, for leukocytes may not be strongly mobilized even when it seems certain that a secondary infection exists. It is clear, however, that the smear technique is often more informative than cultures, since it not only reveals the presence of bacteria but also indicates whether the tissue is reacting. The fact that pathogenic staphylococci and streptococci are almost universally present in exudative, inflammatory lesions of the skin greatly reduces the value of culture alone for the diagnosis of secondary infection.

STERILIZATION OF SKIN BY ARTIFICIAL MEANS

It is impossible to sterilize the skin completely. Part of the flora is inaccessible from the surface because of its deep position within follicles and skin folds.

The bacterial population may be reduced either by mechanical removal, such as scrubbing, or by chemical disinfection. It is easy to be misled when the bacterial population is sampled following treatment with some antiseptic agent. Even if few or no organisms are recovered, this does not mean that they have been destroyed. It may signify only that the bacteria are adhering firmly and cannot be removed easily, or that the chemical antiseptic, for example, mercurial compounds, may simply have formed a relatively sterile coagulum on the surface, under which bacteria may be found in abundance. When the hands are washed in certain of the quaternary ammonium antibacterial agents, subsequent bacterial counts of the treated areas are very low. However, if after this treatment the surface is washed with soap, large numbers of organisms will be released into the wash water, indicating that they were simply being held on the surface. Quaternary salts do not form a protective film under which the bacteria take haven; they change the electric charge of the surface so that the bacteria are strongly attracted. The keratinized scales of the stratum corneum normally have a negative charge and will migrate to the anode in an electrophoretic chamber. Bacteria are also negatively charged; consequently, there is normally an electrostatic repulsion between the skin's surface and its bacteria. Certain quaternary ammonium salts reverse the charge to positive and set up an electric attraction for the negatively charged bacteria. Strong alkalies, such as soap, will reverse the charge to negative again, and release the bacteria.

A reduction of the bacterial flora may be needed only for a short time, during venipuncture for example, to reduce the chances of implanting an organism into deeper tissues or of contaminating the sample, as when blood cultures are being undertaken. Ethanol at 70 per cent concentration is very effective, and its protein-precipitating action makes dispersal of microcolonies unlikely. The antibacterial action ends with evaporation of the alcohol. Longer periods of activity are needed for a response on the hands of a surgeon and for prophylaxis against infection of mild trauma. A variety of preparations are available. A lack of selectivity is advantageous for the surgeon who must reapply the formulation daily for many years. Iodine has been promoted for this purpose but some of the more persistent agents, such as hexachlorophene or chlorhexidine, are widely accepted. These and similar preparations are often used in a way which favors cumulative effects. It can be shown that the reduction from repeated use of these preparations may enhance the effect of alcohol degerming in reducing the skin carriage of microorganisms.

Ecologic effects of antibiotic or chemotherapeutic agents used to treat skin infections or merely to reduce bacterial numbers have become more prominent since awareness of this possibility became common. Topical treatment of a secondary skin infection prolonged after the destruction of the inciting organism may be followed by colonization and infection by a resistant pathogen. Tinea pedis may thus be transformed into Pseudomonas intertrigo; hidradenitis suppurativa infected with S. aureus may become intractable when these organisms are replaced by Proteus; acne vulgaris may have additionally acquired gram-negative folliculitis as a result of treatment. The use of antibacterial agents as deodorants or "sanitizers" may also be a cause of ecologically mediated infections, although the agents used tend to be partially effective only; thus, disaster is frequently avoided. The history of the treatment of severe burns is an example of how first overcoming one potential pathogen, S. aureus, made necessary the avoidance of a second pathogen, Pseudomonas, which has led to current problems with Candida albicans.

The problem of the patient whose immune system has been compromised emphasizes the difficulties of keeping the skin free of any potential pathogen since, in this circumstance, species normally resident may become dangerously pathogenic. Over use of antibacterial agents may then increase the chances of infection.

REFERENCES

Baird-Parker, A. C.: A classification of micrococci and staphylococci based on physiological and biochemical tests. J. Gen. Microbiol. *30*:409, 1963.

Baird-Parker, A. C.: The classification of staphylococci and micrococci from worldwide sources. J. Gen. Microbiol. *38*:363, 1965.

Leyden, J. J., and Marples, R. R.: Ecologic principles and antibiotic therapy in chronic dermatoses. Arch. Dermatol. *107*:206, 1973.

Lowbury, E. J. L., and Lilly, H. A.: Use of a 4% chlorhexidine detergent solution (Hibiscrub) and other methods of skin disinfection. Br. Med. J. *1*:510, 1973.

Maibach, H. I., and Hildick Smith, G.: Skin Bacteria and Their Role in Infection. New York, McGraw-Hill Book Co., 1965.

Maibach, H. I., Marples, R. R., and Taplin, D.: Cutaneous bacteriology. *In* Rook, A., (ed.): Recent Advances in Dermatology. Edinburgh, Churchill Livingstone, 1973, pp. 1–32.

Marples, M. J.: The Ecology of the Human Skin. Springfield, Illinois, Charles C Thomas, 1965.

Marples, R. R., and Williamson, P.: Effects of systemic demethylchlortetracycline on human cutaneous microflora. Appl. Microbiol. *18*:228,

Marples, R. R., Downing, D. T., and Kligman, A. M.: Control of free fatty acids in surface lipids by *Corynebacterium acnes*. J. Invest. Dermatol. *56*: 127, 1971.

Marples, R. R., Heaton, C. L., and Kligman, A. M.: *Staphylococcus aureus* in psoriasis. Arch. Dermatol. *107*:568, 1973.

Noble, W. C. (ed.): Microbial skin disease. Br. J. Dermatol. 86 (Supplement 8): 1972.

Rook, A., and Champion, R. H., (eds.): Bacteriology of skin. Br. J. Dermatol. *81*[Supplement 1]:1, 1969.

Section II

BACTERIAL INFECTIONS OF THE SKIN

Howard I. Maibach and *Peter Hacker*

Cutaneous bacterial infections may be divided into primary and secondary types, and this distinction is useful clinically. *Primary infections* tend to have a characteristic morphology and course, are incited initially by a single organism, and arise in normal skin. *Secondary infections* originate in diseased skin as a superimposed condition, and this results in an acute or chronic intermingling of the underlying skin disease and the infection, which may not follow a characteristic course, and in which the role that bacteria are playing may be difficult to assess. Primary infections are most frequently incited by coagulase-positive micrococci or beta-hemolytic streptococci. These are also the most common invaders in secondary infections, but gram-negative organisms (Proteus, Pseudomonas, *E. coli*) often colonize dermatitic skin, though they do not frequently produce true secondary infection except in special locations such as the external ear, or in certain types of chronic lesions, particularly ulcers. In addition to the types of infection which in most instances are confined to the skin and subcutaneous tissues, there are many systemic bacterial infections for which the skin serves as a portal of entry, usually at some site where the defense of the skin has been breached.

SKIN INFECTIONS

The following classification of the primary skin infections is an attempt to integrate into an organized scheme the numerous clinical entities which pathogenic staphylococci (micrococci) and streptococci excite. It has been devised for practical purposes. Shortcomings and even fallacies are inevitable, for much is yet to be learned about these diseases. In the case of some of the rarer skin infections which have been described under a variety of complex names, knowledge is so meager as to cause hesitation in assigning them a definite place in this group.

CLASSIFICATION OF PRIMARY SKIN INFECTIONS

Impetigo

Impetigo and its annular and circinate variants (mostly due to coagulase-positive micrococci and less often to beta-hemolytic streptococci).

Folliculitis (usually due to coagulase-positive micrococci)

1. SUPERFICIAL FOLLICULITIS.
   a. *Staphylococcal* (Impetigo Bockhart).
   b. *Gram-Negative Folliculitis*
   c. *Corynebacterium acnes Scalp Infection*
   d. *Acne necrotica miliaris.*
2. DEEP FOLLICULITIS.
   a. *Sycosis barbae.*
      (1) Lupoid sycosis. A deep variant of sycosis barbae.

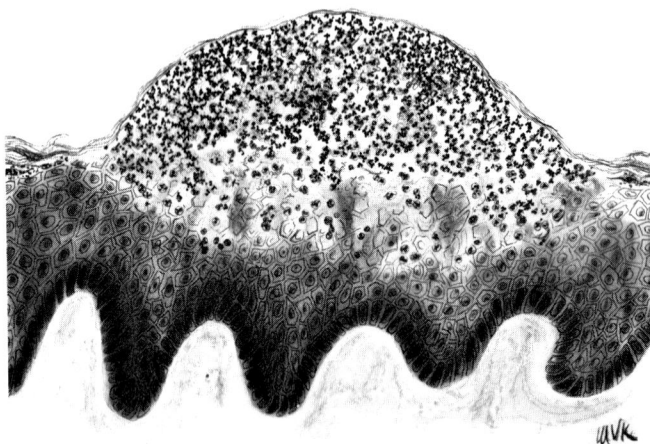

IMPETIGO

Figure 11–1 Schematic representation of the two most common superficial bacterial infections of the skin. The pustule in impetigo starts in a subcorneal location and may enlarge to erode the epidermis. Gram-positive cocci are easily demonstrated in the pus.

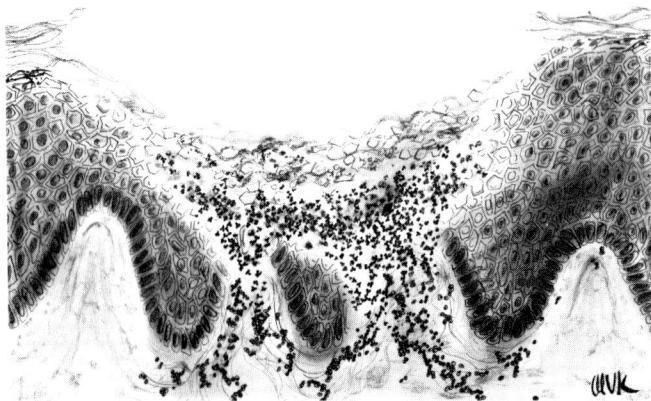

ECTHYMA

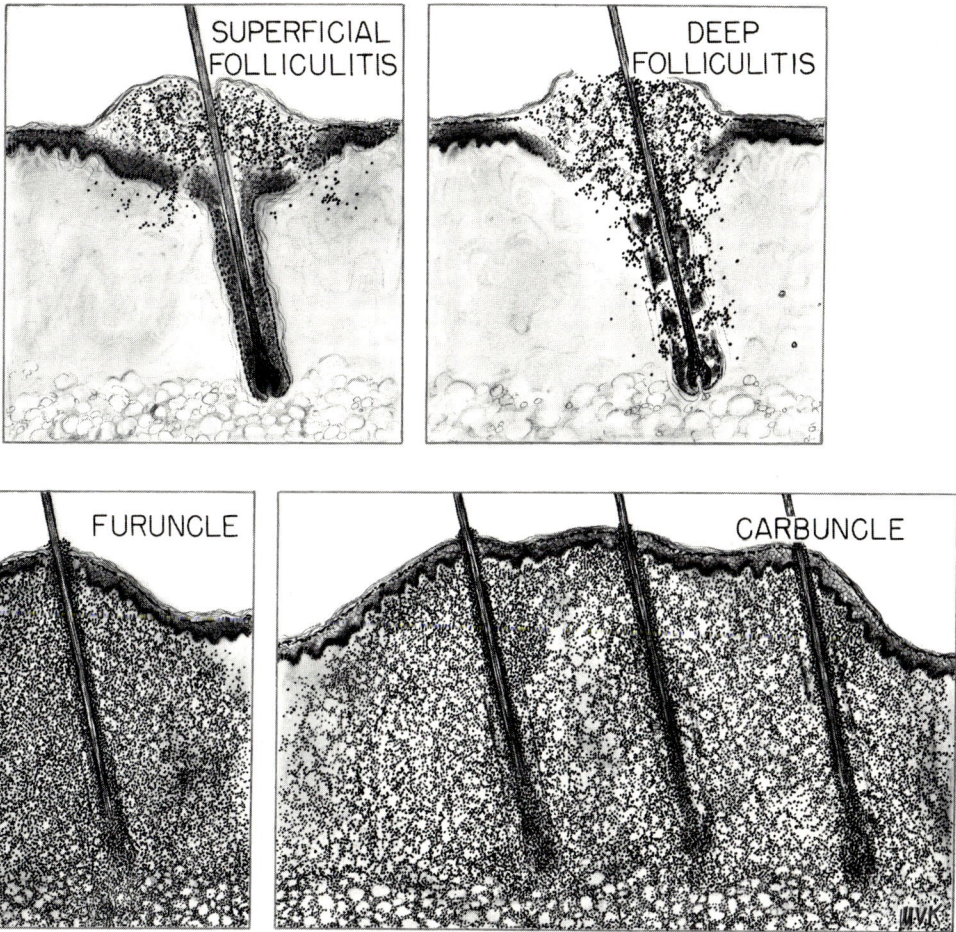

Figure 11–2 Schematic representation of various types of follicular bacterial infections. The organism is usually demonstrated by Gram staining smears of pus.

b. *Perforating Folliculitis of Nose.*
c. *Stye* (hordeolum).
d. *Furuncles* and *Carbuncles.*
3. OTHER FOLLICULITIS SYNDROMES.
a. *Acne varioliformis*
b. *Pyoderma faciale*
c. *Folliculitis decalvans*

Ecthyma

Paronychia

Cellulitis including erysipelas (with the potential sequel of various types of elephantiasis nostras)

Infections of Eccrine Gland Apparatus (Multiple Sweat Gland Abscesses)

Pitted Keratolysis
Botryomycosis
Erythrasma
Trichomycosis Axillaris
Toxic Epidermal Necrolysis (See Chap. 17)

PRINCIPLES OF TREATMENT OF BACTERIAL INFECTIONS

Since certain general principles apply in the management of all types of bacterial infections of the skin, these may conveniently be summarized at the outset. It is important to take advantage of every measure to make the skin as inhospitable as possible to pathogenic bacteria. Cleansing and degerming the skin by simple methods are fully as important as specific antibacterial medication. Soap and water and compresses of bland character are often of great assistance, and a soap substitute containing hexachlorophene may be useful. With measures such as this, many superficial primary infections of the skin may be overcome within a week unless there is some complicating factor. In most instances, the removal of bacteria-laden crusts and debris is a paramount requirement; antibiotic therapy is not an adequate substitute for cleanliness. Bland compresses are exceedingly useful for this purpose. The traditional medicaments in compresses — boric acid, potassium permanganate, aluminum acetate — have feeble antibacterial effects. Saline solutions are, for the most part, just as effective. Certain antibiotics, particularly neomycin (1 gm. per liter), may, in unusually resistant infection, be incorporated into solutions for compressing. The suppressive effect on bacteria may be greater than with ointment vehicles, provided the antibiotic used is stable in aqueous solution. There is little or no place for ammoniated mercury as an antibacterial agent in modern therapy.

Treatment is greatly facilitated by proper diagnosis. The more common bacterial infections, such as impetigo and cellulitis, are often readily diagnosed on morphologic grounds. Atypical lesions require laboratory confirmation. The simplest and most helpful technique is the direct microscopic examination of exudate fluid or pus. Any undiagnosed pustule, vesicle, or bulla should have its contents smeared on a slide and Gram stained. If organisms are demonstrated from an intact lesion, this constitutes convincing evidence of infection (rather than colonization). Specific examples include staphylococci in bullous impetigo, and *Corynebacterium acnes* in atypical acne pustules (such as on the scalp). Several difficult diagnostic problems, such as chronic gonococcemia and meningococcemia, may be clarified with this technique.

Bacterial culture and sensitivity are only occasionally needed in skin infection. *Culture does not replace but supplements direct microscopy.* By the time the culture and sensitivity results are available, the patient generally is near recovery. Systemic infections, resistant organisms, and inadequate blood levels present therapeutic challenge. In most dermatologic infections it is possible to present high enough concentrations of the antibacterial agent to the organism so that the infection will rapidly respond, even though the sensitivity tests reveal resistance.

Drying the Surface

Dehydration has a deleterious effect on most microorganisms; a dry horny layer will afford a more stable mechanical barrier and decrease the number of organisms on the surface. This is also best accomplished by soaks and compresses. The most important aspect of compresses and soaks is the way they are done and, to a lesser degree, the kind of agent used. While some of the commonly used agents have a chemical antibacterial action, the water itself is generally the active agent.

Specific Topical Agents

It may be generally stated that sensitivity studies are not needed for the first line treatment of uncomplicated cutaneous infections. Because of the great concentration of antimicrobial agents achieved by topical application, such therapy is usually effective. If the progress of treatment is below expectation, culture and sensitivity studies are needed.

The hydroxyquinolines exert broad antibacterial, antifungal, and anticandidal action; since they are used as an alternate to the usual topical antibiotics, they are listed here. They may be less effective than some topical antibiotics but will be sufficient in the treatment of many skin infections. As with several of the other agents, they may cause contact sensitization. The most frequently used member of this group is iodochlorhydroxyquinoline (Vioform).

Penicillin ointment is rarely used in this country, since it has been judged a potent sensitizer. Tetracycline and its derivatives (that is, tetracycline cream, U.S.P.) are a useful topical antibiotic with a low incidence of sensitization. Our clinical impression suggests that debridement is not as necessary with the tetracycline as with the neomycin group.

Neomycin is frequently used in combination with bacitracin and polysporin. Its efficacy must be weighed against its rising incidence of sensitization. This sensitization manifests gradually and is easily missed by the physician unless he constantly considers it and conducts patch tests with the appropriate material (20 per cent neomycin).

Gentamicin is similar in action and sensitizing properties to neomycin; patch testing reveals cross-sensitization with the former.

Erythromycin cream is an effective agent and demonstrates no significant sensitization potential to date.

Bacitracin is effective against gram-positive cocci, and polymyxin B against gram-negative organisms, including *Pseudomonas aeruginosa*. Some of the antibiotics are commercially available in combination form (for example, neosporin), though controlled evidence for the increased efficacy of such combinations is not clear. Among antifungal antibiotics the useful anticandidal topical action of the polyene antibiotics, nystatin and amphotericin B, should be mentioned.

Systemic Versus Topical Antibiotics

When should systemic antibiotics be used for cutaneous infections? A hard and fast rule cannot be made, but a few principles may be cited: systemic signs (that is, fever, malaise) accompanying a cutaneous infection are a definite indication for systemic therapy, a useful and often necessary adjunct. Impetigo is discussed below. Widespread infection is often more easily treated systemically than topically. The likelihood of poor patient cooperation in using topical preparations suggests the practicality of parenteral therapy. Systemic therapy is also suggested in the control of disease in epidemics. Children are often more easily treated systemically than topically.

Systemic Antibiotics

Most cutaneous infections of staphylococcal origin are amenable to erythromycin or tetracycline in conventional dosage. The semisynthetic penicillins are the choice for resistant staphylococci, and penicillin G should be given for streptococcal infections or when specific entities such as anthrax are suspected.

Duration of Therapy

There is no general rule, but as a guide the following may be stated: recrudescence of skin infections is often related to inadequate durations of therapy. Minor cutaneous bacterial infections should be treated topically until clinical response, plus at least three days. More serious infections should be treated systemically until they respond, after which the dosage is halved for another week or so. Topical therapy here should be given at least one more week after systemic agents are discontinued. Infections involving the hair follicles are more resistant to therapy and topical treatment should be continued at least two weeks after clinical response.

The Impetigo Family

Impetigo (Contagiosa)

This disease is caused by coagulase-positive micrococci and by beta-hemolytic streptococci; both organisms may be present. The clinical distinction between impetigo caused by each of these two organisms has been stressed by some observers but is not firmly established. Pathogenic staphylococci predominate in the rarely observed, very early lesions, before serous exudation begins. When the organisms are found in combination, the streptococcus may represent a subsequent invader. A primary streptococcal etiology may be suspected if the erythema at the base of new pustules is intense, but this is not invariable. Lesions present for weeks which tend to be indolent in nature and for which the patient has not sought therapy may be primarily streptococcal at this late stage. This is especially common in groups receiving minimal medical care.

The disease is most common in children. It often affects persons in excellent health, but conditions of ill health, especially if accompanied by anemia and malnutrition, predispose. Tropical climates, poor hygiene, uncleanliness, and circumstances resulting in lowering of standards of sanitation, such as might occur in war time, in concentration camps, and with other crises, increase the opportunity of infection. Epidemics occur under such circumstances, particularly when there is close contact. Impetigo may complicate pediculosis, scabies, chickenpox, eczematous eruptions, and other skin lesions.

As the qualifying term "contagiosa" indicates, impetigo has long been considered to be highly infectious. This is true mainly in infants; the disease is *not* particularly contagious among older children and adults. Efforts to transmit the disease experimentally with infectious material or with organisms isolated from this material have often failed, even under conditions of coincident trauma to the skin. However, recently Singh and Kligman reproduced an impetigo-like lesion by long-term occlusion. The pustule is sterile; therefore, its relationship to the clinical lesion is not clear. The combination of predisposing circumstances which lower resistance to this infection is unknown. The disease is uncommon in meticulous persons who are in good health and who have no preexistent skin disease.

Impetigo begins as a small, reddish macule which soon becomes a vesicle. This is situated just under the stratum corneum and consequently has a thin roof that ruptures readily, presenting a weeping denuded spot. This may occur before the lesion becomes pustular. The serous and purulent fluid dries to form a crust which may become quite thick and which has a stuck-on appearance. This crust is the hallmark of impetigo. If the crust is not removed promptly, the process extends beneath the stratum corneum, with further thickening of the honey-colored scab which, upon removal, reveals a slight erosion. New satellite lesions usually appear in the vicinity, and there may be coalescence. The size of an individual lesion rarely exceeds 1 to 2 cm. The face is the usual location, especially about the mouth and nose, but the hands and other exposed areas are frequently involved. However, the lesions may appear anywhere, and in extensive cases (sometimes referred to as *impetiginous dermatitis*) there may be numerous, large, thickly crusted, dirty lesions over the extremities and trunk. In severe, neglected cases there may be vegetative changes and deeper extension to produce ulcerative lesions. The simple, uncomplicated lesions do not produce any atrophy or scarring.

The process sometimes extends peripherally, with central healing, eventuating in annular, circinate, or gyrate patterns. These are morphologic variants of impetigo but are not pathologically distinct. Untreated, impetigo contagiosa may last for many weeks, with continuous development of new lesions. In children there are often blisters. The developing vesicles do not rupture but enlarge to form bullae, often with great rapidity. The flaccid lesions first contain a clear fluid which later becomes cloudy. The roof of the bulla often seems to collapse rather than rupture, collecting the serous contents into folds. Eventually, the roof desiccates to form a thin crust. Group II coagulase-positive staphylococci practically always incite this variety of the disease, which is more common in infants. "Pemphigus" neonatorum is an archaic misnomer; it is an extensive form of infantile bullous impetigo. It occurs in the postnatal period and is now rarely seen, but prior to the antibiotic era, it was one of the most feared of all infantile infections. Contagious spread throughout the population of a nursery sometimes occurred, and new infections of infants might be noted even after the nursery had been vacated and thoroughly cleaned.

TREATMENT. Adequate treatment terminates impetigo promptly. *Sparkling cleanliness and removal of crusts* are essential. Gentle washing with soap must be repeated frequently (two to three times daily) to prevent reaccumulation of the crust. If the crusts are firmly adherent, warm soaks or compresses may be necessary; physiologic saline or *dilute* soap solutions are useful for this. Topical antibiotics should then be *rubbed in thoroughly* at least three times daily. It is advisable to continue treatment for several days after new lesions have ceased to appear, because the normal bacteria do not reestablish themselves quickly, and pathogenic strains may remain for some time. Impetigo involving folds of skin, for example, the external ears, is particularly prone to recurrence and the development of a chronic infection. In widespread cases attended by systemic reactions—fever, malaise, lymph-

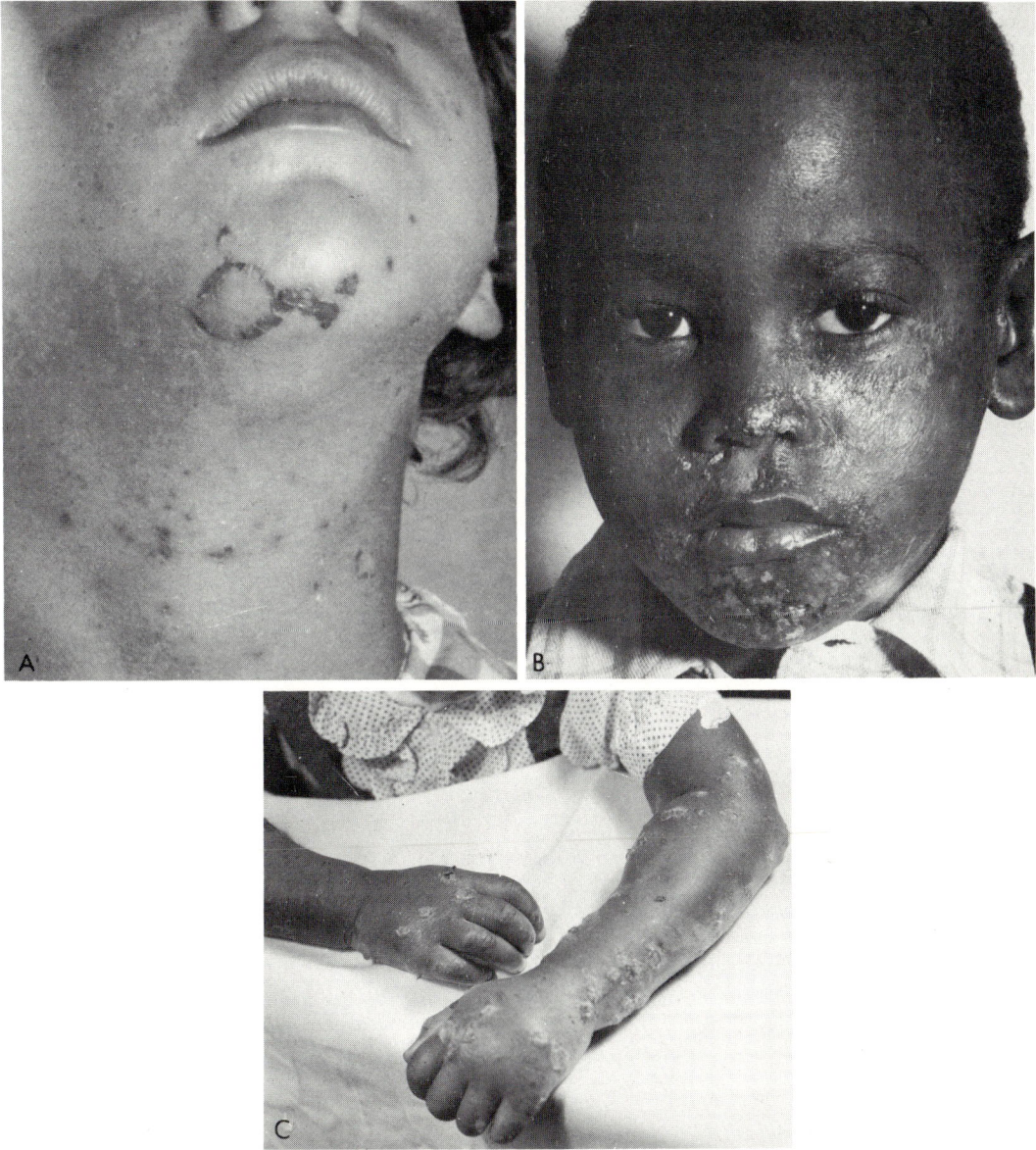

Figure 11–3 Types of impetiginous lesions. *A*, Characteristic primary uncomplicated infection. *B*, Neglected diffuse impetigo. *C*, As complication of papular urticaria. These black and white photographs do not demonstrate the honey-colored crusts that are the hallmark of the disease.

angitis, and so forth—parenteral antibiotic therapy is indicated.

Glomerulonephritis is a feared complication of impetigo. It is emphasized that clinical glomerulonephritis secondary to impetigo is uncommon, except for certain epidemics due to nephritogenic strains of streptococci. Microscopic hematuria probably occurs with a greater frequency but is usually not related to subsequent clinical renal disease. The glomerulonephritis epidemics occur mainly with neglected pyoderma-like lesions in which streptococci become a major pathogen rather than in the classic acute impetigo. Systemic antibiotics appear no more capable of preventing the renal lesion in this disease than they do in the streptococcal pharyngitis leading to the first manifestation of rheumatic fever.

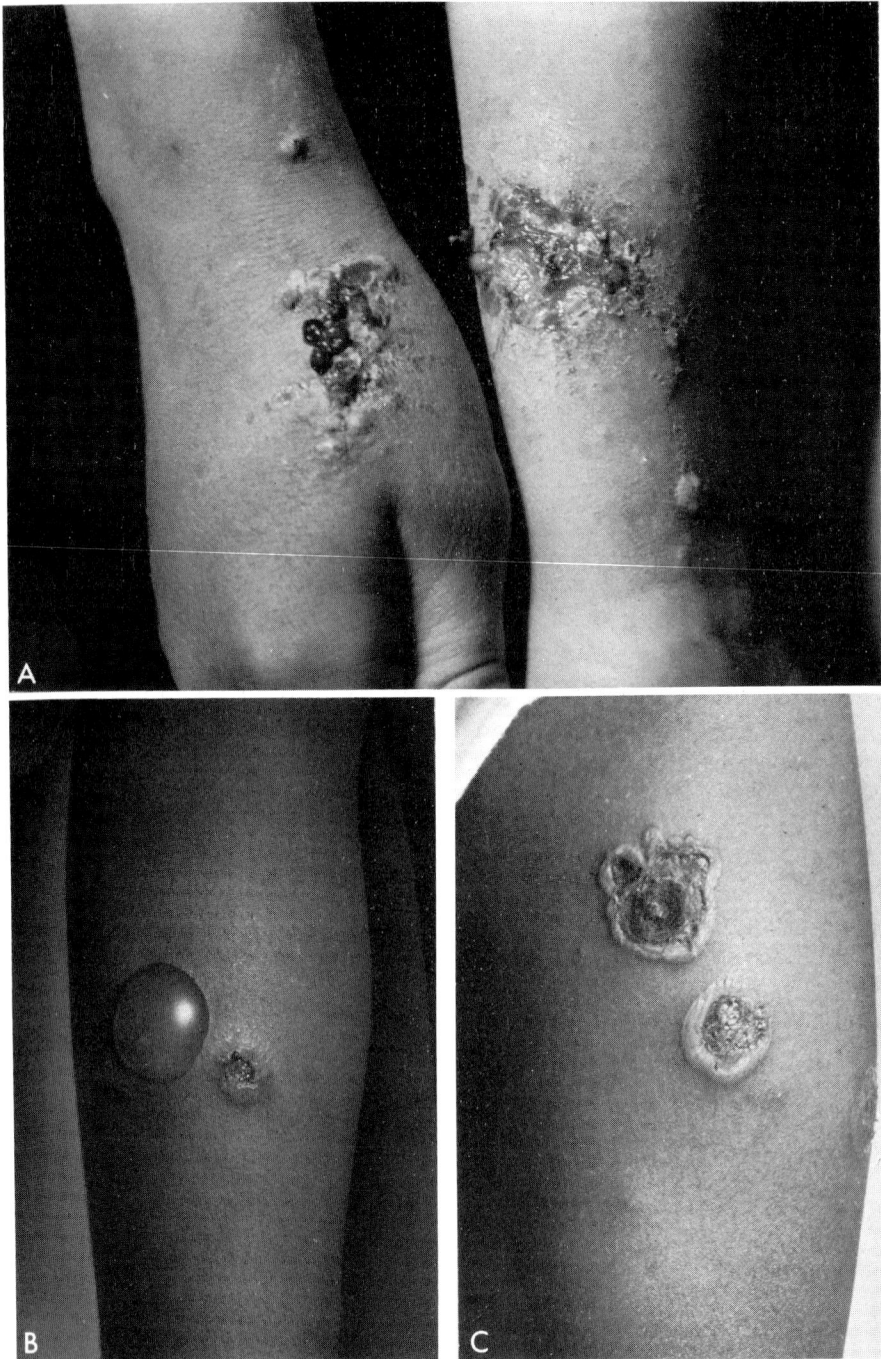

Figure 11–4 *A,* Impetiginous secondary infection in Rhus contact dermatitis. *B,* Early bullous lesion of impetigo. The contents may be serous rather than purulent initially. *C,* Evolution and extensions of bullous impetigo.

Ordinarily bullous impetigo is treated in the same way as impetigo contagiosa. Cleanliness is paramount in preventing and treating the disease. In the early stages, removal of the roofs of the bullae may be an advantageous procedure. In patients with extensive involvement or with bullous impetigo of the newborn, systemic antibiotic therapy is indicated.

Chancriform Pyoderma (Pyoderma Chancriforme Faciei)

This unusual condition represents a clinical entity in which a button-shaped, superficial ulcer appears, closely resembling a syphilitic chancre (Branom et al., 1963; Frain-Bell, 1957; Layman et al., 1954). The lesion is usually on the face, but some genital lesions were reported. The most frequent location is near the eyes. It starts as a papulopustule which then enlarges and becomes chancriform, measuring about 1 to 4 cm. in diameter. It usually involutes in four to eight weeks, leaving a scar. Regional lymphadenopathy is the rule.

Darkfield examination and serologic tests for syphilis are negative. The only consistent positive finding is the isolation of Staphylococcus, usually *S. aureus.*

The lesion responds to the administration of systemic and topical antibiotics.

The most important feature of this condition is the diagnostic difficulty it may cause. Syphilitic chancre, vaccinia, basal and squamous cell carcinoma, chancroid, cutaneous diphtheria, tularemia, impetigo, milker's nodule, primary tuberculosis of the skin, and swimming pool granuloma are part of the differential diagnoses.

Staphylococcal Scarlatina

A scarlet fever–like illness may be caused by certain strains of *Staphylococcus pyogenes.* Toxicity, a bright erythema, and profound desquamation occur in these patients. The illness may be severe. The disease is caused by the erythrogenic toxin possessed by the infecting staphylococcal strains. It may be antigenically different from the streptococcal erythrogenic toxin. Treatment consists of appropriate systemic antibiotics.

Folliculitis

Folliculitis is a pyoderma which originates within the hair follicle. Superficial and deep forms are the chief subdivisions. It is ordinarily initiated by coagulase-positive staphylococci. Under unusual circumstances, however, when the host resistance is impaired, other organisms, such as coliform gram negatives, and possibly even the normal skin micrococci, may be causative.

Superficial Folliculitis

STAPHYLOCOCCAL (IMPETIGO BOCKHART). This disease is essentially a form of impetigo characterized by a small dome-shaped pustule situated at the mouth of the hair follicle. Hair growth is not impaired. The scalp and extremities are favorite sites, the former more often in children. It may be secondary to discharges from wounds, abscesses, and draining lesions. Maceration and lack of cleanliness are promoting factors. A similar condition is occasionally caused by occupational exposure to certain chemicals, notably cutting oils and solvents, but the pustules are largely sterile. Plastic occlusive therapy for other diseases allows significant bacterial multiplication and may lead to folliculitis. Tar therapy on hairy surfaces has a similar effect. The pustules rupture with the formation of a small crust. A possible complication, if treatment is not initiated promptly, is extension of the infection deeper into the hair follicle. In the bearded region or scalp, especially, a chronic infection may result.

Treatment. Soap and water cleansing and local application of topical antibiotics are effective measures. Antibacterial soaps may be of value. Systemic antibiotics are often indicated, especially when the scalp is involved. In treating recurrences, the duration of antibiotic therapy should be increased.

GRAM-NEGATIVE FOLLICULITIS (Fulton et al., 1968). Gram-negative folliculitis mainly occurs as a superinfection in acne vulgaris patients receiving long-term systemic antibiotic therapy. These pustules

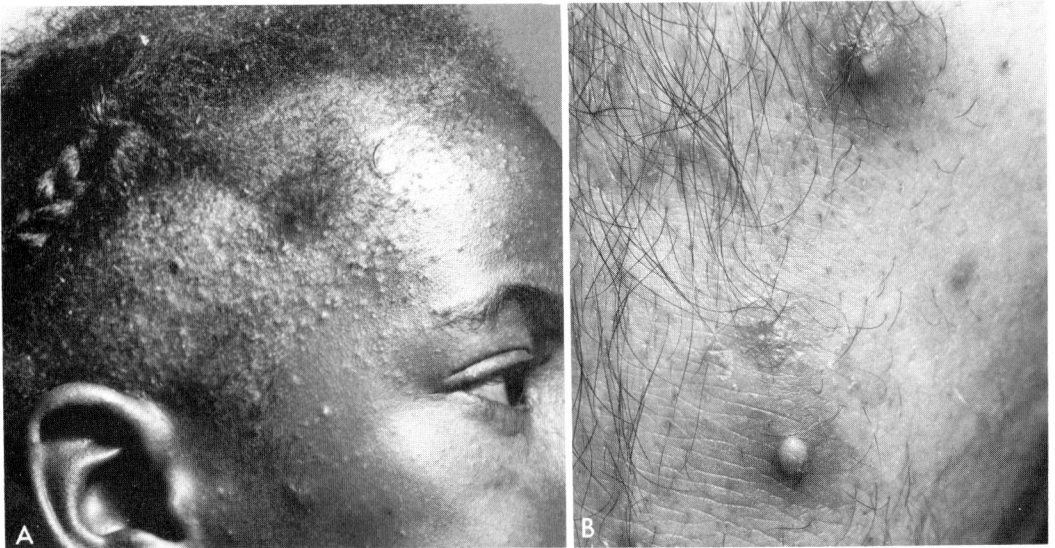

Figure 11–5 *A*, Bacterial folliculitis, becoming chronic. *B*, Admixture of follicular impetigo and furuncle—a common combination.

contain no keratinous plugs and are often concentrated around the nose. The organism is found in the nostril and the pustule. Gram stain of pus usually reveals no gram-negative rods; cultures on appropriate media reveal luxuriant growth of the organism. Therapy is under study at present. A second form of the disease consists of deep nodular cysts, often on the neck. Both forms are often misdiagnosed as an acne flora; a high index of suspicion is helpful for rapid diagnosis.

CORYNEBACTERIUM ACNES SCALP INFECTION (Maibach, 1967). This syndrome has probably been described under numerous names in the literature. The size of the primary lesion is from a pinhead to 3 mm. and it is a dome to flat, white to yellow, follicular pustule. The occiput is more involved than the remainder of the scalp. Scalp erythema is often noted. Men are involved many times more frequently than women. The process may start in the usual acne age; yet most cases seen by the dermatologist will be well past this age. The natural history requires further documentation; many of the patients have been symptomatic into their early fifties. The face may also be involved, especially in the younger patient. Its correct place in the hierachy of acne is not known.

Routine culture is confusing because the causative organism is a fastidious anaerobe.

When the diagnosis is suspected, the pus should be Gram stained. Numerous gram-positive pleomorphic rods are noted. Culture may be performed utilizing nutrient broth, adding dextrose, and using appropriate anaerobiasis. This is only needed when the patient does not respond to therapy as expected.

Tetracycline given orally will abort pustule development. This therapy must be considered in terms of years rather than weeks. The dose is 1 gm. daily; this is tapered to the minimum that will maintain control (generally 0.5 gm.). When this is ineffective, anaerobic sensitivity studies should be performed.

ACNE NECROTICA MILIARIS. This is a rare chronic and recurrent form of folliculitis of the scalp occurring principally in adults. The pustules are tiny, superficial, few in number, and rupture easily, with the formation of a shallow crust. Itching is usually present, and scratching destroys the tiny pustules promptly. The follicular location of the crust and the rapid, though often temporary, response to antibacterial measures is characteristic of the disease. Acne varioliformis is probably a deep variant of this same disease, with which it may coexist. The etiology of these conditions is not known. *C. acnes* scalp infection does not have a necrotic component, yet the two conditions may be similar. In other words, the classic descriptions of acne necrotica were published in the pre-antibiotic era. With antibiotics, the lesions may not develop the necrotic component and thus be identical to *C. acnes* scalp infection.

Deep Folliculitis

Infection extends deeply into the follicle in these instances, and the resultant perifolliculitis is responsible for a more marked inflammatory response than is seen in superficial folliculitis. Single lesions are common and usually trivial. In some instances the folliculitis takes on special characteristics based upon regional location and gives rise to distinct clinical entities.

SYCOSIS BARBAE (BARBER'S ITCH). Sycosis barbae is similar to bacterial folliculitis elsewhere. The primary lesion is a follicular pustule, pierced by a hair. It was commoner when more men wore mustaches or beards and during the pre-antibiotic era. Neglect leads to impetig-

inization and crust formation. Vegetative almost granulomatous reactions are not unknown, especially in the mustache area. If neglected the condition may be fairly persistent and become chronic in that sense. The hair usually does not fall out, nor is its growth retarded. Bearded men may be more prone to attack, a circumstance in marked contrast to pseudofolliculitis of the beard, improperly called sycosis barbae (see Chap. 37), which occurs exclusively in those who shave. Bland compresses, the local application of antibiotics, and administration of them parenterally, usually produce remission of acute pustular sycosis barbae promptly, provided that it is recognized and treated early in its course.

Tinea barbae, or ringworm of the beard, is almost the only condition which might cause diagnostic confusion, but in that infection, the hairs are characteristically loosened or broken off. Moreover, fungal infections of the bearded region are apt to be highly inflammatory, producing nodular suppurating swellings, not discrete

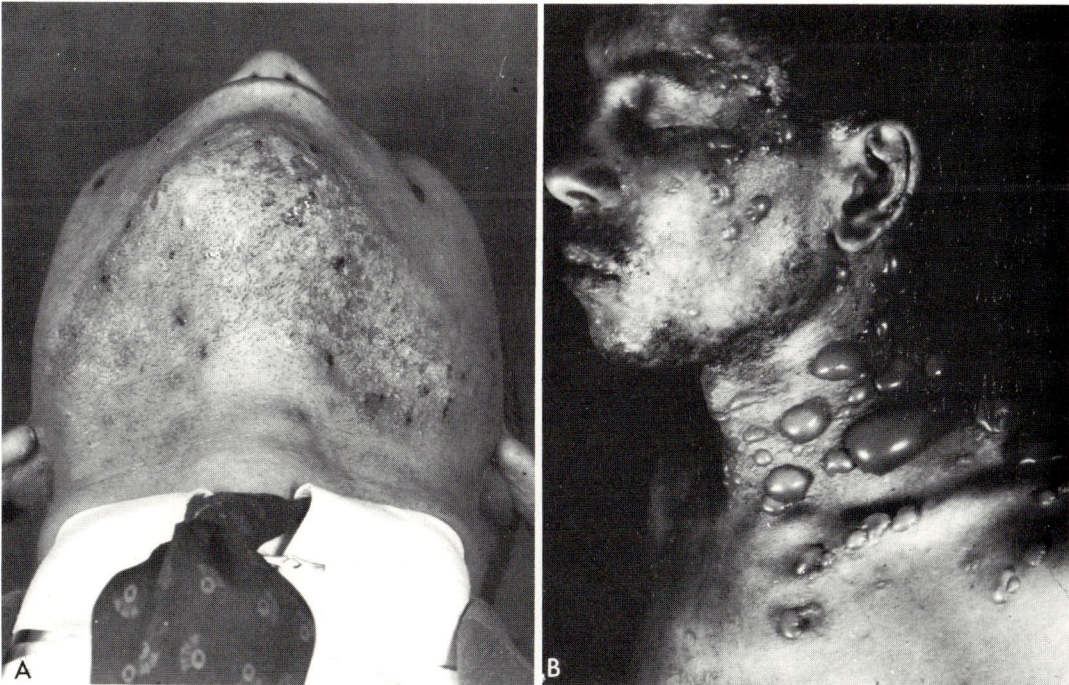

Figure 11–6 *A*, Chronic sycosis barbae in a Negro. Partially obscured by ointment. Topical sulfathiazole therapy was used for several weeks, with resultant sensitization. *B*, Same patient, several months later. The bullous lesions appeared within a few hours after the administration of 0.5 gm. of sulfathiazole orally, in spite of the patient's warning to the physician of his sulfonamide sensitivity.

pustules. Pseudofolliculitis barbae must also be considered.

Lupoid sycosis is probably a chronic scarring form of deep sycosis barbae. Its distinguishing characteristic is a persistent, slowly enlarging circinate patch, occurring anywhere on the bearded area or on the temples, the central area of which shows permanent hair loss and cutaneous atrophy. Follicular papulopustules are present in the "active" border, which slowly advances, while the central area heals with scarring. The atrophy is a consequence of a prolonged, deeply dissecting folliculitis, which destroys the hair bulbs and devitalizes the deeper corium. Pitted scars may be present in the central atrophic zone, the sites of former follicular infections. The disease eventually burns itself out after years. Lupoid sycosis, despite its name, resembles lupus vulgaris or lupus erythematosus only remotely.

When lupoid sycosis begins high on the face, the enlarging lesion may extend into the scalp. This behavior suggests a relationship with folliculitis decalvans, a disease localized to the scalp and usually far less inflammatory in the early stages. The pictures may be quite similar in the advanced stages, clinically and histologically. The disease is rebellious to treatment.

PERFORATING FOLLICULITIS OF THE NOSE. This is an uncommon deep folliculitis of the vibrissae of the external limits of the nares. The early lesion is a pustule in the follicular orifice, a common lesion, often a rather painful one, which usually subsides without sequelae. The distinctive feature in perforating folliculitis, however, is that the process dissects deeply through the tissue and ultimately presents itself as a papule or pustule on the external skin surface. There is, thus, an infected tract extending from the internal to the external surface. The original process in the nose may be inconspicuous and go unnoticed, while the external lesion attracts attention. It may be mistaken for an epithelioma. Therapy directed only at the external lesion fails to bring about cure. The condition may persist for a long time unless its true origin from within the nose is recognized. Epilation of the involved hair, followed by local application of an antibiotic ointment, is ordinarily curative.

STYE (HORDEOLUM). This is a deep folliculitis of the cilia of the lid margin. An erythematous, tender follicular nodule develops which may be capped by a pustule. There is considerable swelling of the perifollicular tissue because of its looseness. Exudate may drain from the lesion and form as a crust along the lid margin.

Warm compresses are helpful to bring about resolution and to promote the removal of exudate before a crust forms. After compressing, the local application of an antibiotic ointment helps speed resolution. With multiple lesions, the administration of an antibacterial agent internally is justified. Errors of refraction as a factor in recurrences have been overemphasized. Chronic low-grade blepharitis, which is often a manifestation of seborrheic dermatitis, is a common antecedent of styes. Hydrocortisone-antibiotic ointments are sometimes very useful in blepharitis with recurrent styes.

FURUNCLES AND CARBUNCLES. These may be discussed together, since a carbuncle may be regarded as an aggregation of furuncles. A furuncle or boil develops in relation to hair follicles and originates either from a preceding folliculitis, or sui generis as a deep seated nodule. A true furuncle is never seen in areas where there are no hair follicles, for example, the palms. The nodule is tender and red. It usually remains tense for two to four days and then becomes fluctuant. The skin thins over the summit and a yellowish point forms. Rupture follows, with discharge of a core of necrotic tissue. Boils are exceedingly painful when they occur in skin which is densely bound down to underlying tissue, for example, over nasal cartilage or in the external auditory canal. A carbuncle is a larger more deeply seated infiltrated lesion which drains through a number of points to the surface, and which, in the pre-antibiotic era, was sometimes fatal. Hair follicles provide the usual pathway of drainage. Furunculosis may be exceedingly chronic and recurrent.

The preferred sites of furuncles are those which are unusually hairy or which are exposed to friction and maceration: the buttocks, neck, face, axillae, and the areas underlying the belt. Lack of good hygiene invites recurrence. Furuncles may complicate a variety of secondarily infected dermatoses, such as pediculosis, scabies, excoriations, and so forth. Systemic factors which lower resistance are uncommonly detectable, including diabetes, obesity, hematologic disorders, cachexia, and malnutrition. Unfortunately, furunculosis commonly occurs in the absence of any apparent local or general predisposing causes. Such individuals may be in perfect health except for recurrent furuncles, and the infection is not uncommon in athletes, for example, football players and wrestlers. Temporary cessation of athletic activity may be necessary to control recurrent furunculosis.

Semisynthetic penicillin or penicillin (in the absence of allergic sensitivity to it) is the drug of choice and should be given parenterally in every case of carbuncles, as well as in severe cases of furunculosis. Local measures alone are indicated if there is only one boil or a few. *Squeezing or too early incision of furuncles is harmful;* the lesion should be allowed to "point," then gently nicked, and drainage established. However, most boils heal effectively without surgical or antibiotic intervention. Medicated wicks and rubber dams may impede healing and increase scarring. Hot wet dressings are helpful. Cleanliness is of paramount importance. The suppurative discharge should be removed as it forms and not allowed to drain over the surrounding skin. Antibiotic ointments may be applied after compressing, though their value is open to doubt, except possibly in preventing the formation of new adjacent lesions. Deep incision, particularly of the cruciate kind formerly recommended for the management of carbuncles, is undoubtedly harmful, because it breaches the dike of reaction which has been built up around the site of infection.

Emphasis should be placed on *resting* the affected skin area in furunculosis, both in terms of restricting motion and avoiding external trauma. Lesions about the nose and upper lip are always to be respected, because of the danger of intracranial extension, with the development of a venous sinus thrombosis. However, this complication, fortunately never common, has become practically unknown with the use of effective antibacterial agents.

The treatment of recurrent furunculosis is difficult and disappointing. Predis-

posing factors which may be uncovered should be corrected if possible: for example, diabetes, poor hygiene, occupational trauma, exposure of skin to hydrocarbons, poorly balanced diets, pyogenic infections in the patient's family, drugs (halogens), hyperhidrosis, and obesity. Every effort must be made to observe strict hygienic principles. The daily use of an antimicrobial soap in order to suppress the transient flora may be helpful, or rubbing the area of recurrence with 70 per cent ethanol or propanol thoroughly one to two minutes daily. The treatment of individual lesions with roentgen rays is *not* recommended. Immunization by means of vaccines or toxoids is a favorite but uncertain measure; controlled studies have shown no clinical improvement (Maibach and Kligman, 1962).

Organisms not usually considered pathogenic may occasionally be the inciting cause of furuncles, particularly if local or systemic disorders have greatly depressed the resistance of the skin to infection. In such cases, cultures may be necessary to direct the proper choice of antibiotic.

Bacterial Interference Therapy ("502 A Therapy"). Most patients with furunculosis have a self-limited disease; occasionally, one person or a whole family will have recurrent furuncles (often with the same strain) over a period of years. Although there is no fixed duration for the term "recurrent furunculosis," bacterial interference therapy is not considered until the patient has had numerous lesions for at least 6 to 12 months.

The basic principle is that in most of these patients it is not possible to rid them of *S. aureus;* however, their colonization level is temporarily inhibited with appropriate systemic and topical antibacterials. At this time, the new strain of Staphylococcus (502 A) is implanted in the anterior nares and other staphylococcal carriage sites (Aly et al., 1974; Maibach et al., 1969; Shinefield et al., 1971). If the 502 A strain is not rejected by the patient, no further furuncles occur.

The 502 A strain is pathogenic; however, it appears far less capable of producing furuncles than the patient's strain. The strain was orginally isolated from a nurse in a pediatric newborn unit who was a heavy carrier but whose strain had not

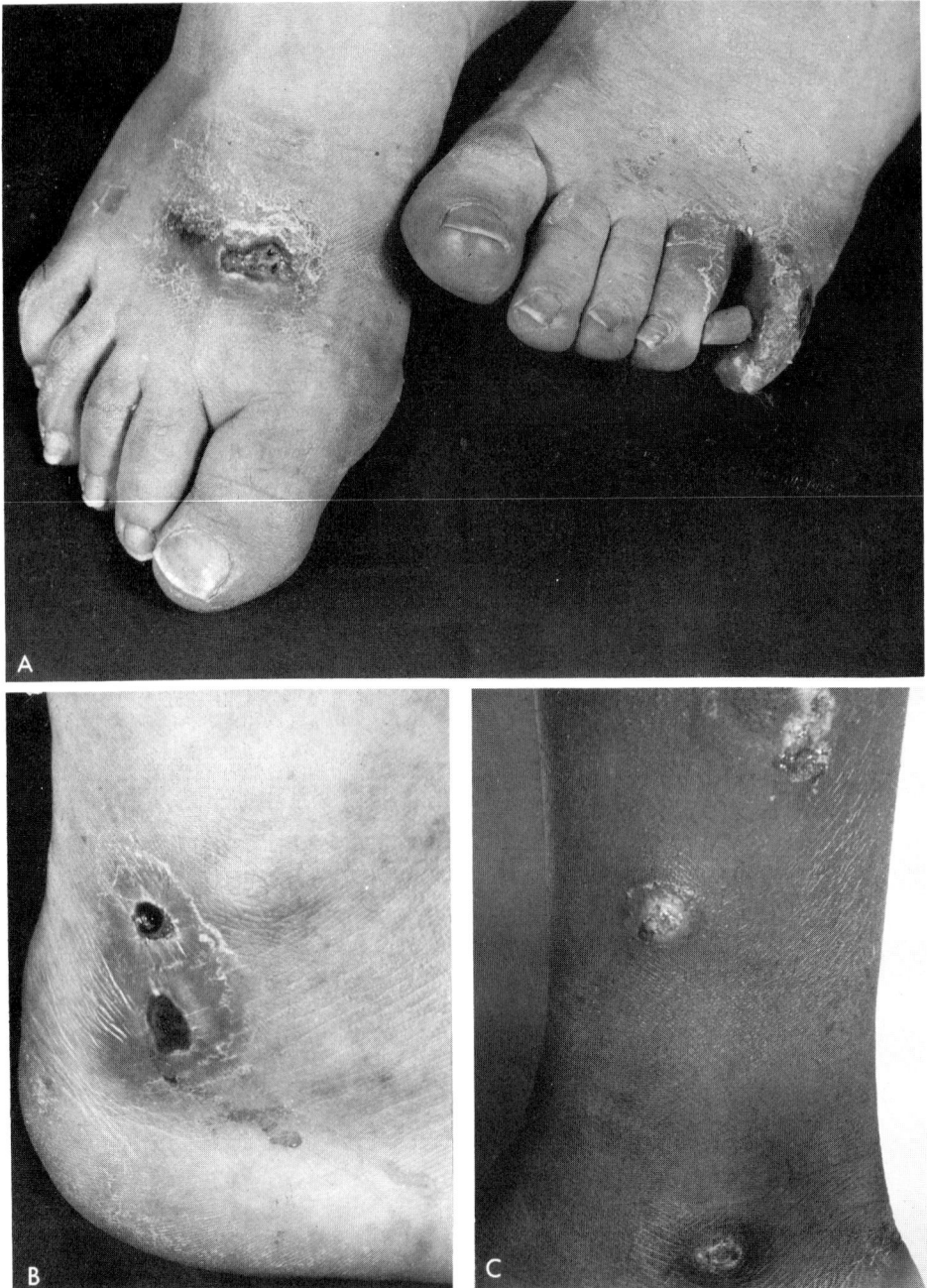

Figure 11–7 *A*, Chronic superficial and ulcerative pyoderma. The factors concerned were (a) fungal infection, (b) trauma from shoe, and (c) uncontrolled diabetes. *B*, Persistent ecthyma, highly suggestive of diphtheria cutis. *C*, "Traumatic infected ulcers" of the lower legs. Raised lesions are present, productive of some scarring.

produced disease in any of the infants during several years of study.

Acne Furunculoid. The term has been coined by the authors to describe a syndrome frequently confused with furunculosis. It occurs primarily in males past the acne age. The primary lesion is an erythematous nodule occurring almost on any part of the body but with greatest frequency on the back. The nodule is often not as warm as a furuncle, and adenopathy is uncommon. "Pointing" is rare. Careful examination frequently reveals other acne lesions such as comedones. The nodules look more like furuncles than acne cysts, thus causing the confusion. Cultures add additional confusion since they are rarely done in an appropriate manner to allow the *C. acnes* to proliferate. Gram stain of pus is most helpful, since it reveals a predominance of Gram-positive pleomorphic rods rather than cocci.

The only therapy of consistent value is appropriate antibiotics such as tetracycline. Therapy is in terms of years rather than weeks. The starting dose is 1 gm. daily; this is tapered as indicated. Anaerobic culture and sensitivity studies may be needed if the patient does not respond to tetracycline.

Job's Syndrome (Bannatyne et al., 1969; Davis et al., 1966). This is a syndrome consisting of recurrent cold staphylococcal abscesses occurring frequently from birth. The organism does not appear to be unusually virulent, suggesting an abnormality on the part of the host. Systemic antibiotic therapy is of some value. Recent evidence suggests that this may be a variant of chronic granulomatous disease.

Other Folliculitis Syndromes

ACNE VARIOLIFORMIS (FOLLICULITIS VARIOLIFORMIS). This uncommon disease is probably a deep variant of acne necrotica miliaris. Indeed, the manifestations may merge with this latter disorder in the same patient; that is, the conditions may coexist. (The term acne for both these conditions is inappropriate.) The lesions are persistent brown papulopustules, usually localized to the brow and scalp, but occasionally involving the nose, cheeks, and even the trunk. The papulopustules, which often have depressed summits, are apparently related to the lanugo follicles. The top of the papule erodes and a crust forms, beneath which there is a necrotic zone. The pathologic reaction is deep, as is evidenced by the formation of a depressed varioliform scar. When the lesions are numerous, scarring may be prominent, particularly on the cheeks and nose, where a reticulated pattern may be produced. Acne varioliformis is not accompanied by much subjective discomfort, but the disease is notoriously persistent.

Pathogenic staphylococci are usually recoverable from lesions of the disease, although it is difficult to assess the etiologic role they play. The basic predisposing causes are unknown. It is not known if acne varioliformis is synonymous with *C. acnes* scalp infection. It is possible that this is an end stage of *C. acnes* infection seen in patients before the antibiotic era.

Locally applied antibacterial remedies sometimes have an immediate resolving effect on the lesions; accordingly, antibacterial measures should be tried first. Recurrence is common however, and treatment may have to be protracted. Many other treatments have been used, particularly those applicable to seborrheic dermatitis, but the results are dubious. Sulfur ointments may prove worthwhile.

PYODERMA FACIALE. This is an uncommon disease which develops acutely in young women who usually have not had any significant evidence of acne; the relation between the two diseases is uncertain. Coagulase-positive staphylococci are often recovered. The predisposing and inciting forces which establish the infection are uncertain. The disease usually develops suddenly in young women in good general health; it is localized to the face. Numerous abscesses and cysts form, and an intense erythema is characteristic. Burrowing is prominent, and sinus tracts link the deep-seated lesions. Untreated, the lesions may last for many months, leaving *severe* scarring. The absence of significant comedones and acneiform lesions elsewhere, as well as the acuteness of this process, differentiates this disease from acne. In addition, the parenteral administration of appropriate antibiotics generally causes moderate to good improvement much more rapidly than in acne. Complete dependence on antibiotics may be unwarranted, for the effect is variable. The type of local therapy is not of primary importance; in general, it should be similar to that for grade IV acne. In some instances, Vleminck solution appears to be a useful agent. Systemic corticosteroids may also be required. If infected sinus tracts persist, they may require opening throughout their length, and this should be done by expert hands.

FOLLICULITIS DECALVANS. This rare disease has something in common with lupoid sycosis, but its true nature is yet to be revealed. Perhaps until there is more knowledge, it is worthwhile to think of it as a species of lupoid sycosis occurring on the scalp. It tends to occur in individuals who have coarse, bristly hair, but the predisposing factors are unknown; it may in truth be more a secondary than a primary infection. The disease begins in a localized area with the formation of a cluster of follicular pustules or papules. Exudation or suppuration soon follows, a crust accumulates, and the hairs are shed. New follicles become involved at the periphery, while centrally the process eventually subsides, with scarring and permanent hair loss. The "active" folliculitis of the slowly extending border and the atrophic healed center are the essential features of the disease. After years, the process becomes quiescent or burned out. Typically, one or more patches are formed, and these extend irregularly at the periphery, sometimes fusing to produce bizarre patterns. The border may not reveal distinct or discrete follicular papules but rather a continuous infiltrated, elevated rim resulting from a deep-seated inflammation in which there is fusion of the inflammatory process in adjacent follicles. Very occasionally, thick comedo-like plugs may be expressed from follicles in which there is an arrested devitalized hair. In severe cases, the whole scalp may be denuded, but tufts of hair usually escape.

Other cicatricial alopecias, such as lupus erythematosus, pseudopelade, localized scleroderma, and favus, must be considered in the differential diagnosis. Biopsy and appropriate cultures are essential to differentiation. Coagulase-positive micrococci are most often recovered but the flora is by no means constant, nor are the organisms always "pathogenic" types. The disease is extremely refractory to treatment. Vigorous parenteral and local antibiotic therapy should be tried in much the same manner as for lupoid sycosis. It is emphasized that the etiologic role of bacteria in this disease is unknown. X-ray epilation is clearly hazardous in view of the atrophy which is a natural part of the disease.

Ecthyma

This condition has certain similarities to impetigo; it begins in the same way, but the process erodes through the epidermis and produces a shallow ulcer. Furthermore, beta-hemolytic streptococci characteristically initiate the disease, although at later stages a variety of other organisms may be isolated. The initial lesion is a vesicle or vesicopustule on an inflamed base. Crusting occurs early and is dry, hard, and firmly adherent. It may become quite heaped up, concealing the underlying erosion. Healing, with variable scar formation, generally occurs in a few weeks. Scratching and hygienic neglect may lead to protraction of the disease and to auto-inoculation into new areas. Children are more susceptible and, because of trauma incident to normal juvenile activity, extension of the lesions is common. The lower legs are affected most commonly (recurrent "traumatic infected ulcers"). It may follow minor forms of injury such as an insect bite or scratch, particularly under conditions of filth. The disease is far more common in warm humid climates. Other antecedent conditions, such as pediculosis, scabies, eczema, and so forth, may be the soil in which ecthyma originates. The vesicopustules of vaccinia, variola, varicella, and zoster may eventuate in ecthyma because of secondary invasion by beta-hemolytic streptococci, though not commonly.

The lesions must be differentiated chiefly from impetigo, in which the crust is not as massive and under which there is no ulcer. It responds readily to therapeutic measures aimed at removing the crust, followed by applications of antibiotic ointments. Warm, bland compresses or gentle soap and water washing are suffi-

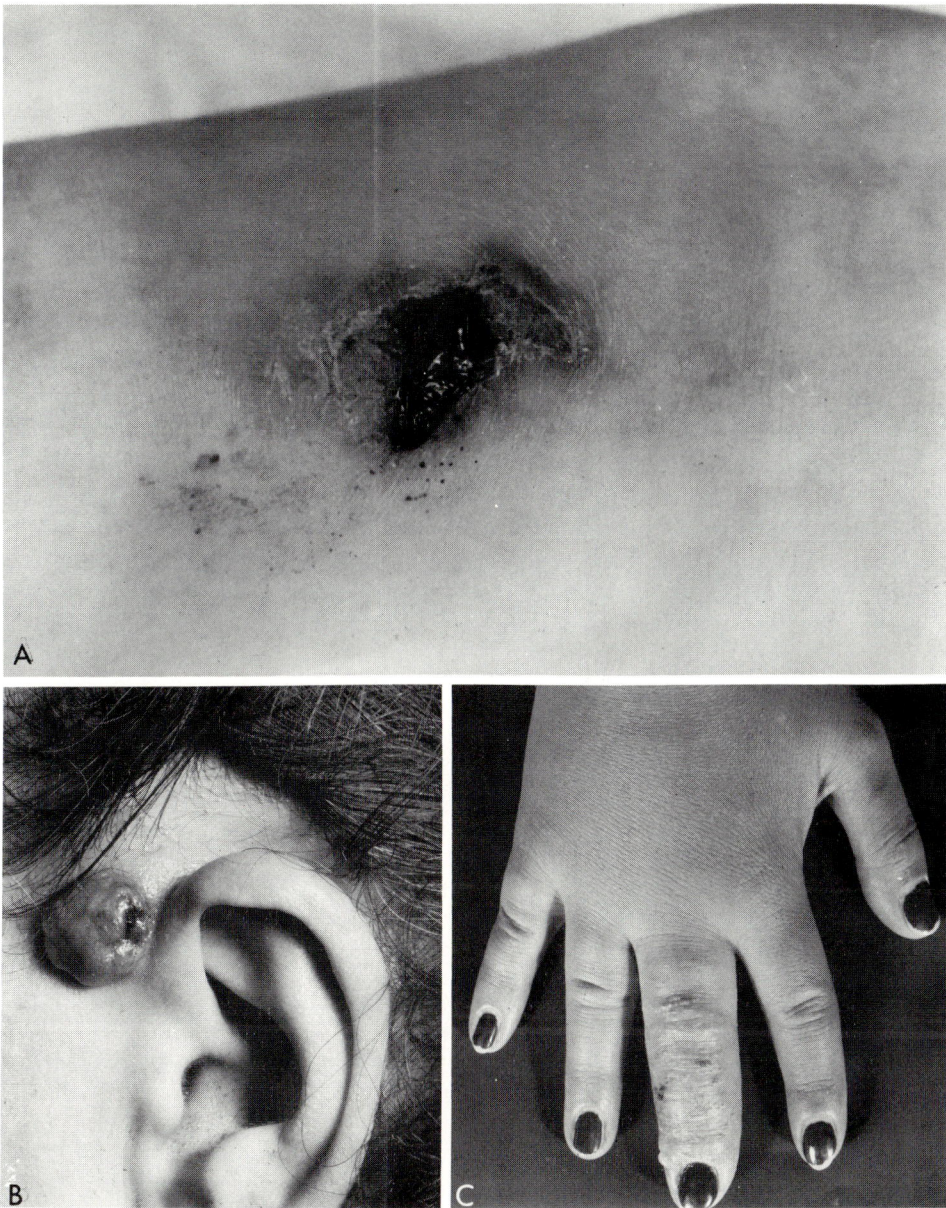

Figure 11-8 *A*, Ecthyma and granulation tissue. The child had been in contact with scarlet fever; several similar lesions developed in other children on the same ward simultaneously. *B*, Pyogenic granuloma. Contrary to the name, this is not bacterial in origin. *C*, Mild dermatitis, recurrent cellulitis, permanent elephantiasis of the finger. An uncommon sequel.

cient for softening and removing debris. Parenteral antibiotic therapy is indicated for disseminated lesions. Attention should be paid to underlying, predisposing causes, and above all, hygienic practices devoted to keeping the skin clean and nontraumatized.

Paronychia

Inflammation of the nail folds (paronychia) surrounding the nail plate is a syndrome, not a specific disease. The nail fold's potential space is an excellent milieu for infection. When due to bacteria, it is appropriately termed pyonychia, signifying a particular type of pyoderma. Pathogenic staphylococci and streptococci are the usual causative microorganisms in acute cases. However, one must look for other bacteria and candida in acute and chronic lesions. Other organisms are associated with chronic cases, but their etiologic relationship is often questionable. The question also arises in persistent cases as to whether infection is primary or secondary. The simplest type of pyonychia is a localized swelling of the lateral nail fold adjacent to the side of the nail. A drop of pus may sometimes be expressed from the tender area. The lesion generally disappears in a few days but may extend all around the nail folds except for the distal edge, a "runaround." The nail folds are red, swollen, tense, and painful. They bulge out over the nail plate. If involution is not rapid, the nail matrix is invariably disturbed, and the nails are consequently deformed to varying degrees. Not infrequently, a small quantity of pus may be pressed from under the posterior nail fold.

The lesion may originate following a simple injury or as a complication of a "hangnail," though usually there is no obvious cause. Chronic paronychia is favored by prolonged immersion in water, by exposure to irritating solutions, and by too vigorous manicuring. It may be an occupational disease in certain industries, particularly canneries, in which workers have their hands in water almost constantly. Housewives and bartenders are likely subjects.

Subungual abscess is an important complication of paronychia. The suppurative process extends in this case beneath the nail, forming a pocket of pus which separates the nail from the matrix and causes it to be loosened and sometimes shed. Transillumination of the finger with a bright light in a dark room may help to detect such hidden abscesses, which definitely require drainage.

Ringworm of the nails is easily differentiated because of the absence of paronychial involvement primarily. Candidal paronychia may resemble the chronic bacterial form closely, but is less tender and not often as purulent.

TREATMENT. Treatment is greatly facilitated by etiologic diagnosis. Gram stain of pus will reveal whether the lesion is primarily bacterial or Candidal in origin. Acute bacterial paronychia due to staphylococci or streptococci is advantageously treated by hot bland soaks combined with parenteral antibiotic therapy. Local application of topical antibiotics ordinarily has a limited value because of lack of penetration. The chronic variety, which is often a secondary type of pyoderma, requires an analysis of the factors which have abetted the infection and which interfere with healing. Exposure to irritating substances and prolonged immersion in aqueous solutions are to be avoided. Every effort must be made to drain loculated pus. The posterior nail fold must be freed as much as possible from the underlying nail plate. This measure is important and too often neglected, for the nail fold may readily become adherent to the nail plate, forming an occluded space which prevents drainage. Trauma and movement are contributory to infection. In many chronic cases due to bacteria, only long-term systemic antibiotic therapy will control the process. Certain cases defy all therapeutic endeavors.

Cellulitis and Erysipelas

Erysipelas is a characteristic type of superficial cellulitis in which an edematous, brawny, infiltrated, sharply circumscribed plaque develops and spreads peripherally. The lesion is hot and bright red, with no obvious central clearing. The border is distinct. The face and scalp are the favorite sites but the infection may occur anywhere else, particularly on the hands and genitalia. Beta-hemolytic streptococci are the causative organisms. The process evolves rapidly, and the affected individuals are sick, with fever, malaise, and general toxic symptoms. In some cases vesicles and bullae may form on the surface of the erythematous skin and are evidences of a more severe infection. A large area may be involved. Erysipelas may originate from a variety of wounds, injuries, ulcers, pustules, and other antecedent conditions which invite colonization by hemolytic streptococci. Cachexia, diabetes, malnutrition, and systemic conditions which lower resistance, especially when accompanied by poor hygiene, promote infection. Drainage from contaminated wounds or suppurative lesions may incite the disease. Sometimes there is no antecedent injury or known predisposing cause. The disease is not ordinarily transmissible (in the form of erysipelas) but was formerly a source of many puerperal infections. It is now uncommon.

Certain individuals have a tendency to develop recurrent erysipelas. The exacerbations occur strikingly in the same area and may, after a period of time, lead to permanent changes typified by elephantiasic swelling. Brawny unremitting edema of the lower legs may arise in this way. Persistent swelling of the lips, cheeks, or other areas is a disfiguring complication of recurrent erysipelas and is known as *elephantiasis nostras.*

Persistent swelling of one or both lower legs, often due to recurrent erysipelas or cellulitis (but also a sequel to chronic venous or lymphatic stasis of diverse origin), may, after a number of years, result in a curious cutaneous pattern which has re-

ceived the designation "elephantiasis nostras verrucosa." The skin over the toes, dorsum of the foot, and the ankles, less often the lower legs, becomes greatly thickened. The verrucous lesions are made up of crowded wartlike growths, which may occur in irregular plaques of different size and shape or may involve a rather large area diffusely. The solitary papillomas often look like fleshy, flattened, smooth growths attached by a slender or broad pedicle but may assume any form, varying in size from 0.5 to 2.0 cm. One or many, they are distributed within the verrucous lesions. Various bacterial species are associated with the lesions, and there may be an associated dermatophytosis. The etiologic role of bacteria and fungi is certain but indirect. Poor foot hygiene is a primary feature in the progression of morbid events in these cases, but it should be remembered that all the changes may be secondary to chronic lymphatic or venous blockage. Prophylaxis must be the keynote of control, for little can be done after the verrucous changes ensue.

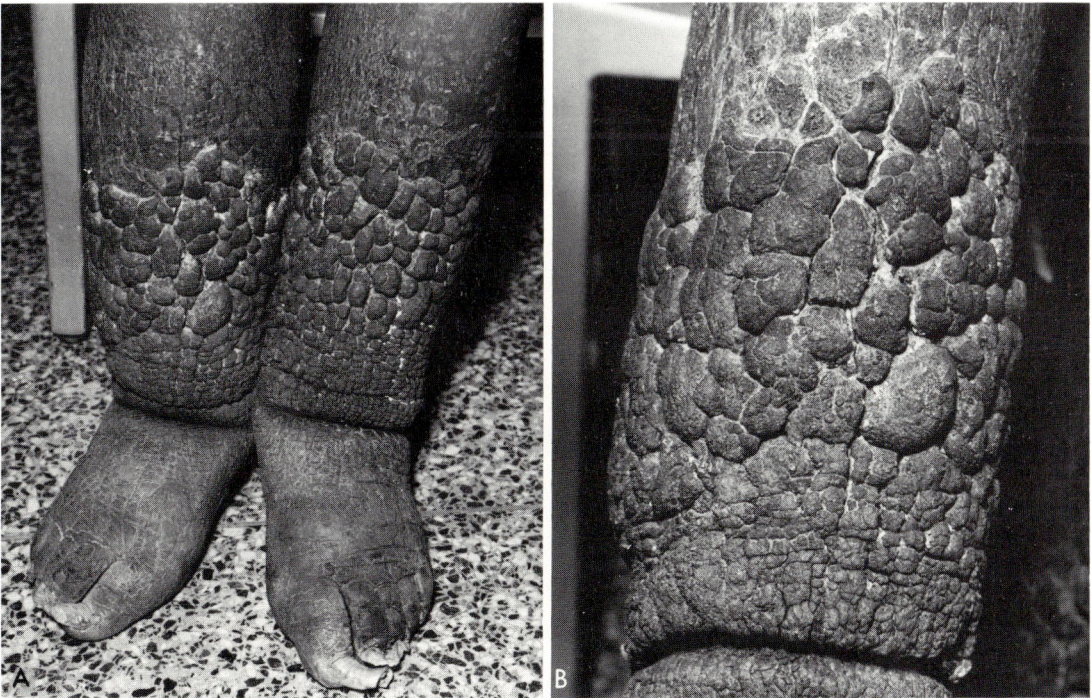

Figure 11-9 Elephantiasis nostras verrucosa secondary to recurrent attacks of thrombophlebitis and cellulitis. A result of long continued neglect.

Erysipelas must be differentiated from erysipeloid, which occurs mostly on the hand and fingers and rarely produces a significant systemic reaction. There is usually no fever and the lesions are not so hot, tender, and fiery red as in erysipelas; a history of contact with fresh seafood is usually obtainable. Ordinary cellulitis may simulate the condition but lacks the sharply marginated pattern. An unusual type of diffuse recurrence of carcinoma of the breast (erysipeloid carcinoma) may give rise to an appearance strongly suggestive of low-grade erysipelas; similar lesions are seen with other tumors that spread via the lymphatics.

Treatment. Attacks of cellulitis and erysipelas may be quickly suppressed by appropriate antibiotic therapy. Penicillin is the agent of choice. Although such treatment is rapidly effective, the patient should be given the benefit of good medical care, including complete bed rest. Cool, wet dressings bring local relief and are particularly indicated when there are bullae. A variety of local medicaments used in the past may be regarded as items of historic interest only. The affected part should be immobilized and elevated. Patients who develop erysipelas on a maternity or surgical ward should be transferred promptly to a less critical area. Certain rites of isolation, including screens, and lysol and mercurial hand solutions, may be regarded as unnecessary persistence of habit.

Erysipelas and cellulitis should be considered dermatologic emergencies, for deaths still occur in the antibiotic era. Dosage should be that used for severe infection. The patient should be watched carefully.

In recurrent infection one should seek the nidus, such as tinea pedis. In some instances, systemic antibiotics given on a long-term prophylactic basis will prevent recurrences.

Necrotizing Fasciitis (Hemolytic Streptococcus Gangrene)

This rare disease is a fulminating infection of the superficial and deep fascia, resulting in thrombosis of the subcutaneous vessels and gangrene of the underlying tissues (Collins and Nadel, 1965; Rea and Wyrick, 1970).

Usually it follows a cutaneous injury, such as a needle puncture, insect bite, or laceration, but sometimes no portal of entry is found. Early in the course, the area becomes hot, edematous, and red, and as it gradually enlarges, a pathognomonic sign develops between the second and the fourth days; the affected skin assumes a blue, dusky tinge. Blisters may be present. The process advances to areas of frank, cutaneous gangrenes, with eventual sloughing. Cutaneous metastatic infections may appear. In the late stages, the involved areas may become painless. The patient is toxic. At this stage, the erroneous diagnosis of a third-degree burn or trauma may be made.

Streptococcus may be demonstrated from the spreading border of the lesion or from the blister fluid. Blood culture will usually also yield the organism. In later stages, a multiplicity of organisms may colonize the necrotic plaque.

The most important part of the treatment is early incision and drainage. The involved part is opened widely at the fascial plane and the gangrenous areas excised with a margin. Skin grafting is done later. Massive doses of antibiotics and vigorous suppurative measures are also indicated.

Mortality rates remain high, in spite of vigorous therapy. This is probably influenced by the underlying disease (such as diabetes mellitus and severe arteriosclerosis) in the patient.

Gram-Negative Infection

The toe web is the site most commonly involved (Amonette and Rosenberg, 1973). This intertriginous site presumably provides the moisture required for such infection. The skin becomes macerated. Wood's light examination revealing a green fluorescence suggests Pseudomonas involvement. Gram staining of ground-up pieces of stratum corneum reveal numerous gram-negative rods. The lesions may require antibiotic therapy; some respond to aeration and compresses.

A more serious syndrome consists of deep, thick-walled bullae of the soles. These are generally misdiagnosed as inflammatory tinea; careful KOH examination is generally negative. If the roof of the blister is prepared for Gram staining, numerous gram-negative rods are seen. Culture and sensitivity should lead to appropriate antibiotic therapy. Topical management, consisting of silver nitrate solution, Castellani's paint, and gentamicin sulfate cream, bed rest, and exposure to air are the best therapy available. Recovery and disability may be prolonged.

Infection of the
Eccrine Sweat Apparatus

Considering the enormous number of eccrine sweat ducts which conduct sweat to the skin's surface, it is altogether remarkable that bacteria so rarely gain ingress into the skin via these tubes. Pure, discretely localized infections of the sweat apparatus are uncommon (or perhaps nonexistent). The bacterial flora play no significant role in the pathogenesis of any of the varieties of miliaria, which is incited when sweat, under an appropriate thermal stimulus, is extravasated into the skin because of closure of the sweat pore. Miliarial lesions, especially those of miliaria rubra, may become secondarily infected, but it is noteworthy that this complication is not frequent. Occasionally, miliaria rubra will be the starting point of a severe pyoderma, usually of the type of impetigo contagiosa (tropical impetigo), but in such cases the sweat retention lesions act largely in a predisposing fashion, damaging the epidermis and weakening its resistance against infection. It is necessary to emphasize that pustular miliaria, which may appear on previously dermatitic skin, especially in the healing stages, is probably not due to bacterial infection; the pustules are usually sterile.

Multiple Sweat Gland Abscesses

Although it is safe to conclude that bacterial infections of the eccrine sweat apparatus are uncommon, some attention must be paid to a syndrome long recognized among European dermatologists which is presumed to be an instance of primary bacterial infection of the sweat glands. The disease is encountered principally in malnourished, weakened infants in poor health; this may account for its rarity in areas where living standards are high and good medical care available. However, normal children may occasionally be affected and there is reason to believe that the disorder may not be such a great rarity: it may go unrecognized in America because it is not considered as a diagnostic possibility. Only infants and young children are susceptible, apparently. The favorite sites are the upper portion of the trunk, the back of the scalp, and the buttocks, though any area may be involved. The lesions begin as flesh-colored or erythematous deep-seated infiltrated nodules, varying in size from that of a small pea to that of a walnut. They are always multiple, tend to emerge in crops, and finally soften, forming abscesses which come to the surface, rupture, and drain a thick creamy yellow pus. Scar formation follows, and recurrence in new areas is to be expected. Some of the smaller lesions may involute without discharging their contents, becoming fibrotic nodules. Typically, the elevated fluctuant, red nodules drain for a period of several weeks before healing. The lesions resemble furuncles, the diagnosis usually made, but close inspection shows that these abscesses are dome-shaped rather than conical, do not have a yellow center through which the abscess points, show no necrotic core or plug which is so typical of furuncles, and do not develop in relation to a hair follicle, though this may be difficult to decide.

Subcutaneous nodules are the hallmark of the disease and generally the only presenting sign. Hot weather is generally not mentioned as a predisposing factor, nor is there a seasonal relationship. Poral closure and sweat retention are not antecedent causative factors, and it seems very unlikely that the organisms, which are usually coagulase-positive micrococci, invade the skin via the ducts. However, some observers have mentioned the simultaneous presence of pustules which on histologic section showed a congregation of inflammatory cells about the sweat ducts, "a periporitis," suggesting that miliaria may sometimes be the starting point of the disorder.

There seems no doubt, however, that the deep-seated abscesses, whatever their true origin, are incited by bacteria and that the parenteral administration of antibiotics should successfully control the infection. Little is to be expected from local medications. Study of the general health of the infant is indicated (Maibach and Kligman, 1962).

Pitted Keratolysis

Definition. This is a superficial skin infection causing asymptomatic pits of the stratum corneum, usually involving the soles of the feet. It was first described by Castellani in 1910 as keratoma plantare sulcatum. In 1930, Acton and McGuire called it keratolysis plantare sulcatum, under which name it was known until 1965 when Zaias et al. renamed it pitted keratolysis.

Etiology. A gram-positive filamentous and coccoidal organism is found in the stratum corneum of the affected skin. Its identification gave rise to difficulties. Acton and McGuire (1930) called it an *Actinomyces keratolytica* species; Taplin, in 1967, identified it as a Corynebacterium species.

Humidity is a frequent aggravating factor. It is often associated with hyperhidrosis. It developed in 53 per cent of 38 volunteers whose feet were continually wet for three days or more.

Clinical Features. Discrete crateriform defects, 1 to 7 mm. in size, are present on the plantar surface, producing a punched-out appearance. The pits may coalesce into irregularly shaped areas of superficial erosion. Sulci are present only in severe cases. Only the horny layer is involved; the pits are produced by a "lytic" process which spreads peripherally. The areas most often affected are the pressure areas of the heels, the ball, the volar pads, and the toes. The involved areas may show a brownish discoloration, giving a "dirty" appearance. The condition is usually asymptomatic; only patients with severe cases experience discomfort. Hyperhidrosis is a common but not essential associated feature.

Laboratory Diagnosis. Gram stain of ground-up stratum corneum will demonstrate the organisms. Biopsy shows the pits confined to the stratum corneum. The filamentous and coccal forms of the or-

ganism may be best demonstrated with Gram stain and are present in the floor and walls of the pits. Culturing of the organism is a research procedure.

Differential Diagnosis. The pits must be differentiated from those seen on the palms and soles in basal cell nevus syndrome.

Treatment. The condition may disappear spontaneously after the patient is removed from the moist environment. Broadspectrum antibacterial agents such as Whitfield's ointment, formalin, and ammoniated mercury are effective.

Botryomycosis (Kansky, 1964; Katznelsen et al., 1964; Waisman, 1962; Winslow, 1959)

The disease is characterized by chronic, suppurating, granulomatous lesions. The specific feature is the presence of granules within the suppurating foci. The granules—which may sometimes be seen without magnification—contain a central mass of bacteria surrounded by a capsule. The causative organism is most frequently staphylococcus, but other organisms, including gram-negative ones, are reported. The pathogenesis of the disease is not clear; it may be the result of a delicate balance between the virulence of the infecting agent and the tissue resistance of the host. The possible role of hypersensitivity is not known. The disease is probably more frequent than the paucity of reports suggests.

The cases fall into two categories: the integumentary form, including muscular and skeletal involvement, and the visceral form. Integumentary botryomycosis presents mostly on the hands, the feet, and the head. The cutaneous features include inflammatory nodules, discharging ulcers, sinuses, and fistulas. Secondary involvement of underlying muscle or bone may occur; less frequently, the cutaneous disease is secondary to osteomyelitis.

Differential diagnoses include actinomycosis and mycetomas.

The granules can be demonstrated on biopsy or smear of the purulent focus; the bacteria will be seen by Gram stain. The capsule is usually PAS positive.

The visceral form of the disease was reported in the lung, liver, and kidney.

There is a recent report of botryomycosis occurring in the lungs of children with cystic fibrosis.

Since antibiotics have difficulty in penetrating the lesions, the therapy of choice is surgical excision in conjunction with antibiotics.

Erythrasma

Definition. Erythrasma is a chronic, superficial bacterial skin infection involving the body folds and toe webs, and sometimes it may be generalized (Hildick-Smith et al., 1964). It was first described by Burchardt in 1859.

Incidence. The condition occurs in all parts of the world, but the wide-spread, generalized form is more common in warmer climates. All age groups are affected. It occurs in both sexes, but the genitocrural form is more common in men.

The disease is more prevalent than previously thought. Colonization without clinical lesion of the groin was found by Sarkany et al. (1962) in 9 out of 25 normal male subjects in Miami and in 5 out of 55 in London.

Toe-web infection was found in 23 per cent of 109 consecutive patients by Sarkany et al. (1962), and in 14.3 per cent of 371 university students by Temple and Boardman (1962). Among 410 school boys, Munro-Ashman et al. (1963) found 17 per cent with coral red fluorescence in the toe webs; in 14 per cent *Corynebacterium minutissimum* was isolated.

Etiology. The causative organism was thought to be a fungus, named *Nocardia minutissima*, until 1961 when Sarkany et al. showed this to be a species of Corynebacterium named *C. minutissimum*. For this organism, Koch's postulates were fulfilled.

Although the toe web infection is common, predisposing factors for the other forms of erythrasma include heat, humidity, obesity, maceration, poor hygiene, and debility. Recently, Montes et al. (1969) found that 9 out of 19 patients with genitocrural or generalized erythrasma had diabetes mellitus.

Clinical Picture. Three forms of the disease are recognized:

1. The classic genitocrural and axillary form. It is seen most frequently on the thighs in contact with the scrotum, but the intergluteal cleft, the axillae, and the folds under the breast may also be involved. The well-circumscribed patches are dry, finely scaling, and slowly spreading. Initially the color is pink; later it may become brown, with fine creases in the skin. It may be asymptomatic or mildly pruritic.

2. Toe web infection. This chronic form is the most common manifestation of the disease. It occurs usually between the fourth and fifth or third and fourth toes. Scaling, fissuring, and maceration occur.

3. The generalized form features well-defined, scaly, lamellated plaques on the trunk and proximal parts of the limbs. It occurs chiefly in warmer climates and is mostly observed in middle-aged Negro women.

Diagnosis

1. Fluorescence. A coral red fluorescence of the lesions under Wood's light is of the greatest diagnostic importance. The fluorescence is caused by a porphyrin produced by the organism but this may have been washed away if the patient has bathed within 48 hours of examination.

2. Direct preparations. Because the organism is bacterial, potassium hydroxide preparations only rarely demonstrate it in the scales. Gram stain preparations of ground-up stratum corneum under high dry or oil immersion microscopy are preferable. The preparations show gram-positive rodlike organisms, filamentous and coccoid forms. The filaments are tortuous and measure 4 to 10 by 1 μ. The coccoid forms are 1 to 3 by 0.5 μ. Both forms are found in all lesions, but the filamentous forms supposedly predominate in groin lesions, whereas the bacillary forms are found on the toe web.

3. Culture characteristics. Culture is rarely required, except as a research procedure. One isolation medium consists of 78 per cent tissue culture medium 199 without bicarbonate, 20 per cent fetal bovine serum, 2 per cent agar, and 0.5 per cent tris-aminomethane (Sarkany et al., 1961). In 24 hours, small, shiny, translucent colonies appear, showing red fluorescence, and, on smear, gram-positive bacillary forms.

Treatment. It is emphasized that most cases represent colonization rather than symptomatic clinical infection and hence require no therapy. The clinical condition without treatment is chronic and may wax and wane for years. Topical antibacterial preparations and keratolytic agents will beneficially affect the lesions of erythrasma. On the foot, extensive washings with antibacterial soap may be all that is necessary. When this is not effective, a systemic antibiotic may be required. A five-day course of erythromycin in the dose of 1 gm. daily is curative in most cases of the classic form of the disease. The condition clears within two to three weeks of the administration of the drug.

Trichomycosis Axillaris (Leptothrix)

This condition is a minor parasitic affection of the axillary and, less commonly, the pubic hairs. It consists of yellow, red, or black concretions on the hair, yellow being the most frequent and black the least frequent color seen. The condition is generally asymptomatic and not contagious. The underlying skin is normal. The involved hairs may be brittle. Invasion and destruction of the hair cuticle and superficial hair cortex have been observed with the scanning electron microscope (Orfanos et al., 1971) but the colonization remains superficial and does not cause the hairs to break off as in ringworm infection. The most frequently associated complaint is coloring of the sweat, to the color of the concretions, and staining of the clothing and may be confused with a dis-order of apocrine sweating, chromhidrosis (Fig. 11–10). There may be a marked axillary odor. The causative agent was shown by Crissey et al. (1952) to be a Corynebacterium species, named *C. tenuis*, but McBride et al. (1968) isolated three different Corynebacterium species from seven cases, often coexisting with each other. The causative bacillus forms dense colonies on the surface of the hair (Freeman et al., 1969) and these are easily visible as discrete colored rather adherent tiny soft nodules distributed irregularly along the shaft or forming a continuous filmy sheath.

Treatment consists of shaving the hairs of the affected area and application of antibacterial soaps and creams.

SECONDARY BACTERIAL INFECTIONS OF THE SKIN

The distinction between primary and secondary infections cannot always be rigid. The cardinal criterion of a secondary infection is that there must be some pre-existing condition, either local or systemic, which diminishes the host's defenses. It is obligatory for the therapist to search for and recognize the primary condition; no such demand may exist in primary infections, where elimination of the bacteria is usually directly curative. Secondary infections usually represent complications of

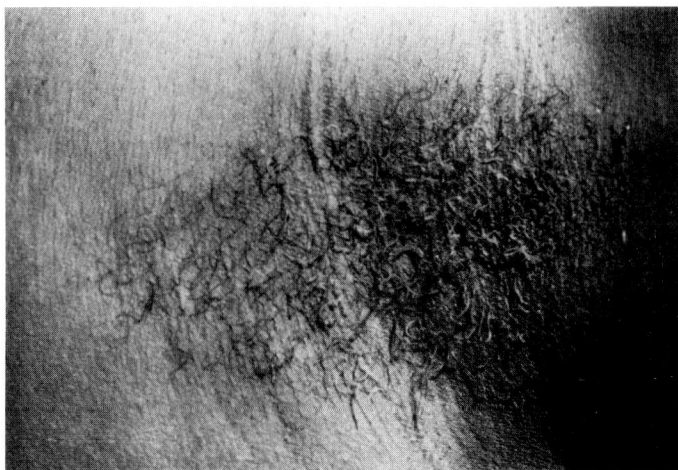

Figure 11–10 Trichomycosis axillaris. Soft nodules are adherent to axillary hairs.

an antecedent cutaneous lesion: a cut, burn, ulcer, a dermatitis—indeed, any significant disturbance of the integrity of the skin. The infection arises in the pre-existing cutaneous lesion, which serves as a portal of entry. While this is the usual circumstance, certain types of secondary infection can occur in apparently normal skin, but *only* when there is an antecedent systemic disease of sufficient seriousness to weaken the host.

In secondary infections, as in primary ones, pathogenic staphylococci and streptococci are the organisms of principal importance, and routine therapy is directed against these. Two factors, above all others, determine whether or not pathogenic staphylococci and streptococci will entrench themselves in diseased skin. These are *chronicity* of the antecedent lesion and *wetness*. Persistent lesions which ooze and weep are extremely favorable sites. Intensely vesicular or bullous eruptions are readily colonized, pathogenic staphylococci in particular being recoverable from 50 to 90 per cent of such lesions if they have been present for a few weeks. However, as has been stressed elsewhere, the mere colonization of lesions by pathogenic organisms is not in itself indicative of the existence of active secondary infection. *Secondary infections cannot be diagnosed solely by cultures.* There must be proof that the host has been damaged in some way, the most obvious local evidence of this being the formation of pus. Smears will demonstrate a leukocytic response as well as the presence of free and engulfed bacteria, the combination forming a valuable basis for diagnosing secondary infections.

Organisms not ordinarily considered pathogenic may be the cause of secondary infections. The principal ones in this group are gram-negative bacilli, chiefly *E. coli*, Pseudomonas, and Proteus. In the very same sense, the possibility of nonpathogenic normal skin residents assuming a pathogenic role cannot be excluded. Attempts at too sharp differentiation of bacteria into pathogenic ("disease producing") and nonpathogenic has led to some confusion; it represents too great emphasis on the bacteria themselves and neglect of the marked variation of susceptibility of the tissues of the host.

The concept of virulence enables one to grasp in proper perspective the role played by the bacteria in inciting disease, making it at once evident that practically all organisms can, under appropriate circumstances, be pathogenic. In short, some are highly virulent, namely, certain streptococci and staphylococci, while others are of lowly virulence, namely, gram-negative coliform organisms. Gram-negative organisms are generally not recoverable from more than about 10 per cent of the general run of skin lesions. Their presence may be without clinical significance. Only persistent, chronic lesions are invaded by gram-negative bacteria, as a rule. Ulcers are particularly vulnerable. Moisture is a determining factor, for these organisms are easily killed by desiccation. Gram-negative organisms thrive under occlusive dressings. They are chiefly responsible for the malodor of ulcerative or eczematous lesions which have been occluded by fixed dressings, especially if these are covered by adhesive tape, plaster or other relatively impermeable material. In general, nothing is to be gained by taking steps to prevent the colonization of such lesions by gram-negative bacteria, provided the *primary* condition is being brought under control by proper treatment.

It must be clear from the very nature of secondary infections that the majority of these will have no characteristic morphology; the clinical features will chiefly reflect the qualities of the primary condition. Hence the secondary infections of preexisting cutaneous lesions are for the most part nondescript and not truly classifiable morphologically, though some are true clinical entities with distinctive characteristics.

CLASSIFICATION OF SECONDARY BACTERIAL INFECTIONS

Nondescript Secondary Infections

Infection complicating any preexisting cutaneous lesion: a burn, abrasion, eczematous eruption, ulcer, fungal infection, insect bite, and so forth. The morphologic changes are those of the underlying disorder, plus minor to gross evidences of infection.

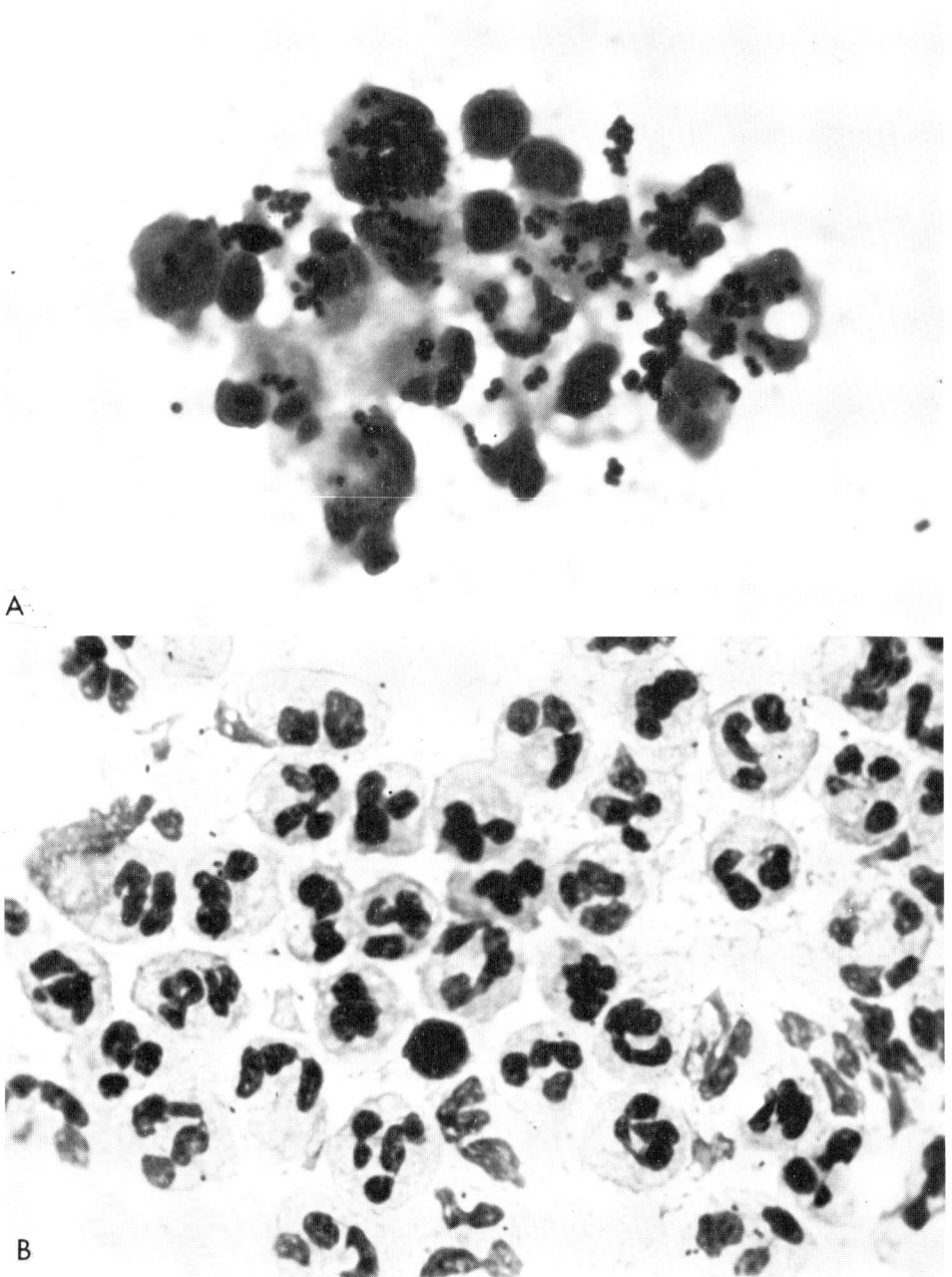

Figure 11–11   The smear technique for diagnosing secondarily infected lesions. *A*, Smear from a case of secondarily infected contact dermatitis. The combination of polymorphonuclear leukocytes and cocci suggests true infection. Many of the leukocytes have engulfed bacteria. *B*, Smear of a sterile pustule. The lack of bacteria tends to rule out an infectious element.

Clinical Entities

Diseases which are clinical entities by virtue of typical morphologic characteristics and course. It is emphasized that in most of these syndromes bacteria play a contributing rather than a primal role in their pathogenesis.

1. SECONDARY FOLLICULITIS.
   A. *The follicular occlusion or retention triad:*
      (1) Acne conglobata.
      (2) Hidradenitis suppurativa.
      (3) Dissecting cellulitis of scalp.
   B. *Keloidal folliculitis (acne keloid).*
2. DERMATITIS VEGETANS (pyoderma vegetans).
3. ACUTE INFECTIOUS ECZEMATOID DERMATITIS.
4. INTERTRIGO.
5. OTITIS EXTERNA (in some cases).
6. PILONIDAL CYST.
7. INFECTED ULCERS of rather specific types (tropical ulcers, phagedenic ulcers, etc.).
8. PSEUDOFOLLICULITIS OF THE BEARD.
9. BLASTOMYCOSIS-LIKE PYODERMA.

Secondary Folliculitis

THE FOLLICULAR OCCLUSION TRIAD: (Acne conglobata, hidradenitis suppurativa, and dissecting cellulitis of the scalp).

These diseases may comprise a generic group. Though not usually classified together, there is reason to believe that they are variants of the same pathologic process, for there are marked clinical and pathologic similarities. The initial and central pathogenic event linking these conditions is an innate tendency toward follicular hyperkeratoses, leading to occlusion of the follicular orifice and *retention* of products normally escaping through it. The clinical features common to all three are multiple comedo formation, abscesses with communicating channels, discharging sinuses, and healing with a marked tendency toward hypertrophic or keloidal scars. Furthermore, two or more of these disorders may coexist in the same person; however, it is usually the first two mentioned in the list.

Acne Conglobata. This is an unusually severe form of acne, the hallmark of which is deep abscesses and draining sinuses. It should be pointed out, however, that the pustular or cystic forms of acne do not usually arise on the basis of secondary infection. That there is an infective component in acne conglobata is rather well confirmed by the definite response of these lesions to vigorous parenteral therapy with antibiotics, although, of course, this does not cure the underlying disease. The management is that of grade IV acne. Marsupialization of sinuses and cysts is often of value.

Hidradenitis Suppurativa. This disease is described in the section on disorders of the sweat glands.

Dissecting Cellulitis of the Scalp (Perifolliculitis abscedens et suffodiens*). The small nodules and draining abscesses which characterize this disease occur on the scalp of young adults predominantly. Men are more frequently involved than women. Typically, the nodules become fluctuant and finally rupture to produce a chronic draining sinus. Drainage may be intermittent. Close inspection often reveals comedo-like plugs or excessive horny material in the follicular orifices, the probable starting point of the disease. The follicular orifices in certain scalp areas may appear deeper than usual, dilated, and choked with keratin. Polytrichia, the apparent emergence of two or three hairs from the same follicle, is a notable feature considerably more evident than in normal persons, though in itself it can scarcely be regarded as an abnormality. Actually, each follicle contains only a single hair but fusion of the follicles near the surface forms a common opening. Though such common orifices are larger than usual, the hairs are crowded within them, increasing the opportunity, especially if there is hyperkeratosis, of actual occlusion. Dandruff may be a prominent incidental finding. There is a notable tendency toward burrowing, so that adjacent draining nodules become interconnected and the skin is undermined. Suppuration is copious. The process waxes and wanes inexplicably. Hair loss occurs to varying degrees and is chiefly a result of healing with keloid-like scar formation. The fibrotic residue is a conspicuous feature. The process is notoriously chronic, new lesions arising in different areas of the scalp. Un-

---

*Fortunately an obsolete designation.

less checked, the process may involve most of the scalp. Frequently there is concomitant acne. Many types of organisms are recoverable, among which coagulase-positive micrococci predominate, especially in the early stages. Different organisms may be present at different times.

Manual epilation of retained hairs, although tedious, is a helpful procedure in managing dissecting cellulitis of the scalp. Halfway or casual measures have no place in the management of this disease; it is all or nothing. Parenteral antibiotic therapy, after determining the in vitro sensitivity of organisms recovered by culture, is decidedly helpful when given vigorously in large amounts during active periods. Antibacterial-induced improvement is often temporary. Not too much can be expected from purely local application of antibiotics. Surgical procedures aimed at securing drainage by laying open interconnected abscesses and releasing pus from fluctuant nodules are imperative. Estrogen therapy to shrink the sebaceous gland has been shown effective but lacks practicality, since feminization ensues.

Dermatitis Vegetans (Pyoderma Vegetans)

The notable feature of this affliction is exuberant granulation tissue. The disorder ordinarily evolves as an unusual reaction to secondary infection of an antecedent eczematous lesion. In short, dermatitis vegetans is not a disease but a peculiar reaction of chronically inflamed skin to a secondary infection. The underlying antecedent dermatitis is often a seborrheic dermatitis or chronic intertrigo. The bright red vegetative granulation tissue is typically superimposed on chronic eczematous weeping patches, particularly in moist areas such as the axillae, groin, genitalia, and lips. However, the lesions may occasionally originate in skin which is apparently normal, in individuals suffering with almost any serious, chronic, general medical disease which lowers resistance.

The early lesions of dermatitis vegetans are small pustules or vesiculopustules tending to form in groups which soon coalesce, extending to form large weeping inflammatory plaques. The pustules are rarely observed, for they rupture readily.

Suppuration and foul odor are characteristic of neglected cases. A massive crust may form, beneath which the piled up granulations are revealed. Unless checked, the process may eventually develop into a rather huge papillomatous and vegetating mass of granulation tissue. A variety of microorganisms are associated with the lesions, among which coagulase-positive micrococci are common. A basically similar process may originate in the mouth and may remain confined to this area. The primary lesions are minute abscesses which involve the buccal mucosa, hard and soft palates, lips, and the gingiva. Secondary changes due to persistence of the disturbance lead to folding of the mucous membrane and the development of a verrucous surface. This variant has been termed *pyostomatitis vegetans*. It may coexist with typical dermatitis vegetans of the glabrous skin, a circumstance probably not due to chance but rather reflecting a true relationship between the two. Serious systemic disease usually underlies pyostomatitis vegetans.

The lesions of dermatitis vegetans respond moderately well to parenteral antibiotic therapy. Large doses must be administered over a long period. Local application of antibiotic preparations may be a helpful adjunct. The secondary infection can usually be suppressed, even though there may be incomplete healing because of persistence of the underlying disorder. Bland hot compresses are indicated for removing crusts and suppurative debris. Fifty per cent urea compresses are also helpful in deodorizing and in cleansing. Cleanliness is essential and crusts must be prevented from forming; the problems of nursing care are great, and a competent nurse can make a greater contribution than the physician in controlling the disease.

Infectious Eczematoid Dermatitis

This syndrome has been so varyingly defined as to be in danger of being rendered meaningless. It has become a diagnostic term utilized for almost any type of persistent eczematous condition in which an infectious element is presumed. The term is reserved herein for the clinical entity described originally by Engman, whose criteria are the only authoritative ones for defining the disorder. Certain definite traits must be present. The condition arises from a primary lesion which is a source of infectious exudate. This may be a boil, a draining ear or nose, an exudative or suppurative dermatitis, an ulcer, surgical wound, or any secondarily infected process which is a more or less persistent source of drainage. The area involved initially is usually in direct contiguity with the primary exudative or discharging lesion, the wet material of which seeps out over the surrounding area and establishes an acute dermatitis. There is a tendency to the formation of circumscribed, eczematous, scaling plaques in which vesicles or pustules may be prominent. These enlarge gradually, but new plaques not uncommonly arise at a distant site. Autoinoculation is characteristic, whereas the same material placed on the skin of another individual usually fails to excite a lesion. A characteristic sign of the disease is a streak of dermatitis along the path of flow of the discharged material. Coagulase-positive staphylococci are the organisms most frequently isolated.

The pathogenesis of acute infectious eczematoid dermatitis is poorly understood. The establishment of new lesions by autoinoculation indicates the possible major role of infection. An allergic component has not been proved. Physical forces are certainly operative, in that the skin over which there is a continuous drainage of wet, suppurative discharge is rendered more vulnerable. The central feature in pathogenesis is the existence of a primary lesion which is a *true infection,* and the disease itself is a complication of this lesion. Infectious eczematoid dermatitis must be differentiated from many eczematous eruptions, including nummular dermatitis, contact dermatitis, seborrheic dermatitis, "autosensitivity" reactions, and so forth. The disease is treated as any other pyoderma, with special attention to bringing about regression of the original lesion. Compresses may be very helpful and should be combined with parenteral antibacterial therapy. Maceration due to the therapy itself is to be avoided. Local application of antibiotics after compressing may be beneficial. Scrupulous cleanliness is required and the patient should be warned about fingering or scratching the lesions.

Intertrigo

The principal etiologic forces in this disease are mechanical, but chronic bacterial infection eventually becomes operative. The lesions are confined to areas where the skin's surfaces are in close contact. Heat, moisture, and sweat retention combine to cause maceration and irritation, especially in areas where the skin is thin. The favorite sites are the groin, the axillae, between the toes, the intergluteal cleft, and wherever, in adipose individuals, the skin is thrown into folds. The region beneath the pendulous breasts of overweight females is a common site. Almost all chubby infants have some degree of intertrigo. Certain types of diaper rash are simply a form of intertrigo. Many of the cases of maceration between the toes, indiscriminately called athlete's foot, are another instance of intertrigo.

In simple cases of intertrigo the skin is red and slightly macerated, but this may progress to marked hyperemia, complete denudation, and erosion. The accumulation of moisture cannot evaporate freely. This moisture initially derives from unevaporated eccrine sweat, but later the inflammation itself contributes to the moisture by "weeping." The population of resident and transient bacteria increases enormously in these areas, and the decomposition of surface constituents may produce an offensive odor. Bacteria are only one of a host of etiologic forces contributing to intertrigo and are probably more important in perpetuating the lesions than in inciting them. In severe cases, bacterial infection or overgrowth usually becomes an important factor, even though there may be no evidence of secondary infection by the usual criteria. Around the inguinal and perineal areas, feces and urine obviously contribute to the maceration and add to the bacterial flora. Occasionally, an overt suppurative process intervenes, sometimes in the form of cellulitis extending from the fissured folds of skin. Impetigo may be a complication, or pustular miliaria may develop suddenly. The disease must be differentiated from monilial intertrigo by appropriate studies, and also from various types of dermatitis,

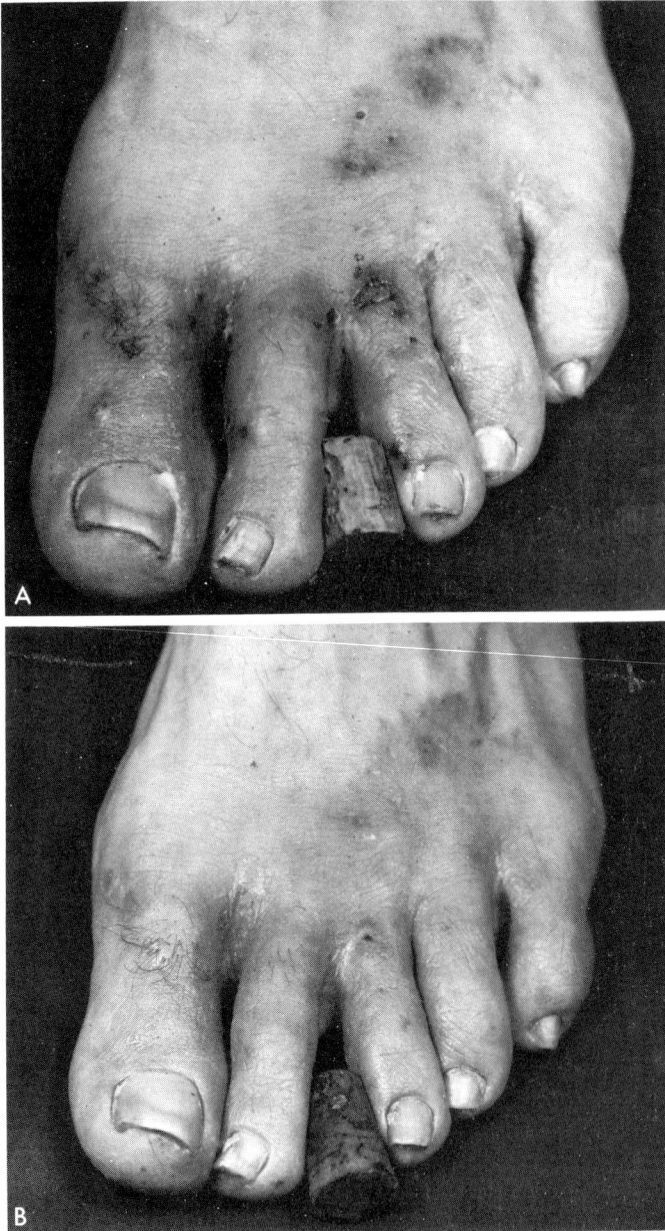

Figure 11-12 *A*, Secondary streptococcal infection arising from chronic intertrigo. *B*, One week after antibiotic therapy and rest.

particularly seborrheic and psoriatic, which may localize in flexural areas. Scaling, usually absent in intertrigo, is a differential point. Scaling between the toes points to fungal infection, not intertrigo.

The aim of treatment is to relieve the mechanical conditions which favor maceration and chafing of apposing surfaces.

A. Physiologic methods to promote drying, combat irritation, and prevent secondary infection.

    1. Thorough cleansing and drying of areas once or twice daily. It is important that all soap be rinsed off. In mild to moderate intertrigo, it is advisable and helpful to rub off macerated skin debris

quite firmly with a dry wash cloth.
2. Liberal use of a simple talc dusting powder (proprietary baby powders are good).
3. Mechanical measures to allow drying and ventilation, for example, "uplift" brassieres, looser drawers, less confining and better ventilated footwear, cotton wisps or pledgets between the toes, and so on.
4. General medical measures in some patients, particularly control of diabetes or reduction diets for obese patients.
5. Avoidance of overuse of occlusive, oily ointments or cosmetic preparations, or of irritant or potentially sensitizing compounds.
6. A cool environment whenever possible. Electric fans directed onto the affected area may be helpful.
B. Pharmacologic measures—in addition to above.
1. Mild to moderate cases.
   a. Topical corticosteroid creams or lotions.

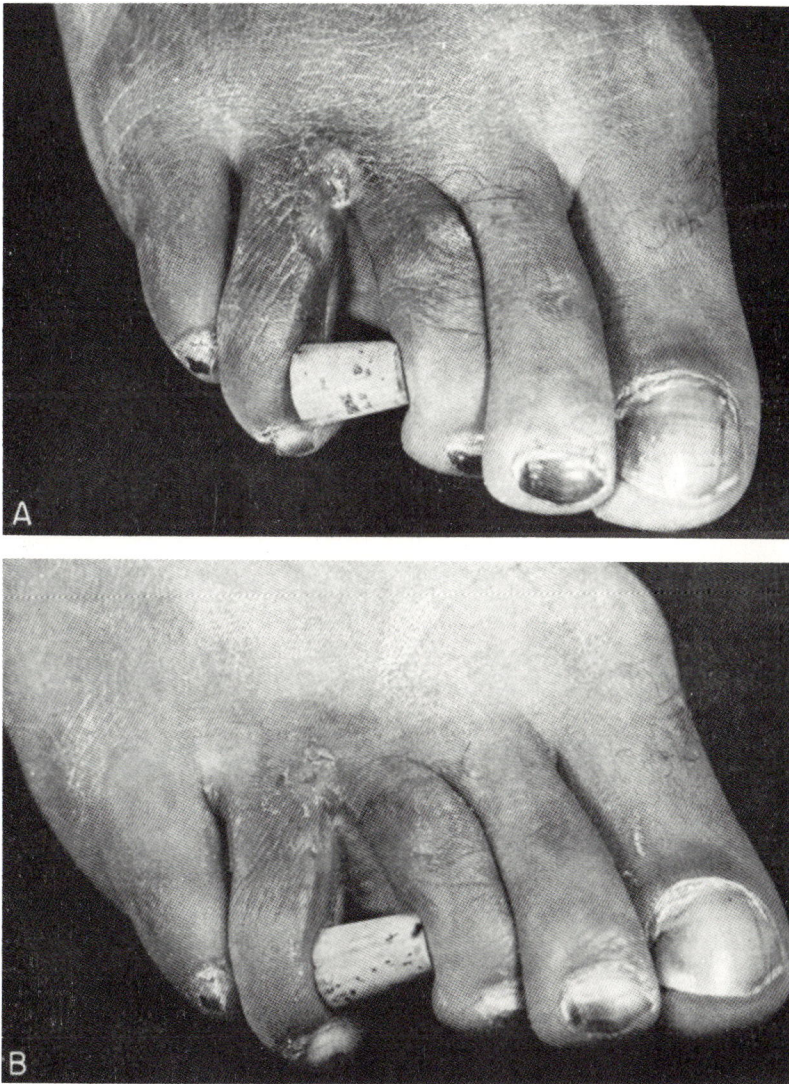

Figure 11–13 *A*, Ulcerated secondary infected fissure. Beta-hemolytic streptococci. *B*, After five days of topical antibacterial therapy. In the pre-antibiotic era, such lesions occasionally led to septicemia and death.

b. Castellani's paint one application daily. The patient
should avoid overusage.
2. More severe cases.
a. Local antibiotic therapy may
be useful if evidence of
secondary infection is
present.
b. Treatment as for impetigo if
there is overt evidence of
superficial bacterial infection.
c. Bland wet compresses.

Otitis Externa

Primary bacterial infection is rarely a
cause; secondary infection is a common
contributory factor.

Pilonidal Cyst

A pilonidal cyst is a congenital lesion in
the midline of the sacral region overlying
the junction of the coccyx with the sacrum.
It may be regarded as a uniquely situated
type of dermoid cyst lined with epithelium and producing hair, sebum, and keratin, which are normally produced by the
epidermis and its appendages. The cyst,
usually single, is seen as a small asymptomatic, congenital dimple over the coccyx.
It either remains undetected or produces
no symptoms until later life, usually between the ages of 17 and 35, when secondary infection occurs. This may in-
augurate a chain of events causing much
distress and severe mutilation of the skin.
The multiplicity of organisms, especially
coliforms, which inhabit the infected cysts
and sinuses clearly points to their playing
only a secondary role. Permanent control
of the disease is not accomplished by antibacterial measures and simple drainage.
Surgical excision is the only curative
method; if it is to be effective and to prevent recurrence, the sinus tracts must be
explored and all viable epithelial elements removed. This is not always simple,
and surgical failures are common.

Ulcers in Which Infection Plays a Role and Which are Clinical Entities by Virtue of Distinct Morphologic Characteristics

It is helpful from a didactic standpoint to
consider in a group all ulcers, whether primary or secondary, in which bacteria have
etiologic significance. In fact, bacteria are
the primary etiologic agents of only a few
ulcerative conditions. Any ulcer, of course,
may become secondarily infected with
bacteria, and most of these will be of the
nondescript type not requiring any further discussion here; common examples
are secondarily infected varicose ulcers
and traumatic ulcers due to burns, chemicals, and mechanical injuries. There are
two main classes of ulcers which have
characteristic clinical and morphologic
features: (1) the infectious gangrenes (primary bacterial diseases), and (2) the
phagedenic ulcers (secondary bacterial infections). The diseases included within
these groups may be classified as follows:
1. Infectious Gangrene
a. Gas gangrene.
b. Hemolytic streptococcus gangrene.
2. Phagedenic ulcers
a. Burrowing phagedenic ulcers (synonyms: Meleney's chronic undermining ulcer, progressive
bacterial synergistic gangrene).
b. Circumscribed phagedenic ulcers
(synonyms: infectious multiple
gangrene of the skin, dermatitis
gangrenosum, gangrenous impetigo).
c. Tropical phagedenic ulcer.
d. Desert sore.

INFECTIOUS GANGRENE. These are primary infections of a decidedly acute nature. They are uncommon in civil practice
but constitute an important aspect of military combat surgery.

Gas Gangrene. The usual organisms
are several species of Clostridium, which
normally inhabit the soil and the bowel.
Clostridium perfringens is the most important of them. The infection is a myositis,
which begins mostly in deep, crushing,
tissue-destroying wounds into which there
is usually incorporated soil, bits of clothing, and other foreign debris.

In a series of cases reviewed by Altemeier and Fullen (1971), the average incubation time was 53 hours. The earliest
sign is pain, followed by tachycardia and
hypotension. Early lesions are typically
white, shiny, and tense, and later ones appear discolored and vesicular (Altemeier
and Fullen, 1971). In the final stage, the
peripheral portions of the wound become

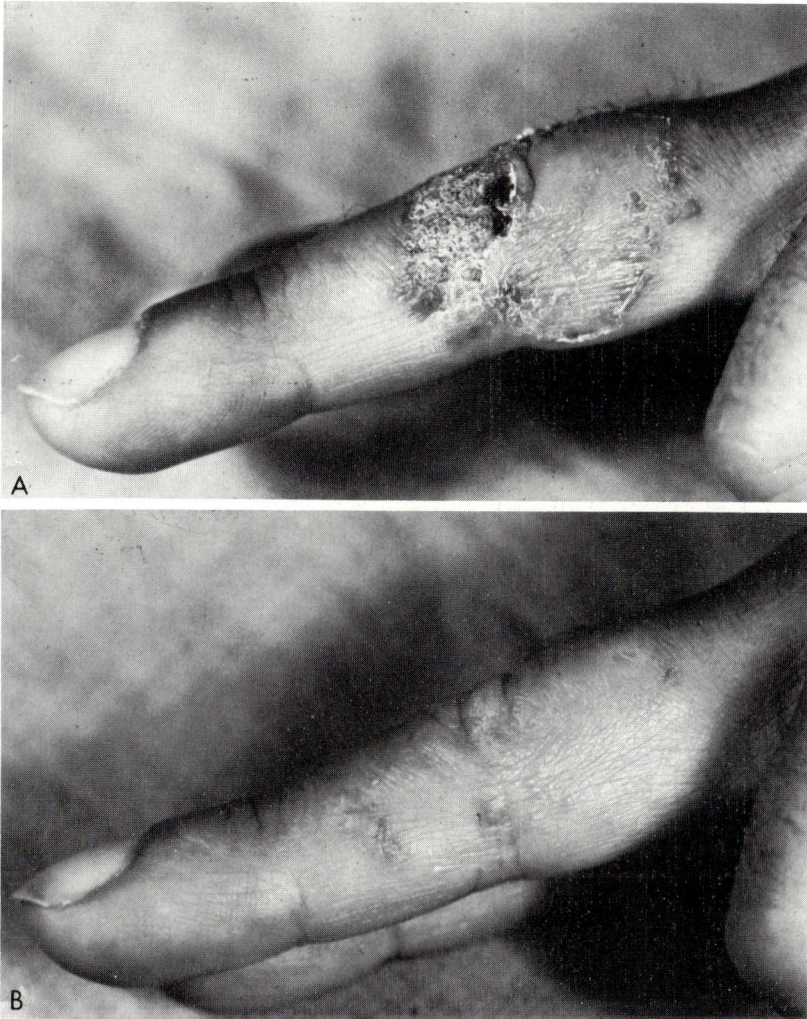

Figure 11–14   Dermatitis repens. *A,* Superficial dissecting vesiculopustular eruption in which infection may be present but is not of primary etiologic importance. Chronic and recurrent. *B,* Improvement after hydrocortisone ointment for one week. This improvement was not permanent.

frankly necrotic and gangrenous. Early skin lesions may show a positive Nikolsky sign. The important sign, crepitation due to accumulation of gas in the tissue, may be elicited by pressure on the margin of the wound. Crepitation may be absent. An x-ray may help to differentiate the gas produced by clostridia from that due to mechanical causes.

Therapy consists of medical and, most important, surgical measures. Penicillin is the antibiotic of choice and is given intravenously in large doses, usually concomitant with tetracycline. Neutralization of the toxin by means of injecting polyvalent gas gangrene antitoxin is done in patients with toxemia. Steroids may be given for septic shock. Hyperbaric oxygen therapy has been used, but its value has not been established. These measures will prove ineffective, however, unless quick and thorough surgical debridement of dead, devitalized tissue is accomplished. The organisms of gas gangrene are the vultures of the bacterial world and will not disperse as long as dead and dying tissue is available to them.

Hemolytic Streptococcus Gangrene. This is a rare disease. Its onset is marked by acute development of pain and swelling

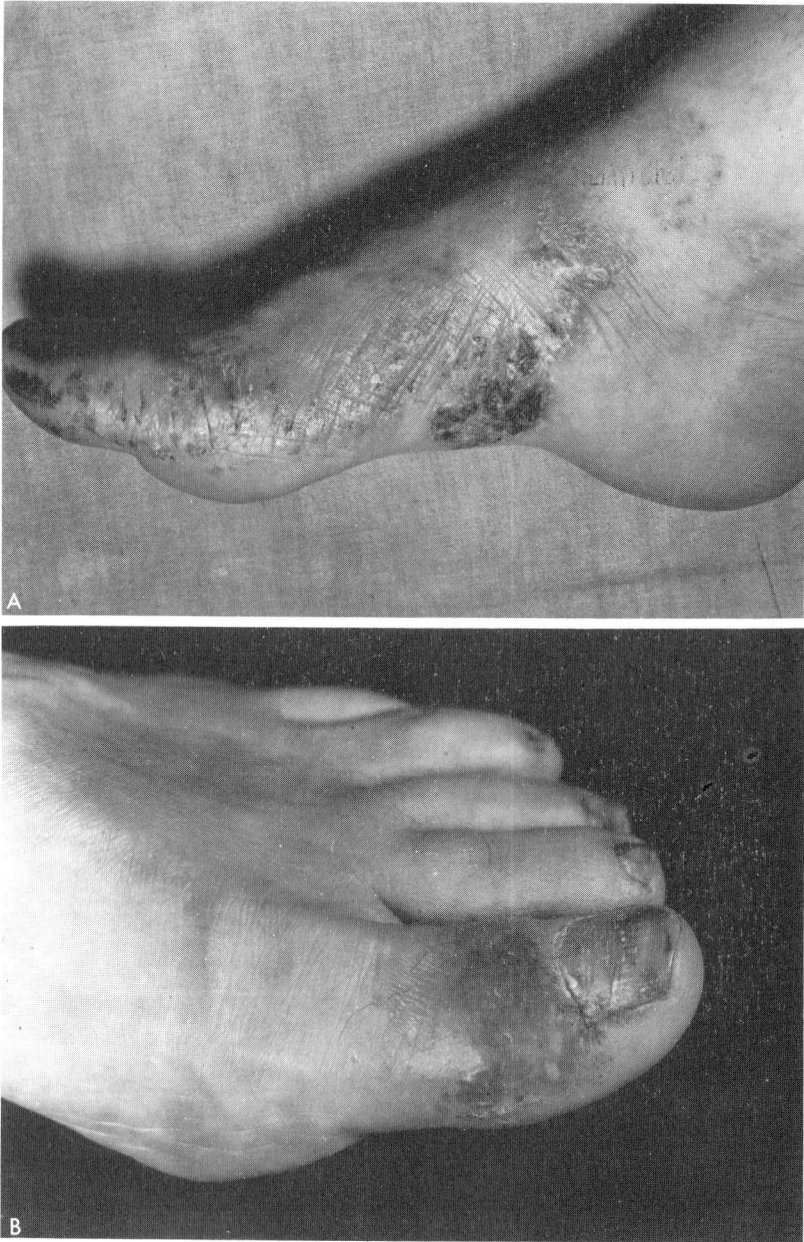

Figure 11–15 *A*, Chronic eczematous dermatitis with low-grade secondary infection. *B*, Trauma from shoe plus superficial streptococcal infection. Attention to both factors is essential to cure.

at the site of some wound or injury. The area becomes hot, edematous, and red, and as it gradually enlarges, a pathognomonic sign develops between the second and fourth day. The affected skin assumes a bluish, dusky tinge which represents the onset of true necrosis. The bluish skin breaks, revealing a large gangrenous plaque which becomes sharply demarcated from the rest of the skin. The disease is basically a gangrene of the subcutaneous tissue, with subsequent necrosis of the overlying skin. It is possible that many cases listed under the name are actually examples of necrotizing fasciitis. If the infection is unchecked, prostration, high fever, and possibly death will follow. Beta-hemolytic streptococci are easily isolated from the spreading borders, but later a multiplicity of bacteria may colonize the necrotic plaque. Penicillin, sulfonamides, or any of the broad-spectrum antibiotics to which the beta-hemolytic streptococcus is susceptible are exceedingly useful in controlling the disease. Vigorous supportive treatment and appropriate surgical measures may be indicated.

PHAGEDENIC ULCERS (with or without gangrenous aspects). Under this heading it seems appropriate to group a host of entities which, in the past, have been largely regarded as independent conditions. It is abundantly clear that many ulcerative lesions which have been separately described at different times under different names, a circumstance which has produced endless confusion and perpetuation of polysyllabic nomenclature, have much in common. If one searches for the singular characteristic of the members of this disorganized collection of clinical conditions, it becomes obvious that they may be consolidated into a single group. The essential qualifications for valid status in the group are:

1. The presence of a necrotizing lesion in which tissue destruction is prominent, hence the name *phagedenic* ulcers. In this respect, attention must be drawn to the casual and inappropriate use of the term gangrene. Tissue death does not qualify a lesion as gangrenous, a common misconception. Many entities regarded as examples of gangrene because of necrotic aspects are falsely named, because gangrene implies a particularly severe and irreversible type of massive destruction, ending in complete devitalization. Of course, the boundary between simple necrosis and gangrene is necessarily indistinct. Furthermore, gangrene can supervene in any ulcerative lesion, but it is then a secondary phenomenon. It is believed that gangrene is not an essential or characteristic aspect of the entities which may properly be included in the phagedenic ulcer group.

2. Phagedenic ulcers are secondary lesions. They do not originate in the normal skin of normal people. Instead, they arise either in a preexisting cutaneous lesion or on the apparently normal skin of individuals who, because of antecedent systemic disease, have very low resistance. A number of bacterial species are encountered in phagedenic ulcers; obviously they are playing a secondary role, taking up their residence in a situation where the host cannot present an adequate defense.

Burrowing Phagedenic Ulcers (synonyms: Meleney's chronic undermining ulcer, progressive synergistic bacterial gangrene). The cardinal characteristic of this type of ulcer is its markedly undermined border along with the tendency to extend insidiously until large ulcerative plaques are formed. However, deep downward extension into the muscles and fascia does not occur. The lesion may be initiated in a number of ways. It may develop at the wound site of an intestinal operation, particularly if this is followed by drainage of purulent material, or from the discharge of a subcutaneous abscess or a ruptured lymph node. These are the types which have been described by surgeons and which are so well known to them under the name of Meleney's undermining ulcer. In addition, the lesion may originate in any type of traumatic wound, including a needle puncture, or it may rarely complicate a furuncle, particularly in individuals in poor health.

The borders of these burrowing ulcers are slightly raised, edematous, and boggy, and usually have a distinct bluish purple color. Beyond this border there is an erythematous areola which fades into normal skin. The central portion of the ulcers is foul and is covered with mucopurulent exudate, removal of which generally reveals a clean, granulating base. The margins are polycyclic or serpiginous and show the distinctive feature of being rolled under and undermined, although this is not a pathognomonic sign. As the ulcer extends, the central portion tends to heal. Such ulcers are ordinarily not gangrenous, but such a complication is not impossible. The elementary lesions developing on the normal skin of weakened persons are groups of discrete pustules which break down, coalesce, and finally ulcerate. There are, of course, no elementary lesions when the process begins in a draining wound or a preexisting skin lesion.

Many different types of organisms have been recovered from such lesions. These include "pathogenic" micrococci and streptococci, as well as gram-negative rods, most of which are not very virulent. Meleney believes that the actual extension of this lesion is due to a concentration of microaerophilic hemolytic streptococci in the border. Although this organism may have been overlooked by other investigators because of their failure to grow cultures under reduced oxygen tension, it is still uncertain as to whether or not it is *constantly* found in this type of ulcer or that the lesion can be precisely correlated with a specific microbial flora.

The treatment of such extensive ulcers requires a vigorous attack on the primary underlying condition. The state of the ulcer is a measure of the general health of the patient, providing an index to the degree of resistance. In certain instances, there may be a specific biochemical defect that is responsible for the vulnerability of the skin to infection: hypogammaglobulinemia.

Vigorous parenteral antibiotic therapy is indicated for the skin lesions. The microflora of the ulcer, particularly in the spreading border, should be accurately determined by refined bacteriologic methods, and the sensitivity of the recovered organisms evaluated. From this, the appropriate antibiotics can be selected. Bland compresses to keep the wound clean and freely draining are helpful. If the process cannot be brought under control and is not too extensive, surgical excision and plastic repair should be considered.

Circumscribed Phagedenic Ulcers (synonyms: infectious multiple gangrene of the skin, dermatitis gangrenosum, dermatitis gangrenosum infantum, gangrenous impetigo). As with the previous groups, the term gangrene for these lesions is inappropriate. What is ordinarily meant is a destructive, necrotizing process usually superimposed upon some preexisting cutaneous lesion in an individual whose resistance has been lowered by ill health. Prior to the modern era, clinicians occasionally had an opportunity to see such circumscribed ulcers as sequelae to varicella and vaccinia, especially in infants who were emaciated and cachectic. In a child with poor resistance, even a simple chickenpox lesion may fail to heal, and because of local devitalization, different types of organisms, among which micrococci and streptococci predominate, may bring about

tissue necrosis, with the formation of a slough. These ulcers tend to remain small, usually not more than an inch or two in diameter, and do not enlarge indefinitely. The borders are well defined, are not undermined, and there is an erythematous areola. The central area contains a mucopurulent slough which may be black, but underneath there is a red granulating base.

Treatment requires an attack on the primary condition. The bacterial organisms are purely secondary invaders. After their sensitivity is determined, appropriate parenteral and local antibiotic therapy may be given.

Tropical Phagedenic Ulcer. This disease is seen mainly among the barefooted people of certain tropical and semitropical countries where the general standards of nutrition, hygiene, and personal care are low. It occurs in young male adults and is almost always found on the lower extremities. The lesion evolves as a complication of some preexisting cutaneous injury — a cut, abrasion, insect bite, burn, or even an antecedent local bacterial infection such as impetigo or furunculosis. In addition, neglect and failure to maintain adequate hygiene, especially following traumatic injuries to the lower extremities, is almost always a factor. Simple hygienic first aid techniques for minor injuries and infections would probably prevent tropical ulcers. The ulcers may be single or multiple and, though usually several inches in diameter, may reach a much larger size. The appearance is quite characteristic, having a remarkably circular outline, with a distinctly elevated and undermined bluish red border. The ulcer has been likened to a cup; a foul smelling mucopurulent slough, often blood-tinged, is generally present in the cavity. Removal of the slough reveals granulation tissue. Unlike other phagedenic ulcers, the process may extend deeply downward to expose tendons, muscles, and even bones, although ordinarily it is not common for the tissues below the deep fascia to become involved. Deep dissection and occasional explosive extension are peculiarities of this process, which otherwise is not greatly different from other phagedenic ulcers. The average case heals in six weeks to three months. The patient's general health often remains surprisingly good.

A variety of microorganisms are recover-

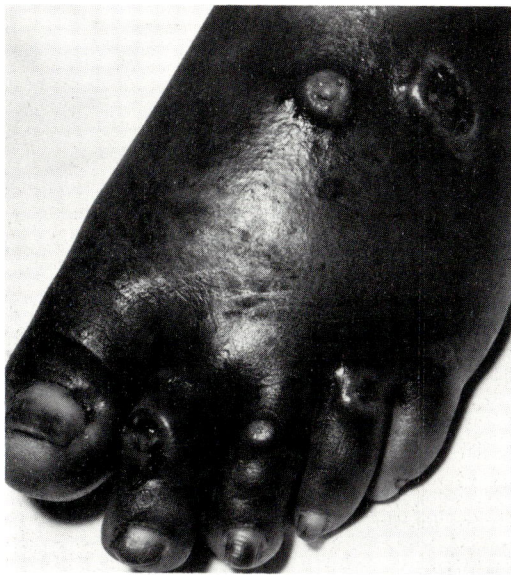

Figure 11–16 Multiple "tropical" ulcers. The extension of such lesions may be phenomenally rapid.

able from tropical phagedenic ulcers. One of these, an anaerobic fusiform bacillus, is constantly present in the flora. Smears of pus taken from early lesions routinely reveal gram-positive fusiform bacilli and occasionally spirochetes which, however, are no longer held to be important in pathogenesis, though in the past. tropical ulcer was regarded as a fusospirochetal disease. The main diseases to be distinguished are cutaneous diphtheritic ulcer, cutaneous leishmaniasis, yaws, leprosy, syphilis, and ecthyma.

The important principles of treatment include rest of the affected part, maintenance of local cleanliness by bland compresses applied frequently enough to keep the wound clean, and the administration of penicillin or other antibiotics. Response to this treatment is rapid and gratifying.

Desert Sore (veldt sore or Barcoo rot). It is uncertain whether this condition, which occurs in South Africa and Australia, is a valid disease. It is certainly not an entity etiologically and probably represents a nondescript infected ulcer developing from some secondarily antecedent neglected lesion. The initial lesions are said to be vesicles and pustules oc-

curring on the dorsa of the hands and forearms, which subsequently evolve into painful, crusted purulent ulcers. These are indolent, multiple, of various sizes and shapes, and may last for weeks or months. The condition is ill-defined and undoubtedly has been confused occasionally with diphtheritic ulcer, ecthyma, and possibly infectious eczematoid dermatitis.

Pseudofolliculitis of the Beard

Exceedingly common as this disorder is, it is altogether remarkable that until recently there has been so much confusion about its pathogenesis, with so little appreciation of its perfectly obvious etiologic factors. Not even a standard name has been adopted, and the one by which most dermatologists knew it, chronic sycosis barbae, has turned out to be a misnomer, for the disease is definitely not a folliculitis and bacteria clearly do not play a primary role.

The disorder occurs predominantly in the beard of Negroes, chiefly in the submandibular region of the neck; it is found only in those who shave, and remission invariably occurs when affected patients give up shaving. The characteristic lesions are erythematous papules, less commonly pustules, containing buried hairs, whose tips can easily be freed up. In affected areas, the hairs are strikingly disoriented, showing no apparent grain and emerging in all directions, with a strong tendency to hug the skin's surface closely. The primary abnormality is the presence of strongly recurved hairs which emerge from curved follicles, shortly reentering the skin and growing downward into it as if to complete a 360-degree circle. The reentrance of such hairs into the skin produces an *ingrown hair*, the sine qua non of the disease.

Strongly curved beard hairs are a racial trait of Negroes, singling them out as particular victims of the disease; Caucasians with similar types of beard hair are not exempt. In fact, a few ingrown hairs are to be found now and then in the beards of most persons. The other factor in pathogenesis which abets the inflammatory reaction provoked by the ingrown hair is an

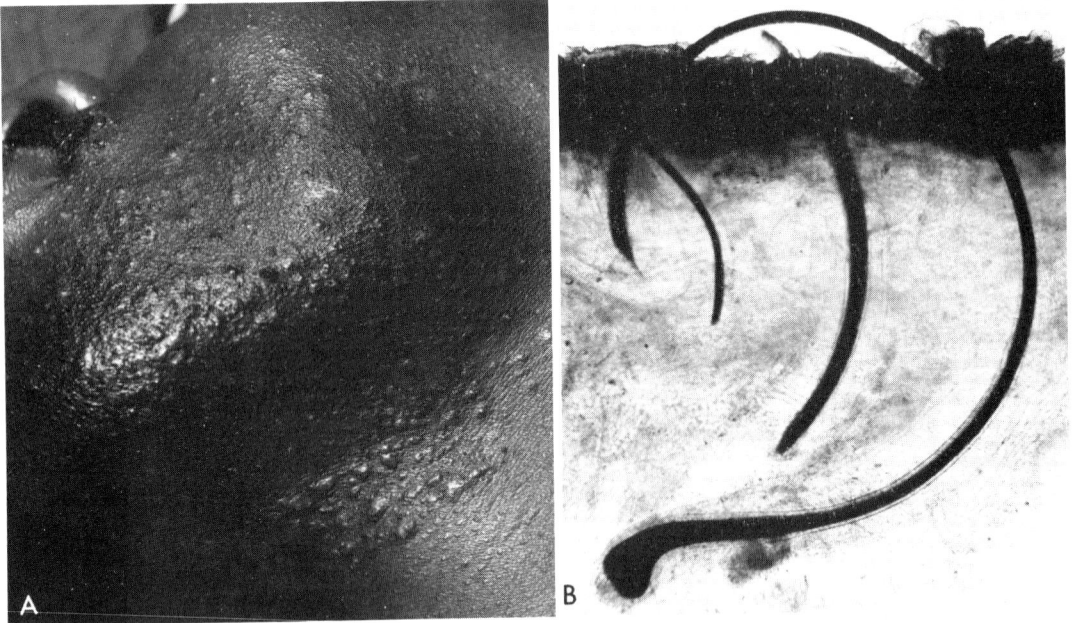

Figure 11–17　Pseudofolliculitis of the beard. *A*, Severe case with numerous papules. *B*, Ingrown hair, transcribing almost a complete circle.

invariable secondary infection by the normal skin micrococci, a phenomenon beautifully illustrating the principle that so-called nonpathogenic organisms, in this case normal resident bacteria, are capable of becoming pathogenic when there is impairment of the host defenses. Organisms generally considered pathogenic are not ordinarily associated with the disorder, but occasionally they are responsible for a superimposed pyogenic infection leading to impetiginization with oozing and crusting.

Shaving is a prerequisite for maintaining the disorder, for a certain percentage of hair tips tightly hugging the surface are missed and these subsequently may form ingrown hairs. Because the hairs emerge practically parallel with the surface, shaving necessarily cuts the hairs obliquely, resulting in sharp tips which doubtless facilitate penetration. Subsequently, some of these sharpened hairs will be missed in shaving and will reenter the skin. On the other hand, if shaving is given up, the hair tips will reenter the skin, to be sure, but as growth continues, the downward penetration reaches a maximum depth of 2 to 3 mm. and thereafter the external segment will form an ever increasing loop,

finally acting like a spring to pull the ingrown tip out, a process invariably resulting in spontaneous involution of the disease. Only short, stiff hairs can reenter the skin, for the long ones simply bend; shaving creates these short hairs. If shaving were really complete all the hairs would be cut just as they emerged and ingrown hairs would be prevented, but this cannot be accomplished with safety or electric razors. A straight razor overcomes this difficulty but creates an equally noxious one of cutting the hairs too short. A really "close" shave requires that the skin be put under tension; when tension is released, some of the hairs retract beneath the surface. These subsequently pierce the follicular wall before emerging. No system or schedule of shaving can cure this disorder but, on the contrary, is the exciting cause of it. Moreover, since bacterial infection is a secondary process, locally applied antibiotic agents often palliate the disease, decreasing the inflammatory component, but can hardly cure it when nothing is done about the primary cause, the ingrown hair.

Chemical depilation offers a practical means of controlling, if not totally curing, pseudofolliculitis of the beard. The precise advantage of chemical depilation is that the exposed tip of the hair is cleanly removed at the skin surface, avoiding the complications of cutting the hair too short, as with a straight razor, or not short enough, as with safety or electric razors. No free tips are available for reentry, either intra- or extrafollicularly. Commercially available lotion type depilatories containing thioglycolates have proved best, for these are the least irritating; even these, however, will not be well tolerated by most skins when used daily. A practical scheme is an application every two or three days. Even though the hair is allowed to grow for two or three days, the cosmetic limitation is usually not embarrassing because the short stubble of Negro hair is not conspicuous against pigmented skin and, furthermore, such hairs hug the surface. Razor shaving is interdicted on the days when the depilatory is not used, for it increases the irritation. The depilating lotion is liberally applied and allowed to remain on the face for 10 to 15 minutes; it is then gently scraped away with a flat stick or a safety razor containing no blade. The concomitant use of antibiotic agents does not improve the results. In mild cases, gentle shaving in the direction of hair growth may be all that is required.

Blastomycosis-like Pyoderma

This disorder is a secondary cutaneous bacterial infection of malnourished individuals in a poor state of health, whose low resistance enables potential pathogens such as coagulase-positive micrococci and beta-hemolytic streptococci to become established. The first lesion generally develops at a site of trauma, but thereafter new ones arise on apparently normal skin. The gross characteristics are practically indistinguishable from cutaneous blastomycosis, displaying peripherally enlarging circinate plaques healing centrally by scar formation. The borders are elevated, fungating, strongly verrucous, and contain a heavy crust, the removal of which reveals numerous abscesses exuding a purulent exudate. A foul odor is produced by the copious suppuration; in this respect the disorder differs somewhat from true blastomycosis.

The patients so far encountered have been chronic alcoholics. Therapy consists of restoring the individual to good health by proper diet and sensible hygienic management, accompanied by vigorous cleaning of the skin (frequent soap and water baths) and by administration of antibiotics and sulfonamides. Large doses should be given. Healing leaves a scar.

REFERENCES

Acton, H. W., and McGuire, C.: Keratolysis plantare sulcatum. Lesion due to Actinomycetic fungus. Indian Med. Gaz. 65:61, 1930.

Altemeier, W., and Fullen, W.: Prevention and treatment of gas gangrene. J.A.M.A. 217:806, 1971.

Aly, R., Maibach, H., Shinefield, H., et al.: Bacterial interference among strains of S. aureus in man. J. Infect. Dis. 1974 (in press).

Amonette, R. A., and Rosenberg, E. W.: Infection of toe webs by gram-negative bacteria. Arch. Dermatol. 107:71, 1973.

Bannatyne, R., Skowron, P., and Weber, J.: Job's syndrome—a variant of chronic granulomatous disease. J. Pediatr. 75:236, 1969.

Branom, W. T., Hyman, A. B., and Rubin, Z.: Chancriform pyoderma. Arch. Dermatol. 87:736, 1963.

Burnett, J. H.: Uncommon bacterial infections of the skin. Arch. Dermatol. 86:597, 607, 1962.

Castellani, A.: Keratoma plantare sulcatum. J. Ceylon Br. Med. Assoc. January, 1910.

Collins, R. N., and Nadel, M. S.: Gangrene due to the hemolytic streptococcus—a rare but treatable disease. N. Engl. J. Med. 272:578, 1965.

Crissey, J. T., Rebell, G. C., and Laskas, J. J.: Studies on causative organism of trichomycosis axillaris. J. Invest. Dermatol. 19:187, 1952.

Davis, S., Schaller, J., and Wedgewood, R.: Job's syndrome. Lancet 1:1013, 1966.

Ferrieri, P., Dajani, A., Wannamaker, L., et al.: Natural history of impetigo. J. Clin. Invest. 51:2851, 1972.

Frain-Bell, W.: Pyoderma chancriforme faciei. Br. J. Dermatol. 69:19, 1957.

Freeman, R. G., McBride, M. E., and Knox, J. M.: Pathogenesis of trichomycosis axillaris. Arch. Dermatol. 100:90, 1969.

Fulton, J., McGinley, K., Leyden, J., et al.: Gram-negative folliculitis in acne vulgaris. Arch. Dermatol. 98:349, 1968.

Gill, K. A., Jr., and Buckels, L. J.: Pitted keratolysis. Arch. Dermatol. 98:7, 1968.

Hildick-Smith, G., Blank, H., and Sarkany, I.: Fungus Diseases and Their Treatment. Boston, Little, Brown & Co., 1964.

Kansky, A.: Botryomycosis. Acta Dermatovener. 44:369, 1964.

Katznelsen, D., Vawter, G. F., Foley, G. E., et al.: Botryomycosis, a complication in cystic fibrosis. J. Pediatr. 65:525, 1964.

Layman, C. W., Balough, C., and Dixon, A.: Chancriform pyoderma. Am. J. Syph. 38:57, 1954.

Maibach, H. I.: Scalp pustules due to *Corynebacterium acnes*. Arch. Dermatol. 96:453, 1967.

Maibach, H., and Hildick-Smith, G.: Skin Bacteria and Their Role in Infection. New York, McGraw-Hill Book Co., Blakiston Division, 1965.

Maibach, H., and Kligman, A.: Multiple sweat gland abscesses. J.A.M.A. *174*:140, 1960.

Maibach, H., and Kligman, A.: Staphylococcus toxoid: A controlled clinical study. Proc. XII Internat. Cong. Dermatol., Internat. Cong. Series 55, Except. Med. Fdn., 1962, p. 1035.

Maibach, H., Marples, R., and Taplin, D.: Cutaneous bacteriology. *In* Rook, A., (ed.): Recent Advances in Dermatology. Edinburgh, Churchill Livingstone, 1973, pp. 1–32.

Maibach, H., Strauss, W. G., and Shinefield, H.: Bacterial interference therapy in the management of recurrent furunculosis. Br. J. Dermatol. *1*:67, 1969.

McBride, M. E., and Freeman, R. G.: The bacteriology of trichomycosis axillaris. Br. J. Dermatol. *80*:509, 1968.

Montes, L. F., Dobson, H., Dodge, B. G., et al.: Erythrasma and diabetes mellitus. Arch. Dermatol. *99*:674, 1969.

Munro-Ashman, D., Wells, R. S., and Clayton, Y. M.: Erythrasma in adolescence. Br. J. Dermatol. *75*:401, 1963.

Orfanos, C. E., Schloesser, E., and Mahrle, G.: Hair destroying growth of *Corynebacterium tenuis* in the so-called trichomycosis axillaris. Arch. Dermatol. *103*:632, 1971.

Rea, W., and Wyrick, W.: Necrotizing fasciitis. Ann. Surg. *172*:957, 1970.

Sarkany, I., Taplin, D., and Blank, H.: The etiology and treatment of erythrasma. J. Invest. Dermatol. 37:283, 1961.

Sarkany, I., Taplin, D., and Blank, H.: Incidence and bacteriology of erythrasma. Arch. Dermatol. 85:578, 1962.

Sarkany, I., Taplin, D., and Blank, H.: Organism causing erythrasma. Lancet 2:304, 1962.

Shinefield, H., Ribble, J., and Moris, M.: Bacterial interference between strains of *Staphylococcus aureus*. Am. J. Dis. Child. *121*:148, 1971.

Singh, G., Marples, R., and Kligman, A.: Experimental Staphylococcus aureus infections in humans. J. Invest. Dermatol. 57:149, 1971.

Stone, O. J., and Mullins, J. F.: Experimental studies on chronic paronychia. Arch. Dermatol. 89:455, 1964.

Taplin, D., and Zaias, N.: Etiology of pitted keratolysis. Report of XII Internat. Cong. Dermatol., Internat. Cong. Series 55, Except. Med. Fed., 1962, p. 593.

Temple, D. E., and Boardman, C. R.: The incidence of erythrasma of the toe webs. Arch. Dermatol. 86:518, 1962.

Waisman, M.: Staphylococcic actinophytosis (botryomycosis). Arch. Dermatol. 86:525, 1962.

Wannamaker, L. W., and Matson, J. M.: Streptococci and Streptococcal Diseases. 2nd ed. New York, Academic Press, 1974.

Winslow, D. J.: Botryomycosis. Am. J. Pathol. 35:153, 1959.

Zaias, N., Taplin, D., and Rebell, G.: Pitted keratolysis. Arch. Dermatol. 92:151, 1965.

Section III

SYSTEMIC BACTERIAL AND NONVENEREAL SPIROCHETAL INFECTIONS

Richard Baughman

SYSTEMIC BACTERIAL INFECTIONS

This heterogeneous group of bacterial infections has in common the ability or probability for systemic dissemination. The skin may simply be the portal of entry, as in bubonic plague, or it may provide diagnosis on clinical grounds alone, as in gonococcemia, when bacteriologic measures fail. The bacteria may produce a powerful exotoxin (anthrax, diphtheria) or endotoxin (meningococcemia). Man may be the sole reservoir (as with meningococcus, gonococcus) or he may be incidentally affected by the vector in a complex animal-vector cycle (for example, plague). The ulceroglandular phases of many of these diseases (anthrax, diphtheria, erysipeloid, glanders, melioidosis, rat-bite fever, plague, *Pasteurella multocida* infection or tularemia) challenge the clinician to recognize and treat before the serious or even fatal dissemination occurs. He must recognize the need for special culture media and handling, and he must be aware of changes in appropriate antibiotic

TABLE 11–1 Systemic Bacterial and Nonvenereal Spirochetal Infections

Bacterial Infections

Gram-Negative:
Neisseria meningitidis—meningococcemia
Neisseria gonorrhoeae—gonococcemia
Pseudomonas aeruginosa
Salmonella infection
Haemophilus influenzae
Brucella organisms—brucellosis
Francisella (Pasteurella) tularensis—tularemia
Pasteurella (Yersinia) pestis—plague
Pasteurella multocida
Bartonella bacilliformis—bartonellosis (Carrion's disease)
Streptobacillus moniliformis—rat-bite fever
Pseudomonas pseudomallei—melioidosis
Malleomyces mallei—glanders

Gram-Positive:
Bacillus anthracis—anthrax
Corynebacterium diphtheriae—diphtheria
Erysipelothrix rhusiopathiae—erysipeloid
Clostridium perfringens (C. welchii)—gas gangrene
Listeria monocytogenes—listerosis

Spirochetal Nonvenereal Infections

Spirillum minus—rat-bite fever
Borrelia recurrentis—relapsing fever
Leptospira species—Weil's disease, pretibial fever

management caused by emergence of resistant strains and availability of new agents. The signs and pathogenicity of these infections cannot be thoroughly interpreted without an understanding of the effects of septic shock, endotoxin, and disseminated intravascular coagulation.

Septic Shock

Septic shock is a dynamic syndrome, induced by infections in which inadequate tissue perfusion results. Although gram-negative bacteremia is the most common cause of the syndrome, it may also result from endotoxin, an exotoxin, direct local bacterial invasion, or mechanical obstruction of blood flow to a vital organ. Predisposing factors include age, debility, burns, cancer, diabetes, transfusions, surgical procedures, and drugs, particularly corticosteroids, broad-spectrum antibiotics, and immunosuppressive agents.

In the early responsive stage of warm shock, the patient is hypotensive but the pulse remains full, the skin is warm and dry, and urinary output is adequate. Without successful treatment of the underlying cause, cold shock ensues, with rapid weak pulse, diaphoresis, pallor, cyanosis, venous collapse, anuria, and a very high mortality rate.

The shock may be due to one or a combination of the following factors: (1) cardiac failure from intrinsic disease or an exotoxin, such as that of diphtheria; (2) volume depletion from severe gastroenteritis, such as that induced by the salmonellae; or (3) peripheral vascular failure.

Therapeutically, prevention by careful attention to predisposing causes and by prompt and vigorous treatment of the infection is the most important step. The central venous pressure must be monitored with or without blood volume determinations in order to assess the cardiac status and the extent of intrinsic or extrinsic volume loss. Blood gases must be monitored with arterial samples in order to direct therapy of the inevitable acidosis, whether metabolic or respiratory. Vasopressors must be used with care: "Tissue perfusion must never be sacrificed for the sake of a rise in peripheral arterial pressure" (Weinstein and Klainer, 1966). The use of antihistamines, corticosteroids, hypothermia, and vasodilators remains controversial.

Endotoxin

Endotoxins exist in the intact cell wall of gram-negative bacteria as protein-lipid-polysaccharide complexes. Lysis of cells releases the active lipid-polysaccharide component whose action is the same, regardless of the inherent pathogenicity of the organism or its antigenic structure. Many phenomena have been attributed to endotoxin (Rosen, 1961), including pyrogenicity, antigenicity, tolerance, lethal shock, and the local or the generalized Shwartzman reaction. Localized vascular damage may evoke a generalized activation of the hemostatic mechanism, leading to disseminated intravascular coagulation.

The human equivalent of the experimental Shwartzman reaction may occur. In animals, the "localized" Shwartzman reaction is produced by the preparatory injection of endotoxin intradermally without reaction. The provoking dose of endotoxin (or even a nonbacterial product) adminis-

TABLE 11–2   Systemic Bacterial and Nonvenereal Spirochetal Infections Involving the Skin

Disease	Organism	Gram Stain	Culture Requirements	Reservoir	Transmission	Portal of Entry	Cutaneous Characteristics	Therapy
Meningococcemia	Neisseria meningitidis	gram neg.	chocolate agar, CO_2	man	airborne	respiratory	purpura	penicillin
Gonorrhea	Neisseria gonorrhoeae	gram neg.	Thayer-Martin VCN	man	sexual contact	mucosa	hemorrhagic vesicopustule	penicillin (TCN)°
Pseudomonas	Pseudomonas aeruginosa	gram neg.	blood agar	man, soil	direct, fomites	skin, catheters	pain, necrosis, color, odor	gentamicin, carbenicillin
Salmonellosis	Salmonella typhi, other salmonellae	gram neg.	selective	man / animals, fowl	food, water	G.I.	rose spot	chloro°° (ampicillin)
H. Influ. cellulitis	Haemophilus influenzae	gram neg.	chocolate agar	man	airborne	respiratory	cellulitis	ampicillin
Brucellosis	Brucella abortus, B. suis, B. melitensis	gram neg.	chocolate agar, CO_2	domestic and wild animals	contact, milk	skin, G.I.	rare	TCN
Tularemia	Francisella tularensis	gram neg.	cysteine blood, thioglycollate	rabbit, muskrat	contact, ticks, flies	skin	ulceroglandular	streptomycin (TCN, chloro)
Plague	Pasteurella pestis	gram neg.	blood agar	rodents	contact, flea	skin, respiratory	buboes	Streptomycin
Pasteurella multocida infection	Pasteurella multocida (P. septica)	gram neg.	blood agar	domestic and wild animals	late or scratch	skin, rarely respiratory	cellulitis, infrequently ulceroglandular	penicillin, tetracycline
Bartonellosis	Bartonella bacilliformis	gram neg.	blood agar, slow	man	sand fly	skin	verruga	penicillin
Rat-bite fever (Streptobacillary)	Streptobacillus moniliformis	gram neg.	blood culture, slow	rodents, wild and laboratory	bite / milk (Haverhill)	skin G.I.	ulceroglandular exanthem	penicillin

(Table 11–2 continued on the opposite page.)

Disease	Organism	Stain	Culture	Reservoir	Transmission	Site	Manifestation	Treatment
Rat-bite fever (Sodoku)	Spirillum minus	Giemsa		rodents, wild and laboratory	bite	skin	ulceroglandular exanthem	penicillin
Melioidosis	Pseudomonas pseudomallei	gram neg.	blood agar	soil, water, domestic animals	soil, water	skin, mucosa	ulceroglandular	(TCN, chloro)
Glanders	Malleomyces mallei	gram neg.	blood agar	domestic animals	contact, fomites	skin, conjunctiva	ulceroglandular	sulfonamide, TCN (chloro)
Anthrax	Bacillus anthracis	gram pos.	blood agar	domestic and wild animals	contact, animal products or inhalation	skin, respiratory	malignant pustule	penicillin
Diphtheria	Corynebacterium diphtheriae	gram pos.	Löffler's, tellurite	man	airborne, contact	skin, oropharynx	ulcer, variability	penicillin, antitoxin
Erysipeloid	Erysipelothrix rhusiopathiae	gram pos.	serum, fortified	fish, poultry, domestic animals	contact	skin	cellulitis	penicillin
Gas gangrene	Clostridium welchii	gram pos.	anaerobic	soil, bowel	direct, fomites	skin, bowel	crepitant cellulitis, necrosis	penicillin antitoxin debridement
Listeriosis	Listeria monocytogenes	gram pos.	blood agar, 1% glucose	man and animals	airborne, food, contact	respiratory, G.I., G.U., skin	variable, purpura	penicillin (TCN)
Leptospirosis	Leptospira ictero haemorrhagiae and other serotypes			farm animals	direct, contaminated food	skin, G.I.	jaundice maculopapular eruption urticaria petechiae	penicillin TCN

°TCN = tetracycline
°°chloro = chloramphenicol

tered intravenously 18 to 24 hours later produces an area of hemorrhagic necrosis at the site of the initial preparatory injection. Pathologic changes consist of severe vascular damage with leaking, formation of fibrin thrombi, and an accumulation of polymorphonuclear leukocytes. If both the preparatory and provoking doses are administered intravenously, the "generalized" Shwartzman reaction produces renocortical necrosis. Pretreatment with systemic corticosteroids may enable a single dose of intravenous endotoxin to induce the entire Shwartzman reaction. If this corticosteroid effect applies to man, the implications are far-reaching in terms of the pathogenicity of gram-negative organisms and the contraindications to systemic corticosteroids.

Disseminated Intravascular Coagulation (DIC)

Disseminated intravascular coagulation ("the fibrination syndrome," "consumption coagulopathy") is defined by Deykin (1970) as "a response to an underlying illness that provokes a generalized activation of the hemostatic mechanism beyond that normally confined to areas of local vascular injury. . . ." The syndrome is best approached as the interaction of two processes: the first is the series of events that lead to the evolution of thrombin; the second is a series of protective mechanisms which attempt to defend against the generalized clotting that would occur if thrombin were left unchecked. Although this combined process may be triggered by many other events (viral and protozoal infections, cancer, heat stroke, transfusion reaction, or amniotic fluid embolization), one of the best worked out models is meningococcemia.

In meningococcemia, the early vascular lesion is characterized by endothelial damage, inflammation, necrosis, and fibrin thrombi. Both direct invasion and liberation of endotoxin are probably important. Some of the interacting events include the following:

1. Vascular injury causes platelet aggregation, initiating the *intrinsic* clotting cascade which leads to the conversion of prothrombin to thrombin.

2. Tissue injury activates the extrinsic pathway of thrombin formation.

3. Particularly in profound hypotension, liver blood flow is reduced by elaboration of bradykinin and by the direct neurotoxic effect of endotoxin. Thus, the ability of the liver to clear and dilute activated clotting intermediates is impaired.

4. Vascular endothelium also activates the conversion of plasminogen to plasmin, the endopeptidose which digests many of the products of clot, including fibrinogen and fibrin.

Thus, clinically, the patient might exhibit evidence of thrombosis (thrombin elaboration with deposition of fibrin in small vessels) or he might exhibit signs of hemorrhage (fibrinolysis), or both.

The ability to diagnose DIC varies with the stage of the process and the diagnostic tests available. Thrombocytopenia is common. Fibrinogen is depressed and the thrombin time prolonged. The shear deformation of erythrocytes traversing damaged vessels leads to "helmet cells" or "schistocytes."

The management of disseminated intravascular coagulation requires the continuing close supervision of the hematologist or clinical pathologist. If the primary condition responsible for the clotting abnormality is reversible, then vigorous attention to the primary cause in conjunction with heparin therapy for the DIC may be lifesaving. However, the role of heparin in specific bacterial diseases such as meningococcemia has not been established.

It is likely that purpura fulminans is another abnormality of this interplay between clotting and fibrinolysis which is, however, not necessarily due to endotoxin. This uncommon syndrome is an acute, nonspecific, hemorrhagic, necrotic process which occurs most often in children following various exanthems. Sequential coagulation studies support the usefulness of heparin in purpura fulminans (Antley and McMillan, 1967).

SYSTEMIC GRAM-NEGATIVE BACTERIAL INFECTIONS

Meningococcemia

Meningococcal disease tends to occur in the winter and spring, in enclosed populations, and in one of three forms: meningitis, acute meningococcemia, and chronic meningococcemia. The causative organism, *Neisseria meningitidis*, is an endotoxin-producing, gram-negative diplococcus which resembles *N. gonorrhoeae* bacteriologically and often clinically (Feldman, 1971). The more common meningococcal meningitis may occur without skin lesions. The less common acute meningococcemia varies from a mild respiratory infection with nonspecific rash to a fulminating septicemia and death within hours. The rare chronic meningococcemia probably represents an unusual host response and may be very difficult to diagnose. Common asymptomatic carriers represent a major problem in diagnosis, prophylaxis, and eradication, particularly in military situations.

Mild acute meningococcemia presents as bronchitis or pneumonitis with a nonspecific exanthem of blanchable, light pink, 2- to 15-mm. macules, or slightly raised edematous papules, which usually appear on the trunk. The eruption and symptoms clear in a matter of hours to two days without treatment, and only subsequently, when the blood culture reveals the meningococcus, is the diagnosis made.

The more characteristic severe acute meningococcemia presents explosively with fever, chills, arthralgias, myalgias, nausea, vomiting, and profound weakness. The eruption is present then or soon thereafter. Meningitis or a profound meningo-

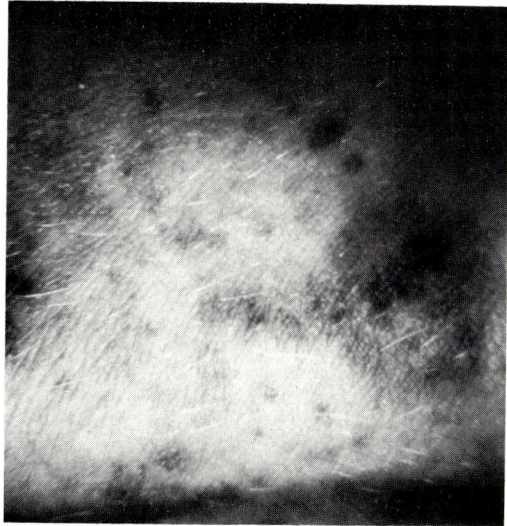

Figure 11–18 Acute meningococcemia, appearing on trunk on day 3, with ecchymotic papules and patches.

encephalomyelitis may or may not occur with the rash. The specific eruption varies from petechiae or edematous petechial papules 1 to 2 mm. in diameter to gross ecchymoses many centimeters in diameter (Fig. 11–18). The trunk and lower extremities are the most common sites, but even mucous membranes and conjunctiva may be involved. The petechiae may form at the center of one of the nonspecific pink macules. In the overwhelming disease, necrotic bullae may advance to ischemic necrosis with sloughing (Fig. 11–19).

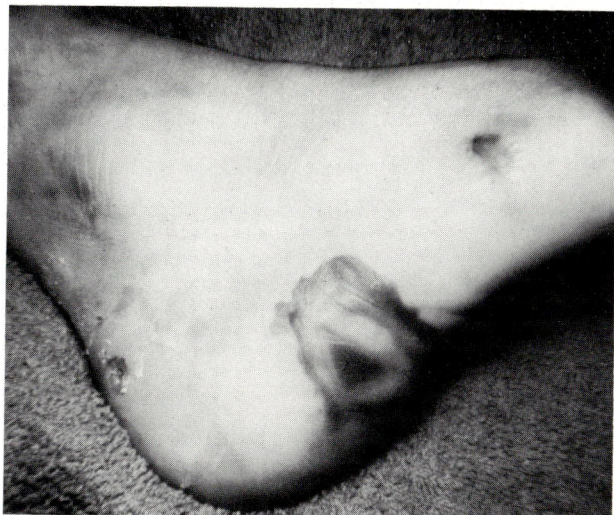

Figure 11–19 Acute meningococcemia after two weeks, showing healing of necrotic ecchymotic bullae.

Death from endotoxic shock may occur within hours of onset.

Chronic meningococcemia is an infrequent but distinct clinical form (Nielsen, 1970). At intervals of one to four days there occur attacks of fever with shaking chills lasting up to 12 hours. The eruption, which is seen in more than 90 per cent of cases, appears coincident with or after the fever, and consists of red macules, usually on the trunk or extensor extremities. These lesions may evolve into tender papules or nodules with a bluish or hemorrhagic center. Other lesions include petechiae, ecchymoses, pustules, or erythema nodosum. Joint pain is common, particularly of the temporomandibular joint and spine. Splenomegaly may be noted. The process may localize, causing fatal complications such as carditis. Blood culture is most likely to be positive during one of the cyclic febrile attacks, but many attempts may be required before a positive culture is obtained.

The differential diagnosis of meningococcal disease includes gonococcemia, subacute bacterial endocarditis, Henoch-Schoenlein purpura, purpura fulminans, acute rheumatic fever, rat-bite fever, staphylococcal and other bacterial septicemias, and Rocky Mountain spotted fever.

Pathologically, in the acute disease, skin findings consist of bacterial invasion of endothelial cells with swelling, formation of fibrin thrombi, vascular damage with hemorrhage, and accumulation of polymorphonuclear leukocytes around the vessels. Later findings depend on the degree of necrosis. In chronic meningococcemia, no organisms or antigenic material can be identified in the endothelial cells, and the thrombi and endothelial swelling are absent.

The organism, *N. meningitidis*, is an aerobic gram-negative diplococcus, best cultured on chocolate agar in a 5 to 10 per cent CO_2 atmosphere. It is differentiated from the gonococcus and nonpathogenic neisseria by fermentation studies. Serologically, there are five groups, based on capsular polysaccharide antigens A, B, C, D, and E, with most cases caused by type B and C, except for periodic epidemics of type A. The bacteria are best cultured from the blood, cerebrospinal fluid, or nasopharynx (the latter particularly in the asymptomatic carrier), but Gram stain or culture from the skin lesions is unlikely to provide diagnostic confirmation. Leukocytosis is common sometime during the course, and early leukopenia is a poor prognostic sign. The cerebrospinal fluid can vary from clear to purulent. The diplococci should be seen on smear and cultured from the spinal fluid in meningitis. Reversible proteinuria, hematuria, and pyuria are common with mild azotemia. Hyperglycemia is commonly seen and is transient. Electrocardiographic charges are usually brief and nonspecific.

Death rates in untreated acute meningococcal disease vary from 20 to 90 per cent. In the fulminant cases particularly, the death rate remains high, even with good treatment. However, cure should be expected in milder forms or in the chronic cases. Early massive parenteral penicillin, 20 million units, or ampicillin at 150 mg. per kilogram is the treatment of choice, starting intravenously. If absolute contraindications to penicillin exist, alternative drugs include Chloromycetin, tetracycline, erythromycin, and the cephalothins. Owing to increasing incidence of resistant strains, sulfonamides are no longer recommended unless specific studies have shown sensitivity. Vigorous supportive therapy is essential, including careful attention to temperature control, fluid and electrolyte balance, maintenance of airway (particularly during seizures), and cardiac status (failure or arrhythmias). Since disseminated intravascular coagulation occurs in meningococcemia, the clotting system must be monitored and heparin therapy instituted when indicated. In the acute disease, adrenal insufficiency cannot be demonstrated by cortisol measurements, even if the adrenal glands are necrotic at postmortem examination (Waterhouse-Friderichsen syndrome). Furthermore, since systemic corticosteroid administration may produce or enhance a Schwartzman-like phenomenon, systemic corticosteroids are not recommended.

Meningococcal disease is most important in enclosed populations, particularly military, where the carrier rate is extremely high. Unfortunately, sulfonamides are no longer effective in prophylaxis, but current clinical trials of vaccines are showing promising results.

Gonorrhea

In the 1960s, there were two major changes in emphasis in cutaneous gonorrhea. First, keratosis blennorrhagica was relegated to Reiter's disease without any probable etiologic relationship to gonorrhea. Secondly, and more important, an increasing incidence of gonococcal septicemia in patients presenting with cutaneous or rheumatic complaints but without genitourinary complaints was recognized.

Gonorrhea is the most common venereal disease. The infection is ordinarily one of mucous membranes and is transmitted by sexual contact; therefore, the usual areas of involvement are the urethra and associated glands in the male and the cervix in the female, with many asymptomatic but contagious cases, particularly in the latter group. Other portals of entry for the gonococcus are the anus and oral cavity. Nonspecific perianal fissures and erosions are associated with gonococcal proctitis. Following direct oral-genital contact, acute inflammation can present as stomatitis, gingivitis, parotitis, pharyngitis, or laryngitis. The character of this inflammation can vary from red, rough edematous patches to yellow linear pseudomembranous exudates. Pustules or clear vesicles may be noted. Gonococcal ulceration of the tongue has also been reported.

Primary cutaneous gonorrhea is rare. Penile abscesses may be seen, particularly on the raphe, with or without urethral disease. These abscesses have no characteristics identifying them as gonococcal except for culture and Gram stain of the pus. Erosive vulvitis is seen with genital gonorrhea in women and molested girls. Gonococcal ecthyma has been reported in the pubic area, but attempts to reproduce this condition experimentally with urethral discharge or pure cultures have failed. In one case, a physician attending a patient with gonorrhea suffered a wound of the thumb and within 30 hours had lymphangitis which evolved into gonococcal septicemia. Because the organisms are difficult to identify in skin lesions of the septicemic state, the examining physician must be aware of these less common primary cutaneous manifestations of gonorrhea, particularly among patients who engage in bizarre sexual practices.

Gonococcal septicemia in its severe or mild form should be recognized clinically by the dermatologist or rheumatologist whom these patients often consult directly. The less common fatal form is associated with endocarditis or meningitis. The more common "benign" gonococcal sepsis occurs most often in women (80 per cent) and homosexuals without genital complaints and accounts for about 5 per cent of cases of gonorrhea. However, the process must not be considered benign, since it may evolve into meningitis, endocarditis, myocarditis, pericarditis, hepatitis, or purulent arthritis. The fact that sexual partners exhibit the same form of the disease more often than one would expect by chance suggests possible strain specificity (Bjornberg, 1970). Within 3 to 21 days of contact, systemic and cutaneous features appear. In women with latent pelvic disease, the septicemia occurs most often during pregnancy and menstruation, or it may follow delivery or gynecologic surgery. Fever, chills, arthralgias, and periarticular tenderness are common. The characteristic skin lesions appear in crops and tend to be few in number (usually fewer than 10) and acral in distribution, especially over the joints. The primary lesion is initially a macule which evolves rapidly into a tender hemorrhagic papule or an umbilicated pustule with a red halo, usually less than 1 cm. in diameter (Fig. 11–20). Rarely, a hemorrhagic subepidermal bulla with necrosis will form an eschar and heal with scarring. The arthritic component of gonococcal sepsis may be a polyarticular arthritis without enough effusion to allow aspiration or a monoarticular involvement with a purulent effusion (Keiser et al., 1968).

The clinical presentation of gonococcemia should be virtually diagnostic, although meningococcemia may present with quantitative variations of some signs and symptoms. The skin lesions in septicemia are probably produced by septic embolization, but rarely do they yield the organism on conventional smear or culture. The Giemsa stain is useful on fixed tissue, and immunofluorescent studies demonstrate antigenic material around blood vessels intracellularly and extracellularly (Kahn, 1969). Similarly, joint fluid rarely yields the organism but a horse serum

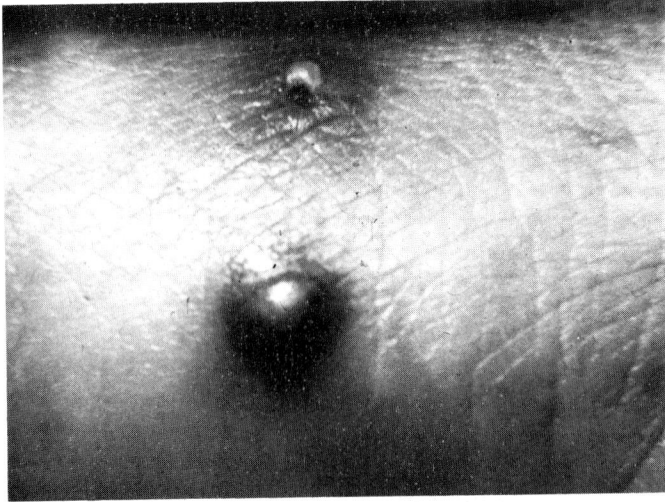

Figure 11–20 Gonococcemia. Acral hemorrhagic vesicopustule and erosion are present.

hyperosmolar medium may grow an L-form (Holmes et al., 1971).

The gonococcus, *Neisseria gonorrhoeae*, is a fastidious gram-negative aerobic diplococcus. Cultural proof of gonococcemia may be difficult, but positive cultures usually come from the blood or swabs from the site of the primary gonorrhea. The clinician must maintain a high degree of suspicion for all possible areas of primary gonorrhea (Metzger, 1970). Material must be plated rapidly on Thayer-Martin VCN medium or chocolate agar.

Parenteral penicillin G in high doses for 7 to 10 days is the treatment of choice. Currecently, 10 million units of aqueous penicillin G daily is recommended to start, even in the absence of meningitis or endocarditis. Constitutional symptoms should resolve within hours or days, and new crops of skin lesions should cease to appear. With the increasing incidence of penicillin-resistant strains of gonorrhea, tetracycline is the next antibiotic of choice, but it is likely that therapy will vary from area to area and time to time.

Pseudomonas

Cutaneous involvement with *Pseudomonas aeruginosa* exhibits a plethora of different expressions, ranging from the severe ecthyma gangrenosum indicative of a systemic catastrophic septicemia to the localized green nail syndrome which is of cosmetic significance only. This gram-negative aerobic bacillus has minimal nutritional requirements and can survive or grow in soil, water, and even topical medicinals, particularly quaternary ammonium amines. In man, it may be cultured from moist intertriginous areas and from stools in a small percentage of normal individuals and a far higher percentage of hospitalized patients. Localized infections usually occur in healthy people whose skin has become burned, irritated, or macerated. Systemic infections occur in hospitalized patients, debilitated from systemic illness, malnutrition, or corticosteroid or immunosuppressive therapy, in whom the pseudomonas has often been "selected" by broad-spectrum antibiotics to which it is resistant. The organism produces many enzymes, including a hemolysin, an inhibitor of the reticuloendothelial system, and a keratinolytic protease which functions optimally in the alkaline environment which the bacterium fosters. It also produces the blue and green pigments pyocyanin and pyoverdin, which impart a greenish white fluorescence under Wood's light which may be diagnostically helpful when present. The bacterium is very sensitive to desiccation and grows poorly in an acid environment.

In Pseudomonas septicemia the skin is most often the portal of entry through loss of barrier function (for instance, decubitus ulcers, thermal burns, surgical wounds, or the psoriatic patch which sloughs from a relative overdose of methotrexate). Maceration and occlusion enhance colonization and penetration. The organism may also enter by way of the lining of the gastrointestinal tract or urinary tract or by erosion through the mastoid from a focus of otitis externa. Recognition of the characteristic skin findings may give the patient some chance of survival if the underlying disease process is not overwhelming. The most specific change in Pseudomonas septicemia is ecthyma gangrenosum, which occurs predominantly in the groin, axillae, and legs. The single or multiple lesions present as vesicles or red macules which become edematous and evolve into necrotic hemorrhagic bullae up to several centimeters in diameter in a matter of hours. Concentric rings of involved and uninvolved skin may be noted at the edge. The necrosis may extend as deep as muscle. Pus is minimal. Signs less extensive than ecthyma gangrenosum include painful grouped hemorrhagic vesicles or vesicopustules, petechiae, painless hemorrhagic cellulitis, or macules resembling the rose spots of typhoid fever (Shanghai fever). Metastatic lesions may involve any system. Smears and cultures of these lesions should yield many organisms.

Pathologically, Teplitz (1965) stresses the unusual nature of the "vasculitis," which consists of perivascular cuffing of organisms with infiltration of the outer layers of arterial and venous walls, relative intimal sparing, a lack of inflammatory response, and lack of intraluminal thrombi. It is therefore more likely that direct bacterial invasion with elaboration of hemolysins and other enzymes is more important than endotoxin in pathogenesis. The peripheral blood smear may also show leukopenia. Greenish fluorescence of urine in severe septicemia is attributed to verdohemoglobin from hemolyzed red cells, which is inadequately cleared by the reticuloendothelial system.

Localized pseudomonas infections usually occur in healthy people in areas of occlusion, maceration, or trauma. Specific syndromes include otitis externa, paronychia with or without green nails, toe web infections, groin infections with or without candidiasis, and pseudomonas pyoderma complicating burns, ulcers, or surgical wounds (Fig. 11–21).

In acute otitis externa, pseudomonas may be the only organism cultured. Clinically, there is no pathognomonic sign, but pain is more severe than that encountered in other forms of otitis externa. The Pseudomonas organism often predominates in the chronic suppurative or eczematous otitis externa in which infection and allergy interact to complicate an underlying dermatosis or a normal canal subjected to trauma or maceration. Erosion into the mastoid area with a resultant meningitis or dissemination occurs rarely.

In paronychial disease, the potential nail spaces beneath the proximal and lateral folds become actual spaces ideal for the growth of pseudomonas and/or *Candida albicans*, particularly in hands subjected to constant wetting or involved with eczematous inflammation. The pigments need not be noted but, if present, may diffuse into the nail, or the bacteria may actually grow in the nail plates (Shellow and Koplon, 1968), presenting discolora-

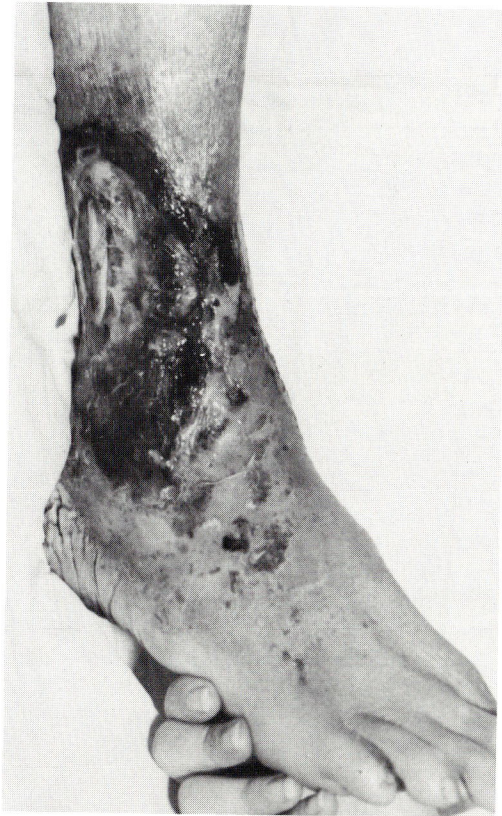

Figure 11–21 Stasis ulcer complicated by pseudomonas infection. The patient had a chronic urinary infection with *Pseudomonas aeruginosa*.

tion diffusely or in horizontal bands reflecting the temporal intensity of infection.

Toe-web infection is frequent, particularly in the military setting where the macerated scaly webs reveal a greenish white fluorescence under Wood's light. Colonization is enhanced by alkalinity and by topical antibacterial agents that suppress gram-positive organisms.

Groin infection with pseudomonas in otherwise healthy young men, particularly athletes, is often unsuspected and therefore causes considerable morbidity before specific therapy is instituted. Pseudomonas and candidiasis may coexist or the candidiasis may precede the pseudomonas. Severe pain, requiring narcotic analgesia, and intolerance of topical medication are the hallmarks of this involvement. Erosions are deeper than those of uncomplicated intertrigo or candidiasis. Alternating $AgNO_3$ wet dressings with a drying lotion containing polymyxin and supporting the scrotum in order to elevate the genitalia from their macerating milieu bring relief within hours or, at most, a few days.

Pseudomonas pyoderma is characterized by a blue-green discoloration of the pus and a mousy odor attributed to trimethylamine. Other signs depend on the predisposing causes.

Treatment of localized infections is directed toward drying, lowering of pH (Burow's solution or acetic acid), and specific antibacterial substances. For the ears, polymyxin B, 500,000 units, may be added to 2 oz. of otic Domeboro, which is instilled every two hours. Unfortunately, the commercially available colistin (Coly-Mycin S otic) also contains neomycin, which is relatively ineffective against pseudomonas and has an unacceptably high incidence of allergic sensitization. In other areas, wet dressings with $AgNO_3$, 0.5 per cent, are very effective, particularly in burns. Sulfamylon also reduces pseudomonas colonization greatly, but its sensitizing potential makes it inappropriate for chronic dermatoses. Gentamicin, 0.1 per cent in a cream, appears to be effective without significant risk of sensitization so far.

Treatment of pseudomonas septicemia achieves variable success depending on the underlying disease. Gentamicin parenterally has been the drug of choice at 3 to 5 mg. per kilogram per day. More recently, carbenicillin has been advocated at 30 gm. daily intravenously (Bodey et al., 1971). Another choice is colistimethate parenterally up to 5 mg. per kilogram per day or polymyxin B, 2.5 mg. per kilogram per day, in the absence of renal failure. If in vitro studies indicate sensitivity, Chloromycetin or tetracycline may be added.

The Salmonellae

Over 600 serotypes of salmonellae have been identified, more than 30 of which have already been proved pathogenic for man. It is best to consider alone *Salmonella typhi*, the cause of typhoid fever, for which man is the only reservoir, and then consider the other salmonelloses as a group. Except for the rose spots of typhoid fever, the cutaneous manifestations of these infections are nonspecific. Typhoid fever is decreasing in incidence, while the other salmonelloses are becoming more common (Aserkoff et al., 1970).

Typhoid fever is transmitted by older chronic carriers, who usually harbor the organism in the gallbladder and also contaminate food. After an incubation period of 3 to 21 days, a severe acute gastroenteritis ensues, with diarrhea, high fever, headache, prostration, and the characteristic leukopenia and splenomegaly. Within a week to 10 days of the onset of fever, the crops of rose spots appear as few (10 to 20), small (1 to 3 mm.), pink papules on the periumbilical area or lower back. These last a few days, leaving hyperpigmentation. The rose spots probably represent capillary seeding of bacteria. Pathologically, macrophages collect around the capillaries. The diagnosis is confirmed by blood or stool cultures or serologic tests. Selective media should be used. The skin may also be involved with fistulous tracts from underlying bone infection or with abscesses in otherwise asymptomatic carriers who disseminate the disease when under stress or when suffering from some other debilitating illness (Burnett, 1962).

Otherwise, salmonellosis is primarily a food-borne illness transmitted by a wide range of animals and animal products, ranging from poultry and dried eggs to pet turtles and medicines of animal origin. The highest incidence occurs between July and October at banquets and picnics or even in hospitals. Of the more than 30 known pathogenic species, *S. typhimurium* is the most common. Salmonellosis is an infection, not an intoxication. The signs, symptoms, and complications (osteomyelitis, meningitis, appendicitis) of the gastroenteritis and/or septicemia are qualitatively similar to *S. typhi* infections, but quantitatively they are less severe, although deaths may occur (Black et al., 1960). Most deaths are caused by gastrointestinal bleeding or perforation.

Chloramphenicol is the treatment of choice for active salmonellosis at 1 gm. every six hours for three weeks, with careful hematologic monitoring. For *S. typhi* carriers, ampicillin is the drug of choice, given alone over a prolonged period or with cholecystectomy.

Haemophilus Influenzae
(Feingold and Gellis, 1965)

Most children are carriers of *Haemophilus influenzae* in the nasal and oral pharynx; infants become susceptible to infection after the third month of life owing to the loss of the protection of the maternal bactericidal antibody. They may develop meningitis, osteomyelitis, or the characteristic facial cellulitis. The organism is a small, pleomorphic, gram-negative, nonmotile, fastidious rod, requiring heme and pyridine nucleotides for optimal growth.

The cutaneous manifestation is seen in children between the ages of 6 and 24 months and is characterized by a solitary bluish red or purplish circumscribed indurated area of cellulitis with an edematous irregular border. There is usually no satellite lymphadenopathy. The face is the usual site of involvement, but less frequently the upper arm is affected. Coryza and fever antedate the appearance of the skin involvement by a few days. Laboratory studies reveal a leukocytosis and a positive blood culture. The condition must be differentiated from streptococcal cellulitis (erysipelas) and staphylococcal infec-

tion. High doses of parenteral ampicillin, 150 mg. per kilogram every six hours, are preferred; other effective antibiotics include cephalothin, tetracycline, and chloramphenicol.

Brucellosis
(Undulant Fever, Malta Disease, Mediterranean Disease)

Brucellosis is primarily a disease of domestic animals (cattle, swine, goats) and less often wild animals (deer, caribou) and occurs worldwide. The disease is sporadic and is diminishing in importance, having reached its peak in the late 1940s. Man acquires the infection through skin contact with infectious material from affected animals, ingestion of raw contaminated milk products or meat, accidental injection when immunizing cattle, or laboratory accidents with virulent cultures.

Undulant fever is an acute or chronic illness characterized by cyclic fevers (up to 105° F.), chills, headache, nightsweats, and extreme weakness. Adenopathy, hepatosplenomegaly, anemia, and leukopenia with lymphocytosis are common. Several species of Brucella (*Brucella melitensis*, *B. suis*, and *B. abortus*) are the etiologic agents of this extraordinarily protean acute or chronic disease. Skin manifestations of the systemic disease are uncommon and lacking in specificity. They occur on less than 5 per cent of patients and range from petechiae to macular or edematous red spots with fine scale on the trunk resembling rose spots (Huddleson, 1943).

The skin is important as a portal of entry, particularly among slaughterhouse workers who handle pigs. Chronic indolent ulcers may develop at the site of an infected abrasion. Histologically, the lesion is granulomatous. Laboratory workers may also become infected by any of the highly invasive species. Another occupational hazard is accidental self-injection by veterinarians inoculating calves against Bang's disease (bovine abortion) with an attenuated live strain of *B. abortus* (Type 19). Much of the symptomatology depends upon the host's prior exposure and immune response. With prior exposure, local and systemic reactions begin within four hours, but without prior sensitization, the systemic disease fails to appear for from 7 to 10 days with bacteremia and a positive skin test to Brucellergen.

Of historic interest is a formerly common affliction of veterinarians reported by Huddleson (1943). Following manual removal of the placentas of infected cows, the skin of the veterinarians' forearms which was in contact with secretions produced one of two reactions: (1) the appearance of an irregular blotchy or confluent blanchable erythema with intense burning lasting four to eight hours, with no residua, or (2) the presentation of small, discrete, elevated, widely separated red follicular papules from 2 to 5 mm. in diameter which may last up to three or four weeks. Although sterile, these lesions were often associated with systemic reaction and could progress to a slough. Because of a rise in titer, these reactions were considered allergic. Although great numbers of older veterinarians experienced this reaction, it is now reported that Bang's disease has been controlled by immunization in the United States.

Brucella produces an endotoxin, but the immunologic response of the host is probably more important in determining the clinical expression. In a highly sensitive patient, intradermal injection of Brucellergen may cause systemic and local reactions at the site of previous involvement. Positive cultures of blood or cutaneous lesions are diagnostic. The cultural yield of this gram-negative coccobacillus is increased by use of chocolate agar under CO_2. Serologic tests are superior to skin tests, which indicate past exposure only. An agglutination titer of greater than 1:100 is significant. It is the 7 S agglutinin which is indicative of active disease, particularly in the chronic form, while both 7 S and macroglobulin agglutinins are present in early infections.

Therapeutically, one or more courses of oral tetracycline, 500 mg. q.i.d. for three weeks, is indicated. In severe or recurrent cases, 1 to 2 gm. of streptomycin may be added intramuscularly for two weeks. If hypersensitivity is considered a significant component, systemic corticosteroids greatly reduce the toxicity.

Tularemia

This disease is widespread in a remarkable number of natural hosts, from which, by direct or indirect means, man may contract the disease. Human infections, most often introduced via the skin, follow contact with infected animals, particularly rabbits and hares; or inoculation may occur through the bite of infected ticks and flies. A recent epidemic in Vermont (Young et al., 1969) involved 47 trappers and handlers of muskrat; in some of these the disease was asymptomatic. Ticks are chiefly responsible for the maintenance of the reservoir of infection among vertebrate hosts. These ticks are capable of transovarian transmission of the disease to their offspring. Fleas, lice, and mites may also be vectors, but ticks of the genus Dermacentor and flies of the genus Chrysops (deer fly) are chiefly responsible for spreading the disease from animals to the human host. Ingestion of contaminated food and water may also cause disease, but thorough cooking of infected animals kills the bacteria. Transmission from man to man is not a problem. Tularemia occurs principally in the North Temperate Zone. *Francisella (Pasteurella) tularensis*, the causative agent, is a fastidious, facultative, intracellular, gram-negative, nonmotile, highly polymorphous organism appearing as globules, bacilliform rods, and tiny filaments.

The ulceroglandular type of tularemia is the most common expression of the disease. The onset is rapid, after an incubation period of only a few (1 to 10) days. Fever, sweats, chills, and aching pains are part of the striking constitutional reaction. Stupor and coma may accompany severe infections. The primary skin lesion develops subsequent to this prostrating onset. It often occurs as a painful papule at the site of a minor injury or insect bite. This papule enlarges rapidly and undergoes necrosis, producing an indolent ulcer with raised edges and a necrotic base. The primary lesion is usually on an exposed extremity, such as a finger or hand (Fig. 11–22), but it may arise in the conjunctiva or even in the nasal or oral mucosa. Regional adenopathy invariably develops shortly after the appearance of the chancre-like primary lesion, usually

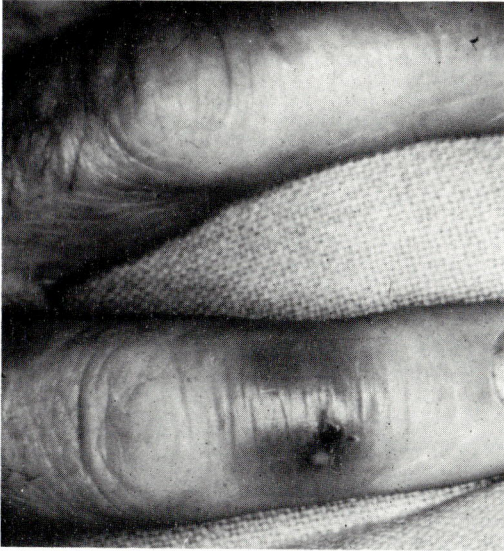

Figure 11-22 Tularemia—early necrotic erosion.

without lymphangitis. In a small number of cases, tender nodules develop along the draining lymphatic channels in a manner suggestive of sporotrichosis. Lymphatic enlargement may occur anywhere in the body following adenopathy of the regional nodes. The enlarged nodes may suppurate. Fever usually lasts for two to four weeks unless new buboes develop; these are accompanied by a recrudescence of fever and symptoms. About 90 per cent of the patients have minor bronchopulmonary changes which are detectable roentgenologically and which account for the frequent symptom of cough and accompanying bronchitic rales. Frank pneumonia is uncommon but serious. The frequent bronchopulmonary involvement simply reflects the bacteremia which is known to be present in the early stages of the disease. At about the second or third week, some 20 per cent of the cases will develop a variable exanthem.

The oculoglandular type of tularemia, represented by a primary lesion in the conjunctiva and adenopathy of the regional nodes, is a clinical analogue of the ulceroglandular type. It is uncommon, as is the purely glandular type, which is represented by buboes without any primary lesion. There is also a typhoid type of the disease which, as the name suggests, has a variable ensemble of symptoms similar to that of typhoid fever. It is rarer and more serious than the cutaneous forms.

The duration of the untreated disease is usually about four months, but the individual variations are great, ranging from two weeks in mild cases to more than a year in those patients who successively develop suppurating buboes and persistent pneumonic lesions. New buboes may appear a year or two later, even after the patient seems to have recovered. The constitutional reactions in this disease greatly overshadow the primary cutaneous manifestations.

Prior to the introduction of antibiotics, the mortality rate was somewhat less than 10 per cent. Involution is the rule when there is no progression beyond the regional lymph nodes and the constitutional reactions are not severe. Recovery is followed by firm immunity. With appropriate treatment, fatalities are now practically nonexistent.

The diagnosis may generally be presumed from the characteristic clinical picture. Confirmation is afforded by a simple agglutination test. Antibodies become apparent after the first week, and the titer is rarely less than 1:640 by the third week. Tularemia also causes an anamnestic rise in brucella titers, but the increase is not of the same magnitude as the tularemia titer. Conventional smears of the lesions are not particularly helpful because of the remarkable pleomorphism of the causative organism, which can scarcely be distinguished from tissue debris by the inexperienced observer. However, fluorescent antibody testing will identify the organism on smear or even on formalin-fixed, paraffin-embedded human tissues (White and McGavran, 1965). Culture is not easily accomplished in conventional media, but growth flourishes on enriched broth.

Pathologically, the reaction in the liver, spleen, and nodes is granulomatous, and caseation may occur. The white blood count is usually low or normal.

Streptomycin at 1 gm. per day is the treatment of choice. Tetracycline or chloramphenicol may also be used but the relapse rate is higher. Penicillin is ineffective. Supportive care includes bed rest, compresses for primary lesions, and the incision of fluctuant lymph nodes, followed by measures to promote drainage.

Plague

The dreaded plague, caused by the gram-negative bacillus *Pasteurella (Yersinia) pestis*, cannot simply be relegated to the historic oblivion of the black death of the Middle Ages. Plague occurs in many parts of the world. Of particular interest, it is now epidemic in Southeast Asia, and endemic foci exist in the southwestern United States (Reed et al., 1970). Man becomes involved incidentally in the rodent-flea-rodent cycle, and the likelihood of human disease is greatly dependent on the species and density of the rodents, the species and density of the fleas, and the susceptibility of the host. There are three major clinical forms of plague in man: bubonic, pneumonic, and septicemic; in addition, there are two epidemiologic presentations, urban and sylvatic.

The most common form presently, bubonic plague, is an ulceroglandular process, and the portal of entry on the extremity is a flea bite or direct contact with an infected animal. Over the past several decades, bubonic plague accounted for about two case reports per year from the United States. The pneumonic plague (black death), involving massive respiratory infection, can be transmitted from man to man. The septicemic form can evolve from either pneumonic or bubonic plague. A wide clinical spectrum (Reiley and Kates, 1970) is seen in Vietnam, where 3500 to 4500 cases per year were reported in the mid 1960s. Pestis minor is a mild form of the disease — mild either because of a less virulent strain or because of partial immunity due to repeated subinfectious inoculation. Asymptomatic pharyngeal colonization also occurs, but the role of these carriers in transmission is unclear.

Epidemiologically, sylvatic plague, as seen in the southwestern United States, is an epizootic among many species of wild rodents whose fleas are relatively poor vectors, and man becomes involved either by direct contact with infected animals or by flea bites. Urban plague is intimately linked to the ecology of the common rat and its flea (*Xenopsylla cheopis*). This flea's amazing vector capacity depends on the blockage phenomenon in which the proventriculus becomes plugged, the valvular action is inadequate, and the recoil drives blood and bacteria back into the victim.

Clinically, the incubation period of bubonic plague is from 2 to 10 days following the bite (usually 4 to 6 days), and the onset of the disease is sudden. The site of the bite may or may not be noted. The hallmark is the bubo, which is usually inguinal or, less often, axillary. The bubo is a large, painful, tender, fixed, matted mass of lymph nodes. The overlying skin is red and feels gelatinous. The bubo may break down and become secondarily infected with gram-positive bacteria. A "carbuncle" may form near the bubo, which in its late stage resembles the "malignant pustule" of anthrax with the centrifugal spread of clusters of vesicles (Letgers et al., 1970). Septicemia occurs early and is accompanied by petechiae of skin and mucous membranes. Leukocytosis may follow an early leukopenia.

The *P. pestis* should be cultured and smeared from aspirates of the bubo or from blood. Immunofluorescence should allow rapid identification. Gram's stain characteristically accentuates both ends of the bacillus like a "safety pin." Virulent strains have a slimy soluble capsule. A guinea pig will also produce buboes when scarified with infected material.

The differential diagnosis of bubonic plague includes many bacterial and nonbacterial ulceroglandular processes. Lymphogranuloma venereum is less acute, painful, and severe. Streptococcal or staphylococcal adenitis should be differentiated rapidly by Gram stain and cultures, that of chancroid should be ulcerated, and that of syphilis and tuberculosis should not be tender. Cat-scratch disease, tularemia, and *P. multocida* infection should show the portal of entry.

Prompt recognition, isolation, and institution of therapy are essential, since septicemia may occur early. The release of endotoxin or a Herxheimer reaction in the septicemic phase has been postulated to explain sudden death during treatment despite bacteriologic cure. Although fibrin thrombi in small vessels have been demonstrated at autopsy, disseminated intravascular coagulation has not been specifically documented.

P. pestis is sensitive to sulfonamides and many antibiotics, although reports from Southeast Asia indicate emerging resistance to sulfonamides and streptomycin. Nevertheless, streptomycin is still the drug of choice, starting at 2 gm. per day for 7 to 10 days. Concomitant tetracycline at 2 gm. per day, chloramphenicol, or sulfadiazine at 4 to 6 gm. per day intravenously (Hoang and Rosendaal, 1968) have also been advocated. Despite in vitro tests which may show sensitivity, penicillin is ineffective. The possibility of endotoxic shock should be anticipated. Prophylaxis with the standard plague vaccine of the United States Armed Forces partially reduces susceptibility and morbidity. Vaccination is advocated for heavily exposed laboratory workers and for those traveling to areas of Asia where plague is endemic, but not for residents of the southwestern United States.

Pasteurella Multocida Infection

Pasteurella multocida (*P. septica*) infection is caused by a small, ovoid, gram-negative, nonmotile, bipolar staining rod which is pathogenic or which may be part of the normal flora of the upper respiratory tract of domestic or wild animals (Schwartz and King, 1959; Tindall and Harrison, 1972). Humans can acquire an infection from the bite or scratch of animals, dogs or cats in particular; this condition, has also been seen in personnel handling experimental animals. A fatal hemorrhagic septicemia has been described in animals.

Although the organism grows readily on nutrient blood agar, it is still not frequently identified. Its bipolar staining mimics that of *Neisseria meningitidis* or *Haemophilus influenzae*. Biochemical and agglutination tests help to identify the organism.

The clinical manifestations in man consist most commonly of a localized cellulitis with or without an accompanying lymphadenitis following an animal bite of the extremities, and rarely a chronic pulmonary infection such as bronchiectasis or a systemic infection. A few hours after being wounded, the patient experiences a cellulitis which, if extensive, is accompanied by lymphadenitis and low-grade fever. The initial lesions may be a painful, inflamed ulcer with a seropurulent discharge, or they may form an abscess. If the wound is deep, it may be complicated by a synovitis or osteomyelitis. A septicemia or meningitis rarely occurs. The infection may resemble clinically other pyogenic cellulitides, erysipeloid, "cat scratch" disease, and other ulceroglandular syndromes such as tularemia.

Although most strains of *P. multocida* are sensitive to penicillin, culture and sensitivity studies should be routinely done; tetracycline is the alternate drug of choice. Healing tends to be slow despite adequate antibiotic therapy (2 to 4 million units of intramuscular penicillin daily) and adequate surgical drainage.

It has been recommended that all domestic animal bites or wounds be routinely and carefully cleansed and the inflicted patient be given adequate systemic penicillin or tetracycline and tetanus prophylaxis.

Bartonellosis
(Carrion's Disease, Oroya Fever, Verruga Peruana)

Bartonellosis is a curious biphasic disease limited to the Andrean valleys of the Peruvian Sierras, with sporadic appearance in Colombia and Ecuador. It is caused by *Bartonella bacilliformis*, a gram-negative, pleomorphic organism which selectively tends to localize in red blood cells and in cells of the reticuloendothelial system.

A striking peculiarty of the disease is its appearance in two distinct stages (Ricketts, 1949):

1. A non-eruptive stage in which the manifestations range from a very mild condition to a severe febrile lethal disease is known as *Oroya fever*. It is essential to recognize that the non-eruptive stage may be completely asymptomatic. In endemic areas as many as 10 per cent of the population may be asymptomatic carriers.

2. The eruptive stage is marked by characteristic hemangioma-like nodules and tumors. These vascular growths are known as verrugas (verruga peruana, Peruvian warts). Verrugas may be the first sign of the disease on those whose antecedent non-eruptive stage was asymptomatic.

These two stages were not recognized as manifestations of the same disease until

Carrion, a medical student, inoculated himself with material from verrugas and developed fatal Oroya fever 21 days later (Schultz, 1968). Markings on Peruvian ceramic pots of the pre-Inca era indicate an early awareness of verrugas. Man is the only known reservoir. The vector transmitting bartonellosis is the sand fly, a member of the genus Phlebotomus. The incubation period is usually 17 to 25 days but may be as long as several months.

Oroya fever is manifested by high fever, chills, and a rapidly progressive hemolytic anemia. Bone and joint pain and prostration are marked. Lymphadenopathy is common. At this stage, the erythrocytes are packed with organisms which may persist for a long time even if the patient recovers. There is a decreased erythrocyte survival time, with increased fragility and sequestration in the spleen. No specific agglutinin or hemolysin has been demonstrated. Leukocytosis is usually mild with a "left shift," and a high white count warns of intercurrent infection. Septicemia of other organisms, particularly salmonellae, is common in fatal cases. Milder cases show only malaise, occasional fever, arthralgia, and a moderate anemia.

The eruptive stage emerges at a variable time after the onset of Oroya fever, sometimes during convalescence, sometimes after clinical remission, and sometimes without any evidence of a preexisting noneruptive stage. The verrugas may arise superficially and be so minute that they are designated as miliary verrugas, or they may occur subcutaneously as hard nodules reaching a size of several centimeters in diameter. The nodules either remain as such or they may erode to the surface, becoming hemangioma-like tumors with irregular contours. The miliary lesions, which are few or numerous (Fig. 11–23), may appear anywhere on the skin or mucous membranes. They are hemispheric, red, raised, and sharply circumscribed (Fig. 11–24). Verrugas bleed easily. The eruption usually lasts from one to six months, and the lesions sometimes occur in waves. No scar is left after healing. Verrugas may involve many other tissues, particularly bone. Histologically, verrugas show an angioblastic proliferation reminiscent of a pyogenic granuloma or an immature capillary hemangioma. With regression, fibrous elements replace vas-

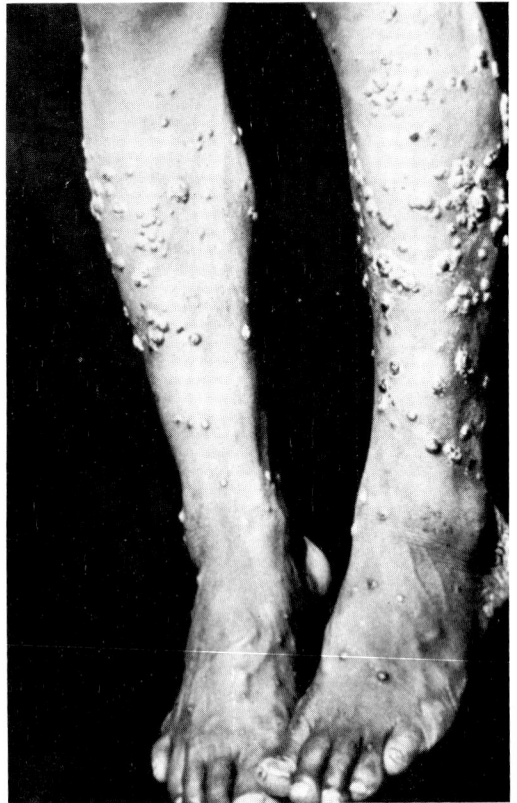

Figure 11–23 Miliary verrugas especially of the extensor surfaces of the extremities.

cular elements. Erythrocytes are normal in this phase of evolving immunity, plasma cells are increased in the lymph nodes, and gamma globulins are increased in the serum. Usually one attack confers complete and permanent immunity.

In the non-eruptive stage, the finding of large numbers of pleomorphic bacteria within the red cells on conventionally stained blood smears establishes the diagnosis, which may be confirmed by blood culture. In the eruptive stage, the gross characteristics of the verruga are pathognomonic. Recovery is the rule in the eruptive stage in contrast to a 40 per cent mortality in acute untreated Oroya fever.

Penicillin and the broad-spectrum antibiotics are effective against *B. bacilliformis*. Streptomycin has also been advocated for the verrugas. Healing of large verrugas may be hastened by surgical excision. Prophylaxis is chiefly concerned with elimination of the breeding places of the insect vector and eradication of the sand fly itself.

Rat-Bite Fever

Two similar but differentiable diseases may follow the bite of a rat, a circumstance which has caused no little confusion. These are sodoku, caused by *Spirillum minus*, and streptobacillary rat-bite fever, caused by the pleomorphic *Streptobacillus moniliformis*. Both may legitimately be called rat-bite fever, and it is remarkable that the two diseases resemble one another so closely. In addition, the *S. moniliformis* may produce epidemic Haverhill fever whose clinical manifestations resemble those of streptobacillary rat-bite fever, but the mode of transmission is raw milk, not the bite of a rodent.

Rat-Bite Fever due to *S. moniliformis*

The general and cutaneous manifestations of this infection may be strikingly similar to sodoku but they differ in the following ways. The incubation period is shorter, usually one to five days but occasionally as long as 10 days. The site of the bite has usually healed by the onset of symptoms and does not break down again as it does in sodoku. True arthritis is more common in streptobacillary disease. Endocarditis and, rarely, pericardial effusion may complicate streptobacillary disease. "False positive" tests for syphilis are less common in streptobacillary disease than in sodoku. The exanthem is a constant expression of streptobacillary disease but its features are variable and not diagnostic.

The gram-negative *S. moniliformis* can be grown from blood culture, in which it forms characteristic "fluff balls" on the bottom of the flask. However, five to six days may be required for growth (Cole et al., 1969), and, if the disease is strongly suspected, penicillin therapy should be started before bacteriologic confirmation is completed. Fluorescent antibody techniques and agglutination are useful in the laboratory. Since untreated endocarditis is uniformly fatal, more vigorous therapy is indicated if heart murmurs, splenomegaly, or Osler's nodes are detected. McCormack et al. (1967) recommend tube dilution sensitivity testing. If the organism is relatively sensitive, the treatment of choice is procaine penicillin G, 4.8 million units daily for four weeks; if less sensitive, 20 million units for six weeks.

Haverhill Fever (Erythema Arthriticum)

The term "Haverhill fever" is applied to an epidemic disease due to *Streptobacillus moniliformis*, but although the symptomatology may be similar to streptobacillary rat-bite fever, inoculation does not occur through a rat bite. The ingestion of contaminated foods is one of the means by which the disease is acquired. The first epidemic in Haverhill, Massachusetts, in 1926 followed the drinking of unpasteurized milk. The onset is acute, with chills, headache, and fever. Arthritis is a striking feature of the disease and involves one or more of the major joints, which become hard, swollen, and tender. Generalized muscle aches accompany the arthritis. A variable exanthem appears in a week or two in almost all cases. It is seen primarily on the anterior and lateral parts of the extremities, particularly around the joints. In severe cases, there is generalization of the rubeola-like exanthem. Often there are flat red papules which vary greatly in size. Petechial hemorrhages may occur in severe cases, particularly on the extremities. The general eruption may later desquamate. The exanthem is likely to appear suddenly when the constitutional symptoms are abating. Subsequently, there is a re-

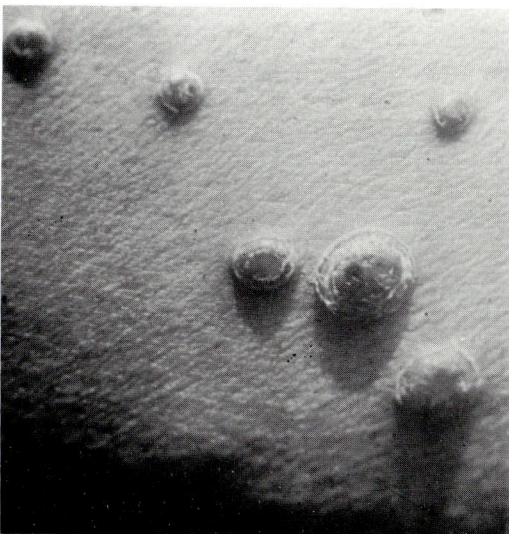

Figure 11–24 Hemispheric, purpuric, scaling, split pea–size nodules (verrugas).

crudescence in which the exanthem becomes more pronounced and the joint signs become reactivated. Other manifestations, such as cough, bronchitis, and dysphagia, may be noted. Generally speaking, Haverhill fever and streptobacillary rat-bite fever have similar manifestations and follow a similar course.

Specific confirmation of the diagnosis is afforded by isolation of the organism from the blood or from joint fluid. Agglutinins for *S. moniliformis* may usually be demonstrated after the second week. Mice are highly susceptible when inoculated with infectious material. The prominence of joint symptoms in streptobacillary infections is a point which differentiates them from sodoku. Recovery is the rule. Eradication of rats and avoidance of unpasteurized milk are the chief prophylactic measures. Penicillin is effective therapy.

Melioidosis

Melioidosis occurs in the tropics of Southeast Asia, particularly Thailand and Malasia, and is caused by *Pseudomonas (Malleomyces) pseudomallei*. The organism is a gram-negative, motile, non-spore–forming bacillus which has some serologic similarity to *Malleomyces mallei*, the etiologic agent of glanders. The reservoir is soil or water, particularly rice paddies, where the organism can survive and grow. Although rat fleas and mosquitoes can transmit the organism experimentally, the usual method of entry is by contact of water with abraded skin or through the mucosa of the gastrointestinal tract, the conjunctiva, or cutaneous abrasions. Infection through laboratory accidents and by contaminated syringes in drug addicts has also been reported. Direct person-to-person transmission is otherwise unlikely. Although the incubation period is generally short, the disease may remain dormant until the host is stressed (by burn or surgery), following which the first signs may appear even after the patient has left the endemic area.

Melioidosis may present as an acute or chronic illness. The acute respiratory infection can vary from mild bronchitis to overwhelming pneumonia and septicemia

with abscesses. Watery diarrhea is frequent. The chronic systemic disease is granulomatous, involving skin, nodes, bones, and lung (where cavity lesions are seen radiographically).

Specifically on the skin, a superficial ulcer may be the portal of entry, with surrounding inflammation and lymphangitis out of proportion to the cutaneous lesion (Sheehy et al., 1967). Miliary septic emboli may then involve the skin, viscera, or both. Lesions are usually multiple: either acutely appearing, coalescing, purulent, necrotic ulcers or chronic, deep-seated, draining sinuses or granulomas. Diffuse cellulitis and tonsillar pustules may also occur (Weber et al., 1969). Urticaria has been reported secondary to chronic pulmonary melioidosis (Steck and Byrd, 1969).

The bacteria may be cultured by standard methods and may be seen on the Gram stain of pus from abscesses. However, bacteria are more difficult to identify in the granulomatous phase, when Giemsa is the stain of choice. Slide agglutination, hemagglutination, complement fixation, and fluorescent techniques are available.

In vitro sensitivities are important in choosing antibiotic therapy (Piggott and Hochholzer, 1970), which is unpredictable and often ineffective. For the chronic disease, tetracycline alone may be sufficient, but with the high mortality rate in the acute disease, high dosage chloramphenicol has been advocated with or without kanamycin or novobiocin. Side effects of these toxic drugs must be carefully weighed against the severity of the disease in each case.

Glanders (Equinia)

Glanders has not been a significant problem in North America since the first quarter of the twentieth century because of effective eradication and sparseness of the principal natural hosts—horses, mules, and asses. The nodulo-ulcerative form of the disease along lymphatics in these animals is called farcy. Humans are quite susceptible, reflected by the ease with which laboratory workers become infected accidentally. Some species of smaller animals are also highly susceptible, particularly the guinea pig, which is the laboratory animal of choice.

The causative organism is a gram-negative bacillus *Malleomyces (Actinobacillus) mallei* which has some clinical and laboratory similarities to *Pseudomonas (Malleomyces) pseudomallei*, which causes melioidosis, although the two organisms can be differentiated biochemically and antigenically. Both direct contact and fomites are important in transmission. The bacillus enters most commonly through an abrasion in the skin, but conjunctival contact, inhalation, and ingestion may also be important.

In man, the disease may be acute or chronic. A few days after inoculation, acute glanders is manifested by the abrupt onset of chills, high fever, and marked prostration. The initial lesion is usually on an exposed area, such as the hands, face, or neck, but the nose and mouth may also be the portals of entry. At the inoculation site there appears a painful swelling which soon breaks down to yield a necrotic, irregular ulcer which produces a purulent offensive discharge. The regional lymph nodes become swollen and tender and not uncommonly break down to form persistent suppurative abscesses. The ulcers may enlarge rapidly; an alarming picture develops when new lesions suddenly arise in many different areas. The early lesions are usually grouped and may pass through a pustular and bullous stage before they terminate in ulceration. Coalescence leads to formation of large, necrotic, foul-smelling ulcers. This skin seems helpless against the onslaught, and gangrenous patches appear. The cutaneous aspect is altogether appalling and ugly. Deep subcutaneous abscesses and infiltrated plaques with draining sinuses develop. Nodules may form along the course of the lymphatics. Hematogenous dissemination produces widespread miliary lesions in the subcutaneous tissues, muscles, lungs, and other viscera. Frequently, there is ulceration of the upper respiratory tract, as well as lung infiltration and splenomegaly. There is a profuse nasal discharge which is thick, tenacious, and foul smelling. Preterminally, there may be a generalized papulopustular eruption. Meningitis, osteomyelitis, and polyarthritis are additional manifestations. Constitutional symptoms progress in severity as new lesions develop on the skin, and ordinarily there is fatal termination in two to three weeks.

The chronic form of glanders is more insidious. The cutaneous manifestations are the same, but the constitutional reactions are less intense. The disease fluctuates, and temporary remissions occur. Mucous membrane involvement is less common than in the acute type. A fatal outcome is frequent in the chronic type after a variable period of months or years of exhausting illness. A mild self-limiting form has been recognized in laboratory workers.

The organisms may be recovered from the lesions as well as from the blood. Intraperitoneal inoculation of infectious material into the hamster or guinea pig is followed by a pathognomonic scrotal swelling, and the organisms may be recovered from the tunica vaginalis. After the second to fourth week, agglutinins and complement-fixing antibodies appear, possessing some degree of cross-reaction with *P. pseudomallei*. A delayed tuberculin-type reaction develops following the intradermal injection of 0.1 ml. of 1:1000 dilution of mallein, an antigen prepared from a culture of the organism. The white blood count may be normal or even depressed.

Therapeutic reports of significant series of patients are lacking. In vivo and in vitro sensitivities vary. Sulfonamides, tetracyclines, streptomycin, and chloramphenicol have been reported as being effective.

SYSTEMIC GRAM-POSITIVE BACTERIAL INFECTIONS

Anthrax
(Malignant Pustule, Malignant Edema)

Anthrax is primarily a disease of domestic animals; it is seen in sheep, cattle, and horses but it may also affect buffalo and other wild animals. It is spread by contact, flies, vultures, and water. It is most frequently transmitted to man via imported animal products, such as hides, furs, and bone meal. The rare pulmonary anthrax is fatal if not recognized and treated early.

The more common cutaneous form may also have severe systemic implications.

The organism, *Bacillus anthracis*, is a gram-positive aerobic bacillus, the spores of which are moderately resistant to heat and chemicals and survive for years in dry earth and for months in hides. The complex exotoxin consists of at least three serologically active components: edema factor (EF, I), protective (immunizing) antigen (PA, II) and lethal factor (LF, III).

Pulmonary anthrax requires a high degree of suspicion for diagnosis in workers who inhale large numbers of spores. Without prompt antibiotic treatment they die of a hemorrhagic mediastinitis or meningitis.

Cutaneous anthrax often follows an abrasion made with contaminated materials. Within a day or two of this inoculation, usually on an exposed part, an inflammatory papule develops which rapidly evolves into a bulla that often contains blood or pus (malignant pustule). Intense infiltration, a very characteristic sign, surrounds the bulla. A ring of vesicles typically forms around the bulla, surmounting the infiltrated zone. The edematous infiltration may become quite extensive (malignant edema). The bulla soon ruptures, leaving a shallow ulcer into which serous fluid issues and dries to form a tough, black eschar (Fig. 11–25). At this stage, the appearance of the lesion is practically pathognomonic. It is painless and consists of an escharotic shallow ulcer surrounded by a zone of infiltration in which there are often numerous vesicles and pustules. Usually, the regional lymph nodes enlarge and may even suppurate. Septicemia may result in hemorrhagic mediastinitis and death, probably owing to the effect of the toxin on the respiratory center of the brain. Occasionally, the malignant pustule fails to develop in its typical localized form; instead, massive edema with bullae, necrosis, and gangrene occur. The gravity of such extensive cutaneous lesions, particularly of the head and neck, cannot be overemphasized because of mechanical and toxic phenomena that may occur.

Finding chains of large, gram-positive rods in smears establishes a presumptive diagnosis which may be confirmed aerobically or anaerobically on conventional

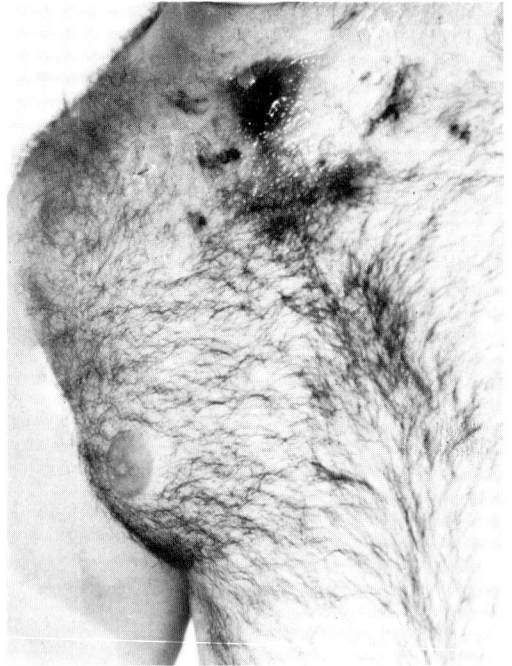

Figure 11–25 Anthrax. "Malignant pustule" is present on upper chest; "malignant edema" extends down chest and arm.

culture media in which virulent strains form a "caput medusa."

With prompt diagnosis and treatment, mortality should be low and the cutaneous lesions should heal with scarring. Parenteral penicillin, 4 to 6 million units daily for two weeks, is the drug of choice. Tetracycline and other broad-spectrum antibiotics may be used, although their onset of effect is somewhat slower. Doust et al. (1968) report reduction of morbidity and mortality with systemic corticosteroids in cases of malignant edema of the chest wall and neck. Public health measures for intercepting and disposing of contaminated materials are most important in prevention. For workers with unavoidable exposure, active immunization is indicated. In experimental primates, survival is enhanced by isoproterenol and mechanical ventilation on a positive pressure respirator (Remele et al., 1968).

Diphtheria

Untreated cutaneous diphtheria can be a mortal disease. The cardiac and neurologic complications of the potent exotoxin are no different from those of the better-known faucial diphtheria. The systemic consequences to the patient are the same, regardless of the site of infection. The usual reservoir of the causative organism, *Corynebacterium diphtheriae*, is the throat of carriers or patients with active faucial or cutaneous diphtheria. Transmission is direct from person to person. The classic lesion of cutaneous diphtheria is a punched-out ulcer. The infection usually does not originate in normal skin. It develops at the site of a preexisting, often trivial, lesion, such as an insect bite, abrasion, burn, or an eczematous eruption of any sort. The disease is largely tropical, although many instances of it have been observed in temperate climates, particularly under conditions of war. Poor hygiene, crowding, maceration of the skin, or repeated multiple abrasions create favorable circumstances for infection, especially under humid conditions. Recent outbreaks have been reported in Texas (Zalma et al., 1970) and in Alabama and Louisiana (Belsey et al., 1969).

The diphtheritic ulcer has typical characteristics which make a correct presumptive diagnosis possible on the basis of clinical examination. The ulcer is shallow, well demarcated, and has a rolled, firm border. It does not dissect down into the deeper tissues. In the very early stage, there is a gray-yellow or brown-gray membrane, which may be peeled off intact, leaving a clean surface. Later, the diagnostic hallmark of the disease appears—a black or brownish black adherent leathery slough or eschar which generally fails to cover the ulcer completely. The eschar is removed with difficulty, revealing an unhealthy base. It is not present in every case, since it may slough off spontaneously. The ulcer is surrounded by a tender inflammatory zone. Very often, there is a rather characteristic bulla which extends 1 to 2 cm. beyond the ulcer. The lesion heals from the outside in, leaving a thin, atrophic, evenly depressed scar. An important diagnostic sign is the anesthesia which may be demonstrated by pin prick in and around the ulcer two to five weeks after onset. This is evidently due to destruction of cutaneous nerves by the toxins of the bacillus. The ulcer is painful in the early stages but is not at all painful later in its course. The lesions heal slowly and may develop anywhere on the body, although the extremities are the most common sites.

A highly characteristic sign of the disease is the repeated formation of a bulla in the scar of a lesion which grossly appears to have healed. The definitive diagnosis is made by cultural isolation of virulent organisms, although the finding of grampositive corynebacteria in smears is suggestive. Löffler's or tellurite agar prevents overgrowth of other bacteria. In older lesions, particularly, demonstration of the diphtheria organisms may be extremely difficult. A high degree of suspicion is required to diagnose a nondescript eczematous type and other variable forms of cutaneous diphtheria which look like more common pyodermas. Such suspicion is justifiably increased under tropical conditions, or if other patients with faucial or cutaneous diphtheria have been encountered in the same geographic area. It is unhappily true, however, that when a wave of cutaneous diphtheria develops in a population, one or more patients will ordinarily progress to fatal heart block or late neuropathies before the suspicions of the attending physicians are sufficiently aroused.

Combined therapy with a suitable antibiotic and specific antitoxin is effective. Penicillin is the antibiotic of choice in a dosage of 2 to 4 million units per day. An alternative is erythromycin at 2 gm. per day. These agents will inhibit the bacteria but will not inactivate the toxins already present. Intramuscular or intravenous injection of 20,000 to 40,000 units of antitoxin derived from horse serum will inactivate the toxin. There seems to be no great advantage in local injections of antitoxin around the lesion. Bed rest and good supportive care are essential. Review of the diphtheria immunization status of all contacts is indicated, although it must be remembered that immunity requires several weeks to develop following the injection of diphtheria toxoid. It must also be emphasized that active immunization protects the host from the systemic effects of the toxin only and does not prevent the development of cutaneous infection or the carrier state. The Shick test indicates lack of immunity to toxin if a local reaction appears within five days at the site of intradermal injection of the toxin.

Erysipeloid

Erysipeloid is essentially an occupational disease of persons who incur abrasions while handling infected organic matter, especially fish, shell fish, meat, or poultry. It occurs principally in kitchen workers, meat dressers, fishermen, and fish dealers (Klauder, 1944). Natural infections appear in a wide range of animals, including swine, sheep, cattle, horses, and fowl. The organism, *Erysipelothrix rhusiopathiae*, a gram-positive, non-encapsulated, non-spore-forming rod, can survive for months in the soil or in decomposed organic material. The disease has three forms: (1) the most common, a localized cutaneous infection lacking important constitutional symptoms, (2) a generalized eruption with occasional systemic symptoms, and (3) a rare systemic form with endocarditis. The organisms have a predilection for skin, endocardium, and joints.

In the mild localized form (Fig. 11–26), erythema and a painful edema develop within one to three days at the inoculation site, which may be a trivial injury. The color is violaceous or purplish red, and the lesion spreads peripherally, with clearing in the center. The margin is slightly elevated and well defined. Vesicles or bullae occur occasionally, and mature lesions may show polycyclic or festooned borders. The hands or wrists are the usual sites of eruption. Relapses are common in untreated cases, and new lesions may appear at remote sites. Fever is generally absent, and there may be no systemic reactions whatever. The localized form usually runs its course in two to four weeks.

Erysipeloid accompanied by a diffuse generalized eruption is a less common type. The lesion may start on the finger and gradually enlarge, spreading along the hand, wrist, forearm, and arm. Over a period of months, practically the entire cutaneous surface may become involved. The lesions have sharply marginated borders, with a tendency to central clearing. Circinate or oval lesions with clear centers may suddenly appear and disappear in various areas. Irregular gyrate patches may form which, through fusion, produce curious patterns. Frequently there are associated constitutional symptoms, of which arthritis, pain, and fever are the more usual. The course is variable; the condition persists for weeks or months, but eventually there is spontaneous recovery.

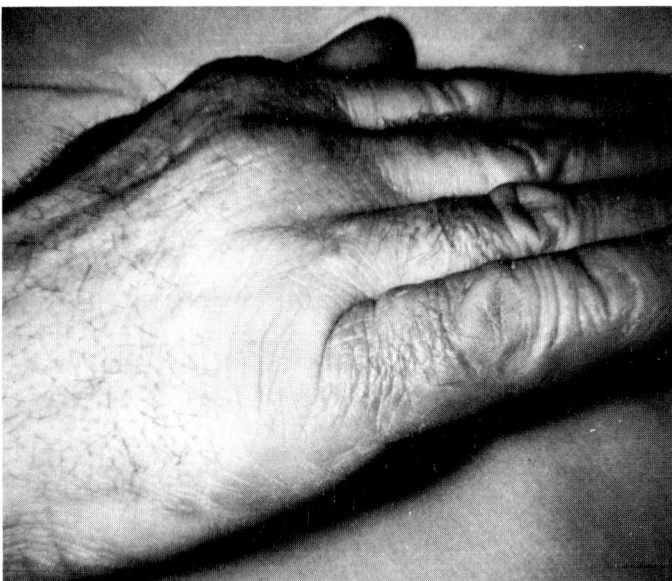

Figure 11–26 Erysipeloid. Two-week-old violaceous patch in a fish handler.

The rare systemic form presents a clinical triad consisting of an eruption, endocarditis, and joint pains. The endocarditis may be fatal. Purpura is a common expression. Discrete macules or red discoid patches occur and coalesce to form large patches. A hemorrhagic necrosis of the ears is uncommon but characteristic. Organisms are present in the blood in the systemic form.

In its ordinary mild form, erysipeloid is chiefly to be distinguished from erysipelas, from which it differs by the lack of constitutional symptoms and a tendency for central healing of the inflammation. Erythema multiforme must be distinguished from the generalized type of erysipeloid. The septicemic form may simulate rheumatic fever. Definitive diagnosis is afforded by culture of biopsy specimens. The organism may rarely be obtained by swabbing the unbroken skin. Infectious material may also be inoculated into mice, from which positive blood cultures are readily obtainable. Penicillin, from 2 to 20 million units per day, is the treatment of choice; the route, dosage, and duration depend on location and severity. The organism is also sensitive to tetracycline and streptomycin.

Gas Gangrene

Gas gangrene evokes thoughts of deep infection by *Clostridium perfringens (C. welchii)* in a military or traumatic setting. However, crepitant cellulitis is, in fact, more often caused by gas-forming coliform bacteria or anerobic streptococci. The spectrum of focal clostridial infection runs from insignificant wound contamination to deep myonecrosis, toxemia, and death. The causative organisms are several spore-forming species of Clostridium which normally inhabit the soil and the bowel. They produce powerful enzymatic exotoxins. The infection is a complication of a deep, crushing, tissue-destroying wound into which there is usually incorporated soil, bits of clothing, or other debris. Within hours of injury the wound becomes swollen, painful, tender, and red, brown, or mottled. As the infection spreads along tissue planes, frank bullae, necrosis, and gangrene occur. The characteristic sign, crepitation due to gas in the tissues, may be elicited by pressure at the wound margin or demonstrated by x-ray; however, neither is constant. Pus is minimal, but a smear from the wound should yield the gram-positive rods.

Bacteremia and septicemia occur rarely with crepitant cellulitis or myonecrosis, occasionally with surgery on the gastrointestinal or biliary tract, and more commonly after septic abortion. The syndrome of gas gangrene sepsis includes hemolysis, tan- to bronze-colored skin, acute renal failure, clotting deficiencies, and hemorrhages (Smith et al., 1971).

Penicillin in high dosage is the antibacterial treatment of choice. Erythromycin and tetracycline may also be used. Neutralization of toxins may be attempted with polyvalent antitoxin. Treatment in a hyperbaric oxygen chamber is aimed at reducing the anaerobic setting in which the clostridia thrive. These measures will prove ineffective, however, unless they are accompanied by surgical debridement of dead tissue.

Listeriosis

Listeriosis (Gray and Killinger, 1966) is an uncommon human infection caused by *Listeria monocytogenes*, a gram-positive microaerophilic bacillus. Animal infections, especially in birds, are common and worldwide. The organism is probably part of the natural flora of man. Animal handlers acquire the cutaneous infection through direct contact. Pregnant women and fetuses have a relatively unusual and unexplainable tendency to acquire the infection. In adults, susceptibility is increased by a debilitated state, prolonged steroid therapy, and an altered cellular immunity due to disease or immunosuppressant therapy.

The small gram-positive rods resemble diphtheroids and are closely related to *Erysipelothrix rhusiopathiae*. The skin lesions and spinal fluid may contain the organisms, and the blood cultures are usually positive. The diagnosis can be further established by animal inoculation and the demonstration of a rising serum agglutination titer. There may be a polymorphonuclear cytosis or monocytosis.

The clinical manifestations of the acute disease in neonates are stillbirths, septicemia, meningitis, and disseminated septic granulomatosis; in adults, the clinical manifestations are septicemia, meningitis, pneumonitis, infectious mononucleosis-like syndrome, urethritis, and oculoglandular syndrome. The differential diagnosis includes toxoplasmosis, cytomegalovirus infection, rubella, disseminated herpes simplex, and systemic bacterial infections. The cutaneous manifestations are variable and depend on the infected host and the mode of acquisition. Infants may have an erythematous papular or a petechial pustular eruption. Veterinarians and other animal handlers develop papular lesions, which become pustular, on the hands and arms with tender axillary adenopathy after one to three days of fever and malaise. The oculoglandular syndrome is characterized by an acute conjunctivitis with preauricular lymphadenitis.

The prognosis is poor in infants and untreated patients but good in adequately treated adults. Those cases resembling infectious mononucleosis have a relatively benign course. Penicillin given intravenously in large doses is effective; tetracycline given intravenously is an effective acceptable alternative.

SYSTEMIC NONVENEREAL SPIROCHETAL INFECTIONS

Rat-Bite Fever due to Spirillum minus (Sodoku)

The disease occurs wherever rats are not controlled and may be transmitted by laboratory rats as well as wild rodents. Following the bite, which usually heals spontaneously, there is an incubation period of several days to a month, usually about 12 days (which is longer than the incubation period for streptobacillary fever). The disease begins suddenly and the clue is the site of the bite. Pain, swelling, erythema, and a nodule develop at this site. The nodule undergoes focal necrosis, producing an ulcer which is surrounded by an edematous zone. Lymphangitis and regional adenopathy follow, and there may be nodular swellings in the inflamed lymphatic channels. General symptoms include fever and an exanthem which is usually generalized but which may be limited to the area close to the bite. The exanthematous eruption is said to resemble syphilis or rubeola. The primary lesions appear as macules, papules, or even nodules which have variable degrees of redness. A significant attribute of these lesions is that they are painful when pressed, though they are not pruritic.

Sometimes there are alarming central nervous system manifestations, such as stupor and coma, followed by death. Pain may be present in the muscles, bones, and joints, but the absence of true arthritis helps separate this infection from the streptobacillary disease.

Without treatment, the disease lasts for weeks or months, showing recurrent periods of activity that are progressively less intense with each recrudescence. The course of the untreated disease was well documented early in this century when sodoku inoculata was attempted in several series as a treatment for general paresis.

The *S. minus* may be demonstrated with ease or with difficulty from the serous fluid at the site of the bite, the exanthem, an enlarged node, or from the peripheral blood smear. Giemsa or silver stains or darkfield examination may be used. The guinea pig is highly susceptible to inoculation with infected material. Eosinophilia is common, and false positive tests for syphilis may be encountered.

In the past, arsenicals were used successfully in the treatment of sodoku, but today penicillin is the treatment of choice. Either procaine penicillin G, 600,000 units intramuscularly, or penicillin V, 1 gm. orally every 6 hours for 10 days, may be used.

Relapsing Fever

Relapsing fever refers to an acute septicemic process caused by one of several species of spirochete of the genus Borrelia. It is characterized by recurrent paroxysms of fever. The borrelia differ from the organisms of the two other genera (Treponema and Leptospira) by their ability to take up aniline dyes. Fewer than one-half of involved patients exhibit a rash. Although the clinical features tend to be similar, epidemiologically it is useful to contrast the tick-borne variety with the louse-borne variety.

Tick-borne relapsing fever occurs worldwide and is reported sporadically in the United States, most recently in Boston (Goodman et al., 1967) and Washington state (Thompson et al., 1969). Many species of ticks serve as both reservoir and vector. These ticks can survive for years without feeding. Transovarian passage of the spirochete also occurs.

Louse-borne relapsing fever is currently endemic only in Ethiopia but the possibility of a devastating epidemic always exists, particularly after war (for example, the epidemic in Turkey and Persia following World War I and that in the Middle East after World War II). *Borrelia recurrentis* is the single species with man as the only known reservoir and *Pediculus humanus* as the vector. The spirochete enters normal or abraded skin after crushing of the louse, not by the louse's bite.

The clinical syndromes are similar for each variety (Southern and Sanford, 1969). The incubation period is usually about one week (4 to 18 days). The onset of the fever is abrupt and can be as high as 105° F., with chills, headache, myalgia, cough, abdominal pain, and vomiting. Hepatosplenomegaly with jaundice may occur. Photophobia and conjunctival suffusion are common. The first febrile episode ends after three to five days, with a crisis and drenching sweats. At this time a generalized or localized eruption appears in fewer than half the cases and lasts usually only a day or two. This eruption may mimic the rose spots of typhoid fever or may consist of macular or papular petechiae. During subsequent febrile attacks, the eruption is unlikely to appear.

The diagnosis is best established by identification of the spirochete in a peripheral blood smear stained by the Wright's or Giemsa technique. A monocytosis may be noted. In the louse-borne variety, over 90 per cent of patients will show a high titer of Proteus OXK agglutinins, while the percentage and titers are far lower in the tick-borne variety.

Untreated, the mortality rate for the louse-borne variety is 40 per cent; it is less than 5 per cent for the tick-borne variety. Therapy lowers the death rate below 5 per cent in the louse-borne, but its effect on the tick-borne variety is hard to assess. Therapeutically, tetracycline is even more effective than penicillin in clearing the spirochetemia, but a Jarisch-Herxheimer reaction is a regular (and occasionally fatal) occurrence. Thus, Bryceson and colleagues (1970) have recommended procaine penicillin 300,000 units the first day followed by tetracycline the next day. Prevention is directed toward control of the arthropod vectors.

Leptospirosis

Leptospirosis is an acute febrile illness with a variety of clinical expressions caused by any one of several serotypes of the spirochete leptospira. The skin may be a portal of entry, particularly through an abrasion, although mucosal or gastrointestinal routes are also important. In a minority of cases, there are cutaneous signs which include jaundice, purpura, urticaria, or less specific eruptions.

Leptospirosis occurs in a broad geographic area, including the United States, and is seen most often in early autumn. It is most common in young men and may be acquired on the farm or in the home, swimming area, or abattoir. In Southeast Asia, leptospirosis was a common cause of mild, self-limited, febrile illnesses among troops (Allen et al., 1968).

The natural reservoir of this spirochete includes a wide range of wild and domestic animals (and occasionally humans) who infect man directly or by "urinary shedding" which contaminates water. Although a particular serotype may show some preference for a certain animal (*Leptospira icterohaemorrhagiae* for rats, *L. canicola* for dogs, and *L. pomona* for cows and swine), these preferences are by no means exclusive.

Clinical syndromes are also not serotype specific. In fact, the general systemic signs and symptoms are more common than the specific syndromes (Heath et al.,

1965) such as Weil's disease (icterohemorrhagic fever) or Fort Bragg (pretibial) fever. After an incubation period of about 10 days (it may range from 2 to 20 days), there occur the abrupt onset of fever (usually 102° F. or higher), anorexia, nausea, vomiting, diarrhea, muscle pain and tenderness, and conjunctival suffusion. The central nervous system is most frequently involved, exhibiting headache and meningeal signs with increased cells and protein in the cerebrospinal fluid. Neurologic signs are nearly always transient.

Hepatic and renal involvement (Weil's disease, icterohemorrhagic fever) are next in frequency and are important prognostic signs, since leptospirosis is rarely fatal in the absence of involvement of these organs in which spirochetes can be demonstrated at postmortem examination. Renal involvement includes pyuria, hematuria, and azotemia. Hepatic necrosis produces jaundice.

Fewer than half of the cases of leptospirosis have cutaneous involvement which varies from nonspecific macules and wheals to purpura. A characteristic symmetrical pretibial eruption with splenomegaly was first described in an epidemic at Fort Bragg (Daniels and Grennan, 1943) and later recognized as spirochetal in origin (Gochenour et al., 1952). The solitary and confluent lesions appear on the fourth day of the illness as warm, slightly raised, poorly circumscribed red patches, 2 to 5 cm. in diameter, which fade in a matter of days. Histologically, only edema and a nonspecific perivascular inflammation are noted.

Leptospira may be identified early and directly in blood smears, or it may be cultured from blood and cerebrospinal fluid early and from the urine later. The diagnosis is usually made by at least a fourfold rise in agglutination or complement-fixation titer but antibodies do not appear until the sixth to twelfth day. Early leukopenia may be followed by variable leukocytosis, with the greatest neutrophilia in the jaundiced patient. Hemolysins are produced in vitro and in vivo. Azotemia is most common also with jaundice.

Prognosis is related to age, with up to 50 per cent mortality in men over 50. Death is rare in the absence of jaundice. Penicillin, 2,400,000 units daily, or tetracycline, 2 gm. daily (Turner, 1969), has been recommended but must be administered in the first four days of the illness if expected to influence the course in this dosage. A Herxheimer reaction is not uncommon. If the renal failure can be managed with dialysis, good recovery of function can be expected.

REFERENCES

Abu-Nasser, H., Hill, N., Fred, H. L., et al.: Cutaneous manifestations of gonococcemia. A review of 14 cases. Arch. Intern. Med. *112*:731, 1963.

Allen, G. L., Weber, D. R., and Russell, P. K.: The clinical picture of leptospirosis in American soldiers in Vietnam. Milit. Med. *133*:275, 1968.

Antley, R. M., and McMillan, W. C.: Sequential coagulation studies in purpura fulminans. N. Engl. J. Med. *276*:1287, 1967.

Aserkoff, B., Schroeder, S. A., and Bradiman, P. S.: Salmonellosis in the United States. A five year review. Am. J. Epidemiol. *12*:13, 1970.

Belsey, M. A., Sinclair, M., Roder, M. R., et al.: Corynebacterium diphtheriae skin infections in Alabama and Louisiana. N. Engl. J. Med. *280*:135, 1969.

Benoit, F. L.: Chronic meningococcemia: Case report and review of literature. Am. J. Med. *35*:103, 1963.

Bjornberg, A.: Benign gonococcal sepsis: A report of 36 cases. Acta Dermatovener. *50*:313, 1970.

Black, P. H., Kunz, L. J., and Swartz, M. N.: Salmonellosis—A review of some unusual aspects. N. Engl. J. Med. *262*:811, 1960.

Bodey, G. P., Whitecar, J. P., Jr., Middleman, E., et al.: Carbenicillin therapy for Pseudomonas infections. J.A.M.A. *218*:62, 1971.

Bryceson, A. D. M., Parry, E. H., Perine, P. L., et al.: Louse-borne relapsing fever. Quart. J. Med. *39*:129, 1970.

Burnett, J. W.: Uncommon bacterial infections of the skin. Arch. Dermatol. *86*:597, 1962.

Cole, J. S., Stoll, R. W., and Bulger, R. J.: Rate bite fever: Report of 3 cases. Ann. Intern. Med. *71*:979, 1969.

Daniels, W. B., and Grennan, H. A.: Pretibial fever. J.A.M.A. *122*:361, 1943.

Deykin, D.: The clinical challenge of disseminated intravascular coagulation. N. Engl. J. Med. *283*:636, 1970.

Doust, J. Y., Sarkarzadeh, A., and Kavoossi, K.: Corticosteroid in treatment of malignant edema of chest wall and neck (anthrax). Dis. Chest *53*:773, 1968.

Feingold, M., and Gellis, S. S.: Cellulitis due to Haemophilus influenzae, type B. N. Engl. J. Med. *272*:788, 1965.

Feldman, H. A.: Meningococcus and gonococcus: Never the twain. . . . Well, hardly ever. N. Engl. J. Med. *285*:518, 1971.

Forkner, C. E., et al.: Pseudomonas septicemia: Observations on 23 cases. Am. J. Med. *2*:253, 347, 1947.

Gochenour, W. S., Jr., et al.: Leptospiral etiology of Fort Bragg fever. Pub. Health Rep. *67*:811, 1952.

Goodman, R. L., et al.: Borrelia in Boston. J.A.M.A. *210*:722, 1967.

Gray, M. L., and Killinger, A. H.: Listeria monocytogenes and listeric infections. Bact. Rev. 30:309, 1966.

Hall, J. H., Callaway, J. L., Tindall, J. P., et al.: Pseudomonas aeruginosa in dermatology. Arch. Dermatol. 97:312, 1968.

Heath, C. W., Jr., Alexander, A. D., and Galton, M. M.: Leptospirosis in the United States. N. Engl. J. Med. 273:857, 915, 1965.

Hoang, M. N., and Rozendaal, H. M.: A modified treatment of bubonic plague. J.A.M.A. 205:124, 1968.

Holmes, K. K., Counts, G. W., and Beaty, H. N.: Disseminated gonococcal infection. Ann. Intern. Med. 74:979, 1971.

Huddleson, I. F.: Brucellosis in Man and Animals. New York, The Commonwealth Fund, 1943.

Hull, T. G.: Diseases Transmitted from Animals to Man. 5th ed. Springfield, Illinois, Charles C Thomas, 1963.

Kahn, G.: Septic gonococcal dermatitis. Arch. Dermatol. 99:421, 1969.

Keiser, H., Ruben, F. L., Wolinsky, E., et al.: Clinical forms of gonococcal arthritis. N. Engl. J. Med. 279:234, 1968.

Klauder, J. V.: Erysipelothrix rhusiopathiae infection in swine and human beings. Arch. Dermatol. 50:151, 1944.

Letgers, L. H., Cottingham, A. J., and Hunter, D. H.: Clinical and epidemiologic notes on a defined outbreak of plague in Vietnam. Am. J. Trop. Med. 19:639, 1970.

Liebow, A. A., MacLean, P. D., Bumstead, J. H., et al.: Tropical ulcers and cutaneous diphtheria. Arch. Int. Med. 78:255, 1946.

McCormack, R., Kaye, D., and Hook, E.: Endocardites due to streptobacillus moniliformis. J A.M.A. 200:77, 1967.

Metzger, A. L.: Gonococcal arthritis complicating gonorrheal pharyngitis. Ann. Intern. Med. 3:267, 1970.

Nielsen, L. T.: Chronic meningococcemia. Arch. Dermatol., 102:97, 1970.

Piggott, J. A., and Hochholzer, L.: Human melioidosis. Arch. Pathol. 90:101, 1970.

Proceedings of the Conference on Progress in the Understanding of Anthrax. In Nungster, W., (Chairman): Federation Proceedings, 263, 1967.

Proctor, W. I.: Subacute bacterial endocarditis due to Erysipelothrix rhusiopathiae. Am. J. Med. 38:820, 1965.

Reed, W. P., Palmer, L. D., Williams, R. C., et al.: Bubonic plague in the Southwest United States. Medicine 49:465, 1970.

Reiley, C. G., and Kates, E. D.: The clinical spectrum of plague in Vietnam. Arch. Intern. Med. 126:990, 1970.

Remele, N. S., Klein, F., Vick, J. A., et al.: Anthrax toxin: Primary site of action. J. Infect. Dis. 118:104, 1968.

Ricketts, W. E.: Clinical manifestations of Carrion's disease. Arch. Intern. Med. 84:751, 1949.

Rosen, F. S.: The endotoxins of gram-negative bacteria and host resistance. N. Engl. J. Med. 264:919, 1961.

Schultz, M.: A History of bartonellosis (Carrion's disease). Am. J. Trop. Med. 17:503, 1968.

Schwartz, M. N., and King, L. J.: Pasteurella multocida infections in man. N. Engl. J. Med. 261:889, 1959.

Sheehy, T. W., Deller, J. J., and Weber, D. R.: Melioidosis. Ann. Intern. Med. 67:897, 1967.

Shellow, W. V. R., and Koplon, B. S.: Green striped nails: Chromonychia due to Pseudomonas aeruginosa. Arch. Dermatol. 97:149–153, 1968.

Smith, L. P., McLean, A. P. H., and Maughan, G. B.: Clostridium welchii septicotoxemia. Am. J. Obstet. Gynecol. 110:135 May 1, 1971.

Southern, Jr., P. M., and Sanford, J. P.: Relapsing fever. Medicine 48:129, 1969.

Spink, W. W.: The Nature of Brucellosis. Minneapolis, Univers ty of Minnesota Press, 1956.

Spink, W. W.: Present status of brucellosis in man: Clinical and diagnostic problems. J. Am. Vet. Med. Assoc. 115:2091, 1969.

Stanley, M.: Bacillus pyocyaneous infections—a review, report of cases and discussion of newer therapy including streptomycin. Am. J. Med. 2:253, 347, 1947.

Steck, W. D., and Byrd, R B.: Urticaria secondary to pulmonary melioidosis. Arch. Dermatol. 99:80, 1969.

Teplitz, C.: Pathogenesis of Pseudomonas vasculitis. Arch. Pathol. 80:297, 1965.

Thompson, R. S., Burgdorfer, W., Russell, R., et al.: Outbreak of tick-borne relapsing fever in Spokane county, Washington, J.A.M.A. 210:1045, 1969.

Tindall, J. P., and Harrison, C. M.: Pasteurella multocida infection following animal injuries, especially cat bites. Arch. Dermatol. 105:412, 1972.

Turner, H. H.: Leptospirosis. Br. Med. J. 1:231, 1969.

Weber, D. R., Douglass, L. E., Brundage, W. G., et al.: Acute varieties of melioidosis occurring in U. S. soldiers in Vietnam. Am. J. Med. 46:234, 1969.

Weinstein, L., and Klainer, A. S.: Management of emergencies. IV. Septic shock—pathogenesis and treatment. N. Engl. J. Med. 274:950, 1966.

White, J. D., and McGavran, M. H.: Identification of Pasteurella tularensis by immunofluorescence. J.A.M.A. 194:294, 1965.

Wolf, R. E., and Bibara, C. A.: Meningococcal infections at an Army training center. Am. J. Med. 44:243, 1968.

Young, L. S., Bickness, D. S., Archer, B. G., et al.: Tularemia epidemic: Vermont, 1968. N. Engl. J. Med. 280:1253, 1969.

Zalma, V. M., Older, J. J., and Brooks, G. F.: The Austin, Texas, diphtheria outbreak. J.A.M.A. 211:2125, 1970.

VIRAL AND
RICKETTSIAL INFECTIONS*

Joseph W. Burnett and *William A. Crutcher*

Viral organisms are capable of producing a wide variety of changes in the skin and mucous membranes of man. Several of these organisms have been known since early antiquity; others have been recognized only in recent years. Until little more than a decade ago, dependence for the diagnosis of a viral disease affecting the skin was perforce placed almost entirely on clinical characteristics. Laboratory procedures, other than histopathologic examination and a few simple animal inoculations, were of comparatively little practical value. The situation has since changed greatly, and the current rate of advance is rapid. This has come about through the study of viruses by means of electron microscope visualization, culture of some viruses on the chorioallantoic membrane of the chick embryo, tissue cultures, special serologic procedures, smear techniques, and special histochemical methods. Some of these procedures are simple enough to be used in routine office and hospital practice. Some require modest special equipment and techniques; others are exceedingly difficult, and can be carried out only in special virology centers, of which there are an increasing number in the United States and elsewhere. In the following summarization of viral and rickettsial infections, reference to laboratory procedures will be confined to those which are relatively ·simple and of undoubted practical value, with only occasional passing mention of procedures which are primarily of research nature.

GENERAL
BIOLOGY OF VIRUSES

Viruses have a greater diversity of structure and composition than originally supposed. While some are pure molecules of ribonucleoprotein, others contain an

---

*Because this chapter was superbly written in Pillsbury et al.: Dermatology, the present authors have kept much of the earlier material. Newer concepts have been added to these sections.

aggregate of complex chemical materials and show internal morphologic differentiation. The essential properties of viruses on which modern classification is based are (1) they are agents of extremely small size capable of passing bacterial filters, (2) they are strict intracellular parasites (which does not differentiate them from rickettsiae), and (3) they do not reproduce by binary fission as do bacteria. This last criterion is one of the important reasons why certain agents previously considered "large" viruses, namely, the organisms of trachoma, lymphogranuloma venereum, and inclusion blennorrhea, have been reclassified as Chlamydiaceae, a group closely related to the rickettsiae. Furthermore, true viruses lack enzyme systems altogether, but the microorganisms of Chlamydiaceae have them in part, on which account the latter group is more susceptible to chemotherapeutic agents than the true viruses. The organisms of Chlamydiaceae differ from viruses in that they are larger, reproduce by binary fission, are more susceptible to chemotherapeutic agents, and display certain tinctorial properties when stained.

Viruses do not reproduce themselves from their own bodies but apparently act as a kind of "template," inducing the host cell to synthesize new virus material along with its normal metabolic products. Somehow the host cell is persuaded to create virus out of its own stores. Shortly after the cell is infected, the virus actually disappears as an infective entity (the eclipse phenomenon) and cannot be recovered by any known means, presumably because it blends with the metabolic machinery of the cell before the cell embarks upon the production of new viral particles. It is known, therefore, that an apparently normal cell can harbor a "something" which under appropriate conditions may start the elaboration of virus particles. The medical significance of this concept is that recurrences of symptomatic viral diseases —for example, recurrent attacks of herpes simplex—need not be explained as a reinfection with fresh virus but rather as persistence of the "virus" in an inactive and undetectable form, harmonized with the cells' normal activities, until some stimulus "activates" the virus-producing system.

When virus is being actively produced,

the cell's appearance is altered in a more or less characteristic way, displaying the so-called inclusion body. The inclusion body is, in some cases, predominantly an aggregation of mature, immature, or imperfectly formed virus particles, as in herpes simplex and warts; in other cases, a variable amount of matrix material of the host cell is mingled with it. In the organisms of Chlamydiaceae in particular, what are so clearly apparent in the light microscope are not pure infective particles but mostly matrix. The inclusion body undergoes a dynamic series of changes in the course of its formation and will, therefore, be visualized differently at different stages of the infection.

Another rather characteristic feature of viral infections is that the primary infection may be completely asymptomatic. The body records the event, however, by building antibodies and by acquiring an immunity just as firm as if clinical disease had occurred. Immunologic status serves to differentiate between primary and recurrent infections, regardless of whether there is recognizable disease or not, for the host has no antibodies at the time of the primary infection. It is for this reason that primary infections with certain viruses, if symptomatic at all, are sometimes extremely severe (for example, herpes simplex).

Since viruses are obligate intracellular parasites, the principal site of attack in the skin is the epidermis, for the corium is mostly a noncellular structure replete with collagen, while the epidermis itself is 100 per cent cellular. An epidermal cell responds to the virus in more than one way: it can be disorganized and lysed, giving rise to the clinical picture of inflammatory changes with vesiculation, or it can be induced to proliferate, forming a localized growth or tumor composed of virus-laden cells.

Viral infections vary greatly in their capacity to produce systemic manifestations. Some (for example, warts and molluscum contagiosum) are entirely dermatotropic. Others (for example, milker's nodules and orf) are capable of limited dissemination, as evidenced by mild systemic symptoms and local lymphadenopathy. Such viral infections as cat-scratch disease, and lymphogranuloma venereum (which is produced by one of the Chlamydiaceae), though ordinarily well localized, are occasionally productive of marked general systemic effects. The most common of all viral diseases, herpes simplex, is usually entirely dermatotropic, but it is capable of producing serious systemic reactions in the course of the initial infection or in persons who are only partially immune. In a number of the virus infections, for example, chickenpox, measles, and smallpox, the viral infection apparently occurs first in the upper respiratory tract and then becomes disseminated, with the production of rather characteristic lesions in the skin and mucous membranes.

The pattern of viral reactions in the skin and mucous membranes varies greatly and includes erythematous lesions, vesicles, pustules, tumors, ulcers, and scars. In a number of such infections, the "trailing" bacterial infection may play a determining role in the systemic reaction or the local changes produced in the skin. The individual viral infections also vary greatly within themselves in respect to their gross clinical manifestations. With warts, for instance, though the pathologic pattern is relatively uniform, the gross morphologic changes differ considerably, from very flat, to sessile, to threadlike lesions, or even to very exuberant multiple moist papules. Molluscum contagiosum has a strikingly uniform gross pattern of reaction. The virus of varicella may produce the clinical syndrome of either chickenpox or zoster, the latter probably representing the response when some degree of immunity is present, though there are still unsolved questions in this respect.

Although the exanthemata are described in most textbooks as having fairly regular patterns of reaction, this may be far from the case. In smallpox, for instance, the characteristics of the skin lesions may differ widely from those which are regarded as typical, and because of this, the initial patients seen in an epidemic may escape diagnosis, even under the observation of physicians with wide experience in contagious diseases. The pattern of reaction in smallpox may also be greatly modified by varying degrees of immunity produced by vaccination.

Viral infections possess another almost unique property in that in many of them the initial infection may be completely inapparent, and large segments of the population may show a specific antibody response to individual viruses in the absence of any history indicating when the initial infection was sustained.

In some of the diseases included in this chapter, proof of the viral etiology is unquestionable and may be demonstrated in a variety of ways. With others, the evidence is strongly presumptive, but absolute proof is lacking. In addition to these diseases, unfortunately, a viral etiology has been ascribed to a variety of other processes, apparently on the basis of inability to prove any other cause and because the hypothesis of a viral etiology is difficult to disprove. With improvement in the variety and precision of virologic methods, it is being shown that a viral etiology of some of these diseases (for example, pemphigus, aphthous stomatitis, and dermatitis herpetiformis) is less likely.

A uniform characteristic of all the true viral infections is their resistance to any antibiotic drugs developed to date. The problem is more difficult than with higher forms, since viruses lack enzyme systems, using those of the host instead. Any attempt to paralyze such systems by chemotherapy would also cripple the host. During the primary infection, reliance must be placed entirely upon the development of antibodies by the host, and upon supportive therapy to prevent complications, particularly secondary bacterial infection. Moreover, recurrent viral infections may appear in the presence of circulating antibodies, possibly because of the intracellular location of the virus. In some of the unusual complications of viral infections, in which there may be an element of tissue sensitization or excessive inflammatory reactions with toxicity, corticosteroid therapy may be of benefit. With infections produced by organisms of Chlamydiaceae and rickettsiae, on the other hand, antibiotic or sulfonamide therapy or both is of great value.

In the following presentations of various viral infections, the greatest emphasis will be placed upon those infections which are primarily dermatotropic. Discussion of the systemic viral infections must perforce be limited principally to the mucocutaneous signs, the chief general diagnostic criteria, and the complications which may occur.

HERPES SIMPLEX

Herpes simplex is one of the most ubiquitous of all the viral infections of man. The virus is relatively large (175 nm.). Almost the entire adult population has sustained infection by it at one time or another, though it may never become apparent clinically. Because the virus is readily obtainable, can be grown easily, and may be visualized in various ways, and because the immunologic responses to it may be studied with relative facility, much has been learned recently concerning the course of the infection.

Infection with herpes simplex virus becomes manifest in one of two ways: the primary infection, which occurs in individuals who have no specific neutralizing antibodies; and recurrent infections, occurring in individuals who possess specific antibodies. Recurrent herpes simplex is an exceedingly common disease, while the primary infection produces recognizable changes in a very small proportion of infected persons.

Recently it has become clear that in addition to variations within strains, there are two major herpes simplex virus subgroups. Type I is usually associated with nongenital lesions whereas type II is the usual form recovered from genital lesions. In addition, type I herpes virus differs from type II in that it does not produce plaques in inoculated chick embryo cells. Furthermore, type I virus causes different-sized pox lesions on chick chorioallantoic membrane and has a different density of DNA (deoxyribonucleic acid) than its counterpart. Once the virus is isolated, differentiation of the two herpesvirus hominis (HVH) types (I and II) can be made by a variety of serologic tests, such as the microneutralization test and immunofluorescent (FA) techniques (Nahmias et al., 1969).

Primary Herpes Simplex Infection

Evidence of herpes simplex is very rare in infants under four months of age because most infants possess passively transferred maternal antibodies until this time.

Until two years of age, relatively few infants possess herpes simplex antibodies and are, accordingly, susceptible to infection. Fortunately, the infection occurs without any clinical manifestations in most infants or children. It may, however, manifest itself in one of the following ways:

PRIMARY GINGIVOSTOMATITIS OR VULVOVAGINITIS. This is a fairly characteristic syndrome which is often falsely diagnosed as Vincent's infection; hand, foot, and mouth enanthem; aphthous stomatitis; or erythema multiforme. It is comparatively uncommon but occasional patients with the disease will be encountered on any large pediatric service. It occurs most frequently between the ages of two and five years, but may be seen in older children and young adults. The disease is characterized by the sudden development of painful oral lesions, with high fever, regional lymphadenopathy, and general malaise. White plaques appear in the mouth and pharynx, often in widespread fashion, and become superficially ulcerated. The gingivae become red, swollen, and painful, a highly characteristic sign. Occasionally, scattered vesicles may be seen which are suggestive of herpetic infection. Fluid balance and nutrition may be seriously disturbed because the mouth lesions are exceedingly painful and the child refuses fluid or food.

The lesions in primary herpetic vulvovaginitis are entirely similar, with the appearance of sharply defined plaques on the vaginal mucosa, usually accompanied by isolated nongrouped vesicles on the surrounding skin. Fever, malaise, and inguinal adenopathy are also present. In vulvar involvement, there may be confusion with gonorrheal infection, thrush, nonspecific vaginitis, unusually severe diaper rash, or even diphtheria. The inflammation persists for a week to 10 days, and recovery will ordinarily be noted within two weeks. The disease may affect the nasal mucosa rarely, or the conjunctiva. The keratoconjunctivitis which may occur as part of the primary herpes simplex infection is alarming in appearance, though fortunately it ordinarily heals without residual corneal damage. There are severe swelling, injection, haziness, and superficial ulceration of the cornea. The eye is ordinarily closed, and there is regional adenopathy.

The diagnosis of primary herpes simplex

infection may be established indubitably if reasonable virologic facilities are at hand. The virus may be isolated from the lesions easily, and the cytologic picture is characteristic, although differentiation from the histologic changes seen in zoster or chickenpox is required. The principal initial changes are in the nucleus, which becomes swollen with viral material, forcing chromatin to the periphery in a ring. Eventually, a characteristic viral-type giant cell forms, which contains several nuclei and may be quite large. The inclusion body of herpes simplex is intranuclear. At the onset of the infection, no virus neutralizing antibodies are demonstrable, but these begin to appear within 5 to 10 days. Their appearance is determined by adding varying dilutions of serum to constant amounts of herpes virus. Samples of blood are examined when the patient is first seen, and again at two-week intervals. An increased antibody titer is diagnostic. Complement-fixing herpes antibodies may also be demonstrated. Occasionally, a primary infection may disseminate to the central nervous system, causing a severe meningitis or encephalitis. In untreated infections, mortality has been reported as high as 60 per cent and serious sequelae are common in survivors. Recently, intravenous idoxuridine at doses approaching 100 mg. per kilogram per day has been given for five days in a slow continuous drip and has apparently reduced both mortality and sequelae. Toxicity includes stomatitis, severe marrow depression with granulocytopenia and thrombocytopenia, and complete alopecia (Meyer et al., 1970).

INOCULATION HERPES SIMPLEX. This type of primary infection is uncommon. It occurs in a patient in whom herpes simplex antibodies are absent and is a result of implantation of the virus into skin which has been abraded or lacerated. There may be some tendency to the characteristic grouping associated with recurrent herpes simplex, but this is not marked; regional adenopathy and some febrile systemic reaction may be noted. When this infection occurs among wrestlers, it is called herpes gladiatorum (Selling and Kibrick, 1964). Another variant is seen frequently in medical and dental personnel in the form of a "herpetic whitlow" on a finger following slight trauma and contact with an in-fected patient (Hambrick et al., 1962). A similar paronychial inoculation may follow nail biting during an attack of primary herpetic-gingivo stomatitis (Miller et al., 1970). Surgical incision wounds have also been reported as sites of primary herpetic infections. The reaction ordinarily subsides without incident, but recurrent herpes simplex at the site may be noted later.

KAPOSI'S VARICELLIFORM ERUPTION. Another form of primary herpes simplex infection is seen in infants with eczema, almost always of the atopic dermatitis type (eczema vaccinatum). The complication is almost always very alarming and may be fatal. It is characterized by the sudden appearance of umbilicated varicelliform lesions distributed principally to the areas of skin commonly involved in atopic dermatitis, especially the upper trunk, neck, and head (Fig. 12–1). Fever may be high, and the patient often appears acutely ill. The vesicles develop a hemorrhagic crust, or sometimes become pustular, and tend to appear in crops for from several days to a week. There is marked adenopathy and local edema. Abortive forms undoubtedly occur and may be attributed to the results of scratching or to secondary bacterial infection, but they are difficult to recognize.

Such abortive forms probably occur almost entirely in atopic patients who have herpes-neutralizing antibodies in their blood. However, such antibodies give no assurance that the symptoms of Kaposi's varicelliform eruption will not be exceedingly severe or that the disease will not recur, although the course is ordinarily less prolonged. A similar type of inoculation may occur in burned patients, resulting in second degree areas converting to third degree loss with a high incidence of concomitant *Pseudomonas aeruginosa* colonization. If the infection is primary, a viremia may result in disseminated visceral herpes, similar to herpes neonatorum, and is frequently fatal. Since burned patients have considerable crusting due to their thermal injuries, secondary viral superinfection is frequently unrecognized. Presence of vesiculation of burn-wound margins followed by rapid extension of third degree, bacterially infected areas, or the occurrence of high fever unresponsive

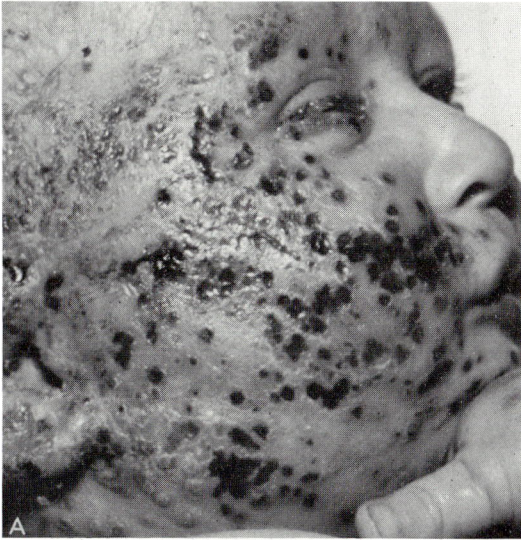

Figure 12-1 *A*, Eczema herpeticum. No herpes neutralizing antibodies were present in this patient; this was the primary herpes infection. *B*, Kaposi's varicelliform eruption due to herpes simplex (eczema herpeticum). *C*, Kaposi's varicelliform eruption due to vaccinia virus (eczema vaccinatum). These two viral complications of eczema are clinically indistinguishable.

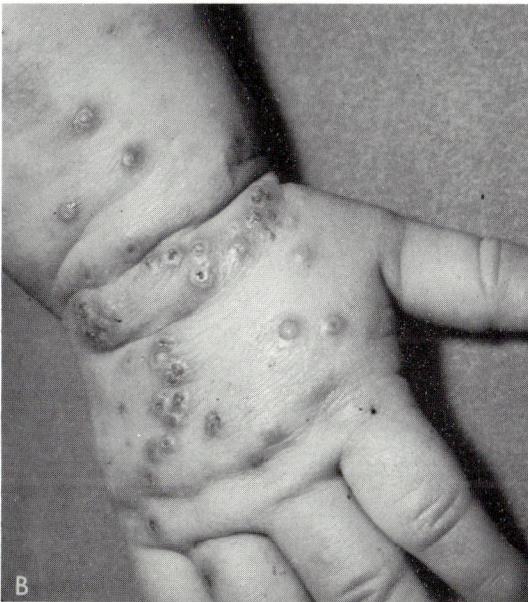

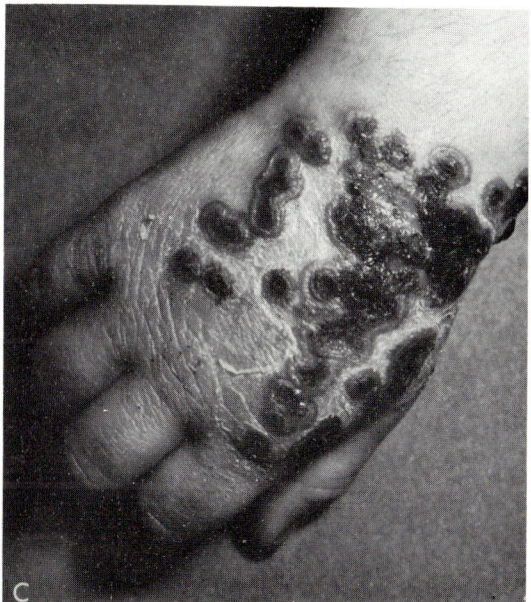

to antibiotics appropriate to cutaneous and systemic bacterial cultures are highly suggestive of this complication. Biopsy of burn-wound margins is important in establishing the diagnosis, and appropriate serology usually confirms a fourfold· or greater rise in neutralizing antibodies if the patient survives (Foley et al., 1970). Several cases of severe or fatal eczema herpeticum have been reported in patients with the Wiskott-Aldrich syndrome. It was speculated that a deficit in cellular immunity allowed virus to persist in the

tissue, inducing at least partial immunologic tolerance (St. Geme et al., 1965).

Vigorous supportive therapy is vital, and may include transfusions, antiviral chemotherapy, and antibiotics appropriate to demonstrated secondary bacterial invaders. Systemic corticosteroids are contraindicated in early phases of primary herpes simplex infections but can be useful to treat complications of encephalitis in which some mechanism of tissue sensitization may be operative. Gamma globulin, even if taken from convalescent serum, is of disputed efficacy but is probably harmless. In neonatal disseminated herpes, disseminated intravascular coagulation may occur, requiring sophisticated hematologic studies and various blood product replacements (Miller et al., 1970). The clinical picture produced by either herpes simplex or vaccinia is indistinguishable grossly. Presumptive evidence of eczema vaccinatum may be obtained on the basis of recent vaccination of the child or contact with another who has just been vaccinated. A definite history of contact with herpes simplex is ordinarily difficult to obtain because this infection is so commonplace.

Fatal viremia can occur in the course of the primary infection with herpes simplex, either in relation to gingival stomatitis or as an infection which is entirely systemic. The latter tends to occur most commonly in premature infants, apparently as a result of infection acquired at delivery. Evidence of the infection begins to appear on the fifth to seventh day, with either fever or subnormal temperature, cyanosis, enlargement of the liver, and sometimes, of the spleen. Multiple lesions are produced in many organs, including the liver, spleen, adrenals, kidney, skin, conjunctiva, and gastrointestinal tract, and the disease is regularly fatal. The pathologic changes in all organs are typical of those produced by herpes simplex.

A simple means of determining the viral character of the infection involves gently scraping the roof or floor of a vesicle with a blade, fixing the smear with alcohol on a glass slide, and staining with Giemsa to demonstrate the multinucleate giant cells. This Tzanck preparation is positive with herpes simplex as well as with herpes zoster or varicella. Vaccinia produces intracytoplasmic inclusions.

Evidence of maternal herpetic vulvovaginitis is an indication for cesarean section in an attempt to protect the child from infection. Occasionally, even that procedure is ineffective, since herpes simplex may be transmitted transplacentally, and these infants may experience vesiculation within several hours after birth (Miller et al., 1970). Another unusual presentation in the neonate is purely cutaneous as grouped vesicles in a zosteriform nerve root distribution (Music et al., 1971).

Recurrent Herpes Simplex

As previously stated, there is evidence that almost all humans eventually sustain infection by the virus of herpes simplex. This may be shown by the presence of herpes-neutralizing antibodies or by the fact that most adults suffer from recurrent herpes simplex occasionally, or will develop lesions of the disease if a sufficient stress is applied (for example, prolonged high fever). The clinical characteristics of recurrent herpes simplex are so well known and commonplace as to require little description. The onset of a lesion is preceded for a few hours or even two or three days by tingling, burning, or itching at the site. In areas where the skin is tense and firmly attached, moderate pain may be experienced. The vesicles of recurrent herpes simplex occur almost invariably in grouped (herpetiform) fashion on an erythematous base. The amount of swelling of the base varies greatly. There may be a single group of lesions or several, sometimes as many as 8 or 10. The individual vesicles are invariably small at the onset, no more than 2 or 3 mm., and do not coalesce. They persist for varying short periods, ordinarily no longer than two days, and the lesion becomes purulent then crusted. Oozing is not marked, as a rule. With very small insignificant lesions, complete involution may occur in four or five days, but in severe lesions, some evidence of it may be present for as long as two weeks, particularly if there has been any secondary infection (Fig. 12–2).

DISTRIBUTION. The lesions of recurrent herpes simplex are seen principally on the lips and perioral region but may occur anywhere. The genital region of both males and females may be affected recurrently (herpes progenitalis); this has at times led to confusion with venereal diseases. Herpes simplex may occur within the oral cavity in the form of grouped vesicles which rapidly rupture; however, this virus is not the cause of recurrent aphthous stomatitis (Fig. 12–3). Recurrent herpes simplex may occasionally appear in a distribution similar to that of zoster, and differentiation may be difficult with the first attack. Erythema multiforme may result as an allergic response to recurrent herpetic infections, and localized skin

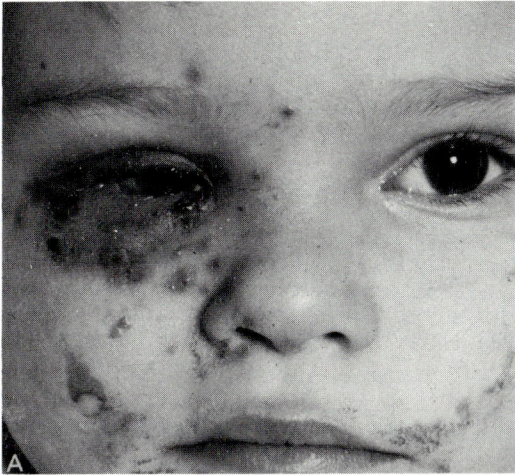

Figure 12-2 *A*, Recurrent herpes simplex of eye and periorbital skin. Topical cortisone or hydrocortisone therapy is *contraindicated* in such lesions. *B* and *C*, Extensive recurrent herpes simplex.

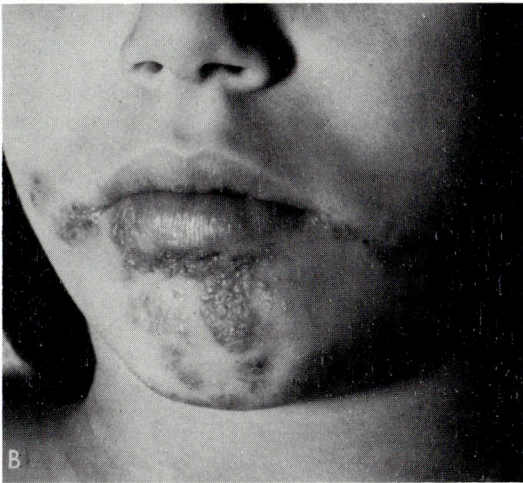

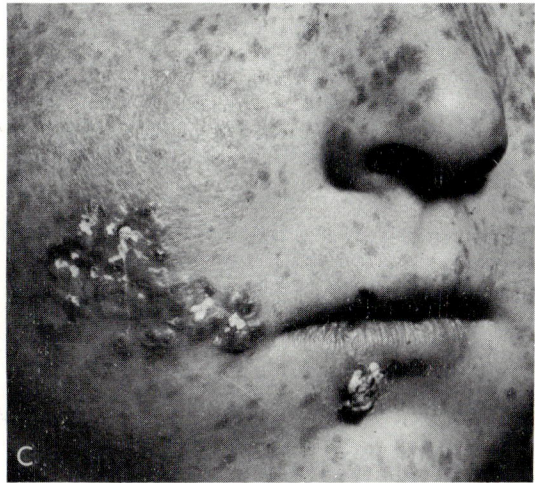

tests with herpes simplex antigen reproduce the clinical and histologic lesions in these patients (Shelley, 1967).

By far the most important type of recurrent herpes simplex is that which affects the eye. The frequency of this type of keratitis has been appreciated only within recent years. It occurs in a variety of forms as a recurrent marginal keratitis and dendritic corneal ulcer. Vesicles may be noted on the eyelids and the palpebral conjunctivae, as well as in the surrounding skin. The corneal lesions may progress to a disciform keratitis.

Prevention of bacterial superinfection is of utmost importance and a broad-spectrum antibiotic in ophthalmic solution should be used. If keratitis is severe or should uveitis appear, careful, frequent tonometric examination is important and

mydriatic and anti-inflammatory therapy is needed. Systemic steroids frequently are useful in disciform keratitis and may be somewhat safer than topical instillation. In the event of marked keratitis or keratoiritis, some physicians have used hourly instillation of idoxuridine (IDU) with prednisolone acetate 1 per cent suspension to arrest viral replication and reduce scarring simultaneously. In the hands of experienced ophthalmologists, results appear promising (Aronson et al., 1970). In recent evaluations, trifluorothymidine appears to penetrate tissue better and to arrest keratitis more rapidly than IDU (Wellings et al., 1972).

Secondary infection of the lesion of herpes simplex occurs infrequently. The reason for this is unknown.

Recurrent herpes simplex sometimes

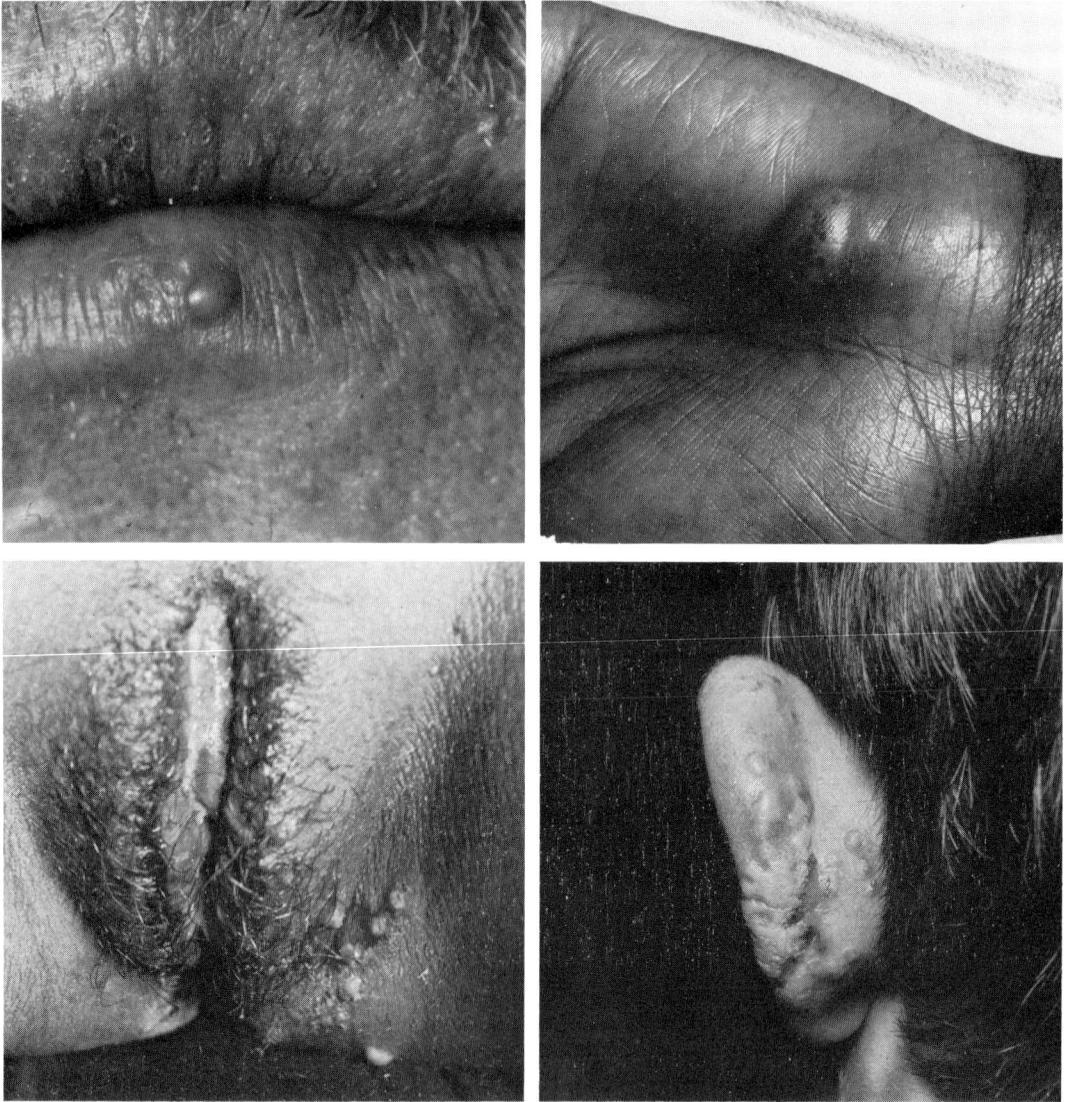

Figure 12–3   Recurrent herpes simplex at various sites. Any area of the skin may be involved.

appears over and over at precisely the same site. Presumably the virus is present in the epithelial cells or nearby neurons in a "latent" phase at all times, and the infection is then reactivated by one of a number of precipitating forces. However, this has not been proved beyond doubt, and it offers an attractive problem for further investigation. Following many recurrences of herpes simplex at the same site, varying degrees of atrophy and scarring may be produced. As a rule, this is of minor cosmetic importance only. Studies are now in progress to determine whether patients

who have sustained repeated attacks of herpes simplex of the cervix are more prone to cervical carcinoma.

The precipitating factors which produce recurrences of herpes simplex are numerous. The influence of the common cold, or fever, is well recognized in the terms "cold sore" and "fever blister." When neurosyphilis was being treated by fever therapy, the development of recurrent herpes simplex was accepted as a complication in almost all patients. During summer months, sunlight is a very frequent precipitating factor. There is good evidence that psychic influences may play a role: for example, the appearance of recurrent herpes simplex during episodes of exhaustion or severe nervous tension, and the apparent occasional effectiveness of psychotherapy in preventing recurrences. The relation of herpes simplex to the menses is observed with fair frequency, but the mechanism involved is obscure. There can be little question that gastrointestinal upsets may sometimes be followed by the development of herpes. Trigeminal sensory root section for trigeminal neuralgia is frequently followed by herpetic vesicles (Carton and Kilbourne, 1952).

TREATMENT. The deficiencies of treatment of viral diseases are possibly nowhere better illustrated than in the case of recurrent herpes simplex, in which the infection is localized and superficial, and yet for which no specifically viricidal compound, even one which is weakly so, is available. All that can be done, essentially, is to assist the infection in running its natural course with a minimum of interference and therapeutic trauma. Several studies have shown that bland topical therapy is better than none at all. A wide variety of drying local preparations, such as plain alcohol, spirits of camphor, or a shake lotion containing alcohol, are satisfactory.

Until recently, only symptomatic treatment, usually consisting of different drying lotions, was available for recurrent herpes simplex. In the last decade, topical idoxuridine has been applied in various vehicles and dose schedules, some including dimethylsulfoxide to aid penetration. More rapid healing seemed to occur, especially if a reservoir or frequent applications were used. Local irritation was a minor problem (Ashton et al., 1971). Photoinactivation of herpes virus has been demonstrated in vitro, and studies of in vivo efficacy are in progress. Since defective viral particles have caused some in vitro cell cultures to lose contact inhibition, a question of potential oncogenicity has arisen. In naturally occurring infections, however, 100 defective viral particles are generated for each infectious one. Some physicians postulate that early control of replication by photoinactivation reduces total exposure to such particles (Jarratt and Knox, 1974).

Vaccines against herpesvirus hominis, types I and II, are reportedly in field trials in the United States and Germany, respectively. Major handicaps in judging effectiveness of any form of treatment have been the variable course of recurrent disease and the effectiveness of suggestion and placebo, as well as active medications, on lesions. X-ray therapy has been used because of its anti-inflammatory effects, which are feeble, and the method has been largely discarded.

PREVENTION. There are no regularly effective means of preventing recurrent lesions of herpes simplex, at least insofar as any immunologic measures are concerned. Repeated vaccination with ordinary smallpox vaccine has long been used, but it has recently been condemned because of the side effects of the vaccination itself. The old hypothesis of "blocking" of the herpes simplex virus is untenable; there is no cross immunity between vaccinia and herpes simplex. Of all the specific excitant agents which have been mentioned, sunlight is the most easily avoidable. Patients with severe recurrences of herpes simplex should be cautioned to use some protective measures on excessive exposure, particularly at the beginning of the summer. Repeated inoculation of the skin with herpes simplex virus has been attempted as a method of prevention. This is without demonstrable good effect in preventing recurrences, and has a further disadvantage in that it may induce recurrent herpes simplex at the vaccinated site. The method has been discarded.

As do many other recurrent afflictions of man, herpes simplex may respond in some degree to a sympathetic attitude and a placebo. Excision of the site of recurrent herpetic infections has been unsuccessful, since subsequent recurrences then occur proximal to the excised area.

VARICELLA AND HERPES ZOSTER

Varicella (chickenpox) and herpes zoster (shingles) are caused by indistinguishable, icosahedral, 180 nm. encapsulated herpes viruses, which produce identical cytopathic changes, complement-fixation reactions, and cross-reacting IgM and IgG antibodies. Epidemics of chickenpox frequently follow exposure to zoster but whether zoster may be triggered to exposure to varicella is still disputed. Varicella is regarded as the primary manifestation of V-Z (varicella-zoster) viral exposure, and the virus is postulated to lie dormant in dorsal root ganglia following sufficient antibody rise, to later recur as zoster, following the sensory nerve root to the cutaneous surface where vesiculation occurs. Recrudescence is believed to occur when antibodies, either complement fixing or perhaps neutralizing, fall below some critical level. Measuring neutralization titers is very difficult because of low V-Z virus yield from present tissue culture systems (Blank et al., 1970).

Chickenpox occurs year round, with a predilection for winter in the more temperate climates. It is highly contagious in the prodromal and vesicular stages, with an 85 per cent incidence of infection by age 9 in urban areas. In rural areas, with fewer large group contacts, 3 per cent of adults are susceptible. During the prodromal and vesicular stages, the transmission is airborne; however, the vesicle can be infectious. Compared with herpes simplex, neonatal passive immunity is slight.

Pathologically, zoster and varicella lesions are identical to herpes simplex in forming intra-epidermal bullae. Infected cells degenerate, swell, and become acantholytic, often containing eosinophilic intranuclear inclusions surrounded by a clear halo and a circle of darkly staining chromatin. Multinucleate giant cells may form. As the lesion evolves, polymorphonuclear cells enter the vesicle, which heals with crust formation. On mucous membranes, the initial vesicles simply rupture and leave superficial, transient ulcers.

Dissemination occurs rarely, but when it does appear, typical inclusion bodies are found in most organs. A pneumonitis is not infrequent and is characterized pathologically by interstitial scattered lesions with nodular hemorrhagic areas. Microscopy reveals the characteristic findings of focal peribronchial necrosis, intranuclear inclusions, and fibrinoleukocytic exudates (Attal and Mozziconacci, 1970).

Clinically, varicella has a natural incubation of 10 to 20 days, with an average of 15 days. A 24-hour prodrome which is characterized by moderate fever and malaise may occur with or precede the exanthem.

Initially, the eruption may be scarlatiniform, with 2- to 4-mm. congested pink papules which usually form a central 3- to 4-mm. vesicle surrounded by an erythematous halo—resembling a "dew drop on a rose petal." Within a day, the vesicle grows turbid with leukocytes, may become slightly umbilicated, then dries and crusts. At first, crusts are firmly attached, but they quickly loosen so that scarring is not noted unless the earlier crust is avulsed. With crusting, lesions become non-infective since the V-Z virus is stable only in vesicular fluid. After 5 to 20 days, average 7 days, undisturbed crusts fall. Lesions present in successive crops. A wide variety of lesions are present during the height of the illness. The distribution is central and is often striking on the face, scalp, and trunk; the proximal extremities may be involved but the palms and soles are spared. Active vesiculation takes place over three or four days, and each crop of vesicles may be accompanied by a fever spike. Mucosae are involved with the vesicles which rupture easily and leave 2- to 4-mm. round white ulcers with an erythematous halo. Involved sites include the hard palate, anterior tonsillar pillars, and sometimes palpebral conjunctiva, vulvar mucosa, the pharynx, and even the larynx (Fig. 12–4).

Systemic symptoms such as moderate fever, headache, malaise, and anorexia precede the eruption by a day or appear concurrently, last as long as active lesions appear, and subside. Nonclassical presentations of varicella occur and may be confusing. One such presentation consists of scattered vesicles which may form polycyclic bullae greater than 1 cm. in diameter. No increased morbidity results, but the differential diagnosis is extended to include bullous diseases of childhood. Another variant includes a scattering of hemorrhagic vesicles with a thin ecchymotic rim at the base of the lesions; this is not to be confused with hemorrhagic varicella.

Hemorrhagic varicella is rare. This serious disease is accompanied by high fever

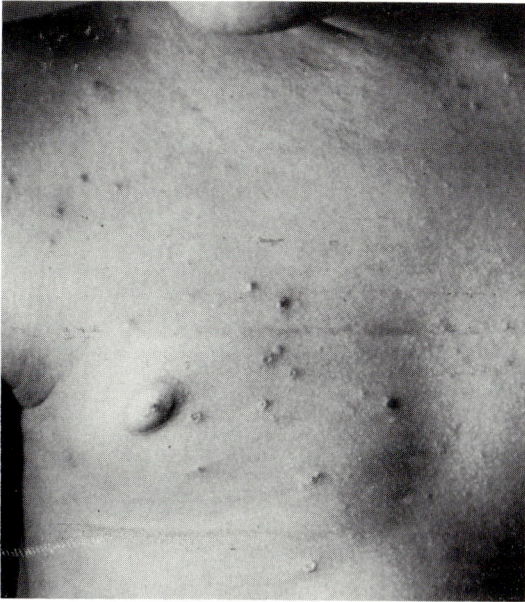

Figure 12-4 Chickenpox (varicella).

and a generalized hemorrhagic diathesis, manifested by hemorrhagic blisters, petechiae, epistaxis, ecchymoses, and hematemesis. Most frequently, it occurs in patients who are immunologically compromised by disease or therapy, or both. Patients who are on chemotherapy for malignancy, renal disease, auto-immune disease, and transplants are predisposed to this frequently fatal variant of this infection. In patients who have possible adrenal suppression, discontinuance or even lowering of corticosteroid is contraindicated (Attal and Mozzieonacci, 1970).

Varicella in the neonate usually results from the transmission of a maternal infection at the time of birth and is frequently benign; unlike herpes simplex, fatal dissemination is unusual. A more serious infection develops if transmission is transplacental; clinical varicella then results within 10 days after birth. Visceral involvement is common and a 21 per cent mortality has been reported (Attal and Mozzieonacci, 1970).

Adult varicella is much more severe than that of childhood. Because of the extended prodrome with severe headache and malaise and the presence of profuse eruption, differentiation from smallpox is sometimes necessary. Complications are more common in adult cases.

In general, complications of varicella are uncommon. Only superimposed bacterial pyoderma occurs frequently, and in developed countries antibacterial chemotherapy has almost eliminated secondary manifestations such as septicemia, bacterial pneumonitis, and osteomyelitis. Since group A beta-hemolytic streptococcal pyodermas can be controlled, there are far fewer cases of glomerulonephritis.

Vesicles located in the bladder may cause transient hematuria; those of the nasal mucosa, epistaxis. Laryngeal edema occasionally requires tracheostomy. Usually, cases of thrombocytopenic purpura are mild, but fatal purpura fulminans has been reported (Attal and Mozzieonacci, 1970). Subclinical varicella pneumonitis is not uncommon and in adults especially may become severe and be complicated by a serious bacterial infection. Neurologic complications are milder and less frequent than those of measles, and usually clear with few sequelae. Local vesicular conjunctivitis and keratitis are common but rarely severe enough to scar. Rare events include mild hepatitis, uveitis, and retrobulbar optic neuritis.

DIFFERENTIAL DIAGNOSIS. Differential diagnosis includes erythema neonatorum which affects 50 per cent of neonates, begins as a diffuse blotchy macular erythema, usually between 36 hours and 4 days of age (occasionally as late as 21 days), and is most marked on the anterior chest, less so on the arms, thighs, and face. Only 10 per cent of cases develop 2- to 4-mm. pustules which may be confused with varicella. Smears of pustules show many eosinophils; eosinophilia may be seen in from 7 to 18 per cent of patients.

Miliaria is common in the first year of life, involving symmetrical crops of papulovesicles about the neck, upper chest, groin, axillae, and sometimes the face. Lesions occur in crops as do those of varicella, but the distribution and morphology without systemic symptoms differentiate the entities (Beare and Rook, 1968).

Impetigo is vesicular in nature but rapidly becomes purulent and frequently crusts. A centrifugal distribution is characteristic, lesions are larger, and honey-colored crusts suggest the correct diagnosis.

Coxsackie A9 may present with fever, malaise, sore throat, and an exanthem. The eruption usually appears in crops concurrently with the fever, progressing from the face or trunk to the extremities and may occasionally involve the scalp, palms, and soles. Vesicles appear on the soft palate, uvula, or tonsils. Primary lesions are 2- to 13-mm. erythematous macules or papules which develop into 1- to 2-mm. vesicles, clearing in three to five days without crusting (Lerner et al., 1960).

Rickettsialpox, carried by a mite parasite of house mice, usually is transmitted during warm seasons. The diagnostic lesion results from the displaced arthropod's inoculating bite and appears as a 0.5- to 2-cm. firm papule which develops a deep-seated vesicle and then crusts. Several cases involved lesions on the face only, and lesions on a sole have been reported. After two to three days, vesicles form on the papules, deeper and firmer than in varicella. These crust and eventually flake off without scarring. Two-millimeter ulcers with bright red halos occur on the tongue, buccal mucosa, palate, and pharynx. If the primary lesion is overlooked, differentiation from varicella may be difficult (Barker, 1949).

The most important differentiation from varicella is variola (smallpox). Misidentification of the latter has, and probably will continue to, cost lives. Diagnosis is by no means simple, as there are varied presentations of smallpox, and most physicians from the western countries have never seen a case. Classic smallpox presents, on an average of 12 days post inoculation, as a fiery red pharyngitis with a moderate to high fever, backache, headache, and rigors, lasting three days. Temperature returns to normal transiently, and on the fourth day a fine, papular, centrifugally distributed exanthem appears, spreading centrally, with or without palm and sole lesions. Vesicles rapidly develop, especially peripherally, and the patient is severely ill. In about three days, lesions become mostly pustular, and gradual improvement occurs. After nine days of the eruption, umbilication is usually prominent in some areas and the lesions start drying and crusting. Modified smallpox,

however, is much more difficult to diagnose. Often the affected individual has a vaccination scar. Symptoms range from none, with simple serum titer rises, to several days of moderate fever, pharyngitis, backache, and headache followed by scattered erythematous papules, sometimes involving the face and arms only in a forme fruste fashion. Vesiculation occurs quickly and may pustulate and crust more rapidly following an attenuated course. Some patients merely develop a few scattered papulovesicular lesions, further complicating diagnosis. Until recently, a positive Tzanck stain for multinucleate giant cells was considered to be reliable evidence for herpesvirus infection, to rule out pox virus. Reliance on such a positive report may lead to a variola epidemic (Heydenreich, 1965).

TREATMENT. At the present time there is no chemotherapy for varicella. Fortunately, the usual childhood infection of chickenpox requires no treatment. The skin lesions should be kept dry so as not to interfere with their normal rapid evolution. If treatment seems indicated for itching, a shake lotion and oral antihistamines may be used. Systemic antibacterial therapy should be reserved for those patients with proved secondary bacterial infection. Prophylactic antibiotics may not only ensure but promote an antibiotic-resistant infection.

Varicella produces almost complete immunity against a second attack of characteristic varicella. Hyperimmune gamma globulin may be administered to debilitated patients after exposure to varicella. A dose of 1.3 ml. per kilogram of body weight is successful in attenuating the subsequent clinical disease.

HERPES ZOSTER

Zoster is the result of a recrudescence of V-Z virus infection. It occurs as frequently among males as females and rises in incidence with advancing age. From birth to nine years of age the annual rate is 0.74 per thousand; from 40 to 49 years, 2.92 per thousand; and from 80 to 89, 10.10 per thousand.

There seems to be no seasonal predilection or correlation with varicella epidemics. A small percentage of cases represent recurrent attacks, often of the previously involved ganglion (Hope-Simpson, 1965). Some predisposition to developing zoster lesions has been demonstrated in Hodgkin's disease and other lymphomas, particularly in anergic patients, and in those who have had recent radiotherapy. In the lymphoma group, absence of varicella-zoster complement-fixing antibodies likewise predisposes to infection. An interesting cluster of varicella and zoster cases in a lymphoma ward even suggested transmission in epidemic fashion among these patients (Schimpff et al., 1972). Zoster has been reported to occur frequently in immunosuppressed renal transplant patients, especially after radiotherapy to inhibit rejection crises (Rifkind, 1966).

Histopathologically, cutaneous zoster lesions are indistinguishable from those of varicella and herpes simplex, previously described. Nerve root changes consist of necrotizing ganglionitis and even cyst formation in severely involved ganglia. Another horn cell damage which is usually much milder than is posterior ganglia is sometimes seen and may account for the occasional paresis in areas of hyperesthesia and paresthesia (Denny-Brown et al., 1944). Early loss of neurofibrils occurs in affected skin even before cutaneous lesions become apparent. With severe neural damage resulting in paresthesia and hyperesthesia, the axon flare following injection of 0.1 to 0.2 ml. of 1:100,000 solution of histamine phosphate is frequently absent. Loss of local neurofibrils is believed responsible for this phenomenon (Muller and Winkelmann, 1969).

Clinically, grouped vesicles appear on an erythematous base in a unilateral dermatomal pattern within one to seven days following onset of pain and hyperesthesia. If the vesiculation follows the pain for one or two days, the eruption clears in about two and one-half weeks, but if lesions erupt over the period of a week, prolonged convalescence may be expected (Burgoon and Burgoon, 1957).

The most frequently affected dermatomes are C2 and L2 and the fifth and seventh cranial nerves. It is interesting to note that on composite segmental distribution diagrams, the affected areas are mostly centripetal, corresponding to the distribution of varicella on the face and trunk. Right-sided and left-sided involvement occurs with equal frequency (Fig. 12–5).

In the usual case, the tense vesicles arise on an erythematous base, become pustular in a day or two, crust, and heal in from two to two and one-half weeks. Secondary bacterial infection or gangrenous changes prolong the healing process. Regional lymphadenopathy is common, as are malaise and a low-grade fever.

Severe, lancinating pain, often with hyperesthetic "trigger points," is common but not invariable. Persistence in the form of intractable neuralgia is a feared complication which may follow zoster in patients over 50 years of age. It is often resistant even to such extreme measures as posterior rhizotomy and cordotomy.

Specific syndromes occur with different zoster-infected ganglia. First-division trigeminal zoster may involve nasociliary distribution, with vesicles on the lateral side of the nose and immediate or delayed appearance of usually benign zoster keratitis through the long ciliary nerves. A temporary or permanent Argyll Robertson pupillary reaction may occur if the ciliary ganglion is involved. Ophthalmic zosters (Fig. 12–6) may also cause extraocular muscle palsies (Blank, 1970).

The Ramsay Hunt syndrome is a zoster of the geniculate ganglion. Sensory fibers from the seventh cranial nerve innervate deep facial tissues; hence, jaw pain simulating a dental abscess is often present. Painful vesicles follow ipsilateral sensory fibers to the uvula, palate, anterior tongue, auricle, and posterior auricular areas. Paresis or paralysis may affect the muscles of facial expression, which also close the eyelids. The levator palpebrae, which is innervated by the fifth cranial nerve, is spared so the eye may remain open (Grant, 1962).

Glossopharyngeal zoster produces pain in the ear and pharynx, with vesiculo-ulcerative lesions of the soft palate and vesicles on the ear. Vagal zoster may cause paresis of the larynx and pharynx as well as cardiac and epigastric distress; there may be vesicles on the base of the tongue, epiglottis, and arytenoids. C2 to C4 phrenic involvement may paralyze the

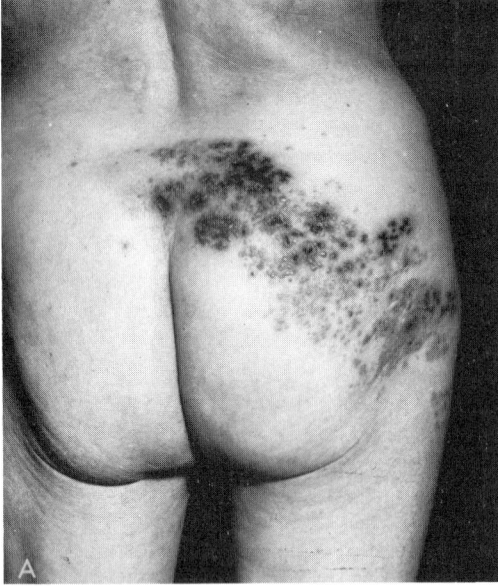

Figure 12–5 *A*, Lumbosacral zoster. *B*, Minimal lesions of zoster. The skin lesions may be slight, or possibly entirely absent. *C*, Diffuse varicelliform lesions following zoster. The patient had Hodgkin's disease.

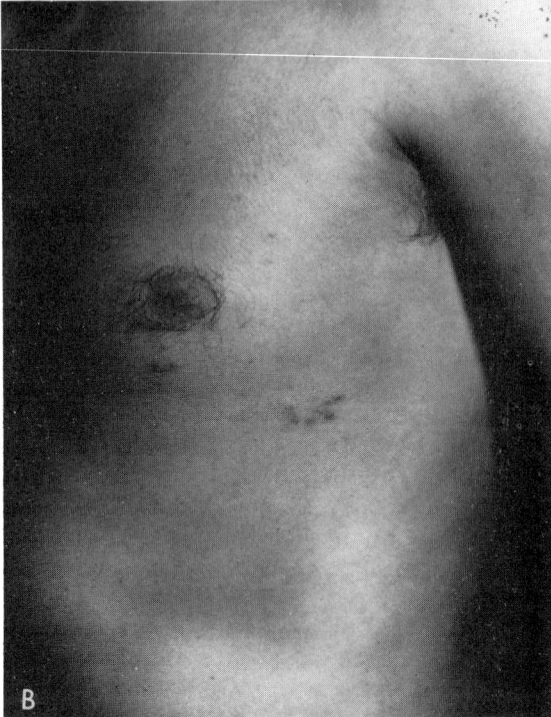

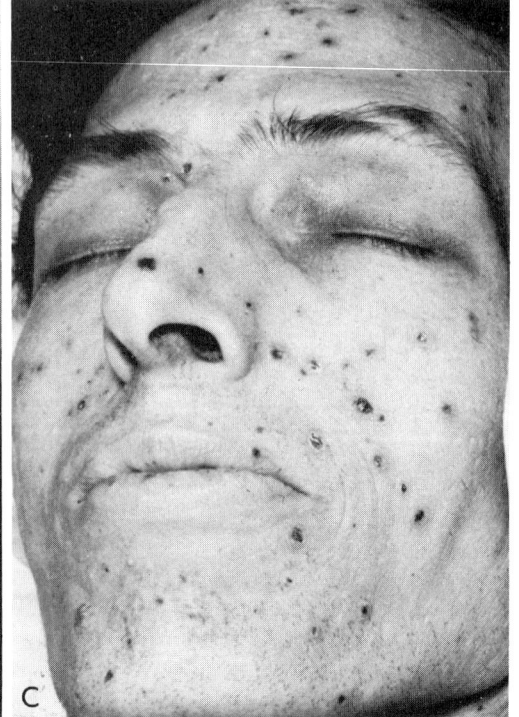

ipsilateral diaphragm. With thoracic zoster, pleural friction rubs may be heard near the involved skin and at times EKG changes have been reported. Lumbosacral involvement may cause symptoms similar to those due to the passage of urinary stones and may result in urinary retention for up to one month (Blank et al., 1970).

Clinical variants of zoster occur. In one instance, the vesicles become hemorrhagic but prognosis is no worse than in the uncomplicated disease. Encephalitis is occasionally reported to follow zoster by two to four weeks, particularly after involvement of cranial nerve ganglia. It is rarely fatal.

Generalized zoster is serious, however. It occurs mainly in patients with Hodgkin's disease, lymphoma, or leukemia. Four to ten days after an initial localized presentation, the patient may become toxic and febrile. Cutaneous vesicles become generalized, and V-Z pneumonitis or encephalitis may develop which is associated with a high mortality rate (Schimpff et al., 1972).

Differential diagnosis of zoster is limited, since the unilateral vesiculation is so characteristic. Herpes simplex may be zosteriform, and such a clinical presentation may be substantiated by tissue culture (Music et al., 1971).

Positive laboratory findings in zoster include the Tzanck preparation which demonstrates multinucleate giant cells. Acute and convalescent complement-fixation titers may be of help in patients with minimal numbers of cutaneous lesions. Viable virus is present in the vesicular fluid for several days and may be cultured on human embryo amnion or kidney cells. Dry crusts yield no infective virus paralleling the course of clinical infectivity.

Therapy of zoster is limited. The un-complicated case in younger individuals should be treated with drying compresses and appropriate pain relief. Hyperesthesia to clothing contact can be dulled with applications of flexible collodion. Since patients 50 to 60 years of age and older have a higher incidence of severe and long-lasting post-herpetic neuralgia, attempts to abort its development with corticosteroids are worthwhile if started very early in the course of the disease. Doses equivalent to at least 40 mg. of prednisone a day for three to six weeks are warranted if not contraindicated (Eaglestein et al., 1970).

Established post-zoster neuralgia may last months or a lifetime. Rhizotomy and cordotomy are usually ineffective and should certainly be preceded by attempts to determine the effectiveness of local nerve block. Local subcutaneous injections of triamcinolone, 2 mg. per ml. of 2 per cent procaine hydrochloride, have been reported to be successful in easing pain if injected into maximally tender trigger areas in 4 to 12 sessions (Epstein, 1971).

Individuals who develop zoster while

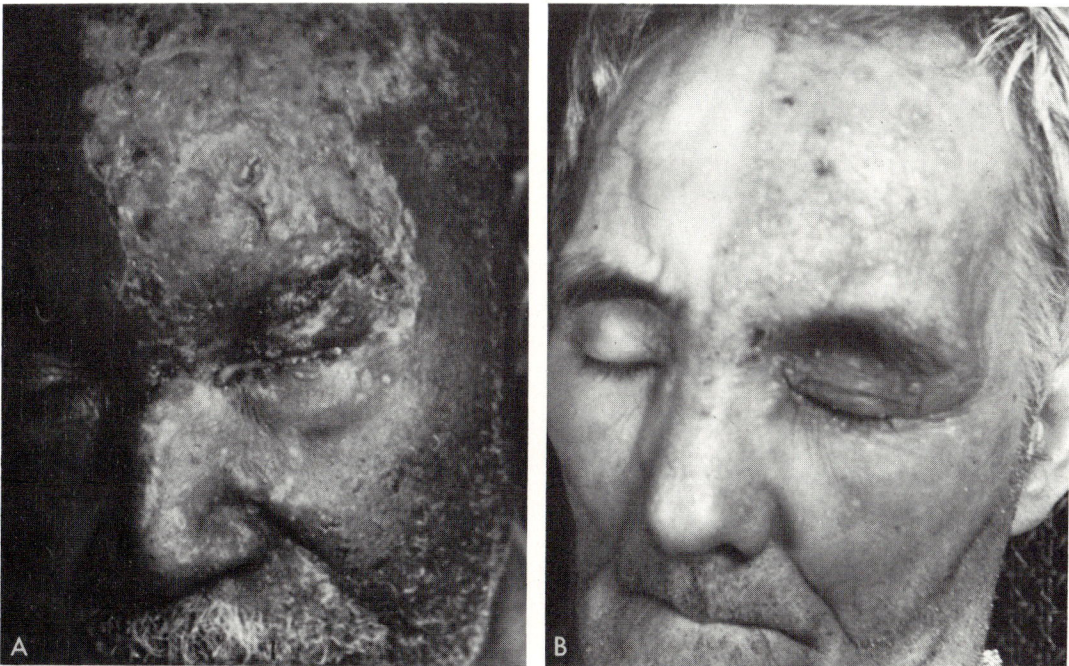

Figure 12–6 Severe zoster in distribution of ophthalmic branch of trigeminal nerve. *A*, Destructive lesions 10 days after onset. *B*, Late scarring and atrophy. Severe neuralgic pain was present.

on steroids are not at any greater risk of complications or dissemination than the general population and should be left on their medication (Attal and Mozziconacci, 1970). Therapy for disseminated zoster associated with malignancy is presently undergoing considerable study. Use of hyperimmune convalescent zoster serum is of debatable value and chemotherapy such as cytosine arabinoside in slow infusions is still experimental.

WARTS

Warts, or verrucae, represent another extremely common viral infection of the skin. Though warts are, by tradition, divided into common (vulgaris) and other types, this differentiation has little usefulness. The wide variations in the shape and size of warts are in part explainable by variations in the local environment of the lesions, but most of the morphologic variations in response to what is apparently the same virus remain a mystery. Warts may be sessile and have a surface that is rough and horny (the most frequently encountered type), threadlike, flat and brownish, or moist and exuberant. The course of this viral infection is completely unpredictable in terms of whether the lesions are single, sparse, or numerous, and whether they will respond to any particular type of treatment or disappear spontaneously. Warts are apparently completely ectotropic, affecting only the skin and the mucous membranes adjacent to mucocutaneous junctions. They may, at times, prove completely incurable, and the methods of treatment are, in general, roundabout and nonspecific. Warts are principally an infection of childhood and young adult life.

Etiology

Proof that an infectious agent is concerned in warts is available in abundance:

1. The auto-inoculation of warts is a commonplace observation. A single initial lesion is frequently followed by development of satellite warts in the area. Warts are inoculated on apposing surfaces of folds of the skin (kissing warts). They frequently occur along scratch marks in a patient with warts, in precise linear arrangement.

2. The presence of a filterable infectious agent in tissue from warts was established almost 50 years ago and has since been confirmed by many investigators.

3. The transmission of warts from man to man may be observed frequently. The development of plantar warts in young adults going away to boarding school or college for the first time is common. In such instances, there may be a clear history of trauma, a splinter, or a cut prior to development of the wart.

The virus of warts has not been convincingly cultivated by any method. Histopathology shows hyperkeratosis and areas of parakeratosis with papillomatosis. In young verrucae, large vacuolated cells may be seen in the stratum malpighii and in the granular layer. Nuclei of these cells are rounded, deeply basophilic, and on electron microscopy contain closely packed aggregates of virus particles. Eosinophilic inclusions which contain no viral elements are occasionally seen in the nuclei or cytoplasm of the epidermal cells. They probably represent a degeneration product of keratin (Almeida et al., 1962).

Morphologic Types of Warts

The following lesions are the chief morphologic expressions of the viral infection of warts. The therapeutic methods used may vary with different types of lesions.

SESSILE LESIONS. Ordinary sessile lesions of the type seen on the extremities, particularly on the fingers. These lesions are raised and have a rough, gray surface as a rule (Fig. 12–7).

FILIFORM OR DIGITATE WARTS. These are most commonly encountered on the face and neck. They may be confused with cutaneous horns or nevoid skin "tags."

PLANTAR WARTS. These warts on the sole, and to a lesser extent on the palm, are prevented by pressure from being elevated. Warts in this location are almost unique in that they may be exquisitely painful if they are on points of pressure. Such a lesion is flush with the surface and may appear to be an ordinary callus, except that the lines of the skin are

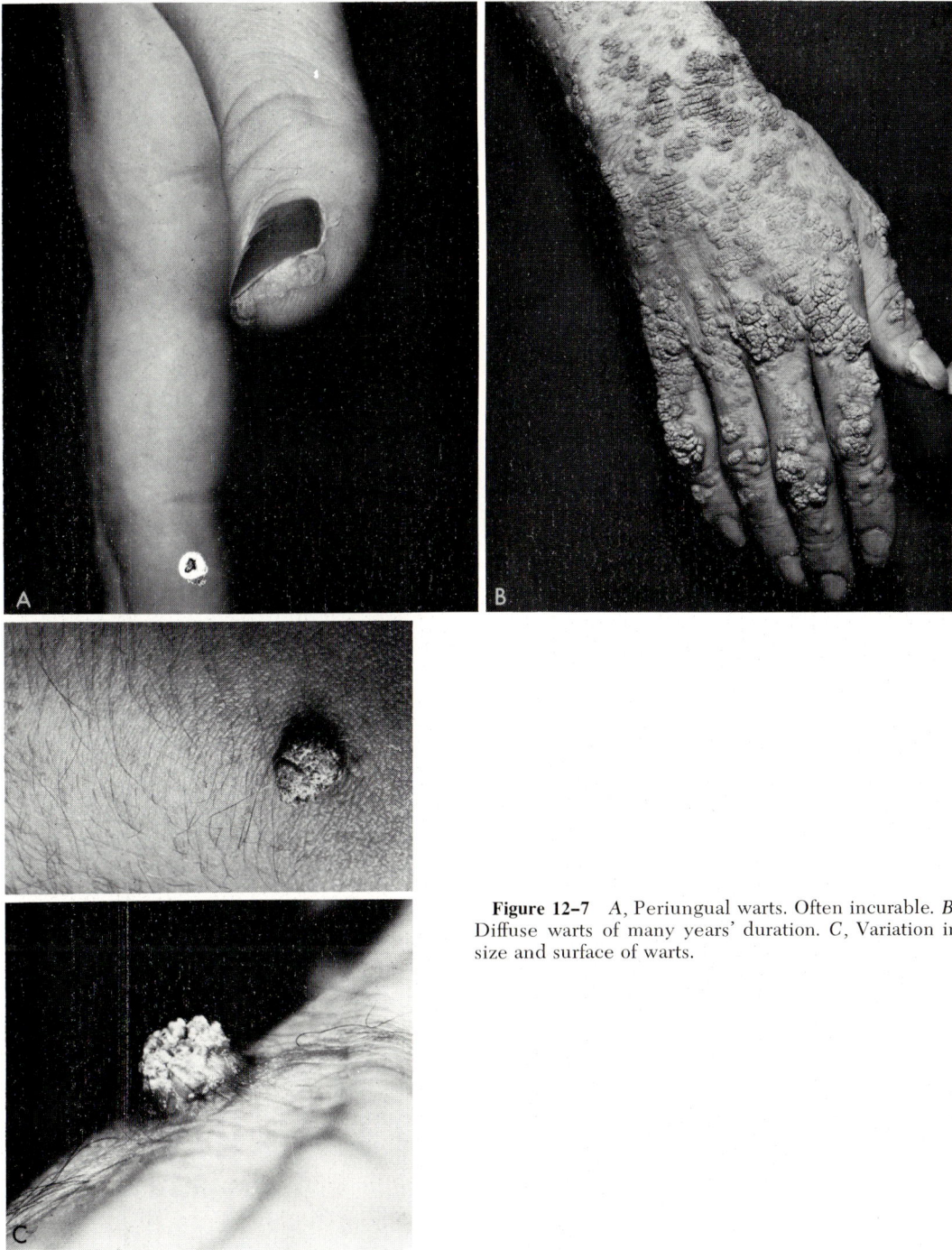

Figure 12-7 *A*, Periungual warts. Often incurable. *B*, Diffuse warts of many years' duration. *C*, Variation in size and surface of warts.

obliterated by the lesion. If the surface of the lesion is shaved off with a razor blade, the wart is easily discernible. Plantar warts may be single or multiple. If multiple, they may be grouped together in mosaic fashion, as many as 40 or 50 together. Dissemination and seeding of wart lesions on the feet may be abetted by hyperhidrosis. The lesions may sometimes show a preference for intertriginous areas and may then be rather exuberant and hypertrophic (Fig. 12-8).

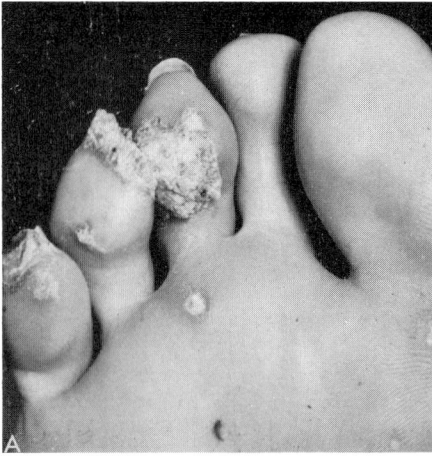

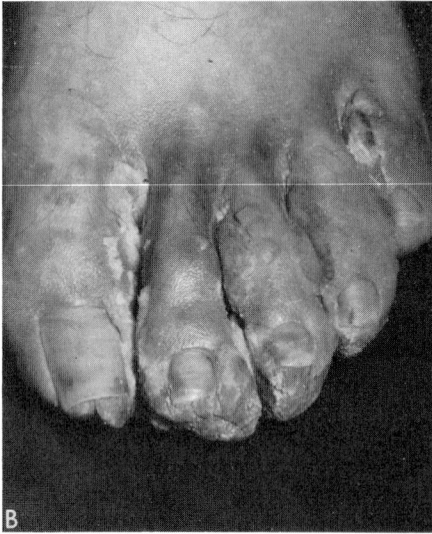

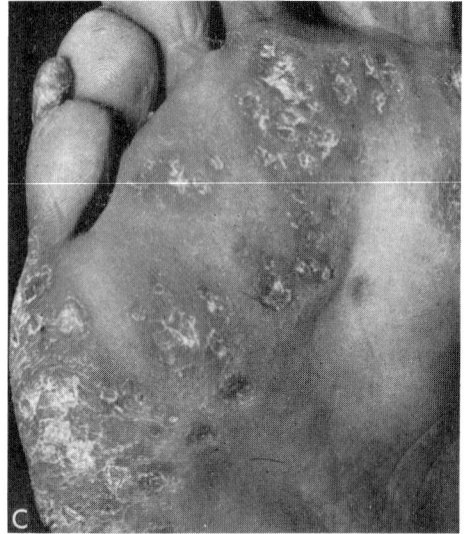

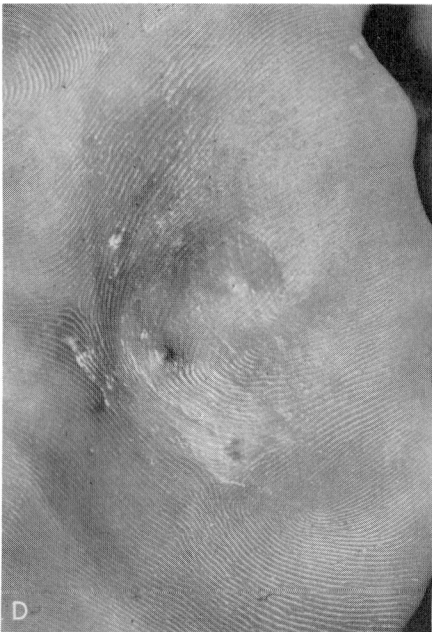

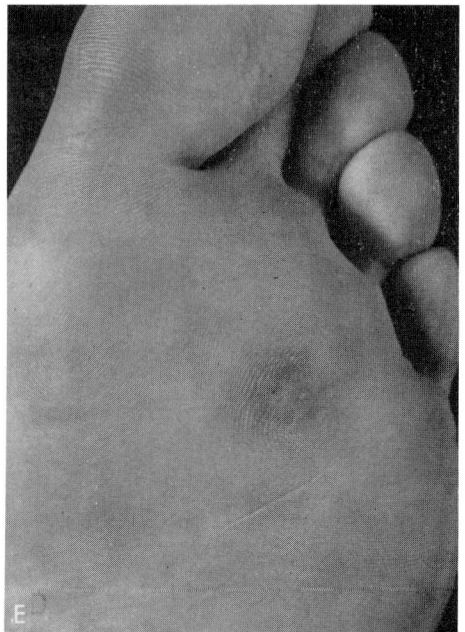

Figure 12–8 *A*, "Kissing" warts on toes and isolated lesions elsewhere. *B* and *C*, Multiple interdigital and mosaic warts of foot (same patient as Figure 12–7*B*). *D*, Appearance of small plantar warts after removal of overlying callus. *E*, Painful scarring at site of plantar warts which had been grossly overtreated with x-rays and electrocoagulation.

FLAT WARTS. Warts sometimes remain entirely flat and may be difficult to distinguish from lightly pigmented nevi. When flat warts occur, they are usually seen in profusion, most commonly in children. The entire forehead or half of the face may be involved, with 50 to 100 such lesions (Fig. 12–9).

MOIST ANOGENITAL WARTS. When the wart virus becomes established in a moist intertriginous area, the resultant papilloma tends to be exuberant and very auto-inoculable. Instead of the usual gray or brownish color of warts, the lesions are pink or white and may have a strawberry-like surface, and the individual lesion may become very large. While they are sometimes venereal in origin, this is by no means always true. Such warts may involve the adjacent mucous membrane of the anus or vulva, but involvement rarely extends inward more than 1 or 2 cm. They may occur on any moist intertriginous surface (Fig. 12–10).

Variations in the Clinical Course of Warts

In addition to their varied morphologic patterns, warts have strange and unpredictable courses in respect to spontaneous disappearance, dissemination, and persistence. The authors have observed each of the following occurrences a great many times:

1. A single wart may appear and persist relatively unchanged for many years. It then ordinarily disappears as the patient ages.

2. A single wart may appear and then be followed in weeks or years by the development of auto-inoculated lesions, either in the form of satellites in the vicinity of the original wart or as distant transplants.

3. In addition to spontaneous disappearance in variable periods of time, warts not infrequently disappear after pure suggestion therapy, particularly in children, or after such therapy is reinforced by some manipulative procedure to one or two of the warts.

4. After removal of one or more warts, the lesions may not recur, or they may reappear within a few weeks, or within a few months to years.

On the basis of these and other observations, it seems clear that any method of treatment which is employed in warts will be successful in a reasonably high percentage of patients because of its psychothera-

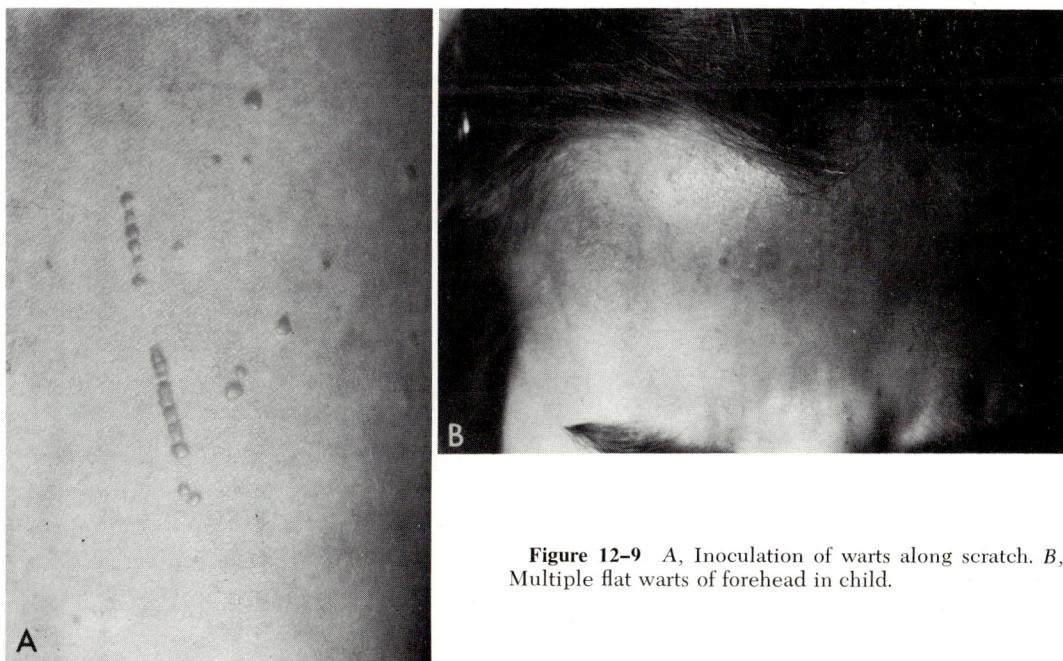

Figure 12–9 *A*, Inoculation of warts along scratch. *B*, Multiple flat warts of forehead in child.

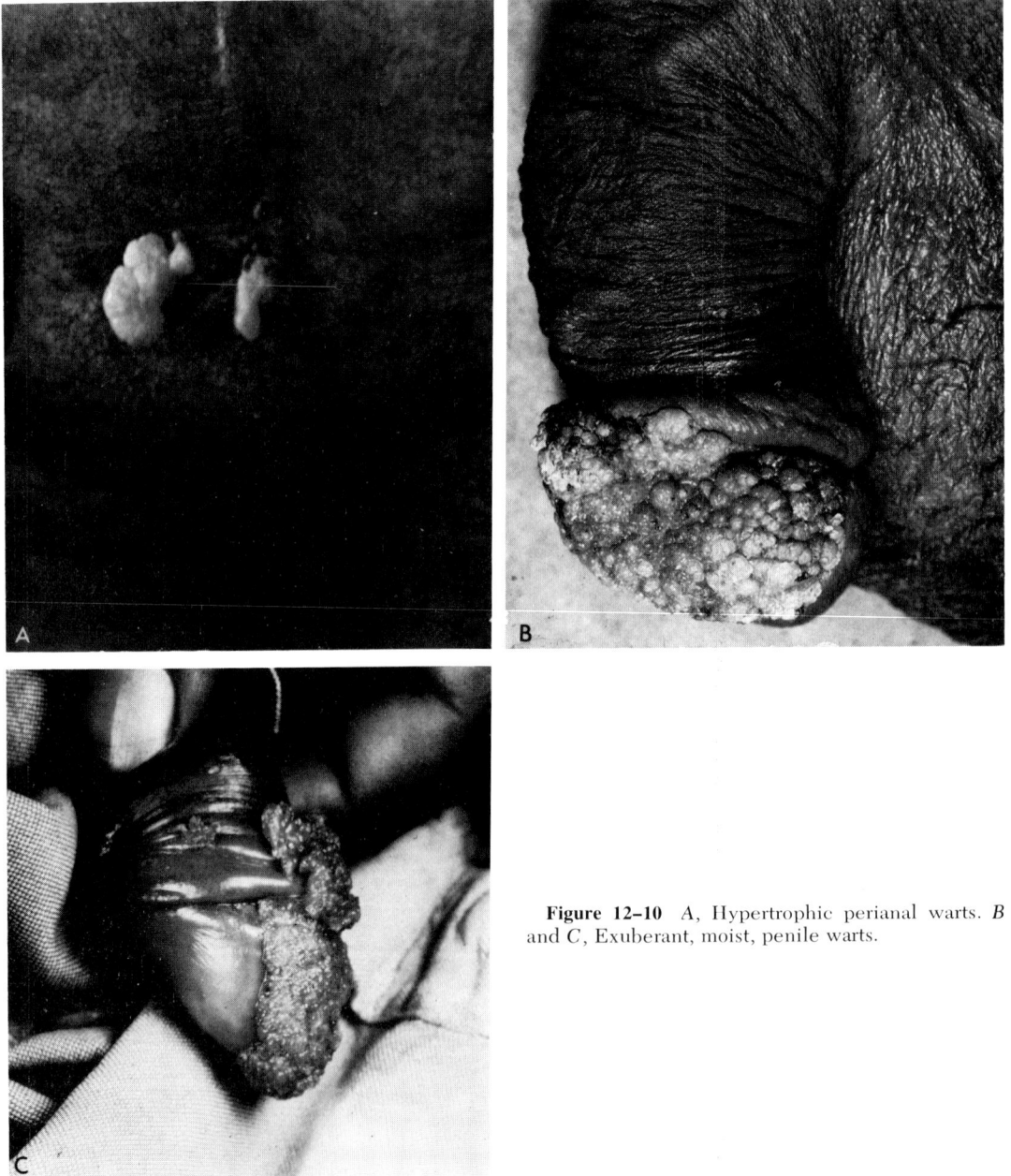

Figure 12–10 *A*, Hypertrophic perianal warts. *B* and *C*, Exuberant, moist, penile warts.

peutic effects alone. In young children or others who are strongly susceptible to suggestion, the use of psychotherapeutic methods alone, with the particular form of "abracadabra" which the therapist chooses, is well worth a trial. If one or two warts have been present for a long time, with no evidence of extension or auto-inoculation, it may be wise just to let them alone. In view of the overwhelming likelihood of uneventful spontaneous disappearance of warts, methods of treatment which produce significant scarring, especially on pressure points on the sole, become completely unjustifiable. In some cases, particularly multiple "mosaic" plantar warts or multiple warts about the nail margins, cure by any means may prove impossible.

Treatment

There is no satisfactory treatment of warts. Recurrences are common and no therapeutic method appears to have any greater success than any other. In ordinary sessile warts of the fingers or elsewhere in adults, provided that they are not too numerous, electrodesiccation or cryosurgery is probably the treatment of choice. It should almost always be done under local anesthesia: an injection of a drop or two of Xylocaine intradermally is all that is necessary. The destruction should not be extensive or deep, for the wart is entirely an intra-epidermal tumor. All that is necessary is to sear the top of the lesion gently until the wart softens, then curette it, and touch any bleeding points of the base lightly. Undue coagulation of the base of the lesion will only produce slowing of healing and undue scarring and would not appear to give any better results in terms of cure.

When cryosurgery is carried out, care must be taken to avoid freezing the digital vessels and nerves on the medial and lateral aspects of the digits. Long-lasting or permanent paresthesias may otherwise ensue. When freezing near the nail matrix, care should be likewise exercised to avoid permanent nail dystrophy.

Cryosurgery may produce hemorrhagic bullae, especially on the plantar surfaces. Describing this to the patient before therapy will avoid many otherwise embarrassing "emergency" calls. It must also be remembered that even cryosurgery can produce scars in some individuals. The number of warts which may be removed at any one sitting will depend to some extent on the stoicism of the patient.

Surgical excision of warts is commonly carried out, but it has distinct disadvantages. It is ordinarily undesirable and unnecessary to do a full-thickness excision of an area of skin to cure a benign lesion which is entirely epidermal. The scarring produced may be very painful, particularly on pressure points of the sole, and on the palmar surface of the fingers. Recurrences of warts in or near the scar or suture points are common.

PERIUNGUAL WARTS.   A wart appearing on the nail fold or under the distal margin of the nailplate should be removed immediately because extension occurs almost inevitably, but care should be taken not to injure the nail matrix. Careful cryosurgery or light electrodesiccation is sometimes successful. Often, however, it is necessary to use or add chemotherapeutic modalities such as 10 to 25 per cent glutaraldehyde solution, 10 per cent formalin ointment, or 0.7 per cent cantharidin in acetone and flexible collodion under tape occlusion (Epstein and Kligman, 1958; London, 1971).

Steady use of these chemotherapeutic agents and frequent paring away of white macerated skin is necessary for success. Allergic and/or irritant reactions to medicaments may limit usefulness.

Treatment of warts of the nail fold are generally difficult, and sometimes unsuccessful.

FLAT WARTS.   Flat warts have no more than cosmetic significance, but they may be quite noticeable and disfiguring when on the face. The individual lesions are easily destroyed. Flat warts are very amenable to psychotherapy, especially in children. This may be reinforced by the use of lotions, of a type similar to those used in acne, which will produce definite exfoliation of the skin, applied as often as twice daily. It is often feasible to undertake very light electrodesiccation of such lesions. If properly done, no scarring will result.

WARTS OF THE BEARDED REGION AND SCALP.   These lesions may be of any type, but are frequently flat or filiform. They are notoriously recurrent in hairy areas, particularly in the bearded region. Such warts may ordinarily be desiccated or frozen lightly without anesthesia, unless they are large. On removal of warts from the bearded region, it is important to have the patient return within a month or two, to detect areas which have been "seeded." Exfoliative lotions may help prevent recurrence. Warts about the mouth, particularly those arising in the angles, may be associated with lesions on the anterior portion of the buccal surface of the cheeks or lips, or even on the tongue. If not too numerous, these may also be destroyed by electrodesiccation if the mucous surface is thoroughly dried. Numerous lesions present a considerable problem, however. They may be treated with a coagulating solution, such as 10 per cent silver nitrate, or with cautious application of 20 per cent podophyllin in compound tincture of benzoin. Extensive warts in the mouth may sometimes prove incurable.

PLANTAR WARTS. The number of treatments which have been suggested for the cure of plantar warts attests to the unsatisfactory character of most of them. Many of them, unfortunately, are capable of producing irreversible scarring which, on pressure points, may be more painful than the original wart. The following are examples of some of the methods of management of plantar warts which are most commonly used:

Chemocauterant Methods. A wide variety of cauterant chemicals have been used in the treatment of plantar warts. None of them is entirely satisfactory, and all ordinarily require repeated application. The following are the most useful:

Repeated Application of 5 to 20 per cent Formalin Solution. This method is particularly applicable to multiple plantar warts. The nightly application of formalin solution produces hardening and drying of the skin surface, following which the warts may shell out. The method has a good psychotherapeutic impact. It may, however, produce excessive primary irritant effects and occasional sensitization.

Phenol-Nitric Acid—Salicylic Acid. This method is representative of a wide variety of cauterant chemotherapeutic methods which have been used in the treatment of plantar warts. It is principally applicable when no more than two or three warts are to be treated. The keratotic surface of the wart is first shaved off, and fuming nitric acid is applied to the wart tissue only. If it produces some burning pain, the psychotherapeutic effects are increased. Following this, phenol is applied, which results in a brown eschar. This is not painful. A salicylic acid plaster, cut to fit the entire hyperkeratotic area, is then applied and firmly strapped in place. In a day or two, pain may result from "liquefaction" of the base of the wart. This is desirable, because the entire wart may then drop out. If this does not occur, it is probably worthwhile to repeat the treatment at intervals of two weeks for six to eight sessions (Fig. 12–11).

Podophyllin and Adhesive Tape. As outlined below, the application of podophyllin is often effective in the treatment of exuberant warts in moist intertriginous areas. It is without effect when applied to warts which have a dry surface. However, if maceration is promoted by the repeated application of adhesive tape of moleskin for several weeks, podophyllin may be effective. After paring down the wart, a 20 per cent solution of podophyllin in compound tincture of benzoin is applied, and then overlain with adhesive tape, preferably of a nonporous water-resistant variety which will increase maceration. Further application may be carried out by the patient at intervals of 48 to 72 hours, with adhesive tape then being reapplied.

The above methods of treatment are simply examples, and many variations have been used, including trichloroacetic acid, silver nitrate stick, and so forth. Much patience is required.

Electrodesiccation. Electrosurgical methods are much less useful in plantar warts than in other types of the viral infection. It should not be employed vigorously on pressure sites, because slow healing and painful scarring almost inevitably result. If used at all after curettage of the lesion, it should be only for the purpose of controlling slight bleeding. The results will be very bad if destruction of the underlying fascia is produced.

X-Ray Therapy. Ionizing irradiation, in tumoricidal doses, is frequently listed as a standard method of treatment of plantar warts. Many instances of annoying or serious sequelae have resulted from such therapy. It obviously should never be used in children because of the possibility of injuring underlying epiphyseal centers. The dose selected should be moderate; the replacement of wart tissue by an atrophic scar produced by x-rays is too high a price to pay for the cure. If the method is employed at all, a single dose of 1000 R sharply screened to a lesion not over 5 mm. in diameter would appear to be the maximum allowable. The authors have discontinued the use of standard x-ray therapy in the treatment of plantar warts.

Surgical Excision. Full-thickness surgical excision of plantar warts is inadvisable, from the standpoint of the immediate risks involved, a low incidence of cure, and the risk of painful scarring. However, simple curettage of the wart to its base

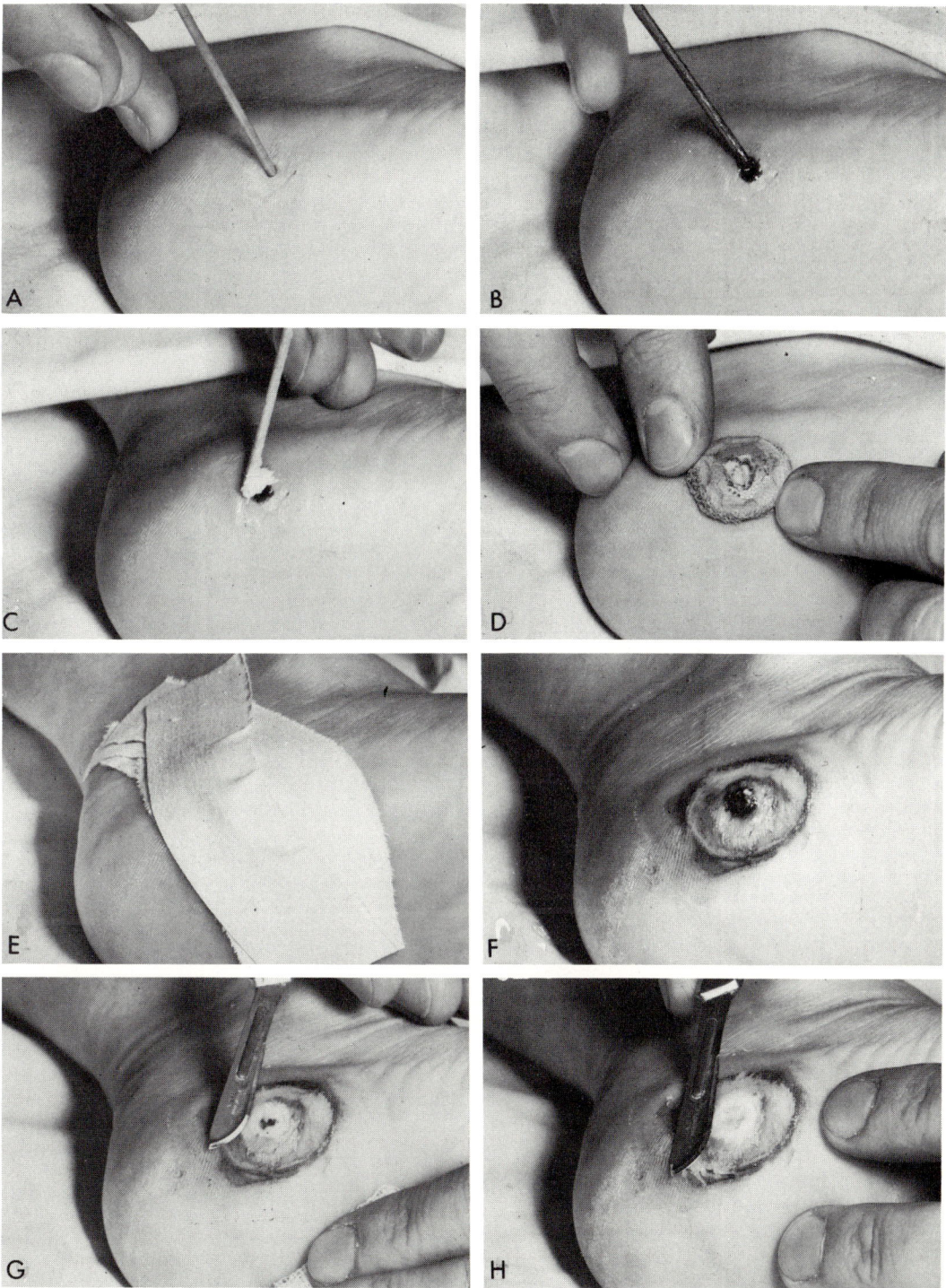

Figure 12–11 Chemocauterant treatment of a plantar wart (Dr. Harvey Blank). *A*, Application of phenol followed by *B*, Nitric acid, and *C*, 30 per cent salicylic acid paste. *D*, Protective moleskin or leather ring and firm adhesive dressing *E*. *F*, Appearance 48 hours later. The wart tissue was removable with ease. *G* and *H*, There are innumerable variations of such therapy which are sometimes successful and often tedious.

and application of a pressure dressing may be curative.

Multiple plantar warts arranged in a mosaic pattern present an exceedingly difficult treatment problem and are sometimes incurable. The simplest initial treatment which offers any hope of effectiveness is probably formalin or glutaraldelyde solution. Large doses of x-ray over the considerable area frequently involved are dangerous and not to be used. Strong keratolytic measures may be required. This may consist of phenol-nitric acid, followed by a salicylic acid plaster, or repeated softening of the area with salicyclic acid, followed by curettage. As many as 15 or 20 treatment sessions may be required, and these are frequently beyond the patience of either patient or physician.

DIFFERENTIATION OF PLANTAR WARTS AND SCARS OR CALLUSES. The most common error in the treatment of plantar warts is a failure to differentiate between warts and scars which occur following treatment. Scars on pressure points, even small ones, build up keratotic tissue very rapidly, and at the central point of this the keratin may be very hard and horny. Such lesions are often exquisitely painful. Continued application of keratolytics or the use of electrodesiccation will only increase the scarring and the tenderness. The keratinous tissue overlying such scars is clear and almost translucent, and the characteristic punched-out area of a wart is not seen at the central portion.

The management of such scars consists in a trial of various means of keeping pressure off the lesion, including bunion rings, arch inserts with cut-out edges, sponge rubber pads affixed immediately posterior to the lesion, and so forth. Painful scars of this type may produce bad habits of walking and standing which may eventually induce a familiar chain of knee and lower back symptoms. Regular shaving off of the hyperkeratotic tissue is necessary and this may ordinarily be done safely by the patient. Excision of the scar and grafting may be attempted, but it is frequently unsuccessful in terms of the eventual result achieved. If there is ulceration following x-ray therapy, however, this may become mandatory as a means of preventing malignant changes. Removal of under-lying metatarsal spurs or even of the metatarsal bone and associated toe has been suggested, but this procedure obviously should be considered only upon the most careful and objective orthopedic advice.

MOIST WARTS. Warts occurring in moist intertriginous areas frequently become numerous and exuberant. Podophyllin is the treatment of choice for these moist warts. It is best used in a vehicle which will tend to keep the active ingredient in place. A 20 per cent solution of tincture of benzoin is satisfactory. Applications are allowed to dry, and the site powdered lightly with talc. The patient is instructed to wash the area thoroughly in five to six hours. Sitz baths are helpful in relieving subsequent discomfort. The treatment should be repeated every week or two. Sexual contacts should be examined to avoid reinfection.

Proctoscopic and vaginal examinations should be done routinely when the adjoining areas are involved to minimize reinfection and further transmission. Resistant condyloma should be excised or electrodesiccated. However, excessive tissue destruction or removal can produce orificial strictures.

If lesions appear or behave atypically, a biopsy should be done to exclude an exuberant squamous cell carcinoma.

MOLLUSCUM CONTAGIOSUM

Molluscum contagiosum is a common pox virus infection of the skin and occasionally of the conjunctiva; it primarily affects children. Spread is by close contact; epidemics in playground and nursery school environments are common. In adolescents and adults, it may be venereally transmitted; the resultant lesions predominate about the pubic area.

Pathologically, the epidermis grows down into the dermis to form saccules containing clusters of virus. The basal layer appears unaffected, but the cells of the first few layers of stratum malpighii have small basophilic or amphophilic inclusions. As the intracytoplasmic inclusions move higher up in the epidermis they stain eosinophilic and enlarge to about 300 by 200 by 100 μ dimensions. The characteristic intracytoplasmic inclusion body, which is composed of mature, immature, and incomplete virus as well as cellular debris, is known as the molluscum body. The nucleus is compressed to the side by the inclusion.

The clinical lesions are discrete, slightly umbilicated dome-shaped papules which usually are fleshy in color but may be pink or gray (Fig. 12–12). Their diameter is commonly 2 to 5 mm. but can be 1.5 cm. In children the distribution is mainly on the trunk, face, extremities, and sometimes the conjunctiva. In the adult, pubic, genital, and perineal areas are favored.

Light microscopic examination of the "core" of the lesions reveals large brick-shaped inclusions which stain easily with Giemsa's or Wright stain.

Differential diagnosis is not difficult but occasionally molluscum contagiosum has been confused with lichen planus, verrucae vulgaris, epitheliomas (for example, basal cell type), chickenpox, and furuncles. Giant molluscum may resemble early keratoacanthomas.

Treatment consists of merely shelling out inclusions with a currette. Light electrocautery or light cryosurgical freezing is also effective. Since the lesions are benign,

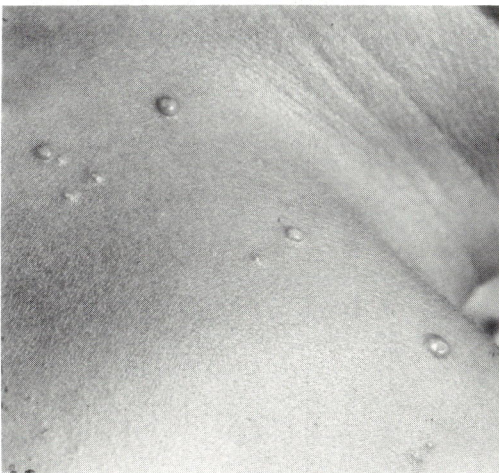

Figure 12–12 Molluscum contagiosum. Multiple small papules. Shiny, light yellow color. Characteristic dell at summit. Cured by expression of contents as for large comedones.

vigorous potentially scarring procedures are discouraged.

SMALLPOX (Variola)

Smallpox is one of the most ancient of all the infectious scourges of man. At the present time, however, most physicians in most countries must derive their knowledge of smallpox from the printed page rather than from practical experience. The fact that smallpox has disappeared as an endemic disease does not allow it to sink below the diagnostic horizon of any physician, because sporadic epidemics of it are constantly occurring here and there. It is obviously of the utmost importance that the first case or cases of the disease in any community be diagnosed promptly, in order that the well-defined and effective means of controlling further spread be carried out at once. The diagnosis of smallpox upon clinical grounds alone may be difficult, but the virologic methods of detecting the disease have reached a level of practical helpfulness, and are increasingly available throughout the world. The following summary is not intended to be complete in respect to all the variants of smallpox and the complications which may arise, but consists only of the chief diagnostic components of the disease.

The following general principles in respect to smallpox should be kept in mind:

1. There is abundant evidence that strains of smallpox virus occurring in nature have varying virulence. If an individual strain produces an epidemic, it tends to produce a disease of comparable virulence in all those infected, though this will be dependent to some extent upon the general state of health and nutrition of the individual patient. For this reason, smallpox has been divided into "major variola" and "minor variola" (alastrim). If an epidemic of smallpox arises and the course in the initial patient seen is severe or mild, it is likely that similar severity or mildness will obtain in unvaccinated individuals who may become infected subsequently.

2. The cutaneous manifestations of smallpox may depart very greatly from those ordinarily associated with this viral infection. They may be hemorrhagic or

may resemble erythema multiforme, and thus they may escape correct diagnosis even by very competent physicians with wide experience in infectious diseases. This occurred in the epidemic in New York City in 1947, in which the patients initially seen were not diagnosed, and the beginnings of the epidemic were not recognized until the disease developed in individuals who had been in contact with the original patients.

3. Smallpox produced by a highly virulent strain may produce the mild disease, varioloid, in persons with partial immunity from a previous vaccination. The infection in this disease, if transmitted to unvaccinated persons, will prove severe.

The mean period of incubation of smallpox is 12 days, but it may vary from one to three weeks. The prodromal symptoms develop suddenly, with headache, backache, high fever, chills, malaise, and sometimes vomiting. The skin is ordinarily clear for three to four days, but there may be a transient macular rash which, if pronounced, is apparently a bad prognostic sign. The characteristic exanthem is papular and tends to be most marked on the face and extremities, with involvement of the palms and soles. This latter feature is a distinguishing point from varicella. With the appearance of the exanthem, the temperature may become normal and the patient feels much improved. The papules become vesicular, but there are no continued showers of new lesions as in varicella. After five to ten days, the lesions become pustular, through either local tissue destruction or secondary bacterial infection. The fever again rises, and leukocytosis develops. In the ordinary course of the disease, crusting of the pustules occurs in most or all of the lesions within two weeks.

The above sequence of signs and symptoms could hardly escape the attention of any physician if smallpox is considered even momentarily. However, it would appear that among populations where vaccination has been carried out routinely and where epidemics of smallpox are uncommon and of limited extent, the classic eruption of smallpox will be seen rarely. Hemorrhagic or erythema multiforme–like eruptions may well be more common, or hemorrhagic lesions may supervene on a process which initially was characteristic. The picture may be one of general hematopoietic depression, and "black" smallpox may be fatal within a few days.

The chief complications of smallpox are bacterial bronchopneumonia, secondary pyogenic infection of the skin, corneal ulcers, and encephalitis. The bacterial infections may be largely controlled by adequate antibiotic and supportive therapy, though this will have no effect upon the viral infection itself. The mortality of smallpox varies widely from under 1 per cent to as high as 50 per cent.

MINOR VARIOLA (alastrim). Minor variola has an incubation period which is somewhat shorter than that of classic smallpox. The prodromal stage is similar but generally much milder. The mortality rate is below 1 per cent, but occasional hemorrhagic cases may occur, and the virus infection may therefore not seem to run "true" in every patient.

VARIOLOID. Varioloid is essentially virulent smallpox occurring in an individual with partial immunity. The prodromal phase is mild to almost absent, and the eruption may be minimal or absent, appearing principally upon the forehead, forearms, and hands. There is ordinarily no secondary febrile phase, and the disease may offer some difficulty in differentiation from varicella. The importance of the syndrome lies in the fact that when the infection is transmitted to nonvaccinated persons, fulminating smallpox may result.

Laboratory Methods of Diagnosis

The methods of confirming or disproving the diagnosis of smallpox have reached a point of much practical usefulness, and the physician should not hesitate to take advantage of such facilities as may be available, in any case in which the signs and symptoms may indicate the possibility of smallpox. These tests utilize tissue culture and serologic and ultramicroscopic techniques. Preparation of crusts, vesicle fluid, or scrapings from vesicle bases may confirm smallpox or identify vaccinia or herpes virus infections by electron microscopy within minutes of collection (Blank et al., 1970). Inoculation of chorioallantoic membranes should be performed as a suitable back-up measure in seriously suspected variola cases.

Infectiousness

Smallpox is among the most highly contagious of all infectious diseases of man. The virus is abundant in secretion from the nose and throat, since lesions are frequently found on the palate, pharynx, and trachea. The virus of smallpox is very stable. It may remain viable after a year at room temperature, and large amounts are present in crusts which are shed while the patient is convalescing. The most stringent precautions in respect to fomites are justifiable.

Treatment

No specific agent against smallpox has been developed. The prophylactic use of systemic antibiotic therapy to prevent complicating bacterial infection, particularly pulmonary or cutaneous, is not justified until actual secondary infection has been proved. Hyperimmune gamma globulin is of value in the early stages of the disease. Corticosteroid therapy would appear to be of value in the encephalitis which may follow smallpox or vaccination.

Prophylactic Control

Among all the more recent advances in therapeutic and prophylactic medicine, Jenner's development of vaccination against smallpox still stands as a giant accomplishment. If the population of a community is effectively vaccinated, epidemics of smallpox cannot occur. The rarity of the disease may, however, lead to failures to detect improper methods of vaccination or the use of impotent vaccines. The precise technique of vaccination is of much importance; the multiple puncture technique is to be preferred. It is important that ether or acetone be used for cleansing the skin prior to vaccination, not alcohol or an antiseptic which will remain on the skin, because this may inactivate the vaccine. The principal contraindication to vaccination is in patients with eczema, where the procedure carries the risk of Kaposi's varicelliform eruption.

Isatin beta thiosemicarbazone is an effective oral prophylactic drug against variola if administered during the prodromal stage. Vaccination of lymphoma patients, particularly if they are on corticosteroid therapy, may result in their death from disseminated vaccinia. Present United States Public Health Service policy contraindicates routine vaccination of the civilian population.

VACCINIA

Though vaccinia and cowpox ordinarily are considered to be due to the same virus, there is increasing evidence to indicate that the strains of vaccinia available today have, through influences which are not thoroughly understood, become changed from the original strains of cowpox from which the virus was presumably derived. These variants are of much interest to virologists, but the reason for differentiation need not concern the general physician. The interpretation of reactions to vaccinations and certain complications of importance will be summarized briefly.

Vaccination

The inoculation of vaccinia virus into the skin of a patient with no immunity results in the characteristic primary vaccination reaction. About the fourth day, a red papule appears on an erythematous base. This increases in size and becomes vesicular within a week after vaccination. It becomes pustular in two to three days more and then gradually dries, with the formation of a crust which drops off within three to four weeks. The local reaction is prolonged and complications are more likely to ensue if the site is not kept dry and exposed to the air. Mild general malaise and occasional fever may occur at the height of the reaction, and regional lymphadenopathy is common. The resultant scar remains somewhat erythematous for a month or two. It should be small and relatively inconspicuous if the vaccination has been properly done by the multiple puncture method.

Vaccination affords protection from

smallpox within three weeks, and the immunity will remain adequate for up to seven years. Vaccination of an individual who is partially immune results in the vaccinoid reaction in which a pustule and some erythema occur in one week, and from which a slight atrophic scar may result. The course is that of a diminutive and abortive primary reaction. The typical immune reaction is characterized by the formation of a small, slightly inflamed papule within two days after vaccination, which may persist and enlarge slightly after one week and then disappear without a trace. Complete absence of any reaction whatever strongly indicates that the vaccine is impotent or has been inactivated by improper preliminary sterilization of the site.

The chief variations and complications of vaccinia are as follows: a vaccination take is occasionally associated with a nonspecific toxic erythematous rash, usually occurring at the height of the take or, much more rarely, a generalized vaccinia. The latter ordinarily involutes quite promptly without scarring and is of no great importance in otherwise healthy persons.

Vaccination, however, is not without complications, some of which may be serious. Incidence of serious reaction to primary inoculations is highest under one year of age, least high during the second year, and reportedly then rises with advancing age. Side effects diminish significantly in healthy individuals who are revaccinated.

The most common reaction is a nonspecific toxic exanthem occurring at the height of the vaccination. In healthy individuals, generalized vaccinia may occur, is rarely serious, involutes promptly, and leaves no scars. In immuno-incompetent or immunosuppressed patients, it can be severe or even fatal.

Eczema vaccinatum (Kaposi's varicelliform eruption) may occur in an atopic patient who is vaccinated or in one who comes in close contact with a person who has been vaccinated. Approximately 10 per cent of these patients who appear to be free of eczema develop vaccinia in clinically appearing normal skin.

Vaccinia necrosum or progressive vaccinia is seen mainly in immuno-incompetent or immunosuppressed patients. It

may be first recognized from 7 to 49 days post-inoculation. Disseminated lesions may occur in this often relentlessly progressive disease, and treatment with isatin beta thiosemicarbazone and vaccinia immune globulin may be beneficial and reduce the spread of the disease by one-half. The mortality rate may be as high as 30 per cent.

Post-vaccinial central nervous system disease or encephalitis, which is rare, can result in death or permanent brain damage. It begins between 6 and 19 days post-vaccination with a fever which often is followed by convulsions. Most patients lapse into a coma during the illness. About 50 per cent of patients have normal cerebrospinal fluid and at postmortem examination may exhibit only diffuse swelling of the cerebral cortex. Treatment is supportive.

Other complications may include congenital vaccinia with stillbirth, transiently false positive serologies, and development of reaction states (erythema nodosum leprosum) in patients with Hansen's disease.

In the United States, these reactions annually cost seven to eight lives. Because there has not been an outbreak of smallpox in the United States since 1949, and because the rate of complication of primary vaccination including death is 74.7 per million persons, suspension of revaccination has been advocated by the United States Public Health Service. This guideline does not apply to medical or military personnel who may encounter the disease without prior alert or to travelers to areas where smallpox is endemic (Lane et al., 1969).

Accidental vaccination in non-immune individuals is by no means uncommon, and is most likely to occur among school or play groups of children when a considerable number of vaccinations are being carried out. If a massive inoculation has occurred, or if the lesion appears on a mucocutaneous junction, it may sometimes be rather puzzling diagnostically. However, the identity with vaccination will ordinarily be apparent if the possibility is considered and if inquiry is made as to the child's contacts. Secondary bacterial infection in the vaccination wounds is unusual but does occur. Epitheliomas have occurred in vaccination scars in later life.

Kaposi's Varicelliform Eruption

This complication of eczema in infants or in adults may be produced by the virus of either herpes simplex or vaccinia, and the clinical course is indistinguishable. It has been described elsewhere.

It is clearly obvious that vaccination against smallpox should not be undertaken in persons with chronic dermatitis of any severity, nor even in persons who have extensive disturbances of the integrity of the skin from other causes. In children having eczema with an up and down course, the decision as to whether or not to vaccinate may be a difficult one. In many instances, it will be concluded that the risk of vaccination to the patient far exceeds the risk of smallpox. Such children are, unfortunately, sometimes excluded from school because they do not have a vaccination certificate, but it is the authors' belief that such exclusion is unjustified under ordinary circumstances.

Probably the most serious complication of vaccination is encephalitis, which is rare in any event, but exceedingly so if vaccination is carried out in early childhood or if the procedure is a revaccination. The patient develops headache and fever, various signs of focal nerve involvement, and, later, convulsions and unconsciousness. The mortality rate is high. Corticosteroid therapy may be helpful.

Stillborns have been a common result of congenital vaccinia. For this reason, smallpox vaccination should best be withheld during pregnancy.

Biologic False-Positive STS

It was strikingly demonstrated during World War II that a significant proportion of patients with vaccination "takes" would develop a biologic false-positive serologic test for syphilis. In some series the incidence was as high as 20 to 30 per cent. In such patients the TPI (*Treponema pallidum* immobilization) test will be negative, and the STS ordinarily becomes nonreactive within two to four months.

Prevention

Isatin beta thiosemicarbazone is an effective oral prophylactic agent against vaccinia. Investigations are now in progress in an attempt to develop an attenuated vaccinia virus capable of protecting against smallpox without producing a transmissible disease in humans.

DISEASES CONTRACTED FROM ANIMALS

In addition to cowpox, a number of human diseases may be contracted from animals. In some of these the viral etiology has been proved beyond a doubt, while in others it is presumed. It is convenient to consider these diseases as a group, though the clinical characteristics of them vary widely.

Cowpox

The term cowpox is being reserved increasingly for the natural disease occurring in cows. To the best of the authors' knowlege, it does not occur in the United States, but it is observed occasionally in Great Britain and Holland as an epidemic infection of the teats and udders. In such outbreaks a history of exposure of the cow to a recently vaccinated farmhand is rare, and the disease may be regarded as distinct from vaccinia or smallpox.

Cowpox is confined in man to persons who have been in contact with infected teats and udders. Lesions occur most frequently on the hands but may appear elsewhere, for example, on the face or forearm. It is characterized by a painful, firm, inflammatory nodule, which may be associated with regional lymphadenopathy and some fever and malaise. The lesions tend to be more severe and hemorrhagic than those seen in vaccinia and may not heal for many weeks.

Cat-Scratch Disease

Cat-scratch disease is a benign infection usually occurring in persons under 20, often children, two-thirds of whom report being scratched within a period of one to four weeks prior to the clinical manifestation of the disease. The seasonal incidence is predominantly fall and winter. The precise etiologic agent has not been identified but is presumed to be a member of the family Chlamydiaceae carried by asymptomatic cats. It has never been isolated nor is there objective evidence of transmission from presumably infected cats. Occasional cases have occurred without cat contact in which dog bites, monkey scratches, or splinter cuts have been implicated.

Cat-scratch disease ordinarily begins with an inflamed papule or pustule usually located on the hand, arm, or leg; in 12 per cent of patients, it appears as a conjunctivitis. After one to two weeks, regional lymphadenopathy develops and usually lasts two weeks to two months but may persist for six months. In one-third to one-quarter of the patients, systemic manifestations of fever and malaise develop. Headache, cough, parotid swelling, splenomegaly, a nonpruritic macular or morbilliform eruption, Parinaud's oculoglandular syndrome, or encephalopathy with grand mal seizure may occur. The clinical presentation is usually regional lymphadenopathy only, the primary lesion having resolved prior to the patient's presentation. An elusive history of cat contact with a relative's or neighbor's kitten may often be the best history obtained from a child patient. The affected lymph nodes are often tender and may become fluctuant and spontaneously drain purulent material (Fig. 12–13).

The only abnormal laboratory finding is an elevated sedimentation rate during the acute lymphadenitis. Skin tests may be performed with antigen which is aspirated from infected nodes, is standardized against other skin test material, and is injected (0.1 ml.) intradermally. A tuberculin-type delayed hypersensitivity reaction occurs if positive and may measure up to 1.5 cm. in diameter and become centrally necrotic. Different lots may react differently; therefore, pooled antigen sources probably give the best chance for eliciting positive results. About 90 to 95 per cent of patients with a clinical diagnosis will show positive reactions. In control series of patients with no cat contact, 98 per cent have negative intradermal tests. Conver-

sion to a positive intradermal test takes place about 30 days post infection (Margileth, 1968).

The histopathology of the involved lymph node is characterized by an initial reticuloendothelial hypoplasia which progresses finally and diagnostically to tuberculoid granulomas and to stellate abscess formations. At this final stage, the histopathologic differential diagnosis is tularemia and lymphogranuloma venereum, and in earlier stages, Hodgkin's disease, tuberculosis, or even sarcoid (Johnson and Helwig, 1969).

Diagnosis can be made on the basis of four of the following five criteria:

1. An appropriate history of animal contact (usually a cat).
2. Aspiration of culturally proven sterile pus from a node.
3. Lymph node biopsy consistent with the disease.
4. A positive skin test (N.B., there is a small percentage of false positives and up to 10 to 20 per cent false negatives with a single batch of antigen).
5. A typical cutaneous lesion and appropriate adenopathy.

The clinical differential diagnosis of this disease includes lymphogranuloma venereum, typical and atypical mycobacterial infection, hidradenitis suppurativa, bacterial and viral lymphadenitis, tularemia, brucellosis, histoplasmosis, coccidioidomycosis, toxoplasmosis, infectious mononucleosis, and benign and malignant tumors of the lymph nodes, especially Hodgkin's disease.

Treatment is nonspecific, consisting mainly of reassurance, analgesics for pain, and aspiration of suppurative nodes. The latter is easily accomplished when necessary with an 18- or 19-gauge needle. Reaspiration may be necessary on occasion. Surgical drainage sometimes results in sinus tract formation. Antibiotics, especially tetracycline, have been administered but are of questionable efficacy.

Ecthyma Contagiosum

This disease is a pox virus infection primarily of sheep, occurring naturally as an inflammatory vesicular and pustular eruption of non-woolbearing areas such as the mouth, lips, nostrils, and groin. The in-

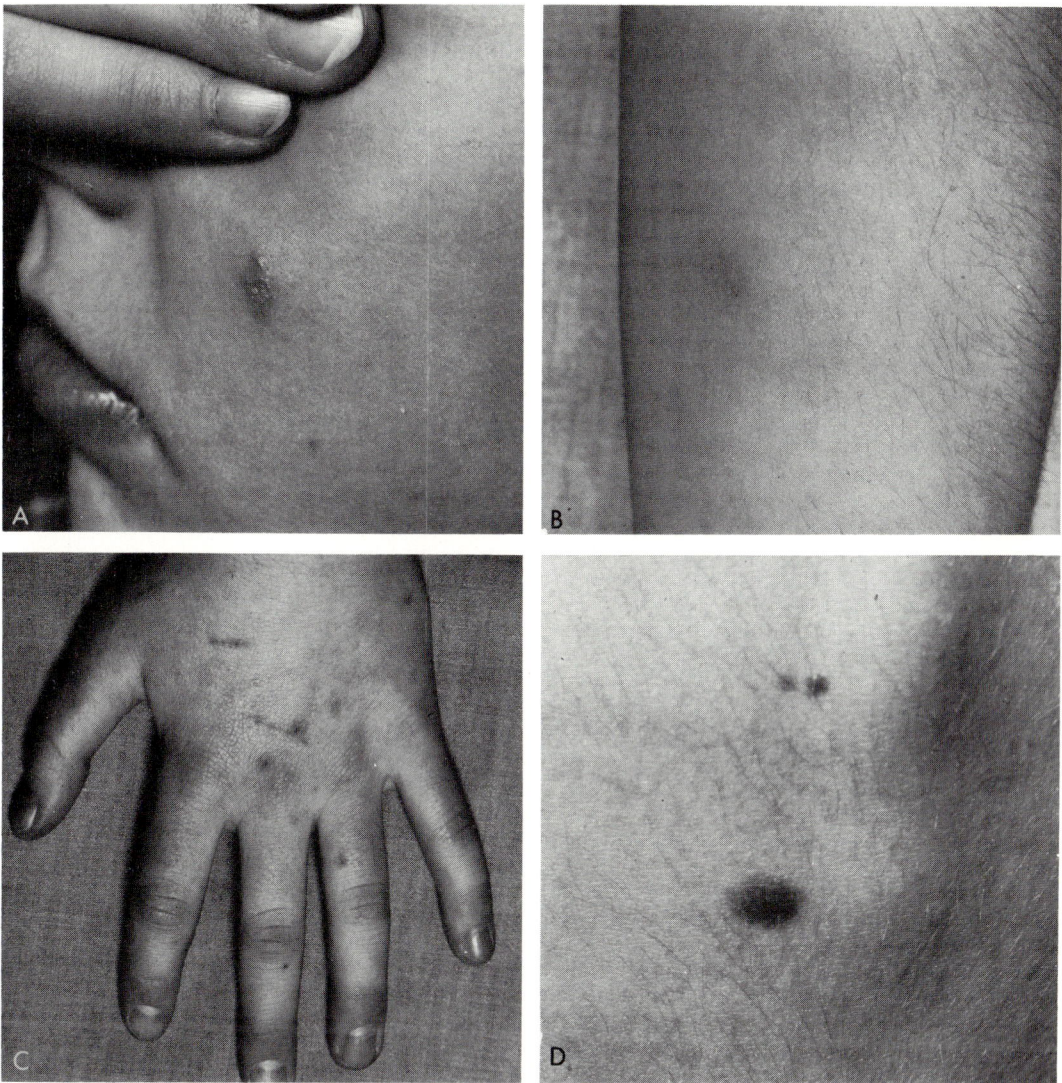

Figure 12–13 Cat-scratch disease. *A*, "Primary" lesion on cheek. *B*, Positive skin test (same patient). *C*, Scratches from family cat. *D*, Papular lesions of back (same patient).

fection is widespread and important economically owing to weight loss and failure of infected lambs and young ewes to grow properly. Mortality rates reach 50 per cent if lesions become secondarily infected with bacteria or parasites. Immunity is established following primary infection, and vaccination is carried out in some areas. Goats may be infected, and laboratory infections have been achieved in rabbits, guinea pigs, and embryonated chicken eggs.

Man is occasionally infected, usually fol-lowing direct contact with infected sheep, but rarely after handling lumber or clothing which has been in contact with infected animals. Ordinarily, one to three lesions develop but up to ten have been reported.

Microscopically, the lesions are papillomatous with pseudoepitheliomatous hyperplasia extending into the dermis from the rete pegs.

Electron microscopic study has revealed cigar-shaped virus particles 325 nm. long and 135 nm. thick in the cytoplasm.

The clinical course of infection is characteristic in both man and sheep, lasting from 14 to 72 days, usually 35 to 40 days. An initially erythematous macule becomes papular in a week, then develops a targetoid red center surrounded by a white rim with an erythematous halo during the second week. By the third week, the lesion becomes eczematous and nodular. During the fourth week, a thin, dry, yellow crust with small black dots composed of pyknotic follicle cells forms and then undergoes successive sloughs with gradual reduction in size until it clears. The sloughs are more frequent in human than in sheep infections. Systemic symptoms are unusual, consisting of an occasional lymphadenitis and rare fever with disseminated lesions. Conjunctival lesions can occur. Lesions resolve without scarring.

Diagnostically significant complement-fixing and neutralizing antibodies have been demonstrated but are not used clinically.

At various stages the differential diagnosis includes vaccinia, cutaneous malignancy, verruca, and an infected keratoacanthoma.

Treatment is nonspecific and although a vaccine is available its use in humans is not warranted (Leavell et al., 1968).

Milker's Nodules

Milker's nodules is caused by a pox virus contracted from infected cow teats or calf muzzles. It is seen among those who have handled infected cows or calves.

On histopathologic examination the nodule shows acanthosis, spongiosis, long thin retes extending into the dermis, multilocular subepidermal vesicles and increase of dermal capillaries. The associated infiltrate is nonspecific and is composed of lymphocytes, histocytes, and plasma cells which invade the dermis. Vacuolated epidermal cells often contain intracytoplasmic eosinophilic inclusions similar to those seen in vaccinia and variola; intranuclear inclusions have been reported (Evins et al., 1971). On electron microscopic studies, cigar-shaped viruses 310 nm. long and 140 nm. wide have been seen in the cytoplasm of infected cells.

Clinically, single or multiple erythematous papules or nodules which measure about 0.5 to 1.5 cm. in diameter, and are firm and nonfixed, become ulcerated and crusted, and heal in about six weeks. Regional adenopathy is common. Unlike the lesions of cowpox, these lesions are usually painless (Fig. 12–14).

Differential diagnosis is the same as that for ecthyma contagiosum.

Laboratory confirmation of infection is made with electron microscopic examination of crusts of the lesions, which have remained positive for virus as long as 30 days (Davis and Musil, 1970).

Treatment is not necessary unless bacterial superinfection occurs.

Some authors feel that ecthyma contagio-

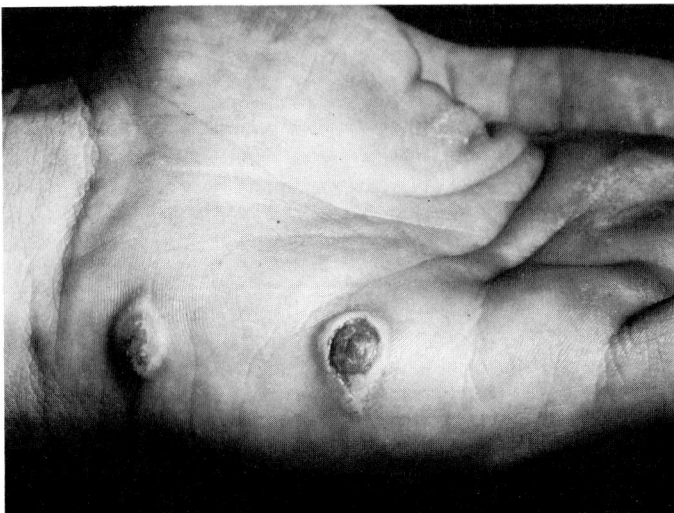

Figure 12–14   Milker's nodules.

sum and milker's nodules may be caused by the same virus (Nagington et al., 1965).

Monkeypox

Since the eradication of smallpox in western and central Africa in 1970, a new uncommon pox disease has been recognized. The disease apparently has been endemic in wild monkey colonies and is usually found in back-country areas where contact with these creatures has been documented or highly suspected. There seems to be no age or sex predilection in man. No person-to-person spread has been documented or suspected. Clinically, the disease presents with a prodrome of fever, malaise, headache, and sore throat followed in one to five days by a single crop of diffusely scattered vesiculopustular lesions in a generalized distribution, including palms and soles. Corneal lesions occur and lymphadenopathy may be prominent. Lesions crust and heal with or without pitted scars in an interval ranging from four days to four weeks. Prior smallpox vaccination appears to grant immunity (Foster et al., 1972).

Laboratory examination has shown characteristic small necrotic hemorrhagic pocks on chorioallantoic membranes and large plaques on Vero cell cultures. Rabbits inoculated intradermally develop large necrotic reactions, a generalized exanthem, and a marked systemic illness in contrast to mild reactions when challenged with vaccinia or variola (Lourie et al., 1972).

The only differential diagnosis is essentially variola which monkeypox resembles very closely clinically.

Treatment has been supportive. No fatalities have been observed.

Vesicular Stomatitis

Vesicular stomatitis is a viral illness of cattle and horses which is occasionally contracted by humans who are in close contact with infected animals.

Within two to eight days after contact the patient may experience fever, malaise, myalgia, nausea, vomiting, and pharyngitis. A vesicular exanthem may appear, as well as submucosal lymphoid hyperplasia, and herpes simplex–like lip lesions.

Laboratory confirmation may be obtained by complement fixation and neutralizing antibody studies of acute and convalescent serum and also by the intracerebral inoculation of three-week-old mice.

The differential diagnosis is essentially that of herpangina. Treatment is symptomatic and the outcome is usually favorable (Fields and Hawkins, 1967).

EXANTHEMS

Many viral illnesses are accompanied by symmetric, erythematous eruptions called exanthems. These rashes are composed of macules, papules, pustules, vesicles, or petechiae. An infectious agent occasionally may be recovered from the cutaneous lesions. Some exanthems have a histologic picture reminiscent of the cytopathic effect produced by the virus on cultured cells. The microscopic morphology of other eruptions consists of a perivascular infiltration of lymphocytes and mononuclear cells.

The main clues to the cause of the exanthem are the primary lesion within the exanthem, the time of appearance of the eruption relative to the onset of the disease, the distribution of the eruption, and the other symptoms produced by the infection.

In Table 12–1, the various diagnostic possibilities are grouped according to the primary lesion of the exanthem. Special attention should be focused upon treatable diseases or highly contagious, potentially lethal infections.

Drug eruptions can mimic any viral exanthem. Subacute bacterial endocarditis, typhoid fever, and rickettsioses should always be considered in the diagnoses of petechial eruptions in febrile patients. When the patient's eruption is symmetric, monomorphous, and maculopapular, secondary syphilis must be considered. Variola must be excluded in patients with monomorphic vesicular or pustular eruptions. Finally, scarlet fever must be considered in the differential diagnosis of all erythematous macular rashes.

TABLE 12–1   DIFFERENTIAL DIAGNOSIS OF EXANTHEMS

Vesiculopustules	*Maculopapules*	*Urticaria*	*Petechiae*
Drug eruption	Drug eruption	Varicella (urticaria	Drug eruption
Herpes simplex	Secondary lues	around vesicle)	Bacterial endocarditis
Variola	Scarlet fever	Coxsackie A5, A9	ECHO 9
Vaccinia	ECHO 9, 16	Infectious hepatitis	Coxsackie A5, A9
Varicella	Coxsackie A5, A9, A16,	Mononucleosis	Mononucleosis
Generalized zoster	B5	*Mycoplasma pneumoniae*	Rubella
Rickettsialpox	Reovirus 2	Hepatitis	Thrombocytopenia with
Coxsackie A and B	Erythema infectiosum		many acute infections
Reovirus 2	Gianotti-Crosti syndrome		
Mycoplasma pneumoniae	Rubella		
ECHO 4	Rubeola		
Orf	Hepatitis		
	Infectious mononucleosis		
	Arborvirus (dengue)		
	Rickettsioses		

The diagnostic techniques that should be employed are listed in Table 12–2. When the physician is unable to obtain prompt facilities for culturing an infectious agent, the clinical specimen should be stored in the cold, in liquid nitrogen if possible. Simple refrigeration is usually sufficient for a few hours, but freezing under temperatures as low as possible would better ensure viral stability for several days. In general, the specimen should be kept in sterile isotonic fluid or as a dissected crust rather than in aqueous solutions. Sterile acute phase sera should always be obtained and either refrigerated or frozen until arrival at the clinical laboratory.

Clinical differentiation of the viral exanthems continues to be interesting and challenging. The "classical exanthems" are listed in the order in which they were described: measles (first disease), scarlet fever (second disease), rubella (third disease), Dukes' disease (fourth disease), erythema infectiosum (fifth disease), exanthema subitum (sixth disease) (Shapiro, 1965).

Some of the newer, recognized exanthems are also described below.

Measles (First Disease)

Measles is a highly contagious worldwide endemic myxovirus infection affecting nearly all humans at some time in their lives. Severe bacterial infections frequently follow the disease, accounting for the high rate of morbidity and mortality, most pronounced in underdeveloped or underprivileged environments; these infections are now treatable with the advent of antimicrobial therapy. In advanced countries, the mortality rate is about 2 per 100,000 cases. In underdeveloped lands, it may run over 500 per 100,000 cases. Measles presents clinically in a classic fashion.

Incubation is usually 10 to 11 days, varying from one to two weeks. About six to seven days post contact, a fever of 38° C. associated with mild upper respiratory infection symptoms may appear, lasting 24 hours. This may represent the first viremia.

The invasion phase, lasting four days to one week, is characterized by systemic toxicity, with high fever, chills, malaise, sweating, prostration, headache, oculonasal catarrh, conjunctivitis, photophobia, coryza with mucopurulent discharge, diarrhea, and a dry, hacking, persistent cough refractory to antitussives. The fever course is biphasic, with an initial one- to two-day rise, a fall to normal for a day, followed by a rise occurring with the onset of the exanthem. Very helpful to diagnosis is the exanthem, which begins as an intensely erythematous suffusion or even petechial eruption on the soft palate concomitant with the invasion phase. One to two days later, Koplik's spots appear insidiously as several tiny, blue-white spots surrounded by a bright red irregular halo on the buccal mucosa adjacent to the second molars. Their number rapidly increases, extending over the buccal mucosa and becoming confluent; they appear as a myriad of white spots on a red background as the rash be-

clinical infection; however, strong evidence has accumulated that this merely raises the incidence of subclinical infections, scarcely desirable for pregnant women in whom detection of first trimester infection is vital if therapeutic abortion is to be considered.

Several attenuated strains are now available for vaccination and although antibody titers are not as high as those following natural infection, results appear promising. A side effect of the attenuated strains is a high incidence of arthritis and carpal tunnel syndrome in adult females (Cooper and Krugman, 1969).

Dukes' Disease (Fourth Disease)

In the late nineteenth century, differentiation of exanthematous eruptions was very important since confusion with scarlet fever meant six to eight weeks of unnecessary quarantine and considerable parental anxiety while watching for potentially fatal nephritis or endocarditis. By 1900, measles, scarlet fever, and rubella were recognized entities; however, given only these three categories, many infectious, exanthematous epidemics could not be clearly classified, which resulted in wild reports of second and third infections with each disease (Shapiro, 1965).

Dr. Clement Dukes, an astute morphologist and clinician, observed concurrent exanthematous epidemics in private English schools and separated true rubella from scarlet fever and from a "fourth disease" on both clinical and epidemiologic criteria. This fourth disease was characterized by an abbreviated, usually mild prodrome consisting at worst of "headache, anorexia, drowsiness, chilliness and even considerable backache" of several hours, followed by a diffuse, bright rosey red, slightly raised eruption which quickly covered the body within a few hours. Dr. Dukes avoided any mention of discrete lesions or configurate patterns and noted that the suffusion spread more rapidly than scarlet fever, but in the same manner. A velvety red pharynx with moderate edema was present, as was conjunctivitis, generalized "hard, tender, pea sized" adenopathy, a virtually normal tongue, and a fever of 98.4 to 104° F. for several days, with only moderately quickened pulse,

mild malaise, and quite variable desquamation. Scaling was fine, not in sheets as in scarlet fever, and varied from nonexistant to severe, involving even the palms and soles and lasting "many weeks," as long as in scarlet fever. Renal disease was never observed and recovery was complete. Spring and summer epidemics were observed from 1892 to 1900 and demonstrated a lack of cross immunity between scarlet fever, rubella, and fourth disease (Dukes, 1900).

In retrospect, this entity was most likely a viral exanthem of the Coxsackie-ECHO group, but recent studies of these agents have not revealed a suitable exanthem.

Today, fourth disease represents an interesting historic example of careful morphologic examination and discerning clinical evaluation which was, unfortunately, too early for modern laboratory classification.

Erythema Infectiosum (Fifth Disease)

Erythema infectiosum is a contagious disease of children 5 to 15 years old, and is probably due to an enterovirus infection. It spreads rapidly within households and slowly outside family groups, and there is evidence of asymptomatic cases which influence the spread of disease.

Incubation is probably 5 to 10 days, with an average of eight days. A prodrome, which rarely occurs, consists of several days of low-grade fever, malaise, mild nausea, occasional vomiting, some diarrhea, and abdominal cramping. Most often, the disease begins with its exanthem which starts on the cheeks as 3- to 5-mm. erythematous, blanchable, slightly raised papules which become confluent over the course of a few hours and give the uniformly bright red "slapped" cheek appearance. The involved skin becomes hot, tight, and smooth to the touch. The rash stops abruptly at the nasolabial fold, spares the base and bridge of the nose, forehead, eyelids, and chin, and assumes a butterfly wing malar distribution.

After two to three days it begins to fade but often recurs several times, especially after exertion or excitement. During this period of facial recurrences, the exanthem involves the extremities, regularly affecting the posterolateral forearm and usually the dorsal hand and sparing the elbow, flexures, and the palm. It often extends up the posterior arm to the shoulder and progresses centripetally. The buttocks and legs, especially the anterolateral thighs, are affected; the soles are spared. The chest is rarely involved. Lesions have an advancing erythematous areola. The eruption develops a characteristic lacelike pattern through the coalescence and irregular clearing of the lesions. It lasts one to two weeks and frequently has successive exacerbations and remissions, on the body as well as the face. There appears to be no enanthem or residual pigmentation, scaling, complication, or sequelae. Generalized adenopathy is present but unimpressive.

Laboratory abnormalities often show a slight lymphocytosis and a definite eosinophilia. The histopathologic picture is of intracellular edema in the malpighian layer with a histiocytic infiltrate. The superficial vascular plexus exhibits endothelial swelling and a perivascular mononuclear infiltrate.

The differential diagnosis includes many of the viral exanthems, especially rubella and exanthema subitum. The characteristic distribution on the face, the lacelike pattern of clearing, and the cyclic pattern of exacerbations make this disease clinically more readily appreciable.

Since the course is mild, only reassurance and occasional symptomatic treatment are necessary.

Exanthema Subitum
(Roseola Infantum; Sixth Disease)

Exanthema subitum or "sixth disease" is a short-lived exanthem of children six months to two years of age. The agent has not been recovered and the mode of transmission is unknown. Epidemics are rare but have been seen in maternity hospital nurseries. It is postulated that many subclinical or undiagnosed cases occur, and some feel that the disease is nearly obligatory during the first two years of life. Maternal antibody appears to play a role in immunity, as clinical infection before six months of age is unusual.

The incubation period ranges from 5 to 15 days, with an average of 12 days. The first clinical sign of infection is a sudden temperature spike to about 39° C. usually persisting for three days and occasionally fluctuating during this time.

Systemic signs may include a slight anorexia, an episode or two of vomiting or diarrhea, and restlessness. Convulsive seizures may be associated with the fever.

Physical examination may reveal disseminated or cervical and occipital shotty adenopathy, splenomegaly, or a mild meningismus. One-third of the cases may develop a mild pharyngitis. Defervescence is abrupt and is followed within a day by the exanthem, which first appears at the nape of the neck and then spreads to the trunk with emphasis on the posterior aspect; it rarely affects the extremities and even then only with a patchy proximal distribution. The face is spared. Primary lesions are discrete or confluent macules, 2 to 4 mm. in diameter, which are pale pink in color, resembling rubella, and are of variable intensity. They last several hours to a day and resolve without recurrence, pigmentation, or scale.

The main neurologic complications are febrile convulsions with occasional residual seizure disorders, meningitis with cerebrospinal fluid abnormalities, or even encephalitis, stupor, and usually transient mono- or hemiplegia with a Babinski sign. Usually, rapid and complete recovery occurs, although EEG abnormalities may persist in a few cases.

Laboratory examination is characterized typically by agranulocytopenia in 8 to 30 per cent of cases, with a mild leukopenia of 3000 to 7000. Early in the course of exanthema subitum, however, a transient granulocytosis may occur. Differential diagnosis most frequently includes rubella (however, the distribution of lesions and the time course are clearly different) and drug eruptions, which may be difficult, since home remedies or prescription items are frequently administered in the prodrome of many viral illnesses. Exanthems due to adenoviruses may be differentiated by their usual accompanying conjunctivitis or upper respiratory infection symptoms, but those due to echoviruses may be more difficult. Treatment is only symptomatic, with careful attention to seizure control if necessary (Blattner, 1969).

New Viral Exanthems

The leading cause of viral exanthems is infection by enteroviruses, a subgroup of picornaviruses which includes Coxsackie and ECHO agents. In temperate climates, infections are most prevalent in the later summer and fall; however, they occur year round in the tropics. Epidemics often spread in communities by a fecal-oral route, first horizontally among children, then vertically to older members of the family groupings. The virus first multiplies in the throat and ileum; a viremia follows in three to seven days, after which antibody appears and the virus is restricted to local multiplication which is probably eventually controlled by interferon. Children are more frequently clinically affected than adults and boys more so than girls, although rates of infection are the same in both sexes. Sources of infection appear to be human reservoirs, since no other species has ever been found to carry enterovirus. Certain virus infections are known to produce several types of exanthem and more than one type can produce a particular exanthem. General systemic manifestations of this group may include the following: fever, malaise, nausea, vomiting, diarrhea, hepatitis, upper respiratory infection or pneumonia, peri- or myocarditis, conjunctivitis, photophobia, nephritis, meningitis, encephalitis, neuropathies, myalgias, lymphadenopathy, splenomegaly, parotitis, spontaneous abortion, generalized infections in the newborn, herpangina, various enanthem eruptions, and a variety of scarlatiniform, urticarial, maculopapular, vesicular, petechial, purpuric, and erythema multiforme–like eruptions (Cherry, 1969).

HAND, FOOT, AND MOUTH SYNDROME. Coxsackie A16 is the agent responsible for the hand, foot, and mouth syndrome, one of the clearest symptom complexes resulting from enterovirus infections. It was first described in the mid 1950s and has apparently become more common recently, as the proportion of positive serologic titers has been increasing. Infections are more common in late summer and in the fall, spreading rapidly among children, with up to 50 per cent vertical transmission in family units. Although similarities exist between this syndrome and the agent of the zoonosis hoof and mouth disease in cattle, also a picornavirus, the latter is acid labile, differentiating it from the human enterovirus.

The incubation period of hand, foot, and mouth disease is four to six days. An enanthem develops in 90 per cent of cases and involves the tongue, palate, uvula, anterior tonsillar pillars, gingival mucosa, or any combination of these. The initially macular lesions evolve rapidly to vesicles, then ulcerate. They vary in size from several millimeters to 2 cm. in diameter and last one to six days. In two-thirds of patients, an exanthem follows the enanthem by less than a day, the basic lesion consisting of 3- to 7-mm. superficial gray vesicles on an erythematous base, frequently with one or more elongated oval lesions which affect the dorsal hands and feet or even palms and soles, the buttocks, or occasionally the legs, arms, and face. Usually these lesions heal over a period of two to seven days by absorption of fluid, but they may on occasion rupture and crust. Reports of finding inclusions or giant or balloon cells in scrapings and in biopsy material are meager (Froeschle et al., 1967). In any event, there is certainly a marked cytologic difference between these vesicles and those found in varicella-zoster and herpes virus infections. Other manifestations of the disease include submandibular and/or cervical adenitis in one-fifth of patients, and coryza, cough, or diarrhea in another tenth. Nausea and vomiting occasionally occur, as may a more severe but short-lived malaise.

Other Coxsackie viruses have caused sporadic outbreaks of hand, foot, and mouth disease. Culturally proved Coxsackie A5 infection has produced a clinically indistinguishable eruption, as well as an atypical variant consisting of scattered yellow vesicles 4 to 5 mm. in diameter which spread centripetally to the trunk with maculopapules over the buttocks. Coxsackie A10 has also given this picture, but in its atypical form may manifest associated ulcerative lesions near or on the labia and an anterior and posterior oral cavity enanthem. Other sporadic cases have been associated with Coxsackie B1 and B3 infections.

ECHO 16 INFECTIONS. ECHO 16 infections (Boston exanthem) follow a three- to eight-day incubation period, with an onset characterized by fever, anorexia, and mild pharyngitis. Some patients develop multiple, small, punched-out ulcers on the tonsillar pillars and soft palate during this stage. Others develop cervical, occipital, or posterior auricular lymphadenopathy. Characteristically, the eruption begins as small (0.4 to 1.5 cm. in diameter), discrete, pink macules, evolving into slightly raised papules first on the face and upper chest, then spreading centrifugally; they are extensive enough in some cases to involve the palms and soles. It is nonpruritic and lasts for from one to five days. Systemic symptoms are of sudden onset and more pronounced in adults, consisting of chills, fever of 101° to 104° F., myalgias, headache, conjunctivitis, sore throat, and abdominal pain, but the rash is less frequent than in children.

ECHO 9 INFECTION. ECHO 9 is a common pathogenic virus frequently associated with exanthems. The infection spreads rapidly through susceptible populations and has an incubation period of five to seven days. Adults suffer more than children from the constitutional symptoms of fever, headache, nausea, vomiting, and myalgia. Cough, coryza, pharyngitis, a nuchal rigidity, cervical lymphadenopathy, abdominal pain, and photophobia also frequently occur.

The exanthem is more common in children, with an incidence of up to 50 per cent. It is usually concurrent with fever, but may precede it by a few days in some cases. The eruption is generalized, usually rubelliform, starting on the face and neck and rapidly spreading to the trunk, extremities, palms, and soles. Petechiae may accompany the rash or may even present as the sole cutaneous sign and may suggest meningococcemia when aseptic meningitis is also present. Cutaneous manifestations frequently clear without residua in three to five days, although rarely vesiculation and crust formation may accompany resolution. Treatment is nonspecific but when petechial eruptions accompany meningitis, one must often treat the patients for a presumed meningiococcemia.

COXSACKIE A9 INFECTION. Coxsackie A9 is another common pathogen, frequently associated with aseptic meningitis in small sporadic outbreaks. The exanthem, although quite frequent, is nonspecific. Often it is a discrete, erythematous maculo-papular eruption starting on the face and neck then spreading to the trunk and extremities. It lasts one to seven days. Patients frequently have not been very ill and develop the rash while afebrile. A chickenpox-like syndrome characterized by a fever up to 103° F. for from 3 to 4 days with centrifugal spread of 1- to 2-mm. vesicles on erythematous bases (Lerner et al., 1960) may occur. The lesions do not crust, however. Urticarial lesions have also been reported, and in one case a diffuse, purpuric eruption simulating meningococcemia was seen.

ECHO 4 INFECTIONS. ECHO 4 infections have caused several epidemics of aseptic meningitis which have been associated with up to 15 per cent occurrence of an exanthem, usually in children. The eruption appears one to three days after onset of the prodrome and lasts one to two days. It begins as a macular, nonpruritic eruption on the trunk or occasionally the face, becomes partially confluent, and extends to the extremities. Occasionally, maculopapular, rubelliform, and petechial components have been described.

COXSACKIE B5 INFECTION. Coxsackie B5 is a common pathogen, often associated with encephalitis, myocarditis, pericarditis, peritonitis, paralytic disease, orchitis, vesicular pharyngitis, hepatitis, nonspecific febrile illnesses, and, in neonates, encephalitis and myocarditis. Clinically, there is often cervical or occipital lymphadenopathy or both. Considerable variation has been noted in the exanthem. A well-detailed series describes the eruption which appears within 36 hours of defervescence and consists of fine macules and papules over the face and neck which spread to the trunk and extremities in 4 to 24 hours. The eruption is most pronounced over the head and neck, sparing the palms and soles (Cherry et al., 1963). Only a small percentage of B5 infections actually have an exanthem. Occasionally, exanthems have occurred during outbreaks of other enterovirus infections, some of which will be described below.

COXSACKIE A4 INFECTION. Coxsackie A4 may present with a prodrome of anorexia, salivation, pharyngitis, fever, and coryza. A herpangitic enanthem regularly occurs, lasting 1 to 10 days. The exanthem begins with or after defervescence, consisting of 2- to 5-mm. macules or slightly raised papules over the face and trunk. These may resolve in one to four days or may evolve into crops of yellowish, opaque vesicles, 5 to 10 mm. in diameter, which appear over the trunk, spreading to the extremities but sparing the palms and soles. The vesicles resolve in one to two weeks without pruritus, scaling, or crusting, and leave a tan-brown hyperpigmentation.

COXSACKIE B1 INFECTION. Coxsackie B1 is associated with a variety of eruptions. Prodromes of fever, headache, aseptic meningitis, and, rarely, a rubelliform eruption have been described. Other manifestations include roseola infantum–like rashes, blotchy macular lesions in neonates, maculopapular eruptions, and occasionally a syndrome similar to hand, foot, and mouth disease. Herpangitic exanthems occur.

COXSACKIE B3 INFECTION. Coxsackie B3 infection involves an exanthem in perhaps a quarter of affected children but this has not been reported in adults. The illness starts with headache, fever, and diarrhea, sometimes presenting with hepatosplenomegaly. Most series report a maculopapular eruption but petechial lesions resembling meningococcemia are not uncommon and hand, foot, and mouth–like syndromes are reported.

ECHO 2 INFECTION. ECHO 2 often begins with a prodrome of rhinorrhea, fever, cervical adenopathy, and pharyngitis. A rubelliform exanthem is common, beginning on the abdomen and back then spreading to the chest, face, and neck. It may turn a coppery tone within a day or two, and usually lasts two to seven days. Complications may include fatal paralytic neurologic manifestations.

ECHO 5 INFECTION. ECHO 5 was described as a result of an epidemic in a nursery in which all affected babies had fever, one-third had diarrhea, and another third presented a faint pink macular eruption which was most prominent over the extremities but also was present over the face and the trunk. The rash develops, lasts two days, and clears without scaling.

Systemic symptoms in adults are more severe and consist of malaise, fever, severe headache, nausea, and vomiting; however, only 3 per cent have an exanthem, although when present it lasts longer than in infants.

ECHO 6 INFECTION. ECHO 6 is a common cause of aseptic meningitis but has only rarely been associated with exanthems. Those reported are commonly of morbilliform or maculopapular nature but instances of purely macular, papulopustular, and bullous erythema multiforme lesions have been reported.

ECHO 11 INFECTION. ECHO 11 infection usually affects young children but does not have a typical presentation. Aseptic meningitis, poliomyelitis, gastroenteritis, upper respiratory infection, and croup all have been associated with infections, and an exanthem is not infrequently reported. The infection may be recurrent, with the virus isolated up to three weeks later in some urticarial or vesicular cutaneous lesions (Cherry et al., 1963).

ECHO 17 INFECTIONS. ECHO 17 infections are characterized by fever and diarrhea with occasional aseptic meningitis. Perhaps one-third of patients have an exanthem which may be transient erythematous blush or may involve maculopapular, papular, or papulovesicular lesions. Several herpangitic enanthems have been observed (Cherry and Jahn, 1965).

ECHO 25 INFECTIONS. ECHO 25 infections usually present with fever and pharyngitis, but one-third of those infected develop an exanthem and one-seventh a herpangitic enanthem. Occasionally, an aseptic meningitis occurs. The eruption often begins during defervescence after three days of fever and consists of a discrete maculopapular eruption over the trunk which lasts two to three days and clears without scaling. Some patients show a more confluent morbilliform pattern, however. Vesicular eruptions also occur.

INFECTIOUS MONONUCLEOSIS

Mononucleosis is a disease of unproved etiology, presumably viral, usually affecting young adults between the ages of 15 and 25. There is no sexual or racial predilection in man. Transmission is apparently by direct contact with a low degree of contagiousness characterized by many small outbreaks. Clinically, the early course is marked by fever of up to 104° F. which may remain steady or oscillate unpredictably. Usually, the body temperature hovers at about 100 to 101° F., and the fever is accompanied by myalgia, cephalgia, malaise, and asthenia. Pharyngitis occurs in 85 per cent of cases, usually after four to seven days, then resolves over another week. One-fifth of patients manifest pharyngeal exudates, some even mimicking a tender diphtheritic membrane. Adenopathy is best appreciated in the cervical region where several adjacent groups are usually markedly swollen and tender and out of proportion to the sore throat; they may be accompanied by axillary or, rarely, inguinal node enlargement (Duhamel, 1970; McCarthy and Hoagland, 1964).

Splenomegaly is present in two-thirds of the cases, but only three well-documented cases of fatal splenic rupture have been reported despite widespread fear of this complication (Penman, 1970).

Hepatomegaly is common and icteric hepatitis is reported in 5 to 10 per cent of cases. Usually, hepatitis is associated with the pharyngitis. However, asymptomatic jaundice may be the only clinical evidence of serologically confirmed mononucleosis (Duhamel, 1970; McCarthy and Hoagland, 1964).

Encephalitis with or without meningism is a rare but not always benign complication which has caused at least five well-documented deaths. Four fatal cases of Landry-Guillain-Barré neuropathy have also been recorded (Penman, 1970). In well-controlled series the incidence of exanthem has been low—about 3 per cent. Nondiagnostic macular erythemas, urticaria, and faint scarlatiniform eruptions are reported (McCarthy and Hoagland, 1964). Recently, a palm and sole eruption consisting of macules and papules was described as the only cutaneous manifestation of mononucleosis (Petrozzi, 1971).

A palatal enanthem appears between the fifth and seventeenth day in 25 per cent of cases. Usually it is composed of discrete, nonblanchable, bright red petechiae, 0.5 to 1.0 mm. in diameter, which fade to a brownish hue in two days. When this eruption occasionally coalesces, lesions tend to be larger and less sharply demarcated. The petechiae tend to occur at the junction of the hard and soft palates. Upper eyelid edema occurs in 50 per cent of cases and frequently narrows the lid aperture (McCarthy and Hoagland, 1964).

In most cases spontaneous recovery occurs in 10 to 20 days. Convalescence is often prolonged in patients with severe asthenia, and relapses are possible (Duhamel, 1970). Recently attempts have been made to associate mononucleosis and childhood leukemias, but these reports are not substantiated (Fraumeni, 1971, and Editorial, Lancet 1971). The histopathology of the lesions is nonspecific.

Laboratory examination reveals a leukocytosis of 15,000 to 30,000 cells per cubic millimeter. Large hyperbasophilic monocytes, 15 to 20 microns in diameter, with indented kidney-shaped nuclei are present in the blood. These may be found in such a multiplicity of viral diseases that a mononucleosis syndrome has been postulated (Duhamel, 1970). Monocytes represent 5 to 30 per cent of the differential and present slightly contorted and indented atypical forms. Total mononuclear forms represent 60 to 80 per cent of the differential.

The Paul-Bunnell test shows that the patient's serum agglutinates sheep erythrocytes at higher titers of up to 1 to 600 to 2000, whereas normal sera are not positive above a 1 to 20 dilution.

Biologic false positive serology has been reported in between .66 and 20 per cent of patients (McCarthy and Hoagland, 1964).

The cutaneous eruption must be differentiated from other febrile states associated with generalized morbilliform, scarlatiniform, and urticarial eruptions. The palatal enanthem must be differentiated from the lesions seen in rubella, secondary syphilis, meningococcemia, and that seen on the palates of heavy smokers (McCarthy and Hoagland, 1964).

Usually, treatment is symptomatic and nonspecific. In patients with severe constitutional reaction or central nervous system involvement, prednisone, 15 to 20 mg. a day for 8 to 12 days, results in rapid improvement. The Paul-Bunnell-Davidson test is not reversed by this regimen.

VIRAL HEPATITIS

The first urticarial exanthem associated with hepatitis was described in 1843 by Graves; arthritis was an accompanying factor. Dermatologic interest in this syndrome of urticaria associated with hepatitis was reignited when Alpert et al. (1971) reported 18 patients with this syndrome. They presented with a serum sickness prodrome of arthritis of one to several weeks' duration accompanied by concurrently arising Australian antigen serum titers and urticaria for several days; these manifestations were followed shortly by transaminase elevation and frequently icterus. In the acute arthritis phase of this disease, the serum complement, C4 levels, was severely depressed and the hepatitis-associated antigen titers were high; these immunologic changes led to the postulation that this serum sickness syndrome is caused by circulating immune complexes. Yellow hives have been described early in such cases, and it appears that icterus may be appreciated clinically in these lesions before it is found elsewhere (Alpert et al., 1971; Lockskin and Hurley, 1972). Patients with the classic symptomatic viral hepatitis may develop at its onset a scarlatiniform eruption which is limited to the trunk and proximal extremities, spares the face, and fades within a week (Prestia and Lynfield, 1970). Drug-induced hepatitis is usually not associated with cutaneous eruptions or arthralgias.

COLORADO TICK FEVER

Colorado tick fever is an acute viral disease affecting individuals of both sexes and all ages who are bitten by the infected tick, *Dermacentor andersoni*. Due to exposure factors, most patients have been male and most cases have been reported in the vector range of western states during April to August. The incubation period is 1 to 14 days. The onset is abrupt, with headache, myalgia, and, in 50 per cent of cases, a moderate fever which runs a biphasic "saddleback" course, characterized by a two- to three-day remission midway in the disease. An exanthem has appeared in 12 per cent of cases but is not characteristic. Various cases have shown generalized morbilliform eruptions while others have been petechial, involving primarily the extremities and occasionally the palate. In 5 per cent of cases, mostly children, encephalitis, meningitis, and meningoencephalitis, occasionally fatal, have been reported. Usually there are no central nervous system sequelae in the great majority who recover.

Laboratory findings include a leukopenia of 2000 to 3000 cells per cubic millimeter and a complement-fixation titer which rises at least fourfold from acute to convalescent sera.

Treatment is nonspecific and supportive.

The chief differential diagnosis is Rocky Mountain spotted fever, owing to the seasonal and geographic exposure similarities and similar prodromes. The eruption rarely suggests rickettsial infection, however. Other viral exanthems such as Coxsackie, ECHO, rubella, and rubeola may resemble tick fever at times. In an occasional petechial case, meningococcemia may be considered (Spruance and Bailey, 1973).

GIANOTTI-CROSTI SYNDROME

Acrodermatitis papulosa infantum or Gianotti-Crosti syndrome is a benign disease of young children. It is presumably of viral origin, with a week's prodrome consisting of fever, malaise, and upper respiratory symptoms. The eruption affects the face, extremities, and buttocks, first as erythematous papules, which later coalesce to form nummular patches or even purpuric groups of confluent papules. The eruption has a pityriasiform scale, or in some cases crusts, and is markedly pruritic. Resolution takes one to two months.

Systemic signs include diffuse lymphadenopathy and hepatosplenomegaly, while laboratory examination is unremarkable.

Histopathologic changes include orthohyperkeratosis, a spongiotic, almost acanthotic, malpighian layer with considerable intracellular edema and occasionally vesiculation, and a perivascular lymphohistiocytic infiltrate with papillary dermal edema. Capillary endothelial cells may be dilated and edematous.

Therapy is symptomatic.

Differential diagnosis includes infectious mononucleosis, early erythema multiforme, lichenoid drug eruptions, and lichen planus (Romiti, 1967).

DENGUE VIRUSES

The dengue family of viruses, which are classified as group B arthropod-borne viruses, are transmitted to man by Aedes mosquitoes. These infections produce illnesses with maculopapular or hemorrhagic eruptions. Korean hemorrhagic fever, a serious disease which occurred in the United Nations forces in the Korean conflict was caused by one of the dengue viruses.

Mycoplasma pneumoniae has been found to produce a generalized vesiculopustular eruption involving the palms and soles. Small red erosions were present on the palate. Less firm evidence associates this organism with morbilliform, scarlatiniform, petechial, urticarial, papulovesicular, and scaly erythematous eruptions.

VIRAL TREATMENT

Presently, viral chemotherapy stands in much the same position as did bacterial chemotherapy in the early 1940s. The medical world is on the threshold of a new era as a result of advances in understanding viral replication and some of the agents affecting specific steps. Briefly, replicative steps include:

1. Attachment—or adherence of virus to the host cell wall.
2. Penetration—or entrance into the host cell.
3. Uncoating—or baring of the viral nuclear protein.
4. Transcription—or coding of messenger RNA by DNA viruses in preparation for translation.
5. Translation—or viral protein and enzyme synthesis using commandeered host mitochondria.
6. Replication—or synthesis of viral daughters' nucleoprotein chains.
7. Assembly—the assembly of viral component parts to form mature virus particles.
8. Release—or the freeing of daughter virus from the host cell.

So far, useful, clinical, antriviral chemotherapy has utilized agents inhibiting penetration, replication, and protein synthesis (Hirschman, 1971).

Alpha adamantanamine (amantadine,

Symmetrel) inhibits influenza A virus penetration if administered several hours before inoculation. Protection is not complete, as humoral immunity can later be demonstrated against the inoculated strains. If influenza actually develops, it is milder than in untreated controls. Dosage is from 4 to 9 mg. per kilogram for 10 to 14 days. Side effects such as dizziness, confusion, and psychotic reactions have occurred, especially among elderly patients. Further trials are necessary before the drug can be released for general use.

5-iodo-2'-deoxyuridine (Stoxil, idoxuridine) slows viral replication by two mechanisms. First, it inhibits thymidilic acid synthetase, depleting the pool of thymidine triphosphate necessary for DNA synthesis. Second, it may be metabolized to IDUR triphosphate and incorporated into nuclear protein helixes. The subsequent abnormalities result in nonfunctioning nuclear proteins which interfere with viral replication decoding processes. Clinically, IDUR is used to treat herpetic keratitis and is being evaluated for use in herpetic encephalitis.

Cytosine arabinoside (1-β-d-orabenofuranosylcytosine) also inhibits nucleic acid synthesis by DNA core viruses. It acts by inhibiting reduction of cytidilic acid to deoxycytidine triphosphate which can be reversed by deoxycytidine. Clinically, it is being evaluated for use in progressive varicella-zoster infections and cytomegalic inclusion disease. Toxicity is significant, however, consisting of hematopoietic depression, stomatitis and alopecia. Its value is presently in dispute (Stevens and Merigan, 1971). Adenine arabinoside appears to be better tolerated, complicated only by nausea. It is under investigation as a replication inhibitor against varicellazoster, herpesvirus hominis, and cytomegalic inclusion disease infections.

Viral protein synthesis inhibitors include N-methylizatin β-thiosemicarbazone, rifamycin, and probably interferon. Methisazone (Marboran) is clinically useful during the prodromal stage of smallpox, significantly reducing incidence, morbidity, and mortality among those exposed to the disease. Dosage is 200 mg. per kilogram initially, followed by 50 mg. per kilogram every six hours for eight doses. Vomiting is a frequent side effect. Jaundice may occur, and a dermatitis responsive to antihistamine therapy has been reported. Preliminary studies are evaluating its usefulness in vaccinia. Recent studies have indicated that it inhibits replication of adeno-, picorna-, myxo-, and paramyxoviruses, perhaps representing a broad-spectrum antiviral agent. Rifamycin inhibits bacterial and mitochondrial RNA polymerases and pox and adenovirus replication, and blocks polypeptide precursor cleavage in vaccinia virus protein synthesis. Oral administration does not prevent vaccination in volunteers but topical administration can significantly reduce the incidence of vaccination reaction and lower seroconversion titers. Toxicity is slight, which may encourage clinical studies of rifamycin as an antiviral agent.

Interferon is believed to act by inhibition of viral protein synthesis. At present, however, clinically useful interferon stimulators are not available (Stevens and Merigan, 1971).

Development of vaccines against viral illnesses continues but this has mainly been concentrated on the stable, classic exanthems, since their antigenic properties do not change from season to season, quickly rendering vaccines obsolete. Efforts have been made to further attenuate vaccinia and rubella strains specifically. Major obstacles to extension of this work into the adenovirus group have been the rapid changes observed in antigenic characteristics of the wild strains. Recently, extravenous, potentially oncogenic viruses have been found in many monkey tissue viral cultures, causing practical difficulties in preparation. The threat of "slow virus" infection complications or auto-immune reactions has also hampered studies with primate cell cultured vaccines.

Immunoglobulin therapy prepared from pooled plasma has proved helpful in preventing or attenuating infections caused by measles, infectious hepatitis (but rarely serum hepatitis), rubella, mumps, vaccinia, variola, and varicella-zoster viruses. Desirability of attenuating potential infection to a subclinical unrecognizable degree should be carefully considered, especially before treating pregnant females who have been exposed to rubella. Subclinical infections in the mother may still result in fetal anomalies (Rytel, 1972).

ENANTHEMS

Mucous membrane eruptions have been noted either alone or concurrently with exanthems for centuries but only recently has progress been made in understanding their etiology. Advances in viral culture, serology, and in light and electron microscopy have divided herpetic gingivostomatitis, aphthous ulcers, and herpangina into separate entities. Paramyxovirus-like particles have been found in Koplik's spots of measles. Even the time-honored acceptance of palatal petechiae without hoarseness as diagnostic of "strep" throat has been shattered by culture techniques (Dyment et al., 1968).

Clinically, however, enanthems are frequently nonspecific, and literature abounds with conflicting descriptions based on small series or reviews of rapidly outdated papers. The task of rigidly controlling large series with appropriate cultures, serology, light and electron microscopy, photography, and clinical observation and follow-up is immense, technically and financially, but must be accomplished if one expects to eventually diagnose enanthems by clinical observation, should that be possible.

Of the common enanthems, Koplik's spots of measles are the most specific, appearing as tiny blue-white dots surrounded by an erythematous halo one or two days after the first systemic symptoms. The spots are located adjacent to the second molars initially but rapidly spread over the buccal mucosa and soon become a myriad of light spots on a red background as the exanthem begins. Mucosal lesions resolve about the second or third day of the rash. Recent histopathologic studies have revealed multinucleate giant cells in the lesions, and electron microscopy has shown viral microtubular aggregates (Dirk et al., 1970).

Another less specific aspect of measles enanthem is an erythematous or even petechial palatal eruption which coincides with the start of the invasion phase and precedes Koplik's spots by one or two days. This must be differentiated from the lesions of streptococcal sore throat, meningococcemia, mononucleosis, rubella, secondary syphilis, and heavy smoking.

Hand, foot, and mouth syndrome produces mucosal lesions which are first macular but rapidly vesiculate then ulcerate, healing in one to six days. Lesions may be located on the tongue, palate, uvula, anterior tonsillar pillars, or gingival mucosa. The exanthem, described previously, follows the enanthem by a day.

Primary herpes simplex gingivostomatitis is one of the most common vesicular and ulcerative diseases of the oral and gingival mucosa, frequently occurring in six-month-old to six-year-old children without seasonal predilection. A one- to four-day prodrome is common, consisting of a 102° F. to 105° F. fever, malaise, anorexia, and sore throat, followed by vesiculation and ulceration of the tonsils, anterior tonsillar pillars, soft palate, and mouth and lips; it may involve the gingiva. Lesions are painful with a gray shaggy base. They slowly enlarge, then resolve in 4 to 12 days. Adult infections seem milder than those of childhood and frequently affect the gingival margins. They are accompanied by erythema and edema which may or may not proceed to vesiculation and ulceration, spreading throughout the mouth. Serologically confirmed cases have sometimes consisted of sore throat, cervicitis, adenopathy, exudate, headache, and fever only (Ship, 1965).

Herpangina is a papular, vesicular, or ulcerative eruption on the anterior tonsillar pillars, tonsils, soft palate, and pharyngeal mucosa associated with a febrile illness in the summer or fall. Children and adolescents are more commonly affected than adults. Although the syndrome was well described in the 1920s, it was 30 years later before the role of Coxsackie A viruses was proved. Since that time, advances in tissue culture have encouraged further study, showing that Coxsackie B and certain ECHO viruses may produce the same picture. The syndrome is now regarded as a nonspecific manifestation of enterovirus infection which must be differentiated from herpetic gingivostomatitis (Cherry and Jahn, 1965). The latter occurs year around and usually is preceded by a more severe prodrome. Since herpes simplex is easily cultured and can be demonstrated by a Tzanck smear, differentiation is frequently possible. Cases of concurrent Coxsackie and herpetic infections have been reported, however, in which the exact etiology of ulcerations is uncertain (Forman and Cherry, 1968).

Varicella as previously described commonly presents a vesicular enanthem. The vesicles rupture, leaving punctate, red-rimmed, usually asymptomatic ulcerations. The total clinical picture is usually unmistakable and confusion with herpetic gingivostomatitis or herpangina is unlikely. Likewise, herpes zoster is frequently easily differentiated due to its unilateral dermatomal distribution and typical grouped configuration. Glossopharyngeal ganglion distribution produces pain in the ear and pharynx, with unilateral soft palate vesiculo-ulcerative lesions and an auricular eruption. A puzzling presentation may occur with vagal ganglia disease in which partial paralysis of the larynx and pharynx and cardiac and epigastric distress may or may not be associated with vesicles on the base of the tongue, epiglottis, and arytenoids. Varicella-zoster lesions are Tzanck positive, as are those of herpes simplex. Although rare in the United States, smallpox is a common viral exanthem which also presents an enanthem. Vesiculo-ulcerative lesions are abundant in the palate, pharynx, and larynx.

A common disease which is rarely reported to cause an enanthem or exanthem is acute epidemic parotitis. In several serologically confirmed cases, one or a few tiny mucosal vesicles formed then ruptured on the buccal mucosa and anterior tonsillar pillars (Cherry and Jahn, 1966). As mentioned in the differential diagnosis of measles exanthem, rubella may present a nonspecific petechial eruption on the soft palate. These lesions may slightly precede or may accompany the exanthem and are known as Forchheimer's spots (Kibrick, 1964).

The main nonviral mucous membrane lesion that may be confused with viral enanthems is aphthous stomatitis. Young women seem to have a higher incidence of these lesions, which may be precipitated by trauma, stress, chemical irritants, or, in older women, hormonal changes. The clinical lesion consists of painful, single or multiple, oral erosions with a gray base surrounded by a thin erythematous ring. Frequently, generalized edema of oral mucous membranes or the tongue is seen. Lesions may be found on the buccal and labial mucosa, buccal and lingual sulci, soft palate, pharynx, larynx, gingiva, head of the penis, or in the vagina or on the labia. Healing occurs in 10 to 14 days but may be delayed for five weeks or more. The deep lesions of periadenitis aphthae sometimes scar. Histologically, a moderate lymphocytic infiltrate first appears near epithelial ductal orifices of minor salivary glands, then becomes a mixed cell infiltrate as ulceration occurs. Lymphocytes again predominate in several days as healing begins, and after several weeks numerous plasma cells can be found.

A skin test with an extract of streptococci has been reported positive in 30 reported patients with clinical aphthous stomatitis, but only 2 of 10 controls manifested a delayed hypersensitivity response. Pleomorphic streptococci were found histologically in 95 per cent of affected individuals but in only 40 to 47 per cent of control populations.

Palliative therapy is possible with tetracycline suspension gargles q.i.d. They promote more rapid healing, but resistance may develop in two to two and one-half years, correlating with in vitro streptococcal sensitivities. Locally applied corticosteroid preparations are reported to accelerate healing, and local cauterization frequently relieves discomfort. No effective preventive therapy has been found (Graykowski et al., 1966).

Streptococcal pharyngitis is associated with approximately a 75 per cent incidence of palatal petechiae, but 25 per cent of sore throat controls without evidence of streptococci also had these lesions (Dyment et al., 1968). Similar lesions have been reported in infectious mononucleosis, secondary lues, and even after smoking tobacco.

Large oral ulcerations with gray bases, appearing as giant aphthae, may represent Behçet's syndrome involving oral mucosa, external genitalia, and the uveal tract, or any one of these locations at a particular time. Histologically, this disease is characterized by an obliterative vasculitis with secondary ulceration which may be widespread at times, affecting the musculoskeletal, respiratory, and central nervous system (Monacelli and Nazzaro, 1966). The painful erosions of pemphigus and occasionally benign mucous membrane pemphigoid, bullous pemphigoid, and familial benign chronic pemphigus are rarely a serious differential problem. Likewise, lichen planus, erythema multiforme, and systemic lupus erythematosus present characteristic clinical pictures. The diphtheritic membrane should also be mentioned but, again, it is characteristic in appearance and rare in the United States.

Reiter's disease may include small superficial mucosal ulcerations, or 0.2- to 2-cm. grayish papules which often coalesce into plaques with a surrounding reddened, granular mucosa (Hamner and Graykowski, 1964). The accompanying triad of urethritis, arthritis, and uveitis usually clearly establishes the diagnosis.

See Table 12–3 for a differential diagnosis of enanthems.

RICKETTSIAL DISEASES
(Zdrodovskii and Golinevich, 1960)

Rickettsiae are small pleomorphic bacteria which take the form of short rods or cocci, existing singly, in pairs, in short chains, or in filaments. They are obligate intracellular parasites, often living symbiotically with arthropods, frequently passing to new generations of these hosts transovarially. When transmitted to an unnatural host such as man, they may produce disease. Some rickettsiae, such as those of the typhus group, grow in cellular cytoplasm, while those of the spotted fever group frequently infect the nuclei.

A characteristic of the genus is a predilection for old tissue cultures in which metabolic activity is waning. This may account to some extent for the increased virulence of the organisms in debilitated or older patients. Likewise, rickettsial growth is enhanced at cooler temperatures. Chick embryo cultures incubated at 32° C. are more productive than those held at 40° C. This may explain the occasional gangrenous changes in cooler, often acral areas of the human body, namely, those of the toes, fingers, nose, earlobes, scrotum, and vulva. Both aging and cooler tissues have in common a slowing of cellular metabolism which predisposes to parasitic infestation. Similarly, cellular metabolic inhibitors such as cyanide stimulate rick-

TABLE 12–3 A DIFFERENTIAL DIAGNOSIS OF ENANTHEMS

Viral Enanthems Disease	Etiology	Intra-oral Location of Lesion	Associated Cutaneous Lesions	Morbidity of Enanthem	Duration of Enanthem	Diagnostic Aids
Herpes simplex stomatitis Primary	Herpesvirus hominis	Generalized, extensive, often includes gingival vesicles or ulcerations	Occasionally perioral vesicles	Moderate to severe	10–14 days	Tzanck preparation, electron microscopy for herpesvirus, viral cultures
Recurrent	Herpesvirus hominis	Lips, occasionally soft palate or tonsillar region vesicles or ulcerations	Often vesicles occur adjacent to the vermilion border	Moderate to severe	3–10 days	Same as for primary herpes simplex stomatitis
Varicella	Varicella-zoster virus	Diffusely scattered vesicles or ulcerations	Centripetal vesicles	Moderate	7–10 days	Tzanck preparation, electron microscopy for V-Z virus. Viral cultures
Herpes zoster	Varicella-zoster virus	Unilateral and dermatomal vesicles or ulcerations	Often involves cutaneous surface innervated by the effected nerve (e.g., Ramsay Hunt syndrome)	Severe pain	Usually 2–3 weeks	Tzanck preparation, electron microscopy for V-Z virus. Viral cultures
Herpangina	Coxsackie and ECHO viruses	Papular, vesicular, or ulcerative lesions on the tonsils, tonsillar pillars, soft palate, and pharyngeal mucosa	Occasionally an exanthem	Mild to moderate	1–7 days	Community epidemiologic experience; summer, fall season; systemic symptoms; acute and convalescent sera; viral cultures
Hand, foot, and mouth syndrome	Coxsackie A5, A10, A16, B1, and B3	A few diffusely scattered vesicles or ulcerations	Tender, oval, gray vesicles with an erythematous rim on palms, soles, or buttocks	Mild to moderate	1–6 days	Same as for herpangina
Measles	Paramyxovirus	Koplik's spots (blue-white dots adjacent to the second molars) later diffusely spread over the buccal mucosa on an erythematous background	Classic morbilliform exanthem	Moderate	3–6 days (classic for only 1 or 2 days just prior to exanthem)	Mucosal biopsy shows multinucleate giant cells; electron microscopy of mucosal biopsy demonstrates myxovirus tubules; above all however, clinical course
Rubella	Paramyxovirus	Forchheimer's spots (punctate petechiae) on the soft palate	Classic rubelliform exanthem may be present	Mild	2–3 days of the late prodrome–early exanthem phase	Acute and convalescent serology and the clinical course
Epidemic parotitis (mumps)	Paramyxovirus	Rarely tiny vesicles or ulcerations on the anterior tonsillar pillars or buccal mucosa, ductal injections, swelling, and ulceration	Classic parotid swelling	Mild	1–3 days	Clinical course, acute and convalescent sera
Smallpox	Pox virus	Diffusely scattered vesicles and ulcerations	Classic centrifugal vesicles	Moderate	3–10 days	Electron microscopy for poxvirus, viral culture, clinical disease
Colorado tick fever	Arborvirus	Hard palate petechiae	Nonspecific exanthem	Mild	Inadequate data	Complement-fixation serology, history of tick exposure, clinical course

(Table 12–3 continued on opposite page)

Aphthous ulcers	Pleomorphic streptococci	Single or multiple ulcerations with a gray base and erythematous hole on buccal and labial mucosa and sulci; soft palate, pharynx, larynx, gingiva	Penile and vaginal ulcers	Moderate to severe	10–14 days	Skin test with streptococcal extract, clinical response to tetracycline mouth washes
"Strepthroat"	Streptococcus	Palatal petechiae	Occasionally scarlet fever	Moderate to severe	7–10 days	Throat culture, ASO titer
Mononucleosis	Unknown	Palatal petechiae	Toxic erythemas and urticarial exanthems	Mild to moderate	2 days	Heterophile agglutination
Secondary lues	Treponema pallidum	Palatal petechiae, white mucous plaques on a red base, bald patches on the tongue	Macular or papular exanthem generalized including palms, soles, scalp	Mild	1–6 weeks	Serology, such as VDRL, Hinton, FTA-ABS, TPI, biopsy, or proper dark-field examination
Meningococcemia	Neisseria meningitidis	Palatal petechiae, diffusely scattered or exudative pharyngitis	Diffusely scattered septic emboli and rarely disseminate intravascular coagulation (DIC)	Mild	1–2 days	Clinical signs and symptoms; bacterial culture of CSF, blood, pharynx; Gram stain of cutaneous lesions and CSF
Diphtheria	Corynebacterium diphtheriae	Membranous pharyngitis	Occasional ecthyma at the site of inoculation or superficial tender membranous dermatitis. The lesions may be anesthetic at times	Severe	7–14 days	Clinical signs and symptoms. Shick test, pharyngeal and wound smears and cultures
Moniliasis	Candida albicans	Scattered or diffuse easily removable white membranous stomatitis	Erosions in moist flexor creases	Mild to moderate	Days to years	KOH microscopic examination, culture
Rickettsial infections Rocky Mountain spotted fever	Rickettsia rickettsii	Palatal petechiae	Generalized hemorrhagic papules progressing centripetally	Mild	14–21 days	Weil-Felix OX-2 and OX-19, complement fixation after 11 days
Epidemic typhus	R. prowazekii	Rarely, palatal petechiae	Centrally distributed hemorrhagic macules	Mild	12–14 days	Weil-Felix OX-19 and complement fixation positive in 10 to 12 days
Miscellaneous dermatoses – bullous erythema multiforme, pemphigus, benign mucous membrane pemphigoid, bullous pemphigoid, Behçet's syndrome, lichen planus, lupus erythematosus, Reiter's disease, smoker's palatal petechiae						

ettsial growth, as do nutritional deficiencies (for example, of riboflavin). Certain dyes which increase cellular oxidative metabolism inhibit infection.

Pathologically, the organisms invade endothelial cells and smooth muscle cells surrounding capillaries and small blood vessels. As bacteria multiply, the vessel lumens become occluded and may rupture, leaving purpuric vasculitic lesions in the skin, brain, heart, and other organs. Strains such as Macchiavello's and Nocht's have proved useful in routine laboratory work, and Romanovsky's method with Giemsa's solution, although laborious, is excellent for showing internal structure of rickettsiae.

Clinical diagnosis remains the most important aspect of rickettsial treatment. The diseases respond well if appropriate therapy is instituted early—within the first week of infection. This is usually before serologic tests are helpful. Often, the exanthem appears just in time to aid early diagnosis if it is characterized and followed carefully in its evolution. Therapy of choice is either chloramphenicol or tetracycline group drugs, each at a dose of 2 to 3 gm. a day after initial loading doses. Some authors prefer tetracyclines since chloramphenicol may induce a fatal pancytopenia. Response to treatment occurs in one to two days, represented by a halt of the disease process in the stage at which treatment was instituted. Therapy should continue three to five days beyond defervescence to avoid relapse. If treatment was started after the sixth day of illness, immunity develops normally and relapse does not occur. To ensure against relapse, cases treated early may be given a short second course of antibiotic six days after original therapy has been discontinued. In dealing with rickettsial infections, it is important to realize that sulfonamides consistently enhance the disease process!

Serologic aspects of rickettsial diagnosis are summarized in Table 12–4. Cultured procedures using embryonated eggs are not discussed, as these provide a great danger of infection to laboratory personnel and are uneconomic or impractical in most clinical situations.

Comparisons of clinical findings and serologic tests for rickettsial diseases are also summarized in Table 12–4 in an attempt to make differentiation of often similar and confusing disease patterns somewhat easier.

EPIDEMIC TYPHUS

Epidemic typhus is transmitted principally by body lice and occasionally by head lice. The causative organism is *R. prowazekii*. The lice may become infected at any stage of their development by feeding on a person with typhus during the period of fever; the organisms multiply in the gut and are found in large numbers in the louse feces. The lice eventually die because of obstruction of the gut. As the skin of a pediculous victim becomes contaminated with this infected fecal material, the rickettsiae enter through the many abrasions which are ordinarily present.

The infection becomes manifest in one to two weeks after inoculation of the skin and is ordinarily characterized by a rather abrupt onset with mild prodromal symptoms. The onset is characterized by headache, chills, generalized pain, and sometimes marked weakness and insomnia. The fever and headache increase, and the rash appears in from four to seven days. It is macular and somewhat variable, with ill-defined discrete lesions 0.5 cm. or less in size. The lesions are first seen on the trunk and then spread to the rest of the body, with the exception of the face, palms and soles. There is conjunctival injection and photophobia. The eruption increases in intensity, becoming red or purple, and the lesions can no longer be obliterated by pressure. Frank hemorrhagic changes in the lesions are a serious prognostic sign.

The systemic findings in untreated cases are those of overwhelming toxicity. Pulse irregularities indicate myocardial damage, and there may be hypotension. The patient is very weak and often stuporous or even comatose. Psychic disturbances such as delirium and hallucinations are characteristic.

An initial leukopenia is noted and there is no eosinophilia. The spleen is often palpable. As the infection progresses, anemia develops, and there may be evidence of nephritis. A fatal outcome occurs with hemorrhagic tendencies in the skin lesions, cyanosis, profound coma, increas-

TABLE 12–4 SEROLOGIC ASPECTS OF RICKETTSIAL DIAGNOSIS

Disease	Species	Vector	Reservoir	Distribution and Season
I. Spotted fever				
A. Rickettsialpox	*Rickettsia akari*	Mites (Allodermanyssus)	Domestic rodents (rats, mice) and mites	Recognized in urban areas of the U.S.A. and U.S.S.R.; usually summer epidemics
B. Rocky Mountain spotted fever	*R. rickettsii*	Ticks (Amblyomma, Dermacentor, Ornithodoros, Rhipicephalus)	Ticks (transovarially), small rodents, possibly dogs	Western and northern United States, Cape Cod and eastern seaboard states, Canada, Mexico, Brazil, Colombia; usually a summer illness
C. Rickettsial fevers				
1. *R. conorii*	1. Dog tick (Rhipicephalus)	1. Dogs, rodents, ticks	Maritime districts of Europe, Africa, Mediterranean basin, Portugal, Spain, southern France, Italy, Roumania, Greece, Morocco, Algeria, Tunisia, Egypt, Black Sea basin, Turkey, Crimea, Caspian basin, Kenya, India, Asia, Australia; usually a summer illness
2. North Queensland tick typhus	2. *R. australis*	2. Tick (Ixodes)	2. Rodents, ticks	
3. North Asian tickborne rickettsioses	3. *R. sibericus*	3. Tick (Dermacentor and Haemaphysalis)	3. Rodents, ticks	
II. Typhus group				
A. Epidemic typhus	*R. prowazekii*	Body louse (pediculosis corporis and pediculosis capitis)	Infected humans, either with a primary attack or Brill's disease	Potentially worldwide. It is most prevalent in the Balkans, Asia, North Africa, Middle East, Mexico, and Andean areas of South America. Crowding and poor hygiene in impoverished areas in cold weather lead to winter and spring epidemics
B. Brill-Zinsser disease	*R. prowazekii*	None	The rickettsiae reside in the individual in a latent state following recovery from a primary infection	Worldwide with no seasonal predilection
C. Endemic typhus	*R. mooseri*	Rat flea (Xenopsylla cheopis)	Rats	Worldwide; in the U.S.A. sporadic cases occur in the Gulf and South Atlantic seaboard states, usually in summer months

(Table 12–4 continued on the following page.)

TABLE 12-4 SEROLOGIC ASPECTS OF RICKETTSIAL DIAGNOSIS (Continued)

Disease	Species	Vector	Reservoir	Distribution and Season
D. Scrub typhus	R. tsutsugamushi	Larval red mites (Trombididae) and rat fleas	Rodents, Trombididae mites	The disease occurs in sharply delimited ecologic habitats of eastern and southeastern Asia, northern Australia, India, and the adjacent islands. Areas of Japan are involved especially during river flooding, with consequent movements of parasitized rodents
III. Q fever	R. burnetii	Airborne	Ticks, sheep, goats, cattle	Worldwide; endemic in California, primarily affecting veterinarians, dairy workers, and farmers, with occasional epidemics in diagnostic laboratories, stockyards, meat-packing plants, and wool-processing factories

Inoculation	Incubation	Presenting Signs and Symptoms	Cutaneous Signs	Systemic Signs and Symptoms
Mite bite; a firm red papule forms one week prior to the fever, vesiculates, crusts, then heals in three weeks with a small pigmented scar	7–10 days	Lymphadenitis occurs in the region of inoculation. In about one week a fever develops with morning remissions, accompanied by headache, myalgia, rigors, and sweats	In two to three days a generalized macular, even papular eruption occurs, sometimes involving palms and soles. The lesions are 2 to 10 mm. in diameter, and often *vesiculate* in one to two days but are in a single stage of development. Crusts form and fall in 7 to 10 days. Occasionally only pinhead size diffuse vesicles are present	The regional adenitis is followed by fever, rigors, sweats (for one week), headache, myalgia, the exanthem, a leukopenia of 2500 to 5000 per cubic mm., and rarely by splenomegaly
Rickettsialpox				
Rocky Mountain spotted fever Tick bite (no eschar forms) Inoculation of crushed tick particles when excoriating Laboratory infection is common	3–12 days (average 7 days)	There is an abrupt onset of high fever, chills, headache, myalgia, arthralgia, nausea, and vomiting. Photophobia and epistaxis may occur	Blanchable 2- to 6-mm. macules appear over the wrists, forearms, and ankles at two to six days, involve the palms and soles, then progress *centripetally* in 24 hours to trunk, scalp, and face. Lesions often evolve into nonblanchable papules with petechial hemorrhage in three days and may coalesce and slough over bony prominences. The Rumpel-Leede test is positive. Gangrenous lesions may occur on the scrotum or vulvae (almost pathognomonic) or on fingers, toes, nose, or earlobes	A diffuse vasculitis occurs which may include photophobia, meningoencephalitis, and coma, or seizures, tachycardia, hypotension, azotemia, hepatosplenomegaly, myositis, and neuritis

(Table continued on opposite page)

Mediterranean fever A tick bite which leaves an eschar ("tache noir"); one or several lesions	1. 5–7 days 2. 7–10 days 3. 2–7 days	One or several reddish, indurated, centrally crusted papules are usually present at the onset of the two-day fever course and are accompanied by lymphadenopathy and a headache	One or several reddish, indurated, centrally crusted papules may occur on the body. In three to four days a morbiliform eruption appears on the forearms and trunk, then generalizes *centrifugally*, often involving the palms and soles. Inoculation in the conjunctiva results in a conjunctivitis and chemosis. The exanthem may become petechial, with petechiae on the palate. Occasionally a furry tongue may be present	Headaches, bradycardia, lymphadenitis, occasionally splenomegaly and constipation characterize the illness
Epidemic typhus Excoriation inoculates dried louse feces containing rickettsiae. No inoculation site is identifiable	5–23 days; usually 10–12 days.	There may be a two- to three-day prodrome of headache and malaise or direct onset of the high, usually unremitting, fever with rigors. An exanthem appears in five to six days	A central macular erythematous eruption frequently begins in three to six days near the axillae, spreading to the trunk and later to the extremities. It rarely involves the face, palms, or soles. Lesions often become petechial, resolving over 12 to 14 days and occasionally include palatal petechiae. *Papules are not present.* Gangrene of toes, nose, fingers, earlobes, scrotum, and vulvae occurs in severe cases	The disease is characterized by an initially high fever for 9 to 11 days which remits a spiking pattern over one to three days. The exanthem appears in about three days. The sympathetic nervous system is affected in the first week, the medullary centers in the second week, and the medulla and cerebrum predominate in the third week. A moderate leukocytosis and splenomegaly are common. Albuminuria is common but azotemia may be the first herald of a severe course. Bradycardia and cardiovascular collapse may prove fatal
Brill-Zinsser disease No reinoculation is necessary, as the disease represents reactivation of a latent infection	Years	There is a gradual onset of moderate fever with malaise and chills	Scattered areas of a morbilliform eruption may appear	A mild course similar to epidemic typhus occurs.
Endemic typhus Excoriation inoculates infective rat flea excrement	6–14 days	A gradual onset of malaise, headache, nausea, and vomiting is followed in several days by a moderate fever. Sudden onset occurs and may mimic a mild case of epidemic typhus	In five to seven days 2- to 5-mm. macules or small papules appear on the trunk and lower limbs. The face is involved in 18 per cent, the palms in 50 per cent, and the soles in 16 per cent of cases. Petechiae rarely develop, and the eruption fades in 6 to 10 days	The illness is similar to a mild course of epidemic typhus. The fever lyses in 10 to 14 days, often fluctuating as it breaks

(Table 12–4 continued on the following page.)

TABLE 12–4 SEROLOGIC ASPECTS OF RICKETTSIAL DIAGNOSIS (*Continued*)

Inoculation	Incubation	Presenting Signs and Symptoms	Cutaneous Signs	Systemic Signs and Symptoms
Scrub typhus A mite bite on a protected area of skin forms a painless crusted ulcer which lasts three weeks	6–21 days; usually 10–12 days	Malaise, headache, dizziness and anorexia are followed in one to three days by a rigor and sudden onset of a spiking moderate to severe fever. Often a painless crusted mite bite is found	A painless crusted ulcer with an erythematous halo usually appears at the site of inoculation accompanied by regional lymphadenitis during the first week of the disease. In six to seven days a diffuse macular, sometimes papular, exanthem appears on the anterior trunk, then spreads to the back and extremities. The face, palms, and soles are rarely involved. Lesions remain blanchable, do not evolve into petechiae, and resolve in three to seven days	A spiking moderate to high fever lasting two to three weeks is accompanied by headache and cerebral symptoms which may include delirium and neuropsychiatric disorders. Conjunctival hyperemia and an exanthem are characteristic. Pneumonitis and splenomegaly frequently occur. The leukocyte count initially falls then returns to normal a week later. Cardiac arrhythmias, cardiovascular collapse, and renal and hepatic dysfunction are uncommon. Cerebrovascular and gastrointestinal thromboses may occur
Q fever Pneumonic via aerosols Oral via infected milk	2–3 weeks	The disease presents with a rigor and is characterized by a two- to three-day rise in a spiking moderate fever with severe headaches, myalgia, nausea, and vomiting	None	A spiking moderate to high fever lasting two weeks is accompanied by severe headaches, myalgia, anorexia, and pharyngitis. Retro-orbital "sore eyes" are common, as are a relative bradycardia and occasionally hepatosplenomegaly. A dry cough with slight amounts of blood-tinged frothy sputum occurs and is mild compared with the striking roentgenographic picture

Course	Laboratory Tests				Prophylaxis	Differential Diagnosis
	Weil-Felix			Complement Fixation		
	OX-2	OX-19	OXK			
Rickettsialpox The disease is mild, with complete spontaneous recovery in three weeks. Fatalities are rare.	Negative	Negative	Negative	53 per cent are positive in 6 to 10 days; 92 per cent are positive by 21 to 30 days	Rodent extermination Residual miticides	1. Chickenpox Rocky Mountain spotted fever Coxsackie A9 exanthem Smallpox
Rocky Mountain spotted fever The disease is severe, lasting 14 to 21 days with a 25 per cent mortality rate if untreated	Positive between the tenth and fifteenth day	Positive between the tenth and fifteenth day	Occasionally positive at low titers	Positive by 10 days and lasts 6 to 8 years	Tick avoidance Killed rickettsia vaccine repeated yearly attenuates the disease	Meningococcemia Measles Murine typhus Brill's disease Enteroviral exanthem Typhoid fever Henoch-Schoenlein purpura Secondary syphilis Mononucleosis with

		...valescence	...valescence			Differential Diagnosis
...treated	Negative			(about 1:2... 1:160) and become positive on the eleventh day of the disease		...urine typhus / Brill's disease / Enteroviral exanthems / Drug eruption / Henoch-Schoenlein purpura / Secondary syphilis / Meningococcemia
Epidemic typhus — The disease is often severe in patients over 40 years of age. Mortality rates for untreated cases have ranged from 6 to 40 per cent	Negative	Positive at 10 days	Negative	19 S globulin titers become positive at 12 to 18 days at dilutions of less than 1:100	Improved personal hygiene. Insecticide delousing of the population. Immunization reduces the mortality rate	Murine typhus / Relapsing fever / Smallpox / Malaria / Typhoid fever / Measles / Yellow fever / Meningococcemia / Viral exanthems / Drug eruption
Brill-Zinsser disease — The mild febrile disease lasts five to eight days and is rarely fatal	Negative	Titers of 1:200 or less may appear in seven to eight days	Negative	7S globulins, indicative of recurrent infection, appear in six to eight days. Titers may exceed 1:1000	Prevention of epidemic typhus	Measles / Viral exanthems / Endemic typhus
Endemic typhus — The mild febrile disease lasts 10 to 14 days and is rarely fatal except in the aged	Negative	Positive at 1:200 or greater dilutions at 13 to 19 days	Negative	Positive at one week in diagnostic titers	Flea control by use of residual insecticides. Rodent control after flea control has been instituted.	Rocky Mountain spotted fever / Epidemic typhus / Brill's disease / Scrub typhus / Viral exanthems / Drug eruption
Scrub typhus — The disease lasts two to three weeks and varies in severity with the locality in which it is contracted. Mortality rates range from less than 1 per cent in the Pescadores Islands near New Guinea to 30 per cent in areas of Japan	Negative	Negative	Positive in 14 to 21 days in 50 per cent of cases	Unreliable unless local strain antigen is used	Mite avoidance. Clearing land then spraying with residual insecticides lowers rates of infection	Measles / Other Rickettsial diseases / Typhoid fever / Dengue fever / Leptospirosis / Malaria / Infectious hepatitis with exanthem / Drug eruption / Viral exanthems
Q fever — The disease lasts about two weeks and is rarely fatal	Negative	Negative	Negative	Positive in 10 to 20 days	Immunization of exposed populations. Pasteurization of milk. Strict animal pen hygiene. Control of infected animals	Influenza / Atypical pneumonia / Typhoid / Hepatitis / Leptospirosis / Meningitis / Sand fly fever / Dengue fever / Malaria / Rickettsial diseases / Psittacosis-lymphogranuloma-like diseases / Coccidioidomycosis

ing evidence of impairment of renal function, hypotension, and pneumonia. There are many other less common findings. The disease is not easy to diagnose in its early phases, and the eruption is by no means characteristic.

Prevention

If louse infestations are prevented, epidemic typhus cannot occur. A vaccine derived from the growth of organisms on the chick embryo yolk sac is effective; though it may not prevent the disease completely, it ameliorates it greatly.

Treatment

The broad-spectrum antibiotics should be given in large doses. Treatment early in the course is important, and an initial large "loading" dose is advisable. In suggestive acute febrile illnesses in regions where typhus might conceivably be expected, it is obvious that such therapy might justifiably be given before the diagnosis of typhus is established beyond doubt.

Serologic Tests

The agglutination test using Proteus OX19 has been widely used. It becomes significantly positive within five to eight days after the onset of the infection, and continues to rise for the next week. A complement-fixation test using rickettsiae obtained from infected yolk sac suspensions is also useful, though not always available, and is specific for the epidemic disease. Other tests are of interest to laboratory workers, including precipitin tests, toxin-antitoxin reactions, and neutralization tests.

BRILL'S DISEASE

Brill's disease, first noted in New York City, has also been encountered in other populous areas and probably represents a recrudescence of epidemic typhus in a patient in whom the infection is latent. In the majority of cases it is not characterized by any cutaneous lesions, and its severity is less than that of the initial infection of epidemic typhus. There seems to be some question as to its incidence, but it must be rare and probably will disappear entirely as epidemic typhus becomes controlled on a worldwide basis.

MURINE TYPHUS

This form of typhus has been distinguished from epidemic typhus only since World War I. It derives from animal reservoirs in rats, mice, and squirrels and may be spread by rat lice, fleas, and body lice.

It is not likely that an inexperienced observer could differentiate this disease from epidemic typhus, but the eruption differs in that it occasionally involves the palms, soles, and face, which is not true in epidemic typhus. The causative organism is *R. mooseri*, and the incubation period is similar to that of epidemic typhus. The onset is less abrupt, the symptoms are in general less severe, and the disease ordinarily persists for not more than two weeks. The eruption is first entirely due to vasodilatation, consisting of macular or papular lesions which tend to be somewhat larger than those of epidemic typhus, up to 1 cm. It rarely becomes hemorrhagic. Evidence of involvement of the nervous system, myocardium, or kidneys is much less common than in epidemic typhus.

The Weil-Felix test with Proteus OX19 becomes positive within three to six days after the onset of the disease, and complement-fixation or agglutination tests with washed antigen are useful in arriving at the correct diagnosis. The broad-spectrum antibiotics are effective. The disease may be controlled by the elimination of rats, and the use of DDT.

TRENCH FEVER

Trench fever, caused by *R. quintana*, was extraordinarily common in the louse-infested troops in Europe during World War I. It occurred chiefly among German troops in World War II. The disease seems entirely confined to central Europe and the Balkans.

On the basis of the published reports, not personal experience, it would appear that some three-quarters of the patients have a roseolar eruption of the trunk which appears at the onset of fever and persists for only a day or two. The incubation period is variable and may be as long as two months. The onset is abrupt, with the usual symptoms of a fairly severe systemic infection. In isolated instances, it may be impossible to differentiate the disease from other short-term infections of viral or bacterial origin. There are no laboratory methods which are of aid in making a diagnosis; the Weil-Felix agglutination test is negative. The spread of the disease can be controlled by louse disinfestation. Presumably the broad-spectrum antibiotics are indicated in treatment, but their effectiveness has not been determined.

SPOTTED FEVER (Rocky Mountain Spotted Fever)*

Rocky Mountain spotted fever is an endemic febrile disease caused by *R. rickettsii* which is of much interest and importance to physicians practicing in North and South America. It is well known to the laity as a medical risk encountered during the tick season, and there are few physicians in the United States who have not been called frantically by a patient who has sustained a tick bite. Prior to the availability of broad-spectrum antibiotics, the disease had, with certain strains of rickettsiae, an extremely high mortality in adults and a somewhat lower though very significant lethal effect in children.

Spotted fever is spread by ticks of various types: the wood tick, dog tick, Lone Star tick, and so forth. It is maintained in nature in rabbits and small rodents, but large domestic animals are not susceptible. If the tick is infected, it remains so throughout its life. It is of practical importance that little danger is attendant upon the bite of a tick if it is removed within an hour or two. The infection is apparently reactivated and its virulence increased after the tick has had a blood meal, and this requires six or more hours.

The incubation period of spotted fever is from two days to a week with virulent infections and somewhat longer with milder ones. After the usual prodromata of infection, the disease has an abrupt onset with chills, generalized pains, and marked prostration. The conjunctiva are involved and there may be photophobia, along with flushing of the face, occasional nose bleeds, and gastrointestinal symptoms. The fever reaches its height rapidly and may be very high, persisting for two or three weeks. Neurologic involvement is prominent in severe infections, with convulsions, disorientation, evidence of meningeal irritation, and loss of sphincter control. The typical eruption occurs between the third and seventh days, first about the wrists and ankles, then becoming generalized, with involvement of the palms and soles. As with other rickettsial infections, the lesions may be obliterated by pressure at their onset, but not as the eruption increases in intensity. The development of purpura is characteristic of spotted fever. With certain strains, the sequelae may be severe, with particular reference to those of the nervous system, and the mortality may be as high as 80 per cent in adults.

The disease may be difficult to distinguish from murine typhus, though the geographic origin will be helpful. Laboratory procedures are useful; with the Weil-Felix test, equivalent titers are obtained with Proteus OX19 and with OX2, and specific agglutination and complement-fixation tests may be performed with washed suspensions of the organism.

The disease may apparently be interrupted at any time in its course by treatment with the broad-spectrum antibiotics. The best method of prevention is to avoid being bitten by ticks. Repellent dusting powders and lotions are only moderately effective in this regard, and most individuals refuse to use them routinely. Clothing which is snug at the ankles, sleeves, and neckline probably furnishes the best protection, but this is impractical during the usual warm weather of the tick season in North America. Inspection and prompt removal of ticks after exposure, particularly in children, is well worthwhile, be-

---

*It is of interest that Howard Taylor Ricketts transmitted the human disease to experimental animals and described the responsible organism. He died in 1910 of a rickettsial infection (epidemic typhus). The name of this group of organisms is a fitting memorial to this outstanding martyr to the advancement of science.

cause of the unlikelihood that the rickett-siae will be transmitted until the tick has had a blood meal. Every woodsman has his favorite method of removing ticks. The insect should not be crushed between the fingers in removal. Touching the end of it with a match-head which has just been extinguished will sometimes cause the tick to loosen its grip on the skin. Tweezers or paper may be used to grasp the blood-filled bulbous insect. If portions of the insect's head remain in the skin, there may be some local reaction. Ticks may easily escape detection in the scalp, and children, especially, should be inspected carefully after exposure.

Various geographically localized forms of typhus are transmitted by ticks, includ-ing African tick typhus, North Queensland tick typhus, Russian tick typhus, and Indian tick bite fever.

RICKETTSIALPOX

This rickettsial infection is of consider-able interest because it may be confused with chickenpox and possibly has a fairly wide distribution in the eastern United States, although it was recognized as a separate disease only during the past dec-ade. An initial lesion is ordinarily detect-

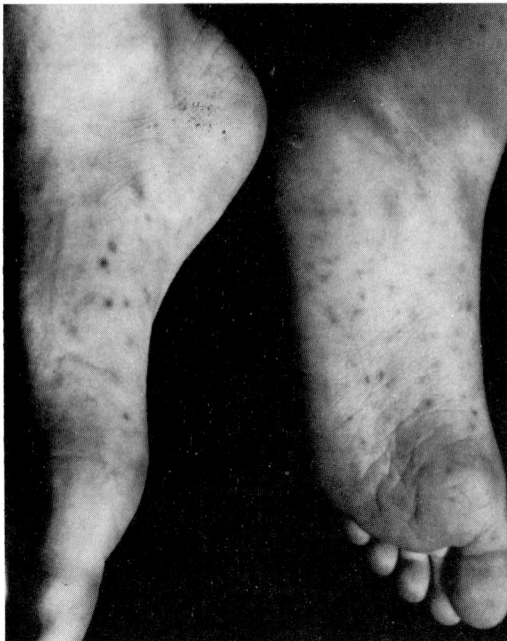

Figure 12–15   Rocky Mountain spotted fever.

able where a mite, *Allodermanyssus san-guineus,* has bitten the patient. This mite may be found on the ceilings and walls of overheated quarters, and the house mouse is a temporary animal reservoir. Within about ten days after the bite, a papule forms, then becomes vesicular, and de-velops into a lesion 1 or 2 cm. in diameter which to some extent resembles a vaccina-tion take. There may be considerable ten-der regional adenopathy. Within a few days after the appearance of the initial lesion, evidence of systemic infection de-velops, with chills, fever, prostration and severe frontal headache. The fever may persist for up to ten days and then grad-ually falls. With the onset of fever or a few days later, a generalized eruption may oc-cur consisting of individual erythematous papules which then become vesicular at the summit and is surrounded by a zone of erythema. These lesions are smaller than the primary lesions. The course is, in gen-eral, relatively mild, and the rickettsial infection is suppressed by broad-spectrum antibiotic therapy. The Weil-Felix test is negative in this disease.

SCRUB TYPHUS
(Tsutsugamuchi Disease)

Scrub typhus, a rickettsial disease en-countered in Australia and Asia, assumed considerable importance during World War II. It is transmitted through mites of the chigger mite family. A primary lesion appears at the site of the bite, followed in a week or so by a generalized maculopap-ular eruption and constitutional symptoms similar to the other rickettsial infections.

REFERENCES

Ackerman, A. B., and Suringa, D. W. R.: Multinucle-ate epidermal cells in measles. Arch. Dermatol. *103*:180, 1971.

Almeida, J. D., Howatson, A. F., and Williams, M. G.: Electron microscope study of human warts; sites of virus production and nature of the inclusion bodies. J. Invest. Dermatol. 38:337, 1962.

Alpert, E., Isselbacher, K. J., and Sheer, P. H.: The pathogenesis of arthritis associated with viral hepa-titis. N. Engl. J. Med. 285:185, 1971.

Aronson, S. B., and Moore, T. E.: Anti-viral proper-ties of idoxuridine during steroid treatment of herpes stromal keratitis. Ann. N.Y. Acad. Sci. *173*: 96, 1970.

Artenstein, M. S., and Demis, D. J.: Recent advances

in the diagnosis and treatment of viral diseases of the skin. N. Engl. J. Med. 270:1101, 1964.

Ashton, H., Frenk, E., and Stevenson, C. J.: Herpes simplex virus infections and iodoxuridine. Br. J. Dermatol. 84:496, 1971.

Attal, C., and Mozziconacci, P.: Measles: Clinical features. In Debre, R., and Celers, J., (eds.): Clinical Virology. Philadelphia, W. B. Saunders Co., 1970, pp. 320–335.

Attal, C., and Mozziconacci, P.: Varicella-herpes zoster infections. In Debre, R., and Celers, J., (eds.): Clinical Virology. Philadelphia, W. B. Saunders Co., 1970, pp. 389–401.

Barker, L. P.: Rickettsialpox. J.A.M.A. 141:1119, 1949.

Bayer, W. L., Sherman, F. E., Michaels, R. H., et al.: Purpura in congenital and acquired rubella. N. Engl. J. Med. 273:1362, 1965.

Beare, J. M., and Rook, A.: The Newborn. Textbook of Dermatology. Vol. 1. Philadelphia, F. A. Davis Co., 1968, pp. 112–137.

Bedson, H. S.: The laboratory investigation of vesicular skin rashes. Publ. Health, (London) 85:171–174, 1971.

Blank, H., Davis, C., and Collins, C.: Electron microscopy for the diagnosis of cutaneous viral infections. Br. J. Dermatol. 83:69, 1970.

Blank, H., Eaglestein, W. H., and Goldfaden, G. L.: Zoster, a recrudescence of V-Z virus infection. Postgrad. Med. J. 46:653, 1970.

Blattner, R. J.: Exanthema subitum. In Nelson, W. E., Vaughan, V. C., and McKay, R. J., (eds.): Textbook of Pediatrics. Philadelphia, W. B. Saunders Co., 1969.

Burgoon, C. F., and Burgoon, J. S.: The natural history of herpes zoster. J.A.M.A. 164:265, 1957.

Carton, C. A., and Kilbourne, E. D.: Activation of latent herpes simplex by trigeminal sensory root section. N. Engl. J. Med. 246:172, 1952.

Cherry, J. D.: Newer viral exanthem. Adv. Pediatr. 16:233, 1969.

Cherry, J. D., and Jahn, C. L.: Herpangina: the etiologic spectrum. Pediatrics 36:632, 1965.

Cherry, J. D., and Jahn, C. L.: Exanthem and enanthem associated with mumps virus infection. Arch. Environ. Health 12:518, 1966.

Cherry, J. D., Lerner, A. M., Klein, J. O., et al.: Coxsackie B5 infections with exanthems. Pediatrics, 31:455, 1963.

Cherry, J. D., Lerner, A. M., Klein, J. O., et al.: ECHO 11 virus infections associated with exanthems. Pediatrics 32:509, 1963.

Cooper, L. Z., and Krugman, S.: The rubella problem. Disease-a-Month, February, 1969.

Davis, C. M., and Musil, G.: Milker's nodule. A clinical and electromicroscopic report. Arch. Dermatol. 101:305, 1970.

Debre, R., and Celers, J., (eds.): Clinical Virology. Philadelphia, W. B. Saunders Co., 1970.

Denny-Brown, D., Adams, R. D., and Fitzgerald, P. J.: Pathologic features of herpes zoster. Arch. Neurol. Psych. 51:216, 1944.

Dirk, W. R., Suringa, M. D., Lincoln, J., et al.: Role of measles virus in skin lesions and Koplik's spots. N. Engl. J. Med. 283:1139, 1970.

Duhamel, G.: Infectious mononucleosis. In Debre, R., and Celers, J., (eds.): Clinical Virology. Philadelphia, W. B. Saunders Co., 1970, pp. 676–687.

Dukes, C.: On the confusion of two different diseases under the name of rubella. Lancet 2:89, 1900.

Dyment, P. G., Klink, L. B., and Jackson, D. W.:

Hoarseness and palatal petechiae as clues in identifying streptococcal throat infections. Pediatrics 41:821, 1968.

Eaglestein, W. H., Katz, R., and Brown, J. A.: The effects of early corticosteroid therapy on the skin eruption and pain of herpes zoster. J.A.M.A. 211:1681, 1970.

Editorial: Infectious mononucleosis and acute leukemia. Lancet 1:688, 1971.

Editorial: Medical News: Photoinactivation may find use against herpesvirus. J.A.M.A. 217:270, 1971.

Epstein, E.: Triamcinolone-procaine in the treatment of zoster and postzoster neuralgia. Calif. Med. 115:6, 1971.

Epstein, W. L., and Kligman, A. M.: Treatment of warts with cantharidin. Arch. Dermatol. 77:508, 1958.

Evins, S., Leavell, V. W., and Phillips, I. A.: Intranuclear inclusions in Milker's nodules. Arch. Dermatol. 103:91, 1971.

Fields, B. N., and Hawkins, K.: Human infection with the virus of vesicular stomatitis during an epizootic. N. Engl. J. Med. 277:988, 1967.

Foley, F. D., Greenawald, K. A., Nash, G., et al.: Herpesvirus infection in burned patients. N. Engl. J. Med. 282:652, 1970.

Forman, M. L., and Cherry, J. D.: Exanthems associated with uncommon viral syndromes. Pediatrics 41:873, 1968.

Foster, S. O., Brink, E. W., Hutchins, D. L., et al.: Human monkeypox. Bull. W.H.O. 46:569, 1972.

Fraumeni, J. F.: Infectious mononucleosis and acute leukemia. J.A.M.A. 215:1159, 1971.

Froeschle, J. E., Nahmias, A. J., Feorino, P. M., et al.: Hand, foot and mouth disease (Coxsackie A16) in Atlanta. Am. J. Dis. Child. 114:278, 1967.

Fulginiti, V. A., Eller, J. J., Downie, A. W., et al.: Altered reactivity to measles virus. J.A.M.A. 202:101, 1967.

German, L. J., McCracken, A. W., and Wilkie, K. McD.: Outbreak of febrile illness associated with ECHO virus type 5 in a maternity unit in Singapore. Br. Med. J. 1:742, 1968.

Gold, E.: Serologic and virus isolation studies of patients with varicella or herpes-zoster infection. N. Engl. J. Med. 274:181, 1966.

Gordon, J. E.: Control of Communicable Diseases in Man. 10th ed. New York, American Public Health Association, 1965.

Grant, J. C. B.: Grant's Atlas of Anatomy. Baltimore, Williams and Wilkins Co., 1962, p. 657.

Graykowski, E. A., Barile, M. F., Lee, W. B., et al.: Recurrent aphthous stomatitis. J.A.M.A. 196:637, 1966.

Hambrick, G. W., Cox, R. P., and Senior, J. R.: Primary herpes simplex infection of fingers of medical personnel. Arch. Dermatol. 85:583, 1962.

Hamner, J. E., and Graykowski, E.: Oral lesions compatible with Reiter's disease: A diagnostic problem. J. Am. Dent. Assoc. 69:560, 1964.

Herrmann, E. C., Person, D. A., and Smith, T. F.: Experience in laboratory diagnosis of enterovirus infections in routine medical practice. Mayo Clin. Proc. 47:577, 1972.

Heydenreich, J. S. S.: An outbreak of smallpox in an urban area. S. Afr. Med. J. 39:463, 1965.

Hirschman, S. Z.: Approaches to antiviral chemotherapy. Am. J. Med. 51:699, 1971.

Hope-Simpson, R. E.: The nature of herpes zoster: A long term study and a new hypothesis. Proc. R. Soc. Med. 58:1, 1965.

Horsfall, F. L., and Tamm, I.: Viral and Rickettsial Infections of Man. 4th ed. Philadelphia, J. B. Lippincott Co., 1965.

Jarratt, M., and Knox, J. M.: Photodynamic action: Theory and application. Progr. Dermatol. 8:1, 1974.

Jawetz, E., Melnick, J. L., and Adelberg, E. A.: Review of Medical Microbiology. 7th ed. Los Altos, Lange Medical Publications, 1966.

Johnson, W. T., and Helwig, E. B.: Cat scratch disease. Histopathologic changes in the skin. Arch. Dermatol. 100:148, 1969.

Kibrick, S.: Rubella and rubelliform rash. Bact. Rev. 28:452, 1964.

Lane, J. M., and Millar, J. D.: Routine childhood vaccination against small-pox reconsidered. N. Engl. J. Med. 281:1220, 1969.

Lane, J. M., Ruben, F. L., Neff, J. M., et al.: Complications of smallpox vaccination, 1968. N. Engl. J. Med. 281:1201, 1969.

Leavell, U. W., Jr., McNamara, M. J., Muelling, R., et al.: Orf. J.A.M.A. 203:657, 1968.

Lerner, A. M., Klein, J. O., Levin, H. S., et al.: Infections due to Coxsackie virus group A, type 9 in Boston, 1959, with special reference to exanthems and pneumonia. N. Engl. J. Med. 263:1265, 1960.

Lockskin, N. A., and Hurley, H.: Urticaria as a sign of viral hepatitis. Arch. Dermatol. 105:570, 1972.

London, I. D.: Buffered glutaraldehyde solution for warts. Arch. Dermatol. 104:96, 1971.

Lourie, B., Bingham, P., Evans, H. H., et al.: Human infection with monkeypox virus: Laboratory investigation of six cases in West Africa. Bull. W.H.O. 46:633, 1972.

Macrae, A. D., Field, A. M., McDonald, J. R., et al.: Laboratory differential diagnosis of vesicular skin rashes. Lancet 2:313, 1969.

Margileth, A. M.: Cat scratch disease: Nonbacterial regional lymphadenitis. Pediatrics 42:803, 1968.

McCarthy, J. T., and Hoagland, R. J.: Cutaneous manifestations of infectious mononucleosis. J.A.M.A. 187:193, 1964.

Meller, G. D., and Tindall, J. P.: Hand-foot-and-mouth disease. J.A.M.A. 203:107, 1968.

Meyer, J. S., Bauer, R. B., Rivera-Olmos, V. M., et al.: Herpes virus hominis encephalitis. Arch. Neurol. 23:438, 1970.

Miller, D. R., Hanshaw, J. B., O'Leary, D. S., et al.: Fatal disseminated herpes simplex virus infection and hemorrhage in the neonate. J. Pediatr. 76:409, 1970.

Monacelli, M., and Nazzaro, P.: Behçets Disease. Basel and New York, S. Karger, 1966.

Muller, S. A., and Herrman, E. C.: Association of stomatitis and paronychias due to herpes simplex. Arch. Dermatol. 101:396, 1970.

Muller, S. A., and Winkelmann, R. K.: Cutaneous nerve changes in zoster. J. Invest. Dermatol. 52:71, 1969.

Music, S. I., Find, E. M., and Togo, Y.: Zoster-like disease in the newborn due to herpes-simplex virus. N. Engl. J. Med. 284:24, 1971.

Nagington, J., Tee, G. H., and Smith, J. S.: Milker's nodule virus infections in Dorset and their similarities to orf. Nature 208:505, 1965.

Nahmias, A. J., Josey, W. E., and Naib, Z. M.: Infection with herpes virus hominis Types I and II. Progr. Dermatol. 2:7, 1969.

Nahmias, A. J., Josey, W. E., Naib, Z. M., et al.: Perinatal risk associated with maternal genital herpes simplex virus infection. Am. J. Obstet. Gynecol. 110:825, 1971.

Neimann, N., DeLavergne, E., and Olive, E.: Herpes. In Debre, R., and Celers, J., (eds.): Clinical Virology. Philadelphia, W. B. Saunders Co., 1970, pp. 457–474.

Netter, R.: Varicella-Zoster: Virological Features. In Debre, R., and Celers, J., (eds.): Clinical Virology. Philadelphia, W. B. Saunders Co., 1970, pp. 402–415.

Payne, F. E., Baublis, J. V., and Itaboshi, H. H.: Isolation of measles virus from cell cultures of brain from a patient with subacute sclerosing panencephalitis. N. Engl. J. Med. 281:585, 1969.

Penman, H. G.: Fatal infectious mononucleosis: a critical review. J. Clin. Pathol. 23:765, 1970.

Petrozzi, J. W.: Infectious mononucleosis manifesting as a palmar dermatitis. Arch. Dermatol. 104:207, 1971.

Prestia, A. E., and Lynfield, Y. L.: Scarlatiniform eruption in viral hepatitis. Arch. Dermatol. 101:352, 1970.

Rifkind, D.: The activation of varicella-zoster virus infections by immunosuppressive therapy. J. Lab. Clin. Med. 68:463, 1966.

Romiti, N.: The Gianotti-Crosti syndrome. Dermatol. J. Lat. Am. 2:41, 1967.

Rytel, M. W.: Currently available drugs for prophylaxis and therapy of viral infections. Drug Therapy 2:25, 1972.

St. Geme, J. W., Jr., Prince, J. T., Burke, B. A., et al.: Impaired cellular resistance to herpes simplex virus in Wiscott-Aldrich syndrome. N. Engl. J. Med. 273:229, 1965.

Schimpff, S., Serpick, A., Stoler, B., et al.: Varicella-zoster infection in patients with cancer. Ann. Intern. Med. 76:241, 1972.

Selling, B., and Kibrick, S.: Outbreak of herpes simplex among wrestlers (herpes gladiatorum). N. Engl. J. Med. 270:979, 1964.

Shelley, W. B.: Herpes simplex virus as a cause for erythema multiforme. J.A.M.A. 201:153, 1967.

Shapiro, L.: The numbered disease: First through sixth. J.A.M.A. 194:680, 1965.

Ship, I. I.: Viral and viral-like diseases of the mouth. Postgrad. Med. 38:499, 1965.

Shklar, G.: Oral reflections of infectious diseases. Postgrad. Med. 49:87, 147, 1971.

Sigel, N., and Larson, R.: Behçet's Syndrome. Arch. Intern. Med. 115:203, 1965.

Simon, H. J., and Sokoi, W.: Staphylococcal antagonism to penicillin G therapy of hemolytic streptococcal pharyngeal infection. Effect of oxacillin. Pediatrics 31:463, 1963.

Spruance, S. L., and Bailey, A.: Colorado tick fever. Arch. Intern. Med. 131:288, 1973.

Stevens, D. A., and Merigan, T. C.: Approaches to the control of viral infections in man. Rational Drug Therapy, 5:1, 1971.

Wellings, P. C., Awdry, P. N., Bors, F. H., et al.: Clinical evaluation of trifluorothymidine in the treatment of herpes simplex corneal ulcers. Am. J. Ophthalmol. 73:932, 1972.

Zdrodovskii, P. F., and Golinevich, H. M. (translated by B. Haigh): The Rickettsial Diseases. New York, Pergamon Press, 1960.

CHAPTER
13

SUPERFICIAL AND
DEEP MYCOTIC INFECTIONS

Donald L. Baxter

MISCELLANEOUS SUPERFICIAL FUNGAL INFECTIONS

TINEA VERSICOLOR

Tinea versicolor is an easily diagnosed, common, and relatively trivial disorder of noninflammatory nature. It is extremely chronic and usually symptomless. The complaints of patients are usually based on the cosmetic changes which it produces. The disease is noncontagious but is seen with greater frequency in laborers, athletes, servicemen, and other occupations where exposure to heat, humidity, grease, and dirt may be increased. Although common enough in all climates, it is seen most frequently in hot, humid tropical regions, where as many as 50 per cent of the population may be affected.

The typical lesions of tinea versicolor are multiple macular patches, of all sizes and shapes, varying in color from whitish to fawn-colored to brown. The nonpigmented variety have been designated as *achromia parasitica*, but there is no reason for a separate term for it. The qualifying term "versicolor" is apt, in consideration of the varying color of the lesions. The portions of the skin most frequently affected are the upper trunk, front and back. However, the lesions commonly extend on to the proximal portions of the extremities, to the lower abdomen, and sometimes to the neck and face. Scaling is not a marked feature, but scratching of the lesion invariably yields a fine branny scale which contains numerous organisms.

The lesions of tinea versicolor often become confluent, acquiring curious patterns. They may be visualized easily with the aid of a Wood's light, and this sometimes shows that the involvement is much more extensive than might be suspected from ordinary clinical inspection. The areas of involvement frequently show rather marked changes on exposure to sunlight. Some of the patches may become darker, while others, because of failure to tan, become more conspicuous by contrast. This latter occurrence is the feature of the disease which most frequently causes affected patients to seek medical advice.

Direct microscopic examination of scrapings reveals a combination of fungus elements which is diagnostic: (1) filaments having a tendency to break into short segments of various sizes, and (2) grapelike clusters of round cells which occasionally

bud. There is a resemblance of the grapelike clusters of round budding cells found in tinea versicolor to those shown by *Pityrosporum orbiculare*, a normal skin resident. This organism has been isolated on cultures from patients with the disease and its identity with *Malassezia furfur* established (Keddie and Shadomy, 1963). When cultures of *P. orbiculare* are inoculated onto the skin of patients receiving systemic corticosteroids, the disease may be reproduced (Burke, 1961). This finding suggests that the disease results from an

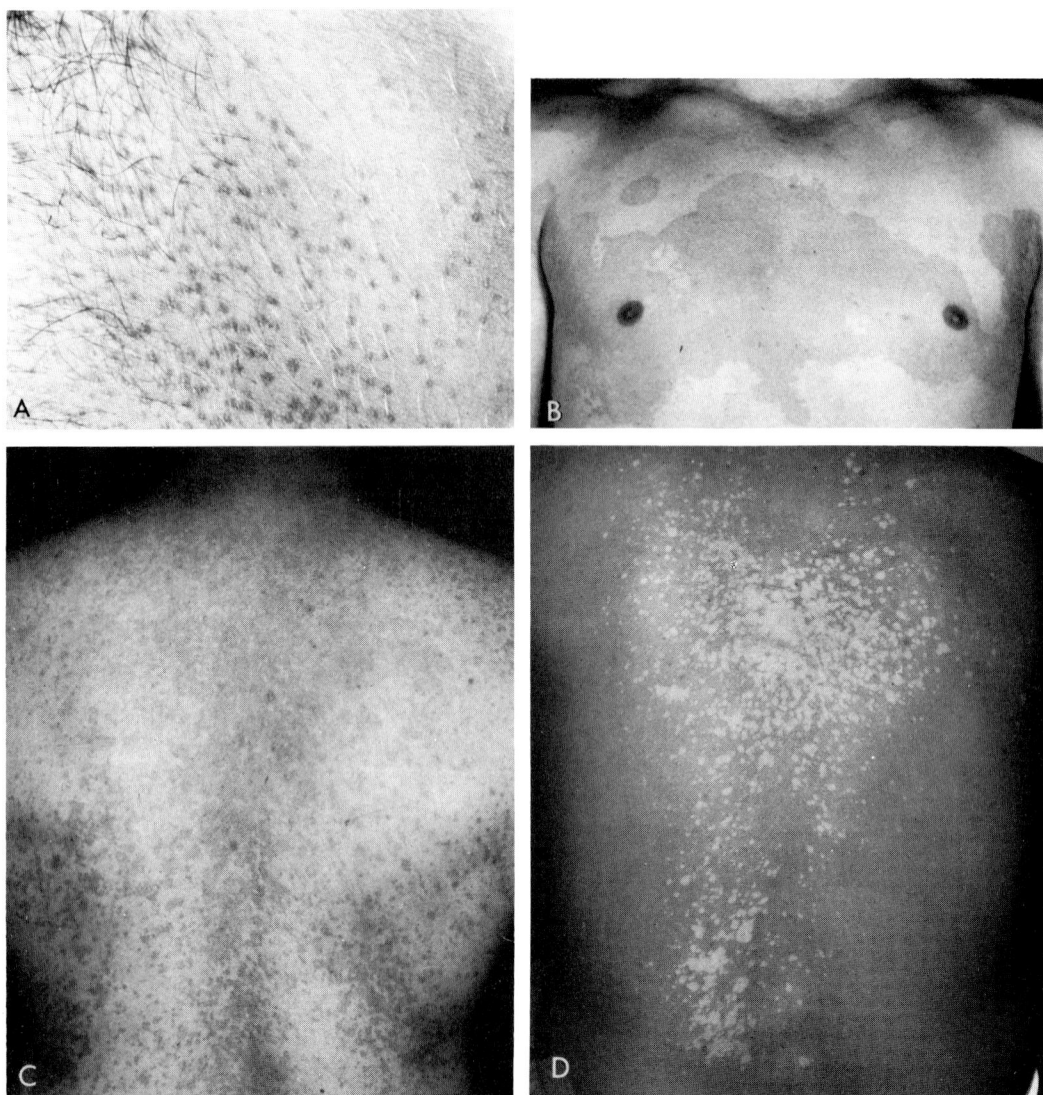

Figure 13–1 Tinea versicolor. *A*, Early lesions with hyperpigmented macules spreading from hair follicles. *B*, Extensive coalescent involvement. The darker areas are affected. Even wider distribution was demonstrable by Wood's light examination. *C*, Widespread macular scaling patches. *D*, Depigmentation at sites of lesions, contrasting sharply with surrounding tanned skin.

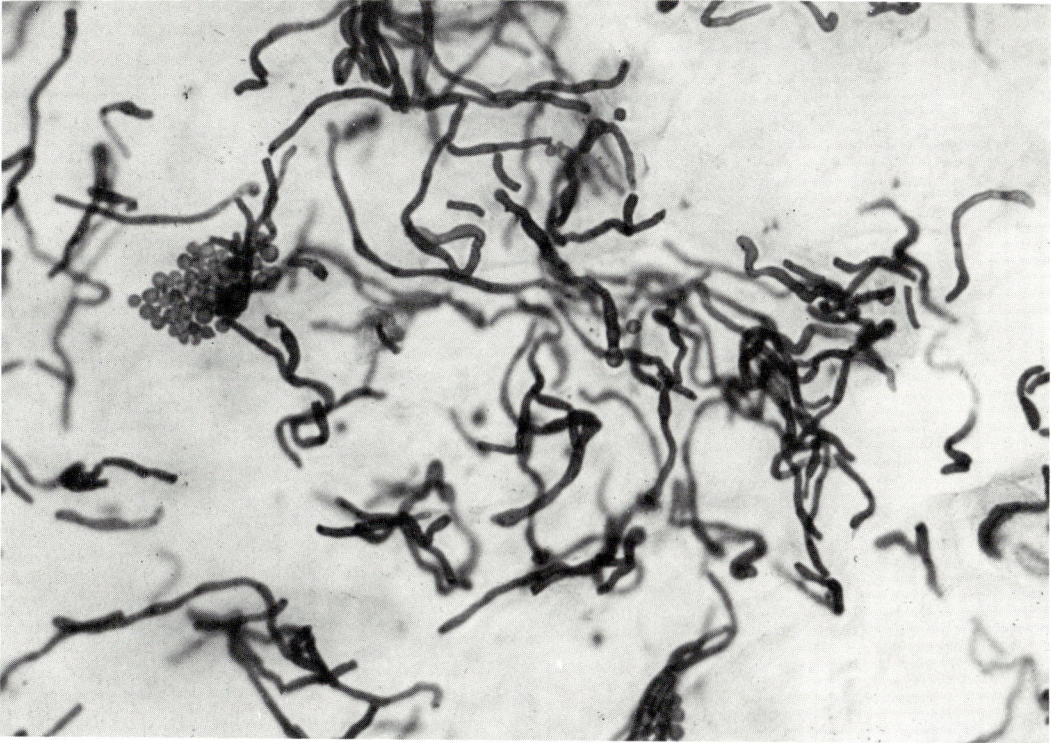

Figure 13–2 Hotchkiss-McManus stain of tinea versicolor fungi.

overgrowth of an organism in the normal flora to which there is no inflammatory response. Because of generic precedence, the correct name of the fungus causing tinea versicolor is *Pityrosporum furfur.*

Treatment and Prognosis

Tinea versicolor responds readily but temporarily to a considerable variety of topical medicaments. Almost any of the common fungicides are useful, including particularly the daily application of solutions or creams containing sodium thiosulfate, haloprogin, tolnaftate, or 9-aminoacridinium 4-hexylresorcinolate. These usually cause prompt disappearance of the patches; the rapidity of the response may be increased by cleansing with a suspension of selenium sulfide (Albright and Hitch, 1966) or thorough brush scrubbing with soap and water. In patients who already show a contrast between relatively depigmented and heavily tanned skin, the appearance will not, of course, be improved until the contrast is lessened by the passage of time. Recurrence is ordinarily the rule on cessation of topical treatment and patients should be advised to retreat individual lesions as they recur in order to avoid widespread involvement.

If the process is discovered in the course of a routine examination, and if the patient is not aware of it, it is best for the physician to say nothing. For most patients who note the "disease," reassurance as to its harmlessness is usually all that is necessary, though they should be informed of the possible contrast in pigmentation which may occur after exposure to sunlight. The disease is very chronic and long-standing, but sometimes disappears in middle to old age.

TINEA NIGRA

As the name indicates, this minor fungal infection is characterized by patches which are strikingly dark and which have been described as looking like spattered silver nitrate stains. The lesions occur on

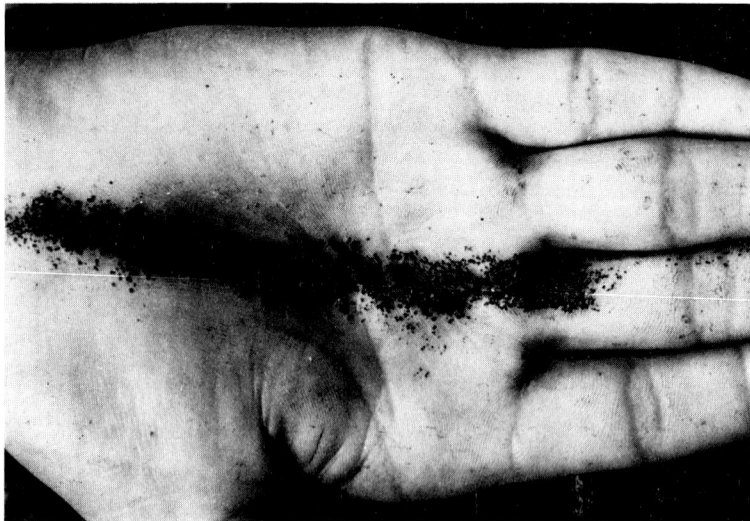

Figure 13–3   Tinea nigra. The resemblance to stains of silver nitrate is obvious.

the palms, sides of the fingers, the wrists and, very rarely, other areas of the skin. The disease is encountered in South America, principally in Brazil, though occasional cases have been reported from Cuba and the southern portions of the United States. The causative organism is *Cladosporium wernecki*. A similar, if not identical, fungus infection caused by *C. mansoni* has been reported in southeastern Asia. The process is very slightly contagious and is apparently acquired from exogenous sources in nature, a trivial injury sometimes marking its onset. There is no particular age or sex incidence. The clinical appearance is striking and almost pathognomonic; the diagnosis may be easily confirmed by the finding of brown to dark green branching filaments in scrapings. *C. wernecki* is easily cultured from scrapings inoculated onto Sabouraud's agar or medium containing cycloheximide. Topical treatment with Whitfield's ointment, tincture of iodine, or creams containing sulfur and salicylic acid produces rapid involution. Oral administration of griseofulvin is usually ineffective.

PIEDRA

Two entities have been described under this heading: piedra (black piedra), an affection of hairs of the scalp occurring principally in South America and certain tropical areas, and trichosporosis (white piedra), an uncommon condition of man and animals of worldwide distribution.

In piedra, small, hard, brown to black, adherent nodules are formed on the shafts of scalp hairs. Infection may be related to climate or communal factors and does not depend on age, sex, race, or occupation. The disease may be contagious and once established may spread to involve the entire scalp. The nodules are composed of the stromata of the ascomycetogenous fungus, *Piedraia hortae*. The microscopic appearance of the nodules is characteristic with masses of brown fungus cells about the hair shaft. Within these masses are hyaline loculi containing ovoid asci about 25 microns in length. Within each ascus there are two to eight single-celled, twisted ascospores packed in the form of a helix. Cultures are easily obtained on Sabouraud's agar or on medium containing cycloheximide and antibacterial antibiotics, but the culture is not as characteristic as the direct examination of nodules, since asci usually are not produced in cultures. If untreated, the disease may persist for years. Removal of the affected hair by clipping or shaving is usually curative. Recurrences are not uncommon if the patient resides in an endemic area.

Trichosporosis is characterized by soft, mucilaginous, white to light brown nodules which develop within and on hairs of the scalp, beard, mustache, and genital areas. The nodules may vary from microscopic to visible size and contain masses of thick-walled, rounded, yeast-like cells which are easily demonstrated on microscopic examination. *Trichosporon cutaneum* may be cultured on Sabouraud's agar, but unlike *P. hortae* this fungus usually is inhibited when inoculated onto medium containing cycloheximide. In the past, trichosporosis has been confused with piedra since *T. cutaneum* may also be recovered from patients with the latter condition. *T. cutaneum* is a common contaminant of skin, and the diagnosis of trichosporosis should not be made in the absence of the typical microscopic features on direct examination of nodules.

RINGWORM INFECTIONS

The diseases in this group, called the Tineas, are due to various species of dermatophytes. While it would be logical to describe the varied clinical manifestations of infection by these fungi according to the particular species concerned, the changes produced by the same fungus in different areas of the body frequently differ so greatly as to make a regional approach the most useful one.

RINGWORM OF THE SCALP

Tinea capitis is an important and widespread disease constituting a significant public health problem in many areas. Though it does not ordinarily produce much disability or even great discomfort, except in markedly inflammatory infections, it is cosmetically disfiguring, and the daily life of the affected patient is often greatly inconvenienced by regulations promulgated by school health authorities and immigration officials.

Tinea capitis is produced only by species of Microsporum and Trichophyton. Although various organisms may produce clinical manifestations which are indistinguishable, and clinical classification may be developed from the principal organisms concerned, this need not be complex. So much has been written about the disease as to make the subject highly confusing, and it has seemed best, in the following section, to err on the side of simplicity, at some risk of incompleteness of discussion.

The species concerned in tinea capitis are:

MICROSPORUM
(1) *M. audouini*—epidemic, urban tinea capitis (common).
(2) *M. canis*—sporadic, often contracted from domestic animals (moderately common).
(3) *M. gypseum*—highly inflammatory (very rare).
(4) *M. ferrugineum*—(rare in the United States, but endemic in Japan and adjacent areas).
(5) *M. distortum*—(very rare).
TRICHOPHYTON
Ectothrix
(1) *T. mentagrophytes*—inflammatory tinea capitis (common).
(2) *T. rubrum*—(very rare).

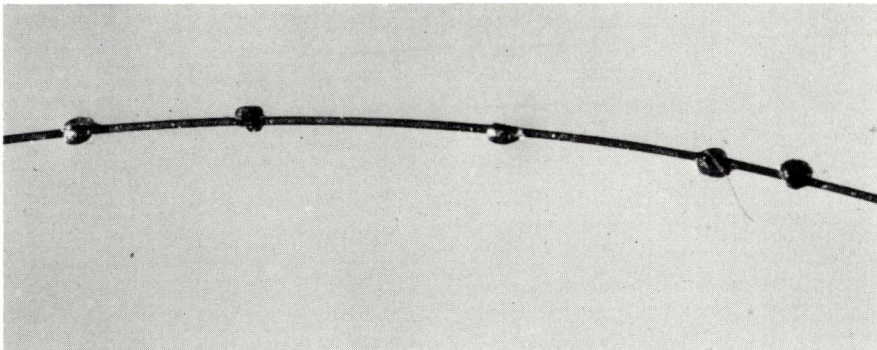

Figure 13-4 Piedra nodules on hair shaft.

Endothrix

(1) *T. tonsurans* – exceedingly chronic, often familial type, found principally in the southwestern United States.

(2) *T. violaceum* – cause of "black dot" ringworm (uncommon in the United States, but more frequent in eastern Europe and the Far East).

(3) *T. schoenleini* – cause of favus (rare in United States, relatively common in Eastern Europe).

Tinea Capitis Due to M. Audouini

Epidemiology

M. audouini produces the most common type of tinea capitis in the United States. It is primarily a disease of city children. Though the infection is easily transmitted, it would appear that a high proportion of children are resistant to it. In "epidemics" of the infection, it is rare to encounter it in over 5 per cent of the pediatric population. In a large city where the infection is endemic, less than 1 per cent of the children are infected, as a rule. Though the incidence is high in siblings of infected children, it is by no means uncommon for sibling contacts to escape. The infection is very rare in adults, and is likely to be of shorter duration than in children. It is commonest in children between the ages of three and eight.

The resistance to *M. audouini* infection shown by adults has been attributed to a higher content of fungistatic fatty acids in the sebum after puberty. This thesis is not completely proved but has earned wide support because it is logical and attractive. Sebum, whether obtained from a pre- or postpubertal subject, is fungistatic *in vitro*, and it is remarkable that the spores germinate so readily in this milieu *in vivo*. The forces which govern immunity to the infection are still poorly understood. The fungistatic potency of the sebum of children who remain uninfected despite deliberate exposure is not greater than that of children who acquire the disease. It is widely believed that the infection undergoes spontaneous remission at puberty, but this does not by any means occur

rapidly, and in long standing cases of tinea capitis, the rate of spontaneous cure at puberty is probably no more rapid than it is in younger children.

Transmission of the infection occurs most readily under conditions of crowding and poor hygiene, and it is therefore seen more frequently in children from families whose economic advantages are not great. This is by no means always true, however. Males are infected from 5 to 10 times more frequently than females, apparently because of the shortness of the hair and the ease with which the spores can reach the scalp. When female children become infected, the initial lesions are commonly noted where the scalp is exposed in the part line of the hair.

It has been demonstrated experimentally that minor trauma to the scalp is necessary to implant the spores sufficiently to germinate. Dropping of spores on the scalp surface without any trauma does not produce infection. Direct contact is the most important source of contagion. Contaminated barber's instruments may transmit the disease readily, since the spores are implanted in the scalp with associated minor trauma. Combs may also transmit the disease. Much has been made of the role of theater and auditorium seats in transmitting the infection, but it is believed that this has been exaggerated.

Diagnosis

Broken off hairs and partial alopecia are the cardinal signs of tinea capitis. The infected areas are round or oval, sometimes irregularly so, and often fuse to form gyrate patterns. It is uncommon to encounter ringworm of the scalp which is confined to a solitary patch; ordinarily at least two or three are present. It is also uncommon to see involvement of more than one-half of the total scalp surface. The individual patches are rarely larger than 6 to 8 cm. in diameter. The first patch is ordinarily the largest and is the last to disappear.

In the early phases of the ringworm infection, while the patch is enlarging, the features of the lesion are in all respects similar to ringworm infections of the glabrous skin. The border is "active" and slightly elevated, while the central area shows only scaling. The term "gray patch ringworm" describes the disorder admirably because the scaling is conspicuous and dense in most cases. Fungal filaments may be recovered in profusion from the active border of the lesion but are absent in the central area. When the patch reaches its maximum size, fungal filaments disappear. In some individuals, in addition to the distinct patches of partial alopecia, infection of a variable number of single hairs may be detected irregularly through the scalp. The infection is asymptomatic as a rule, though occasional patients complain of moderate itching.

The Wood's light is an essential diagnostic tool in tinea capitis. Hairs infected with *M. audouini* show a bright blue-green fluorescence. The Wood's light, which emits ultraviolet irradiation in the range of 3300 to 3600 Ångström units, is invaluable for the detection of the infection early in its course and for determining the extent of involvement. Similar fluorescence is exhibited in infections caused by *M. canis, M. ferrugineum,* and *M. distortum.* Other types of tinea capitis fail to fluoresce or do so only weakly.

Culture is necessary for species identification. Microscopic examination of infected hairs in potassium hydroxide shows an ectothrix arrangement of small spores (external spore sheath), but the appearance of *M. audouini* infections is identical with that of *M. canis, M. ferrugineum, M. distortum,* and some *M. gypseum* infections. While culture of the causative organism is useful and satisfying, it is by no means always essential to diagnosis, especially in areas where *M. audouini* is endemic and accounts for more than 95 per cent of all cases of tinea capitis.

Tinea capitis due to *M. audouini* is a highly refractory disease. It was formerly thought to undergo spontaneous involution rarely. In patients with widespread involvement of the scalp, spontaneous involution cannot be expected for very long periods, and the extent of involvement is apparently a measure of low resistance to the infection. In patients who develop only two or three patches, however, a higher degree of immunity would seem to be operative, and the outlook for spontaneous involution within a few months is better.

Tinea capitis due to *M. audouini* is characteristically noninflammatory at the outset (Graham et al., 1964), most cases remaining so throughout the course of the disease. However, inflammation may develop later in a variable percentage, reported as high as 30 per cent in some regions and as low as 5 per cent in others. The fully developed inflammatory change is a boggy tumefaction called a *kerion.* In infections in which inflammation is noted, it will ordinarily be seen initially throughout the involved sites, following which a nodular induration develops in one or more areas, becomes elevated, and produces a raised tender mass. Folliculopustules appear over the surface of the lesion, and these coalesce and rupture, with release of exudate. The hairs are spontaneously shed, and temporary baldness results. The appearance of the inflammatory change is such as to lead to an anticipation of permanent alopecia, but this is uncommon and usually is the sequel to severe secondary bacterial infection.

The onset of a kerion is associated with the development of allergic sensitization to the fungus, and the development of such a lesion is an almost certain indication of spontaneous cure. Kerions ordinarily heal slowly within a period of four to six weeks, or even longer, but this may be shortened by treatment with griseofulvin. Following resolution of a kerion, hair growth may not become apparent for from two to five months, but the eventual regrowth is almost invariably excellent.

Pathogenesis

The understanding of the course of *M. audouini* tinea capitis has been greatly advanced by studies in which humans have been inoculated experimentally (Kligman, 1952, 1955), permitting the collection of precise and detailed clinical and pathologic information during the entire course of the infection. These observations are variously applicable to other types of superficial ringworm infections, and may be summarized as follows:

The incubation period of the infection is brief; the spores which have lodged in the stratum corneum or in the hair follicles germinate within a few days and shortly produce a

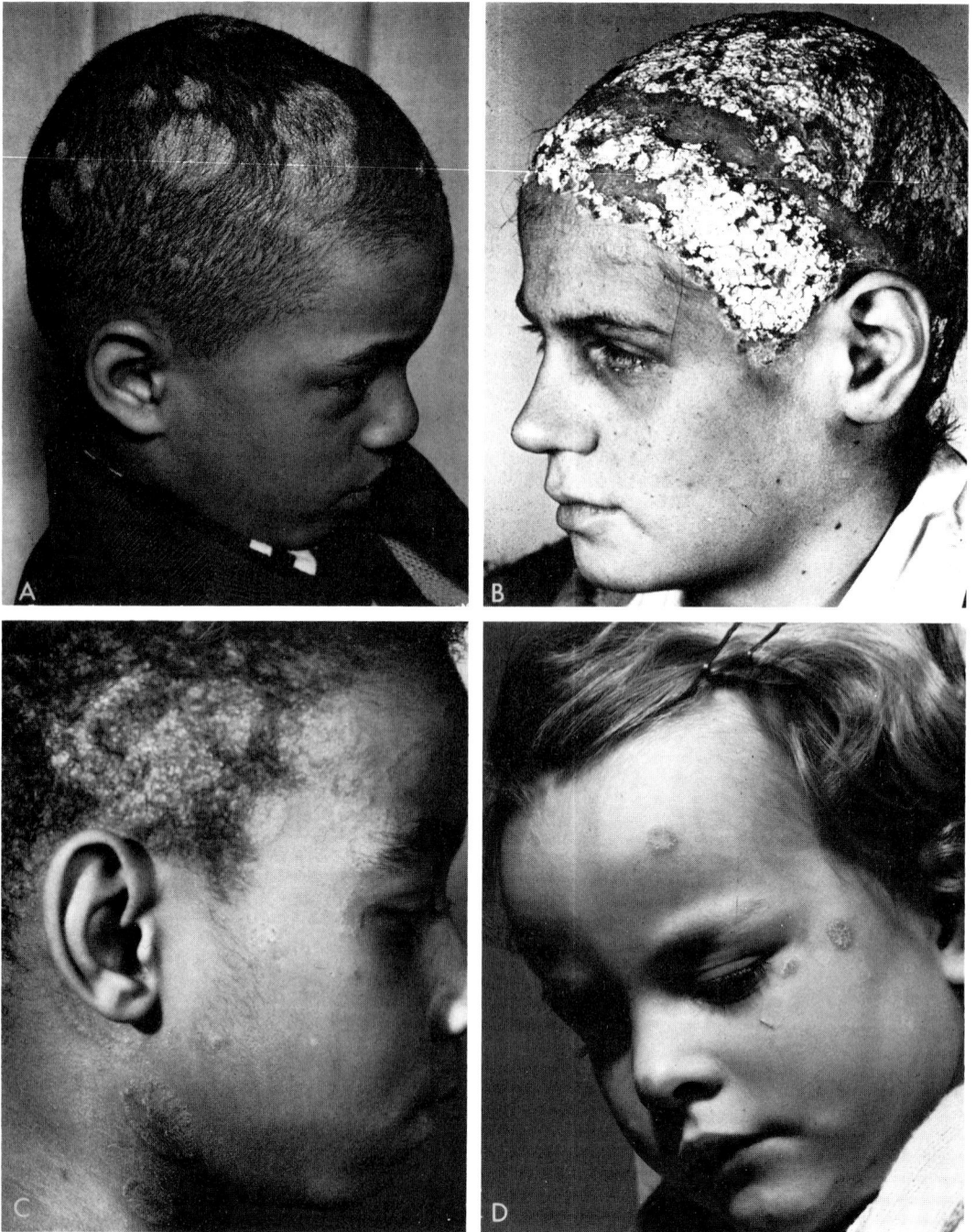

Figure 13–5   *A*, Characteristic widespread tinea capitis due to *M. audouini. B*, Favus. A rare disease in the Americas. *C*, Tinea capitis with circinate lesions on face and neck. *D*, Round scaling patches on glabrous skin in child with tinea capitis. Such lesions on nonhairy areas respond to treatment much more promptly than in the scalp.

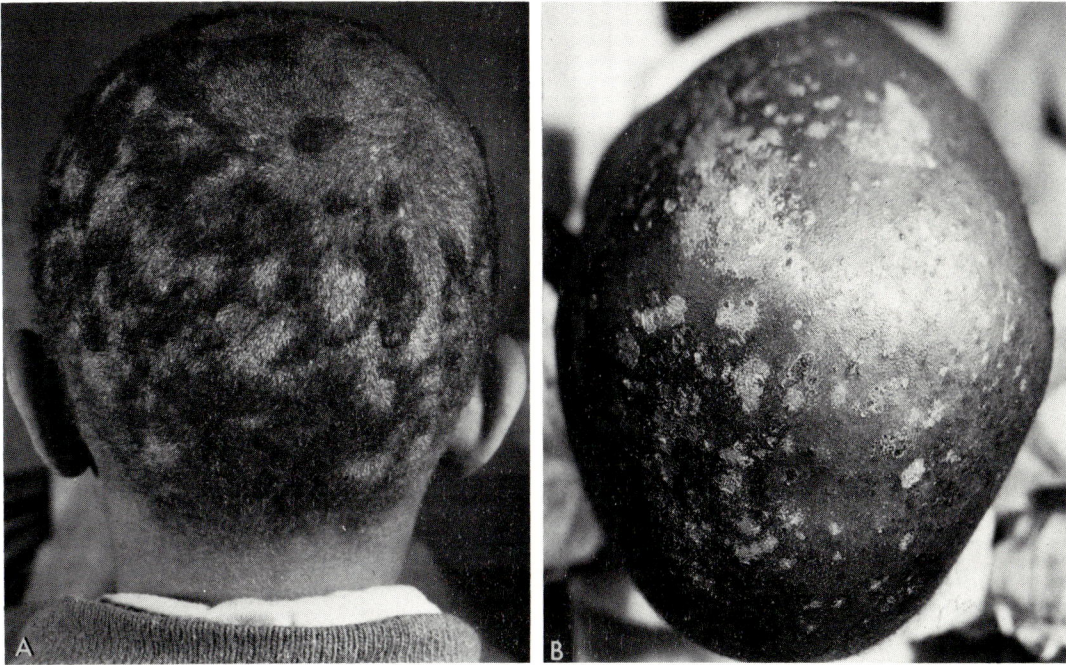

Figure 13–6 *A*, Widespread persistent *M. audouini* infection. *B*, Appearance after x-ray epilation. The white scales mark the sites of infection.

mass of fungal filaments in the follicular orifices. The filaments entwine the hair, not invading it initially, and grow down into the follicle on the hair surface. Invasion of the hair shaft occurs within six or seven days after inoculation, and fluorescence develops at this time. The fluorescent material, which may be extracted from the hair in boiling water, would seem to be a product of the growth of the fungus within the hair. The initial invasion of the hair shaft occurs at the midpoint of the intrafollicular portion and is not immediately visible on the surface.

During this period, fungal elements have been proliferating in the stratum corneum, and the infection has extended radially away from the point of inoculation, with invasion of more and more hair follicles. At the end of two weeks, the fungi have extended down along the hair follicle to their deepest and final position, and an external sheath of spores has been formed. Shortly thereafter, the rich growth of fungi within the hairs produces digestion and disorganization of the keratin, and the hairs begin to break off.

An understanding of this sequence of events has clinical application, because it indicates clearly that no evidence of tinea capitis may be expected until more than three weeks after inoculation, and the

signs of the infection may not be noted by parents until six weeks or more after inoculation. In some patients, particularly girls, tinea capitis of moderate extent may escape detection for several months.

Most but not all of the hairs in a patch of ringworm are infected. The club or resting hairs remain uninvolved, and apparently are not a suitable substrate for the growth of the parasite. An individual patch of tinea capitis rarely continues to enlarge for more than three months, after which time the surface infection regresses and the fungi disappear from the stratum corneum, leaving an infection which is entirely confined to the hairs. It is possible to determine whether or not an individual lesion is still spreading, either by finding hyphae in surface scrapings at the margin or by demonstrating a fluorescent band in normal hairs plucked from the periphery. If new lesions are to appear elsewhere in the scalp, they will ordinarily do so within three or four months after the initial inoculation. After this time the infection becomes stabilized, and no new lesions appear. The reason for the refractoriness of some portions of the scalp to infection is not known; it apparently is not related to an acquired immunity, because the original infection may persist for months or even years thereafter. After the infection becomes stabil-

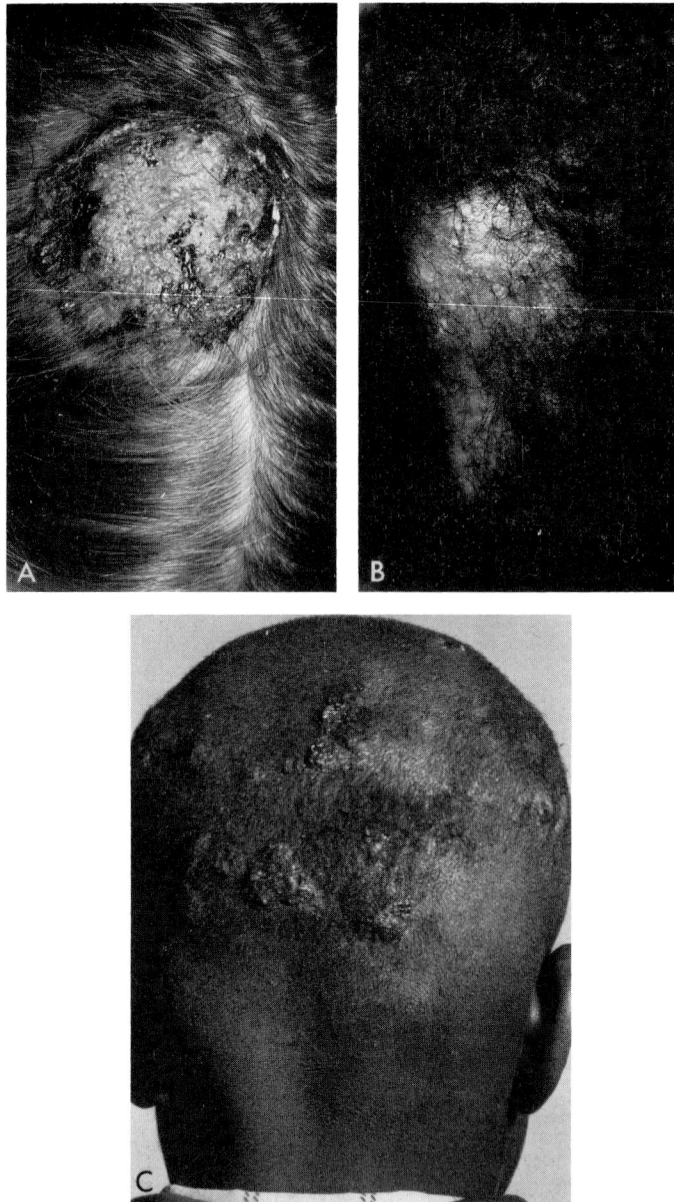

Figure 13–7 Inflammation and scarring in tinea capitis. *A,* Typical kerion. Bacterial infection is *not* responsible. *B,* Scarring and permanent alopecia after severe kerion. This sequel is uncommon. *C,* Moderate inflammation in scattered patches of *M. audouini* infection. This is a certain sign of imminent spontaneous cure.

ized, it may remain so in the individual hair for long periods, but in a small percentage of the hairs, the fluorescence is gradually lost and involution occurs, insofar as the particular hair is concerned.

One factor which will terminate the infection in an individual hair is well established. When an individual hair enters the resting stage of its life cycle, with formation of a club hair, the growth of *M. audouini* ceases, and the infection disappears. This biologic peculiarity probably does not hold for other types of tinea capitis, especially the endothrix trichophyton infections. Since scalp hairs grow from two to six years before entering a resting phase, this time range would appear to set an upper limit for the duration of infection by *M. audouini*. When the hair emerges from its resting phase, it cannot be reinfected. The noninfectibility of resting hairs is well shown by the short course of occasional *M. audouini* infections of the cilia of the eye, where the growing phase of the hair is only a few months long. On the glabrous skin, also, the short hairs ordinarily grow for only about six months and then rest for a similar period, and *M. audouini* infections in this area are therefore relatively brief. These biologic facts offer one explanation for the unique persistence of fungal infections of the scalp, in that more than 95 per cent of the hairs in this area are in a growing phase, and this phase persists for a very long time.

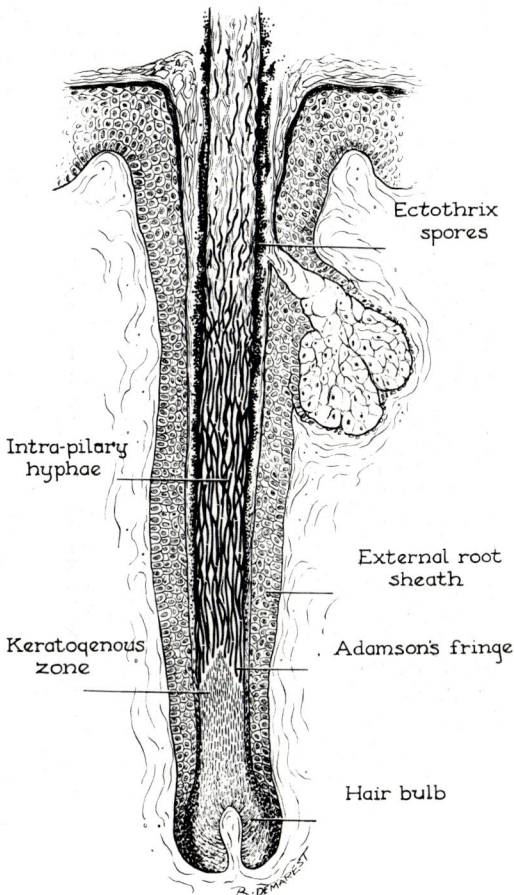

Figure 13–8 Diagrammatic representation of an *M. audouini* infected hair illustrating the main features of the host-parasite relationship characteristic of all types of tinea capitis. The fungal filaments do not extend into the bulb of the hair but terminate abruptly in contact with hair matrix cells which still retain their nuclei. Only the *fully* keratinized portion of the hair shaft is invaded.

A rather remarkable phenomenon is observed in relation to the growth of the fungal parasite within the hair. The fungal elements rapidly reach a lower level which corresponds to the upper limit of the keratogenous zone of the hair matrix, a point about 0.5 mm. above the papilla, where the cells, though almost completely keratinized, still retain their nuclei. This zone, and the hair bulb itself, is *never* invaded, well demonstrating that ringworm fungi are necrophilic and cannot proliferate in viable or semiviable tissue. In tinea capitis, each infected hair may be looked upon as a separate fungal colony, confined entirely to the dead portion of the hair. There the growth of the fungi downward and of the hair upward remains in perfect balance. Should the fungus fail to extend downward at the same rate as hair growth, it would be pushed outward and discarded. The living matrix of the hair remains completely uninvolved, and this explains why permanent hair loss is not noted in tinea capitis due to *M. audouini* except in unusual instances where intense inflammation intervenes. The site of the lower fungal growth down in the hair shaft is known as Adamson's fringe. In this area the fungus and the living host are pitted against each other in perfect antagonistic balance, an almost unique biologic phenomenon.

In addition to the growth of the fungi within the hair, the filaments close to the cuticle send out short external branches which break up into chains of cuboidal, thick-walled spores (arthrospores), forming the so-called ectothrix spore sheath. Each infected hair is therefore surrounded by innumerable spores, but these are dormant and not active cells. They have nothing to do with maintaining the infection in a particular hair, but serve to disseminate the disease.

Treatment

The oral administration of griseofulvin has revolutionized the treatment of tinea capitis (Blank and Roth, 1959; Blank et al., 1959). This antibiotic is incorporated in the hair as it is formed, providing a fungistatic barrier which upsets the delicate balance between downward invasion of the fungus and the outward growth of the hair. The diseased hair is cast off as a result of normal hair growth. Griseofulvin is generally administered in a dose of 20 to 40 mg. per kg. per day and is continued for six to eight weeks. Absorption of the drug is enhanced if it is given with meals. Somewhat less effective is a single oral dose of 8 to 12 gm. which may be repeated in one month if the infection persists.

Certain measures are probably worthwhile to carry out as adjunctives which may shorten the course for treatment with griseofulvin. These are as follows:

(1) *Clipping the hair short in boys*, for facilitating shampooing and the application of whatever topical agent may be used. In girls, close cutting of the hair is often traumatic psychologically to both the patient and the mother, and need not be insisted upon. It is probably best to shampoo the scalp twice weekly. There is no need for daily shampooing unless the lesions become inflammatory and oozing.

(2) *The application of a mild antifungal agent.* This may kill off some of the fungal elements on the surface and may decrease the dissemination of spores. A 1 per cent solution of tolnaftate or haloprogin may be applied twice daily or the area may be treated with preparations containing sulfur and salicylic acid.

X-RAY EPILATION. Although x-ray epilation is curative in almost 100 per cent of cases of tinea capitis, there is seldom, if any, indication for its use since the introduction of griseofulvin. It should be restricted for the rare patient who is unable to take griseofulvin because of drug intolerance or allergy.

TREATMENT OF INFLAMMATORY TINEA CAPITIS. As stated above, inflammatory ringworm infections regress spontaneously, with the exception of certain endothrix infections. In nearly all patients with inflammatory tinea capitis, resolution is more rapid if griseofulvin is started as soon as the diagnosis has been established. In such patients, it is important to keep the scalp clean, to promote drainage, and to prevent secondary bacterial infection. Daily shampooing or the application of warm soapy compresses may be helpful in this regard. There is no objection to the regular application of antibacterial ointment, though the value of this is uncertain in either preventing infection or curing it after it has occurred, because it is ordinarily well below the skin surface. In some patients, fever and cervical adenopathy may be noted, and this is ordinarily a justification for systemic antibacterial therapy. Occasional inspection of the skin surface to detect the development of "ids" is advisable, because these are seen more commonly in patients with kerion.

Rather marked inflammation may persist for a month or more, but it then ordinarily subsides gradually. While it is helpful to open small superficial pustular lesions, wide incision is not recommended. Deep extension of secondary bacterial infection should, however, be watched for. The prognosis for hair regrowth in kerion is excellent, even in the face of a rather alarming local inflammation. If, however, the hair has not shown evidence of regrowth within six months, it is fairly clear that the hair matrix has been destroyed, and nothing further can be done. Such areas are, however, ordinarily of limited extent, and may be obscured by proper combing.

PROPHYLAXIS AND CONTROL OF EPIDEMICS. The question as to whether infected children should be admitted to school while they are under treatment is an extremely difficult one. It is our belief that they should be admitted, since the risk of transmission is probably not too great, provided that antifungal agents are used regularly. Presumably, infected children should be restricted as to play and physical contact with other children, but any parent or teacher will agree that this is a hopeless injunction if it must be enforced for prolonged periods. Thorough shampooing of uninfected children after each haircutting may reduce the possibility of infection from barber shops.*

Contact between siblings in the home is even more difficult to prevent. While precautions to prevent common use of towels, combs, clothing, etc., can be carried out to some extent, a completely rigid regimen is impossible because the infected child must endure a general shrinkage of personality, both bodily and spiritually, until he occupies no space freely and has few human prerogatives. Under such circumstances, the physician and parents do the best they can, relying on the regular application of antifungal agents to the scalp and reasonable efforts to prevent gross cross-contamination.

---

*The only effective method of sterilizing hair clippers without damaging them is to place the head of the instrument in very hot petroleum oil for several minutes. Barbers, however, find this method too difficult for practical use.

Tinea Capitis Due to M. Canis

Tinea capitis due to this organism is more easily dealt with than *M. audouini* infections, because the course of the disease tends to be much shorter and there is greater likelihood of an inflammatory response. *M. canis* infections are indistinguishable from those due to *M. audouini* in terms of the clinical features, direct microscopic findings in the hair and fluorescence. Epidemics do not occur, except among small groups of persons who are intimately associated. The chief source of contagion is domestic animals, particularly kittens, hence the term "zoophilic" infection. The disease in an infected kitten may be inconspicuous and demonstrable only by examination by the Wood's light. *M. canis* infections occur sporadically in relation to the distribution of infected animals, and a history of animal contact is ordinarily obtainable. Widespread epidemics of the infection do not occur, apparently because it is too short-lived to maintain a large human reservoir for prolonged transmission from human to human. It has been suggested that the virulence of the organism deteriorates after several passages through humans, but there is no certain proof of this, and the theory seems improbable. The infection persists much longer in the cat than in man. In humans, children comprise the susceptible population, and adult infections are rare.

Zoophilic fungi are regarded as producing more highly inflammatory lesions in man than do anthropophilic fungi, but this is not always true. *M. canis* infections may remain noninflammatory throughout their course and be indistinguishable in all particulars from typical cases of *M. audouini* infection, save for the shorter duration. The disease regresses shortly after the onset of the inflammatory changes, but the brief duration of the infection cannot be attributed entirely to this characteristic. Even if inflammation does not supervene, cure ordinarily occurs spontaneously in from two to four months. In infections in which inflammation is present from the onset, the disease persists for only five to six weeks, and its contagiousness is low. Inflammation may occur at any time during the course. In patients in whom there is no inflammation whatever,

regression may not be noted in this period, but persistence for more than nine to twelve months is rare.

The differentiation of such infections from those due to *M. audouini* requires cultural identification of the organism. The treatment is essentially the same as for *M. audouini* infections, keeping in mind that spontaneous involution is much more likely to occur. In spite of the tendency for spontaneous involution, treatment with griseofulvin should be started as soon as the diagnosis has been established.

Tinea Capitis due to M. Gypseum

This infection is uncommon. When it occurs, intense inflammation and severe kerions are the rule. The organism is easily recoverable from soil, where it grows as saprophyte. When it grows in the human skin, spontaneous involution occurs uniformly, though two to three months may be required for the inflammation to subside completely, and hair loss in the involved area is a frequent sequel. On direct examination of the hairs, the appearance is similar to that seen in *M. canis* and *M. audouini* infections, but the Wood's light reveals no fluorescence. Definitive diagnosis requires culture. Treatment is entirely similar to that outlined for inflammatory *M. audouini* infections.

Tinea Capitis due to Trichophyton Mentagrophytes

Tinea capitis caused by this organism, which is invariably associated with inflammation and intense kerions, is rare. The causative organism, a zoophilic species, is the organism most commonly recovered from fungal infections of the feet, but it is important to recognize that foot strains are quite different, morphologically and physiologically, from those which incite inflammatory tinea capitis or infections of the skin and beard. Tinea capitis caused by this fungus is encountered principally in rural areas, in farmers who have been in contact with infected cattle, horses, dogs, and other species, some of them wild.

These animal strains are highly infective and virulent, incite inflammatory reactions in man, and are quite pathogenic for laboratory animals. The ordinary "athlete's foot" strains seem well adapted to the human skin, do not incite deep highly inflammatory reactions, and are not notably pathogenic for animals. In the rare instances of tinea capitis due to this species, the infection is evidently acquired from animal contacts and not as a result of extension from the feet of the patient or of other individuals. The medical history of the patient should include questioning regarding animal contacts. The kerions produced by this organism are not distinctive, resembling those caused by other ringworm species. Culture is required for definitive diagnosis, and the granular colonies are highly distinctive. Microscopic examination of hairs reveals an ectothrix arrangement, with rather large spores and chains outside the hair, as well as intrapilary filaments. There is no fluorescence on examination with the Wood's light. The preferred treatment is griseofulvin, as for kerion due to *M. audouini*.

Tinea Capitis due to T. Tonsurans

This disorder is highly prevalent in Mexico and the southwestern United States. In recent years there has been a significant increase in the incidence of this disease in urban areas in the more northern parts of the United States, especially among the Latin American population of New York and Philadelphia. It is characterized by extreme chronicity and by ready escape from detection, even in large medical centers.

Trichophyton tonsurans is anthropophilic, man being the only known reservoir of infection. Contagiousness is not great except under conditions of prolonged intimate contact. In families, however, most or all of the group acquire the infection. Responsible mycologists and dermatologists greatly fear the possibility of the disease becoming endemic in the U.S.A. Furthermore, adults are susceptible to the infection, though it occurs more commonly in children. Most cases of tinea capitis *in adults* throughout the world are caused by endothrix species of Trichophyton (*T. tonsurans, T. violaceum,* and *T. schoenleini*).

Signs and Symptoms

The manifestations of tinea tonsurans are more uniform and characteristic in children than among adults, but variability in the clinical picture is noteworthy with this infection. The only constant sign, one of considerable diagnostic value, is the broken off hair or "stub," which is a cardinal clue to the disease. In children, the clinical picture is one of irregular, slowly extending patches of partial baldness, which are not always oval or rounded, but often polygonal or angular in outline. This is in contrast to the characteristic round patches of Microsporum infection. In tinea tonsurans, the margins are often indistinct, with fingerlike projections, and, frequently, many normal hairs are seen within the patch. A fairly distinctive feature is the tendency for infected hairs to break off at the scalp surface, producing an appearance of "black dots" resembling the infection due to *T. violaceum*. This is not a constant finding, however, for the hairs may fracture at various distances from the scalp. Scaling is a fairly regular feature, though variable in amount, and may conceal the dots or inconspicuous stubs of broken off hairs. When hair loss is not a prominent feature, the disorder closely mimics seborrheic dermatitis or psoriasis, and the most competent dermatologist may fail to recognize the infection.

Pruritus may be marked in tinea tonsurans, but it is not a feature of Microsporum infections. Scaling may be minimal, and occasionally there is a mild folliculitis around the periphery of the patch. When the disease is of long duration, the hairs in the central area of involvement may recover and regrow, while the lesion spreads at the periphery. The disease is not recognizable by examination under the Wood's light, the infected hairs standing out only as lusterless whitish stubs. Inflammatory changes are not uncommon, and frequently progress to the formation of a definite kerion or inflammatory nodules, folliculitis, or plaques of impetiginous dermatitis. Unlike Microsporum infections, inflammation is not found in all the

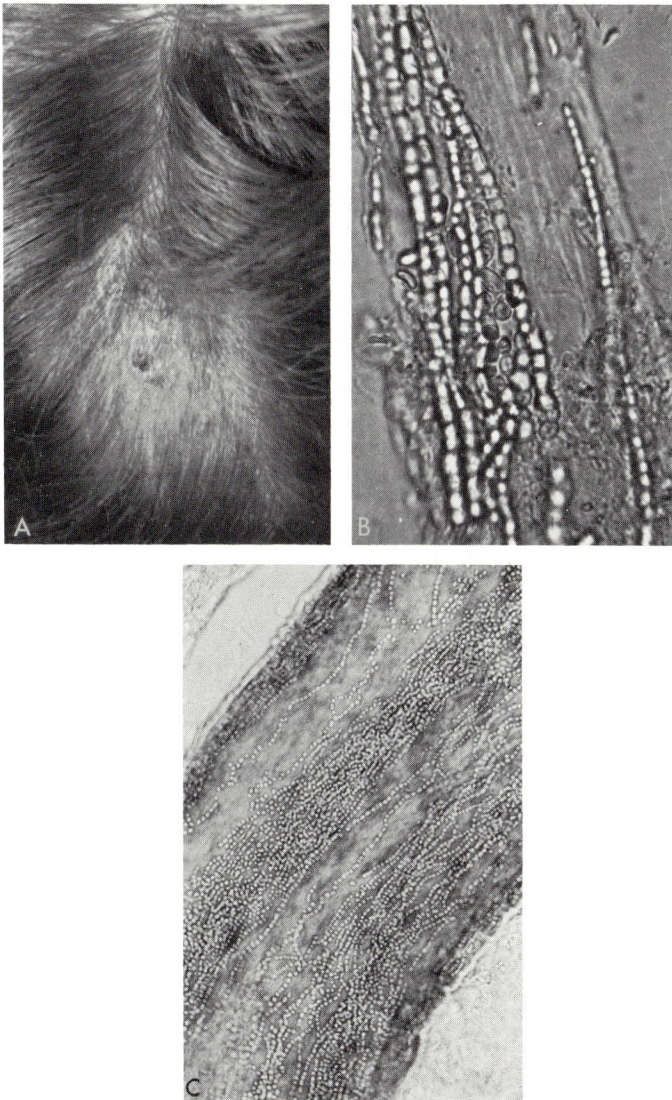

Figure 13–9 "Endothrix" tinea capitis due to *Trichophyton tonsurans*. A, Nondescript lesion resembling seborrheic dermatitis. B and C, Mycelia and spores within hair shaft. Chains of spores indicate a Trichophyton infection.

areas. Frank kerion formation appears always to presage spontaneous cure. The course of the disease is notoriously unpredictable; while regression within six months may be noted, it may persist indefinitely for many years, and chronicity is an outstanding trait. It may persist well into adult life, and occasionally for a lifetime. In patients in whom the disease has been present for 10 or more years, it is always noninflammatory, mimics many other affections of the scalp, and is rarely diagnosed unless cultural studies are done. It has been confused with simple bacterial folliculitis, cicatricial alopecia, seborrheic dermatitis, psoriasis, and even discoid lupus erythematosus. In chronic infections with this organism, infections of the skin elsewhere often develop and regress after variable periods. Onychomycosis may be noted. These lesions, especially if recurrent, may point to the scalp as the primary source of the infection and may lead to the proper diagnosis.

In obtaining material for direct examination and culture, the stubs or "black dots" may have to be removed with a needle after they have been located by careful search. Potassium hydroxide preparations demonstrate swollen hairs containing filaments and/or chains of large rectangular spores of variable length. The spores, which are entirely within the hair, may be densely packed in a mosaic arrangement. The microscopic appearance of the hair simulates that seen in *T. violaceum* infections, as does the clinical picture at times. Treatment is essentially the same as for infections with *M. audouini*. Griseofulvin may need to be administered for 8 to 12 weeks and recurrences are not uncommon.

Tinea Capitis due to T. Violaceum

Tinea capitis due to this fungus is characterized by a chronic noninflammatory course and by a distinctive "black dot" appearance resulting from the tendency of infected hairs to break off at the surface of the scalp. The fungus is anthropophilic; there is no significant animal reservoir. As is the general pattern with such fungi, the infection in the skin is relatively noninflammatory. The infection is rare in America, the British Isles and western Europe, but it has become endemic in some regions where low living standards and poor personal hygiene are the rule. A principal focus in the past was in eastern Europe. The contagiousness of the infection is low, and, in the absence of any known animal reservoir, it is passed solely between humans. Though children are most susceptible to the infection, adults have no marked resistance to it. The disease is very chronic and may last for decades.

The most typical manifestations of *T. violaceum* infections are seen in children and consist of patches of baldness containing "black dots." With the passage of time, the patches become less distinct, and infection may be demonstrable only in a few scattered hairs. Mild superficial folliculitis may develop occasionally, but this is insufficient to produce spontaneous epilation and arrest of the disease. The infection is capable of producing atrophy and permanent loss of hair.

Because of the black dot appearance, which may occur also in *T. tonsurans* infection, it is not possible to distinguish these two types of tinea capitis definitely on clinical grounds. *T. tonsurans* is an endothrix infection, and microscopic examination of the hairs reveals an abundance of fungal spores entirely within the hair shaft. Fluorescence is absent in both types, and culture is necessary to establish precisely the particular type of infection. Griseofulvin is necessary for cure.

Tinea Capitis due to T. Schoenleini

This fungus produces a distinctive and remarkable type of tinea capitis called *favus*. The infection is now rare in most parts of the world; its persistence in tiny foci is apparently dependent upon conditions of poor hygiene, intimate contact and, possibly, malnutrition. It is of interest from the medico-historical standpoint, because it was a principal medical disqualification for immigration into the United States during the peak of such admissions in the late 19th and early 20th centuries. It was previously endemic principally in eastern Europe. The only known focus of the disease in the U.S.A. at present is in the mountains of Kentucky, where settlers of Scottish descent live under the most backward conditions, and where the disease has persisted for generations after having been brought over by the original immigrants something over a century ago. The disease is most commonly acquired in childhood by direct contact with other infected persons, and persists into adult life. Adults have no immunity, as is true with all endothrix infections.

The conspicuous and diagnostic feature of favus is a yellow, cup-shaped crust composed of a dense mat of mycelia and epithelial debris, the scutulum. The concavity of this cup faces upward and is pierced by a hair, around the orifice of which the cup has developed. As the infection progresses, the scutula enlarge and merge to form massive prominent yellowish crusts. The odor of these crusts is reputed to be that of mice or of cat urine. The crusts may be extraordinarily extensive, involving the entire scalp and, sometimes, other portions of the body. The infection does not interfere with the hair structure as markedly as in other types of fungal infection; the hairs are often of normal length and hairs stubs are not a prominent feature. Fluorescence may occur in some cases, but it is variable, more prominent if the hair is light in color. It is a greenish gray in color and is definitely less intense than that seen in hairs infected by Microsporum. While spontaneous involution of the infection has been observed to occur within a few months to a year, the usual duration is several decades.

Cutaneous atrophy and permanent hair loss are common sequelae, though not inevitable. Atrophy is not related to any acute inflammatory phenomenon but progresses insidiously through the years, finally producing the characteristic appearance of "burned out" favus, in which tufts of hair persist grotesquely among the scarred areas. Even in this phase, however, the fungus may persist in hairs which appear relatively normal. Accurate diagnosis at this phase of the disease requires considerable clinical acumen and very careful mycologic study, since it may simulate cicatricial alopecia due to other causes. In common with other endothrix infections, favus may present an atypical and bizarre appearance which makes it exceedingly difficult to differentiate from seborrheic scaling or psoriasis. Hair loss may, at times, be inconspicuous. As might be expected in any chronic infection to which little immunity is developed, involvement of the glabrous skin or the nails occurs quite commonly. The characteristic yellow cup may or may not be present in cutaneous lesions, while the nail infection is indistinguishable from that produced by other species of fungi. In extensive favus infections, the appearance is bizarre and revolting.

In patients suspected of having favus, a definitive diagnosis may be made by direct microscopic examination of the hair, prior to culture. A pathognomonic change is seen in the form of rectangular cells within the hair, some of which apparently degenerate and are replaced by air, with production of a "bubbly" appearance. It is also quite characteristic that the fungal elements within the hairs are relatively scarce, which is probably the reason why so few hairs become disintegrated and broken off. Wood's light examination may be helpful in picking out infected hairs, though the fluorescence is weak. Griseofulvin is necessary for cure.

Tinea Capitis due to T. Verrucosum (T. Faviforme)

This fungus is zoophilic and causes an extremely inflammatory type of ectothrix tinea capitis which often results in cicatricial alopecia. The infection is most commonly contracted from cattle, and is therefore seen most frequently in farmers. It produces massive kerions which heal spontaneously, though the course may extend over several months and considerable tissue damage may occur. The treatment is similar to that for other types of inflammatory tinea capitis.

Infected hairs may be difficult to detect because they are rapidly shed by the inflammatory process. Microscopic examination of them reveals an *external* spore sheath consisting of chains of rather large rectangular cells which may be considerably disarranged. Culture is necessary for diagnosis but may not be interpretable easily, because *T. verrucosum* grows in three different cultural variants: (1) ochraceum, (2) album, and (3) discoides. These colonies differ considerably and have been a source of some confusion in proper identification and classification, but there appears to be little doubt that they are derived from a single species and are capable of inciting the same type of disease in man. Enriched media, containing either blood or thiamine, may aid in isolation because the organism requires extra growth substances for artificial cultivation.

TINEA BARBAE

Though inflammatory eruptions of the bearded area are common, they are rarely caused by fungi. However, zoophilic fungi residing in wild or domestic animals may provide a source of infection, and the disease is seen most frequently among farmers. The infection resembles various types of tinea capitis in many respects, apparently because beard hairs are similar to scalp hairs in that they grow rapidly and have a life cycle characterized by a long growing phase.

Tinea barbae may be divided into three types: (1) inflammatory, (2) superficial ringworm type, and (3) sycosiform.

INFLAMMATORY TINEA BARBAE. *T. mentagrophytes* and *T. verrucosum* are the predominant organisms, at least insofar as the U.S.A. is concerned. The typical lesions are essentially kerions—nodular, boggy, exudative circumscribed tumefactions which are studded with pustules. Suppuration is a prominent feature, and secondary bacterial invasion is common. Marked crusting may occur, and the odor of the lesions may be foul. The hairs in the affected areas either are epilated spontaneously or break off. Healing occurs spontaneously in from one to two months, often with atrophy and permanent hair loss. The diagnosis may be established by examining infected hairs in KOH preparations, but culture is required for definitive diagnosis. Treatment is with griseofulvin and is similar to that outlined for the kerions of tinea capitis.

RINGWORM TYPE TINEA BARBAE. The lesions in this variant are similar to those noted on relatively nonhairy skin and are characterized by annularity, an "active" border, and central clearing. Occasionally, ringworm infections of the face may resemble lupus erythematosus (Gilgor et al, 1971) or other dermatoses (Shapiro and Cohen, 1971). The causative fungi vary, including any which produce tinea capitis. Involvement of the hairs is variable and often inconspicuous. The lesions ordinarily reach maximal size within a month or two, then resolve spontaneously. Filaments are easily demonstrable in scrapings from the infected border, and the hairs, if infected, have an appearance similar to scalp hairs infected by the particular fungus concerned. Griseofulvin is curative and complete clearing may be expected in 3 to 4 weeks or less. The application of solutions or creams containing tolnaftate or haloprogin or of a sulfur-salicylic acid preparation may aid in bringing the infection to a speedier termination.

SYCOSIFORM TYPE TINEA BARBAE. This is a rare type, indistinguishable clinically from chronic bacterial folliculitis. A considerable portion of the bearded region may be involved, and the individual lesions are seen as follicular pustules, with a hair in the center. Evolution of the infection produces crust formation. The hairs either break off and leave stubs or are epilated. If epilation occurs, it is a distinguishing point from bacterial infections, in which the affected hairs are

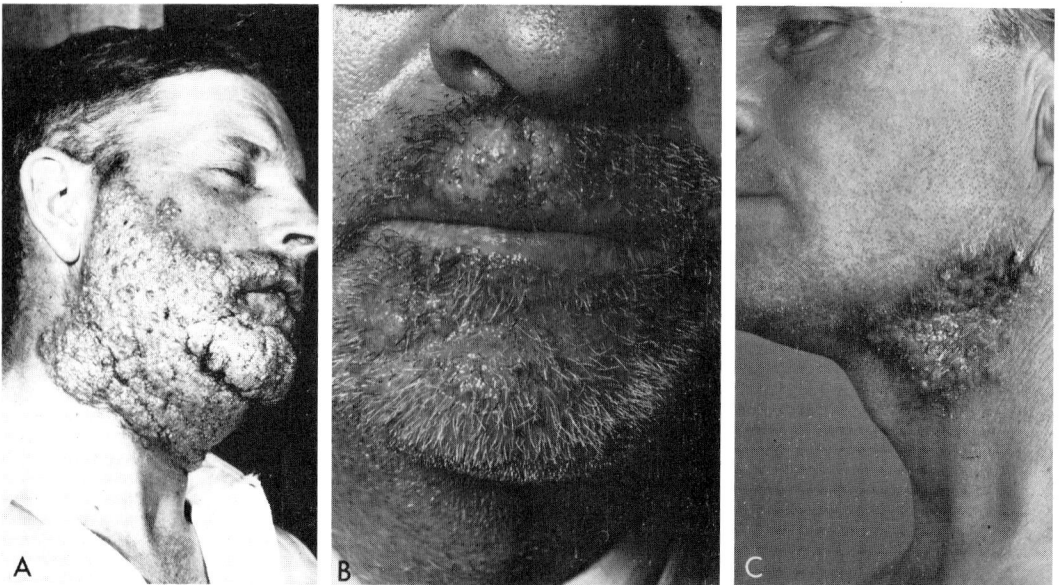

Figure 13–10   Tinea barbae. Various clinical types. Now uncommon. Note nodular masses.

removable only with difficulty. The causative fungi are *T. violaceum* and, less often, *T. rubrum*. Microscopic examination of the hairs establishes the diagnosis promptly, and is probably advisable as a routine measure in all resistant cases of chronic folliculitis of the beard, in spite of the fact that fungi are uncommonly the etiologic factor. This type of tinea barbae is extremely chronic, and topical therapy is of uncertain value. Griseofulvin is necessary for cure.

RINGWORM OF THE FEET
(Dermatophytosis, "Athlete's Foot," Tinea Pedis)

This is the most common type of ringworm infection. It is a penalty of civilization and the wearing of shoes—it is uncommon in primitive races accustomed to going barefoot. The infection has been the subject of overpopularization in medical and lay literature. Misconceptions and myths concerning its transmission, prevention, and treatment are rife. All this has led to much misdiagnosis of ringworm infection of the feet and to the assumption that almost all inflammatory dermatoses affecting this portion of the body are due to fungi. While there are many unanswered questions concerning ringworm infections of the feet and much to be desired in prevention and treatment, certain facts are known.

The majority of shoe-wearing adult males acquire fungal infections of the feet; the changes produced by this infection may be inconsequential to marked. Dermatophytosis of the feet is exceedingly rare in children, and any inflammatory eruption of the feet in a child is almost always due to some other cause. The infection is uncommon in adult females. Many theories have been advanced to explain this low incidence in these age and sex groups, but the basic reason for the marked comparative "immunity" has not yet been established. The various factors which may lessen infection include the practice of going barefoot, the wearing of less occlusive footgear, better hygiene, lessened sweating in females and, possibly, intrinsic antifungal properties within the skin which are related to age and sex. Numer-

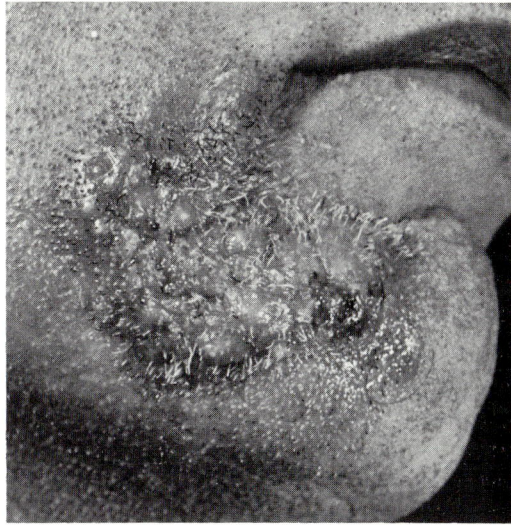

Figure 13–11 Sycosiform type tinea barbae. Crusting and follicular pustules are similar to bacterial infections of the beard.

ous surveys of the feet of young adult males in respect to the presence of infection have disclosed intertriginous changes in between 40 and 80 per cent. This incidence is highest in semitropical to tropical climates, provided that the subjects wear shoes.

It is traditionally accepted that if a fungus is isolated from an inflammatory eruption of the feet, the dermatosis is *ipso facto* caused by the fungus concerned. This is a gross oversimplification of the problem. In many inflammatory foot disorders, the changes seen are demonstrably due to factors other than the fungi themselves, though in some instances these organisms are unquestionably the principal factor. While it is convenient and satisfying to demonstrate the presence of a fungus in a foot eruption and to assume that all changes on the foot are related thereto, this may lead to neglect of etiologic forces which are of far greater importance. Under such circumstances, the application of an antifungal agent may not only not cure the eruption, it may intensify it.

Although fungi are present on the feet of the majority of young adult males, the means by which they reach there are far from well understood. In particular, misconceptions have arisen regarding transmission and reinfection, and these have led to prophylactic measures of unproved value, sometimes almost ludicrous in their complexities. Young men appear to acquire the infection if they are susceptible, regardless of any precautions which they may take and irrespective of participation in athletics and exposure to gymnasiums, swimming pools, and the like. There is a considerable degree of inevitability in respect to the growth of superficial fungi on the skin of young men.

A few facts regarding the acquisition of fungal infections of the feet and episodes of reinfection are known, and these make some of the hypotheses regarding acquisition and prophylactic treatment of the disease untenable. In the first place, attempts to recover pathogenic fungi from areas in which they are presumed to be lurking in abundance, e.g., shower stalls, bathrooms, swimming pools, and gymnasiums, ordinarily end in failure. The most thorough search and innumerable cultures are required. In the second place, conjugal infections are so rare as to make it likely that they have occurred purely by coincidence. This is in striking contrast to the situation obtaining in ringworm of the scalp, where transmission of infection among siblings is common. A third fact is that, with the notable exception of granular strains of *T. mentagrophytes* isolated from servicemen in southeast Asia, ringworm infections of the feet are quite difficult to produce experimentally save under very particular conditions (Baer, 1966), in spite of gross continuous exposure to the organisms and maintenance of poor hygienic conditions on the feet which would seem almost certain to make the skin susceptible. In the very few instances in which this has been accomplished, the infection is ordinarily short-lived. From the evidence to date, one must assume the existence of a "factor X" in the acquisition of fungal infections which is either completely unknown or the importance of which has not been fully appreciated. The striking fact remains that the disease definitely is a penalty of civilization and is dependent upon one of several factors related thereto. Man has not, either orthopedically or dermatologically, fully adapted himself to the wearing of shoes.

As is the case in respect to the acquisition of ringworm infections of the feet, it is clear that much remains to be learned regarding reinfections, though a few facts are reasonably clear. Many practices have arisen in an effort to prevent reinfection. Prophylactic foot baths and sprays are still available in many locker rooms, though their value in preventing infection or reinfection is completely unproved.

Fungi are occasionally recoverable from footgear, but ordinarily only with difficulty. The boiling of socks does not give assurance of killing off all the fungi which may be present; in any event, if the socks are to be worn by the same individual, the procedure is unnecessary. The supposed advantages of white socks are probably mythical, except insofar as contact dermatitis from dyes may be prevented. Fungi in shoes may be killed off by exposing the shoes to formalin vapor but, again, this is probably worthless if the same person is wearing the shoes all the time. The most important point in relation to relapses of fungal infection is that, once it becomes established, the individual remains a carrier insofar as his own skin is concerned, though the gross appearance of the skin and nails may be completely normal. It is not possible for the infection to remain completely dormant on the surface in the form of spores, because some growth of the fungus is necessary to maintain itself in the stratum corneum; otherwise it would be cast off rapidly. Evidence is constantly being accumulated that in bona fide fungal infections of the feet, several areas may be affected other than the one in which gross inflammatory changes are seen. This is particularly true of the nails, and fungi are recoverable from nails which appear in every respect normal. It is only with the passage of considerable time, in many cases, that the nails take on the appearance which is regarded as characteristic of fungal infections.

Another important fact in respect to ringworm infections of the feet is that the diagnosis cannot be made with absolute certainty on the basis of the clinical findings, except in some instances of *T. rubrum* infections. Though inflammatory changes associated with fungal infections have certain sites of predilection on the foot and an appearance which is suggestive, these are by no means sufficient to prove that a fungus is chiefly responsible for the objective changes. In particular, intertriginous inflammation is not pathognomonic of superficial ringworm infection; it can result from a variety of causes.

Diagnosis of Tinea Pedis

Ringworm of the feet occurs in three principal forms: (1) intertriginous inflammation, (2) vesicular and bullous lesions, and (3) dry squamous inflammation. Gradations and admixtures of these three types occur frequently. The first two tend to be inflammatory and recurrent. The squamous type is comparatively noninflammatory and extraordinarily persistent.

Intertriginous Ringworm

The chief changes in this type consist of maceration, sogginess, scaling and fissuring in the interdigital spaces, with accompanying malodor and pruritus. Scaling is the most characteristic and almost invariable sign of ringworm, helping to differentiate ordinary forms of intertrigo. The fourth interspace is most commonly involved, but in more extensive cases all the interdigital spaces show inflammation. The preference for involvement of these intertriginous areas would appear to be due to occlusion, with constant moisture, maceration, and some degree of mechanical irritation. Intertriginous ringworm of the feet is rarely seen in persons who, on standing barefoot, show wide spreading of the toes. The first interspace is the largest anatomically and is the least often involved. Extension to the undersurface of the toes and the adjacent portion of the sole occurs frequently, and this may continue on to the ball of the foot. In these areas, the initial lesion is seen to be groups of small vesicles, which are rarely apparent in the interspaces themselves. The dorsal surfaces of the toes and feet are not commonly involved in a "pure" ringworm infection, a useful point in differentiating the condition from contact dermatitis due to footgear or applied medication. Intertriginous ringworm may be associated with the dry squamous type, with frankly vesicular lesions elsewhere. In a low-grade

subacute form, the intertriginous lesions may persist for months or years, always presenting some desquamation and maceration, with recurrent pruritus. The condition almost invariably becomes worse with warm weather. Even during cold weather, undue exposure to heat from a radiator or an automobile heater may produce a prompt exacerbation. The inflammation is particularly prone to persist unabated in persons with hyperhidrosis, in whom the sweating is dependent upon emotional forces rather than thermal.

When acute flare-ups of intertriginous ringworm occur, the organisms may not be recoverable because they are being cast off rapidly. Aside from the itching, the malodor, and the constant temptation to apply this or that new topical medicament, the most serious complication is secondary bacterial infection, which rises most frequently in fissures. The pathogenic bacteria may become an irremovable part of the bacterial flora of the region, capable of producing recurrent infection, sometimes leading to lymphedema and elephantiasis nostras.

Intertriginous inflammation of the toes may persist frequently in the absence of fungi. This may be part of a more generalized process, such as an extensive seborrheic dermatitis or psoriasis, or it may be due entirely to factors of maceration and irritation, to which fungi are making no contribution. It is probable in some cases that the initial inflammation was produced by fungi, which were then cast off, and the process perpetuated by other factors. In many cases of intertriginous inflammation of the toes, the determination as to whether or not fungi are present is a matter of academic interest only. Even if found, the extent to which they are contributing to the inflammation may not be clear. The supportive treatment is similar in any event. Bacterial cultures are sometimes helpful, though the mere recovery of pathogenic strains is, again, not proof that they are contributing to the eruption. In performing studies for fungi, copious amounts of scales should be collected. If vesicles are present in the border, the roofs of these furnish a good source.

Intertriginous fungal infections of the feet are chiefly associated with *T. menta-*

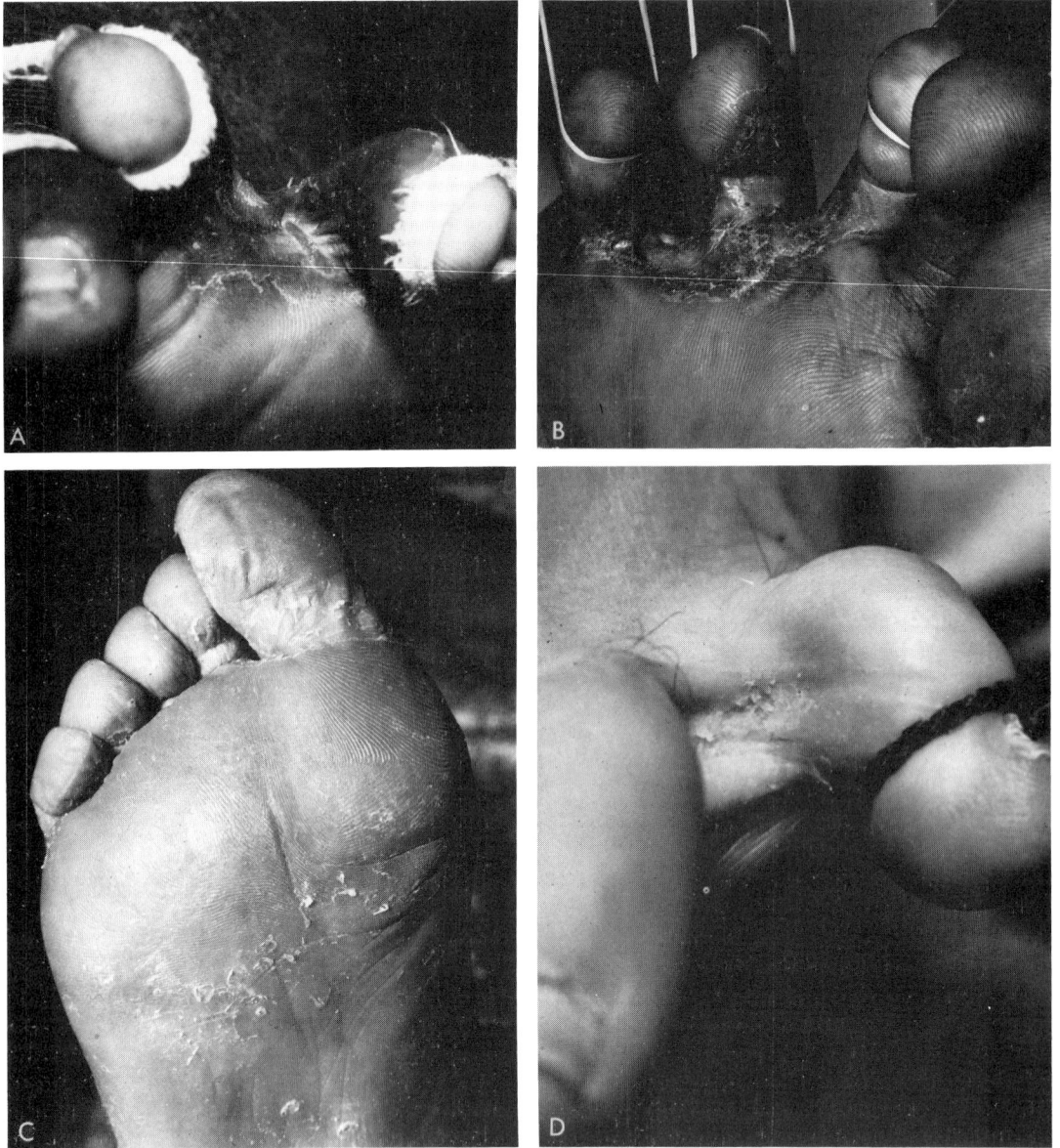

Figure 13–12 Various clinical manifestations of fungal infections of feet. Scaling is a constant feature of subacute or chronic lesions.

grophytes, though the strains of this species are distinctly different from those which uncommonly cause tinea capitis. *T. rubrum* and *Epidermophyton floccosum* are less commonly recovered from intertriginous inflammation of the toes. *Candida albicans* is not infrequently cultured, but its significance in producing the disease in question is often difficult to assess, and it seems certain that true candidiasis

of the interdigital surfaces of the toes is uncommon. The objective changes produced are, moreover, rather different.

TREATMENT. Griseofulvin in oral doses of 500 mg. twice daily with meals for two to three weeks or the topical application of creams or solutions containing tolnaftate or haloprogin (Olansky, 1972) may be curative if nails are not involved. Recurrences are extremely common due to host susceptibility. Adjunctive treatment of intertriginous ringworm of the feet is essentially that of intertrigo in general.

The most effective methods of adjunctive treatment are simple, and may be outlined as follows:

Dryness. This is the most important single factor in successful treatment. It may be achieved in several ways, which are variously adaptable to the particular patient in question. These include *the most meticulous and careful drying of the toes after bathing* or on removing the shoes. It is helpful and safe to do this with a crash wash cloth, with friction sufficient to remove scales and macerated skin (except, of course, in very acute flare-ups). Aeration of the feet is also helpful. This may be accomplished in decreasing order of effectiveness by (1) having the patient go barefooted as much as possible, (2) instructing him to wear sandals whenever feasible and/or (3) wearing "ventilated" shoes, especially during warm weather. The wearing of any rubber soled shoes, particularly sneakers, or shoes of nonporous leather, e.g., cordovan, or poromeric synthetic materials, is decidedly harmful. Decreased moisture and protection from mechanical rubbing may be accomplished by inserting absorbent cotton (cotton wool) or similar soft material into the affected interspaces. If this is allowed to remain until it becomes soggy, however, more harm than good will result. A finely ground nonabrasive dusting powder is also helpful, and it is possible that those which contain nonirritating antifungal agents are superior, though by no means markedly so. A powder composed of microporous cellulose, talc, and parachlorometaxylenol is particularly useful and less occlusive than powders containing fatty acids. Dusting of the toes should be carried out on arising and, in some instances, more frequently. If the powder is at all abrasive, and many powders are, or if it tends to become caked, the effect is more harmful than helpful. A change of socks more than once daily may be advisable to promote dryness, and these should be of an absorbent material, not of nylon.

Rest Is Essential in severe intertriginous ringworm. It is discouraging to note how patients continue to traumatize the skin by full activity in the face of rather marked inflammation, often by athletic or other activities which are not essential. The skin receives no opportunity to restore itself to integrity. This is of particular importance if marked fissuring is present or if there is the slightest suggestion of secondary bacterial infection. As the acute manifestations subside, a gradual increase in activity is allowable, but this should be kept within reasonable limits.

Removal of Macerated Debris. In some instances of intertriginous fungal infections of the feet, the accumulation of debris is such as to make it impractical for the patient to remove it himself. Under such circumstances, careful curetting away of this material by a physician or nurse is very helpful. Two precautions should be observed: (a) The tops of any large bullae which form should *not be cut off entirely*, especially on thick skin which is subjected to the trauma of walking. The contents should be drained, and the roof of the bulla removed later when the underlying epidermis has had an opportunity to heal, usually in three or four days. (b) If the macerated tissue is adherent, care should be taken not to tear off strips into adjacent normal skin. After curetting, Castellani's paint should be applied.

Soaks and Wet Dressings. Acute flareups of intertriginous ringworm are best treated with foot soaks of any innocuous material, e.g., Burow's solution for twenty minutes, three to four times daily. The skin should be carefully dried after each soak. A shake lotion may be used sparingly to advantage. Topical hydrocortisone is often helpful, though not frequently necessary, and is best applied in liquid shake lotion form. In this phase the application of heavy greasy ointments is inadvisable, because they simply increase the "gunkiness" of the skin. Emulsion type ointment vehicles are allowable, however. Particular observation should be made for the onset of secondary bacterial infection, in the form of either a superficial pyoderma or cellulitis. Should this occur, it should be dealt with promptly.

Topical Antifungal Preparations. Subacute or chronic types of intertriginous fungal infections of the feet are helped by therapy which is a little more stringent. Of all the compounds having antifungal effects *in vitro,* preparations containing tolnaftate, haloprogin, or fatty acids are probably the most useful because they rarely cause irritation. *Ointments should not be applied before shoes are to be worn.* They produce discomfort at times and may increase maceration. A very bland dusting powder is allowable, or a lotion containing 3 per cent salicylic acid in 70 per cent alcohol, or Castellani's paint. As the process passes over into a chronic phase in which the evidences of inflammatory reaction are very minimal and the accumulation of macerated tissue greater, somewhat harsher remedies are helpful. Ointments containing salicylic acid in maximum percentage, ordinarily of 3 per cent, are useful.

Measures to Prevent Relapse. The advisability of wearing fresh, dry absorbent socks has been emphasized above, as has the advisability of shoes which allow aeration and which do not promote hyperhidrosis. There is no necessity to boil the socks. The value of white socks as compared to dyed ones would seem to have been overemphasized. Attempts to sterilize the shoes are probably useless because the skin ordinarily furnishes an adequate source of reinfection if it is to occur. Patients who are insistent upon a precaution of this sort should be instructed to place the shoes in a tight box in which an open container of formalin is present, and to expose the shoes to this vapor for from 24 to 48 hours. Under no circumstances should a pledget soaked with formalin be placed in the toe of the shoe; this will frequently result in irritation and sensitization of the skin. In warm weather, or if the patient has hyperhidrosis, alternate wearing of different pairs of shoes on successive days is advisable, because this gives one pair of shoes an opportunity to become dry.

Vesicular Ringworm of the Feet

This manifestation of ringworm often accompanies the intertriginous type and is frequently an evidence of increased sensitization to the organism. The lesion may actually contain fungi, or it may be a dermatophytid, i.e., a sensitization reaction in the absence of fungi within the lesion. The most common sites of involvement by vesicular ringworm are the instep portion of the sole and the heel and ball of the foot. In severe cases, the whole sole may be involved, though the process does not commonly extend over the dorsum of the foot, except in combat troops serving in tropical climates where the feet become macerated and abraded under the boot laces by silt-laden water from swamps and rice paddies (Allen et al, 1972). Such involvement has been extremely common in southeast Asia and is caused by a highly virulent granular strain of *T. mentagrophytes* endemic to that area. Vesicular ringworm may occur suddenly, often with the onset of very warm weather. Deep-seated vesicles of variable size and number develop; these are not characterized by erythema at their onset. They frequently fuse to form bullae or multilocular blisters, which contain a yellowish gelatinous fluid. Vesicles which occur in areas with very thick stratum corneum may appear to be papular and frequently resolve with the formation of a hard keratotic button which persists for a long time. The rupture of vesicles and bullae leaves a sensitive, red, eroded area at the border of which new blisters often form. Pruritus is severe. The demonstration of fungi in the lesions is medically satisfying but is not an essential procedure; considerable search may be necessary to recover the organism in very acute cases.

T. mentagrophytes is the most common organism involved in acute vesicular fungal infections, though *T. rubrum* may be recovered, in spite of its general tendency to produce chronic lesions of low-grade inflammatory type. *E. floccosum* is an occasional causative agent. Vesicular ringworm of the feet is frequently associated with vesicles or bullae on the hands, though these are almost always dermatophytids, and fungi are not recoverable from them. In acute flare-ups, the severity of the process on both the feet and hands may be equal.

The chief condition which is to be differentiated from vesiculobullous dermatophytosis is contact dermatitis. Failure to recognize this possibility has led to much mistreatment and disability, because the application of rather strong active "antifungal" medicaments to a contact dermatitis can result only in further exacerbation.

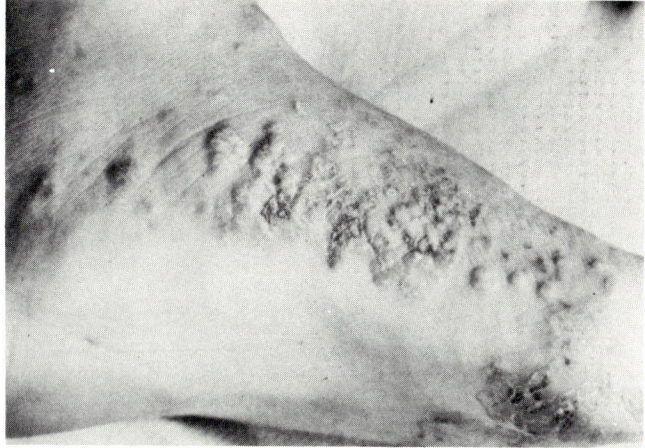

Figure 13–13 Vesicular ringworm of the foot. Vesicles over ball of foot and instep are fusing to form multiloculated bullae.

In contact dermatitis, however, the soles are rarely involved, and the most acute manifestations will practically always be seen on the dorsal surface of the toes and foot. Other conditions which may simulate ringworm infections are acute dyshidrotic eruptions, reactions to drugs, and pustular psoriasis or "bacterids."

Griseofulvin is effective in the treatment of acute vesiculobullous fungal infections. Adjunctive treatment is exactly the same as that which is advisable for acute contact dermatitis. One point of difference is that greater care should be taken to evacuate the contents of aggregated vesicles and bullae which occur under the thick skin of the sole or palm. This is often followed by prompt relief of itching and/or pain. *The entire top of the bulla should not removed.* Rest is essential. Bland soaks should be used two to three times daily, followed by talc or a shake lotion. If there is definite evidence of secondary bacterial infection, systemic antibacterial antibiotics are indicated. During warm humid weather, the patient's progress will be increased if he can remain for a time in a cool, air-conditioned environment. The subsequent treatment as the process subsides is exactly the same as that outlined for subacute chronic intertriginous infections. In any patient who has sustained an acute disabling flare-up, little urging will be required to induce observance of reasonable precautions in regard to foot hygiene. Creams containing corticosteroids and iodochlorhydroxyquin may be helpful in the less acute cases in which continued vesiculation may be chronic and very troublesome.

Squamous Ringworm of the Feet

This type of ringworm infection ordinarily follows a course which is quite dissimilar to that of the more common intertriginous or vesicular types. It is most frequently caused by *T. rubrum,* an organism which does not produce an inflammatory reaction of sufficient degree to induce disposal of it by the skin. The infection is characterized by diffuse scaling, often of a fine, branny character, relative lack of inflammation, and extreme chronicity. Though the mildly inflammatory changes may seem to involve certain areas to the exclusion of others, the process usually becomes diffuse over the entire plantar surface and may extend partially over the sides of the foot in what has aptly been called a "moccasin" distribution. There may be associated intertriginous involvement of the toes. The scale is adherent and silvery white, and is most marked in skin furrows. The color is dull red, if there is any color at all, and moderate hyperkeratosis is often present. The infection often escapes detection because the "normal" foot acquires many evidences of the wear and tear to which it has been subjected through the years. It may be difficult to differentiate from ichthyosis, congenital keratosis plantaris, or psoriasis. If very marked hyperkeratosis and thick callous formation are present, this is probably not

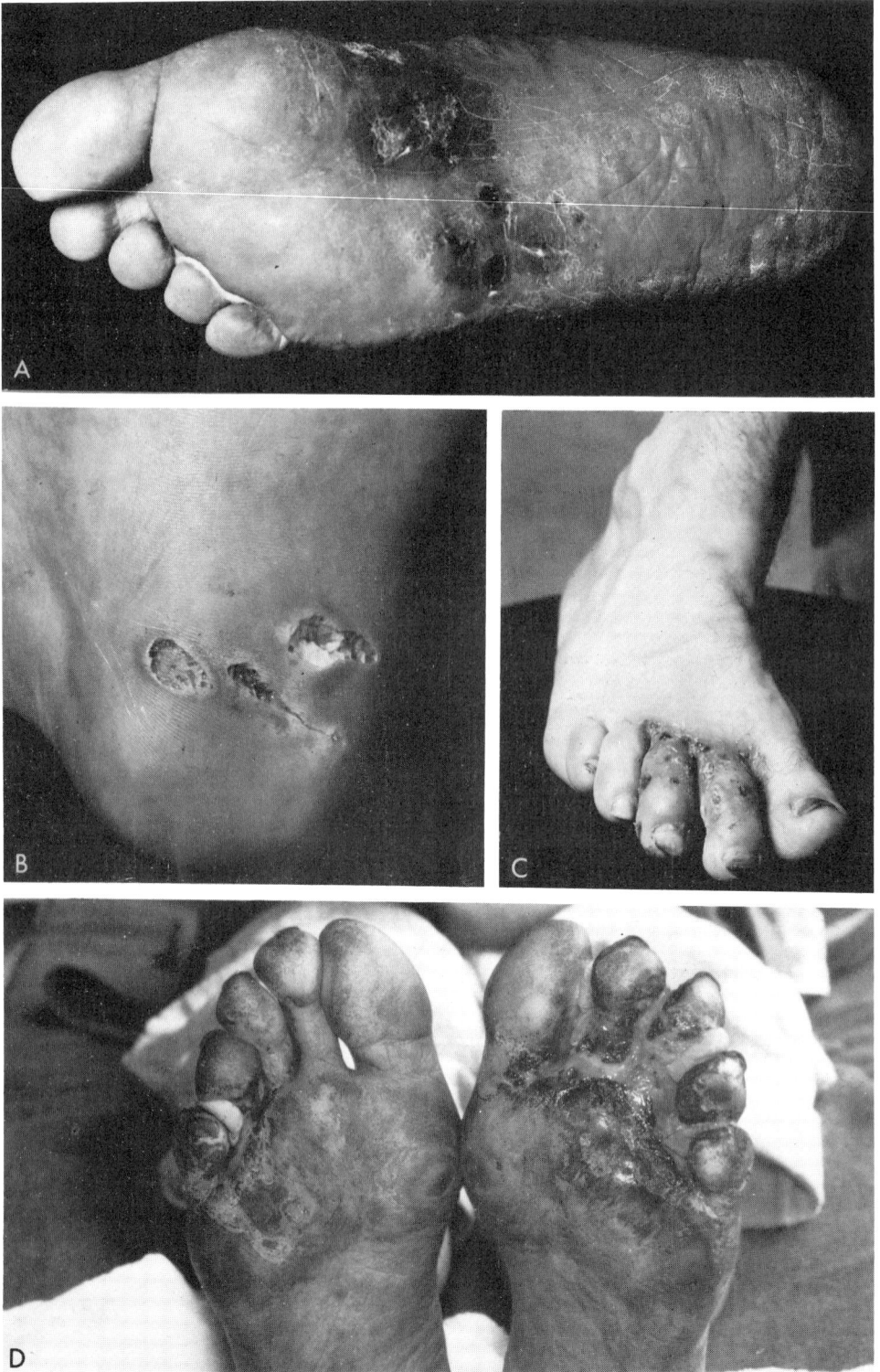

Figure 13–14 Severe disabling acute dermatophytosis. Bacterial secondary infection present in *C* and *D*.

due entirely to the fungal infection itself. Hyperhidrosis may be present, but this is often of a localized variety, and the affected portions of the foot may appear excessively dry.

In many patients, the involvement is relatively restricted, though fungi may be recoverable from skin which appears normal. Involvement of the dorsal surface of the foot is not particularly uncommon, in contrast to other types of foot ringworm. The scaling may extend up the posterior aspect of the heel and even involve the ankle, producing erythematous and moderately eczematous plaques with poorly defined borders. Small vesicles or pustules may sometimes develop in these plaques and may prove extraordinarily persistent. These are not commonly seen on the plantar surface in such infections, however.

The majority of individuals with chronic squamous tinea pedis do not, fortunately, acquire lesions elsewhere on the body, despite a steady contaminating shower of organisms. Nevertheless, the process may sometimes be transmitted to the hands. It seems entirely possible that the use of manicuring instruments on both the feet and hands may be a source, since the conditions are theoretically ideal for producing an infection elsewhere, with a combination of mild trauma and an organism to which the affected individual is known to be susceptible.

The presence of a *T. rubrum* infection may be suspected upon the basis of the low-grade clinical changes seen. Changes

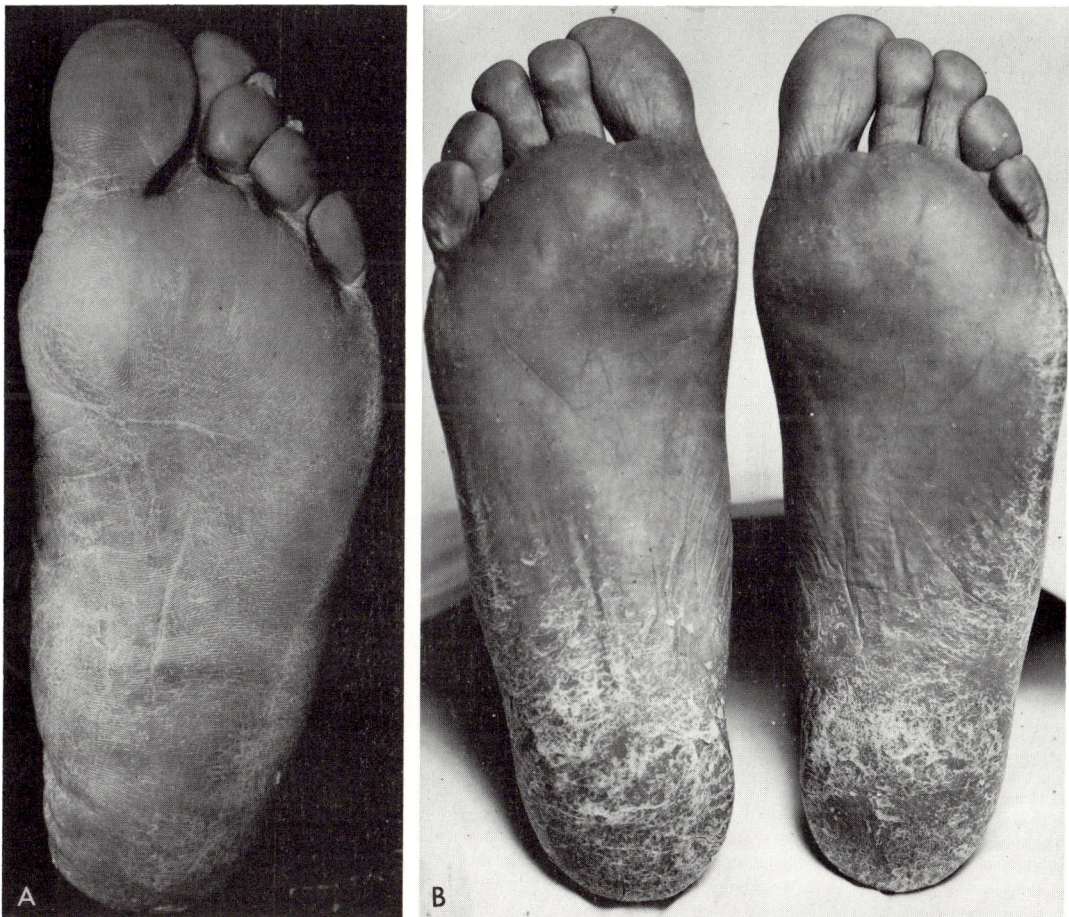

Figure 13–15 *A*, Dry squamous *T. rubrum* infection. Note flat foot; orthopedic and vasomotor abnormalities are sometimes factors in the chronicity and severity of fungal infections of feet. *B*, Hyperkeratotic chronic symmetric tinea pedis.

in the toenails develop slowly but may be troublesome by reason of marked thickening or curling up of the distal border. Regular care by a podiatrist may be helpful. In occasional instances in which the nail is greatly distorted and troublesome by reason of catching on the socks or digging into adjacent skin, removal of the nail and destruction of the matrix may be considered, but necessity for this will be uncommon.

Fungi are easily demonstrable in the scales, provided that sufficient material is collected. Misdiagnosis may result, however, by reason of mistaking an artefact, the "mosiac fungus," for true fungal elements. In cleared thick preparations of skin, especially, refractile elements are seen to follow the intercellular spaces between the cornified cells. These are regularly and easily demonstrable in normal plantar stratum corneum. The artefact has been the subject of much discussion, and it is unfortunate that it was ever related to true fungal elements within the skin, because it is completely without significance in this regard. Mistaken interpretation of it

can result only from inexperience in simple mycologic techniques, but this has occurred frequently.

One rather characteristic immunologic phenomenon which may be demonstrated with *T. rubrum* infections is that following the intradermal injection of trichophytin, an immediate wheal-type reaction is seen, in addition to the delayed tuberculin-type reaction.

TREATMENT. Griseofulvin in adequate dosage is the treatment of choice in chronic squamous *T. rubrum* infections of the feet and may be curative if continued long enough. Unfortunately, recurrences are quite common and resistant strains of *T. rubrum* are occasionally encountered. The topical application of preparations containing haloprogin or tolnaftate may result in clearing of mild infections if nails are not involved. Moderate exacerbations of inflammation may be dealt with as in other types of ringworm. Hyperkeratosis may require the regular use of salicylic acid preparations, sometimes in concentrations as high as 6 or 8 per cent, but this should be done with care. It is important that the

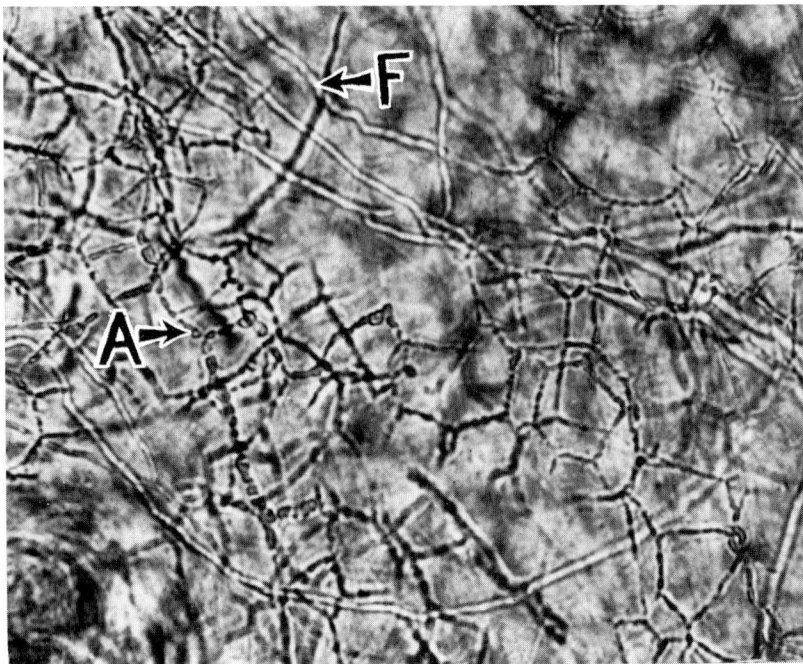

Figure 13–16 Fungi and mosiac artefact in KOH prepared skin scraping. F indicates the rather clear, linear hyphae of fungi. A indicates the darker mosaic artefact; it outlines the keratinized cells. Note irregularity in size and shape of mosiac elements.

patient realize that the disease is relatively harmless and that transmission to others is unlikely to occur.

RINGWORM OF THE HANDS

Fungal infections of the hands are by no means rare, but inflammatory eruptions in this region are so diagnosed with much too great frequency. The disease has so much in common morphologically and clinically with infections of the feet that it need not be considered in any great detail. There are two main types: (1) the inflammatory vesicular, and (2) the noninflammatory squamous. The former is very uncommon in temperate climates, though dermatophytids associated with infections on the feet are common. Vesicles occur, usually in clusters and frequently multiloculated, principally on the palms but rarely on the dorsal surfaces. The distinction from dermatophytids or dyshidrotic eruptions will rest upon mycologic studies, but these are not ordinarily necessary. *T. mentagrophytes* is the usual organism recoverable from the acute vesicular type. The course is toward spontaneous healing, provided the hands are not subjected to constant chemical or traumatic irritation, either occupational or therapeutic. It is of particular importance that a diagnosis of fungal infection of the hand not be made too lightly, with neglect of other more probable sources of inflammation in this region. The most common source of chronicity is the replacement of the fungal infection by a chronic eczematous process, due to the fact that the hands are constantly subjected to such a wide variety of external insults. The treatment of acute vesicular fungal infections of the hands is identical for similar infections of the feet.

The squamous type of fungal infection of the hands resembles the lesions on the feet closely and is ordinarily caused by the same organism, *T. rubrum*. The palms and palmar aspects of the fingers are the sites of predilection. The infection is accompanied by a diffuse, fine, branny, adherent scale, which is especially noticeable in the furrows. The underlying skin may seem quite normal or only slightly erythematous, but may become markedly thickened and hyperkeratotic with, sometimes, the de-

velopment of painful fissures. In a majority of instances of this infection, only one hand is involved, and this is a curious phenomenon, because the opportunities for inoculation of the other hand are obviously continuous. Hyperhidrosis is common, but is not always present. Scaling is not always confined strictly to the palmar surface, and scrapings from skin which appears normal may sometimes reveal fungi. Involvement of the nails is variable, but it eventually occurs in a majority of cases, though it is uncommon to observe dystrophy of all the fingernails.

In addition to the dry, moderately scaling type described above, *T. rubrum* infections of the hands may occasionally be manifested by infiltrated thickened erythematous scaling plaques, distributed in haphazard fashion on the palm or dorsum of the hand, rarely on the fingers. In such instances, the distinction from contact dermatitis, neurodermatitis, and nummular eczema may be difficult, unless scrapings are examined for fungi. *T. rubrum* infection may produce other reaction patterns, and at times the manifestations are so minimal as to cause the infection to be overlooked completely. It is probable that this type of infection on the hand is much more common than is generally realized.

Treatment

Griseofulvin is effective in the treatment of *T. rubrum* infections of the hand, but must be continued until all evidence of infection has cleared. Adjunctive therapy with preparations containing haloprogin, tolnaftate, or salicylic acid may be helpful.

Dermatophytids of the Hands

Allergic reactions to fungal infections occur most frequently on the hands. These lesions are called "ids." The typical picture is that of dyshidrosis, which is essentially a reaction pattern produced by various etiologic mechanisms. It is not possible to distinguish a true fungal infection of the palms from an allergic dermatophytid on morphologic grounds; this must rest on whether or not the fungi are found

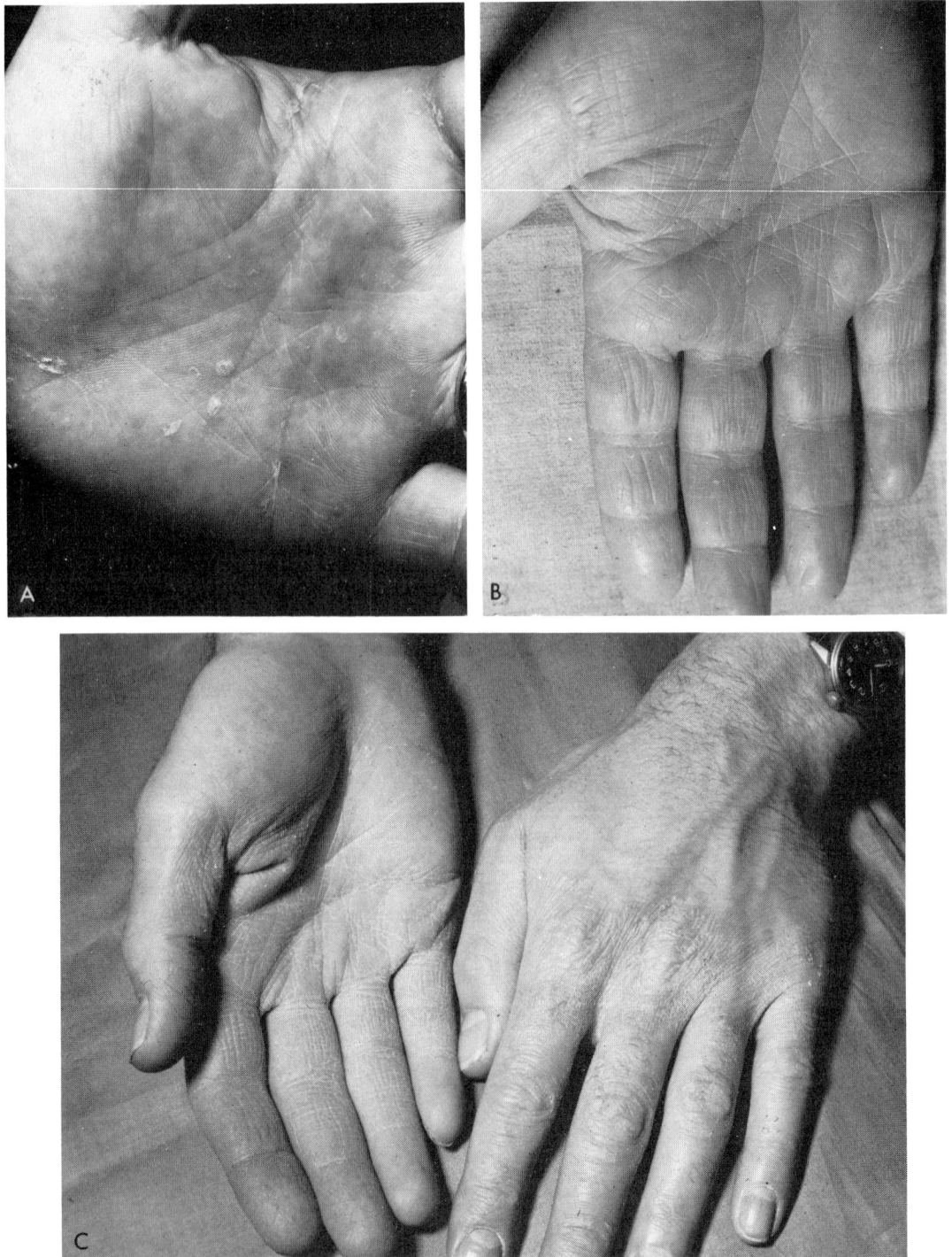

Figure 13–17 *T. rubrum* infections of hands. Frequently unrecognized as fungal infection. Modest inflammation, frequent involvement of nails, and persistence are characteristic.

in the lesions. The diagnosis of dermatophytid is too frequently invoked in respect to hand lesions. The criteria for such a diagnosis are not easily fulfilled, and the evidence is almost always circumstantial, not absolute (see p. 1187). The eruption is most frequently seen in conjunction with exacerbations of inflammatory fungal infections of the feet. A diagnosis of dermatophytid should not be made simply on the finding of a chronic inflammatory eruption of the feet in association with a dyshidrosiform eruption of the hand. It is frequently stated that in such cases adequate treatment of the process on the feet will result in involution of the lesions of the hands, but this is by no means always true.

RINGWORM OF THE GLABROUS SKIN
(Tinea Glabrosa, Tinea Circinata, Tinea Corporis)

Superficial ringworm infections of areas other than the scalp, hands, feet, and groin express themselves in widely differing and often bizarre morphologic variations. Such lesions may run the gamut from vesicles resembling herpes simplex, through scaling eczematous lesions, to massive granulomas which may be mistaken for skin cancer. All areas of the smooth surface of the skin may be involved; all of the fungi belonging to the ringworm group may incite these diseases; every age group is susceptible; and such infections are encountered in all areas of the world. It is convenient to discuss tinea cruris and tinea imbricata separately because, though both of these are variants of tinea glabrosa, they have special characteristics which permit fairly sharp clinical differentiation.

Ringworm infections of the glabrous skin are much more common in hot humid climates and reach their peak incidence in the tropics and subtropics. There can be no question that heat and moisture are strongly contributory to such infections. In addition, in many tropical regions, poor personal hygiene, poor nutrition, and debilitating systemic diseases are additive factors. In temperate climates, such infections are seen far more frequently during the hot summer months. While the lesions ordinarily tend to remain localized and are not very numerous, suitable conditions of climate may bring about extraordinarily widespread involvement of the skin in persons suffering from systemic diseases such as diabetes, leukemia, and various endocrine disorders.

It is worthy of emphasis again that superficial fungal infections are not solely dependent upon a meeting of a pathogenic species and normal human skin. It is difficult to transmit such infections experimentally, and healthy persons in temperate climates have marked inherent resistance. It would seem that it is only under special environmental conditions or a background of systemic disease that such fungi are

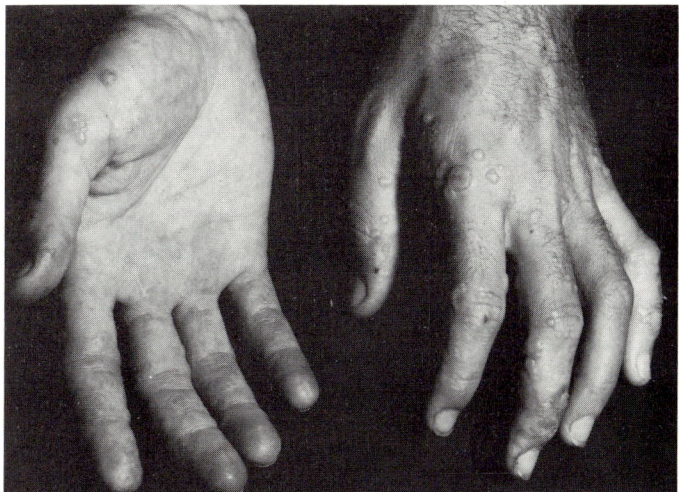

Figure 13–18 Dermatophytid of hands. Vesicular eruption resembling dyshidrosis, occurring coincidentally with acute fungal infection of feet. No fungi demonstrable on hands. Rapid involution occurs with subsidence of foot lesions.

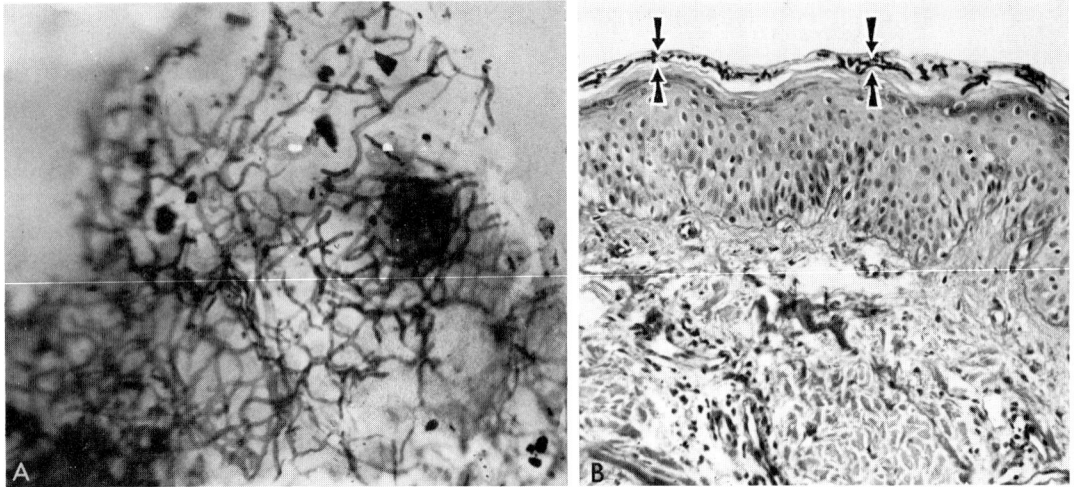

Figure 13–19   Fungi demonstrated by Hotchkiss-McManus method. *A,* Abundantly shown in skin scrapings. *B,* Fungal filaments are seen in the stratum corneum of a biopsy specimen. The superficial ringworm fungi involve *only* dead keratinous tissue.

able to gain a foothold. Glabrous ringworm infections occur particularly in four groups: (1) persons who may be repeatedly exposed to infected domestic animals, such as kittens and cattle, (2) persons with chronic fungal infections of the feet or nails, (3) persons who are in close and regular contact with humans suffering from certain types of fungal infections, particularly individuals with tinea capitis, from whom the amount of spore dissemination is enormous, and (4) servicemen serving in tropical climates under conditions of less than optimal hygiene in which the skin may be continuously wet and a particularly virulent strain of dermatophyte may be present in the environment. In southeast Asia, infections have been caused by a virulent strain of *T. mentagrophytes* which has been isolated from hair clippings of rats sharing the same bunkers and elevated ground with the soldiers. In patients with tinea corporis, it is worthwhile to inquire regarding these possible sources of infection.

Ringworm infections of the glabrous skin mimic a wide variety of other dermatoses, and it is almost impossible to make such a diagnosis with assurance on the basis of the morphologic changes alone. In particular, such infections may resemble seborrheic dermatitis, pityriasis rosea, some types of psoriasis, and various granulomas. In temperate climates, a diagnosis of ringworm infection of the skin made on the basis of a ring-shaped lesion will be more often erroneous than correct, and such a diagnosis should always be confirmed or negated by the simple procedure of examination of scrapings taken from the *border* of the lesion.

Glabrous ringworm infections are, by and large, relatively self-limited, or at least easily cleared by a variety of treatment methods. In temperate climates, a marked inflammatory reaction is often indicative of spontaneous resolution, but in tropical ringworm of the glabrous skin, such lesions may evolve into chronic follicular and perifollicular granulomas which require prolonged treatment with griseofulvin to effect a cure.

Clinical Variants of Tinea Glabrosa

The morphologic patterns produced by superficial ringworm infections of the glabrous skin are so varied as to have led to their designation as separate and distinct diseases. This is unnecessary and confusing. The following are the main types of clinical expression of such infections.

ANNULAR LESIONS, "CLASSIC" RINGWORM.   This is the lesion which has led to the term *ring*worm (Tinea circinata), but it is by no means the most common expression of such infections. The lesion begins as an erythematous papule; this then enlarges to form a ring with a center which is relatively normal and a sharply defined "active" border. The border may be elevated, red, and infiltrated, and often contains small vesicopapules. The lesions may be single or numerous, but ordinarily only one or a few lesions are seen; this is in contrast to other types of annular lesions such as pityriasis rosea. It is uncommon to see a patch of annular ringworm larger than 10 cm. in diameter, though

adjacent lesions may fuse, with resultant large gyrate plaques. Smaller rings form within the larger one occasionally, but this is not typical and is more characteristic of certain types of "fixed" erythema eruptions. In annular ringworm infections, skin which has recently been the site of infection tends to be resistant for a period of several months. On reaching its maximum size, annular ringworm may persist for a few weeks and then undergo spontaneous regression. The only symptom is moderate pruritus. Such lesions are feebly contagious. Almost all of the

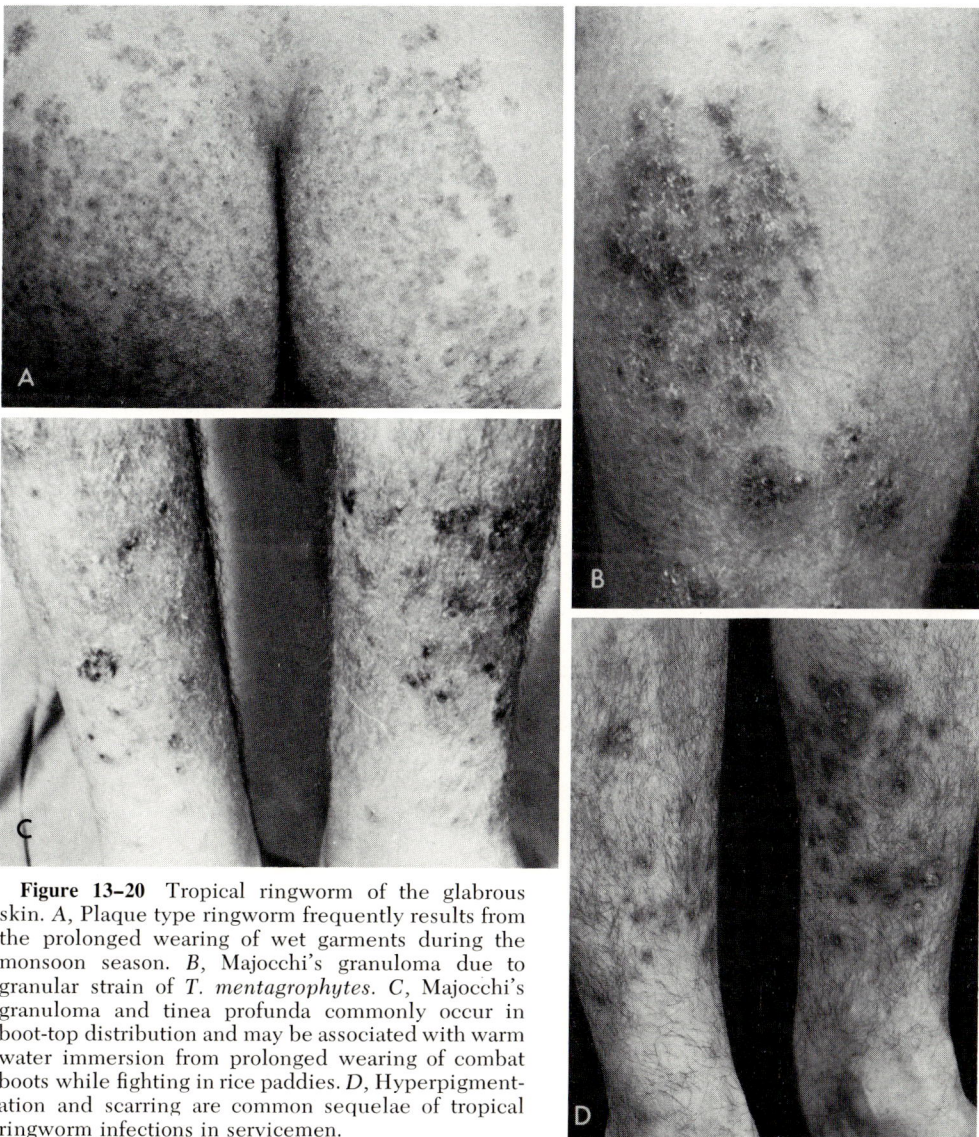

Figure 13–20 Tropical ringworm of the glabrous skin. *A*, Plaque type ringworm frequently results from the prolonged wearing of wet garments during the monsoon season. *B*, Majocchi's granuloma due to granular strain of *T. mentagrophytes*. *C*, Majocchi's granuloma and tinea profunda commonly occur in boot-top distribution and may be associated with warm water immersion from prolonged wearing of combat boots while fighting in rice paddies. *D*, Hyperpigmentation and scarring are common sequelae of tropical ringworm infections in servicemen.

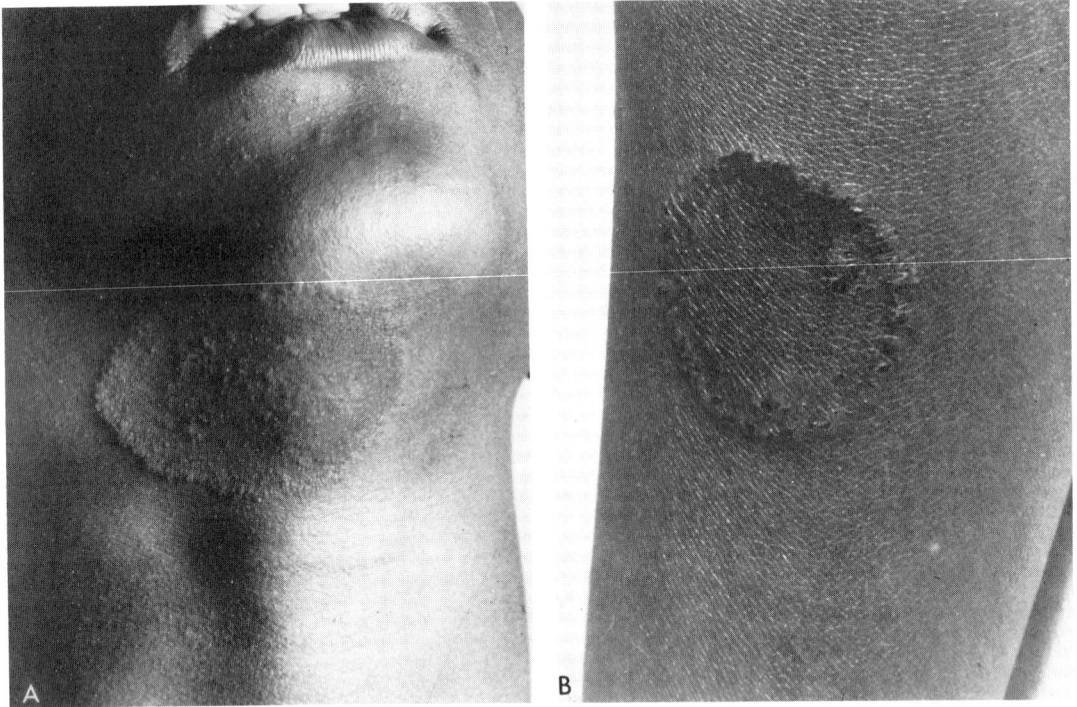

Figure 13–21   Tinea circinata of the classic "ringworm" type.

dermatophytes are capable of producing this type of lesion, but in the U.S.A. the most common causative organisms are *M. audouini*, *M. canis*, and *T. mentagrophytes*.

In healthy persons living in temperate climates, this type of ringworm infection is responsive to treatment with griseofulvin or topical preparations containing halo-progin, tolnaftate, or salicylic acid.

ECZEMATOUS ANNULAR RINGWORM. The characteristic feature of this morphologic response is the lack of central clearing. The lesions are round, but scaling, redness, and slight infiltration are present throughout the lesions. Endothrix Trichophyton species most frequently cause this type of infection, which is relatively uncommon. The treatment is similar to that outlined for ordinary annular ringworm.

CRUSTED TYPE. The prototype of this morphologic response to ringworm is favus, which is extremely rare in the U.S.A. Scutula and crusted masses similar to those occurring in the scalp develop on the glabrous skin. Other more common species of dermatophytes occasionally produce lesions which form thick crusts, but this is a bizarre and unusual manifestation. The response to topical treatment is slow at best, and griseofulvin should be given in adequate dosage for four to six weeks.

HERPETIFORM TYPE. This is a decidedly inflammatory vesicular type of ringworm which is ordinarily due to a zoophilic species. The primary lesion is a mound of fused vesicles. This ordinarily ruptures, leaving a red, eroded base on which a crust may form. New vesicles may form in the periphery, but the lesions do not achieve a diameter greater than 2 cm. as a rule, and the outlook is for spontaneous involution. Hyphae are found in abundance in the vesicle, but the clinical expression is so bizarre as, ordinarily, to lead to disregard of the possibility of a ringworm infection.

PLAQUE TYPE. In some fungal infections, a lack of spontaneous healing and chronic extension of lesions may result in the formation of large scaling plaques. *T. rubrum* is the chief offender. The plaques may resemble those of seborrheic dermatitis or of psoriasis with minimal scaling. They enlarge eccentrically, forming arciform and gyrate patterns. The borders are sharply defined, and the lesions are dull red, with slight infiltration and scaling throughout. Diabetes and leukemia are diseases which may furnish a favorable soil for such a fungal infection, but in most instances no outstanding predisposing factor will be disclosed, other than the usual climatic one. Infections of the nails and feet are commonly associated. Griseofulvin should be given for several months or until all clinical evidence of infection has cleared. Recurrences are quite common, and resistant strains are occasionally encountered. In such cases, preparations containing haloprogin or tolnaftate may be helpful.

KERION TYPE (TINEA PROFUNDA). The prototype of this manifestation of fungal infections of the glabrous skin is the kerion which is seen much more frequently on the scalp. The lesion is ordinarily due to a zoophilic organism and is most frequently acquired by farmers exposed to cattle infected with *T. verrucosum*, or servicemen exposed to granular strains of *T. mentagrophytes* in tropical climates. The lesion is intensely inflamed; it consists of an elevated, sharply circumscribed, rather boggy tumor, with a bright red exuding granulating surface. Follicular pustules are a prominent feature, and the lesion may stink. The appearance may simulate a highly anaplastic tumor. At times the entire mass becomes fluctuant and necrotic. The suppuration is an evidence of reaction to the fungus itself and is not initially due to secondary bacterial infection, though this may occur later as the lesion ulcerates and is quite common in tropical climates. Such lesions may heal spontaneously within a few months and produce scarring. In tropical climates, spontaneous healing seldom occurs and the lesions may resist all treatment until the patient is evacuated to a temperate climate or hospitalized in an air-conditioned room. Conservative therapy such as bland compresses two or three times daily is indicated. The clinical course may be shortened and scarring minimized by the early administration of griseofulvin. If there is clear evidence of secondary bacterial infection, the use of an appropriate systemic antibacterial therapy may be required.

MAJOCCHI'S GRANULOMA. This distinctive manifestation of ringworm infection is essentially a *granulomatous folliculitis* and *perifolliculitis*. Although it has been known for many years, it has only recently been "rediscovered" and observed with some frequency. In part, this is due to the availability of improved methods for visualizing ringworm fungi in biopsies. The lesion is far less inflammatory and acute than kerion and develops in the form of nodules or infiltrates in a plaque of chronic low-grade eczematous ringworm or following the more acute phase in tropical ringworm infections. The nodules lead to the designation "granuloma."

The affected patients are most frequently women who shave their legs. The primary focus of infection is ordinarily a diffuse *T. rubrum* infection of the feet. Indefinite and often rather indistinct scaling patches develop on the lower half of the lower leg, and the inflammatory nodules develop in the borders of these. The nodules rarely exceed a centimeter in diameter and are flat or only slightly elevated. If the lesion is observed early, it may be seen to be centered by a hair. The lesions are ordinarily unilateral. The nodules are neither painful nor pruritic, do not progress to suppuration, and persist for varying periods from three to four months. They may then become slowly absorbed or undergo necrosis and heal with a depressed scar. As a rule a few nodules are present in varying stages of development and regression. The etiologic agent is *T. rubrum*. Patients with Majocchi's granuloma are, rather surprisingly, usually negative to trichophytin insofar as any delayed tuberculin type reaction is concerned. This is strong evidence against the possibility of the nodular lesions being "ids." Histopathologic examination reveals a characteristic foreign-body type granuloma, and if the sections are stained by the Hotchkiss-McManus method, globoid or rectangular fungal elements are seen to occur in chains. These segmented fungal filaments were originally present in ectothrix arrangement about a hair. The basic process is a mycotic folliculitis and, apparently, a portion of the follicle becomes disrupted and a fragment of infected hair with its accompanying fungal elements is displaced into the corium, there exciting a foreign body response. This response may be due either to the fungal cells or to hair fragments. The hair fragment is ordinarily resorbed in time, but the fungal elements may remain viable for prolonged periods, though showing evidence of steady degeneration. This occurrence has been cited by some as an exception to the general law that the superficial ringworm fungi grow only in dead tissue, i.e., are necrophilic. It is our belief that the phenomenon is not an exception to this rule, since the fungus apparently does not proliferate significantly in the corium but is passively sequestered there and persists for a time. It is reasonable to assume that shaving may be a factor in producing the process by promoting the formation of ingrown hairs and the deposit of fungal elements and hair in the corium.

Majocchi's granuloma is not well known, even among experts, and various erroneous diagnoses such as blastomycosis, tumors, or tuberculosis may be made.

Treatment with griseofulvin is curative and may prevent scarring. Discontinuance of shaving is helpful, but fastidious women cannot ordinarily be induced to do this. It is possible that the use of chemical depilatories instead of shaving might reduce the incidence of granulomas.

Tinea Cruris
(Eczema Marginatum)

Tinea cruris is an exceedingly common type of fungal infection in males. It is relatively uncommon in females, but its incidence is increasing with the wearing of tight-fitting slacks and pantyhose. It is

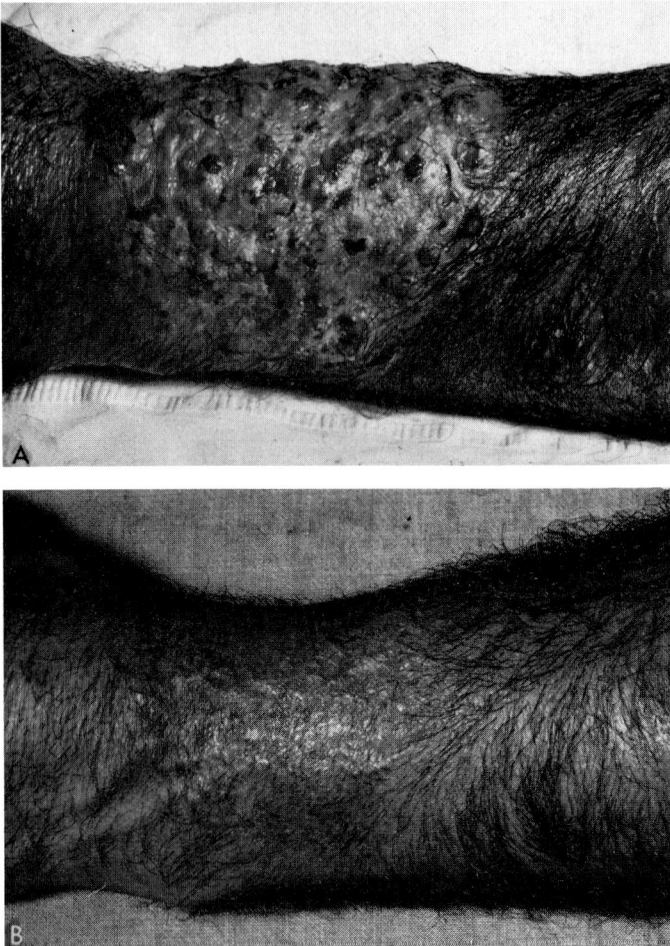

Figure 13–22 Tinea profunda. An inflammatory fungal infection (*T. faviforme*) acquired from a cow. *A*, Three weeks after onset. Almost no constitutional reaction. *B*, Eight weeks later. Spontaneous involution occurred; wet compresses and rest were the only treatments.

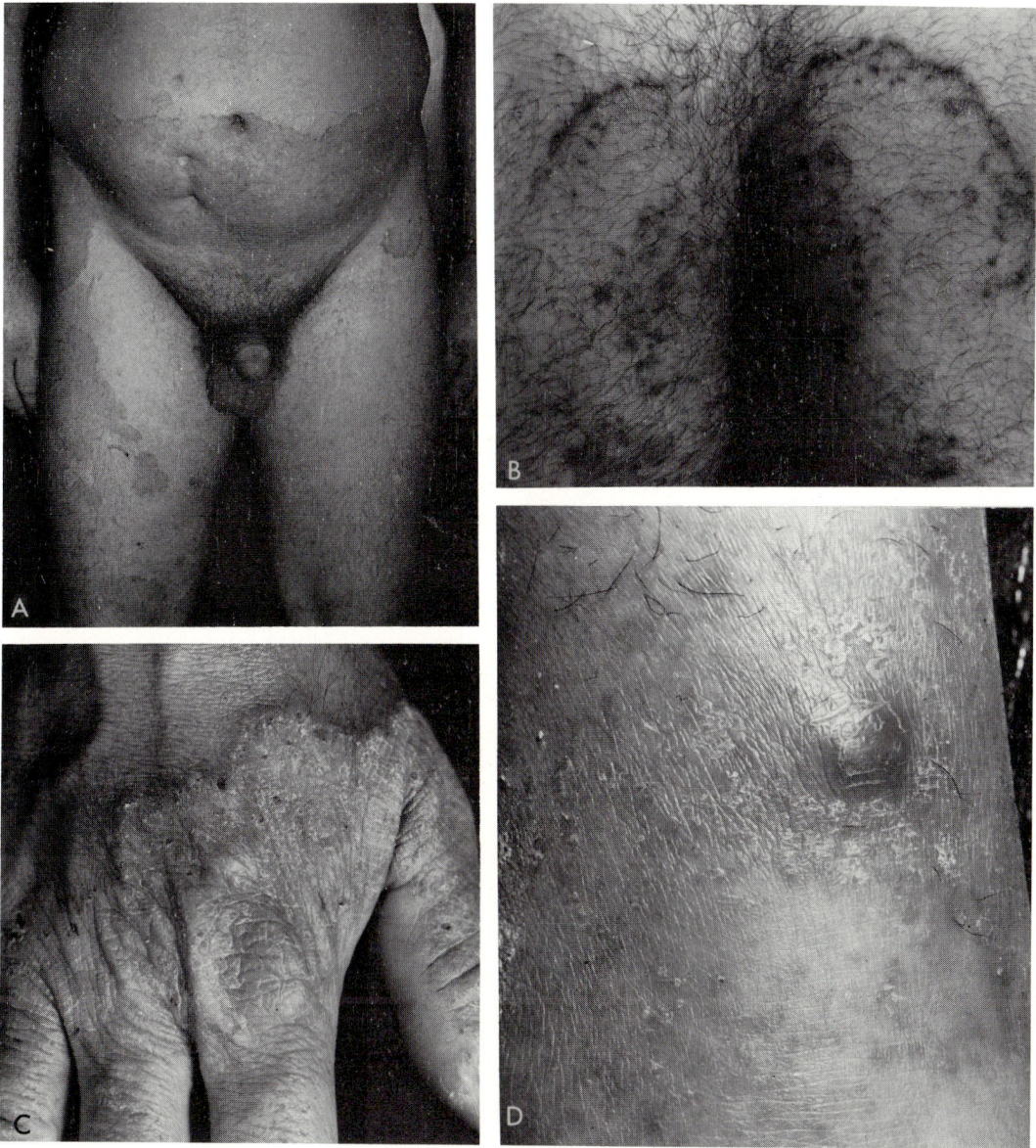

Figure 13–23 *T. rubrum* ringworm. *A*, Extensive involvement seen principally in warm, humid climates or in individuals with various systemic illnesses. *B*, Circinate lesions of buttocks. This degree of symmetry is unusual. Note advancing border and recrudescence at central portions. The intervening portion is temporarily resistant to infection. *C*, Hand lesion. The patient had noted recrudescence each summer for many years. During cold weather the skin appeared almost normal. *D*, "Majocchi's granuloma" of lower leg due to *T. rubrum*. Note surrounding scaling, betraying fungal infection.

essentially an intertriginous infection starting in the crural and/or perineal folds, with extension onto the upper inner surfaces of the thighs and, occasionally, onto the external genitalia or posteriorly over the perineum. The disease is not, of and by itself, seriously disabling as a rule, but it is frequently rendered so by inappro-

priate irritating treatment. The male genitalia, especially the scrotum, are exceedingly susceptible to primary irritants or sensitizers, and when an eczematous reaction is produced, it tends to persist for much longer than in most other areas of the body. Itching of the male genitalia is often marked, as compared with other

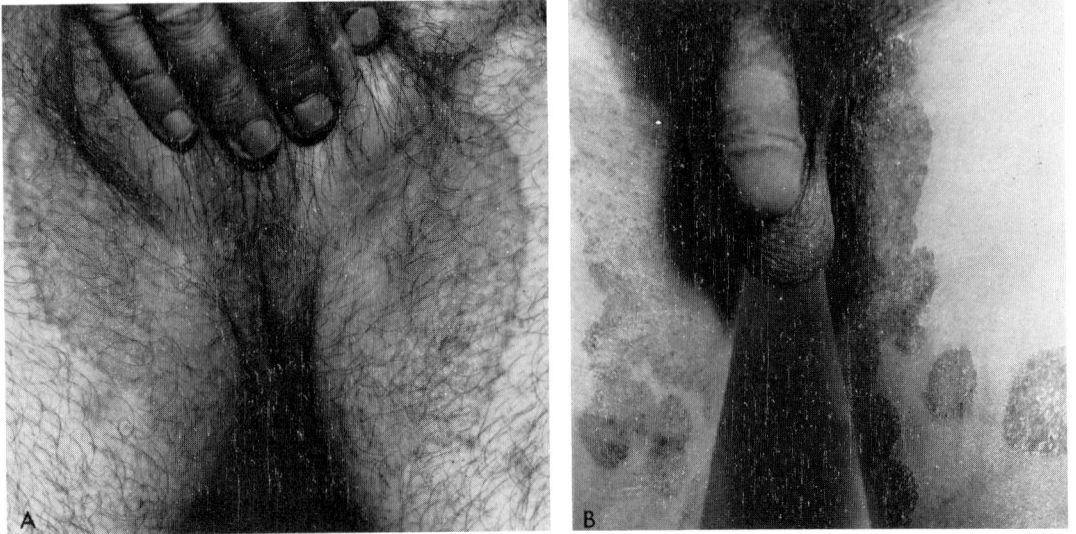

Figure 13-24   Tinea cruris. *A,* Chronic long-standing lesions. *B,* More extensive involvement of type seen most frequently in the tropics.

portions of the skin, and scratch dermatitis or chronic neurodermatitis are frequent sequels of inflammation in the region. Moreover, the region is highly vulnerable to sweat retention and miliaria, which is sometimes of pustular character.

Tinea cruris is ordinarily assumed to be produced most frequently by *E. floccosum,* but this may not actually be the most common offender; both *T. rubrum* and *T. mentagrophytes* are frequently responsible. The changes produced by these different organisms are roughly similar, though *T. mentagrophytes* infections tend to be more acute and self-limited, while *T. rubrum* is, as always, productive of less inflamed chronic lesions. The involvement is ordinarily bilateral, with half-moon shaped circinate lesions on each upper inner thigh, extending out from the crural fold. Central clearing may or may not be present. The color may vary from red to brown, and scaling is not a prominent feature because the area is moist. Erythrasma may be confused with this type of ringworm infection, but it is characterized by complete lack of inflammation, the absence of an "active" border, and an orange-red to coral-pink fluorescence under the Wood's lamp. Seborrheic dermatitis, candidiasis, and psoriasis frequently occur in this area and more often than not

are confused with tinea cruris, though the clinical manifestations are rather dissimilar. The presence of a ringworm infection may easily be proved by examination of scales for filaments.

Once well established, tinea cruris tends to be recurrent. There are several factors which unquestionably favor relapse. These are:

1. High environmental temperatures and sweating, whether of thermal or emotional origin. Prickly heat is a frequent accompaniment of tinea cruris, and is markedly pruritic in this area. It is, in essence, the adult equivalent of a diaper eruption.

2. The wearing of athletic supporters or shorts which produce binding or chafing in the crotch ("jock strap itch"). Snug fitting shorts may have the same effect, acting through mechanical chafing and occlusion. Prolonged wearing of a wet bathing suit is one of the surest means of reviving tinea cruris.

3. Obesity. Established tinea cruris is much more difficult to relieve in obese persons than in thin ones. There is constant mechanical irritation of apposed surfaces, decreased opportunity for aeration and drying of the skin, increased sweating, and more difficulty in adequate hygiene, particularly in respect to rinsing soap off

the skin thoroughly. Moreover, some unfortunately obese persons cannot inspect the area except through the use of some periscopic device, and the patient may not be aware of recrudescence of the infection except through an increase in itching. Reducing diets are essential in the management of some patients with persistent tinea cruris. In these patients, particularly, the possibility of diabetes should be considered.

The diagnosis of tinea of the anus and perianal region is frequently made, but is infrequently justified. Ringworm infections are not a common source of pruritus ani. If bona fide tinea cruris occurs in the area, it is usually in the form of a circinate lesion on one side of the anus; if it is bilateral, it is almost invariably asymmetric. Such infections may occasionally spread out over the buttocks. They are most frequently due to *T. rubrum*.

Treatment

The average moderate tinea cruris, if recognized promptly, can be relieved with ease. Griseofulvin or preparations containing haloprogin or tolnaftate may be curative in two to three weeks. A preparation containing 2 to 3 per cent each of salicylic acid and sulfur incorporated in an emulsion-type base is useful. It should be applied at night. If any grease-type preparation is applied in the morning, it is often rather uncomfortable. Some fatty acid preparations, notably those containing undecylenic acid, are rather irritating when applied to the male genitalia and are not advised. Castellani's paint is a useful alternate method of treatment, though messy in respect to staining underclothing.

In very acute eruptions in the groin, whether due to tinea cruris itself or to applied medication, mild sitz baths should be used, followed by an extremely bland dusting powder or shake lotion. Aeration and rest are sometimes essential. In less severe phases in ambulatory patients, the avoidance of any tight fitting athletic equipment or clothing is crucially important. Drawers should be loose and absorbent; nylon drawers are unsatisfactory because they are clammy and nonabsorb-

ent. The area should be kept dry, both mechanically and through the use of powders. Care should be taken not to allow powders to cake in the folds. Soap should be rinsed off thoroughly; the use of a soap substitute is sometimes justified. When tinea cruris occurs during hot weather, exposure to an air-conditioned environment, even if for just a few hours daily, is helpful in relieving the invariable associated sweat retention. Strenuous athletic activity, particularly swimming, should be avoided for a time. Secondary bacterial infection is not common but should be watched for and dealt with promptly, because it may extend rapidly.

On subsidence of the acute phase, the patient should be made clearly aware of the recurrent nature of the process. Relapses can be prevented by the observance of simple precautions, without too complicated a hygienic regimen or significant restriction of physical activity.

Tinea Imbricata (Tokelau)

This distinctive variety of widespread ringworm of the glabrous skin is a tropical disease and occurs only in some regions in the southwest Pacific, Africa, and Central America (Schofield et al., 1963). Constant high heat and humidity are ordinarily necessary for its development. If these are present, the disease may be almost endemic in a given community, though individual susceptibility to the infection is the most important determining factor; it does not seem to be highly contagious. The early lesion is annular, with a circle of scales at the periphery, the scales being attached along one edge rather characteristically. Therefore, a new and larger scaling ring forms, with a zone of apparently normal skin between the rings. This phenomenon occurs successively, with the pathognomonic appearance of concentric circles, which may reach as many as 10 per lesion. The distance between the rings increases, targetwise, toward its periphery. Confluence of separate lesions may form bizarre polycyclic patterns which may involve almost the entire cutaneous surface. The inflammatory reaction is not marked as a rule, but intense itching may

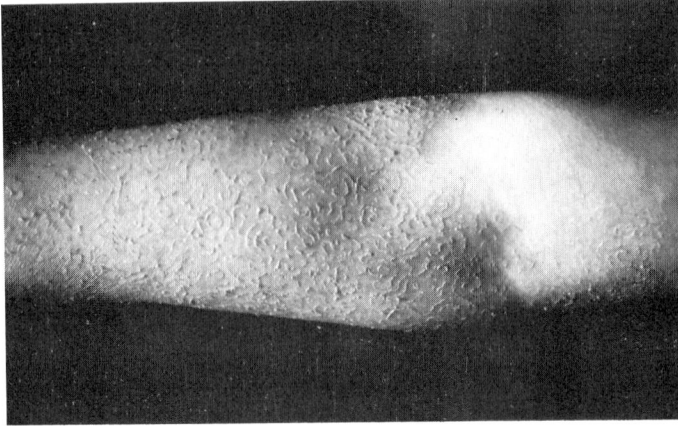

Figure 13–25 Tinea imbricata. A widespread bizarre fungal infection encountered almost entirely among native populations of certain tropical regions.

be noted, probably in part due to sweat retention. As the disease persists chronically, the concentric pattern may become obscured with the development of an appearance not unlike that seen in ichthyosis. It is said that eosinophilia is frequent. One organism, *T. concentricum*, is apparently the responsible agent. Fungal filaments are easily visualized in scrapings.

Griseofulvin is usually curative. Topical medication is relatively ineffective. Removal to a cooler climate would undoubtedly be helpful, but this is not possible in the native populations most frequently affected.

DERMATOPHYTIDS

The known facts and theories concerning the mechanism of "id" reactions associated with infections by ringworm fungi have been considered elsewhere (Chap. 3). The clinical manifestations of dermatophytids are varied, and many other dermatoses may be simulated. Since the clinical picture of an id is often not pathognomonic, and since no test is available which confirms this possibility with absolute certainty, the diagnosis must often rest on clinical judgment and is subject to some margin of error. There can be little question that the diagnosis of dermatophytid is made too frequently; it serves as a waste basket for the diagnosis of puzzling eruptions for which no cause other than a focus of fungal infection elsewhere in the skin can be uncovered.

The minimal requirements for a presumptive diagnosis of dermatophytids are:

1. A primary focus of fungal infection, usually one which is acutely inflammatory. The most common source of undoubted id reactions is kerion in children. In adults, the most common primary source is an inflammatory vesicular or bullous fungal infection of the feet. Chronic noninflammatory localized ringworm infections rarely are a source of dermatophytids, though such a diagnosis is frequently made on this trivial basis. A positive trichophytin test is essential to the diagnosis of a dermatophytid; it may be ruled out categorically if the test is negative.

2. A lesion suspected of being a dermatophytid does not, of course, contain fungi.

3. Some relation between the waxing and waning of the primary fungal infection and the "id" respectively should be apparent. If their clinical course in respect to exacerbations is completely independent, the diagnosis of dermatophytid is unlikely.

Clinical Variants of Dermatophytids

Fungal id reactions, like drug eruptions, are morphologically versatile. The following are reaction patterns more commonly seen in id eruptions:

VESICULAR IDS OF THE HANDS. The pattern is one of dyshidrosis and may consist of small recurrent vesicles to large acute bullae. The palms and the inner sides of the fingers are most markedly involved.

PAPULAR IDS. These are small erythematous papules, often grouped follicular lesions, which appear on the trunk particularly. This type is most frequently associated with kerion of the scalp.

ERYSIPELAS-LIKE ID OF THE LOWER EXTREMITIES. This is an uncommon type of id, difficult to differentiate from recurrent bacterial infection. The picture is that of a recurrent superficial cellulitis, the duration of which is brief. The existence of this type of id has been denied by some, but it would appear to be a valid entity.

ERYTHEMA ANNULARE CENTRIFUGUM. This is one of the almost innumerable variants of erythema multiforme which *occasionally*, though by no means always, may be a dermatophytid. The lesions are of annular urticarial nature, and irregular concentric rings may be seen. The eruption may be very mild and is easily overlooked in some cases. The primary lesion is an erythematous papule which enlarges peripherally to form a ring, the border of which is red and rather hivelike, while the central region is often yellowish and shows a fine branny scale. At times, the lesion may be reproduced by the intradermal injection of trichophytin into uninvolved skin. However, when trichophytin is injected into the center of an annular dermatophytid, a negative or anergic response may be elicited.

VASCULAR RESPONSES. The following reaction patterns may be representative of allergic sensitivity to ringworm in some cases: (a) erythema nodosum, (b) erythema multiforme (rare), (c) indefinite macular rashes. The hypothesis that migratory thrombophlebitis or thromboangiitis obliterans are id reactions is unproved, in our opinion. It has been suggested that urticaria may be an id at times, but if it is, the association must be rare indeed.

MISCELLANEOUS. Pityriasis rosea-like and eczematous eruptions on the trunk have been described as id reactions. This causation is probably rare; the diagnosis must be made cautiously and strictly on

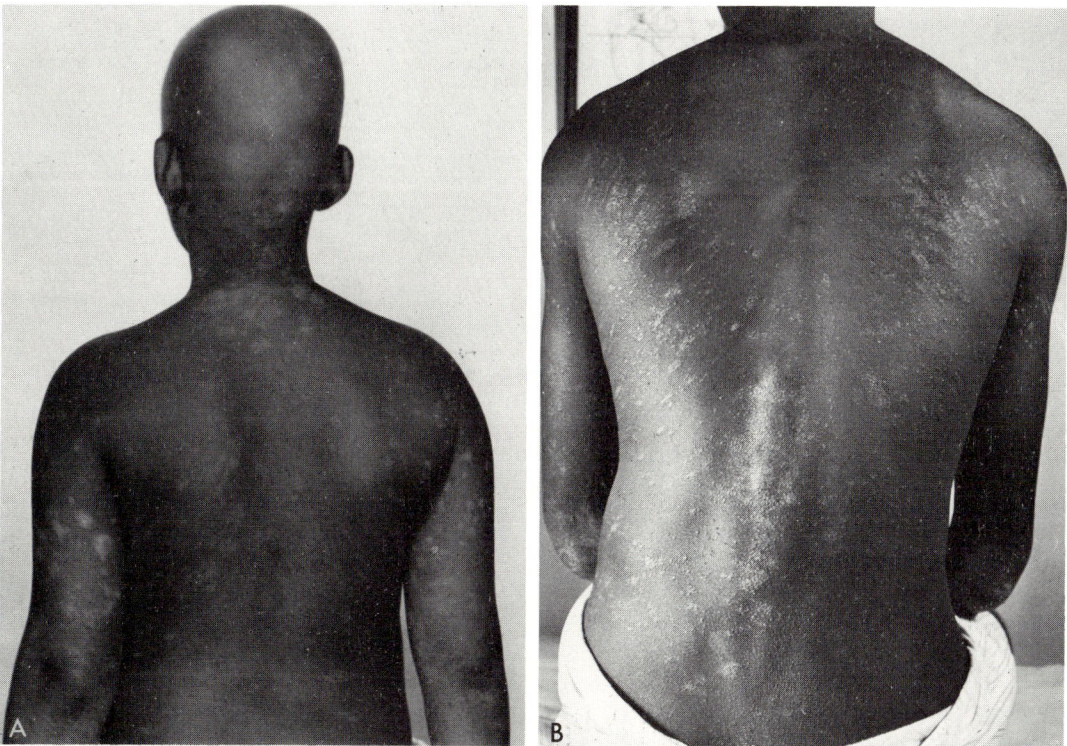

Figure 13–26 *A*, Pityriasis rosea-like "id" following x-ray epilation for tinea capitis. *B*, Grouped folliculopapular "id" developing during course of inflammatory *M. audouini* tinea capitis. Spontaneous cure occurred.

the merits of the findings in the individual patient.

FUNGAL INFECTIONS OF NAILS

Invasion of the nail apparatus by fungi produces changes of varying degree which are indistinguishable in respect to the causative fungus. A variety of other dermatoses affect nail growth and are frequently misdiagnosed as fungal infections. However, the clinical features of these nail conditions are ordinarily sufficient to distinguish them. The fungus which causes nail infections most commonly is *T. rubrum*. Next in importance is *T. mentagrophytes*, though it infects the toenails most commonly, rarely the fingernails. Other species of dermatophytes, including members of the genera Microsporum and Epidermophyton, cause nail infections uncommonly, with the possible exception of *T. violaceum*, which has been reported as the responsible agent in fingernail infections by observers in some Far Eastern countries. Candidiasis of the nails, a condition of different etiology and course, is considered elsewhere.

Ringworm infections of the toenails are an exceedingly common condition in races accustomed to wearing shoes. It is almost inevitable in persons who have had recurrent attacks of athlete's foot or who suffer from the chronic squamous type of foot ringworm caused by *T. rubrum*. It is encountered most frequently in adult males, though it is by no means uncommon in females. Ringworm of the toenails is of little medical importance, since it causes no subjective distress unless the distortion is very marked, with resultant impingement of the nail margin on the soft tissues. The average older male pays no attention to fungal infections of the toenails and accepts gradual distortion as an inevitable process of aging. In females accustomed to wearing open-toed shoes and to zealous cosmetic care of the toenails, changes due to fungal infection are ordinarily noted quite promptly and are a cause of some mental distress.

Griseofulvin may be curative, but must be given over a period of six months or longer. Treatment failures are common, especially in patients with peripheral vascular disease. Topical antifungal compounds are completely ineffective in reversing the changes and do not have any demonstrable effects in preventing progression of the infection. Nails which become distorted and ridged may be trimmed and filed off, and well-trained chiropodists perform an expert and useful service in this regard. Patients with ringworm of the toenails should wear nonocclusive shoes; they should go barefooted as much as possible, since much of the distortion may be due to mechanical pressure. The nails should be cut squarely across, not rounded. Mechanical trauma to the soft tissues and resultant occasional paronychial infections will have to be dealt with appropriately as they occur. In some patients, orthopedic therapy may be necessary to relieve conditions produced by overcrowding or overlapping of the toes.

Avulsion of the nail plate alone will not result in cure of fungal infections of the toenails, but when accompanied by treatment with griseofulvin, the course of treatment may be shortened to 3 or 4 months.

Ringworm infections of the fingernails are, understandably, a source of much psychic trauma because of the cosmetic implications of the disease. The infection ordinarily remains limited to one or a few nails for a time, or sometimes indefinitely. In patients in whom there is a distortion of all ten fingernails simultaneously, some other cause is more likely. Ringworm infections of the fingernails are practically always due to *T. rubrum*, at least in the U.S.A. Careful examination of the skin surface will ordinarily reveal a focus of the infection on the hands, feet or elsewhere. Associated *T. rubrum* infections of the skin of the hands may produce minimal changes, such as very slight erythema and small scaling patches. In such infections, the lesion may extend directly up over the nail folds.

The amount of solid scientific information regarding the pathogenesis of diseases of the nails is relatively small, and the diagnostic classifications available are frequently uninformative (see Chap. 26). The term "ringworm of the nails" is not the most satisfactory one for fungal infections of this structure, because the hard keratin of the nail plate is not the primary

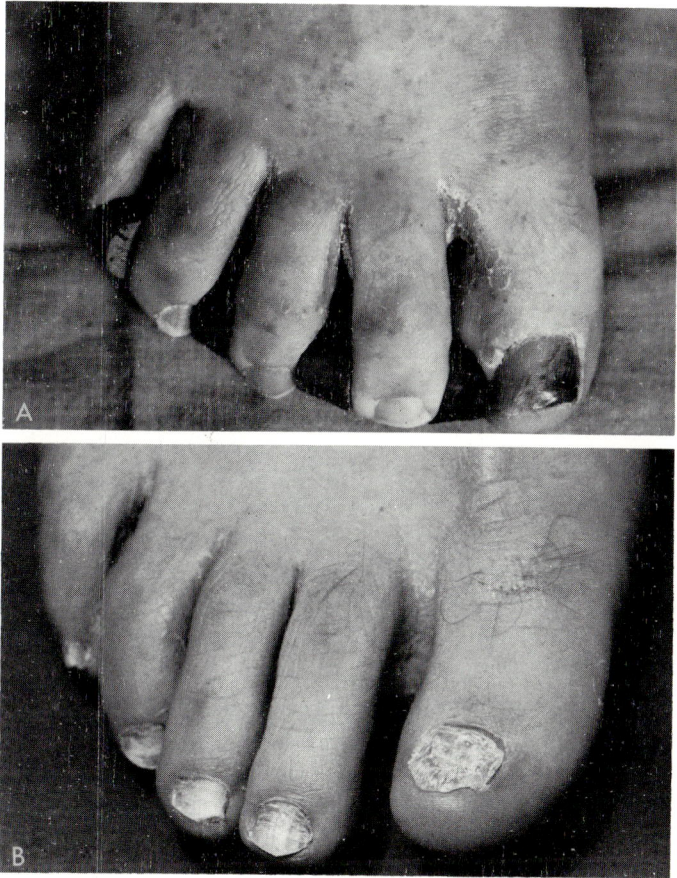

Figure 13–27 *A,* Chronic fungal infection of all interspaces. The great toenail is serving as a dependable source of reinfection. *B,* Friability of toenails due to fungal infection.

site of attack. An understanding of the normal progression of ringworm infections of the nail organ is helpful in diagnosis and treatment. The infection of the nail organ proper ordinarily begins in the lateral nail grooves, which normally contain considerable amounts of soft keratin in the gutter between the nail fold and the nail plate (see Figure 13–28). The infection may spread into this gutter by direct extension, or fungal elements from some other focus on the body may be implanted.

Ringworm infections of the nail organ vary greatly in their manifestations (Zaias, 1972), from changes which are hardly detectable to the full-blown infection in which the nail plate is almost completely disintegrated. The infection may be entirely confined to the lateral nail groove, failing to invade the substance of the nail plate at all, or doing so to a very trivial degree. This is the most minor expression of ringworm of the nail organ, and it is usually overlooked. It is frequently encountered in patients with extensive ringworm infections of the palm.

Further extension of the infection occurs from the lateral grooves *underneath the lateral borders of the nail* into the keratin produced by the nail bed. It then extends upward into the lower surface of the nail plate. The infection frequently becomes static at this point, progressing no further over a period of years, and resulting only in white or yellow discoloration of the lateral borders of the nail and minor disorganization of the involved portion of the nail plate. If the affected zones are firm and intact, the changes do not ordinarily cause much concern to the patient.

With further progression of the disease, the fungus extends farther into the lower portion of the nail plate, and a disturbance of the nail bed results, transforming it

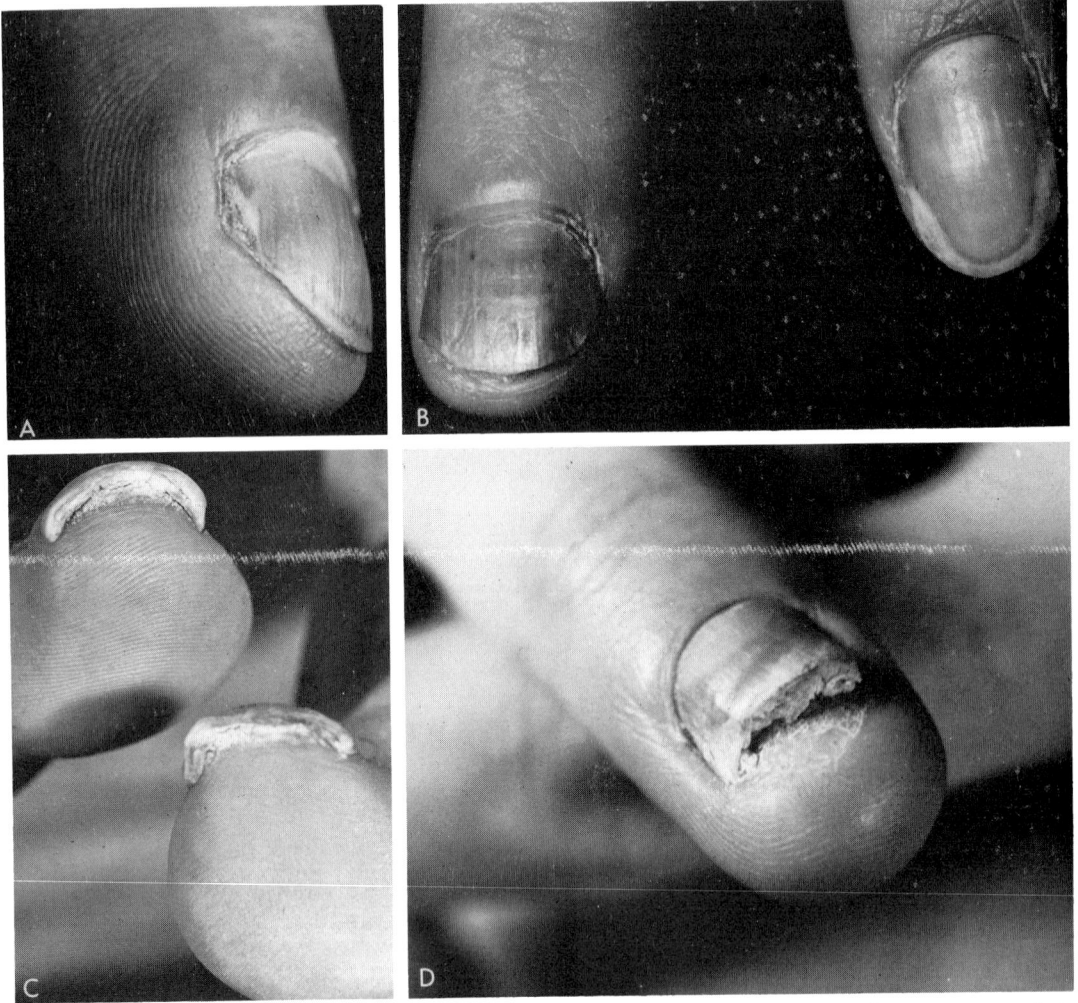

Figure 13–28 Fungal infection of nails. *A*, Early involvement at lateral margin. The infection is *primarily in the underlying nail bed;* the nail itself is invaded secondarily. *B*, Long-standing (left) and early (right) onychomycosis. *C*, Piling up of subungual kerototic debris is the cardinal sign of onychomycosis. *D*, Separation, disintegration and partial loss of nail plate.

into a thickened membrane which synthesizes keratin rapidly. This stimulation of the nail bed epithelium to produce soft keratin is the most characteristic change in well-defined ringworm infections of the nail, since it produces an accumulation of variable amounts of subungual hyperkeratosis. This change may, however, be produced in other diseases and is not pathognomonic for ringworm infection. The fungus proliferates abundantly in this subungual mass, serving as a mycotic reservoir for extension of the infection farther into the nail plate. The progression from this point on is variable. The nail bed may become very hyperkeratotic, lifting up and separating the nail plate. The keratinous debris may fuse with the over-riding nail plate and give the impression that the nail itself is greatly thickened.

The nail matrix remains uninvolved, and this is characteristic of the biologic course of all superficial ringworm infections, because these fungi are incapable of invading living tissue. The destructive changes in the nail occur after it is formed, not because of any primary disturbance in its growth. In some instances the nail plate may be very widely separated from the bed, and the curved nail becomes troublesome mechanically. Destruction of the nail plate usually occurs distally in the beginning, but may extend all the way to the proximal portion.

Primary invasion of the nail plate is rare, but may occur in *white superficial onychomycosis* (leukonychia trichophytica). In this curious entity, opaque, well-demarcated, soft white spots appear in the surface of the nail plate. These are found to contain masses of fungal filaments. *T. mentagrophytes* has been most frequently cultured from this condition, but *Cephalosporium* and *Aspergillus* species and *Fusarium oxysporium* have also been reported. The fungus appears to invade the nail plate on its surface forming punctate colonies which gradually enlarge and may coalesce to involve the entire surface.

Another unusual variant of onychomycosis is seen in *proximal subungual onychomycosis*. This condition is characterized by the formation of white areas extending distally from under the proximal nail fold. The lesion is not on the surface of the nail plate, but rather in the deeper layers of the nail. Scrapings from the nail plate reveal abundant hyphae if the outer layers of the nail plate are first removed. The point of entry would appear to be under the proximal nail fold. As the nail grows, the white areas are carried distally with the nail plate. This uncommon variant of onychomycosis has been reported more often in the European literature. *T. rubrum*, *T. megnini*, *T. schoenleinii*, *T. tonsurans*, and *T. mentagrophytes* have been recovered on culture.

In summary, it is important to realize that most fungal infections of the nail organ primarily affect the nail bed and invade the nail plate only secondarily. The matrix remains uninvolved. Simple removal of the nail plate does not rid the region of the primary source of the fungal infection. It is clear from this that in making scrapings for direct examination or culture from the nails, it is important to obtain the subungual keratinized debris and not material from the nail surface, because only in advanced cases will the fungus penetrate upward through the entire thickness of the nail and be recoverable from the surface. Fungi may be demonstrable only with difficulty in undoubted infections, because they may be sparsely distributed through the keratinous debris, and the sources of contaminating material are numerous. Cultures should be planted on media containing cycloheximide and antibacterial antibiotics in order to suppress overgrowth by fungal and bacterial contaminants. In our own experience, *T. rubrum* is the organism most frequently recovered. Our experience with *T. violaceum* infections is limited, but it is believed that the pathogenesis and extension of the infection with this organism are quite similar to those seen with *T. rubrum*.

Secondary Mold Infections

A great deal of confusion and debate has arisen from the fact that the keratinous tissue of diseased nail organs furnishes an ideal substrate for the growth of numerous microorganisms. A number of organisms which are usually considered to be saprophytic molds, especially species of Aspergillus, have been incriminated as etiologic agents of onychomycosis. *It is our belief that the only fungi which can incite the typical manifestations of onychomycosis are the dermatophytes or ringworm fungi.* There is no indication that the saprophytic molds are capable of attacking keratin and causing its dissolution. They are only opportunistic residents growing in a favorable habitat. Unfortunately, the cause of many dystrophic changes of nails is obscure, and the finding of any microorganism, however nonpathogenic it may be, may lead to its incrimination as the cause of the changes present. A nail which is diseased from other causes invites dermatophytes as well as mold organisms; this constitutes a *secondary* type of ringworm. Under these circumstances, even the recovery of a pathogenic dermatophyte may not furnish absolute proof that the basic nail changes are due to a fungal infection.

An example of secondary onychomycosis is seen in ringworm infections of nails which are diseased from psoriasis, in which the dermatosis produces hyperkeratosis of the nail bed. In such instances, there is a co-existence of psoriasis with the fungal infection and, indeed, the latter may sometimes persist when the psoriasis has subsided. The two diseases closely mimic each other insofar as the nail changes are concerned, and at times differentiation may be extremely difficult.

Treatment

Griseofulvin must be given for many months to produce clearing of ringworm infections of the nails. Treatment failures are common, especially when the toenails are involved. This may be due to the slower rate of growth of toenails and the increased moisture of the subungual keratinous debris which enables the fungal infection to maintain a state of equilibrium with the growing nail. We are not aware of any topically applied preparation which has the slightest influence on ringworm infections of the nails. This is to be expected, because the primary site of infection is under the nail plate. Efforts may be made to remove the nail mechanically or by chemicals which dissolve keratin, but it is ordinarily impossible to do this to a degree sufficient to expose the causative fungi. The application of a drying agent such as 2 per cent thymol in chloroform several times daily under the nail plate may be helpful.

Under some circumstances, surgical avulsion of the nail may be curative, but it frequently fails. The best results are obtained if only one or two nails are involved and griseofulvin is given post-operatively until the nail has regrown.

The technique of surgical avulsion is outlined in Figure 13–29. It is important to realize that simple removal of the nail plate will not necessarily remove a major portion of the fungi. The nail bed must be carefully curetted, along with the lateral grooves, and all keratinized debris removed. Following removal, preparations containing haloprogin or tolnaftate may be applied two or three times daily.

SYSTEMIC FUNGAL INFECTIONS
(The Deep Mycoses)

The systemic fungal infections are produced by organisms which, unlike the superficial ringworm fungi, are capable of extending into living tissue rather than being confined to dead keratinous tissue. The clinical manifestation of this group of fungal infections are exceedingly diverse. The following diseases are included:

Candidiasis
Coccidioidomycosis
Blastomycosis (North American Blastomycosis)
Paracoccidioidomycosis (South American Blastomycosis)
Histoplasmosis
Actinomycosis
Nocardiosis
Sporotrichosis
Phaeosporotrichosis
Cryptococcosis (torulosis)
Chromomycosis (Chromoblastomycosis)
Mycetoma (Madura foot)
Rhinosporidiosis
Aspergillosis
Phycomycosis

CANDIDIASIS
(Moniliasis)

Though candidiasis is primarily a cutaneous or mucous membrane disease, it occasionally produces systemic involvement. There can be little question that the disease is diagnosed far more frequently than is justified. Confusion and error have arisen, and the etiologic role of Candida in many conditions which are accepted as examples of candidiasis is highly questionable. The following principle is of paramount importance in the interpretation of this group of diseases:

Candida albicans *exists most commonly as a harmless colonist on abnormal skin or normal and abnormal mucous membranes, and in the gastrointestinal tract. Isolation of the organism from a disease process means, of and by itself, little or nothing. Even when Candida are present in profusion, their pathogenic role is doubtful, because the organism readily seeds itself in many preexistent pathologic processes. The virulence of Candida is extremely limited. In all instances of supposed candidiasis, it is obligatory to search for the underlying primary disorder, whether of local or systemic nature.*

C. albicans is not the only member of the genus Candida which on occasion

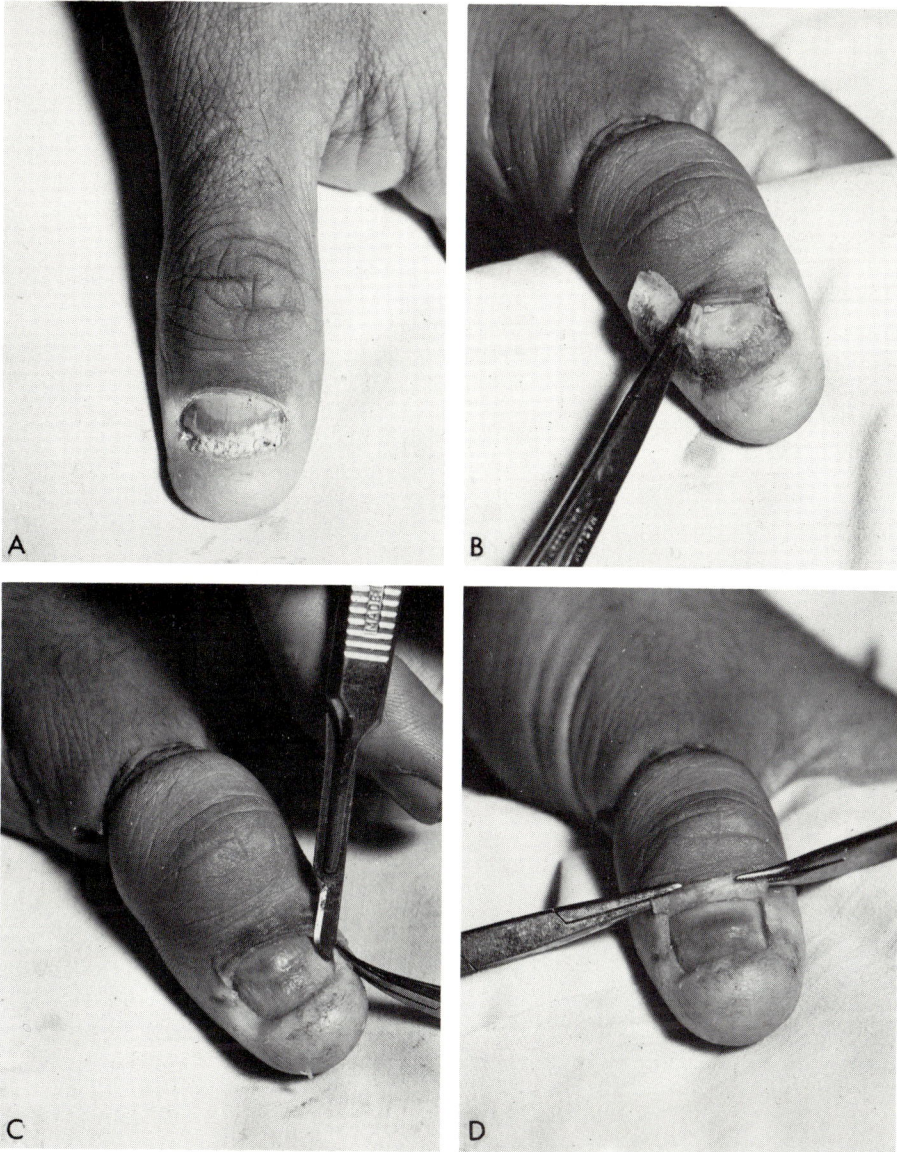

Figure 13–29 Surgical avulsion of thumb nail infected with *T. rubrum.* (All the other fingernails and the hands were uninvolved.) *A,* Pre-operative. Distal end of nail disorganized; nail bed has produced a mass of keratinized debris which abounds with fungi. *B,* Nail plate has been grasped with a small pointed hemostat and simply "rolled" off its moorings revealing the semi-lunar whitish mount of tissue, the matrix. It is uninfected and care is taken to leave it alone. Distal to the matrix is the fungus-laden kerototic product of the nail bed. All of this must be removed by scraping with a scalpel. *C,* Nail bed has been scraped clean, including the lateral gutters, a favorite place for the fungus to hide. The aim is to remove all the horny material but no more, a delicate objective requiring experience. *D,* The posterior nail fold has been retracted and small shreds of deeply lodged nail plate removed. Griseofulvin should be given post-operatively until the nail has regrown.

may acquire some pathogenicity. A host of other Candida species are resident organisms in the body, and some of these, under special predisposing circumstances, may incite disease. *C. albicans* heads the list in frequency, followed by *C. tropicalis.*

The several clinical expressions of candidiasis may most conveniently be divided into the following groups: (1) candidiasis of the mucous membranes, (2) candidiasis of the skin, (3) chronic mucocutaneous candidiasis, and (4) systemic candidiasis.

Candidiasis of the Mucous Membranes

THRUSH. This disorder is the proto-type of mucous membrane candidiasis and, with vulvovaginal candidiasis, constitutes the most common expression of the infection. The hallmark of the disease is the development of creamy white patches on any portion of the mucous membranes of the mouth, usually sparing the pharynx. The patches are composed of a soft creamy or crumbly material, are generally not very adherent, and often reveal a red base when removed. They may suggest a membrane but cannot be detached as a membranous film. There may be only a few scattered patches on the tongue, gums, palate, and buccal membrane, or through confluence, the mouth may be covered with a dense white, creamy coating, especially on the tongue. In extensive cases, the patches may extend into the trachea, upper bronchi, and even into the esophagus. Cracks and fissures of the corners of the mouth, *perlèche*, may be coated with the creamy material. True candidal perlèche is usually associated with evidence of the disease elsewhere in the mouth. Perlèche existing alone is *rarely* due to *C. albicans*, and the diagnosis is not valid unless the creamy material, the signal finding of candidiasis, is present. In all varieties of mucous membrane candidiasis, the creamy white patch, which on microscopic examination is seen to be comprised *predominantly* of budding cells and filaments, is a condition *sine qua non* for diagnosis. The white patches are actually almost pure colonies of the fungus. The organism is situated mostly *on* and not in the tissue of the mucous membrane. The organism may abound in the "normal" mouth, but this is not tantamount to a diagnosis of candidiasis. In particular, one should be aware of this source of error if the patient has received wide spectrum antibiotics, for then the mouth, whether it appears normal or not, will teem with the organism. There is no evidence that any of the various inflammatory types of mouth lesions, the red beefy tongue of intense glossitis, the atrophic shining papilla-less tongue of chronic glossitis, painful red stomatitides, acute pharyngitis, etc., are expressions of candidiasis, even though there may sometimes actually be evidence of thrush. True candidiasis of the mucous membranes is a relatively uncommon complication of antibiotic therapy; the cause of inflammatory oral reactions to these agents is unknown.

Thrush, formerly common in sick, weak infants a few days after birth, and in elderly individuals in poor health, must now be regarded, at least in the U.S.A., as a rather infrequent disease. This may well be a direct result of improved nutrition, better medical care, and a generally healthier population. When thrush does occur in a young infant, immediate inquiry into the general health is indicated, and the mother should be examined for vulvovaginal candidiasis. Thrush in the newborn is a not infrequent complication of vulvovaginal candidiasis at the time of delivery.

VULVOVAGINAL CANDIDIASIS. The above analysis of the pathogenicity of *C. albicans* and the criteria of true infection of the oral mucous membranes hold equally well for vaginal disturbances. The pertinent facts are:

1. The organism is often present in the *normal* vagina. Its incidence is increased in pregnancy, diabetes, and in women taking oral contraceptives or antibiotics. The organism, therefore, may be a normal resident, and asymptomatic carriers are frequently encountered.

2. There is an increased incidence of candidiasis in individuals with pathologic changes in the vagina and cervix; patients with discharges of whatever origin harbor *C. albicans* more frequently. It is hard to say how often *C. albicans* is a harmless colonist thriving in a milieu made favorable by preexisting disease. An associated trichomonas infection may be a promoting factor, in which case the fungus should not be considered the *cause* of the discharge. The coexistence of these two organisms is common.

3. A white or yellow curdy discharge, sometimes likened to watered-down buttermilk, containing a dense mass of budding cells and filaments, is the only reliable sign of true candidiasis of the vagina. It may be difficult or impossible to tell how much of the inflammatory reaction is actually related to some preexisting disease which prepared the way for the candidal infection. Usually, in addition to the rather thin discharge, there is redness and

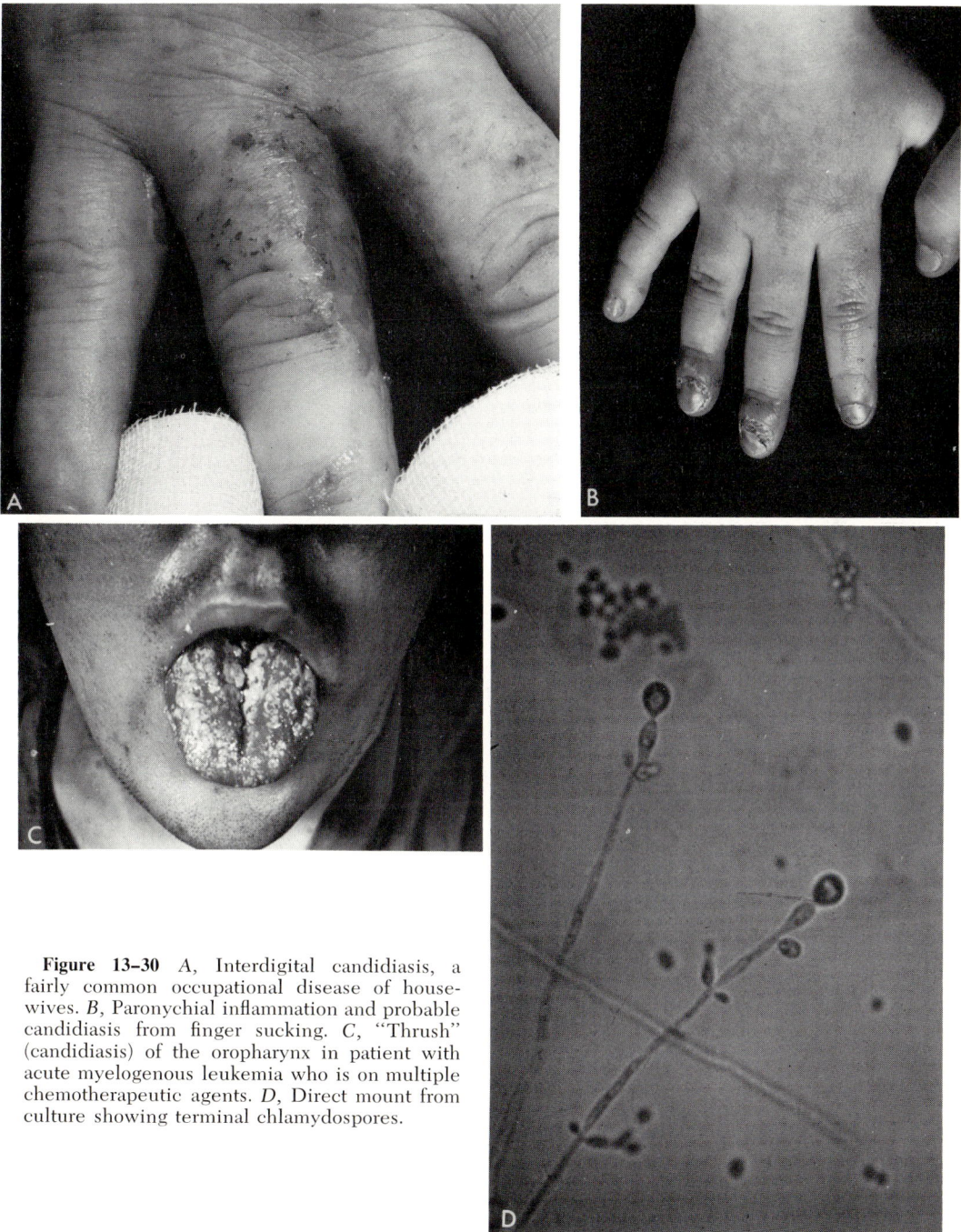

Figure 13–30 *A*, Interdigital candidiasis, a fairly common occupational disease of housewives. *B*, Paronychial inflammation and probable candidiasis from finger sucking. *C*, "Thrush" (candidiasis) of the oropharynx in patient with acute myelogenous leukemia who is on multiple chemotherapeutic agents. *D*, Direct mount from culture showing terminal chlamydospores.

smarting of the vagina, and examination often reveals curdy flakes attached to the vaginal wall or in the discharge. *Itching of the vulva is a constant complaint.* The vulvar region frequently becomes red, swollen, and intensely pruritic, but this often does not reflect actual invasion of the skin by the fungus so much as a secondary effect due to the vaginal discharge. However, a true candidal intertrigo may develop. The vulva, perineum, and inguinal crease may show an acute macerated, eroded, red, weeping dermatitis with flaccid satellite pustules or erosions. Pregnancy is a definite predisposing factor, as is diabetes. Asymptomatic individuals who harbor *C. albicans* may suddenly develop candidiasis when they become pregnant or when there is some alteration in the integrity of the vagina as when, for instance, a pessary is worn. The healthy vagina rarely acquires candidiasis when the organism is introduced experimentally; if it does, the infection is trivial and self-limited. Newborn babies may acquire the infection via passage through the infected birth canal. Conjugal transmission of the disease to the male has been reported, particularly in the uncircumcised, but it is difficult to assess the validity of such instances or their frequency. Candidiasis in the male has been represented as balanitis, balanoposthitis, monilial intertrigo, and a dermatitis of the scrotum and perineum. Such lesions cannot be accepted unreservedly as candidiasis because of contact with an infected spouse, unless the usual diagnostic criteria are satisfied by the demonstration of budding cells and filaments in scrapings from the affected area. Whenever true candidal balanoposthitis occurs in the absence of an infected sexual partner, diabetes must be suspected.

Cutaneous Candidiasis

The varieties included under this heading are (a) candidal intertrigo, (b) candidal paronychia (and associated nail dystrophy), and (c) candidiasis of the glabrous skin.

CANDIDAL INTERTRIGO. Again it is necessary to emphasize that the mere recovery of *C. albicans* from an intertriginous lesion is not tantamount to a diagnosis of candidiasis. Clinical findings, plus the demonstration of *large* quantities of the fungus in scrapings from the lesions, provide the chief criteria for diagnosis. The most characteristic manifestations of candidal intertrigo are well-defined, weeping, eroded lesions with a scalloped border, usually having a collar of overhanging sodden scales and an intensely red base. Greater confidence may be placed in the diagnosis if there are, outside the main intertriginous plaque,

satellite flaccid vesicopustules, which are thought to represent the primary lesions. The chief sites of involvement are the groin, the axilla, the intergluteal cleft, and the inframammary region. It will be seen that seborrheic dermatitis also commonly localizes in such sites, a circumstance which has led to great confusion, for *C. albicans* may, of course, colonize the lesions of that disorder. Furthermore, ordinary intertrigo may support the residence of *C. albicans*. *C. albicans* may often be isolated from intertriginous macerated lesions of the foot, resembling athlete's foot, posing the perplexing problem of its pathogenic status. In "true" cases, most or all of the interdigital spaces are involved and the lesions commonly extend onto the dorsum of the foot, unlike ordinary athlete's foot. From ancient times, physicians have been intrigued by a special type of candidal intertrigo occurring on the webs between the fingers, usually between the third and fourth fingers, perhaps localizing especially in this site because anatomically this interspace is narrower and is more prone to retain water. This variant is honored by the mellifluous name of "erosio interdigitalis blastomycetica." It is most often encountered in those who have their hands in water a good deal—housewives, bartenders, etc.

CANDIDAL PARONYCHIA (WITH ASSOCIATED NAIL DYSTROPHY). While it is probable that there is a definite paronychial entity due to *C. albicans*, uncertainty and doubt accompany any effort to define it decisively. Nail dystrophy or deformity in so-called candidal onychomycosis is a purely secondary process, subsequent to chronic paronychia. *C. albicans* has no keratinolytic enzymes and does not disorganize nail substance. The ridges, furrows, and discoloration of the nails are not different from the nail-plate defects induced by any type of chronic paronychia and are brought about through damage to the *matrix*. Naturally, a disturbance in the matrix is reflected in the formation of an abnormal nail, but it is significant that the nail is usually hard, has good luster, though it may present a brownish discoloration, and does not crumble away or disorganize as in true onychomycosis. If the matrix is severely injured, the nail defects will be more marked. The fungus is not ordinarily found in the substance of the nail plate except when its formation has been so faulty as to permit penetration of the organism into the porous interstices. The absence of subungual keratosis, another characteristic sign of true onychomycosis, reflects lack of involvement of the nail bed.

Paronychial involvement always antecedes the nail changes in candidiasis and is not particularly distinctive from chronic paronychial inflammation due to other causes. The paronychial tissue is swollen, red, and relatively nontender. It does not become fluctuant, though from time to time a drop of pus may exude or be expressed from under the nail fold. The nail folds of several fingers are usually involved; the condition is persistent. Whether *C. albicans* is the true cause of this disorder or is a secondary invader, perhaps aggravating the basic inflammatory process, is a legitimate question to which there is no conclusive answer. Other chronic paronychias of unknown origin clinically indistinguishable from candidiasis are common, and they would unhesitatingly be labeled candidiasis if culture yielded *C. albicans*.

CANDIDIASIS OF THE GLABROUS SKIN. Judged from the viewpoints presented above, the entities in this group can be considered only as questionable expressions of candidiasis (Maibach and Kligman, 1962). "Water bath dermatitis" is the name given to a disorder produced by excessive immersion in baths or by prolonged exposure to occlusive wet dressings. The skin becomes macerated and eroded, has a red base and satellite pustules. At best, this is an expression of secondary candidiasis due to injudicious treatment. It is said that a somewhat similar condition may emerge, especially in intertriginous areas, following the prolonged local application of wide spectrum antibiotics to a preexisting dermatitis. So-called generalized cutaneous candidiasis, usually observed in the newborn, is a vague disorder with widespread lesions of an eczematous exudative or vesiculopustular nature accompanied by more certain evidence of candidiasis in the form of thrush of the oral cavity or glossitis. There is some resemblance to seborrheic dermatitis or psoriasis, and one wonders whether this or some other widespread eruption, perhaps congenitally determined, is not the primary condition providing a favorable "soil" for Candida to become established. In most cases there is associated vulvovaginal candidiasis of the mother and the infection was acquired during transit through the candidal birth

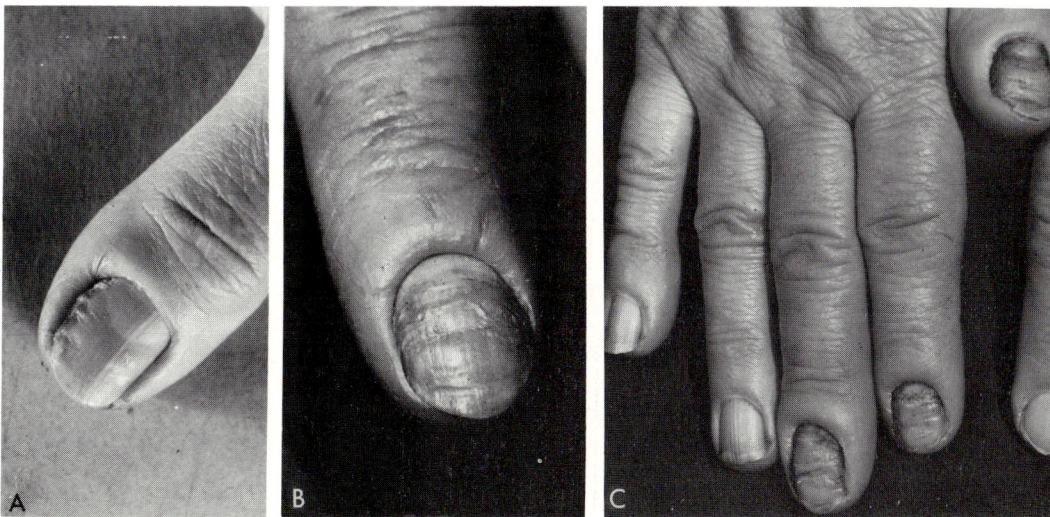

Figure 13–31 Candidal paronychia with secondary changes in the nail plate. Injury or disease is a usual prerequisite to infection (for example, physical trauma, frequent immersion of hands). Paronychial changes are ordinarily absent in ringworm of the nails.

canal. This type of generalized cutaneous candidiasis is usually responsive to treatment in the absence of associated congenital defects. Only rarely does it progress into chronic mucocutaneous candidiasis.

Chronic Mucocutaneous Candidiasis

Chronic mucocutaneous candidiasis is a progressive candidal infection which usually is associated with some constitutional defect, especially congenital thymic disorders affecting lymphocyte function (Chilgren et al., 1967). The disorder may have its onset in the neonatal period, but more often begins later in infancy or early childhood. It has been reported rarely in adults with thymoma (Maize and Lynch, 1972). It may begin as thrush, candidal paronychia, or intertrigo, but is unusually resistant to the customary treatment measures. The candidal infection spreads to involve the scalp and glabrous skin. The eruption consists of horny plaques of variable size, often with distinct papules covered with a thick, scaling crust. Coalescence of individual lesions leads to formation of bizarre, hyperkeratotic, crusted masses from which hornlike or knoblike structures protrude, sometimes reaching the striking length of 1 to 2.5 cm. Removal of the horny crusts reveals underlying granulation tissue. Scarring and loss of hair are common sequelae. The disease is refractory to treatment, but systemic candidiasis develops rarely; death may result, or the general health remain unimpaired. Innumerable fungal elements

of *C. albicans* proliferate in the crust, but generally fail to invade the living portion of the skin. Endocrinopathy is sometimes observed and usually consists of hypoparathyroidism (Montes et al., 1972), hypoadrenalism, or diabetes.

Defective cutaneous expressions of cell-mediated immunity are observed consistently (Canales et al., 1969); for example: anergy to skin testing with oidiomycin, tuberculin, mumps, diphtheria, and so forth; resistance to cutaneous sensitization with dinitrochlorobenzene; and failure to reject cutaneous homografts. Paradoxically, the lymphocytes from patients with chronic mucocutaneous candidiasis respond in vitro to phytohemagglutinin, antigens from *C. albicans*, and allogenic cells. The administration of dialyzable transfer factor or the lymphocytes from healthy donors may restore cutaneous reactivity to oidiomycin and other delayed hypersensitivity antigens (Chilgren et al., 1969). Clearing of the lesions results when cutaneous cell-mediated immunity has been restored. These observations suggest that chronic mucocutaneous candidiasis results from a deficiency of migration inhibitory factor or the presence of an inhibitor to this factor or other mediator of delayed hypersensitivity. A genetic basis has been suggested by the occasional finding of cutaneous candidiasis and cutaneous anergy in siblings. In adults, chronic mucocutaneous candidiasis may be due to thymoma-induced defects in cell-mediated immunity since similar observations have been made in the few patients reported with this condition.

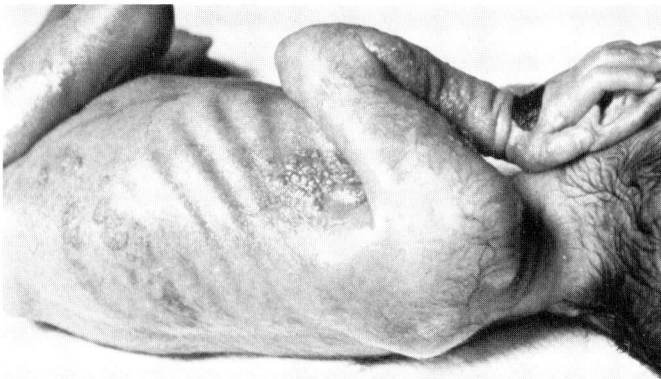

Figure 13–32 Generalized cutaneous candidiasis of the newborn. The child was delivered prematurely. The mother suffered from recurrent vulvovaginal candidiasis.

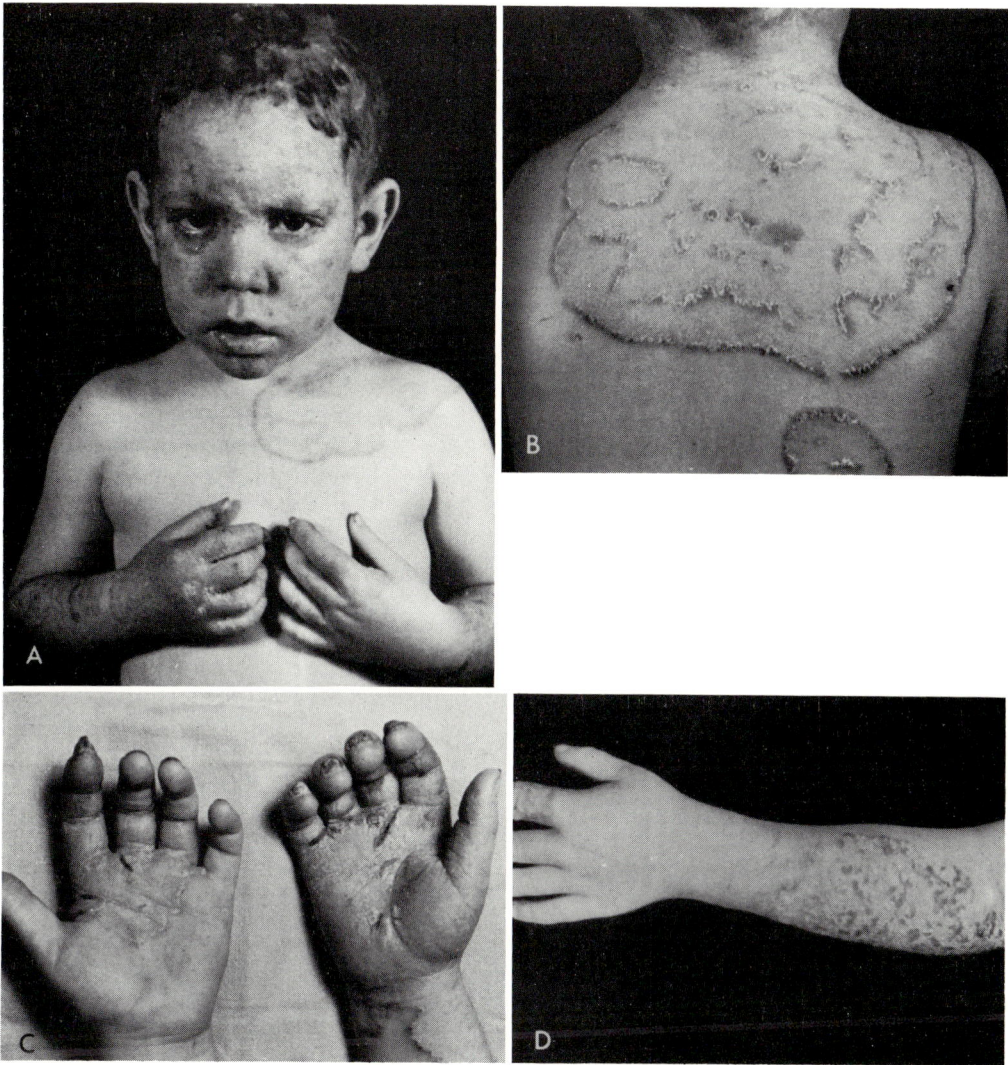

Figure 13–33 Chronic mucocutaneous candidiasis. *A*, Horny plaques and hyperkeratotic crusted masses on scalp. *B*, Coalescence of lesions to produce bizarre polycyclic plaques resembling ringworm of the glabrous skin. *C*, Thickened palms may resemble psoriasis or pityriasis rubra pilaris. *D*, Psoriasiform plaque on the arm. *Candida albicans* was demonstrated in profusion on biopsies, scrapings, and cultures from all lesions.

Systemic Candidiasis

Systemic expressions of candidiasis are not rare. Bronchopulmonary and pulmonary candidiasis are considered to be the most frequent types and may develop as a complication of chronic primary pulmonary disease, especially in patients with diabetes who are taking systemic corticosteroids and wide-spectrum antibiotics (Louria et al., 1962).

Candidemia, with or without dissemination to internal organs, has become an in-creasing complication of cardiac and renal surgery, and of long-term therapy with immunosuppressive agents, antimetabolites, and wide-spectrum antibiotics. In addition to *C. albicans*, other species of Candida are frequently recovered on culture. Direct access of the fungus to the circulation is facilitated by the use of indwelling polyethylene catheters for intravenous infusions. Disseminated visceral candidiasis may result from the septicemia. The gastrointestinal tract, lungs, and kidneys are affected most frequently. Other rare expressions of systemic candidiasis include endocarditis, meningitis, and bone and joint lesions. The underlying predisposing factors must always be sought in all forms of systemic candidiasis.

Allergic Reactions in Candidiasis

Fallacies flourish in respect to the role of allergic reactions in the diagnosis, symptomatology, and pathogenesis of candidiasis. There is no convincing evidence that allergic mechanisms are of any significance. Skin testing is valueless in diagnosis. Many individuals without candidiasis react to candidal allergens possibly as a result of sensitization from saprophytic *C. albicans* in the gastrointestinal tract, while others with definite evidence of the disease fail to react. Oidiomycin, the allergenic material used for skin testing, has fallen into disuse. Candidids, moniliids, or levurids, thought to be analogous to dermatophytids, have never been conclusively demonstrated and cannot be accepted as clinical entities. Primary foci of candidiasis are not known to generate allergic responses elsewhere. The concept of levurid should be abandoned.

Diagnosis

It has been emphasized in the preceding paragraphs that the diagnosis of candidiasis in its serious forms is by no means simple. Laboratory tests do not suffice, and clinical findings are often inconclusive. No single item, but rather an ensemble of supporting data, enables one to arrive at the diagnosis, though even this will often be *presumptive* rather than final. In synoptic form, the helpful criteria for establishing a diagnosis include:

1. Demonstration of a sizable quantity of budding cells and filaments in material taken from the lesion itself, or in biopsy specimens.

2. Isolation by culture.

3. Correspondence of the lesions with the typical manifestations considered characteristic of bona fide candidiasis. Unhappily, there is great room for argument as to what the typical expressions of certain entities are.

4. Exclusion of other diagnoses.

Skin tests have no value in confirming or excluding the diagnosis. Serologic reactions do not furnish positive evidence for diagnosis (Taschdjian et al., 1967), though in occasional instances the lack of agglutinins may help exclude it. The blood of most adults contains anticandida agglutinins in low titer; in extensive cases of candidiasis, particularly the systemic forms, the presence of large numbers of organisms may provide an intense immunologic stimulus so that the titer may exceed 1:160, a level rarely exhibited by normal sera (Kozinn et al., 1969). Accordingly, if the titer in a suspected extensive case (excluding purely local forms such as thrush) is within the normal range, that is, 1:40 or below, candidiasis becomes an unlikely possibility. On the other hand, high titers are not certainly diagnostic, for a profuse growth of *C. albicans* as an innocuous colonist will excite a similar significant antibody response.

Treatment

The remedies recommended for candidiasis are legion. Here, too, the evidence for a satisfactory therapeutic response is often highly questionable, especially since the disease being treated may not even be candidiasis.

The most reliable principle in therapeutic management is correction of the underlying factors which have made the individual vulnerable to this parasite. The importance of identifying predisposing situations such as malnutrition, antecedent local or systemic disease, excessive exposure to moisture, etc., cannot be overemphasized. In this disorder, pre-eminently, the forces within the host that have provided the opportunity for invasion may be recognized in a high percentage of cases, and the therapeutic attack necessarily must be focused on strengthening resistance by means of maintaining the health of individual tissues and of the patient as a whole.

The polyene antibiotics nystatin and amphotericin B are the treatment of choice for candidiasis (Butler, 1966). Both are available in a wide variety of topical preparations and in combination with topical antibacterial antibiotics and corticosteroids. Unfortunately, neither of these antifungal antibiotics is absorbed from the gastrointestinal tract sufficiently to be of value in the oral treatment of systemic infection. Because of maceration which usually precedes or accompanies superficial candidal infection, preparations in an ointment base are to be avoided.

In *thrush,* nystatin is administered by oral suspension which may be dropped directly on the tongue. A dose of 100,000 units four times daily for 7 to 10 days is often curative. In refractory cases the oral mucosa may be treated with a 0.5 per cent aqueous solution of gentian violet which is swabbed onto the affected area two or three times daily. Stronger concentrations of gentian violet may be irritating and are no more effective.

Nystatin may be administered as a vaginal tablet in *vulvovaginal candidiasis.* One tablet containing 100,000 units should be inserted intravaginally twice daily for 7 to 14 days. In refractory cases gentian violet may be used in the form of an intravaginal gel which is inserted with an applicator. When recurrences are frequent and especially in women taking oral contraceptives or long-term antibacterial antibiotics, it may be necessary to suppress the gastrointestinal reservoir of *C. albicans* in order to prevent reinfection. Nystatin oral tablets may be given in a dose of 500,000 to 1,000,000 units two or three times daily. Occasionally, it may be necessary to keep such patients on maintenance dosage of 500,000 units daily.

The treatment of *candidal intertrigo* is essentially identical to treatment of intertrigo of other etiology. It is mandatory that the predisposing factors promoting maceration be corrected. Only water-miscible preparations of nystatin or amphotericin B should be used, since ointment vehicles may serve to perpetuate the maceration. There is seldom, if ever, any indication for combinations of nystatin with antibacterial antibiotics and corticosteroids if a correct diagnosis has been made. Such preparations not only suppress the bacterial antagonists of *C. albicans* but also are potentially sensitizing and may lead to superimposed allergic contact dermatitis to one or more of the many ingredients.

In *candidal paronychia,* no treatment is effective unless the hands are kept dry.

Exposure to water should be avoided and a separate cotton glove should be worn underneath any other protective glove. Cotton-lined rubber gloves are not much better than ordinary rubber gloves, since the lining cannot be removed for laundering and is easily saturated with perspiration which causes further maceration of the nail folds. A solution of 2 per cent thymol in chloroform may be applied under the nail folds two or three times daily and after each time the hands have been wet. Only water-miscible preparations of nystatin or amphotericin B should be used and these should always be applied toward the distal end of the finger. When hand creams and other medications are applied in a proximal direction, they tend to become impacted in a pocket between the proximal nail fold and the nail plate.

The treatment of *candidiasis of the glabrous skin* is essentially the same as for candidal intertrigo.

The intravenous or prolonged oral administration of amphotericin B may result in clearing of *chronic mucocutaneous candidiasis* (Montes et al., 1971). Recurrence invariably occurs when treatment is discontinued and the nephrotoxicity of amphotericin B may preclude its continued use (Butler et al., 1964). The administration of dialyzable transfer factor or lymphocytes from healthy donors may reverse the cutaneous anergy in this disease, with complete clearing of all cutaneous and mucosal lesions.

In *systemic candidiasis,* treatment should first be directed to the underlying disease, and, where possible, iatrogenic factors predisposing to candidemia should be corrected; for example, infected intravenous or urethral catheters, tracheostomy tubes, and so forth. Indications for specific antifungal therapy include the following: a persistent or rising titer of 1:320 or greater in the agglutination test, a positive precipitin test, the presence of Candida sp. on smear, culture, or biopsy of visceral tissue or body cavities, and a clinical course typical of systemic candidiasis. Intravenous amphotericin B should be started at a dose of 0.25 mg. per kg. and this is increased gradually as tolerated up to 1 mg. per kg. daily. Each dose is given by slow intravenous infusion and the patient should be monitored closely for a rising blood urea nitrogen or anemia. Febrile reactions, anemia, and nephrotoxicity are common and dosage must be individualized according to clinical response and signs of toxicity (Utz, 1964).

COCCIDIOIDOMYCOSIS

The pathogenesis of this disease has much in common with histoplasmosis. The causative organism (*Coccidioides immitis*) is a soil saprophyte, geographically restricted to hot, dry areas. The inhalation of its spores, especially common when there are dust "storms," establishes a pulmonary infection. The primary disease in the lung is usually asymptomatic, but may be accompanied by signs of an acute febrile respiratory illness which, however, resolves spontaneously in the overwhelming majority of cases. Most persons living in an endemic area acquire the disease unknowingly, having no recollection of the time of the infection, but give indisputable evidence of having been previously infected, by reacting positively to an intracutaneous injection of coccidioidin, a filtrate of the fungal growth.

Although primary pulmonary coccidioidomycosis is overwhelmingly a self-limited, benign disorder, a small number of symptomatic cases (0.1 to 1.0 per cent) may go on to develop lesions in other systems, particularly in the skin, brain, and bones, but actually in almost any body organ. *This complication is 5 to 10 times more frequent in Negroes and Filipinos* than in whites. Extrapulmonary extension institutes the *progressive* form of the disease which may, in persons of low resistance, be a disseminated, generalized infection leading to death. Where resistance is greater, there may be only one or several circumscribed lesions in other organ systems, in which case the prognosis is not nearly so grave. Usually, the progressive form of the disease becomes apparent within the first few months of symptomatic infection, reflecting a steady amplification of the primary lesion, with little or no immunity. Occasionally there is a "latent" period of relatively good health between the onset of infection and the first sign of dissemination. Moreover, it is essential to appreciate that occasionally cutaneous lesions may suddenly appear in a person otherwise well, as a result of spread from an asymptomatic pulmonary focus. Usually, however, extrapulmonary dissemination (progressive coccidioidomycosis) occurs in individuals who have symptomatic pulmonary disease and whose primary lesion is therefore evident.

Coccidioidomycosis is endemic in the arid southwestern U.S., in California principally, but also in western Texas, Arizona, New Mexico, Utah, and Nevada. The only other known areas of endemicity, of far less significance, are certain regions of Mexico, Argentina, Paraguay, Venezuela, Honduras, and Guatemala. These areas conform to the geologic Lower Sonoran Life Zone and are characterized by semiarid low altitudes with hot summers, infrequent freezes in winter, and an association with certain plants and rodents. Sporadic cases have been reported in travellers returning from endemic areas (Harrell and Honeycutt, 1963).

Rodents and domestic animals in the endemic area acquire the infection in the same manner as man. The disease is not transmitted from man to man or from animal to man. The spores of the mold growing in nature are highly infectious, as the frequency of infections, some fatal, among *laboratory workers* will attest. Transmission of the disease by spores on contaminated fomites has been reported (Rothman et al., 1969). Progressive coccidioidomycosis is more common in males than in females, and Negroes have a far greater susceptibility than whites.

The initial primary pulmonary infection of coccidioidomycosis may be symptomless or may produce an acute respiratory infection which is occasionally severe and prostrating; it is characterized by fever, pleural pain, unproductive cough, malaise, headache, backache, myalgia, anorexia, and night sweats. In about two to three weeks after the onset of symptoms, some 20 per cent of such patients develop erythema nodosum lesions over the pretibial areas, and occasionally elsewhere. This is frequently accompanied by arthropathy and eosinophilia, pointing to an allergic sensitization. In some cases, erythema multiforme may develop independently or be accompanied by erythema nodosum. Individuals with acute pulmo-

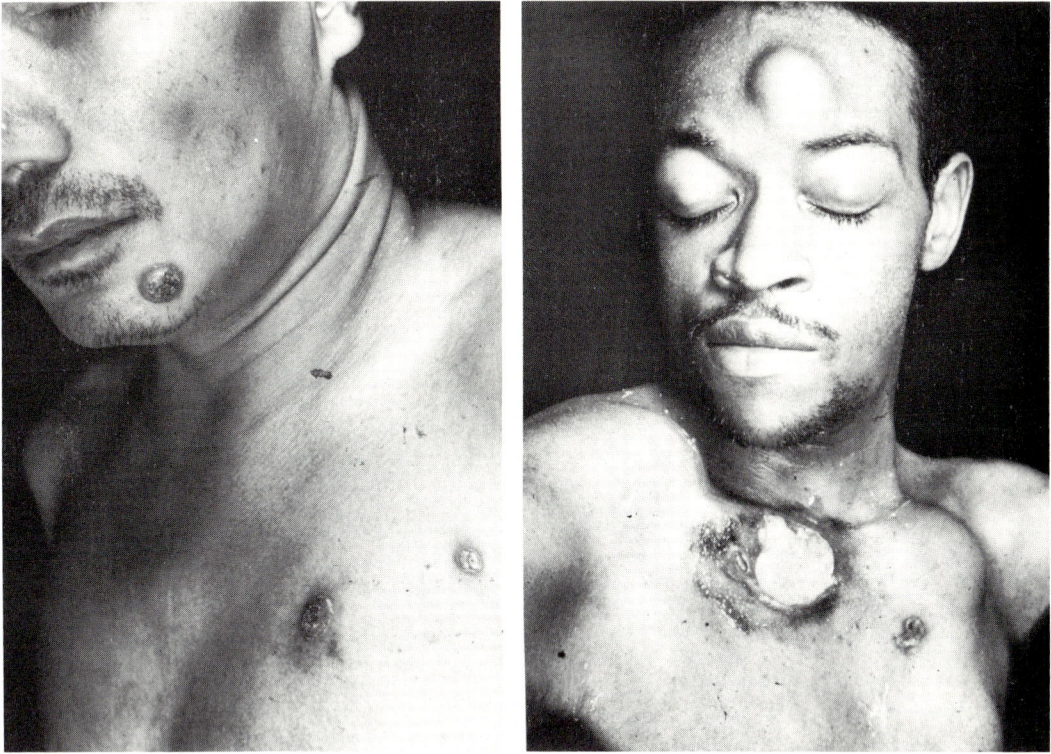

Figure 13–34 Disseminated late coccidioidomycosis. Negroes have a very low resistance to the disease.

nary coccidioidomycosis also occasionally develop a transient nonspecific toxic erythema which may be urticarial, scarlatiniform, or morbilliform in appearance.

If progression of the infection takes place, the skin is one of the favorite sites, sometimes being the only organ in which extrapulmonic lesions develop. The lesions are granulomas but do not, on the whole, have highly distinctive characteristics which permit their immediate recognition. Subcutaneous masses develop and break down to form either abscesses draining a thick mucoid pus or chronic necrotic ulcers. The lesions are often multiple and frequently fuse, producing extensive, ugly ulcerations. One of the more typical developments is for the ulcers, after a period of months, to undergo vegetative or papillomatous changes, sometimes acquiring a distinctly verrucous or roughened surface. Neoplastic growth may be simulated. Less often, nondescript papules and pustules may develop. The presence of coccidioidal skin lesions demands a thorough search for evidences of infection in other organs, as

well as comprehensive general medical study.

PRIMARY CUTANEOUS COCCIDIOIDOMYCOSIS, in which the lesion is thought to result from exogenous implantation of the organism into the skin, is, contrary to former teaching, a medical rarity. The skin is very rarely the portal of entry. Almost all of the cases which have been represented as primary skin infections are in reality unusual instances of hematogenous spread from an inapparent pulmonary focus. It is easy to understand how the emergence of one or two circumscribed cutaneous granulomas in an otherwise healthy patient may be attributed to exogenous introduction of the organism into the skin, especially if the patient is able to recall some previous trauma at the site. However, true primary cutaneous coccidioidomycosis is a distinctive entity, following a course altogether different from that of the usual case of localized cutaneous coccidioidal granuloma. The unique feature of true cases of external inoculation of the skin is the development of a primary complex, *chancriform syn-*

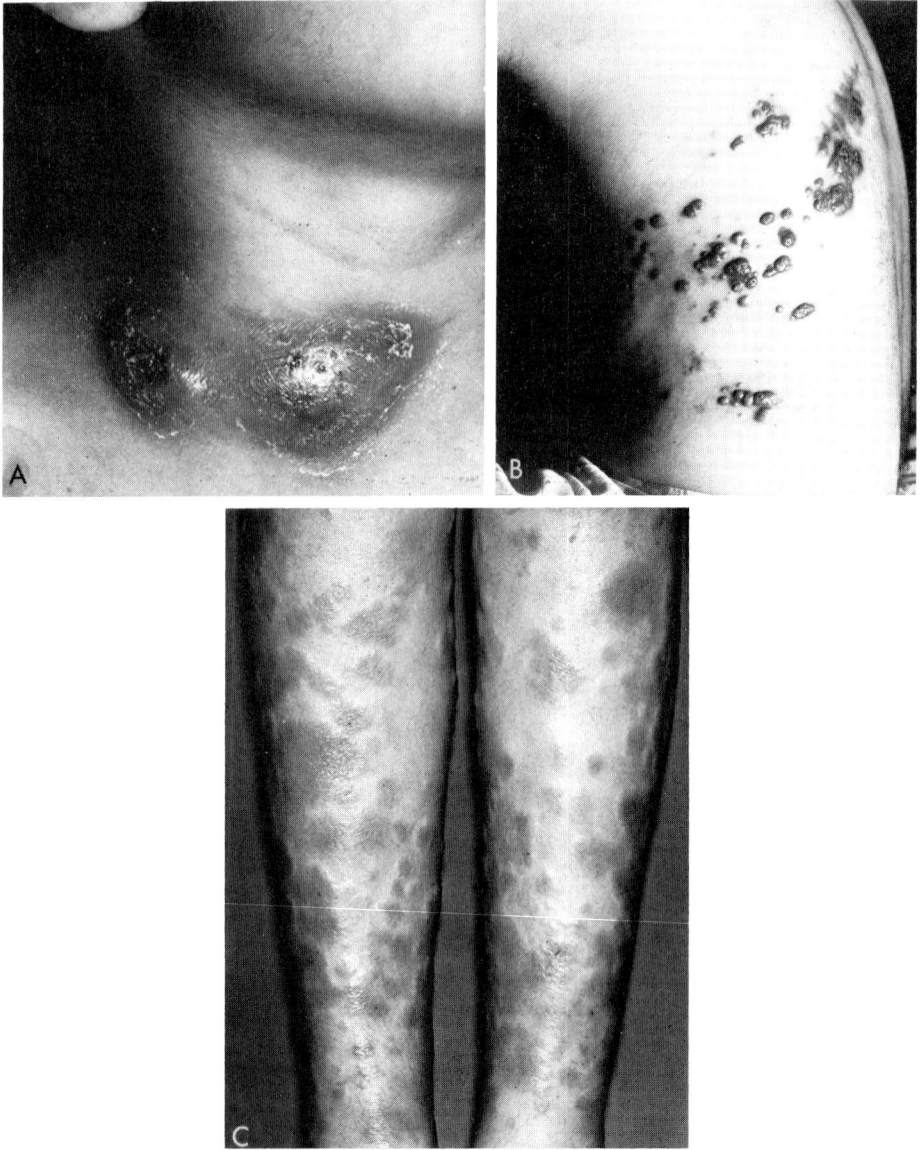

Figure 13–35 Coccidioidomycosis. *A*, Inflammatory granulomatous lesions of neck in disseminated disease. *B*, Multiple extensive nodules of lateral thorax in disseminated disease. *C*, Erythema nodosum in primary pulmonary phase.

drome (Wilson, 1963). A chancre develops at the site of inoculation and this is shortly followed by regional adenopathy. Multiple nodules may form along the course of the lymphatics draining the area. Spontaneous resolution in a short time may be anticipated. A history of injury will ordinarily be elicitable; there is no history of a recent pulmonary infection. All this stands in sharp contrast to localized coccidioidal

granuloma produced by hematogenous dissemination from an endogenous lung focus. In that case, a chronic draining, torpid lesion develops and shows no tendency to heal. There is no adenopathy; a history of trauma is not usually elicited; the lesion may or may not be on an exposed area; and there will usually be evidence, subjective or objective, of a recent pulmonary infection. The pathogenesis of localized cutaneous coccidioidomycosis is in exact parallel with localized cutaneous blastomycosis, in which disease the cutaneous lesions usually represent spread from an inapparent focus, and not exogenous inoculation.

Except for localized forms of progressive coccidioidomycosis, the disease is very serious, especially if there is widespread dissemination, perhaps more than 50 per cent of the cases ending in death if untreated. Pulmonary involvement usually dominates the clinical picture, but every organ of the body may be riddled.

Diagnosis and Prognosis

The coccidioidin skin test is invaluable in epidemiologic studies and for diagnosis. For routine testing, 0.1 ml. of 1:100 coccidioidin is injected intradermally, although higher dilutions (1:1000 to 1:10,000) may be indicated in acute cases in which extreme hypersensitivity may be suspected. In the highly sensitive subject there may be undesirable focal reactions, or an attack of erythema nodosum may be precipitated by the test. Immediate reactions should be disregarded in reading the test; the significant reaction is of delayed tuberculin type. Sensitivity generally develops within a few weeks after the initial pulmonary infection. The diagnosis of coccidioidomycosis is ordinarily excluded if there is no sensitivity to coccidioidin. There are two qualifications to this statement, however. One is the anergy which develops in gravely ill individuals with disseminated disease just before death, and the other is a curious biologic phenomenon which is peculiar to coccidioidomycosis. As the disease disseminates and the condition worsens, sensitivity to coccidioidin frequently diminishes. Serial coccidioidin tests in a patient with a disseminating infection may frequently show that increasingly concentrated solutions are required to elicit a positive reaction. Diminishing reactivity to coccidioidin is, therefore, a clinical index of reduction of the host's defenses and an indication for treatment with intravenous amphotericin B.

Individuals who are sensitive to coccidioidin may react to histoplasmin and, rarely, to blastomycin. The cross reactions, however, are generally weaker than the coccidioidin test. In clinical practice all three antigens are frequently used at the same time, but the phenomenon of cross reactivity is not a source of much confusion, because these three infections are usually distinguishable on clinical grounds and have different geographic distributions. Repeated skin testing with coccidioidin does not induce sensitivity, but may induce antibodies reacting with yeast phase antigen from *Histoplasma capsulatum.*

Precipitins appear in the blood of individuals with coccidioidomycosis in the early phase of the acute pulmonary infection, being detectable even in mild cases. These tend to decline and disappear as the patient recovers. The precipitin test is an important confirmatory procedure, and in the case of pulmonary infections will indicate infection much oftener than is possible by cultures. Complement fixing antibodies develop somewhat later; they are detectable in most cases of severe primary pulmonary coccidioidomycosis, but may be absent or minimal in asymptomatic or mild cases. A rising complement fixation titer presages progression and dissemination of the infection. Thus, this test gives evidence of the degree of involvement and shows a correlation with the clinical course; a rising or persistently high titer is a bad prognostic sign.

A definite diagnosis is made by demonstrating the characteristic endosporulating spherules in sputum, smears or biopsy specimens, or by culture of the fungus. Special precautions are necessary to avoid laboratory accidents due to airborn spread of arthrospores. Culture tubes should be opened only under a suitable hood or after first flooding the surface of the colony with saline. The organism is easily isolated from or visualized in cutaneous granulomas. The cutaneous lesions of coccidioidomycosis must be differentiated from tuberculosis, neoplasm, other fungal infections, syphilis, glanders, and tularemia.

The majority of infections with coccidioidomycosis are self-limited and do not require specific antifungal treatment. Pulmonary resection may be indicated for solitary pulmonary granulomas or persistent cavitary lung disease. In progressive or disseminated disease, especially in Negroes and Filipinos, and as presurgical treatment for pulmonary cavities and nodules, parenteral amphotericin B is the drug of choice. Intravenous infusion of amphotericin B must be individualized and the patient monitored closely for signs of nephrotoxicity, hepatotoxicity, hypokalemia, and anemia.

BLASTOMYCOSIS
(North American Blastomycosis)

The causative organism of this disease, *Blastomyces dermatitidis*, doubtless originates exogenously, and has been recovered repeatedly from soil, as have practically all other pathogenic fungi. The disease is confined almost entirely to the United States, where its occurrence is sporadic (Busey, 1964). A few cases have been observed in Canada. It is rather uncommon and is not transmissible from man to man. There are no clear-cut endemic areas where a significant percentage of persons acquire the infection asymptomatically, as in histoplasmosis and coccidioidomycosis. As is the case with other systemic mycoses, adult males acquire the infection much more frequently than adult females and children. Though laborers are affected principally, there is no definite occupational relationship. Infections have been reported in dogs, with a greater frequency among sporting and hunting breeds (Menges et al., 1969). An intimate contact with soil appears associated with both human and animal blastomycosis. The formation of a localized cutaneous plaque of distinctive morphology is the most characteristic expression of blastomycosis. There is also a rare systemic disorder, usually originating as a pulmonary infection, which may become disseminated and involve many organs, particularly the skin, bones, and viscera (Vanek et al., 1970). Localized cutaneous blastomycosis has, until recently, been thought to originate from exogenous implantation of organisms into the skin, but this view has had to be revised. The localized plaque represents a metastasis from a pulmonary focus which may be unrecognized. As in other pulmonary my-

coses, it is definitely established that circumscribed lung lesions may be completely asymptomatic. Roentgenologic study of the lungs of patients with localized cutaneous blastomycosis frequently reveals pulmonary residua, and this procedure should be a routine part of the examination of any patient suspected of having blastomycosis.

Localized cutaneous blastomycosis arising from a pulmonary focus, the most common expression of the disease, follows a course which is different from the *chancriform syndrome* seen in physicians and laboratory workers who have accidentally inoculated themselves with Blastomyces organisms. The disease which eventuates from a *known* inoculation into the skin has nothing in common with the usual case of cutaneous blastomycosis (Landay and Schwarz, 1971). It has the following distinctive characteristics:

1. A primary complex (chancre) forms rapidly. A lesion occurs at the site of inoculation, followed shortly by enlargement of the regional nodes, perhaps with some constitutional reaction.

2. The primary lesion and the enlarged nodes heal spontaneously, after cutaneous inoculation, and the disease involutes completely.

3. Cases of accidental inoculation therefore represent a distinctive entity which may legitimately be termed *primary cutaneous blastomycosis*, in contradistinction to the usual expression of the disease which, from the standpoint of pathogenesis, is best called *secondary localized cutaneous blastomycosis*. Primary cutaneous infection follows an *injury*, but such an event is generally not elicited in the history of patients with the secondary type of disease. Furthermore, secondary localized cutaneous blastomycosis does not by any means always begin on an exposed part, as might be expected if the organism reached the skin exogenously.

The above sequence of events is entirely analogous to that of cutaneous coccidioidomycosis, which also was for many years thought to be an exogenous infection, until the observation of accidental inoculations proved otherwise. There is a striking parallel in the historical development of the knowledge of these two diseases.

SECONDARY LOCALIZED CUTANEOUS BLASTOMYCOSIS generally appears as a papule or nodule, which subsequently ulcerates and discharges purulent material. Usually there is only one lesion, and a history of antecedent injury is not elicitable. The face, wrists, hands, and feet are most commonly involved, but lesions may appear anywhere on the skin. The lesion enlarges eccentrically at the periphery and tends to clear centrally, leaving a dense scar. Extension is slow but relentless, and after many months the lesion tends to acquire an arciform or serpiginous outline. The borders are sharply elevated and distinctly verrucous, with a violaceous margin. *Miliary abscesses* are invariably found in the abruptly sloping border. Organisms are present in the tiny pus droplets which may be expressed from the abscesses. As the verrucous border advances, the central region remains as an atrophic scar. Experienced observers can identify blastomycosis almost at a glance, especially if the border is examined carefully. In the ordinary case of localized cutaneous blastomycosis, native immunity is high, and the lesion is restricted to a single site, whereas in systemic blastomycosis poor immunity permits the development of *multiple* lesions in the skin and other organs. In disseminated blastomycosis, the cutaneous lesions often originate as multiple subcutaneous nodules which later ulcerate.

Diagnosis

The diagnosis of cutaneous blastomycosis is confirmed by collecting material from the miliary abscesses and demonstrating round budding organisms in a potassium hydroxide mount or a McManus stained smear. Careful search is indicated, for organisms are often sparse. Cultures should, of course, be made. Biopsies from the *border* of the lesions may also be diagnostic. Roentgenologic examination of the lungs is indicated in every case. Aspirates of unruptured subcutaneous nodules in disseminated cases are excellent sources of culture material.

The organism of blastomycosis is weakly antigenic. Complement-fixing antibodies are ordinarily not present in patients with a single cutaneous lesion. They are inconstantly detectable in relatively low titer when there is marked systemic involvement; the titer more or less parallels the severity of the disease. Cross reactivity with Histoplasma antigen is a constant finding, but usually poses no problem because the diseases are so readily differentiated on other grounds. Individuals with cutaneous blastomycosis usually develop a delayed tuberculin-type

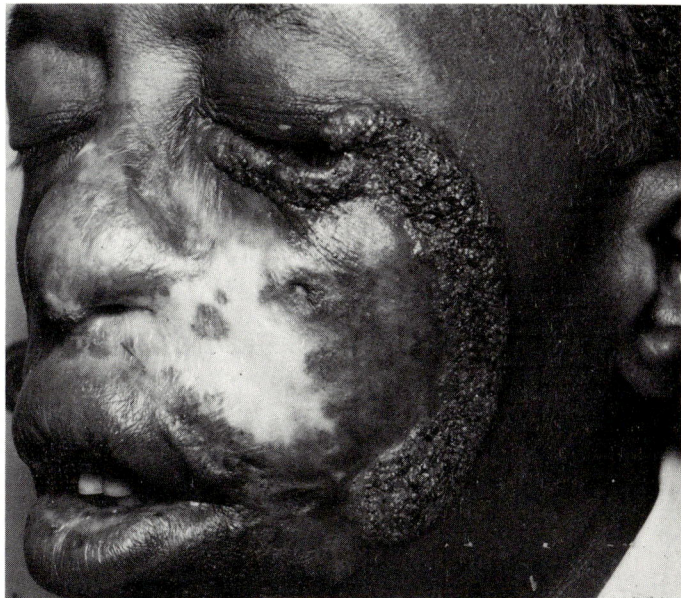

Figure 13–36 Blastomycosis. Long-standing, relentlessly progressive. General health unimpaired.

reaction to the intradermal injection of 0.1 cc. of 1:100 blastomycin, a filtrate of the cultured organism. Such reactions are also characteristic of systemic blastomycosis, except in the terminal stages of the disease, when a general anergy develops. There is cross reactivity to histoplasmin, and to a lesser extent to coccidioidin. In general, the blastomycin skin reaction has presumptive diagnostic value because it is rarely positive in patients who do not have blastomycosis, the exceptions being cross reactions in individuals with past or present histoplasmosis or, to a much lesser extent, coccidioidomycosis. There are no endemic areas of blastomycosis in which large numbers of people acquire a mild or asymptomatic disease as in histoplasmosis or coccidioidomycosis, and the contacts of patients with blastomycosis do not have a higher incidence of cutaneous reactivity than the average population, emphasizing the sporadic nature of this disease. It is well to remember, however, that there is every reason to believe that occasional cases of asymptomatic pulmonary infection do occur, resulting in a primary complex, which probably more often than not undergoes spontaneous resolution, with or without leaving roentgenographically detectable sequelae.

Cutaneous blastomycosis must be differentiated from tuberculosis, neoplasm, drug eruptions (particularly those due to iodides and bromides), syphilis, granuloma inguinale, and other deep-seated fungal infections. Chronic granulomatous pyoderma may be a particular source of confusion.

Treatment

Only two drugs are available for treatment of blastomycosis: Amphotericin B and the stilbamidine derivatives. Amphotericin B is given by slow intravenous infusion, and treatment must be individualized to reduce nephrotoxicity, hepatotoxicity, hypokalemia, and anemia. The initial dose is 0.25 mg. per kg. of body weight. The dose is gradually increased to a maximum daily dose of 1 gm. per kg. Toxicity may be reduced by alternate day dosage after obvious clinical regression has been observed. Progressive clearing of lesions has been reported in patients re-

ceiving oral amphotericin B after initial intravenous treatment. The mechanism for this is not clear. Although oral amphotericin B is well tolerated even in large doses, absorption from the gastrointestinal tract is poor and blood levels remain low or undetectable.

Stilbamidine is one of the aromatic diamidines which have long been successfully used as trypanocidal agents. Propamidine, pentamidine, and 2-hydroxystilbamidine are related compounds with known antifungal activity, of which the last, though less effective, may supplant stilbamidine because of its lower toxicity. Curiously enough, although most of the deep fungi are sensitive in vitro to these agents, blastomycosis is to date the only mycotic disease in which the clinical response is clear-cut.

Stilbamidine is a white crystalline powder which is soluble in water. The solution is unstable unless kept in the dark. The degradation products are toxic. Fresh solutions must be used and should be dispensed in dark glass or paper-covered bottles. The drug is sometimes hepatotoxic or nephrotoxic, but this reaction is uncommon unless the function of these organs is already impaired. Elementary liver and kidney function tests should be done before stilbamidine therapy is started, as well as during therapy. Moderate impairment is not an absolute contraindication to treatment but is an indication for smaller doses over a longer period of time.

The drug is removed from the blood stream rapidly. The maintenance of antifungal levels, therefore, requires intravenous infusions continued over a period of hours daily. Experience has not been sufficient as yet to determine precisely the optimal regimen of administration. A total amount of 4 to 6 gm. of stilbamidine has proved adequate for most cases. Six to 10 gm. of 2-hydroxy-stilbamidine is probably required because of the lower antifungal potency of this drug.

Stilbamidine may be administered in two ways: (1) Daily infusions may be given for a period of a month or more until the total dose is reached, or (2) the total dose may be divided into two or three courses, consisting of two-week periods of daily infusions, interrupted by two-week rest periods. The former is perhaps preferable. The initial doses must be small, and the maximum dose per day should not exceed 150 mg. An acceptable program is as follows:

First day: 50 mg. intravenously in 100 cc. of 5 per cent glucose solution, infused over a period of one hour.

Second day: 100 mg. intravenously in 100 cc. of 5 per cent glucose solution, infused over a period of one hour.

Third day and thereafter until the total dose is reached: 150 mg. in 500 cc. of 5 per cent glucose solution, infused over a period of three to four hours.

Improvement is ordinarily seen in a few weeks with either amphotericin B or stilbamidine, and this may become progressively more apparent after therapy is stopped. Additional courses of treatment may be required after a suitable rest period has elapsed. The drugs are usually suppressive rather than completely curative. The localized cutaneous type responds more favorably than the active pulmonary or disseminated disease. The latter disease may require repeated courses, and relapses are common.

With stilbamidine, *trigeminal neuralgia, which may appear months after cessation of treatment, is a distressing and very frequent side reaction.* The principal symptoms, which are usually entirely sensory, are paresthesias and hyperesthesias of the face. These may persist for months or even indefinitely. The use of 2-hydroxystilbamidine does not prevent this complication but may lessen its incidence.

Iodide therapy and desensitization procedures probably no longer have a place in the treatment of blastomycosis. They should not be given as an adjunct to stilbamidine therapy. Excision and plastic repair of a localized cutaneous lesion is possible in the early stage of the lesion and is preferable to the definite risks associated with stilbamidine therapy.

PARACOCCIDIOIDOMYCOSIS
(South American Blastomycosis)

This disease is limited to South America. Most cases have been observed in Brazil, but cases have been reported in all South and Central American countries except Chile, Guyana, and French Guiana. The endemic areas are humid, tropical regions where the average annual temperature is between 63 and 70° F. The causative organism, *Paracoccidioides brasiliensis,* probably lives on vegetation or in the soil as a saprophyte, but the single report of isolation from the soil is not conclusive. Primary infection probably occurs through direct implantation of the organism into the skin or mucous membranes; consistent with this is the high incidence of the disease in adult male rural workers. The disease is not contagious from man to man.

Although the manifestations of the disease are diverse, resulting in subdivisions into many types, one denominator is common to all types, namely, *lymph node enlargement.* There is no clear-cut distinction between primary and disseminated paracoccidioidomycosis. In disseminated cases, the skin, as well as many other organs, may be the site of numerous granulomatous ulcerative lesions. The disease most often originates in the mucous membrane of the mouth, on the tongue, gums, palate, cheeks, lips, and, occasionally, on the nasal mucosa. A smooth, firm ulcer dotted with punctate hemorrhages is formed. This enlarges and deepens rapidly, producing a brawny hard mass which is quite characteristic. New ulcers originate in the mouth and these, too, extend rapidly, often destroying most of the mucosal surface and spreading out on the skin of the mucocutaneous junctions around the lips and nose. Shortly after infection, regional adenopathy, an inevitable and characteristic development, becomes apparent. The lymph nodes of the neck are generally the first to enlarge and, after reaching massive proportions, undergo necrosis and rupture, producing draining sinuses. Through hematogenous dissemination, other internal and peripheral lymph nodes become diseased. Rupture of axillary, inguinal and other nodes onto the skin creates additional draining sinuses. Lung involvement resembling tuberculosis occurs in over 70 per cent of the cases, but is seldom seen without associated mucocutaneous and lymphatic involvement. Hepatosplenomegaly is a frequent finding. In grave cases, dissemination results in lesions throughout the body, involving the viscera, central nervous system and myocardium, as well as numerous regions of the skin and subcutaneous tissues.

The thick-walled, yeastlike organisms, with their diagnostic multiple buds, may readily be found in biopsy specimens or in curettings from the mucous membrane lesions. Aspiration of pus from lymph nodes is a fruitful means of obtaining material for microscopic examination and culture.

Most patients with South American blastomycosis react with a tuberculin-type response to an intradermal injection of a filtrate from the fungal growth. The results are somewhat inconstant, however, and the degree to which skin testing can be relied upon for diagnosis is still undetermined. There is reciprocal cross reactivity between the antigens of this organism and *Blastomyces dermatitidis,* though this offers no practical complications because these diseases have independent geographic distributions. The value of the complement fixation test still remains to be established, though there can be no doubt that antibodies are generally formed in extensive infections. The specificity of the test leaves something to be desired, for such antibodies may also be found in normal individuals, though perhaps in lower titers.

The disease is notoriously chronic and may end in death if dissemination occurs. Localized forms appear to respond fairly well to sulfonamide therapy. Four to 6 gm. of sulfadiazine or sulfamerazine may be given daily and continued for a period several weeks after all active signs of the disease have disappeared. Sulfonamides are often only suppressive rather than curative in disseminated cases. Repeated courses may be required. Amphotericin B has produced rapid regression in mucocutaneous lesions and a good response in several cases with visceral involvement. Iodide therapy and immunization procedures with killed vaccines have no proved value.

LOBO'S DISEASE (*Keloidal Blastomycosis*). This chronic localized disease occurs in the northern and Caribbean part of the South American continent and overlaps the endemic area of paracoccidioidomycosis. Lesions may be localized to the feet, legs, buttocks, face, or other areas and begin as intracutaneous nodules which become verrucous and crusted, spreading slowly by peripheral extension or auto-inoculation. Lymphatic and visceral involvement is not seen and the disease tends to be chronic. The causative organism, *Loboa loboi,* has not been cultivated on artificial media, but may be demonstrated without difficulty in biopsies from the cutaneous nodules. Although this disease has been considered in the past to be a variant of paracoccidioidomycosis and the organism bears some resemblance to *P. brasiliensis* in biopsy material, it is probably a separate entity. Excision of localized nodules may be curative.

HISTOPLASMOSIS

This is one of the most protean of all diseases, having a wide variety of clinical expressions ranging from an innocuous, asymptomatic pulmonary infection to a progressive, disseminated fatal disorder in which no tissue is exempt. The largest number of cases are asymptomatic, benign, self-limited pulmonary infections which may leave calcified residua in the lungs. The pulmonary disease, which may also be symptomatic, earns its medical importance because of the difficulty of distinguishing tuberculosis and other diseases of serious import, such as carcinoma. The pulmonary disease is endemic in the Mississippi and Ohio River valleys, in certain areas of which more than 80 per cent of the population have acquired the infection at some time in their lives, as revealed by cutaneous reactivity to histoplasmin. Elsewhere in the U.S. the disease is seen to a lesser degree. Endemic foci exist also in South America, Africa, and Asia. The disease is extremely uncommon in Europe, although positive soil cultures have been reported.

The causative organism, *Histoplasma capsulatum,* exists as a saprophyte in nature. Its spores are highly infectious for humans as well as for many small animals; for example, dogs, cats, rats, mice, and skunks. The fungus has been repeatedly isolated from soil. Inhalation of the airborne mold spores is the usual route of infection. The disease is not transmitted from man to man or from animal to man. Focal epidemics have occurred among groups of men exposed to atmospheres containing an abundance of spores, as in incidents following exploration of certain caves, demolition of old buildings, and cleaning out of sites rich in vegetable debris or fowl excrement. Erythema multiforme and erythema nodosum have occasionally been observed in association with epidemics of primary pulmonary histoplasmosis (Medeiros et al., 1966; Sellers et al., 1965). Infections of laboratory workers are common, though usually not serious. Despite the readiness with which the organism enters the human body, its virulence is relatively low, and immediate mobilization of body defenses generally confines the lesion to the point of entry, resulting in a benign course in the overwhelming majority of infections. The phagocytic cells of the reticuloendothelial system, the wandering tissue cells, as well as those in the fixed depots such as the liver, spleen, lymph nodes, and bone marrow, constitute the vanguard of cellular defense, ingesting the small, oval budding fungal cells until the cytoplasm is literally swollen with masses of the parasite. The disease on this account may be conceived immunopathologically as a reticuloendothelial cytomycosis. In view of the predominantly self limited character of the infection, it would appear that the phagocytes eventually digest and destroy the parasite in most instances. Actually, the tissues of the host seem able to tolerate a considerable crowd of fungus-containing phagocytes without conspicuous interference in organ function. Accordingly, the organism is often discovered incidentally in tissues which give no indication of malfunction, even in persons who are not suspected of having histoplasmosis. There is indication that disseminated cases of histoplasmosis may be asymptomatic, multiple calcifications of the spleen being offered in evidence. The progressive disseminated form of the disease is uncommon (Smith and Utz, 1972). Death is frequent, but not inevitable, in cases with extensive involvement of the liver, spleen, bone marrow, and lymph nodes (the reticuloendothelial system) and the impairment resulting from invasion of these organs: anemia, leukopenia, fever, emaciation, weakness, and so forth (Sarosi et al., 1971). Infants are more susceptible to progressive histoplasmosis.

Primary lesions in the skin are rare but may be seen in laboratory or autopsy workers; these lesions produce the typical *chancriform syndrome* with a characteristic chancre at the site of entry accompanied by regional lymphadenopathy. These infections usually are self-limited and seldom result in disseminated disease. Isolated circumscribed lesions on the skin and in particular the mucous membranes of the mouth and the penis (as well as other organs) are occasionally encountered without evidence of disease elsewhere, but it is not possible on such evidence to conclude that the fungus actually entered at these sites. It is just as likely that such lesions represent peripheral spread from an inapparent pulmonary focus. Focal lesions of this kind may persist for a long time without evident change, and the prognosis is good in such cases. They may be regarded as one of the benign expressions of the disease, analogous to circumscribed pulmonary lesions. Only very occasionally will dissemination occur subsequently.

On the other hand, cutaneous lesions are not infrequent in the uncommon progressive form of histoplasmosis, in which the skin is only one of many organs involved in the generalized infection. The lesions are by no means distinctive or uniform, but most often take the form of persistent punched-out or circumscribed granulomatous ulcers, mimicking other granulomas. Among the less common cutaneous manifestations of the generalized disease are purpura, crops of papules, chronic abscesses, impetiginized dermatitis, and furunculoid and vegetating lesions. In short, the skin lesions which may be encountered in systemic histoplasmosis are exceedingly varied, a fact which should be kept in mind, for a cutaneous lesion may sometimes be the first visible expression of generalization. Special attention should be called to the frequency of mucous membrane lesions, which appear most often as persistent ulcerative granulomas in perhaps one-third of the progressive cases. The first recognizable lesion in generalized histoplasmosis may be an ulcerative process in the mouth or pharynx, with occasional extension to the larynx and esophagus. It is thought, on this account, that the mouth or other mucous membranes, the gastrointestinal tract in particular, may be the most common portal of entry in the systemic disease. Pulmonary histoplasmosis, the commonest type of the disease, rarely undergoes generalization, and disseminated histoplasmosis would appear to originate most commonly in some fashion other than through the lungs. In children particularly, who are far more likely to have generalized histoplasmosis, the frequency of extensive ulcers along the gastrointestinal mucosa, giving rise to diarrhea and other gastrointestinal disturbances, suggests that the organisms may be ingested rather than inhaled. A striking number of cases of generalized histoplasmosis have occurred in association with grave diseases such as the lymphomas and tuberculosis, which evidently reduce the resistance of the host to the point where the usual ability to confine the infection is lost.

Diagnosis

BIOPSY AND CULTURE are the paramount diagnostic tests for mucocutaneous lesions of histoplasmosis. In disseminated cases, adequate material for cultures or smears may be obtained from bone marrow aspiration, lymph node biopsy (or biopsy of other accessible lesions), and the peripheral blood. Cultures of the organism are exceedingly difficult to secure in the circumscribed pulmonary disease, even when the lungs are the site of multiple lesions sufficient to cause acute pulmonary symptoms. The definitive finding in biopsies and smears consists of macrophages loaded with tiny intracellular oval yeastlike fungi. Mucocutaneous lesions are crowded with fungus-laden macrophages, and the diagnosis is readily established if adequate samples are taken.

Sensitivity to histoplasmin is usually established within a few weeks after infection has occurred. The diagnostic implications and limitations of a positive test, which is of the delayed tuberculin type, are similar to those of the tuberculin test. It signifies past or present infection and is a fairly reliable screening procedure. Except in the terminal stages of advanced disease or in acute febrile cases, the diagnosis of histoplasmosis is improbable in the absence of a positive histoplasmin test. The organisms causing coccidioidomycosis, blastomycosis, and histoplasmosis share common antigens, accounting for the cutaneous cross reactivity observed when tests are simultaneously done with each antigen. Histoplasmin is perhaps the least specific of the three; individuals with a strong sensitivity to coccidioidin and blastomycin almost invariably react to histoplasmin, though the reaction to the homologous antigen tends to be stronger, permitting a tentative means of distinguishing the homologous antigen by "titrating" the skin reactions with different dilutions. To a lesser extent, coccidioidin and blastomycin elicit cross reactions in patients primarily sensitive to histoplasmin. Actually, the situation does not create as much confusion as might be thought, because blastomycosis is a very uncommon disease, and coccidioidomycosis has a distinctive geographic distribution different from the endemic area of histoplasmosis. Nonetheless, it is customary to use all three antigens in skin testing patients for a suspected mycosis. Repeated skin tests do not induce cutaneous sensitivity but may induce circulating antibodies in individuals who are skin test negative or may cause a significant rise in titer in those who already have antibodies in their sera (Furcolow, 1963).

SEROLOGIC REACTIONS, when properly interpreted with full recognition of their limitations, may be quite helpful in diagnosis. In all cases, serologic evaluation should be carried out prior to skin testing in order to avoid misinterpretation of the serologic test. In a general way the titers of agglutinins, complement-fixing antibodies, and precipitins reflect the extensiveness of the disease, at least in the early stages. They are low or absent in circumscribed, self-limited, mild or asymptomatic cases, and reach higher levels in more extensive symptomatic infections, especially in the generalized types. Agglutinins and precipitins tend to appear rather early, within the first few weeks, and then to diminish or disappear. Complement-fixing antibodies appear later and are more persistent. A peculiarity of the complement fixation reaction is that the titer may fall as the disease becomes more disseminated and grave; in long-standing systemic disease there may be no detectable complement-fixing antibodies. With any of the serologic tests, titers of less than 1:16 should be viewed with much suspicion. Not infrequently, the sera of normal individuals will yield titers of 1:4 and 1:8. Titers exceeding 1:32 are not in themselves conclusively diagnostic, but are highly suggestive if in conformity with the clinical findings. The serologic reaction may on occasion prove to be the first important diagnostic clue in puzzling cases which do not present a clear-cut clinical picture. The lack of standardized antigens and standard procedures further complicates the interpretation of serologic tests. Moreover, as in skin testing, there is serologic cross reactivity with blastomycin, and to a lesser extent to coccidioidin. In proved cases of histoplasmosis, the cross reacting titer to blastomycin may equal that of the homologous antigen, but fortunately the two diseases are otherwise not too difficult to distinguish.

Treatment

Antifungal treatment is seldom necessary except for progressive disseminated disease or in the presurgical management of solitary pulmonary granulomas or refractory cavity lung disease (Parker et al., 1970). Amphotericin B may be curative, but the known risks of nephrotoxicity, hepatotoxicity, hypokalemia, and anemia must be weighed against the clinical course of the disease, and dosage must be individualized. The drug is given by slow intravenous infusion, beginning with a dose of 5 mg. per kg. of body weight and increasing gradually to a maximum dose of 1.0 mg. per kg. In disseminated disease, treatment is generally continued until a total dose of 4 gm. has been given (Furcolow, 1963). Toxicity may be reduced by alternate day dosage once the patient has shown definite clinical improvement (Tynes et al., 1963).

African Histoplasmosis (Williams et al., 1971). Although infections with *H. capsulatum* are not rare in Africa and resemble histoplasmosis elsewhere, a special form of histoplasmosis has been reported from a wide band extending across the African continent between the Sahara Desert to the north and the Kalahari Desert to the south. The organism causing these infections is *H. duboisii* and is indistinguishable from *H. capsulatum* in its mold phase on culture. In the yeast phase and in biopsy specimens, the budding cells are larger and more closely resemble *B. dermatidis*. They may be distinguished by the narrower point of attachment of the developing blastospore in *H. duboisii*. The yeast phase cells of *H. duboisii* have a single nucleus whereas *B. dermatidis* is multinucleated. In African histoplasmosis, pulmonary lesions are rare. The disease generally presents with multiple subcutaneous and osseous cold abscesses. Pathological fractures are not uncommon. The route of infection and pathogenesis have not been delineated owing to the lack of laboratory facilities in the endemic area.

ACTINOMYCOSIS

This disease is caused by funguslike higher bacteria which are probably related to the diphtheroids. It is included in this chapter because it more closely resembles the mycoses in clinical course, chronicity, and histopathology. The usual etiologic agents are *Actinomyces israelii* (in man) and *A. bovis* (in cattle). Both species are anaerobic or microaerophilic organisms. This requirement limits growth to situations in which the oxygen tension of the tissue is greatly reduced, as in devitalized tissues or occluded spaces, and is the central feature in understanding the pathogenesis and course of the infection. The hallmark of the disease is the formation of granulomatous draining sinuses, from which pus containing "sulfur" granules (which are actually colonies of the organisms) exudes. Involvement of the skin occurs through extension from an underlying focus, not as a result of primary inoculation. Wherever the infection starts, it tends to burrow to the skin surface. The syndrome has such clear-cut characteristics as to make the diagnosis reasonably certain on the basis of simple clinical examination.

The source of the organism is endogenous; it exists as a harmless resident in the mouths of some normal individuals, being found particularly where anaerobic condi-

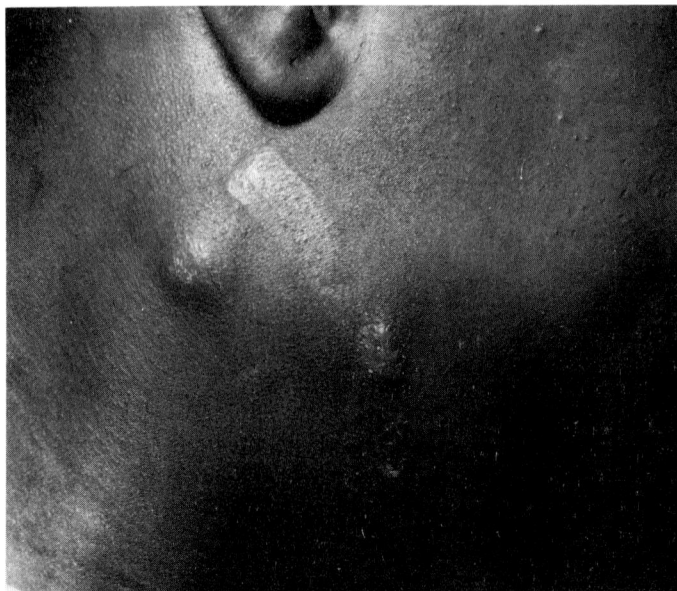

Figure 13–37   Actinomycosis. Early nodular lesions. No drainage or adenopathy yet.

tions favor its growth; that is, in the tonsillar crypts and around carious teeth. Normally it remains innocuously confined to these more or less septic sites unless nearby or distant tissues are devitalized and rendered anaerobic through trauma. This invites seeding of the organism into the pathologic soil. Contagiousness is not a factor, and the disease is not transmissible. Though cattle may acquire the infection, neither they nor the environment they contaminate are sources of infection for other cattle or for man. The long held theory that the disease is acquired by chewing contaminated straws is untenable.

All ages and races are susceptible, though adults are affected most frequently, males twice as often as females. The greater incidence in laborers is probably attributable to poorer oral hygiene, and perhaps this is also why males predominate. The world-wide distribution of the disease is hardly surprising in view of the endogenous source of the organism.

Actinomycosis is classified into three main types according to its localization: (1) cervicofacial, (2) thoracic, and (3) abdominal. Generalized infection is uncommon and is usually due to dissemination from one of the above types. Rarely, isolated lesions may occur in organs such as the liver, brain, kidneys, skin, joints, and so forth.

CERVICOFACIAL ACTINOMYCOSIS.   This disorder is appropriately known as "lumpy jaw" because its usual manifestation is a nodular swelling beneath the mandible. It is the commonest type of actinomycosis, probably accounting for almost two-thirds of all cases. A history of trauma to the jaw, a tooth extraction, or a fracture is almost always elicitable as the antecedent event leading to infection. If the organism is already present around a carious tooth, extraction promotes introduction of the fungus into traumatized tissues under favorable conditions for growth. The hole which is left is a highly inviting anaerobic pocket in which the fungus can gain a foothold, and, once established, can further the tissue necrosis and anaerobic environment. The infection burrows down along the periodontal membrane within the soft tissues and finally appears in the skin beneath the jaw as a firm, red, nontender swelling. Inspection of the mouth may reveal little, for the lesion is "buried" within the soft tissues of the jaw until it reveals itself under the skin. At first the swelling is not characteristic, but soon it becomes woody-hard, and nodules develop within the infiltrated area, giving it a "lumpy" appearance. A purulent exudate is eventually discharged from sinuses in the granulomatous mass.

Less often, the infection originates in

the upper jaw, and it may then burrow insidiously through the contiguous tissues, finally dissecting into the sinuses, orbit, or even the brain. A lesion which begins in the tonsils or in the pharynx may burrow into the neck and extend into the thoracic cage, with varying degrees of involvement of the mediastinum and trachea. Typically, the draining sinuses appear first at the angle of the jaw and involve only the soft tissues initially. If unchecked, the process may later extend into the mandible, finally ending in a full-blown osteomyelitis. Secondary bacterial infection can always be assumed to be adding to the destructiveness of the basic mycotic infection in the later stages. Indeed, *Bacterium actinomycetem comitans*, a bacterium resembling *Hemophilus influenzae,* fusiform bacteria, anaerobic streptococci, and various other anaerobic gram-negative bacteria may play a synergistic role from the very beginning. Patients with lumpy jaw suffer comparatively little pain and continue in good health, except for neglected cases with extensive destruction of the bones, muscles, and soft tissue of the jaw, and possible extension into the neck.

The clinical picture of lumpy jaw is distinctive, and the finding of "sulfur granules" in the pus is diagnostic. These are little yellow grains the size of a pinpoint or less, which have a lobulated outline on microscopic examination. They will often be found within the meshes of a gauze square placed over the draining lesion, or they may sometimes be washed, swabbed or curetted out of the draining sinuses. Occasionally they are grossly absent, but microscopic examination of pus may reveal little clumps of the characteristic filaments.

THORACIC ACTINOMYCOSIS. This is primarily a parenchymatous disease of the lungs, presenting the signs and symptoms of a subacute pulmonary infection, and having many of the characteristics of tuberculosis. Massive infiltrates, usually in the bases, may develop, and the patients are decidedly ill, in contrast to the usual benign course of lumpy jaw. Sooner or later, however, the disease obeys its tendency to burrow through to the surface, eventually presenting itself as multiple draining sinuses of the chest wall. Ugly, extensive, granulomatous, ulcerative lesions may be produced, which continuously discharge an exudate containing the characteristic granules. Thoracic actinomycosis may not be a primary process but rather a complication of bronchiectasis, lung cancer, lung abscess, or any other antecedent pathologic disturbance which could provide favorable anaerobic circumstances for the fungus. In fact, it is unlikely that the disease originates in a normal lung.

ABDOMINAL ACTINOMYCOSIS. This disorder is rarely recognized until the characteristic draining sinuses present themselves on the abdominal wall. The infection usually begins in the ileocecal region, where a mass may be palpated, accompanied by signs of acute or subacute appendicitis. Eventually there may be extension to other intra-abdominal viscera and even perforation into the thoracic cavity. The finding of "sulfur" granules in the draining sinuses is diagnostic.

Immunologic Responses

Antibodies are not consistently nor significantly present in patients with actinomycosis, and serologic reactions consequently have no diagnostic value. Cutaneous reactions to intradermal injections of vaccines of the organism are too variable and inconsistent to be helpful. Cutaneous sensitization is not a regular phenomenon in actinomycosis and is not specific, for normal individuals also react inconsistently. It is highly questionable whether any credence can be placed in the "cures" which have been achieved through administration of Actinomyces vaccines.

Diagnosis

The highly characteristic clinical findings, plus the demonstration of organisms in the pus, ordinarily render the diagnosis of actinomycosis fairly simple. Error may arise, however, due to the uncommonness of this infection and resultant failure to consider it as a diagnostic possibility. Gram stains of the pus, and particularly of the "sulfur" granules, if these can be found, will show lobulated masses composed of delicate, intertwining, gram-positive filaments; these are dense colonies of

A. israelii. Often, but not always, the periphery of the granule will show numerous club-shaped processes at the tips of the filaments. These represent condensations of tissue substance around the ends of the filaments, and because they are radially arranged, the appearance has suggested the name "ray fungus." Instead of fully formed granules, there may be only little clumps of delicate, branching, gram-positive filaments in the pus. These tend to break up into chains of bacillary cells, and this is true of the organism in the granules as well as in culture. The "sulfur" granules and clumps of filaments cannot be microscopically distinguished from those found in mycetoma due to Nocardia or Streptomyces, but distinction from this latter disorder may be made on the basis of clinical characteristics and cultural identification of the organisms. "Sulfur" granules are found readily in biopsy specimens, where they can be visualized in lakes of pus as round or oval bodies from 100 to 300 microns in diameter. They are deeply stained with hematoxylin except in the periphery which is stained by eosin. The filaments, which rarely exceed one micron in diameter, are stained readily by a gram staining method for tissues such as the Brown and Brenn or MacCallum-Goodpasture techniques.

Culture provides a definitive diagnosis. The pus, particularly if the granules can be separated out and washed gently and rapidly in sterile saline, may be streaked over brain-heart infusion agar plates and incubated anaerobically at 37° C. with and without 10 per cent CO_2. Cultures in brain-heart infusion shake tubes and Brewer's thioglycollate broth should also by prepared, for bacterial contamination is a common difficulty. Cultures should not be placed on media containing antibiotics, since growth may be inhibited or prevented by these additives.

DIFFERENTIAL DIAGNOSIS. Cutaneous actinomycosis must be separated principally from mycetoma, tuberculosis, neoplasm, osteomyelitis, amebiasis, granuloma inguinale, and glanders.

Treatment

Antibiotic therapy, vigorously administered, is curative when combined with good general medical and surgical management. Most strains are susceptible to penicillin as well as to the broad-spectrum antibiotics. In vitro sensitivity tests are desirable but may not always be practical. Penicillin is the initial drug of choice. Large quantities must be given, because actinomycosis is suppurative and necrotic, a circumstance which interferes with the attainment of high antibacterial concentrations at the sites of infection. The dose should not be less than 1.2 million units daily, perhaps even 4 to 6 million units daily. In patients who are allergic to penicillin, erythromycin or tetracycline may be substituted. Sulfonamides are far less effective. Antibiotic therapy should be maintained for at least several weeks after all signs of activity have subsided, and usually is continued for a period of 6 to 18 months. Adequate surgical drainage is an essential part of treatment and extensive excision of diseased tissue may be necessary. Good supportive therapy is also required. Iodides have no place in the modern treatment of actinomycosis, and it is highly questionable that they ever did anything more than increase the discomfort of the patient.

NOCARDIOSIS

Like actinomycosis this disease is caused by a funguslike bacterium, *Nocardia asteroides,* which is closely related to the diphtheroids and mycobacteria. It is included in this chapter because of clinical and histopathologic similarities to the systemic fungus infections. Unlike *A. israelii,* *N. asteroides* is not endogenous to man and is always a pathogen when isolated from human sources (Weed et al., 1955). The organism has been recovered from infected domestic animals, but there is no record of spread from animal to man or man to man. *N. asteroides* has been isolated repeatedly from soil samples and is cosmopolitan in distribution. It is gram-positive, partially acid-fast and may be cultivated readily on Sabouraud's agar, brain-heart infusion medium, or media used for isolation of mycobacteria growing at room temperatures or 37° C. under aerobic conditions.

Nocardiosis is usually a primary pulmonary disease (Pinkerton et al., 1971) which resembles tuberculosis in its clinical and x-ray findings. Infection probably occurs through inhalation of contaminated dust. The disease may be characterized by single lesions or scattered infiltrations resembling miliary tuberculosis. Consolidation of an entire lobe, honeycomb cavitation, or the formation of one or more large cavities may develop, and pleural effusion may be massive. The patient may experience malaise, weight loss, low-grade fever, night sweats and pleuritic pain. Cough is initially nonproductive but becomes productive of mucopurulent sputum which may be blood-streaked. Hemoptysis is not infrequent in cavitary lung disease. Because of the obvious similarity of clinical symptoms and x-ray findings and the partial acid-fast staining of *N. asteroides* in sputum specimens, many patients suffering from pulmonary nocardiosis have been initially misdiagnosed as having tuberculosis. The demonstration of branching filaments in smears of sputum is helpful, but a definite diagnosis depends upon the cultural identification of *N. asteroides*. Although this organism may be recovered on media customarily used for the primary isolation of *Mycobacterium tuberculosis*, the differentiation of these two diseases should not be difficult.

In late cases of pulmonary nocardiosis there may be marked pleural thickening accompanied by the formation of thoracocutaneous fistulas. Cutaneous lesions are seen in less than 15 per cent of advanced cases. The most common lesions are abscesses of the chest wall surrounded by granulomatous infiltration of the skin. *Sulfur granules* are seldom seen in the purulent drainage since *N. asteroides* shows little or no tendency to clump together to form granules or microcolonies. In biopsies of nocardial granulomas, the branching filaments are widely dispersed within the granulomatous inflammation. They are not readily seen on routine stains and may be missed altogether unless stained by a modified acid-fast technique, such as the Fite-Faraco stain, or with gram staining methods for tissues.

Primary gastrointestinal nocardiosis occurs less frequently and is probably due to ingestion of food contaminated with *N. asteroides*. The cecum and appendix are occasional sites of primary infection and may present as a tender abdominal mass, but the true nature of the disease is seldom recognized until dissemination has occurred or cutaneous fistulas have developed. Localized infections of skin have been reported at sites of injury, as from a puncture wound caused by a thorn or splinter. The typical *chancriform syndrome* rarely occurs.

Secondary lesions may occur by hematogenous dissemination to brain, kidney, spleen, liver, adrenals, and, rarely, to bone. The brain is the most common site, and lesions may be multiple but more commonly localize to form large abscesses. Symptoms of a space-occupying intracranial lesion may be the initial clinical manifestation. If the primary site of infection is minimal or unrecognized, the diagnosis may not be suspected until after craniotomy and microscopic examination of material from the abscess. The meninges are sometimes involved, but *N. asteroides* is seldom demonstrated in smears or recovered on cultures from the cerebrospinal fluid because of the intense inflammation which surrounds the abscess.

Treatment

Unfortunately, the diagnosis of nocardiosis is seldom established until the disease is far advanced, and the prognosis is poor regardless of treatment. Not infrequently, nocardiosis is secondary to lymphoma, leukemia, or prolonged steroid therapy (Cross and Binford, 1962), and the primary disease also must be treated. The sulfonamides have been most effective. Serum levels should be maintained at 10 mg. per 100 ml., and treatment continued for at least six weeks after clearing of the disease. Streptomycin, the tetracyclines, and other antibacterial antibiotics may have an additive effect and are frequently given in combination with sulfonamides. There is considerable variation in strain susceptibility to the antibacterial antibiotics, and resistant strains are frequently encountered. The selection of antibiotic should be made on the basis of in vitro sensitivity studies whenever possible. Treatment failures are common. Approximately 50 per cent of the reported patients have died with this disease. Surgical incision and drainage of abscesses, and excision and debridement of localized lesions are often necessary. Amphotericin B, griseofulvin, and iodides are ineffective and have no place in the treatment of nocardiosis.

SPOROTRICHOSIS

In its usual form, sporotrichosis is a granulomatous mycosis of the skin and subcutaneous tissues (Fetter and Tindall, 1964), having characteristics so typical that trained observers can recognize it instantly. The disease is world-wide and occurs at all ages, but most often in adult males. It is due to an exogenous fungus, *Sporotrichum schenckii,* which grows saprophytically in soil and on wood. The greater incidence of sporotrichosis in certain regions and in some occupations, particularly among farmers, laborers, and certain types of miners, reflects both an abundance of the organism in the local environment as well as opportunity for appropriate exposure. The organism gains entrance into the skin through a cut or wound inflicted by an object such as a splinter, thorn, piece of rock or glass, etc. which happens to be contaminated with Sporotrichum spores. The organism is a "wound pathogen" which requires a break in the integrity of the skin to produce infection. Infections usually begin on an exposed part, particularly the hands, less often on the face, neck, and feet. Domestic animals (horses, dogs, cats, rats) may acquire the infection in the same way as man, but transmission to man from animals does not occur. The largest number of cases has been observed among the gold miners of South Africa, thousands of whom have become infected following cuts and abrasions sustained in the mines. The luxuriant growth of the organism as a mold on the timbers of the mines is the reason for the high incidence. In such instances the disorder clearly has an occupational origin, and the same consideration applies to horticulturists and agricultural workers who are exposed to a fungus-laden environment. Infections are occasionally reported in children following exposure to vegetation and soil contaminated with the organism (Lynch, 1971). The distribution of the disease can, therefore, be correlated with the climatic and geologic circumstances which permit the growth of the organism in nature. Direct transmission from man to man does not ordinarily occur.

The disease has a variety of clinical expressions in addition to the classic one, and this has fostered an unwieldy classification into many different types. The single most important fact in the pathogenesis of the disorder is the development of a *primary lesion at the site of injury.* This may be a nodule, an ulcer, an infiltrated plaque, acneiform pustules, a verrucous, papillomatous growth, or an abscess. In short, the primary lesion in the early stage may not arouse much suspicion and may be mistaken for an ordinary bacterial infection such as a boil or, in the later stages, a granulomatous process such as luetic chancre or cutaneous tuberculosis. The chancre-like lesion is clinically predominant. The incubation period varies from several weeks to months. Classification of clinical variants is based on the particular way in which the primary lesion evolves or extends, that is, whether it stays "fixed" and grows locally according to one of several patterns, or whether metastatic lesions arise in different patterns.

The most logical classification of sporotrichosis is one which recognizes the natural history of the primary lesion and the different paths along which the infection may evolve, permitting an integrated and dynamic conception of the great variety of clinical manifestations which may emerge. There are three main cutaneous types: (1) the lymphatic, (2) the fixed, and (3) the hematogenous. In addition, extracutaneous sporotrichosis is a well-established entity which may be localized or multifocal.

LYMPHATIC SPOROTRICHOSIS. The development of new lesions via lymphatic spread from the primary chancre is the distinguishing feature of this type. When the initial lesion occurs on an extremity, the metastatic lesions arise linearly along the regional lymphatics, producing the *ascending lymphangitic type of sporotrichosis.* This is the best known "classic" form of the disease and by all odds the commonest. When, less commonly, the infection arises elsewhere, as on the face, satellite lesions are scattered irregularly around the primary lesion as a result of lymphatic spread in all directions, without a distinctive linear pattern.

Since trauma is a prerequisite for infection, it is obvious that most infections will begin on an extremity, usually the fingers or hand. The initial lesion is a nontender, hard, elastic, freely movable subcutaneous nodule which later becomes attached to the skin, assumes a peculiar cyanotic tint, and finally breaks down to produce a chronic ulcer with a necrotic base, the *sporotrichotic chancre*. Within a few weeks, new subcutaneous nodules arise consecutively along the course of the regional lymphatics extending up the fore-

arm in a more or less linear fashion. These nodules, appearing one after the other, enlarge rather rapidly and finally soften and break down, exuding some thin pus. Some become covered with persistent crusts, others continue as draining abscesses or ulcers, and some heal in time. The primary lesion may last for many months and it, too, may finally heal. Long-standing lesions may be difficult to recognize owing to secondary changes, possibly due to bacterial superinfection. Plaques with nodular and vegetative changes may develop. A conspicuous feature of ascending lymphangitic sporotrichosis is the

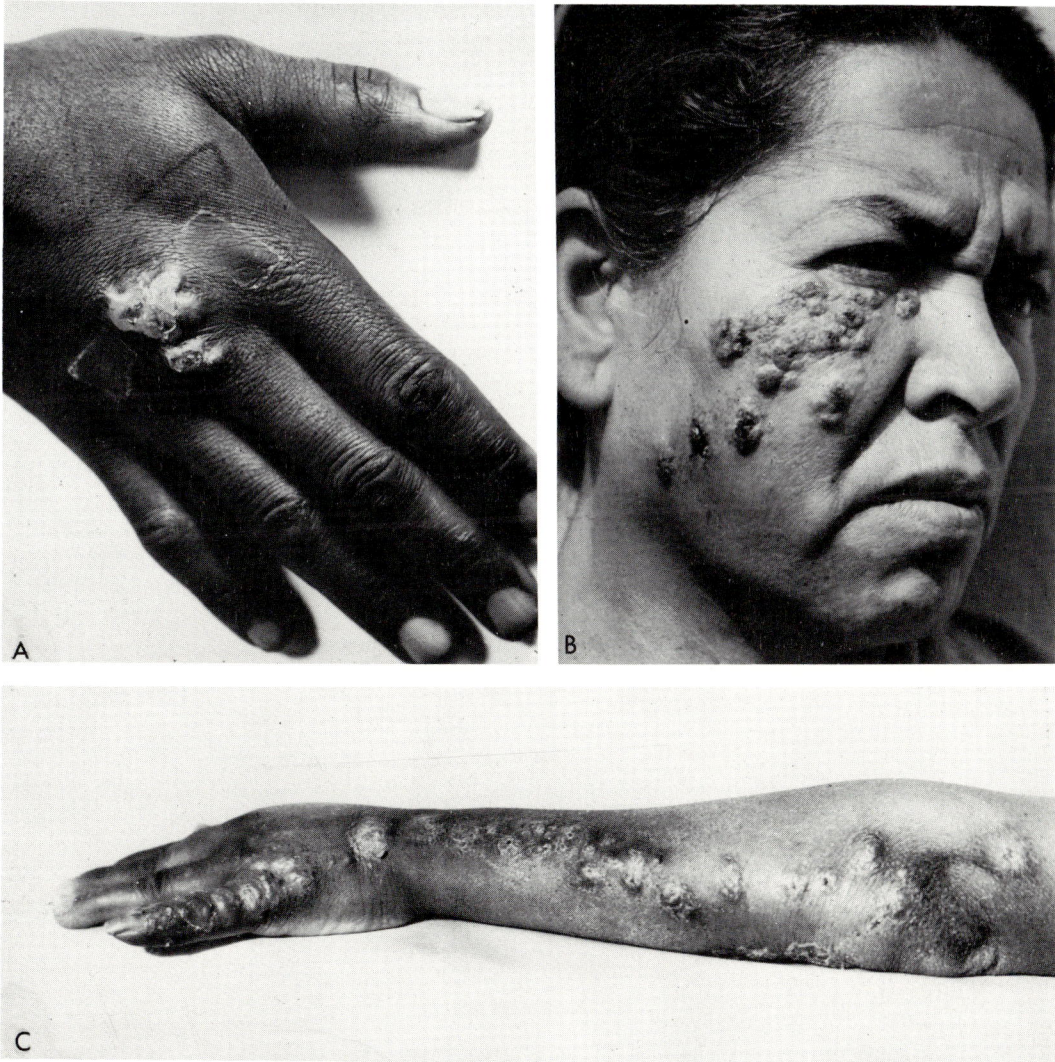

Figure 13–38 Sporotrichosis. *A*, Sporotrichotic chancre. *B*, Gummatous "lymphatic" lesions. *C*, Linearly arranged inflammatory nodules on arm.

great, cordlike thickening of the lymphatics along which the lesions are distributed. Curiously enough, lymph node involvement is the exception, not the rule. The "pipe stem" lymphatics and the linear granulomatous lesions along their path present an unmistakable picture of sporotrichosis, which is unlike any other disease. Furthermore, though the infection may persist for months or years, the general health remains unimpaired, and the individual is not particularly discomforted by the disease.

The satellite metastatic lesions arising in the vicinity of the primary chancre which originates on the face, neck, or elsewhere than on the extremities, have the same characteristics as those already described in ascending sporotrichosis. Irregular clusters of nodules are formed which may eventuate in chronic ulcers or crusted gummatous nodules. The appearance may not suggest sporotrichosis, but rather syphilis, tuberculosis, or other types of granuloma.

FIXED SPOROTRICHOSIS. This type is distinguished by the absence of metastatic lesions; that is, the organism remains confined to the point of entry, producing lesions of variable characteristics. Presumably, this type of the disease reflects a higher degree of immunity of the host. The commonest lesion is a slowly developing ulcer which is usually covered with a thick impetiginous crust, and which may be surmounted by verrucous vegetations. Verrucous, warty plaques, resembling tuberculosis verrucosa cutis, are another form, most often seen on the face. A very uncommon manifestation is an acneiform eruption of the face, presenting papules which break down, finally becoming covered with a crust. The eruption may also resemble a severe pyoderma of the face, a process which would hardly lead one to think of sporotrichosis. Other unusual and deceptive lesions include infiltrated plaques resembling sarcoid, and an erythematous, superficial psoriasiform, scaling dermatitis. The variable morphologic qualities of the fixed types of sporotrichosis are noteworthy.

HEMATOGENOUS SPOROTRICHOSIS. This is a rare form of disseminated sporotrichosis in which the primary lesion may not be recognized or may have occurred in the lungs or other organs. A crop of subcutaneous nodules emerges all over the body at about the same time. These are similar to and follow the same course as the nodules of the lymphatic type, finally ending in chronic crusted ulcers. These patients, who have been seen mostly in France, often have internal foci of sporotrichosis as well, and are gravely ill. Death is a frequent outcome.

COMPLICATIONS OF CUTANEOUS SPOROTRICHOSIS. A serious complication of leaving cutaneous lesions untreated, especially those on the face, is the possibility that the infection may extend deeply into the underlying contiguous tissues, involving important organs in its path of enlargement. Lesions of the nose, mouth, eye, pharynx, and bones of the face have originated in this way, secondary to the primary skin infection.

EXTRACUTANEOUS SPOROTRICHOSIS (Roberts and Larsh, 1971). This type is exceedingly rare. No organ is immune. The internal involvement is generally in association with the hematogenous forms of sporotrichosis, in which the multiple skin nodules furnish the clue to the identity of the internal lesions. Very rarely, localized sporotrichosis may develop in bone, lung, eye, central nervous system, kidney, or other organs. In most instances, visceral lesions are the result of hematogenous dissemination from an unrecognized primary focus in the skin or lungs. Primary pulmonary sporotrichosis has been reported with increasing frequency in recent years (Baum et al., 1969; Mohr et al., 1972). Studies of cutaneous hypersensitivity to sporotrichin suggest that the incidence of asymptomatic infection may be much higher than originally suspected; 58 per cent of nursery workers employed for more than 10 years acquire positive skin tests without history of primary sporotrichosis (Schneidau et al., 1964). It is quite possible that an asymptomatic and self-limited primary pulmonary form of this disease may occur in individuals occupationally exposed to dust contaminated with S. *schenckii*.

Diagnosis

Cultures, preferably from unopened lesions, permit definitive diagnosis, and the fungi are readily grown. On the other hand, the organisms are usually quite scarce in the lesions and cannot be visualized in smears or even in biopsy specimens, though thorough study of a number of sections stained with the periodic acid-Schiff reaction after digestion with diastase may be rewarded by the finding of a few fungal elements. The histopathologic reaction is not pathognomonic but is highly suggestive if a few of the pleomorphic fungal cells are found.

Serologic and sensitivity reactions are adjunctive techniques which may support the diagnosis, but they are rarely essential. Circulating antibodies in the form of agglutinins, complement-fixing antibodies, and precipitins are frequently present, particularly in cases in which there is extensive involvement. The agglutination test is most sensitive and is positive in nearly all patients with pulmonary sporotrichosis (Smith et al., 1971), but no serologic test is entirely reliable. Such tests may be negative in proved cases, especially if the infection is of limited extent. On the other hand, practically all patients with sporotrichosis develop cutaneous reactivity to a heat-killed vaccine or to a polysaccharide prepared from the fungal medium. The reaction is of the delayed tuberculin type. Immediate reactions should be disregarded. Wide experience has shown that an intracutaneous test with 0.1 cc. of 1:2000 polysaccharide is highly specific for sporotrichosis.

Treatment

Iodides are practically a specific chemotherapeutic agent for the usual cutaneous forms of sporotrichosis, but they are apparently ineffective in internal infections and in the disseminated hematogenous cutaneous types. This is the only mycosis in which the curative powers of iodides are beyond dispute. The therapeutic effect is not due to any fungistatic power, but to some unknown influence on the tissue reaction which increases the resistance of the host nonspecifically. Potassium iodide is given in ascending doses up to a point approaching tolerance. The drug should be continued at full doses for a period of one month past the time of apparent heal-

ing, to reduce the likelihood of recurrence. A practical program of administration is to begin with 5 drops of a saturated solution of potassium iodide three times daily. The drops may be added to milk or, less preferably, water, and should be taken after meals. The individual dose may be raised by increments of 1 drop per dose as tolerated until 30 to 40 drops three times daily are given. Gastric reactions are frequent but, unless severe, are not an indication for stopping treatment. If the drug cannot be tolerated by mouth, one gram of sodium iodide may be given intravenously each day. The patient should be observed for evidence of iododerma but, unless this is severe and advancing, it is not a contraindication to further therapy.

Griseofulvin has been reported curative in several patients with primary cutaneous sporotrichosis, but many strains of *S. schenckii* appear to be resistant to this antibiotic. In disseminated and extracutaneous sporotrichosis, especially in the presence of a rising titer with agglutination or complement fixation tests, amphotericin B is indicated. Because of the well-known toxicity of this antibiotic, dosage must be individualized. Amphotericin B is given by slow intravenous infusion beginning with a dose of 0.25 mg. per kg. of body weight which is increased to a maximum dose of 1.0 mg. per kg.

PHAEOSPOROTRICHOSIS

This uncommon disease is characterized by the formation of subcutaneous, intramuscular, or, rarely, osseous abscesses or cysts caused by the dematiacious fungus, *Phialophora gougerotii*. Sporadic cases have been reported from Europe, the Americas, and Africa, and it is quite probable that phaeosporotrichosis is cosmopolitan in distribution in tropical and temperate climates. It is not contagious and probably results from exposure to soil and vegetation. Dematiacious fungi similar to *P. gougerotii* have been isolated repeatedly from these sources. The mode of infection is unknown. Usually there is no definite history of preceding injury. Some cases have occurred in patients suffering from diabetes, tuberculosis, syphilis, or other debilitating disease. The commonest clinical type is a single, deep, subcutaneous or intramuscular cold abscess which may reach several centimeters in diameter. The abscesses are frequently attached to the overlying skin, but ulceration is infrequent. Persistent draining sinus tracts may result from aspiration or biopsy of the lesions, and if the cysts are incompletely excised, recurrent abscesses are frequent. In some patients, regional adenopathy occurs, but unlike sporotrichosis, lymphangitic nodules or abscesses are not seen. Dissemination is rare, but in a few patients, multiple lesions have been described. When dissemination occurs, it is more likely to be by a hematogenous route. The pigmented hyphae and budding cells are easily demonstrated in the thickened wall of the abscess or in aspirated pus, and the organism may be cultured on the usual mycological media. It is not inhibited by cycloheximide and grows well at room temperature. Optimal growth occurs at 30° C. Phaeosporotrichosis differs from the mycetomas due to *P. jeanselmei* in that there is no tendency for *P. gougerotii* to aggregate to form granules in the purulent drainage from the abscesses and sinus tracts. Complete excision of the unruptured cyst or abscess appears to be the treatment of choice.

CRYPTOCOCCOSIS

This disease, due to an exogenous yeast-like fungus, *Cryptococcus neoformans* is world-wide in distribution. The organism has been isolated from many sources including pigeon excreta (Newberry et al., 1967) and soil. Central nervous system involvement is the dominant feature, and neurologic disturbances resulting from invasion of the brain and meninges represent the chief clinical manifestations. The respiratory tract is the probable portal of entry. Pulmonary lesions are frequent, though these are usually inconspicuous both clinically and roentgenologically. Circumscribed lesions occasionally occur in skin, bones, lungs, and elsewhere, unaccompanied by central nervous system involvement. Such isolated localized lesions probably represent spread from an inapparent pulmonary focus. Patients with Hodgkin's disease, sarcoidosis, leukemia, or those receiving systemic corticosteroids or antimetabolites are especially susceptible to this disease.

Cryptococcosis is ordinarily a generalized disease with widespread organ involvement, though the prominence of the central nervous system manifestations eclipses all other signs. The major symptoms are those of a chronic meningitis

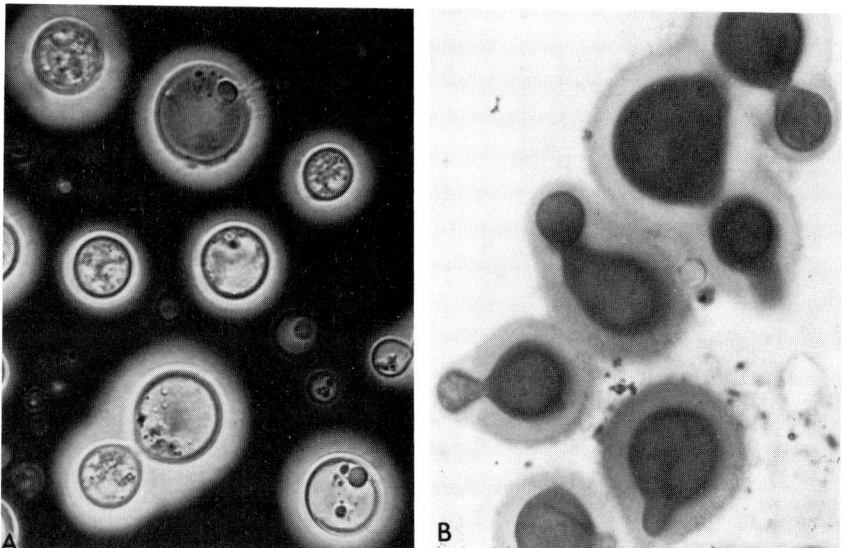

Figure 13–39   *A*, India ink mount of *C. neoformans* showing capsular "halos" around the round, budding, yeastlike cells. *B*, Hotchkiss-McManus stain.

(Edwards et al., 1970), closely simulating tuberculosis. Focal brain lesions produce symptoms suggestive of tumor. Fever is low grade or absent. The health of the patient usually declines gradually until stupor and coma ensue; death results in the majority of cases within six months to a year if untreated. Occasionally, however, the course fluctuates, with periods of complete remission, and many years may elapse before the almost inevitable fatal outcome.

Cutaneous lesions are uncommon (Noble and Fajardo, 1972); they are extremely variable and have no characteristic or unique features. Subcutaneous fluctuant masses, nodules, acneiform lesions and granulomatous ulcers have all been reported. Granulomatous lesions may also occur in the mouth. The initial skin lesions are often acneiform papules situated on an infiltrated plaque which soon tends to break down, producing an ecthymatous ulcer. The margins of the torpid ulcers are sharp, and through enlargement and confluence, large irregular areas of ulceration may result. Localized, soft tumor-like masses may occur as an isolated expression of cryptococcosis practically anywhere, including the skin. Such lesions may remain circumscribed without spread for a considerable period of time, a circumstance which highlights the low virulence of the organism. The surprisingly frequent association of cryptococcosis with other serious systemic conditions such as leukemia, tuberculosis, and sarcoid bears further witness to this; the organism for the most part lacks invasive powers unless the host's resistance has been lowered by previous disease. An investigation should always be made for primary underlying disease or predisposing circumstances.

India ink smears of centrifuged spinal fluid specimens reveal a round budding yeast surrounded by a wide capsule. Similar preparations from material aspirated from cutaneous abscesses and granulomas usually abound in organisms. Cultural isolation is simple, but growth may be inhibited by media containing cycloheximide. Differentiation of *C. neoformans* from nonpathogenic cryptococci depends chiefly on its ability to grow well at 37° C. and to produce lethal meningoencephalitis

when injected intravenously in mice. The lack of tissue reaction to the voluminous mass of organisms is remarkable. The host, on the whole, appears indifferent to the organism, which apparently exerts its deleterious effect through forming space-taking lesions. The organism is weakly antigenic and, accordingly, serologic reactions are absent or of insufficient potency to be useful diagnostically in the majority of cases (Bindschadler and Bennett, 1968; Gordon and Vedder, 1966). Cutaneous sensitivity does not develop.

The variable cutaneous lesions are to be distinguished from other deep fungal infections, tuberculosis, syphilis, acneiform eruptions, and other granulomas. A persistent cutaneous lesion in association with chronic meningoencephalitis is suggestive of cryptococcosis.

Amphotericin B may be lifesaving in this disease, with reduction of overall mortality to less than 20 per cent (Spickard et al., 1963). The antibiotic is administered by slow intravenous infusion beginning at a dose of 0.25 mg. per kg. of body weight and increased gradually to a maximum of 1.0 mg. per kg. Treatment should be continued for at least one month after all cultures are negative. Relapses are common unless the total dose of amphotericin B is greater than 2 gm. In some patients it may be necessary to administer amphotericin B intrathecally. Toxicity to amphotericin B is common and dosage must be individualized. In patients who do not respond to amphotericin B or when this antibiotic cannot be used because of toxicity, 5-fluorocytosine may be of value (Fass and Perkins, 1971; Steer et al., 1972). Localized, circumscribed lesions, whether they occur in the lung, skin, or bones are sometimes amenable to resection, and amphotericin B should be withheld pending evidence of dissemination.

CHROMOMYCOSIS
(Chromoblastomycosis)

Though most cases of this uncommon mycosis occur in tropical and subtropical regions, the disease has been encountered on practically every continent save Asia. Warty and papillomatous excrescences, generally confined to the skin, are the diagnostic hallmarks of the disease, accounting for the apt name "mossy foot." A variety of dematiacious fungi initiate the infection, probably following abrasion or injury by an object contaminated with fungal spores. At least three species have been isolated from nonhuman sources. The causative species are undoubtedly exogenous, existing saprophytically in nature, and only incidentally becoming pathogenic after being introduced traumatically into human tissue. Adult male laborers whose occupation brings them into intimate contact with the soil are chiefly affected. Factors which contribute to infection are lack of shoes, low living standards, and indifference to injuries sustained on the extremities.

The infection usually begins on the leg or foot, but less often the inoculation may occur on some other exposed part. The early lesion is a pruritic papule which enlarges irregularly and slowly forms a nondescript superficial plaque, sometimes resembling a ringworm patch. The lesion is infiltrated, dull red, and sharply defined. The original plaque may continue to extend peripherally, subsequently acquiring the hyperkeratotic and verrucous appearance which characterizes the disorder. More commonly, at intervals, new crops of satellite lesions emerge, principally along the path of lymphatic drainage, resulting in the insidious spread of the eruption in a general upward direction. In the early stages, the appearance is often not highly distinctive and resembles other granulomatous diseases. After many years most of the extremity becomes irregularly enveloped by granulomatous masses. Most of the lesions are greatly elevated, hard, and have a decidedly warty rough surface, an appearance which is all but pathognomonic to the experienced eye. The multiple lesions fuse, forming irregular verrucous masses, leaving patches of normal skin in between. Progression is slow, and the general health remains good. Sometimes, the lesions become papillomatous, and masses of elevated, hard, brownish or reddish nodules surmount the plaques, giving a cauliflower-like appearance. Through secondary infection and neglect, older lesions may ulcerate and exude a foul-smelling discharge, but the lesions are characteristically *dry* and *hard*.

Invasion of the underlying muscle and bone does not occur. Rarely, hematogenous spread to the brain, causing localized brain abscesses, has been reported. The lesions are painless. Spread may cease spontaneously in an early stage, confining the lesions to a small area. There may be complete involution, or in the severest cases, new lesions may emerge over a period of 15 to 20 years. In extensive involvement, the deeper lymphatics eventually become blocked, and elephantiasic enlargement of the extremity results.

Regardless of the causative species, the clinical manifestations and histopathologic findings are essentially similar. Culture affords a definitive diagnosis and is rather easily accomplished. The clusters of brown, thick-walled, septated fungal cells seen in curettings or biopsy specimens are diagnostically conclusive. Five species of closely related fungi, *Phialophora verrucosa, Fonsecaea pedrosoi, F. compacta, F. dermatitidis,* and *Cladosporium carrionii,* have been chiefly linked to the disease. The capacity of these species to form different types of spores in various proportions has incited a great deal of taxonomic confusion leading to the creation of many new generic names, an argument which need not concern us here. In short, a stereotyped pathologic response is excited by a variety of different fungi. Reactions to skin tests are inconstant. The presence of circulating antibodies which may develop in the sera of some cases is of no more than theoretic interest.

The disease must be differentiated from tuberculosis, yaws, syphilis, neoplasms, and other fungal granulomas.

Early diagnosis is the most important element in therapy, for at that stage resection or destruction of the plaque, with plastic repair if necessary, is curative. Time is on the side of the physician, for the advance of the disease is slow. Although the organisms causing chromomycosis may be sensitive in vitro to amphotericin B, the minimal inhibitory concentration is generally too high for intravenous infusion to be effective. In localized lesions, intralesional amphotericin B may be curative (DeFeo and Harber, 1959). It is given in a concentration of 5 mg. per ml.

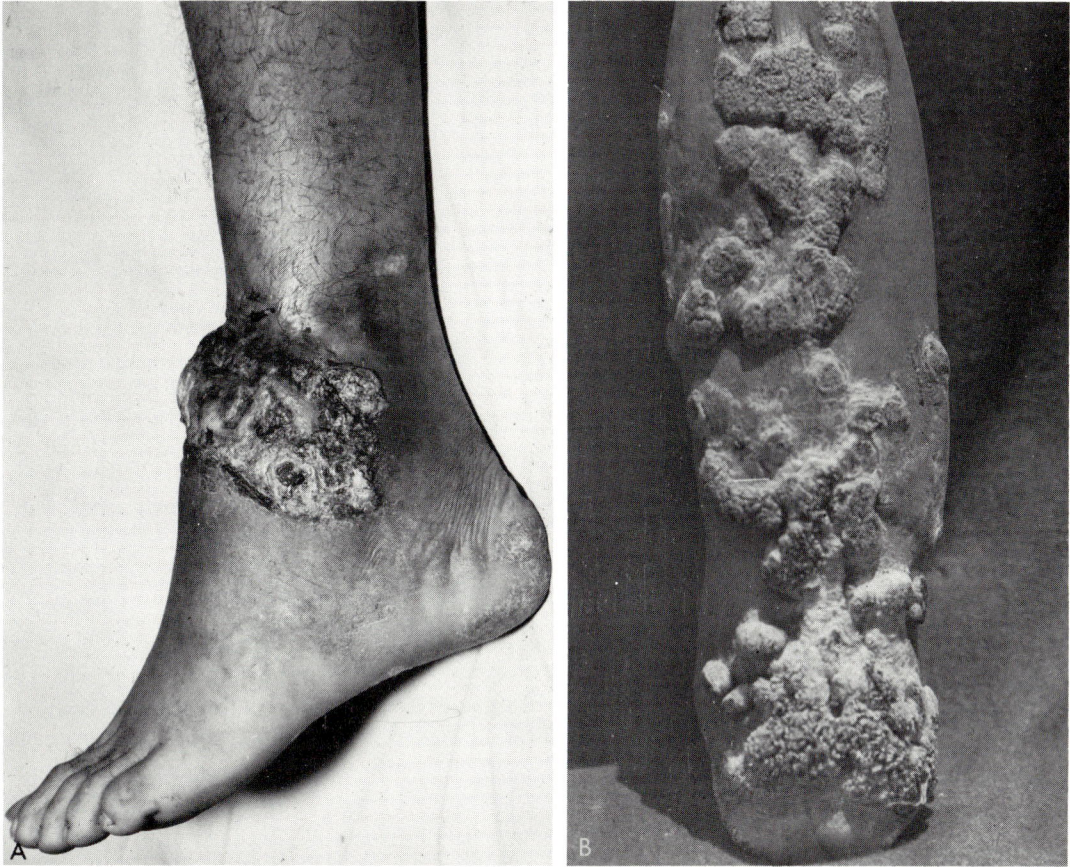

Figure 13–40 *A,* Mycetoma. *B,* Chromoblastomycosis.

in 2 per cent lidocaine which is injected subcutaneously into the lesion. In more superficial lesions, intralesional amphotericin B may be injected by dermojet. Isolation perfusion techniques have also been employed to produce higher tissue levels than can be achieved by intravenous infusion. Variable results have been reported with calciferol, iodides, and thiabendazole (Bayles, 1971) in this disease. Physicians in endemic areas are currently impressed with oral 5-fluorocytosine (Lopes et al., 1971).

MYCETOMA (Madura Foot)

Mycetoma literally means fungal tumor, a name which depicts the chief characteristic of the disorder. There is marked enlargement of the affected part, which is usually, but not always, the foot. Since the "tumor" may occur elsewhere on the body, usually on an exposed part, Madura foot is obviously an inappropriate term. To understand the way in which the disease develops, it is necessary to appreciate that host factors and the circumstances of inoculation play a dominant role in pathogenesis, for the "causative" fungi are ordinarily harmless saprophytes. The assortment of common molds, including such innocuous organs as Aspergillus, Penicillium, Cephalosporium, etc., which are associated with mycetoma are noteworthy for their lack of virulence and are certainly not pathogens in the ordinary sense. These organisms inhabit the soil, flourishing in nature, and only under unique circumstances can they become etiologic agents of disease. The decisive event is an injury which seeds the fungus, probably along with foreign debris, in the skin. The "causative" organisms are "wound" pathogens.

The disease is most prevalent in tropical and subtropical regions, among barefoot laborers with inferior standards of health and hygiene (Abbott, 1956); it is rare in industrialized, highly developed countries. As is the case with other mycoses resulting from an injury with fungus-contaminated objects, male adults acquire the disease most frequently. Mycetoma is not contagious.

The first clinical expression of mycetoma is a rather nondescript papule, nodule, or plaque. The disease evolves slowly over a period of months and years, with occasional arrest and subsequent reactivation. Nodules, the hallmark of the disease, and draining abscesses gradually form near the primary lesion. After many years of slow extension of the infection, the whole foot becomes massively enlarged, studded with nodules and draining sinuses, and finally becomes grotesquely malformed. Partial healing brings about fibrosis and irregular contracture, adding to the deformity. The relentlessly developing destructive process extends deeply into the underlying tissues, invading the muscles, bones, and fascia, causing necrosis and depriving these structures of useful function. The draining sinuses often seem to issue from the summits of nodules. Pain is minimal, and affected individuals manage to hobble along with their deformity for years, without obvious systemic reaction. Metastases to other areas do not occur; the disease, though not undergoing spontaneous involution, remains pretty much confined to the extremity and does not threaten life directly. In the late stages, through neglect, secondary bacterial infection may cause septicemia and death.

The truly diagnostic feature of mycetoma is tiny granules, of pin-point size or less, which may be found in the exuding suppurative fluid. The granules are actually compact fungal colonies made up of dense intertwining masses of filaments. Their color, which may be red, yellow, white, or black, is not a reliable indication of the possible causative species, for the same species may produce differently colored granules (Zaias et al., 1969). The constitution of these granules is of great importance prognostically. Two main classes of organisms are associated with mycetoma: (1) the fungus-like bacteria, the actinomycetes, usually species of Nocardia and Streptomyces, which produce granules indistinguishable from those found in actinomycosis, and (2) the filamentous or weed-mold fungi. Mycetoma due to the former may be termed *Schizomycetoma*, whereas the latter is more properly termed *eumycetoma*. Granules from the schizomycetomas, when gram stained and examined microscopically, are composed of delicate filaments of *bacterial* width, often dissociating into chains of bacillary cells, whereas the granules of the eumycetomas contain filaments of much larger size which need only be examined in ordinary KOH mounts. Perhaps as many as half the cases of mycetoma are schizomycetomas, a circumstance which is fortunate, for these organisms are susceptible

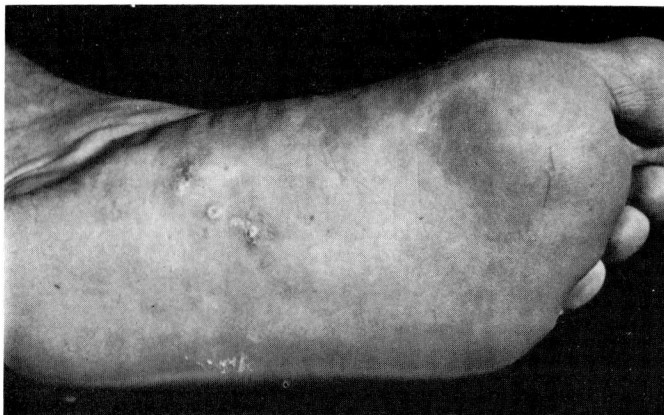

Figure 13–41 Mycetoma. Early pustular lesions. *Allescheria boydii* was recovered on culture and the lesion was cured by excision and skin graft.

to chemotherapeutic agents, whereas there is no effective therapy for mycetoma due to filamentous fungi.

It should be remembered that mycetoma may occur elsewhere than on the foot and presents its pathognomonic characteristics wherever it develops: nodules and chronic sinuses in the drainage of which the diagnostic granules are found. However, swelling is not a prominent feature except when an extremity is involved.

The finding of fungal granules in a lesion clinically consistent with mycetoma is ordinarily sufficient for diagnosis. Microscopic examination of granules or of biopsies will further enable a division into one of the two major classes of mycetoma. Culture will determine the species, which is of little more than academic importance in cases due to filamentous fungi but highly useful in schizomycetoma. The in vitro sensitivity spectrum to sulfonamides and antibiotics can then be determined, providing an opportunity for rational selection of the most effective remedial agents. In North America, *Allescheria boydii* is the species most often encountered in mycetoma, and it has been isolated from the soil. Other species in the filamentous group include *Madurella mycetomi*, *M. grisea*, *Phialophora jeanselmei*, *Cephalosporium recifei*, *C. granulomatis*, *C. falciforme*, *Curvularia lunata*, *C. geniculata*, *Pyrenochaeta romeroi*, *Leptosphaeria senegalensis*, *Neotestudina rosatii*, *Fusarium solani*, *Aspergillus nidulans*, *A. bouffardii*, and *Penicillium mycetogenum*. (Mackinnon, 1954). In the schizomycetomas the following actinomycetes have been identified: *Nocardia brasiliensis*, *N. asteroides*, *N. caviae*, *Streptomyces madurae*, *S. pelletieri*, and *S. somaliensis* (Mackinnon and Artagavetyla-Allende, 1956). Many other species of fungi and fungus-like bacteria have been reported from isolated cases, but the mycology of the organisms has not been fully evaluated.

Early diagnosis is a prerequisite for therapy, especially in respect to preventing the extensive mutilation and destruction of the full-blown process. Sulfonamides are the drugs of choice in schizomycetoma. Large amounts should be given, for suppuration and necrosis are a prominent part of the pathologic reaction, and reduce the efficacy of the drugs. Six to 8 grams of sulfadiazine (or its equivalent in other types of sulfonamides) should be given daily until all active signs of the disease have disappeared, and probably for several weeks after that. The fungus-like bacteria are also variously susceptible to antibiotics such as penicillin, the tetracyclines, and chloramphenicol; one of these may be administered along with the sulfonamide to ensure a successful response, particularly if the organism has been shown before hand to be sensitive to the agent chosen. Diaminodiphenylsulfone has been reported to be effective in some schizomycetomas due to *N. brasiliensis*.

No chemotherapeutic agents are uniformly effective for mycetoma due to filamentous fungi. The results with amphotericin B have been poor. Early diagnosis would in such instances make surgical resection of the lesion possible, with plastic repair if necessary. In late, neglected cases, amputation may become necessary. Locally applied fungicides and iodides by mouth are valueless.

RHINOSPORIDIOSIS

This uncommon disease, due to an exogenous fungus, *Rhinosporidium seeberi*, is endemic in India and Ceylon but occasionally occurs in other parts of the world, including the U.S.A. Water, particularly if stagnant, may be the chief source of the organism. A remarkable number of infections have occurred in certain sand dredging operations in India but only in workers who were actually in the water. Adult males engaged in agricultural labor are chiefly affected. The fungus has not been cultured. Poor personal hygiene, in combination with low living standards, probably contributes to infection. Horses and cattle also acquire the infection.

The typical lesions are polypoid masses of what appears to be exuberant granulation tissue. These growths almost always begin in the nares, the principal site of the lesions, but sometimes the ocular, conjunctival, and lacrimal sacs are involved. Rarely the tumors are found in the upper respiratory tract, in the larynx, pharynx, and tonsils, as well as on the genitalia and glabrous skin. At first sessile and bleeding easily, they later become pedunculated.

The surface of the vegetating growths has a raspberry-like appearance and is seen to be studded with tiny white or yellowish nodules. These are actually large sacs containing innumerable round fungal spores. The slow-growing papillomatous tumors may reach large size and extrude from the anterior nares over the upper lip, or they may hang down as a pedunculated mass into the posterior pharynx. The disease does not impair the general health. The symptoms are those of a space-taking lesion, and obstruction to breathing is the chief complaint. There is a definite resemblance to condyloma acuminatum when the lesions occur around the genitalia. The disease lasts for many years, but spontaneous resolution has occasionally been observed. It is not communicable.

Scrapings from the surface of the tumors show great numbers of the large spores which, in combination with the clinical picture, are diagnostic.

Resection or electrosurgical destruction are the methods of choice. Early diagnosis is important. Recurrence following surgical excision is common unless a wide zone of normal tissue is also removed. No effective antifungal or chemotherapeutic agent is known.

ASPERGILLOSIS

This is an uncommon opportunistic fungal infection caused by a variety of species of Aspergillus. *A. fumigatus* is the most commonly identified pathogenic species, but *A. niger* and an increasing number of species have been reported in recent years. The infections are exogenous and not contagious. Aspergillus sp. are ubiquitous, being found as a common household mold and isolated regularly from a variety of nonhuman sources. The fungus requires reduced host resistance to establish infection. Aspergillosis is generally a complication of severe debilitating disease and occurs in patients suffering from neoplastic disease, tuberculosis (Parker et al., 1970), silicosis, diabetes, and bronchiectasis; it also occurs in patients who are receiving corticosteroid, antibiotic, cytotoxic, or immunosuppressive therapy. The usual route of infection is pulmonary. Cutaneous lesions are rare.

The intracavitary fungus ball is the most common manifestation of aspergillosis and occurs in individuals with cavitary lung disease. The fungus forms a mass of mycelia within a cavity or bronchiectatic bronchus. This may be seen on x-ray as a dense mass within the cavity which changes position when erect and recumbent x-rays are compared. Invasive bronchopulmonary aspergillosis is generally caused by *A. fumigatus* (Vedder and Schorr, 1969). Granulomatous lesions extend into the lung parenchyma and undergo central necrosis with cavitation (Eastridge et al., 1972). Lesions may be solitary or multiple. The fungus extends radially invading blood vessels with hematogenous dissemination to kidneys and other viscera. Sputum is initially mucopurulent and often blood-tinged. Hemoptysis may be moderate to severe. The course of the disease is progressive, with remittent low-grade fever, productive cough, weight loss, toxemia, and death.

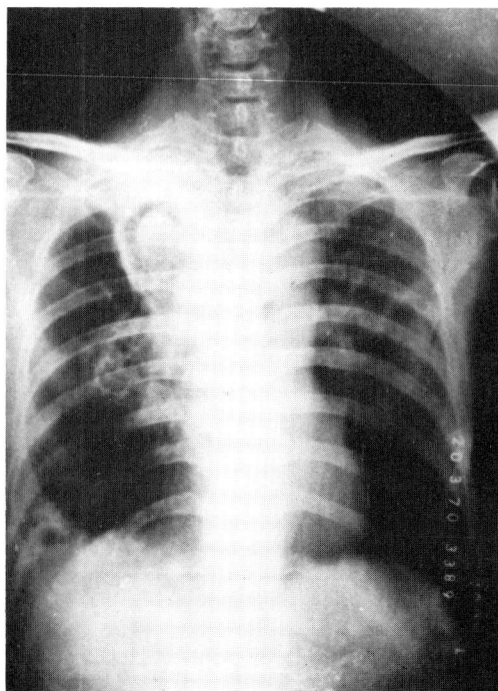

Figure 13–42 Aspergillosis. Intracavitary fungus ball in right upper lobe in patient with cavitary lung disease due to advanced tuberculosis.

Less commonly, an opportunistic infection of the paranasal sinuses may result in symptoms of persistent mucopurulent or blood-tinged nasal discharge, headache, periorbital neuralgia, and unilateral vasomotor rhinitis. The infection may spread by peripheral extension to involve adjacent structures, including orbit, brain, or overlying skin. The face becomes swollen, erythematous, warm, and tender, resembling cellulitis or erysipelas.

Mycotic keratitis (Naumann et al., 1967) is frequently caused by various species of Aspergillus. A great variety of other genera have also been isolated from infections of the cornea, including species of Candida, Fusarium, Fusidium, Gibberelli, Penicillium, Actinomyces, Nocardia, Cephalosporium, Curvularia, and Ustilago. The stroma of the avascular cornea is invaded by the ordinarily saprophytic fungus following trauma. The initial lesion is a gray-white nodule which spreads peripherally to produce corneal opacification. With further extension of the fungus, corneal ulceration occurs. Penetration of Descemet's membrane results in endophthalmitis and loss of the eye.

Various species of Aspergillus have been recovered from the so-called *otomycosis* (Kingery, 1965). In this condition there is colonization of cerumen, epithelial debris, and detritus within the external auditory canal. The resulting mycelial plug may cause irritation and pruritus with superficial erosion and swelling of the external auditory canal, but there is seldom invasion of viable tissue and the tympanic membrane remains intact. Removal of the mycelial plug and detritus, and treatment of the external otitis is curative.

Inhalation of spores of Aspergillus sp. may result in an acute allergic bronchitis and pneumonitis resembling Loeffler's syndrome in patients sensitized to this fungus (Slavin et al., 1970). The condition is characterized by fever, wheezing, cough, and prostration, with recovery in 12 to 36 hours. The fungus may be recovered from sputum during the acute phase, but disappears as the patient recovers. Eosinophilia and urticaria are not uncommon during the acute attacks.

The recovery of Aspergillus sp. on culture is of little value unless the organism can also be demonstrated in pathologic material, since the fungus is so commonly found as a laboratory contaminant. The hyphae are easily demonstrated in tissue sections without special stains and are characterized by segmentation and branching at acute angles. In biopsies or tissues obtained at autopsy from patients with cavitary lung disease or with aspergillosis of the paranasal sinuses where there is an air-tissue interface, one may occasionally identify the characteristic conidiophores as well as filaments of the fungus. Serologic tests have been of limited value in the diagnosis of aspergillosis (Walter and Jones, 1968).

The prognosis in bronchopulmonary aspergillosis is grave. Although there have been several promising reports of recovery following treatment with amphotericin B, treatment failures are common. Intracavitary fungous balls and aspergillomas generally require pulmonary resection (Kilman et al., 1969), since the mycelial mass is not resorbed even if the fungus has been killed.

PHYCOMYCOSIS

Phycomycosis is an opportunistic infection occurring in patients with a variety of debilitating diseases including diabetes, leukemia, lymphoma, cancer, liver disease, anemia, heart disease, and burns; it also occurs in patients receiving corticosteroids, cytotoxic agents, and immunosuppressive therapy. The causative agents are the so-called bread molds and include species of Mucor, Rhizopus, Absidia, Mortierella, and Cunninghamella. These fungi are ubiquitous and are frequently found as common laboratory contaminants. They are incapable of infecting healthy tissue. The portal of entry may be in skin, paranasal sinuses, lung, or gastrointestinal tract in patients with lowered host resistance.

Cutaneous phycomycosis is rare. Patients with severe diabetes mellitus with recurrent acidosis and patients with severe burns are especially susceptible (Bruck et al., 1971). The initial lesion is usually a small area of macular discoloration or dusky erythema which gradually enlarges and ulcerates. Necrosis may be marked and there is usually a profuse, foul-smelling, purulent exudate. The large, non-septate, branching filaments of the phycomycete are easily demonstrated in tissue sections from the granulation tissue in the base of the ulcer. The portal of entry is unclear. Patients with cutaneous phycomycosis seldom give a history of preceding trauma, and similar lesions may arise by hematogenous dissemination from primary foci in the lungs, gastrointestinal tract, or other site.

Phycomycosis may develop in the paranasal sinuses with extension into adjacent structures including bone, brain, orbit, and overlying skin (Groote, 1970). The initial clinical manifestation may be a unilateral retrobulbar mass. The skin of the face may be swollen (Martinson, 1971) and assume a dusky erythematous hue. The cerebral manifestations are not characteristic. Headache, cranial nerve palsies, and cerebral infarction are common. Primary phycomycosis of the lung and gastrointestinal tract may result from the inhalation or ingestion of spores of the phycomycetes. These fungi have a tendency to invade blood vessels and grow into the lumen as though coursing through a conduit. Hematogenous dissemination is common with involvement of distant viscera. The intravascular mycelial plug frequently results in infarctions in brain, skin, lung, spleen, kidney, and other organs.

All methods of treatment fail unless the underlying predisposing disease can be corrected. Reversal of diabetic acidosis may result in spontaneous remission if dissemination has not occurred. When this is not possible or when phycomycosis occurs in association with other diseases, the patient should be treated with intravenous amphotericin B.

SUBCUTANEOUS PHYCOMYCOSIS (Williams, 1969). This uncommon disease has been reported from tropical and subtropical climates in Indonesia, southeast Asia, and Africa. It is caused by several species of phycomycetes which belong to the order Entomophthorales, including *Basidiobolus meristosporus* and *B. haptosporus*. The infection begins as a firm, lenticular, subcutaneous nodule which is freely movable over the muscles but is attached to the skin. Lesions occur more often on exposed surfaces of the extremities. The skin becomes discolored over the nodule but ulceration is infrequent. The nodule may enlarge to 10 to 20 cm. in diameter, and the entire extremity may become involved with massive edema resembling elephantiasis. Dissemination to internal viscera does not occur and general health is not affected. It is thought that the fungus may be introduced by biting insects. The course is chronic but spontaneous remission usually occurs after months or years.

INFECTIONS CAUSED BY ACHLORIC ALGAE (Protothecosis)

Human and animal infections caused by achloric mutants of the green alga, Chlorella, have recently been reported (Klintworth et al., 1968). Three species, *Prototheca segbwema*, *P. wickerhamii*, and *P. zopfi*, have been demonstrated in tissue specimens and identified by culture. Other species of Prototheca have been recovered from feces in cases of tropical sprue, as contaminants (or secondary pathogens) in actinomycosis and paracoccidioidomycosis, as pathogens in domesticated and wild animals, from the mucous flux of trees, and from contaminated fresh and marine water.

Although widespread visceral disease has been reported in animals, the reported infections in humans have been localized to the skin, subcutaneous tissue, and regional lymphatics. The initial lesion is a subcutaneous or intracutaneous nodule or tender red papule. The lesions enlarge, become pustular, ulcerate, and produce a blood-tinged, malodorous, purulent discharge. As the disease progresses, satellite lesions develop and tend to become confluent. The lesions may become verrucous and closely resemble lesions seen in chromomycosis. Metastatic granulomas may occur in regional lymph nodes. The portal of entry is unclear, but most of the reported cases have had a history of exposure to water which could have been contaminated with the organism.

The diagnosis is made by the demonstration of Prototheca in histologic preparations (Tindall and Fetter, 1971). The organisms are spherical and vary markedly in size from 2 to 11 microns in diameter. The larger organisms have thick walls and characteristic internal septations. They are basophilic and gram-positive and stain well with Grocott's methenamine silver stain, colloidal iron stains for acid mucopolysaccharides, and the periodic acid-Schiff reaction. Prototheca grows readily on Sabouraud's agar, blood agar, or brain heart infusion agar at an optimum temperature of 30° to 32° C. The colonies are cream-colored and yeastlike.

The disease is chronic and progressive, with the capacity for metastatic spread to lymph nodes in man and internal viscera in animals. Early excision may be curative. No effective chemotherapeutic agents have been reported.

REFERENCES

Abbott, P.: Mycetoma in the Sudan. Trans. R. Soc. Trop. Med. Hyg. *50*:11, 1956.

°Ajello, L.: Coccidioidomycosis. Tucson, University of Arizona Press, 1967.

Albright, S. D., and Hitch, J. M.: Rapid treatment of tinea versicolor with selenium sulfide. Arch. Dermatol. *3*:460, 1966.

Allen, A. M., Taplin, D., Lowy, J. A., et al.: Skin infections in Vietnam. Milit. Med. *137*:295, 1972.

Baer, R. L.: The biology of fungous infections of the feet. J.A.M.A. *197*:1017, 1966.

°Baum, G. L., and Schwarz, J.: North American blastomycosis. Am. J. Med. Sci. *238*:661, 1959.

Baum, G. L., Donnerberg, R. L., Stewart, D., et al.: Pulmonary sporotrichosis. N. Engl. J. Med. *280*:410, 1969.

Bayles, M. A. H.: Chromomycosis: Treatment with thiabendazole. Arch. Dermatol. *104*:476, 1971.

Bindschadler, D. D., and Bennett, J. E.: Serology of human cryptococcosis. Ann. Intern. Med. *69*:45, 1968.

Blank, H., and Roth, F. J.: The treatment of dermatomycoses with orally administered griseofulvin. Arch. Dermatol. *79*:259, 1959.

Blank, H., Smith, J. G., Roth, F. J., et al.: Griseofulvin for the systemic treatment of dermatomycoses. J.A.M.A. *171*:2168, 1959.

Bruck, H. M., Nash, G., and Pruitt, B. A.: Opportunistic fungal infection of the burn wound with phycomycetes and *Aspergillus*. Arch. Surg. *102*:476, 1971.

°Burgoon, C. F., and Keiper, R. J.: Tinea capitis. Pediatr. Clin. North Am. 8:759, 1961.

Burke, R. C.: Tinea versicolor: susceptibility factors and experimental infection in human beings. J. Invest. Dermatol. *36*:389, 1961.

Busey, J. F.: Blastomycosis: I. A review of 198 collected cases in Veterans Administration hospitals. Am. Rev. Resp. Dis. 89:659, 1964.

Butler, W. T.: Pharmacology, toxicity, and therapeutic usefulness of amphotericin B. J.A.M.A. *195*:371, 1966.

Butler, W. T., Bennett, J. E., Alling, D. W., et al.: Nephrotoxicity of amphotericin B. Ann. Intern. Med. *61*:175, 1964.

Canales, L., Middlemas, R. O., Louro, J. M., et al.: Immunological observations in chronic mucocutaneous candidiasis. Lancet *2*:567, 1969.

Chilgren, R. A., Meuwissen, H. J., Quie, P. G., et al.: The cellular immune defect in chronic mucocutaneous candidiasis. Lancet *1*:1286, 1969.

Chilgren, R. A., Quie, P. G., Meuwissen, H. J., et al.: Chronic mucocutaneous candidiasis, deficiency of delayed hypersensitivity, and selective local antibody defect. Lancet *2*:688, 1967.

°Conant, N. F., Smith, D. T., Baker, R. D., et al.: Manual of Clinical Mycology. 3rd ed. Philadelphia, W. B. Saunders Co., 1971.

Cross, R. M., and Binford, C. H.: Is *Nocardia asteroides* an opportunist? Lab. Invest. *11*:1103, 1962.

DeFeo, C. P., and Harber, L. C.: Chromoblastomycosis treated with local infiltration of amphotericin B solution. J.A.M.A. *171*:1961, 1959.

Eastridge, C. E., Young, J. M., Cole, F., et al.: Pulmonary aspergillosis. Ann. Thorac. Surg. *13*:397, 1972.

Edwards, V. E., Sutherland, J. M., and Tyrer, J. H.: Cryptococcosis of the central nervous system. J. Neurol. Neurosurg. Psychiatry. *33*:415, 1970.

°Emmons, C. W., Binford, C. H., and Utz, J. P.: Medical Mycology. 2nd ed. Philadelphia, Lea & Febiger, 1970.

Fass, R. J., and Perkins, R. L.: 5-Fluorocytosine in the treatment of cryptococcal and candida mycoses. Ann. Intern. Med. *74*:535, 1971.

Fetter, B. F., and Tindall, J. P.: Cutaneous sporotrichosis. Arch. Pathol. 78:613, 1964.

°Fields, B. T., Bates, J. H., and Abernathy, R. S.: Amphotericin B serum concentrations during therapy. Appl. Microbiol. *19*:955, 1970.

°Fiese, M. J.: Coccidioidomycosis. Springfield, Charles C Thomas, 1958.

Furcolow, M. L.: Comparison of treated and untreated severe histoplasmosis. J.A.M.A. *183*:823, 1963.

Furcolow, M. L.: Tests of immunity in histoplasmosis. N. Engl. J. Med. *268*:357, 1963.

Gilgor, R. S., Rindall, J. P., and Elson, M.: Lupus-erythematosus–like tinea of the face (tinea faciale). J.A.M.A. *215*:2091, 1971.

Gordon, M. A., and Vedder, D. K.: Serologic tests in diagnosis and prognosis of cryptococcosis. J.A.M.A. *197*:961, 1966.

Graham, J. H., Johnson, W. C., Burgoon, C. F., et al.: Tinea capitis: A histopathological and histochemical study. Arch. Dermatol. 89:528, 1964.

Groote, C. A.: Rhinocerebral phycomycosis. Arch. Otolaryngol. *92*:288, 1970.

°Gruhn, J. G., and Sanson, J.: Mycotic infections in leukemic patients at autopsy. Cancer *16*:61, 1963.

Harrell, E. R., and Honeycutt, W. M.: Coccidioidomycosis: A traveling disease. Arch. Dermatol. 87:188, 1963.

°Hildick-Smith, G., Blank, H., and Sarkany, I.: Fungus Diseases and Their Treatment. Boston, Little, Brown & Co., 1964.

Keddie, F., and Shadomy, S.: Etiological significance

of *Pityrosporon orbiculare* in tinea versicolor. Sabouraudia *3*:21, 1963.

Kilman, J. W., Ahn, C., Andrews, N. C., et al.: Surgery for pulmonary aspergillosis. J. Thorac. Cardiovasc. Surg. *57*:642, 1969.

Kingery, F. A.: The myth of otomycosis. J.A.M.A. *191*:129, 1965.

Kligman, A. M.: The pathogenesis of tinea capitis due to *Microsporum audouinii* and *Microsporum canis*: I. Gross observations following the inoculation of humans. J. Invest. Dermatol. *18*:231, 1952.

Kligman, A. M.: Tinea capitis due to *M. audouinii* and *M. canis*: II. Dynamics of the host-parasite relationship. Arch. Dermatol. *71*:313, 1955.

Klintworth, G. K., Fetter, B. F., and Nielsen, H. S.: Protothecosis, an algal infection: Report of a case in man. J. Med. Microbiol. *1*:211, 1968.

Kozinn, P. J., Taschdjian, C. I., Seelig, M. S., et al.: Diagnosis and therapy of systemic candidiasis. Sabouraudia *7*:98, 1969.

Landay, M. E., and Schwarz, J.: Primary cutaneous blastomycosis. Arch. Dermatol. *104*:408, 1971.

°Littman, M. L., and Walter, J. E.: Cryptococcosis: Current status. Am. J. Med. *45*:922, 1968.

°Littman, M. L., and Zimmerman, L. E.: Cryptococcosis. New York, Grune & Stratton, 1956.

Lopes, C. F., Cisalpino, E. O., Alvavenga, R. J., et al.: Treatment of chromomycosis with 5-fluorocytosine. Int. J. Dermatol. *10*:182, 1971.

Louria, D. B., Stiff, D. P., and Bennett, B.: Disseminated moniliasis in the adult. Medicine *41*:307, 1962.

Lynch, P. J.: Sporotrichosis in children. Am. J. Dis. Child. *122*:325, 1971.

°Lynch, P. J., Voorhees, J. J., and Harrell, E. R.: Sporotrichosis and sarcoidosis. Arch. Dermatol. *103*:298, 1971.

Mackinnon, J. E.: A contribution to the study of the causal organisms of maduromycosis. Trans. R. Soc. Trop. Med. Hyg. *48*:470, 1954.

Mackinnon, J. E., and Artagavetyia-Allende, R. C.: The main species of pathogenic aerobic actinomycetes causing mycetomas. Trans. R. Soc. Trop. Med. Hyg. *50*:31, 1956.

Maibach, H. I., and Kligman, A. M.: The biology of human cutaneous moniliasis (*Candida albicans*). Arch. Dermatol. *85*:233, 1962.

Maize, J. C., and Lynch, P. J.: Chronic mucocutaneous candidiasis of the adult. Arch. Dermatol. *105*:96, 1972.

Martinson, F. D.: Chronic phycomycosis of the upper respiratory tract. Am. J. Trop. Med. Hyg. *20*:449, 1971.

Medeiros, A. A., Marty, S. D., Tosh, F. E., et al.: Erythema nodosum and erythema multiforme as clinical manifestations of histoplasmosis in a community outbreak. N. Engl. J. Med. *274*:415, 1966.

Menges, R. W., Doto, I. L., and Weeks, R. J.: Epidemiologic studies of blastomycosis in Arkansas. Arch. Environ. Health *18*:956, 1969.

Mohr, J. A., Patterson, C. D., Eaton, B. G., et al.: Primary pulmonary sporotrichosis. Am. Rev. Resp. Dis. *106*:260, 1972.

Montes, L. F., Cooper, M. D., Bradford, L. G., et al.: Prolonged oral treatment of chronic mucocutaneous candidiasis with amphotericin B. Arch. Dermatol. *104*:45, 1971.

Montes, L. F., Pittman, C. S., Moore, W. J., et al.: Chronic mucocutaneous candidiasis: Influence of thyroid status. J.A.M.A. *221*:156, 1972.

Naumann, G., Green, W. R., and Zimmerman, L. E.: Mycotic keratitis: A histopathologic study of 73 cases. Am. J. Ophthalmol. *64*:668, 1967.

Newberry, W. M., Walter, J. E., Chandler, J. W., et al.: Epidemiologic study of *Cryptococcosis neoformans*. Ann. Intern. Med. *67*:724, 1967.

Noble, R. C., and Fajardo, L. F.: Primary cutaneous cryptococcosis: Review and morphologic study. Am. J. Clin. Pathol. *57*:13, 1972.

Olansky, S.: Double-blind study of a topical antifungal agent in the treatment of human cutaneous fungal infections. Cutis *9*:470, 1972.

Parker, J. D., Sarosi, G. A., Doto, I. L., et al.: Pulmonary aspergillosis in sanatoriums in the south central United States. Am. Rev. Resp. Dis. *101*:551, 1970.

Parker, J. D., Sarosi, G. A., Doto, I. L., et al.: Treatment of chronic pulmonary histoplasmosis. N. Engl. J. Med. *283*:225, 1970.

Pinkerton, J. A., Lawler, M. R., and Foster, J. H.: Pulmonary nocardiosis. Am. Surg. *37*:729, 1971.

°Rebell, G., and Taplin, D.: Dermatophytes, Their Recognition and Identification. 2nd ed. Coral Gables, University of Miami Press, 1970.

Roberts, G. D., and Larsh, H. W.: The serologic diagnosis of extracutaneous sporotrichosis. Am. J. Clin. Pathol. *56*:597, 1971.

Rothman, P. E., Graw, R. G., Harris, J. C., et al.: Coccidioidomycosis: Possible fomite transmission. Am. J. Dis. Child. *118*:792, 1969.

Sarosi, G. A., Voth, D. W., Dahl, B. A., et al.: Disseminated histoplasmosis: Results of long-term follow-up. Ann. Intern. Med. *75*:511, 1971.

Schneidau, J. D., Lamar, L. M., and Hairston, M. A.: Cutaneous hypersensitivity to sporotrichin in Louisiana. J.A.M.A. *188*:371, 1964.

Schofield, F. D., Parkinson, A. D., and Jeffrey, D.: Observations on the epidemiology, effects and treatment of tinea imbricata. Trans. R. Soc. Trop. Med. Hyg. *57*:214, 1963.

Sellers, T. F., Price, W. N., and Newberry, W. M.: An epidemic of erythema multiforme and erythema nodosum caused by histoplasmosis. Ann. Intern. Med. *62*:1244, 1965.

Shapiro, L., and Cohen, H. J.: Tinea faciei simulating other dermatoses. J.A.M.A. *215*:2106, 1971.

Slavin, R. G., Milton, L., and Cherry, J.: Allergic bronchopulmonary aspergillosis: Characterization of antibodies and results of treatment. J. Allergy *46*:150, 1970.

Smith, A. G., Morgan, W. K. C., Hornick, R. B., et al.: Chronic pulmonary sporotrichosis. Am. J. Clin. Pathol. *55*:401, 1971.

°Smith, D. T.: Fungus Diseases of the Lungs. 2nd ed. Springfield, Charles C Thomas, 1963.

Smith, J. W., and Utz, J. P.: Progressive disseminated histoplasmosis. Ann. Intern. Med. *76*:557, 1972.

Spickard, A., Butler, W. T., Andriole, V., et al.: The improved prognosis of cryptococcal meningitis with amphotericin B therapy. Ann. Intern. Med. *58*:66, 1963.

Steer, P. L., Marks, M. I., Klite, P. D., et al.: 5-Fluorocytosine: An oral antifungal compound. Ann. Intern. Med. *76*:15, 1972.

°Sweany, H. D.: Histoplasmosis. Springfield, Charles C Thomas, 1960.

Taschdjian, C. L., Kozinn, P. J., Okas, A., et al.: Serodiagnosis of systemic candidiasis. J. Infect. Dis. *117*:180, 1967.

Tindall, J. P., and Fetter, B. F.: Infections caused by achloric algae. Arch. Dermatol. *104*:490, 1971.

Tynes, B. S., Utz, J. P., Bennett, J. E., et al.: Reducing amphotericin B reactions. Am. Rev. Resp. Dis. *87*:264, 1963.

Utz, J. P.: Amphotericin B toxicity: Combined clinical staff conference at the National Institutes of Health. Ann. Intern. Med. *61*:334, 1964.

Vanek, J., Schwarz, J., and Hakim, S.: North American blastomycosis: A study of ten cases. Am. J. Clin. Pathol. *54*:384, 1970.

Vedder, J. S., and Schorr, W. F.: Primary disseminated pulmonary aspergillosis with metastatic skin nodules. J.A.M.A. *209*:1191, 1969.

Walter, J. E., and Jones, R. D.: Serologic tests in diagnosis of aspergillosis. Dis. Chest *53*:729, 1968.

Weed, L. A., Amdersen, H. A., Good, C. A., et al.: Nocardiosis: Clinical, bacteriologic and pathologic aspects. N. Engl. J. Med. *253*:1137, 1955.

Williams, A. O.: Pathology of phycomycosis due to *Entomophthora* and *Basidiobolus* species. Arch. Pathol. *87*:13, 1969.

Williams, A. O., Lawson, E. A., and Lucas, A. O.: African histoplasmosis due to *Histoplasma duboisii*. Arch. Pathol. *92*:306, 1971.

Wilson, J. W.: Cutaneous (chancriform) syndrome in deep mycoses. Arch. Dermatol. *87*:81, 1963.

°Wilson, J. W., and Plunkett, O. A.: The Fungous Diseases of Man. Los Angeles, University of California Press, 1965.

°Winner, H. I., and Hurley, R.: *Candida albicans*. Boston, Little Brown & Co., 1964.

Zaias, N.: Onychomycosis. Arch. Dermatol. *105*:263, 1972.

Zaias, N., Taplin, D., and Rebell, G.: Mycetoma. Arch. Dermatol. *99*:215, 1969.

°General references

TREPONEMAL INFECTIONS

Leslie Nicholas

TREPONEMATOSES

The treponematoses consist of several diseases due to organisms which cannot be differentiated from each other at the present time. Hudson hypothesized that the treponematoses are only one disease when considered etiologically, the differences in the clinical expressions resulting from environmental factors (temperature, humidity), social adjustments, and various host-parasite relationships (especially body temperature).

Until further information becomes available, it seems advisable to continue to identify species of treponemes which are pathogenic for vertebrates according to the clinical syndromes (syphilis, jaws, pinta, endemic syphilis, and bejel) they produce. In two species, subspecies should probably be recognized in the genus Treponema.

These so-called pathogenic treponemes naturally inhabit primates only, with the exception of *T. cuniculi* which is a pathogen of low virulence for rabbits. In addi-

tion to these pathogenic treponemes, a wide variety of nonpathogenic treponemes exist in nature as part of the mixed microbial flora indigenous to many vertebrates, including man. At present there is no adequate means of identifying and classifying these microorganisms except by size, shape, and normal habitat. More refined means of taxonomic identification may be expected from ultrastructural, biochemical, and other biological studies, all of which are delayed by man's inability to cultivate the pathogenic treponemes either on artificial media or in tissue culture.

Cross-immunity experiments in man would tend to support the theory that the

TABLE 14–1 SPECIES OF TREPONEMA

Species	Subspecies
T. pallidum	T. pallidum, variant: endemic, nonvenereal
T. pertenue	T. pertenue, variant: cynocephalus
T. carateum	
T. cuniculi	

various pathogenic treponemes are not identical, since *T. carateum* may protect against *T. pallidum* and *T. pertenue*, *T. pertenue* may protect against *T. pallidum* but not against *T. carateum*, and *T. pallidum* does not protect against either *T. pertenue* or *T. carteum*. Thus, perhaps in the future, it will be possible to immunize man with the organism isolated from one of the treponematoses and thereby provide a moderate, or possibly sufficient, degree of protection against the other treponemal diseases.

The pathogenic treponemes appear as fine threadlike spirals composed of 8 to 20 closely wound and rigid coils (Fig. 14–1). The organism is 6 to 15 microns long and 0.09 to 0.18 microns in diameter. The movements are characteristic, consisting of (1) a rotary motion on its longitudinal axis, (2) quivering movements which permit forward or backward travel, and (3) flexion with maintenance of the coils. These pathognomonic movements can be appreciated by examining under darkfield microscopy fresh, unfixed secretions (1) taken from surface lesions or (2) aspirated from enlarged lymph nodes. Treponemes can also be demonstrated by the direct fluorescent antibody technique when there are no facilities for immediate darkfield examination.

Electron microscopy provides much detail, including an axial bundle in those preparations in which the spirals were intact, and a capsular structure (periplast) surrounding the internal substance of the treponemes. The earlier electron microscopic pictures showed flagella-like structures which are now interpreted as artefacts created by rupture of the axial bundle.

SYPHILIS

Syphilis is capable of producing a more varied group of manifestations in the skin and mucous membranes than any other infectious disease, with the possible exception of tuberculosis. It may also mimic a wide variety of other systemic diseases — infectious, neoplastic, and degenerative. The truly competent syphilologist, and there have been relatively few, was perforce possessed of ability in the fields of internal medicine, dermatology, neurol-

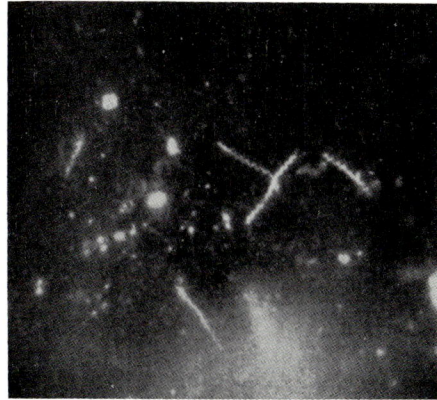

Figure 14–1 *Treponema pallidum* from chancre. Darkfield × 1000. (From Stokes, J. H., Beerman, H., and Ingraham, N. R., Jr.: Modern Clinical Syphilology. 3rd ed. Philadelphia, W. B. Saunders Co., 1944; collection of Dr. Noguchi.)

ogy, ophthalmology, urology, gynecology, and immunology. Until 1945–48, syphilis was an infectious disease of great magnitude throughout the world. Since that period, its incidence fell precipitously until July, 1958, when the downward trend reversed — not only in the United States but in many countries throughout the world. In the United States, for the fiscal year ending July 1, 1970, the number of reported cases of infectious (primary and secondary) syphilis was 20,186, almost twice the 1960 incidence of 12,471. In England and Wales, between the years 1960 and 1969, the number of new patients attending venereal disease clinics increased by 78 per cent.

The reasons for this increased incidence are not known but various factors have been implicated: the changes in attitudes and morals, increased promiscuity, more homosexual activity, increased tourism, greater population migration, and most recently, the widespread use of cyclic contraceptive medications and intrauterine devices with corresponding diminution in popularity and use of the condom. Further resurgence of syphilis is possible by any of the following mechanisms: (1) The emergence of a penicillin-resistant strain of treponemes, or a strain which might even resist all currently available antibiotics. Fortunately, there has been no indication whatever of this since penicillin therapy for syphilis was introduced in

1942. (2) Increased allergic sensitization of the population to various treponemicidal antibiotics. This has already occured in relation to penicillin. (3) Failure to recognize the earliest manifestations of syphilis because of lack of experience in syphilology among the younger physicians. Since 1946, it has been increasingly difficult to give any practical training in clinical syphilology to medical students and resident physicians. The development of fully trained syphilologists is now impossible because of this decreased amount of clinical material.

Transmission

When *T. pallidum* invades the host by placental transmission from the mother, the infection is called *congenital syphilis.* All other infections with *T. pallidum* are *acquired syphilis.* The latter is due almost invariably to the moist contact associated with any variety of sexual activity. Extragenital infection may result from sexual or nonsexual activity, an example of the latter being the digital infection of physicians. Indirect transmission from toilet seats, door knobs, and so forth does not occur.

Acquired Syphilis

Stages and Phases

To encompass the natural history of acquired syphilis, one may employ either of two basic classifications. The older one is clinical; the more recent one is epidemiologic; and a combination of the two provides the maximum efficiency.

The clinical classification is composed of four stages:

1. The *primary stage* is characterized by the presence of a chancre, usually with regional lymphadenopathy.

2. The *secondary stage* is known for its widespread, often symmetric eruption, mucous membrane lesions, and generalized lymphadenopathy.

3. The *latent stage* is the period when there are neither symptoms nor signs of any infection, and the diagnosis is based on reactive serologic tests for syphilis. Latency, or inactivity of the disease, may not be diagnosed until after the cerebro-

spinal fluid is examined and found to be normal. If the patient has an abnormal cerebrospinal fluid, he is classified as having asymptomatic neurosyphilis.

4. The *tertiary stage* encompasses all late clinical changes, many of which may be preceded by prolonged asymptomatic periods during which considerable tissue destruction occurs.

The epidemiologic classification is based on the amount of time elapsed since *T. pallidum* entered the patient. The dividing line between the *early phase* and the *late phase* was originally four years, but now two years is preferred in most clinics. The reasoning behind this classification is that early syphilis (less than two years duration) is infectious, tends to relapse, is seldom scarring, and should provide excellent yield to careful epidemiologic investigation. On the other hand, late syphilis (more than two years duration) is rarely infectious (except to the unborn child through the infected pregnant woman), rarely will develop infectious relapse, is often destructive and scarring, and on epidemiologic investigation produces neither source nor spread cases.

The combination of these two classifications permits the common use of the following terms:

1. Early lesion syphilis includes primary and secondary syphilis and infectious relapses.

2. Early latent syphilis is latent syphilis of two years or less.

3. Late latent syphilis is latent syphilis of more than two years duration.

4. Late manifest syphilis includes tertiary lesions and all other symptomatic and asymptomatic manifestations, two or more years after the original infection.

Diagnosis of Early Syphilis

THE PRIMARY LESION. The chancre of syphilis appears, on the average, three weeks after the skin has been inoculated. Considerable variations in time do exist, however, and this primary incubation period may be as short as 10 days or as long as 90 days, a fact which must be remembered when performing adequate epidemiologic investigation. The morphologic appearance of the chancre is usually suggestive but not diagnostic. It tends to be rather indurated, relatively clean (Fig. 14–2 A), as compared to chancroid, and gives rise to a nontender, nonfluctuant, rather firm regional lymphadenopathy (bubo). Wide deviation from this pattern may be noted, however; multiple chancres are unusual (Fig. 14–2 B), and the chancre may coexist with chancroid, lymphogranuloma venereum, granuloma inguinale, or nonvenereal diseases such as herpes simplex and scabies. *It is essential that all ulcerative genital lesions be suspected of being syphilis until proved otherwise.* The primary lesion of syphilis may appear anywhere on the skin surface; the most frequent extragenital chancres are on the lip, mouth, fingers or breasts (Fig. 14–3). In these locations the associated node may be very large and is ordinarily unilateral. In the female, a chancre which does not appear externally may pass unnoticed and is detected only by speculum examination. Many female patients, however, may not appear for study until the chancre has subsided spontaneously or has become so mixed with secondary lesions as to make it unrecognizable. In the male homosexual, any anal lesion, even the smallest fissure or ulcerated hemorrhoid, must be viewed with suspicion, especially if associated with inguinal lymphadenopathy.

The essential procedures in the study of ulcerative genital lesions can be outlined quite clearly. Expert darkfield examination is not as easily obtainable as it was prior to 1945. Demonstration of treponemes with the darkfield microscope is a simple enough procedure, but it is by no means free from error if an improper site is selected for obtaining material or if the examination is done by an inexperienced technician. The material selected for darkfield examination should be obtained from the deeper portions of the lesion. The surface should be wiped off gently or, if it is greatly contaminated, should be cleansed with saline soaks. Following scraping of the surface, a serous sample is obtained by squeezing, with as little admixture of red cells as possible. In some instances it may be deemed advisable to obtain material from deeper portions of the lesion or from a neighboring bubo by needle aspiration. Ulcerative lesions of the mouth are an untrustworthy source; it is impossible to distinguish the treponemata of syphilis from many other spirochetal organisms in the mouth flora. A similar error may occur in relation to lesions about the anus, though material from this area may be accepted if expertly obtained.

A serologic test for syphilis (STS) is obtained on the first visit, along with the

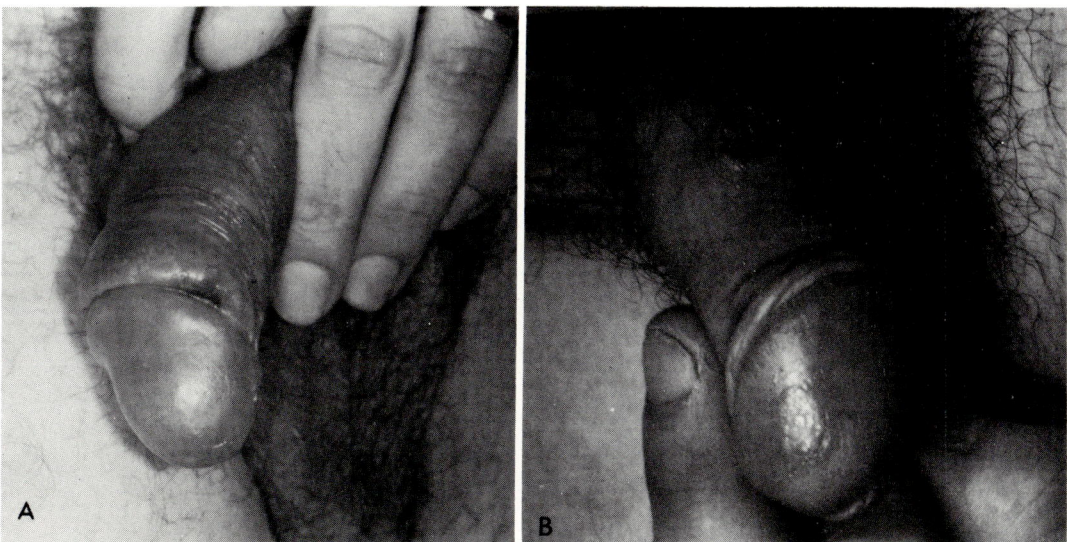

Figure 14–2 Darkfield positive chancres of syphilis. *A,* Painless solitary ulceration of coronary sulcus of penis. *B,* Unusual multiple chancres of shaft and glans penis.

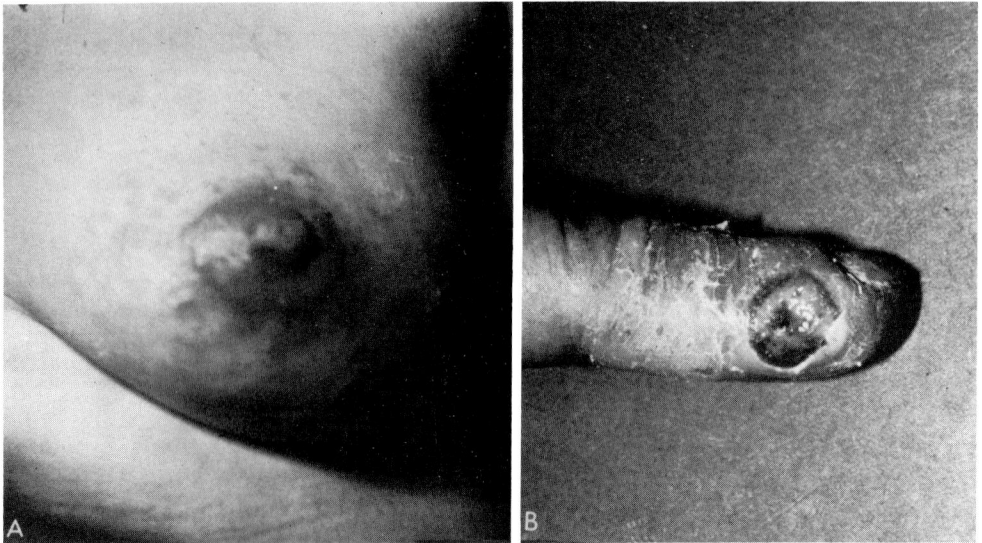

Figure 14-3 Extragenital chancres. *A*, Chancre of nipple. (Courtesy of Dr. Herman Beerman.) *B*, Painful digital chancre of man whose wife has darkfield positive secondary syphilis. (Courtesy of Dr. Louise E. Tavs.)

darkfield examination of serum from the presenting lesion or lesions. If the initial darkfield examination is negative, it should be repeated on three consecutive days. No local application other than saline soaks should be made. It is obvious that neither penicillin nor other broad spectrum antibiotics should be administered during this period. If, however, there is clinical evidence for chancroid, it is permissible to administer a sulfonamide, since this has no effect upon the organism of syphilis. If the darkfield examination is negative, one must depend upon further observation of the patient and repetition of the STS. The STS should be repeated once weekly for one month, and the patient inspected for the development of any mucocutaneous lesions. If the STS is to become reactive, it will ordinarily do so within this period in the presence of syphilis, provided the test is properly performed. To guard against late development of seroreactivity, it is wise to repeat the STS on four further occasions at monthly intervals. In the absence of some compelling reason, further serologic follow-up thereafter will not be worthwhile.

A significant source of error in the past has been the acceptance of a single reactive STS as diagnostic of syphilis in the presence of a darkfield negative ulcerative genital lesion. This is a slim reed upon which to lean for the diagnosis of such a serious disease. The STS should be repeatedly reactive and, in the presence of early syphilis, it will ordinarily show a considerable rise in titer within two to three weeks. A slight delay in diagnosis at this time is not crucial, and speed should not be regarded as a reason for accepting inadequate evidence for the disease.

SECONDARY LESIONS. The mucocutaneous lesions of early syphilis occur in wide morphologic variety. These are seen within a few weeks after the occurrence of the primary lesion. The interval from the first manifestation of the chancre to the appearance of the secondary eruption is called the secondary incubation period. The initial lesions may be minimal and hardly detectable, and may be relatively evanescent, disappearing within two or three weeks, even though the disease is untreated. In many patients with untreated early syphilis, however, the mucocutaneous lesions may be prominent from their onset, or may gradually develop into very extensive lesions of varying morphologic patterns.

A description of all types of secondary

lesions would include a major portion of morphologic dermatology. Certain lesions are much more suggestive of syphilis than are others, however. The chief characteristics are as follows:

1. By and large, the mucocutaneous lesions of early syphilis tend to be symptomless.

2. Frankly vesicular or bullous lesions are not due to syphilis (except occasionally in infants). Pustular lesions may be seen occasionally, but tend to be less acute, and are not grossly suggestive of bacterial infection as a source.

3. Dry macular or papular, slightly inflammatory lesions on the palms and/or soles (Fig. 14–4*A*) are strongly indicative of syphilis if they occur as part of the usual ensemble, and may be almost pathognomonic to an experienced observer.

4. In the presence of an ensemble of a subsiding genital lesion, regional or generalized adenopathy, absence of high fever, and painless eroded lesions of the mouth or multiple, moist wartlike lesions in the anogenital region, a diagnosis of syphilis will prove almost inescapable.

5. Among the most characteristic of all mucocutaneous lesions of early syphilis are those which are annular (Fig. 14–4*B*), seen much more frequently in Negroes than in whites. Such lesions are rather bizarre at times and ordinarily produce hyperpigmentation at the center. Although they may be mimicked by other diseases, an experienced dermatologist can recognize such lesions with a high degree of accuracy.

6. "Moth-eaten" alopecia (Fig. 14–5) and iritis may be associated with the secondary mucocutaneous lesions and lymphadenopathy. Demonstration of treponemes in lesions of secondary syphilis is easily accomplished, especially if carried out within a week or two after the appearance of the lesions. The material may be obtained in much the same manner as a scraping would be done for the bacillus of leprosy, but as a rule it is only necessary to abrade the surface slightly, wait for the bleeding to subside, and then obtain some of the serous discharge.

The lesions of secondary syphilis may be confused with many nonsyphilitic dermatoses, including, particularly, grouped follicular eruptions, chronic widespread acneiform lesions, pityriasis rosea (although this requires a very low order of dermatologic ability), psoriasis, sarcoid infiltrations of the skin, and various types of nonscarring alopecia. However, these variations are now an aspect of clinical dermatology which has largely disappeared, and a recounting of them in too great detail would serve no useful purpose here.

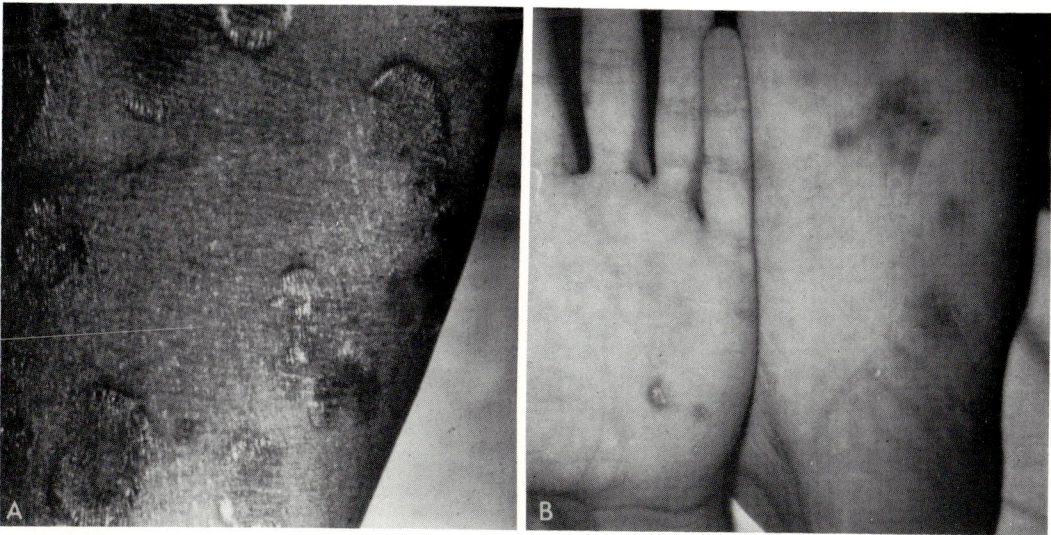

Figure 14–4 Secondary syphilis. *A*, Annular lesions always suggest syphilis in differential diagnosis. *B*, Papular ham-colored lesions of the palm and sole.

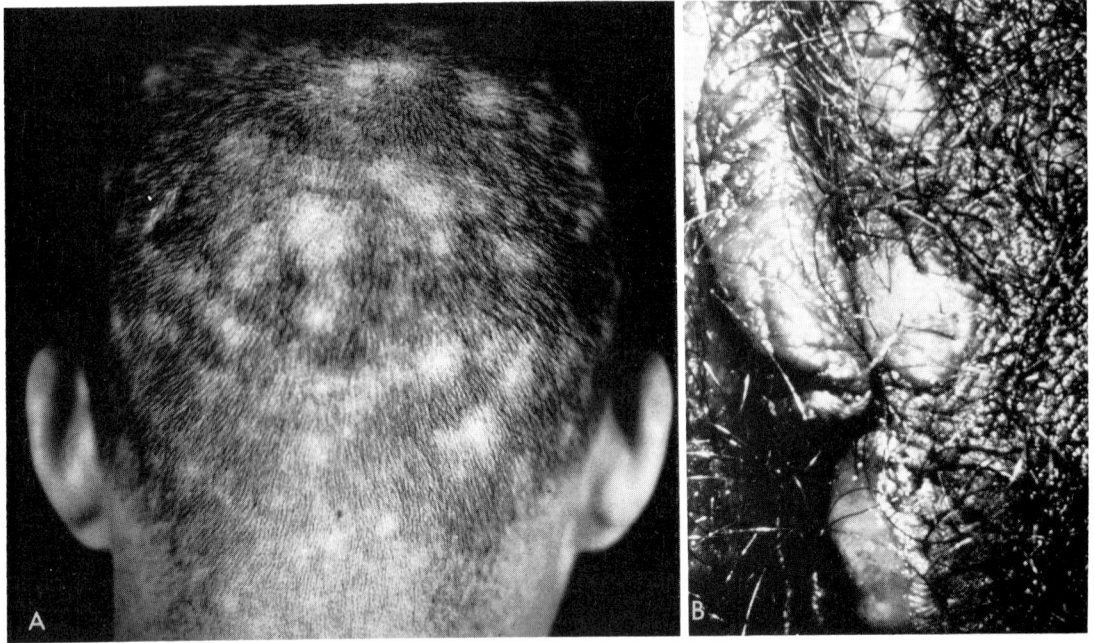

Figure 14–5 Secondary syphilis. *A*, Moth-eaten alopecia is a transient nonscarring type of loss of hair. (From Carson, T. E., and Johnson, D. W.: Venereal Disease in the Military. *In* Nicholas L., (ed.): Sexually Transmitted Diseases. Springfield, Charles C Thomas, 1973.) (Reproduced by permission.) *B*, Condylomata lata occur in moist intertriginous areas and are teeming with *T. pallidum*.

Constitutional reactions, ordinarily mild, are very common in early syphilis. They consist principally of headache, malaise, low-grade fever, and sometimes arthralgia. The more severe and significant reactions include iritis, marked generalized lymphadenopathy, evidence of periostitis, or even meningitis.

Late Syphilis

As stated at the outset of this chapter, no attempt will be made herein to outline the diverse and numerous evidences of late syphilis affecting the various organ systems and the special sense organs. Late syphilis has undergone an even more rapid disappearance from the medical scene, at least in the United States, than has early syphilis. Some patients with long-standing late organic damage due to syphilis remain, but these present principally general medical, cardiovascular, and neurologic problems for which specific treatment for syphilis will be of little or no avail. In any event, the wellspring of late syphilis seems to have dried up at its source.

A few statements will suffice concerning late syphilis affecting the skin and mucous membranes. Although the appearance of a gumma affecting the skin and subcutaneous tissues is highly characteristic, the diagnosis should not depend entirely upon the morphologic changes but should include the usual studies which might be applied to any destructive granuloma of the skin, including complete general medical study of the patient and biopsy of the lesion. Gummas affecting the skin and subcutaneous tissues are characteristically indolent and deeply infiltrated. If there are multiple lesions, these are often few in number and strikingly asymmetric (Fig. 14–6 *A*). Grouping of gummatous nodules is common, for reasons which still are not understood. Ulceration of such nodules often produces a punched out appearance at the rather scalloped border of the lesion. Treponemes are not demonstrable in the nodules. Coalescence of the lesions produces arciform and serpiginous outlines which are highly characteristic. These lesions may persist for years, with gradual extension at one border and healing in other areas. The scarring produced is noncontractile, and this has been emphasized as a distinguishing feature from the contractile scarring of lupus vulgaris. Late syphilis involving the mucous membranes of the nose and throat may produce extensive destructive changes. Perforation of the palate is an almost pathognomonic lesion of syphilis in the absence of any history of injury, operation, malignant tumor, or chrome poisoning.

Patients with tabes dorsalis (locomotor ataxia), late neurologic parenchymal syphilis, may develop, because of the absence of pain sensation, not only indolent ulcers of toes and feet (Fig. 14–6 B) from pressure but also destruction of weight-bearing joints and adjacent bones (Charcot joints) from the constant trauma of use.

Late syphilis of the skin and mucous membranes is not infrequently associated with involvement of bones. Patients with such a condition, in spite of extensive ulcerative and destructive changes, often show no evidence of other organic involvement, particularly on the cardiovascular or nervous systems. As such, they constitute a group known as "benign late syphilis" because, though the lesions may be disfiguring and sometimes partially disabling, the infection has no significant effect upon the life span of the individual affected. Gummas of the skin and mucous membranes, in the absence of secondary infection and necrosis of underlying bone or cartilage, frequently respond to mild, older methods of treatment, including

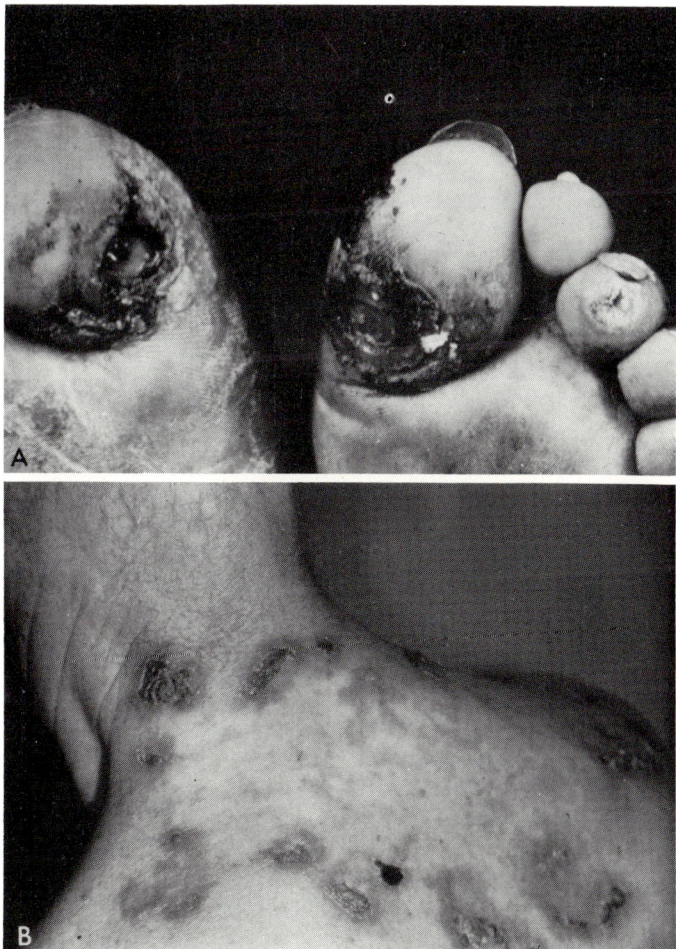

Figure 14–6 Late syphilis of the skin. *A*, Bilateral perforating ulcers in a patient suffering from tabes dorsalis. (Courtesy of Dr. Herman Beerman.) *B*, Nodulo-ulcerative lesions which developed in a patient who failed to return for treatment 35 years previously when he had a darkfield positive chancre.

such outmoded therapy as mercury or iodide by mouth. Penicillin is the treatment of choice, both because of its antisyphilitic effects and the antibacterial effects on secondary infection. In most patients with gummas affecting the skin or mucous membranes, a single injection of as little as 2,400,000 units of benzathine penicillin G will be adequate in the absence of concomitant evidence of involvement of other organs.

Even a brief discussion of late syphilis cannot be concluded without emphasis upon the fact that the destructive involvement of the nervous system and the cardiovascular system constitutes the most significant and serious development of all types of late syphilis. Occasional patients will inevitably slip through the diagnostic screen in regard to syphilis and will escape the prophylactic effects of antibiotics given for other reasons. It may also be expected that the index of suspicion of physicians who have received their training during the past 25 years, in respect to the formerly well-known and highly characteristic lesions of cardiovascular and neurosyphilis, will continue to decrease.

Congenital Syphilis

As a result of the detection of syphilis in pregnant women and treatment given as soon as possible during pregnancy, great strides toward the elimination of congenital syphilis were made during the heavy metal treatment era. By 1940, it could almost be said that, in patients subjected to an adequate program of prenatal care, congenital syphilis could be completely eliminated. Penicillin is still more effective in this regard and has the advantage that, even if treatment is given late in pregnancy when the fetus is already infected, active congenital syphilis after birth may be completely prevented. In pregnant women so treated, provided their subsequent course is satisfactory, infection of the fetus will not occur in later pregnancies.

Syphilis in the Newborn and Young Infant

Since the methods of preventing transmission of syphilis from the mother to the fetus are, for all practical purposes, 100 per cent effective, active early congenital syphilis in the newborn and young infant has become an exceedingly rare disease among populations to whom adequate medical facilities are available. For this reason, the clinical manifestations of congenital syphilis will be outlined only briefly.

MUCOCUTANEOUS LESIONS. The mucocutaneous lesions of congenital syphilis are comparable to those produced by the infection acquired in adult life, with the exception that the lesions may occasionally be bullous. This is in accord with the tendency of other dermatoses to produce bullae more readily in infancy than in older skin, because of the ease with which the infant's skin is separated at the dermo-epidermal junction. As in early acquired syphilis in the adult, mucocutaneous lesions appear in a variety of forms, but the most common are papules or even plaques. The lesions may be extraordinarily profuse at times, and treponemes may be recovered from them easily and in great numbers. Infants with such lesions, prior to treatment, are highly infectious. A bronze color of the lesions was emphasized in the older literature, but this is not a regular feature, at least on the basis of the author's experience. As with many other inflammatory lesions in the infant, a yellowish or brownish cast may be present at times because of the large amount of pigmented lipophyllic materials in the skin. It is also stated in classic descriptions that infants with widespread mucocutaneous lesions of syphilis are ordinarily marasmic and ill. While this may be true at times and was undoubtedly true several decades ago because of the generally high proportion of underweight or marasmic infants, it is certainly not in accord with this author's own experience. A well-fed and otherwise healthy child may withstand, for a time, the early overwhelming spirochetemia without serious inconvenience.

The x-ray changes, which consist of a typical osteochondritis and periostitis in the long bones, are characteristic in early congenital syphilis. If the infection is untreated, progress toward a typical combination of increased and decreased bone density may be seen. The picture is almost pathognomonic to experienced eyes, but should not be relied upon solely for the diagnosis, since confirmatory evidence of the infection is always present in patients thus infected. The lymphatic system may be markedly affected in early congenital syphilis, with generalized lymphadenopathy and often marked splenomegaly. As in the acquired infection in adults, a diverse combination of signs and symptoms related to involvement of other organ systems has been encountered, but these signs and symptoms are now of interest chiefly to medical historians.

CONGENITAL VS. ACQUIRED SYPHILIS IN INFANCY. While the distinction between infantile syphilis acquired in utero and that acquired after birth is now chiefly a matter of academic interest, it is quite clear that when signs of syphilis appeared in infants in the past, it was often too readily assumed that the infection was maternal in origin. When the signs appear within the first few weeks of life, the odds are overwhelming that the disease was acquired in utero or during passage through the birth canal; however, in infants of over three or four months of age, consideration must be given to the possibility that the infection was acquired from a source other than maternal. The care of infants and the custom of evidencing affection for them offer many opportunities for transmission of the infection from an adult.

Late Congenital Syphilis

Congenital syphilis is capable, if untreated, of producing a wide variety of signs and symptoms in late childhood or adult life. A number of these symptoms are so characteristic as to be pathognomonic to the experienced eye and have been termed congenital syphilitic "stigmata." These various signs are, in this author's experience at least, now of interest only as items of medical history and will be listed without any attempt at full description.

OSSEOUS AND DENTAL SYSTEMS. Untreated congenital syphilis is capable of producing marked aberrations in the growth and development of bones and teeth. The characteristic osteochondritis accompanying early congenital syphilis has been referred to above. Although the late changes produced by this involvement of germinal centers may vary widely, certain changes are outstanding. These include (1) changes in the skull, including, particularly, prominent frontal bossae, palatal destruction and perforation, and destruction of the nasal cartilage, producing the characteristic stigma of "syphilitic saddle nose"; (2) various changes in the shoulder girdle, including clavicular thickening and characteristic "wing-type" scapula; and (3) tibial changes consisting of thickening and anterior bowing, the "saber shin." These are among the more characteristic changes, but x-ray studies in late congenital syphilis have revealed a variety of other abnormalities.

The dental changes in late congenital syphilis are among the most pathognomonic of all signs of the disease. Interference with one of the germinal centers of the permanent upper central incisors produces the well known Hutchinsonian incisor (Fig. 14–7), in which there is enamel-covered notching at the center of the bite margin and anteroposterior and lateral thickening which produces a "grain of wheat" appearance. When all criteria are present, this sign is pathognomonic. It never develops, however, if adequate treatment was given to the infant prior to

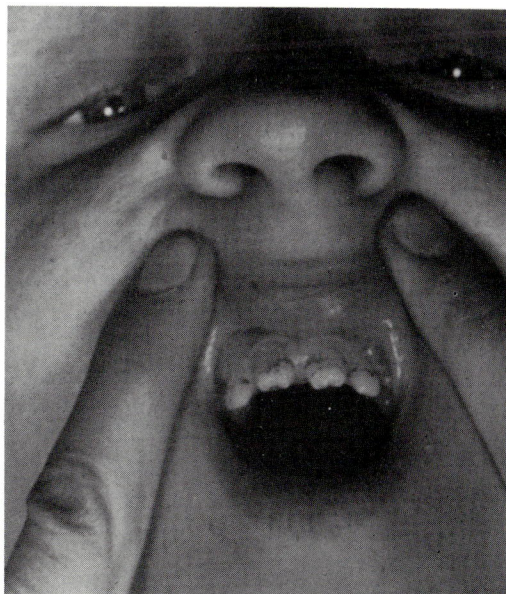

Figure 14–7 Hutchinson's teeth of late congenital syphilis.

his third month of life. Another characteristic dental sign is the disturbance in the six-year molars, with aberration of the cusps, producing a "mulberry" appearance. These teeth are subject to very early decay. The germinal centers of other teeth are frequently affected, but ordinarily not in a pattern which can be distinguished from changes produced by other disease states.

The most feared sequel of congenital syphilis is a characteristic interstitial keratitis inflammation. This occurs in late childhood, the teens, or even in the twenties. It represents a curious late phenomenon, probably a localized disturbance of tissue-immune reactions, but it is not due to direct invasion of the cornea by treponemes. Treatment for the condition is nonspecific; corticosteroid therapy, which has replaced fever therapy, is generally favorable. Interstitial keratitis due to syphilis was one of the leading causes of blindness until three decades ago and followed a relentless relapsing course in many patients, with eventual production of impenetrable corneal clouding. Photophobia is marked, and the changes within the eye itself are diagnostic.

The combination of interstitial keratitis, Hutchinsonian incisors, and eighth nerve deafness constitutes the Hutchinsonian triad, one of the most famed and characteristic pathognomonic groups of signs in all of medicine.

MUCOCUTANEOUS SYSTEM. Evidence of late congenital syphilis due to primary involvement of the skin or mucous membranes is conspicuous by its absence. Such involvement ordinarily occurs by extension from underlying bone or cartilage, and under such circumstances it could be marked. Characteristic skin gummas do not occur in congenital syphilis.

NEUROSYPHILIS. Neurosyphilis has always, fortunately, been uncommon in congenital infection. However, when paresis or taboparesis occurs, its manifestations are severe and disabling. The response to treatment with older methods, including fever therapy, has been minimal and does not approach the results obtained in neurosyphilis due to acquired infection in the adult. Congenital neurosyphilis now appears to be a syndrome of the past.

CARDIOVASCULAR SYSTEM. Syphilis acquired in utero does not produce the characteristic cardiovascular changes seen in late acquired syphilis.

Laboratory Diagnosis

The laboratory diagnosis of syphilis may be considered in four categories: (1) darkfield examinations, (2) serologic tests, (3) spinal fluid examination, and (4) histologic studies.

Darkfield Examinations

These techniques include (1) the conventional direct darkfield examination, (2) the indirect darkfield, or examination of the material aspirated from the enlarged regional lymph node, and (3) the fluorescent antibody darkfield (FADF) examination.

The conventional direct darkfield examination requires the ordinary white light microscope with a darkfield attachment. The clinician must obtain from an abraded primary or secondary lesion a specimen of serum which is adequate, preferably not secondarily infected. The material must be examined promptly, before any drying might occur. The morphology and motility of *T. pallidum* must be familiar to the examiner, since both are needed for an accurate diagnosis.

The indirect darkfield is performed on material aspirated from an enlarged lymph node. After 0.1 to 0.2 ml. of physiologic saline solution is injected into the enlarged node, the tip of the 25-gauge needle is twisted about and then suction is applied. The aspirated material is examined as an ordinary darkfield procedure. This method of examination is more rewarding when the aspirated node is the satellite node draining a chancre rather than one which is part of the generalized lymphadenopathy of secondary syphilis.

The chief indications for this procedure are when the suspected chancre is (1) inaccessible, as under an edematous phimotic prepuce or above the anorectal line, (2) secondarily infected, or (3) located in the mouth on the gingival, lingual, or buccal surface where the presence of *Treponema microdentium* might defy differentiation from *T. pallidum*.

The FADF is an experimental immuno-fluorescent staining technique developed for identification of *T. pallidum* in stained smears of lesion exudate or other material. This technique requires that the serum air dry on the slide and then be fixed in acetone for ten minutes, which permits storage and/or shipping of the slide to the laboratory for processing with conjugated specific antibody and examination under ultraviolet light microscopy.

In summary, a darkfield examination of some type is indicated when the clinical lesion suggests syphilis in the primary or secondary stage. When serum is not available, the surface of the lesion may be abraded, or the regional node may be aspirated. Darkfield microscopy of lesions of late syphilis (over two years' duration) is neither rewarding nor indicated.

Serologic Tests

The most rewarding use of serologic tests for the diagnosis of syphilis requires the correct interpretation of the results and the proper choice of test to be performed. One must remember that the various serologic tests are judged by their sensitivity and specificity. Sensitivity is defined as the percentage of positive results obtained with the test on syphilitic serums, while the specificity of a serologic test is defined as the percentage of negative results obtained in a nonsyphilitic population.

T. pallidum, comparable to a mosaic of antigens, following invasion of a human host, causes the production of multiple antibodies of two basic types:

1. Nonspecific antibodies (reagins) which are directed against lipoidal antigens of the treponeme, or against a lipoidal antigen that results from the interaction of host and parasite. Tests for reagins are best called nontreponemal tests, but are usually referred to by the less specific term serologic test for syphilis (STS). The cardiolipin-lecithin antigens used in the nontreponemal tests are found in a number of normal tissues, and it is perhaps not surprising that these tests are sometimes "falsely positive" (reactive even though the patient does not have syphilis).

2. Specific antitreponemal antibodies, which are measured by a variety of trep-onemal tests. The treponemal tests use one of a variety of preparations of the treponeme itself as the antigen, and a reactive test is usually a quite specific indication of past or present infection by treponemes.

NONTREPONEMAL TESTS. These tests are of two general types: flocculation and complement fixation. The Venereal Disease Research Laboratory (VDRL) slide test and the Rapid Plasma Reagin Card (RPRC) test are the most commonly used flocculation tests. The Kolmer test, a modification of the original Wassermann reaction, was the most common complement fixation test employed until 1970, when most authorities agreed that determination of a single, reproducible nontreponemal test is of much more benefit than performance of more of the related tests, as was formerly practiced. The VDRL and RPRC tests remain popular because they are easily performed and quantitated, and are inexpensive. They remain the standard for screening purposes, and for following the serologic response to treatment.

Most laboratories report the result as the highest dilution of a patient's serum that still gives a positive test. A titer reported as 1:32 or 32 dil. means that the serum was reactive in a dilution of 1:32 but not in a dilution of 1:64. The quantitative titer of nontreponemal antibodies may be helpful in diagnosis, but change over a course of time is more informative than the level of antibodies present at a given moment. Since reagin is not detectable during the 7 to 10 days after the chancre appears, the STS may be nonreactive, or the titers may be low or high in primary syphilis. The titers are commonly high in secondary syphilis and in late syphilis with gumma formation (1:32 or higher), and are otherwise variable. False positive reactors ordinarily have titers of 1:8 or below, although, rarely, higher titers are found. A fourfold or greater change in the quantitative titer is necessary to demonstrate a noteworthy change in the level of reagin-type antibody in a patient's serum, since twofold changes in titer are commonly due to technical factors.

An occasional negative reaction may be encountered when a test for reagin is performed with undiluted serum containing very high titers of reagin; as many as 1 per cent of patients with secondary syphilis have a nonreactive test with undiluted serum, which is reactive on further dilution of the serum (the "prozone" phenomenon). The physician should note that many laboratories do not routinely perform quantitative tests (that is, they do not dilute the patient's serum) unless the test is reactive with undiluted serum.

The reagin titer diminishes within a year to a nondetectable level if the individual is treated for syphilis in the primary or early secondary stage. The longer the infection has persisted, the less the chance for serum reversal following therapy. However, as many as 30 per cent of patients with ophthalmologic and/or neurosyphilis will become seronegative with no therapy or with inadequate therapy.

TREPONEMAL TESTS. Although the VDRL and related nontreponemal tests are useful, they may be falsely positive in a substantial number of persons. The proportion of reactive nontreponemal tests that are falsely positive has been variously estimated at 3 to 40 per cent, depending on the type of test employed and, especially, on the incidence of syphilis in the population of patients studied. For this reason a number of methods have been devised to test for antibodies that are specific for syphilis. The antigens employed are (1) whole body *T. pallidum* (viable or nonviable), (2) chemical fractions derived from *T. pallidum*, or (3) chemical fractions derived from the nonpathogenic Reiter treponeme.

The *T. pallidum* immobilization (TPI) test, devised in 1949 by Nelson and Mayer, measures the ability of antibody and complement to immobilize a suspension of living treponemes extracted from rabbit testes, as viewed under a darkfield microscope. The test is expensive and cumbersome, and at present is performed in only a few laboratories in the United States. The presence of antibiotics in a serum specimen will invalidate the test, since the antibiotics will also inactivate motile treponemes. Lack of standardized procedures and difficulties inherent with a complicated bioassay of this type have resulted in relatively poor reproducibility of results. Reactivity to the TPI test develops slowly; two-thirds of the patients with primary and

one-third of those with secondary syphilis have a nonreactive TPI. The TPI, like other treponemal tests, is reactive in the nonvenereal treponematoses (bejel, yaws, and pinta).

Another treponemal test that was temporarily in vogue is the Reiter protein complement fixation (RPCF) test. This test uses the cultivatable, nonpathogenic Reiter strain of treponeme as the antigen. Although cheaper and more easily performed than the TPI, the RPCF test has fallen into disfavor because it has proved in time to be less sensitive and less specific than the initial evaluations.

The most important recent developments in testing for syphilis have resulted from the application of immunofluorescent methods. The fluorescent treponemal antibody (FTA) test employs dried Nichols strain *T. pallidum* (which must still be grown in the testis of a rabbit) on a glass slide as antigen, to which a patient's serum is added. If antitreponemal antibody is present, it is detected by addition of fluorescein isothiocyanate-labeled antihuman gamma globulin, with subsequent visualization of the complex by fluorescent microscopy.

The FTA test has undergone a number of modifications, the test used today being the fluorescent treponemal antibody-absorption (FTA-ABS) test. A 1:5 dilution of the patient's serum is absorbed with an extract ("sorbent") of a culture of the nonpathogenic Reiter strain, to remove group antibody directed against antigens common to *T. pallidum*, the Reiter strain, and certain nonpathogenic oral and genital treponemes that are normal saprophytes in man. The absorption step was added after it was learned that the original FTA, which used a 1:5 dilution of serum and was sensitive in all stages of syphilis, was often reactive in normal controls. The false reactions could be removed by dilution of the patient's serum 1:200 before the test was performed, but the test then suffered from lack of sensitivity in patients known to be syphilitic. The present FTA-ABS test appears to have the best features of both older versions: it is reactive in most cases of syphilis, even in the primary stage, and so far has been falsely positive in only a limited number of patients, most of whom have had diseases associated with abnormal globulins. These cases should be recognized by the technician because the fluorescence has a "beaded" appearance. The FTA-ABS test for syphilis has generally replaced the TPI, and is the standard treponemal test in most state health laboratories.

CLINICAL APPLICATION. In general, the use of the serology laboratory depends first on whether or not the patient has any clinical, historical, or epidemiologic evidence of syphilis. Without any data in any of these categories, the patient whose initial STS is reactive presents a diagnostic problem. The STS (quantitative) should be repeated to rule out technical errors, mistakes in reporting, and so forth. When the second test is reported reactive, and the patient still denies previous disease as well as prolonged antibiotic treatment for syphilis or any other condition, and no clinical features have developed, the FTA-ABS test should be ordered. Recent antibiotic therapy will not alter the FTA-ABS test, whereas the presence of antibiotics in the serum would affect the TPI test.

If the FTA-ABS test is reported reactive, the patient has or has had a treponemal disease (venereal syphilis, endemic syphilis, yaws, bejel, or pinta). A cerebrospinal fluid study is then indicated so that the extent of involvement can be determined before starting therapy.

If the FTA-ABS is reported nonreactive, the patient neither has nor had syphilis or any other treponematosis. He is a biologic false positive reactor (BFP or BFR). If this state exists for less than six months, it is considered an acute BFP, and is due to a large variety of infections, mostly viral diseases. A BFP of more than six months duration, called a chronic BFP, is often indicative of a collagen disease which may be diagnosed by repeatedly performing a lupus erythematosus (LE) prep, antinuclear antibody test, rheumatoid factor test, albumin-globulin (A-G) ratio and immunoelectrophoresis. Leprosy is probably the only infection which can cause a chronic BFP.

The patient with clinical, historical, or epidemiologic evidence of syphilis must be studied in order to make a diagnosis. If the initial STS is reactive, the STS (quantitative) may be repeated and appropriate

therapy instituted. Should the clinical data include lesions of primary or secondary syphilis, they should have been evaluated by darkfield examination at the time of the initial testing. If the historical data include accurate description of adequate previous treatments, clinical judgment will be required in order to differentiate a reactive test due to residual antibody following therapy from a reactive test due to reinfection. The FTA-ABS test will perform neither of these functions.

The patient with clinical, historical, or epidemiologic evidence of syphilis may, on the other hand, have a nonreactive STS. The blood serum of this individual should be subjected to the FTA-ABS test because he may have either early primary syphilis (in which the reagin has not yet reached the reactive level) or late syphilis (in which the reagin fell—with or without therapy—below the reactive level). Surely, the early syphilis case might be diagnosed by repeating the reagin test one or more times, but time may be saved by employing the fluorescent technique.

For the diagnosis of congenital syphilis, a special technique must be applied so as to rule out reactivity with reagin or treponemal antibodies which were maternal in origin prior to transplacental migration. Since IgM does not pass the placental barrier, the demonstration of IgM in the newborn should make the diagnosis of congenital syphilis. A practical way to do this is to perform the FTA-ABS test with one modification: the use of tagged antihuman IgM rather than tagged antihuman globulin (IgM–FTA-ABS test). Of course, if this is not available, the quantitative reagin test repeated monthly will show a decrease in titer to nonreactivity by the end of the third month of life in all cases of "passive reaginemia."

Indications for FTA-ABS Testing. Treponemal testing is of greatest value in (1) assisting in the diagnosis in STS nonreactive patients who epidemiologically should have the disease, (2) helping to distinguish a valid reactive STS from a biological false reaction, and (3) helping to establish a correct diagnosis in STS nonreactive patients who have clinical evidence of syphilis, particularly late syphilis.

Indications for VDRL or RPRC Testing. Although the treponemal tests are valuable, testing for reagin should be continued for several reasons.

1. They are invaluable as screening tests because of their economy and relative ease of performance.

2. A reactive test for reagin is confirmatory when correlated with history and clinical evidence of syphilis.

3. A reactive nontreponemal test is highly significant when used in conjunction with epidemiologic investigation.

4. A reactive STS is almost diagnostic of syphilis when it is reactive in high or rapidly increasing titer (although occasionally a BFP occurs in high titer).

5. A good quantitative test for reagin is an excellent diagnostic tool when used for babies suspected of congenital syphilis.

6. Finally, for the observation of the serologic response following treatment, repeated quantitative determinations should be made with tests that measure reagin rather than with tests that measure treponemal antibodies, because treponemal antibodies do not change substantially after therapy.

SPINAL FLUID EXAMINATION. In all cases of primary and secondary syphilis, the spinal fluid should be examined between the sixth and twelfth month following therapy. This is considered superfluous by many physicians, particularly when the diminution in serologic titer progresses satisfactorily in the post-treatment follow-up of individuals whose original diagnosis was early syphilis. This is probably correct if the therapeutic agent was a form of repository penicillin administered in adequate dosage. However, all penicillin-allergic patients and others treated with alternate drugs should be subjected to a spinal fluid examination.

In all other cases of acquired syphilis, the spinal fluid should be examined before making the diagnosis in order to determine and then institute proper therapy. Without a spinal fluid examination, it is impossible to make a diagnosis of asymptomatic neurosyphilis. Early cases of paresis may be missed. The presence of late involvement of the aorta, the skin, or any of the organs or viscera is no longer considered assurance that there may not be concomitant active disease in the central nervous system.

The minimal examination of the spinal fluid must include a cell count within one hour of obtaining the fluid, quantitative protein determination, and a serologic test. The latter is concerned with the specificity of the infection; the cell count and protein are reflections of the activity of the process. At the present time, it would seem that the FTA test, with or without absorption, had best be considered an experimental tool, since there is inadequate correlation between these reactions and neurosyphilis (either in the clinical or the neuropathologic pictures).

Histologic Studies

The fundamental pathologic changes in syphilis are a predominantly perivascular, coat sleeve–like infiltrate composed of lymphocytes and many plasma cells, and endarteritis and endophlebitis. Special staining shows the treponemes in the dermis to be in and around the walls of the capillaries and lymphatics in the cutaneous lesions of early syphilis. In late syphilis, common additional findings are a tuberculoid infiltrate and caseation necrosis. The finer points of differentiation of the various lesions of the different stages of syphilis are clearly described in textbooks of pathology and dermatopathology.

Treatment

Penicillin

Penicillin is the drug of choice in the nonallergic patient. In primary or secondary syphilis, or for preventive treatment of sexual contacts of syphilis, a single intramuscular injection of 2,400,000 units of benzathine penicillin G is curative in the great majority of cases. Other acceptable schedules include procaine penicillin G in a dose of 600,000 units intramuscularly once daily for 10 days, or procaine penicillin G with 2 per cent aluminum monostearate in a dose of 2,400,000 units intramuscularly on the first day, with an additional 1,200,000 units in each of three subsequent injections three days apart. In latent syphilis with a known normal spinal fluid, the same treatment is used as in primary or secondary syphilis. In late syphilis, 6,000,000 to 9,000,000 units of penicillin should be given (2,400,000 units of benzathine penicillin G weekly for three weeks, to total 7,200,000 units; or 1,200,000 units of procaine penicillin G with 2 per cent aluminum monostearate at three-day intervals for six injections, after the initial injection of 2,400,000 units to make a total dosage of 9,600,000 units). Treatment of syphilis in pregnancy is the same, depending on the stage. Treatment of congenital syphilis is accomplished with a single injection of benzathine penicillin G in a dose of 50,000 units per kilogram of body weight.

Other antibiotics are indicated if the patient is allergic to penicillin.

Tetracycline

Oral tetracycline in a total dose of 30 gm. administered over 10 to 15 days is approximately as effective as penicillin in early syphilis. Tetracycline has not been extensively evaluated in late syphilis, but it is recommended that a total dose of 60 to 80 gm. should be administered for late stages of the disease. Since tetracycline may cause staining and other adverse effects on teeth and bone, it should not be used in pregnancy or in treatment of children less than six or seven years of age.

Erythromycin

Erythromycin is active against *T. pallidum*. A total dose close to 400 mg. per kilogram is required in early syphilis. The more reliably absorbed propionyl sulfate salt of erythromycin, which is occasionally hepatotoxic, is effective in total doses of 20 to 30 gm. Erythromycin does not have adverse effects on the fetus. Erythromycin has not been well evaluated in late syphilis.

Cephaloridine

Cephaloridine causes little pain when administered by intramuscular injection, and can be given with reasonable safety to the penicillin-allergic patient. A small percentage of patients who are allergic to penicillin will have an allergic reaction to cephalosporin antibiotics as well. Cephaloridine is approximately 5 to 10 per cent as active as penicillin G against *T. pallidum*. Cephaloridine crosses the placenta well and gives serum levels in the fetus equal to those obtained in the mother. Cephaloridine may therefore be considered alternate injectable therapy for the penicillin-allergic patient with syphilis, but further studies are needed to assess its efficacy and safety, particularly in pregnancy. A dose of 0.5 to 1.0 gm. intramuscularly once a day for 10 days is probably effective.

Follow-up Study

The patient with primary or secondary syphilis should be followed clinically and with periodic quantitative STS for one year. Other forms of syphilis should be followed for two years. The STS will usually become nonreactive 6 to 12 months after treatment of primary syphilis, or 12 to 24 months after treatment of secondary syphilis. The state public health authorities should be notified of all cases of syphilis, particularly early infectious syphilis, so that epidemiologic investigations can be instituted.

YAWS

Yaws is a treponemal infection characterized by a clinical picture which is similar to that of early syphilis in some respects, but which does not produce serious late manifestations in organ systems other than the skin and bones. It is apparently dependent upon factors of hygiene, race, and climate for its transmission and persistence and possibly for its different clinical course. The evidence for an essential difference in the treponeme which causes the disease and in the immune responses evoked is as yet incomplete. Though instances of superinfection of yaws or syphilis have been reported, it must occur very uncommonly, and attempts to produce experimental inoculation of yaws in patients with late syphilis result in failure. Yaws produces a specific reactive STS, and the treponemal tests (both FTA-ABS and TPI) are reactive. In view of the fact that the treponeme which causes the disease is indistinguishable from that of syphilis, justification for continuing to designate it as *Treponema pertenue* might be questioned. The organism cannot be cultured in vitro.

Clinical Findings

The *primary lesion* (mother yaw) appears within three to four weeks after the organism enters the skin. From a small papule it enlarges to a lesion which is ordinarily much larger than the chancre of syphilis. The inoculation may occur in skin which grossly appears normal or it may arise in an already existent ulcer, in which case the primary lesion may be quite large. Darkfield examination of the primary lesion will yield an abundance of treponemes.

The infection is ordinarily nonvenereal, and children are commonly infected. The disease is not transmitted congenitally.

The *secondary lesions* of yaws appear somewhat more rapidly than is noted in the case of syphilis. These lesions are comparable to the primary lesion (Fig. 14–8 A) and may be exceedingly numerous and widespread. Involvement of the mucous surfaces of the mouth and at mucocutaneous junctions is common. All of these lesions yield treponemes in abundance for identification under darkfield microscopy. In spite of the exuberance of the lesions, they are not destructive and heal without scarring, or with only some depigmentation and occasional atrophy. The morphologic patterns may be striking, particularly in respect to annularity and coalescence.

As is the case with syphilis, the clinical appearance of yaws may vary greatly and often resembles common dermatoses of other types. The general tendency is toward an exuberance rarely attained by the

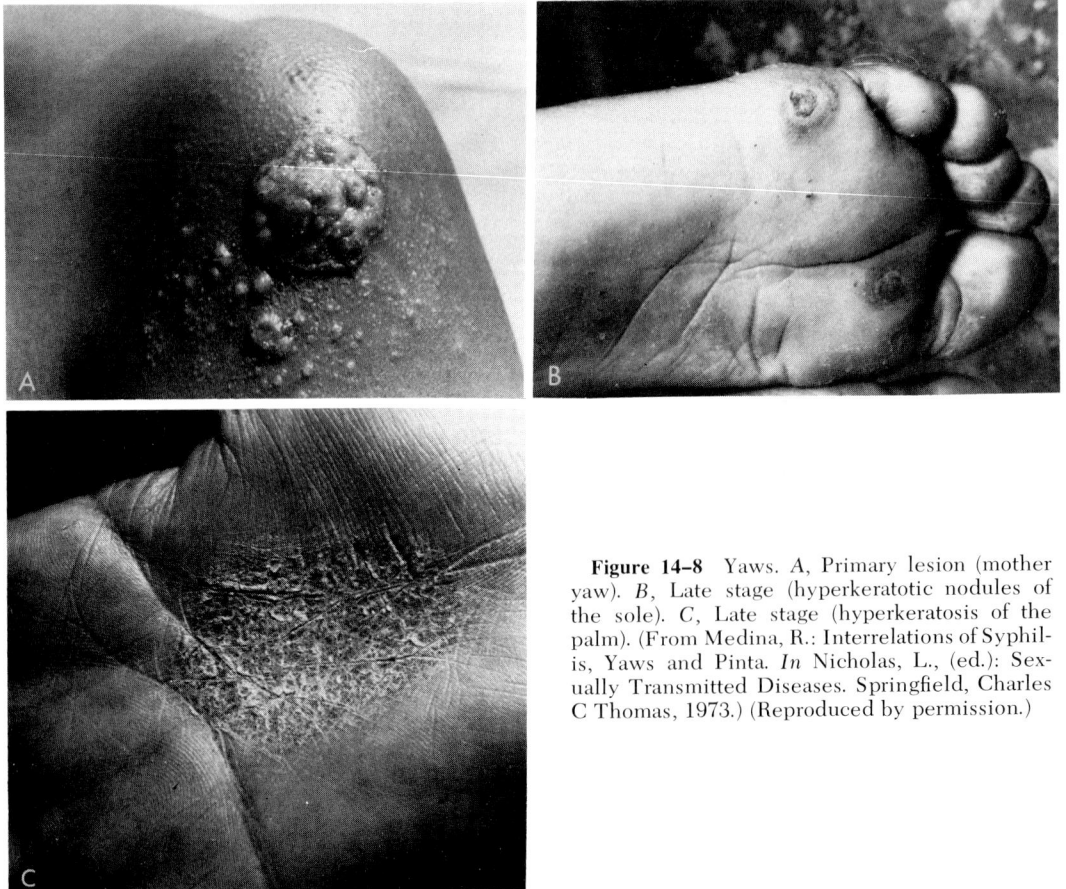

Figure 14–8 Yaws. *A*, Primary lesion (mother yaw). *B*, Late stage (hyperkeratotic nodules of the sole). *C*, Late stage (hyperkeratosis of the palm). (From Medina, R.: Interrelations of Syphilis, Yaws and Pinta. *In* Nicholas, L., (ed.): Sexually Transmitted Diseases. Springfield, Charles C Thomas, 1973.) (Reproduced by permission.)

secondary lesions of syphilis. Palmar and plantar lesions may be severe.

Yaws is characterized by systemic manifestations rather frequently, particularly in relation to involvement of the osseous system. This is most extreme in children, and extensive periostitis and rarefaction may be seen in many bones. Low-grade fever, malaise, and generalized lymphadenopathy may be encountered. Some disability may result from trauma to palmar and plantar lesions.

During the first two or three years of the infection, the course is one of numerous relapses, although the lesions remain non-destructive. Spontaneous cure may then occur, or lesions of the tertiary stage may occur from three to many years later. The incidence of spontaneous cure is not known, nor are accurate figures on the average length of latency available. It is definitely established that the course in children may be more rapid; nevertheless, late yaws is seen most frequently in adults.

Late yaws is characterized by chronic and destructive involvement of the skin and bones. The lesions in the skin are entirely comparable to gummas and are apparently indistinguishable histologically. Nodules break down into indolent ulcers, which individually may reach a size of 10 to 15 cm. in diameter. As in late syphilis, healing occurs in some areas while further extension is noted elsewhere. The scarring produced is ordinarily atrophic and as a rule becomes deeply pigmented eventually. It may be so extensive as to produce marked contractures. Late lesions of the palms and soles (Fig. 14–8 B and C), as in the case with syphilis, follow a somewhat different morphologic pattern, with extensive thickening and superficial ulceration and variegated patterns of annular lesions. These lesions may be difficult to differentiate from secondary yaws. Considerable disability may arise in hands or feet long affected by tertiary yaws.

Involvement of bone is a striking feature of tertiary yaws. This may at times be extensive, though ordinarily only one or a few bones are affected. The characteristic course is one of periosteal stimulation and rarefaction together. When involvement of bones close to the surface occurs, nodular and ulcerative extension into the subcu-taneous tissues and skin results not infrequently. Tertiary yaws occurring in bones of the hand and foot is particularly disabling, and may produce marked deformity and dysfunction. The process produces extensive destruction in the palate and nasopharynx, and this can lead to very severe mutilation. It seems certain that almost every bone in the body is capable of involvement in late yaws, and the changes may be similar to those seen in congenital syphilis, such as saber tibia and thickening of the clavicles.

The tertiary stage may persist for a number of years, and the activity then gradually dies off. The end result is often one of scarring, depigmentation, hyperpigmentation, and a variety of types of impairment of function of bones and joints. Symptoms referable to the osseous system are common, and pain may be extreme at times.

Other Visceral Involvement

Although changes in the spinal fluid have been reported in association with yaws, they are relatively evanescent, and no characteristic involvement of the nervous system occurs. There is no suggestion of specific involvement of the cardiovascular system.

The disability produced by yaws is therefore related to pain and misery, widespread and conspicuous ulcerative lesions of both the secondary and tertiary phases, and more or less extensive destructive involvement in the osseous and cutaneous systems. The patient, while not directly killed by the infection, is obviously greatly inconvenienced and sometimes severely mutilated, and all this, occurring endemically in a population subjected to a wide variety of other diseases, constitutes a serious medical problem. Possibly no better example of the variation in medical care available to populations throughout the world can be cited, because yaws, like syphilis, should be susceptible to almost complete elimination. This has been brought about in some communities.

Treatment

The lesions of yaws can be healed promptly and progression of the disease arrested in a high proportion of cases by a single injection of penicillin. Probably best is an injection of 2,400,000 units of benzathine penicillin G. In case of penicillin allergy, oral tetracycline in a total dose of 30 gm. administered over 10 to 15 days is effective.

Gondou is apparently a special type of yaws in which marked proliferative changes occur in the maxilla. It has the status of a separate disease in the older literature, but its identity with yaws now seems clear. In advanced cases, surgical resection of the bone is necessary and produces excellent cosmetic results.

PINTA

Pinta is a treponemal infection, characterized by bizarre pigmentary changes, which is encountered almost exclusively in the hot lowlands of the American continent and in Cuba. The treponeme which produces it is indistinguishable morphologically from the organism which causes syphilis, yaws, and bejel. The most common designation of the causative organism is *Treponema carateum*. It regularly produces a reactive STS which is specific in character, thus the treponemal tests (FTA-ABS and TPI) are likewise reactive. Although the disease has long been known, its treponemal origin was not established until three decades ago.

Pinta affects almost exclusively the colored races living in the zones where it is endemic, although it has been reported in the white race, also. Whether this is related to some peculiar racial susceptibility is not known. The transmission and growth of the organism in man is apparently dependent upon hot, humid climatic conditions. It occurs most commonly where people are congregated in villages. Transmission apparently occurs by direct contact; in children of parents with pinta, infection is the rule rather than the exception. The number of individuals in the world affected by pinta was probably well over a million at one time; however this number was substantially reduced as effective antibiotic therapy became available to the communities in which it is endemic.

As with other treponemal infections, pinta is divided into three stages. How-

ever, particularly in the secondary and tertiary phases, the change would seem to be relatively imperceptible, and there is no period of latency. The initial lesion of pinta is ordinarily not noted by the patient, information concerning it having been obtained principally from experimental inoculation of the causative treponeme. The incubation period is similar to that of other treponemal infections, namely, one or more weeks. The initial lesion (Fig. 14–9 A) may be one or several, and ordinarily occurs on uncovered portions of the body, particularly the extremities. It is papular, without ulceration, and slowly increases in size and becomes thicker. The lesion scales and shortly develops striking pigmentary changes, principally shades of brown and red.

Dissemination of the lesions (Fig. 14–9 B) to other portions of the skin occurs in two or more months; these lesions are entirely comparable to the initial one, which does not disappear. The lesions may be few or numerous, and though distributed mainly to the lower extremities, may affect any portion of the cutaneous surface. The borders of the lesions are sharply defined and are annular. Scaling is the rule, sometimes amounting to hyperkeratosis. The color changes are bizarre and vary, from loss of pigment to a slate-blue color and shades of brown or red. The color changes are probably related to the fact that many diseases of the skin show varying colors in naturally pigmented skins which are not apparent in white skins, but pinta is extraordinary in its capacity for producing bizarre dyschromic changes (Fig. 14–9 C and D). The positive STS develops more slowly than is the case in other treponemal diseases, but the eventual incidence of seropositivity is apparently 100 per cent.

The pintids of the early disseminated phase apparently persist for some years, following which some of them may disappear and while the others progress into the late cutaneous changes. It is a curious fact that, while the earlier lesions are entirely asymmetric, late lesions tend to adopt a symmetric distribution and are much more generalized. This is in contrast to the secondary lesions of syphilis which are ordinarily symmetric and often generalized, while late gummas are asym-

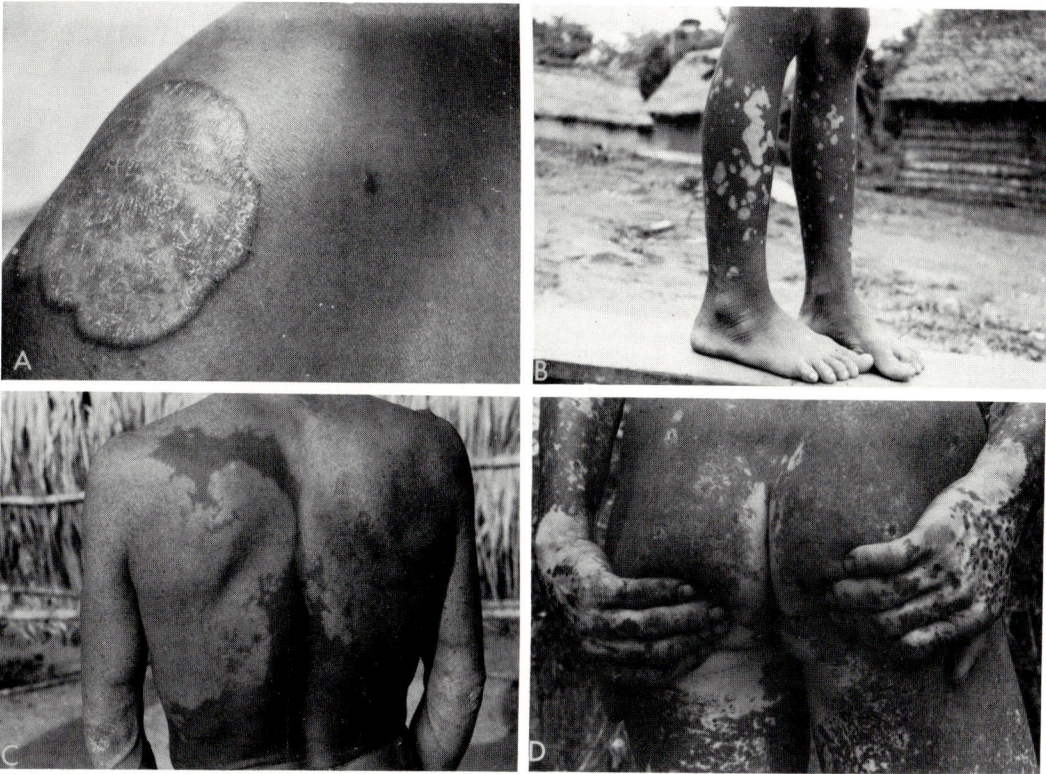

Figure 14–9 Pinta. *A*, Initial macule. *B*, Erythematous secondary lesions. *C*, Hypochromic lesions. *D*, Achromic lesions. (From Medina, R.: Interrelations of Syphilis, Yaws and Pinta. *In* Nicholas L., (ed.): Sexually Transmitted Diseases. Springfield, Charles C Thomas, 1973.) (Reproduced by permission.)

metric and usually rather sparse. The late lesions of pinta develop even more bizarre color changes, and atrophy occurs quite frequently. Alopecia and dystrophic nail changes may be produced.

Visceral changes related to pinta are exceedingly rare if, indeed, they occur at all. Treponemata are demonstrable from the lesions of pinta for many years, in contradistinction to the finding in syphilis. Individuals known to have late syphilis can be inoculated with pinta while the reverse is not the case; that is, pinta protects against syphilis. Reinfection does not occur in late pinta.

Differential Diagnosis

It is obvious from the foregoing description that pinta may frequently resemble other dermatoses, particularly those which are associated with scaling and/or achromic changes. These include, especially, super-ficial fungal infections, various types of eczema, psoriasis, and vitiligo. The definitive method of differentiation is based upon the demonstration of treponemes, which are readily obtainable from the lesions of pinta except in extremely late cases.

Treatment

Penicillin is the treatment of choice for pinta, and a single injection of 1.2 to 2.4 million units of benzathine penicillin G is apparently adequate. Serologic reversal may not be expected in late cases.

BEJEL

Bejel is a treponemal infection produced by an organism indistinguishable from *T. pallidum.* It is found only among the Arabs of the Syrian desert. It has many points of similarity with yaws. Its epidemiology is precisely that of yaws, in that the disease affects families and communities and is acquired nonvenereally, usually in childhood. The skin lesions are similar to those of yaws, and there is a lack of late involvement of the central nervous or cardiovascular systems. The infection produces a specifically reactive STS. The treatment is similar to that for yaws.

REFERENCES

Beerman, H., and Nicholas, L.: Syphilis. *In* Tice-Harvey's Practice of Medicine. Vol. 3. Hagerstown, Maryland, W. F. Prior Company, 1964, pp. 329–449.

Hudson, E. H.: Treponematosis in perspective. Bull. W.H.O. 32:735, 1965.

Nicholas, L., (ed.): Sexually Transmitted Diseases. Springfield, Illinois, Charles C Thomas, 1973.

Stokes, J. H., Beerman, H., and Ingraham, N. R., Jr.: Modern Clinical Syphilology. 3rd ed. Philadelphia, W. B. Saunders Co., 1944.

NONTREPONEMAL VENEREAL INFECTIONS

Orlando Canizares

INTRODUCTION

The factors responsible for the current greater incidence of venereal disease are changes in the organisms, host, and environment (Willcox, 1972). Changes in the behavior of the organism result from altered virulence, antibiotic therapy, and alteration in drug sensitivity; those in the environment are due to an increased number of susceptibles and a greater mobility of the population. Factors contributing to changes in the host include improved nutrition and hygiene, the present relaxed attitude and behavior conditioned by a permissive society which encourages promiscuity, a reduction of fear of venereal disease and pregnancy, and changes in sexual practices. The outlook for successful control of venereal diseases is not very bright owing to the likelihood of greater population mobility, continuation of permissiveness, and the continued appearance of drug-resistant strains. In view of the overwhelming influence of human behavior, the only recourse for the practicing physician is to diagnose and treat as early and as quickly as possible. In addition, one must be aware of the fact that syphilis and gonorrhea constitute but a fraction of the whole venereal problem. The other sexually transmitted diseases of dermatologic interest are caused by bacteria other than gonococci, and by viruses, protozoa, fungi, and parasites (see Table 15–1).

GONORRHEA

Definition

Gonorrhea is an acute or chronic contagious infectious disease caused by *Neisseria gonorrhoeae*. In men, it causes urethritis and local complications of the genitourinary tract. In women, it causes urethritis, cervicitis, and local complications which may lead to sterility. Extragenital primary infections (rectal, oro-

TABLE 15-1 Sexually Transmitted Diseases in Man

Causes	Organisms	Diseases
Spirochaeta	*Treponema pallidum*	Syphilis
Bacteria	Gonococcus	Gonorrhea
	Haemophilus ducreyi	Chancroid
	Donovania	Granuloma inguinale
Viruses	Mycoplasmataceae	Nongonococcal urethritis
	Clamydiaceae°	Lymphogranuloma venereum
	Herpes simplex Type II	Herpes progenitalis
	Poxvirus	Molluscum contagiosum
Protozoa	*Trichomonas vaginalis*	Trichomoniasis
Fungi	*Candida albicans*	Candidiasis
	Epidermophyton floccosum	Tinea cruris
	Trichophyton rubrum	
Parasites	*Sarcoptes scabiei*	Scabies
	Phthirus pubis	Pediculosis

°The agent of lymphogranuloma venereum, *Miyagawanella lymphogranulomatosis*, is now classified as belong to the Family Chlamydiaceae, genus Miyagawanella. These are minute bacteria which lack many synthetic enzymes, and, unlike all other bacteria, cannot synthesize ATP.

Genus Chlamydia includes TRIC (trachoma inclusion conjunctivitis) agents and *C. trachomatis.*

Genus Miyagawanella includes *M. lymphogranulomatosis* and *M. psittaci* (psittacosis or "parrot fever").

pharyngeal) occur in both sexes. Gonococcal septicemia may lead to involvement of the joints, meninges, endocardium, and skin. In children, it may result in vulvovaginitis, and in newborns and adults it may produce ophthalmia. Gonorrhea is almost always acquired by sexual intercourse. Newborns may contract the infection during birth and children may become infected through accidental contamination with infected articles of clothing or bedding.

Historical Review

The differentiation between syphilis and gonorrhea was made by Benjamin Bell in 1792 and confirmed by the lifetime studies of Phillippe Ricord from 1831 to 1861. The causative organism, the gonococcus, was discovered by Neisser in 1879. Leistikow, in 1882, and Bumm, in 1885, cultured the organism and successfully produced experimental infections in men.

The gonococcal complement-fixation test was developed by Muller and Oppenheimer in 1906. The direct fluorescent antibody technique was developed by Deacon et al. in 1960. The indirect fluorescent antibody test was introduced as a diagnostic tool in 1965. In 1966, Thayer and Martin introduced the selective antibiotic medium. Skin lesions and arthritis in gonorrhea were first described by Vidal in 1893. The association of gonococcemia with the syndrome of fever, arthritis, and skin lesions was described by Silvestrini in 1903. The history of the treatment of gonorrhea ranges from the early sandalwood oil, potassium permanganate irrigations, and "vaccines," to the sulfanilamides and penicillin. As penicillin-resistant cases continue to appear, a host of new antibiotics continue to be tried.

Epidemiology

There is a recent worldwide increase in new cases of gonorrhea, many of which are reinfections often involving teenagers. Important epidemiologic factors responsible for this increase are a changing pattern of morals, promiscuity and homosexuality, mass migrations of people, reservoir of infection in women, and the improper reporting of cases, which hampers the effectiveness of health officers.

Present day gonorrhea differs from that of the pre-antibiotic era. The effectiveness of modern treatment reduces the duration of the disease and invites frequent reinfections in some individuals. In men, late complications of epididymitis, prostatic abscesses, and urethral strictures are rare. In women, signs of gonococcemia and arthritis are relatively common. Gonorrhea, previously found almost exclusively in lower socioeconomic groups, is now also commonly encountered in individuals in higher economic levels. The highest incidence is found in young people between 20 and 24 years of age. The ratio of infection, male to female, is 3:1; women often have asymptomatic infections.

Etiology

The gonococcus, *N. gonorrhoeae*, is a gram-negative, coffee bean–shaped diplococcus with flat sides which are almost in opposition. It is found intracellularly in smears made with purulent discharge. Cultures are best grown in the Thayer and Martin antibiotic selective medium.

The organism can be identified by the demonstration of a strongly positive oxidase test and by the evaluation of the fermentation reactions; the gonococcus ferments glucose but not maltose or sucrose.

Transgrow medium allows the growth of the organism while in transit to a distant laboratory. Animal inoculations, including those in anthropoid apes, have been unsuccessful. The gonococcus does not produce immunity.

Pathology

The favorite tissue target of the gonococcus is the mucosal columnar epithelium of the urogenital tract. Invasion elicits a profuse polymorphonuclear reaction in the submucosa. All structures with this type of epithelium are more susceptible to infection, while those with transitional and stratified epithelium are relatively resistant. As a result, in the male, the spongy urethra, which is lined by columnar epithelium (except at the fossa navicularis), is first affected. Later, Littre's and Cowper's glands, and the prostate, seminar vesicles, and epididymes may be involved. In women, part of the urethra, Skene's and Bartholin's glands whose ducts are lined with columnar epithelium, the cervix, and the fallopian tubes are often involved. The vulva, vagina, and the uterus are less frequently affected. In both sexes, the bladder is relatively resistant to invasion by the gonococcus but the rectum may be involved. As suppuration subsides, fibrosis often develops, leading at times to urethral stricture in males and to obliteration of the fallopian tubes and sterility in females.

Clinical Manifestations

GONORRHEA IN MEN. The incubation period (Table 15–2) is usually two to five days. At first there is a slight burning of the urethra on urination and then a mucoid discharge develops. The discharge rapidly becomes profuse, purulent, and whitish yellow, gradually turning yellowish green. At this time, urination and erections are painful. Constitutional symptoms are minimal or absent but can be severe. The external urinary meatus and surrounding

TABLE 15–2 AVERAGE DATE OF ONSET OF VENEREAL DISEASES AFTER INFECTIVE SEXUAL INTERCOURSE

(A COMPARATIVE STUDY TO ASSIST IN THE DIAGNOSIS OF "MIXED" INFECTIONS)

Weeks / *Days*	1st (1 – 7)	2nd (14)	3rd (21)	4th (28)	5th (35)	6th (42)	7th (49)	
Syphilis		chancre	adenitis				secondaries →	
Gonorrhea	▓							
Chancroid	▓	bubo						
Lymphogranuloma venereum		primary	bubo					
Granuloma inguinale				▓				
Abacterial nonspecific urethritis		▓						

tissues are erythematous and swollen. Palpation of the anterior urethra is painful. Involvement of the posterior urethra, rare at present, occurs at about the third week and leads to multiple complications. Clinically, it is manifested by pain at the end of urination and at defecation, and by a sensation of weight at the perineum.

Involvement of the posterior urethra may be roughly detected by the Thompson two-glass urine test (a small amount of urine in the first glass and the remainder of the urine in the second glass). A hazy appearance of the urine in the first specimen and clear urine in the second glass indicates anterior urethritis; this is the usual finding in early cases. Cloudiness of the urine in both glasses is indicative of posterior urethritis. The addition of a few drops of acetic acid will clear a urine which is hazy because of an excess of phosphates. The almost constant involvement of the ducts of the urethral glands of Littre and the lacunae of Morgagni causes casts of the ducts, which appear as threads in the hazy urine, adding diagnostic value to the two-glass test.

In patients with a long prepuce and poor hygiene, gonococcal balanitis may develop, causing ulceration about the frenum. In addition, *abscesses of Tyson's glands* may appear at this site; initially these lesions are nodose, and later they may resemble a syphilitic chancre. *Thrombosis of the dorsal vein* of the penis and *acute lymphangitis* of the dorsum of the penis occur rarely and are painful. Periurethral abscesses cause painful inflammatory nodules near the frenum, the root of the penis, and upper scrotum. These suppurate and may break down, forming sinuses. *Inguinal lymph nodes* may be enlarged but are rarely tender and almost never suppurate. Abscesses of Cowper's glands may develop; they are usually unilateral, exceedingly painful, and detectable by bidigital palpation (the index finger in the rectum and the thumb in the perineum) and may cause perineal sinuses.

Acute prostatitis is, at present, uncommon. It is encountered in patients with involvement of the posterior urethra and is manifested by a sensation of weight in the perineum, frequent and painful urination, and low-grade fever. Digital rectal examination elicits an enlarged tender prostate. Prostatic abscess causes severe local and systemic manifestations until it extends to involve the urethra or the rectum. Epididymitis is rare and usually unilateral, is manifested by pronounced local inflammatory signs, and is associated with a hydrocele and fever. Chronic urethritis is found in neglected cases of gonorrhea and is due to the localization of the gonococcus in well-defined foci.

Sequelae of gonorrhea which may follow the various acute processes are fibrotic urethral strictures of annular or tubular type, chronic prostatitis, chronic epididymitis, and seminal vesiculitis; all are serious but fortunately rare at present.

GONORRHEA IN WOMEN. Acute gonorrhea in women is much less dramatic than in men; in about one-half of the cases it is asymptomatic. Urethritis is the most common initial manifestation. It is characterized by a burning sensation on urination, but urethral discharge is scanty and the external urinary meatus is only occasionally inflamed. The adult female vagina, which is lined with stratified epithelium, is resistant to the gonococcus. There is often an associated trichomonal vaginitis with profuse purulent vaginal discharge. This association should be kept in mind, and the proper laboratory investigations for both diseases should be performed simultaneously.

Acute cervicitis is usually secondary to urethritis and is the next most frequent expression of the infection in the female. It is usually asymptomatic but there may be low back or lower pelvic pain. A yellowish discharge may be the first sign. On examination with a speculum, there is a mucoid or mucopurulent cervical discharge, and the external os is edematous, eroded, and bleeds easily. *Chronic cervicitis* is manifested by granular erosions and retention nabothian cysts.

Bartholinitis, inflammation of Bartholin's glands, may be the first sign of the disease or it may develop from a urethritis or cervicitis (Rees, 1967). A large painful mass appears on the lower part of either labia majora which, if untreated, suppurates and breaks down through the mucosal side of the labium majus, discharging a yellowish or brownish foul pus. *Chronic bartholinitis* or recurrent abscess may occur.

Vulvitis is rare in the adult, but cystitis may occur.

Salpingitis is manifested by spasmodic, acute lower abdominal pain associated with unilateral or bilateral tenderness to deep palpation in the iliac fossae, low-grade fever, and leukocytosis; when an abscess develops, a tender fluctuating mass may be felt. Pelvic peritonitis may ensue. Bilateral salpingitis usually causes sterility.

ANORECTAL GONORRHEA (Owen, 1972). In the male, anorectal gonorrhea manifests itself almost exclusively as gonococcal proctitis which is almost always due to homosexual practices and, rarely, the breakdown of a prostatic abscess into the rectum. In women, anorectal involvement develops in about one-third of cases; it is usually caused by spread of the infection from the genitals but may be the result of anal coitus. In both sexes, rectal involvement is usually asymptomatic. There may be pruritus ani, constant urgency to empty the bowel, discomfort on defecation, and bloody mucopurulent stools; thrombosed hemorrhoids may be found. Proctoscopic examination shows a swollen, red, easily bleeding mucosa which is often bathed in a mucopurulent discharge. Perianal or ischiorectal abscesses or anal fissure may be found. Ulceration of the skin is more common in men than in women. Perirectal involvement and ulceration suggest a possible simultaneous lymphogranuloma venereum. Perianal verrucae acuminata are not uncommonly observed.

GONORRHEA IN CHILDREN. Gonococcal infection of children is rare; girls are more often affected than boys. In girls, the most common manifestation is acute *vulvovaginitis.* Most infections are due to accidental contaminations with infected articles of clothing or bedding; rarely it may be due to rape or sexual promiscuity.

The vagina of young girls is susceptible to the gonococcus because it is lined, until puberty, with columnar epithelium. After puberty, the epithelium becomes stratified, and the vagina is then resistant to the gonococcus. Acute vulvovaginitis is manifested by burning and itching of the vulva, with severe pain at urination. The vulva is red and swollen. The redness may extend toward the groin and upper inner thighs; a yellow-green purulent discharge is abundant. Rectal involvement is common and is manifested by inflammation of the anus and anal discharge. Complications are rare.

In boys, gonorrhea is less common than in girls. It is more prone to develop as a result of abnormal sexual practice or sexual promiscuity than through accidental inoculation.

The incubation period and clinical picture is the same as that for gonorrhea in adults. The gonococcal urethritis should be distinguished from the common balanoposthitis of boys resulting from phimosis. Conjunctivitis may be found in both boys and girls.

OPHTHALMIA NEONATORUM (Brown et al., 1966). Ophthalmia neonatorum is a serious but preventable infection which, if unrecognized and untreated, will cause blindness. The infection usually occurs during the passage of the newborn through the genitals of the infected mother. Generally, symptoms become apparent 48 hours after delivery. One or both eyes may be affected. There are edema of the eyelids, red and granular conjunctivae, and a profuse purulent exudate in which the gonococcus may be found; corneal ulcers may develop. Prophylactic measures consist first of cleansing the eyelids and eyelashes with a weak antiseptic. This is followed by instillation into the conjunctiva of one or two drops of time-honored 1 per cent silver nitrate solution. Chemical conjunctivitis is avoided by washing after a few minutes with saline solution. Other silver preparations and a solution of penicillin (10,000 units of crystalline penicillin per milliliter) have also been advocated.

The present increase of gonorrhea requires that prophylactic treatment of all newborns be strictly enforced. If a purulent discharge develops shortly after birth, treatment should be started immediately.

Other Extragenital Primary Gonococcal Infections

Primary gonococcal infections of the oral mucosa, pharynx, and tonsils are found in homosexual males and in women who practice fellatio. In stomatitis, the affected mucous membrane may show edematous rough patches or linear yellowish pseudomembranes which bleed easily when scraped off (Schmidt et al., 1970). In cases of pharyngitis, multiple discrete clear vesicles are found in the oropharynx and there are areas of exudate in the tonsils; there is minimal, tender cervical adenopathy (Metzger, 1970).

"Amniotic infection syndrome" is a common form of neonatal gonorrhea. It develops when the fetus swallows infected amniotic fluid. Handfield and his colleagues (1973) found gonococci in oropharynx or orogastric aspirates of neonates who appeared septic at birth.

Gonococcal conjunctivitis of the adult is rare. It results from careless direct contamination of the eye by fingers and towels soiled with gonococcal discharge. Early diagnosis and treatment result in complete recovery. Undiagnosed or neglected cases may result in blindness.

GONOCOCCEMIA.   Gonococcemia may develop in acute genital or extragenital gonorrhea and in the gonococcal carrier stage in both women and men. The main signs and symptoms are chills, fever, malaise, myalgia, migratory polyarthralgia, tenosynovitis, and skin lesions. In arthritis, the early "bacteremic stage" with positive blood cultures is followed by a "septic joint stage" with positive synovial fluid cultures or joint destruction. Cell wall–deficient gonococci may be isolated from apparently sterile septic joints (Holmes et al., 1971). One or more joints may be painful, swollen, and red. Tenosynovitis about the joints is manifested by tender streaks of redness.

The clinical presentation of skin lesions in association with fever and arthralgia has been called the *gonococcal arthritis-dermatitis syndrome*. This is found more often in women in the asymptomatic carrier stage. The skin lesions are few and asymmetric and are usually found near the joints of the extremities. They are often seen at different stages of development, from discrete reddish-violaceous papules with a hemorrhagic center to vesiculopustules with an erythematous halo. Some lesions may present a gray necrotic center on a hemorrhagic base. Pea-sized, purplish, subcutaneous nodules resembling erythema nodosum were observed by Barr and Danielsson (1971). These authors found the gonococcal complement-fixation test to be of diagnostic value during the acute phase of the disease. The finding of gonococci by immunofluorescent techniques confirms the embolic nature of skin lesions. The organism disintegrates early; therefore, cultures are usually negative. The clinical picture of gonococcal arthritis-dermatitis syndrome resembles chronic meningococcemia, and the differentiation is made by bacteriologic studies. Other manifestations of gonococcemia are endocarditis, myocarditis, pericarditis, and meningitis.

Laboratory Diagnosis

The clinical diagnosis of gonorrhea is easily confirmed in men by the finding of gram-negative intracellular gonococci in smears from the urethral discharge stained with Gram's stain. In the average case this finding suffices and treatment should be instituted immediately. Cultures in Thayer-Martin medium are positive in 48 hours; these oxidase-positive, gram-negative colonies ferment glucose but not sucrose or maltose. In women, cultures are essential for the diagnosis. Urethral and cervical smears should be performed in all cases. Anal cultures may be obtained by the simple insertion of a sterile cotton-tipped applicator into the anal canal; this procedure should be used also in suspected homosexual males.

Direct and indirect fluorescent tests may be used for the identification of gonococci in special cases. Transgrow medium has been recommended for the transport and cultivation of *N. gonorrhoeae* when sending the specimen to a distant laboratory. Its effectiveness decreases rapidly after 24 hours, however. The gonococcal complement-fixation test is of limited value, as it is negative in early stages of the disease; it is usually positive in patients with complications. In those patients suspected of septic gonococcemia, blood, pharyngeal, urethral, cervical, and rectal cultures should be taken; they may assist in the location of an elusive primary site.

Diagnosis and Differential Diagnosis

The clinical diagnosis of acute gonococcal urethritis in men should be suspected in the presence of a profuse purulent discharge developing a few days after sexual intercourse. Gonococcal urethritis should be distinguished from the nongonococcal urethritis group, which consists of those conditions due to *Trichomonas vaginalis*, infections of the bladder and kidneys, Candidiasis, and, mainly, the nonspecific (abacterial) type, the nature of which is not known. Abacterial nongonococcal urethritis is transmitted by sexual intercourse; the period of incubation ranges from 8 to 14 days. Clinically, the urethritis resembles that of gonorrhea but is milder and asymptomatic. Prostatitis is common; epididymitis and urethral stricture may occur.

The differential diagnosis of gonococcal arthritis manifested by chills, fever, and migratory polyarthritis in otherwise asymptomatic gonorrhea requires careful investigation. It should be distinguished from other acute arthritides such as acute rheumatic fever, serum sickness, and Reiter's syndrome, and from subacute bacterical endocarditis, rheumatoid arthritis, and collagen diseases. The presence of skin lesions helps in the diagnosis. Meningococcemia and other bacteremias should also be considered.

Treatment

The drug of choice is aqueous procaine penicillin G. As a result of the increasing partial resistance of the gonococcus to penicillin, the dose recommended has been periodically increased. The treatment recommended by Rudolph (1972) and advocated by the United States Public Health Service is as follows:

Men and women are given 4,800,000 units of aqueous procaine penicillin G I.M. divided into two doses. It is administered during one visit with 1 gm. of probenecid (this potentiates penicillin by retarding its renal excretion) given orally at least one-half hour prior to the initial injection. Ampicillin (3.5 gm.) and probenecid (1 gm.) given simultaneously may be administered to men and women orally.

ALTERNATIVE TREATMENT. For patients in whom penicillin or ampicillin with probenecid is contraindicated, men may receive 2 gm. of spectinomycin dihydrochloride pentahydrate in one intramuscular injection and women may be given 4 gm. of spectinomycin dihydrochloride pentahydrate in one intramus-

TABLE 15–3 SUMMARY OF TREATMENT OF VENEREAL DISEASES

	Syphilis	Gonorrhea	Chancroid	Lympho-granuloma Venereum	Granuloma Inguinale	Abacterial Nonspecific Urethritis
Sulphonamides			1	1		
Penicillin	1	1				
Streptomycin		2			1	
Tetracycline		2		2	2	1
Erythromycin	2					2
Spectinomycin		2				
Ampicillin		2				

Effective   1=Drug of choice   2=Alternative drug

Moderately effective (in gonorrhea, high degree of resistance)

cular injection (Pedersen et al., 1972). Men and women may receive orally, when necessary, tetracycline hydrochloride (1.5 gm. in an initial dose followed by 0.5 gm. four times daily until a total dose of 9 gm. has been taken).

The administrations of 4,800,000 units of penicillin is assumed to abort any co-existing incubating syphilis. Thus, follow-up serologic tests for syphilis are not needed. However, patients treated with ampicillin, spectinomycin, and tetracycline should have a follow-up serologic test for syphilis each month for four months.

Complicated gonorrhea requires larger doses of aqueous procaine penicillin G. Patients with gonococcal epididymitis should receive at least 2,400,000 units daily for seven days. Treatment for gonococcal salpingitis and gonococcal arthritis consists of rest in bed and 10,000,000 units administered intravenously as a slow drip daily for 10 to 14 days. Alternative treatment is tetracycline, first dose 1500 mg. followed by 500 mg. four times daily for two weeks. Meningitis and endocarditis are treated with 10,000,000 to 20,000,000 units of aqueous procaine penicillin G daily, the former for two weeks and the latter for four to six weeks.

The treatment of gonococcal ophthalmia neonatorum requires immediate hospitalization. After the eyes have been cleansed of purulent material, 2 drops of aqueous solution of crystalline penicillin (10,000 units per millimeter) is instilled in each eye every 5 minutes for 30 minutes, followed by 2 drops every 30 minutes for 3 hours, and thereafter 2 drops every hour and later every 2 hours for five days. If the cornea is damaged, the pupils should be dilated with atropine sulphate twice daily. Aqueous procaine penicillin G, 50,000 units per kilogram of body weight should be injected intramuscularly daily for five days.

CHANCROID

Synonyms

Soft chancre, ulcus molle, Ducrey's infection.

Definition

Chancroid is an auto-inoculable infectious venereal disease caused by *Haemophilus ducreyi*. It is manifested by painful ulceration, usually of the genitals, and is often accompanied by suppurative regional adenopathy.

Historical Review

Chancroid was differentiated from syphilis by Bassereau in 1852. In 1889, Ducrey described the causative organism. Nicolle, also in 1889, reproduced the disease experimentally in monkeys. Ito, in 1913, prepared the first vaccine from culture. Koch's postulates have been satisfied by the experimental studies of Greenblatt and Sanderson (1938). The introduction of sulfonamides in the treatment of chancroid in 1938 radically changed the course and prognosis of the disease.

Epidemiology and Etiology

Chancroid is usually contracted through venereal contact. The disease has a worldwide distribution but its frequency is greater in large cities, sea ports, tropical regions, and during unusual conditions, such as wars and mass migration of people, which cause shifts in populations. During the Korean war, Asim (1952) found chancroid to be four times more common than syphilis. In the Vietnam war, Kerber and his colleagues (1969) found it to be second only to gonorrhea.

Chancroid is a disease of poverty and ignorance and is usually found in individuals with poor hygiene. It is more common in men than in women, the ratio being about 20:1. Women seldom develop inguinal adenopathy because of anatomic differences in their lymphatic drainage. Ducrey's bacilli have been found in the genitals of healthy women, suggesting the possibility that they may act as carriers of the disease.

H. ducreyi is a short, gram-negative rod with rounded ends. The two ends often stain more deeply than the center, giving the rod a "safety-pin" appearance. The bacillus may be found within the cells but it is usually extracellular and forms characteristic bands in parallel rows ("flotilla," "school of fish"). Culture is difficult and requires special conditions and media containing blood. No immunity develops to infection; repeated attacks are not uncommon.

Pathology

Microscopic examination of the ulcer shows three definite zones. The base of the ulcer, which is the first zone, shows necrotic tissue, fibrin, red blood cells and abundant polymorphonuclear leukocytes. Just below it is the second zone which consists of a wide band of edematous tissue with abundant endothelial cells in different stages of proliferation, numerous newly formed blood vessels, and other blood vessels with degeneration of their walls and thrombosis. The third and deeper zone shows a dense infiltrate in which plasma cells and lymphocytes predominate. Ducrey's bacilli are rarely demonstrated in the tissues. (Although the histologic changes are rather characteristic, biopsy is not a practical routine procedure.)

Clinical Manifestations (Storey, 1970)

The incubation period of chancroid is short, less than six days, usually two to three days. The early lesion is a tiny erythematous macule which rapidly becomes a pustule and breaks down within hours, causing a small ulceration with an erythematous halo. The lesion is usually attributed by the patient to trauma or a "hair cut" during intercourse. The early stages of the disease are seldom observed by the physician. As the ulcer increases in size, it becomes irregular in outline, with ragged, well-defined, elevated, and undermined borders. The base of the ulcer is covered with a purulent grayish exudate which, when removed, presents a granulomatous appearance. The ulcer is surrounded by an erythematous halo. Pain is a constant finding; at times, the mere friction of clothing or irritation from urine is intolerable. Careful palpation will show a lack of infiltration of the base; hence, the name soft chancre. This finding contrasts with the hard, infiltrated, and painless syphilitic chancre.

H. ducreyi has a preference for the skin; mucous membranes are seldom affected. In men, the sites of predilection are the prepuce, especially at its internal surface, the coronal sulcus, frenum (Fig. 15–1 *A*), and shaft of the penis. In women, the chancre is usually located on the labia majora, fourchette, or clitoris. Rarely, it may be found at the vaginal orifice, or on the cervix, or even intraurethrally, causing a scanty discharge. The lesions may also be found rarely on the perineum, abdomen, or thighs. Anal lesions may resemble a fissure surrounded by hypertrophic vegetations and may be mistakenly diagnosed as hemorrhoids.

The ulcer may remain single but usually becomes multiple through auto-inoculation. Lesions in the inner surface of the prepuce cause considerable edema resulting in phimosis. Extragenital ulcers may occur on the fingers, lips, breast, and even tongue. In these locations the diagnosis is often missed. Chancroidal lymphangitis of the dorsum of the penis, accompanied at times by localized foci of suppuration (bubonulus), has been described.

A most important and rare *clinical variant* is the so-called *phagedenic chancroid* which is characterized by a rapidly destructive ulcerative process which spreads serpiginously to involve the skin not only of the genitals (Fig. 15–1 *B*) but also of the abdomen and thighs. Fusospirochetes are abundant in the smears.

Other clinical variants include tiny lesions, at times follicular, (dwarf chancroid) or a single large ulceration (giant chancroid). The transient chancroid, the small self-healing ulcerations followed by adenopathy mentioned in older literature, was probably lymphogranuloma venereum. The rare papular and nodular varieties resemble syphilitic lesions.

Significant *inguinal lymphadenitis* (Fig. 15–1 *C* and *C*) is observed in about one-third of the cases. The other patients may have a slightly enlarged and tender inguinal lymph node or no lymph node involvement.

The inguinal bubo usually develops one or two weeks after the appearance of the ulcer. It occurs on the side of the ulcer but occasionally may be bilateral. A single lymph node is usually enlarged and it is extremely painful to the touch. When sup-

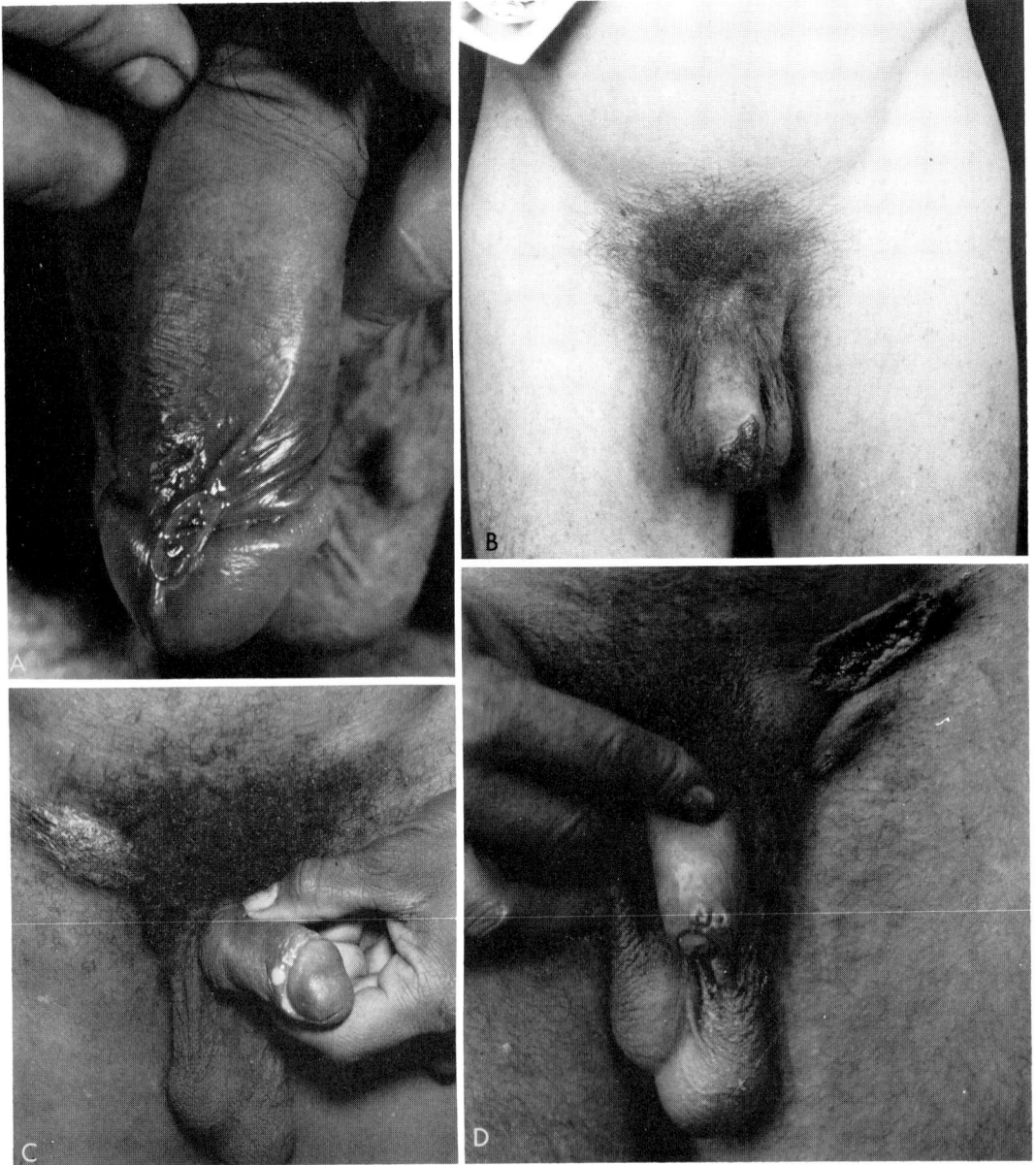

Figure 15–1   *A*, "Soft" chancres of chancroid, one involving the frenum, a site of predilection. (From Cani-zares, O.: Modern Diagnosis and Treatment of the Minor Venereal Diseases. Springfield, Illinois, Charles C Thomas, 1954.) *B*, Rapidly progressive destructive type of chancroid, the so-called phagedenic variant. *C*, Multiple ulcers of chancroid with satellite fluctuant bubo. *D*, Multiple chancroid ulcers of the penis associated with unilateral, multiple, tender, suppurative inguinal lymph nodes; several of the nodes are draining through ulcerations of the skin (fistulas).

puration develops, the overlying skin is red, thin, and tender and the mass has all the characteristics of an acute abscess. The overlying skin never becomes thickened and edematous as in the bubo of lympho-granuloma venereum. If untreated, the mass may break down, forming an irregu-larly shaped, draining sinus. Inoculation of the skin around the sinus may cause ex-tensive ulcerations. Pain is severe through-out the whole course of the lymphadenop-athy; palpation of the area should be performed with extreme care. There appears to be no relation between the severity of the ulceration and the inguinal lymphadenopathy. Small ulcers may cause large buboes, and multiple large ulcerations may not be accompanied by lymphadenopathy. Bacteriologically proved chancroidal bubo without mucocutaneous ulceration was reported by Gougerot (1925).

The associated constitutional manifestations are mild, even in cases of severe and extensive ulceration; however, the lymphadenopathy is often accompanied by malaise and fever which seldom exceeds 102° F.

Chancroid is often acquired simultaneously with other venereal diseases. If associated with gonorrhea, the clinical signs of both diseases develop about the same time since both have a short period of incubation. When chancroid coexists with syphilis, the ulcer, if untreated, will present first as the "dirty" ulcer characteristic of chancroid. In two or three weeks it will become painless, cleaner, and infiltrated—the characteristics of the usual syphilitic chancre. Successive darkfield examinations following saline compresses to cleanse the ulcer will allow an earlier diagnosis. Lymphogranuloma venereum, granuloma inguinale, and chancroid are encountered rarely concomitantly.

The course of chancroid is usually chronic with little tendency to spontaneous healing. Extensive chronic cutaneous ulcerations as a result of broken-down buboes are exceptional.

Laboratory Diagnosis (Strakosch et al., 1945)

SMEARS FOR HAEMOPHILUS DUCREYI. The value of this test depends greatly on the skill and the experience of the technician. Material should be taken with a wire applicator or the flat end of a sterile toothpick from under the undermined borders of the ulcer. Surface smears are worthless. After fixing by heat, the slide is stained with the Barrit's modification of the Unna-Pappenheim pyronin–methyl green stain. The organisms stain bright red and the pus cells, blue green. The *H. ducreyi* are demonstrable in the stained smears in about one-third of the cases; smears of the aspirates of unruptured buboes or of the auto-inoculated ulcers have a higher yield of positivity on staining for the organism. Deacon (1964) has shown that *H. ducreyi* may be identified in smears by the fluorescent antibody staining technique.

Culture of *H. ducreyi* requires a special medium containing defibrated rabbit's blood, dextrose, cystine, and beef-infusion agar. Best results are obtained in an environment of moisture at 28 to 32° C. Growth develops in 48 hours as small, convex, clear dew drop–like colonies. Culturing is more successful when the inoculum consists of pus aspirated from unruptured buboes rather than from material from the chancroidal ulcers which is usually heavily contaminated with other bacteria; a positive culture is obtained in 50 to 90 per cent of cases. Culturing is of little practical value because of the inherent technical difficulties.

OTHER LABORATORY PROCEDURES include the intradermal test with Ducrey vaccine (Ito-Reenstierna test) which gives a papular reaction in 24 hours when buboes have developed but may be negative at the onset of the disease. Ability to react to the vaccine persists for years after infection. The value of this test is now debatable; the vaccine is no longer commercially available. *Auto-inoculation* of pus on a healthy area such as the arm may yield a pure culture of the causative organism. For practical and medicolegal reasons, this method is not a routine procedure. *Biopsy,* although giving a fairly characteristic microscopic picture, is of little practical value; it is indicated only in ulcers of long standing to rule out malignancy.

The preceding discussion shows that the laboratory diagnosis of chancroid leaves much to be desired. In practice, the diagnosis is often made "by exclusion," that is, ruling out other venereal diseases, especially syphilis, and by the therapeutic response. This approach probably will continue until an effective and simple diagnostic test is devised.

Diagnosis and Differential Diagnosis

Single or multiple painful ulcerations of the genitals developing one or two days after sexual intercourse suggest the diagnosis of chancroid. The possibility of chancroid is even stronger if there is an associated painful lymphadenopathy.

Chancroid should be distinguished from a syphilitic chancre which is usually single, painless, infiltrated, and not ulcerated but eroded. The diagnosis should never be made on clinical grounds alone. Darkfield examination for *Treponema pallidum* repeated in three successive days and serologic tests for syphilis should be performed in all genital ulcerations of sudden onset. Even the most typical case of chancroid may be a mixed infection (Lomholt, 1972).

Other conditions to consider in the differential diagnosis of chancroid are the primary lesion of lymphogranuloma venereum; herpes simplex progenitalis; genital pyoderma, primary or secondary, such as in scabies and traumatic changes; eroded lesions of erythema multiforme bullosum or fixed drug eruptions; and ulcus vulvae acutum (Lipschütz's ulcer) which may follow systemic infections such as typhoid fever and virus pneumonia or be part of an incomplete Behçet's syndrome.

The chancroidal lymphadenopathy should be distinguished from that caused by pyogenic organisms, lymphogranuloma venereum, and syphilis. The possibility of an inguinal bubo of mixed causation should always be kept in mind. The lymphadenopathy of tularemia, cat-scratch disease, and plague (in endemic areas) is considered rarely in the differential diagnosis of chancroid; that of lymphomas and malignancy is usually not inflammatory and is chronic.

Treatment

Prophylactic administration of 2 gm. of sulphonamides within three hours of sexual contact often prevents infection. Locally, plain soap and water after intercourse does not prevent infection.

LOCAL TREATMENT. In mild cases, local treatment is unnecessary. In extensive lesions, soaks with potassium permanganate (1:10,000) are helpful. Local application of an ice bag may relieve the pain of the lymphadenopathy. Suppurating buboes should be aspirated with a No. 16 to 18 needle attached to a 10-cc. syringe; repeated aspirations may be needed. The bubo should never be in-cised. If severe phimosis is present, a dorsal slit of the prepuce will promote local drainage; it should be performed after systemic therapy has been started.

SYSTEMIC TREATMENT. The sulphonamides are the drug of choice; they are effective, inexpensive, and do not interfere with the diagnosis of a concomitant syphilitic infection. Sulfadiazine, sulfathiazole, sulfisoxazole (Gantrisin), or a triple sulfa preparation may be used. The first dose, 2 to 4 gm., is followed by 1 gm. every six hours for at least one week, or for two weeks if buboes are present. Long-acting sulfonamides are effective but not recommended except in unusual circumstances because of their potential side effects. The response to sulfonamide therapy is rapid; pain decreases within 24 hours and the ulcer becomes cleaner. Lymphadenopathy never develops after two days of treatment.

Streptomycin is also effective and does not mask a possible concomitant syphilitic infection. It may be administered in daily intramuscular injections of 1 gm. for 5 to 10 days or in a single dose of 5 gm. The possibility of vestibular damage is a serious objection to this medication.

In individuals who are allergic or resistant to sulfonamides, tetracycline or oxytetracycline may be used, although their effectiveness is questionable. Kerber and associates (1969) found that tetracycline alone was effective in only 30 per cent of cases. The dose recommended is 500 mg. every six hours until healing is complete. It should be kept in mind that these medications in small doses may mask a concomitant syphilitic infection. Simultaneous administration of streptomycin with sulfonamides or preferably tetracyclines may be useful in patients who are not healing with sulfonamides alone or who have large inguinal adenopathy. Penicillin has no therapeutic value. Erythromycin is of questionable efficacy and chloramphenicol, although effective, is not recommended because of its potential hematologic toxicity.

Phagedenic component of chancroidal ulcers caused by fusospirochetes should be treated immediately with 1,200,000 units of penicillin daily for one week. In resistant cases, kanamycin intramuscularly or cephalothin intravenously may be used (Marmar, 1972).

GRANULOMA INGUINALE

Synonyms

Granuloma pudendi chronicum; granuloma venereum, sclerosing granuloma, granuloma Donovani, donovanosis.

Definition

Granuloma inguinale is a chronic, infectious, granulomatous disease which involves the genitalia and neighboring tissues and is caused by *Calymmatobacterium (Donovania) granulomatis.* It shows no tendency to spontaneous healing and responds to streptomycin and broad-spectrum antibiotics. Because of its sites of predilection, granuloma inguinale is usually considered a venereal disease (Riberiro, 1972).

Historical Review

Granuloma inguinale was described by MacLeod in India in 1882. In 1905, Donovan found ovoid organisms inside mononuclear cells which he believed to be protozoa similar to leishmania. In 1943, Anderson cultured the causative organism in the yolk sac of the chick embryo. Tartar emetic was introduced in the treatment of granuloma inguinale by Aragao and Vianna in 1913. This was the drug of choice until 1947 when streptomycin was found to be effective.

Etiology and Epidemiology
(Lal and Nicholas, 1970)

The causative organism *Calymmatobacterium (Donovania) granulomatis* (Donovan body) is an encapsulated, straight or slightly curved gram-negative rod 1.5 by 0.5 microns in diameter; it is possibly related to the Klebsiella group. With Wright's stain the capsule takes a pink color and the rod is dark blue or purplish. Characteristically, the poles of the rod are deeper in color, creating a safety-pin appearance (Fig. 15–2 A). Tiny, immature, non-encapsulated forms may be found in specimens taken from the lesions. These bodies are found in thick clusters or in cystic spaces inside the large mononuclear cells and often close to the nucleus.

The organisms have been grown in the yolk sacs of chick embryos and in liquid media containing egg yolk sac material or soya meal and thioglycollate. Electron microscopic examination reveals dense peripherally located cytoplasmic inclusions suggestive of a bacteriophage. Ultrastructure findings characteristic of gram-negative bacteria were consistently found (Davis, 1970).

Granuloma inguinale is more common in men than in women in a ratio of 2 or 3 to 1. The causative organism has been found in the cervix of apparently healthy women, suggesting the possibility that some women may act as carriers of the disease. There is evidence that the agent may have a fecal habitat, suggesting that the disease may be acquired by rectal intercourse.

The highest incidence of the disease is between the ages of 20 and 45, but it has been observed in young children and in the aged. No race is exempt, but Caucasians are seldom affected. It is more common in tropical and subtropical areas but it is not necessarily limited to these regions. In the United States, it is encountered in the South and in cities with a large black population.

Granuloma inguinale does not appear to be very contagious; however, it is not infrequent in marital partners and this suggests that the disease is sexually transmitted in spite of opinions to the contrary. Little is known about immunity in this condition.

Pathology (Davis, 1970)

The histologic picture is that of a granuloma. The epidermis is usually absent over ulcerated lesions and often acanthotic at the margin of the ulcer. In the corium there is a dense infiltrate consisting mainly of histiocytes and plasma cells. There is no caseation necrosis or giant cells and few lymphocytes. Two characteristic features have been described: (1) microabscesses of polymorphonuclear leukocytes scattered throughout the predominantly mononuclear infiltrate and (2) large vacuolated histiocytes which may habor clusters of Donovan bodies which are better appreciated with the use of the Warthin-Starry silver stain. The morphologic characteristics are never as clearly

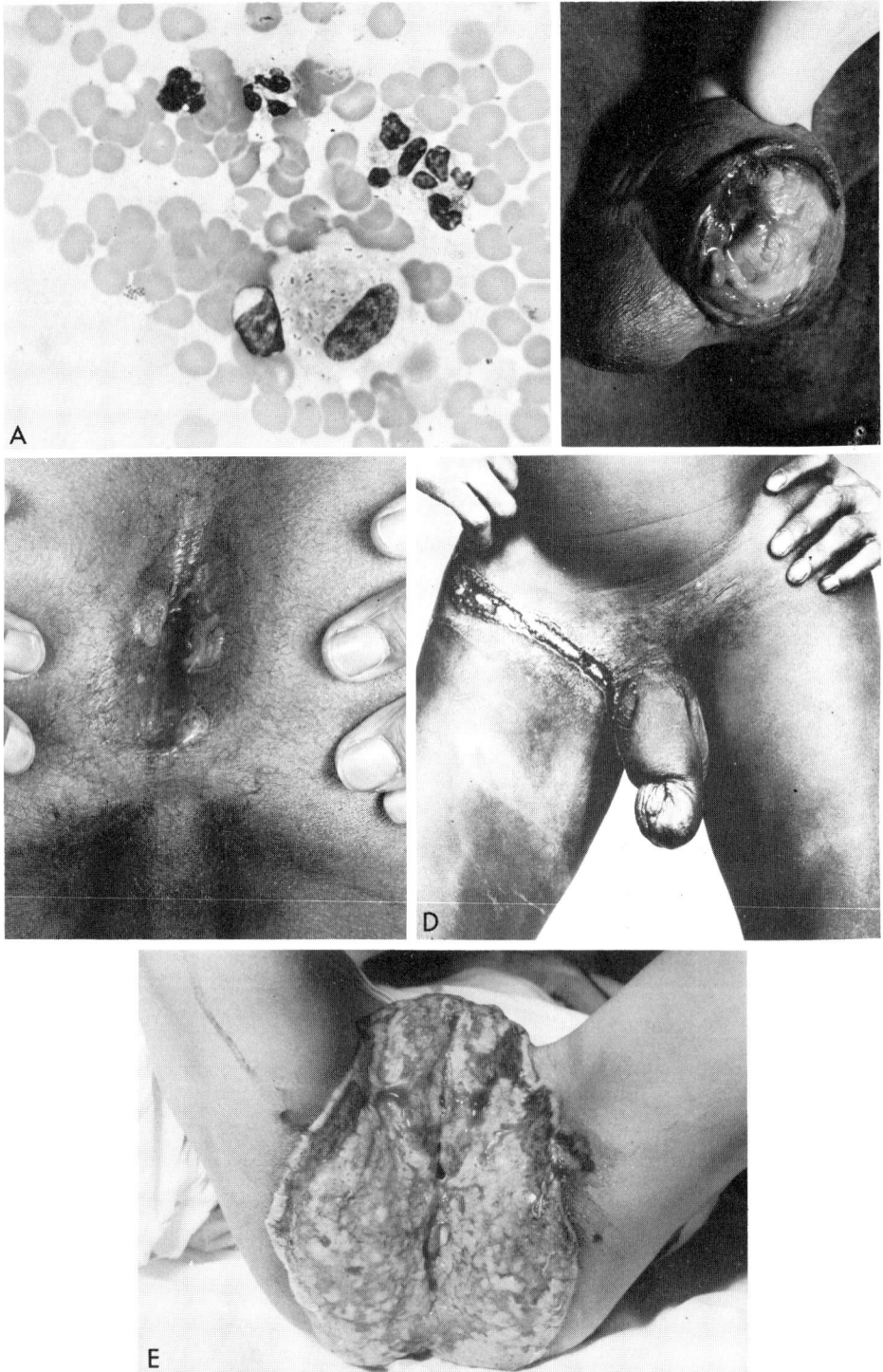

Figure 15–2 *A*, Donovan bodies, gram-negative rods. With Giemsa stain, the poles of the rods stain more deeply and give a "safety pin" appearance. *B*, Painless beefy granulomatous lesion on the head of the penis. *C*, Perianal lesions which may resemble condyloma lata or framboesiform lesions of yaws. (Courtesy of Harry Shatin, M.D., Veterans Administration Hospital, Bronx, New York.) *D*, The cicatrizing type characterized by granulomatous and scarring process with secondary penile lymphedema. *E*, Extensive ulcerovegetative type involving the perineum. (Courtesy of Francisco Kerdel Vegas, Caracas, Venezuela.)

revealed in biopsy preparations as in direct smears. Pseudoepitheliomatous hyperplasia may develop and require differentiation from carcinoma.

Clinical Manifestations (Riberiro, 1972)

The incubation period of granuloma inguinale is difficult to determine; it ranges possibly from 1 to 12 weeks. In experimental infections it was found to be three to six weeks.

In most cases the first lesion appears on the genitals as a soft, painless, elevated, flat nodule with a bright, beefy red, granulomatous surface (Fig. 15–2 B). The sites most commonly affected are the coronal sulcus, the shaft of the penis, and the labia majora. In a few weeks, satellite lesions appear at the periphery and, by their coalescence, well-defined elevated plaques with polycyclic borders develop. The primary and secondary lesions favor the warm, moist folds and creases of the groin, perineum, and intergluteal area. The anus (Fig. 15–2 C) may be involved but the rectum is not invaded. Extragenital lesions are rare; they may be found on the face, neck, hands, larynx, and pharynx.

In the older lesions, the borders are grayish or hypopigmented, elevated, and at times rolled and cord-like. They are never undermined. The center of the lesion is formed by an irregular conglomeration of granulations with patchy whitish epithelialization and erosions, resembling a relief map. The involved area may be bathed in a fetid, often blood-tinged discharge. As a rule there is little discomfort, but extensive lesions may cause pain on walking; these patients have an awkward slow gait with their legs spread apart. There is no specific involvement of the regional lymph nodes. Slight inguinal lymphadenopathy, if present, is caused by secondary infection. Pseudobuboes are subcutaneous granulomatous lesions which are located in the groin and eventually break through the skin to cause typical lesions.

Other clinical variants of granuloma inguinale include: (1) the *cicatricial type,* characterized by hypertrophic scars alternating with active granulomatous lesions. The finding of Donovan bodies below the scars indicates the presence of active lesions (Fig. 15–2 D), (2) the *ulcerovegetating type,* the most common, which develops from the nodular variety (Fig. 15–2 E) and (3) the *hypertrophic type,* which is rare and ranges from vegetating masses to elephantiasis of the affected areas caused by impairment of the lymphatic drainage and not by direct involvement of the lymph channels as in lymphogranuloma venereum. However, both diseases, despite their different responsible pathogenic mechanisms, can present the same hypertrophic clinical picture; for example, in women, granuloma inguinale may cause an esthiomene picture identical to that of lymphogranuloma venereum. The disease process may extend along the female genital tract to the cervix.

Systemic manifestations are minimal. Metastases to the bones (Kirkpatrick, 1970), joints, and viscera have been reported. Common *complications* are urinary tract infections, secondary anemia, and sudden hemorrhage caused by erosion of a large blood vessel. Squamous cell carcinoma may develop in cases of long duration and should be suspected in all vegetating lesions that fail to respond to therapy.

The course of untreated granuloma inguinale is steadily progressive; the disease lasts 10 to 20 years, and death may result from complications of the disease and from cachexia.

Laboratory Diagnosis

The diagnosis of granuloma inguinale is confirmed by the finding of the Donovan body in the lesions; all other laboratory procedures are of little practical value. *Smears for Donovan bodies* should be made by removing a small lesion or a piece from the edge of a large lesion with a scalpel or a punch. A deep portion of the tissue may be crushed between two glass slides. Smears are best made by using the undersurface of the removed tissue and placing it on several slides. After fixing with alcohol, the smears are stained with Wright's or Giemsa stain. Donovan bodies will be found within the mononuclear cells. Routine hematoxylin and eosin stain rarely demonstrates Donovan bodies in tissue. The bodies stain bright red with Giemsa stain and brown to black with silver stains.

Intradermal tests give many false positive reactions; there is no antigen commercially available. Complement-fixation test is often negative in early cases and the titer increases with the duration of the disease. Since successful culturing of the organism is difficult it is not a routine procedure.

Diagnosis and Differential Diagnosis

A typical lesion of granuloma inguinale consists of a beefy red, elevated, well-defined, granulomatous plaque which is easily diagnosed clinically. Early lesions should be differentiated from condyloma lata of syphilis by darkfield examination and serologic tests. Lesions on the glans should be distinguished from erythroplasia of Queyrat and psoriasis. On the labia and shaft of the penis, the erosive, elevated, pyogenic plaques, called pseudo-lues papulosa by Lipschütz, may resemble granuloma inguinale.

Late lesions should be distinguished from lymphogranuloma venereum, ulcerative cutaneous tuberculosis, deep mycotic and eosinophilic granulomas, ulcerative hidradenitis suppurativa, pyoderma gangrenosum, and carcinoma. The possibility of a superimposed carcinoma in a chronic granuloma inguinale should always be kept in mind.

Treatment (Riberiro, 1972)

The drugs of choice are streptomycin and the broad-spectrum antibiotics. Streptomycin (3 gm.) is given intramuscularly (1.5 gm. in each buttock) every six hours for three days in early cases and for 10 days in those with extensive lesions. Broad-spectrum antibiotics are also effective. Tetracycline, oxytetracycline, and clorotetracycline are administered orally 2 gm. daily (500 mg. every six hours) for 10 to 20 days. The masking effect of these medications on syphilis is not a major problem in granuloma inguinale since most cases are seen after the lesions have been present for months. Erythromycin and carbomycin are also helpful. After healing, the patient should be seen every two months for at least one year.

Relapses may occur months or years after treatment. In case of relapse or resist-ance to a medication, retreatment should consist of another antibiotic administered for a longer period of time. Penicillin is indicated only in cases of secondary infection with fusospirochetes. There are contradicting reports as to the value of ampicillin. Thew et al. (1969) found it effective in doses of 1 gm. daily for three to five weeks, while Davis (1970) reported failures with doses of 2 gm. daily. Locally, potassium permanganate soaks (1:10,000) are helpful to control secondary infection and to act as a deodorant. At times, surgery is indicated for reconstruction or excision of a complicating cancer.

LYMPHOGRANULOMA VENEREUM

Synonyms

Lymphogranuloma inguinale, lymphopathia venereum, fourth or fifth venereal disease, Nicolas-Favre disease, climatic bubo.

Definition

Lymphogranuloma venereum is a systemic disease, usually of venereal origin, which is manifested by an inconstant, small, evanescent, primary genital lesion followed by regional lymphadenitis with periadenitis and accompanied by constitutional symptoms (Sigel, 1962). The late rectal and genital involvement is neoformative and suppurative and results in rectal stricture, ulceration, abscesses, and fistulae. The causative agent which is related to the psittacosis-trachoma group has been classified as a *Bedsonia* (genus Chlamydia).

Historical Review

In 1789, Hunter described the inguinal adenopathy which characterizes lymphogranuloma venereum. Some early reports from French colonies mentioned a non-venereal adenopathy attributed to climatic factors, hence the name of "climatic bubo."

In spite of earlier publications, the credit of recognition of the disease as an independent entity belongs to Durand, Nicolas, and Favre who, in 1913, reported the first clinical and pathologic description of the disease which they called lymphogranuloma inguinale. Gamma, in 1924, described large bodies in the cytoplasm of cells from infected lymph nodes. Definite proof of the specificity of this entity was presented by Frei in 1925 with the introduction of human antigen for the test which bears his name. Later, Frei and Kopple found positive skin tests in many patients with rectal strictures and esthiomene, which until then had been attributed to syphilis; thus, they enlarged the clinical concept of the disease. In 1930, Hellerstrom and Wassen transmitted the disease to monkeys by intracerebral inoculation. In 1940, Rake, McKee, and Shaffer cultured the agent in the yolk sac of the chick embryo; this led to the development of a highly purified antigen now used as a skin test and an antigen for the complement-fixation test. Rake and Jones in 1942 studied the developmental cycle of the agent.

Etiology and Epidemiology

The causative agent of lymphogranuloma venereum has been classified with psittacosis and trachoma because of its immunologic and morphologic similarity to the causative agents of these diseases and has been called *Miyagawenella lymphogranulomatosis*. The group of agents are characterized by large elementary particles and are considered to be small bacteria, not a large virus (Moulder, 1962). These agents occupy an intermediate position between the rickettsiae and the viruses (Bedson, 1959). Inclusion bodies within the cytoplasm of mononuclear cells are found in pus aspirated from unruptured buboes and in biopsy material of early and late lesions. The size of the inclusion bodies varies from barely visible to 4.5 microns in diameter and correlates with the different stages of the developmental cycle.

The agent can be cultivated in corneal and HeLa tissue cultures and especially in the embryonated egg. Monkeys and mice are highly susceptible to inoculation; other experimental animals are more resistant to infection.

Lymphogranuloma venereum is almost always contracted through sexual intercourse; there are a few reports of accidental inoculation of the fingers of doctors and nurses. The disease is more common in the tropics but is not rare in temperate climates, especially in large cities. It is more frequent in men than in women and no race is immune. The incidence of lymphogranuloma venereum has recently increased in the United States; this is due in part to returning military personnel infected in Vietnam (Abrams, 1968).

An infected individual is refractory to intradermal or cutaneous reinfection with material containing the agent; only a papular Frei test–like reaction develops. It is not known if this immunity persists after the agent has disappeared from the patient. Clinically recovered experimental animals have been found to be immune to reinfection.

Pathology

Gross examination of a surgically removed lymphatic mass shows several lymph nodes matted together by pronounced periadenitis. A cross-section shows congestion of the glands with yellowish necrotic islands of varying sizes. The larger foci of necrosis are filled with pus. In the early stages, one sees histopathologically small groups of epithelioid cells, with occasional giant cells, scattered in chronic granulation tissue with abundant plasma cells. Later, the centers of these islands of epithelioid cells become necrotic, are filled with polymorphonuclear leukocytes, develop a characteristic angular shape, and are called stellate abscesses. Periglandular fibrosis is a constant and characteristic finding. (Although the histologic picture is not diagnostic, a pathologist's report of "consistent with lymphogranuloma venereum" may be helpful in doubtful clinical cases.)

The microscopic appearance of elephantiasic and papillomatous forms is nonspecific granulation tissue with fibrosis. Rectal tissue shows a granulomatous reaction and chronic lymphangitis of the inner layers of the rectal wall with varying degrees of fibrous tissue proliferation. Biopsies may be done on the old persistent skin lesions to rule out a complicating carcinoma.

Clinical Manifestations
(Abrams, 1968; Sigel, 1962)

The clinical manifestations of lympho-granuloma venereum depend upon the location of the portal of entry and the duration of the disease. The predominant signs occur in the region of the lymphatic drainage from the primary lesion, usually on the genitals but at times in the anorectal area. As a result there are two main varieties of the disease; the early *primary lesion–inguinal adenitis* and the late *anorectal* and *genital* syndromes. This latter variety may develop from the inguinal involvement or from direct implantation of the responsible organism in the anorectal region.

PRIMARY LESION–INGUINAL ADENITIS SYNDROME (Fig. 15–3 A) The *primary lesion* develops one to three weeks after the infective sexual contact. The lesion may be a small, transient, painless papule, a herpetiform vesicle or pustule, or rarely, an ulceration. It occurs usually on the coronal sulcus, prepuce, glans, or shaft of the penis in males. When located inside the urethra, a mucoid discharge develops. The primary lesion (which may be easily missed or unnoticed) is found in about one-fourth of the male patients. In women, the favorite primary sites are the fourchette and the labia minora near the urethral meatus or the lower portion of the vagina. The lesion lasts for a few days and often heals before the development of the

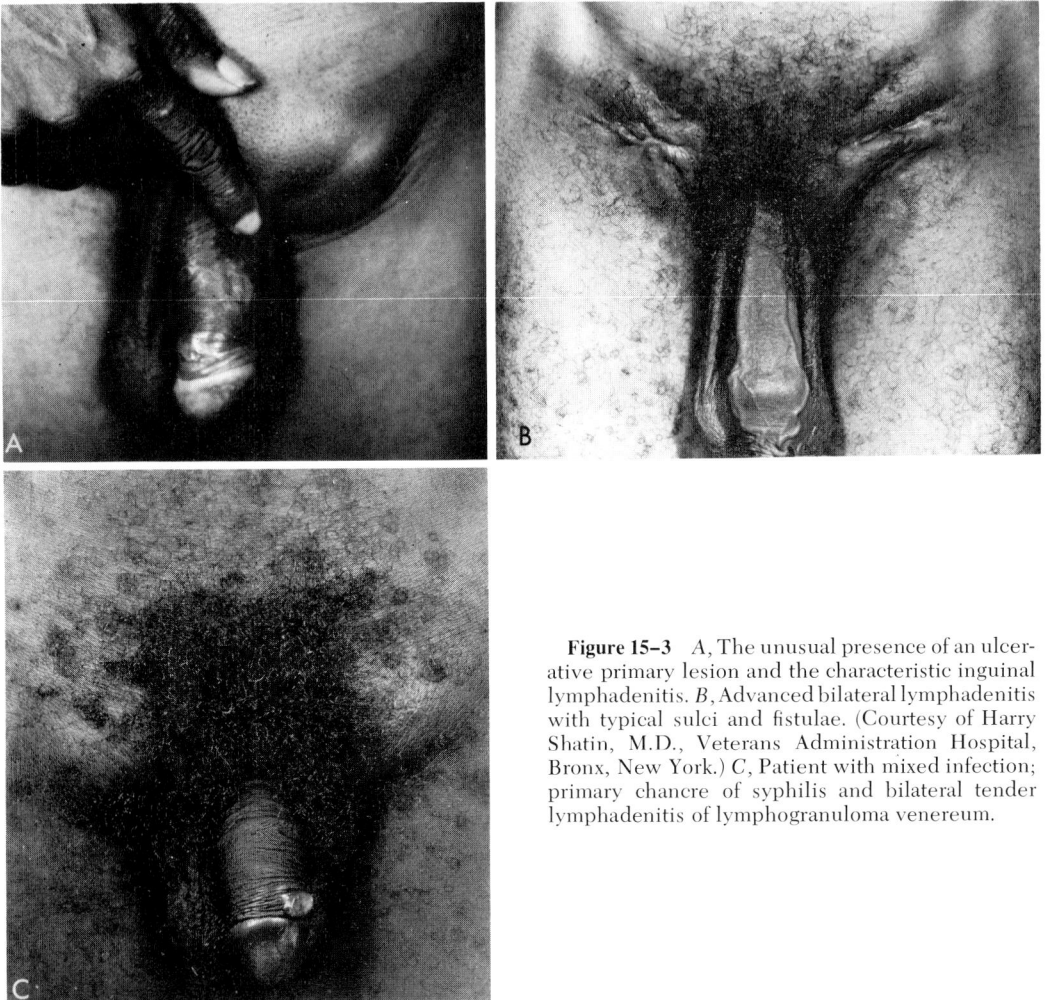

Figure 15–3 *A,* The unusual presence of an ulcerative primary lesion and the characteristic inguinal lymphadenitis. *B,* Advanced bilateral lymphadenitis with typical sulci and fistulae. (Courtesy of Harry Shatin, M.D., Veterans Administration Hospital, Bronx, New York.) *C,* Patient with mixed infection; primary chancre of syphilis and bilateral tender lymphadenitis of lymphogranuloma venereum.

inguinal adenitis; it rarely appears after the onset of the adenopathy.

The *inguinal adenitis* develops about two to three weeks after the appearance of the primary lesion; thus, the period of incubation from the time of the infective sexual contact may be three to six weeks. The adenopathy is often unilateral on the side of the primary lesion but in about one-third of the cases it is bilateral. The lymph nodes are initially discrete, movable, and tender and within one to two weeks become the more typical, firm egg- or fist-sized, moderately tender, oval or elongated mass formed by their fusion. The overlying skin is edematous, purplish, attached to the underlying tissues, and often divided by one or more transversal sulci (Fig. 15–3 *B*); this manifestation constitutes the "purplish wrinkled adenopathy" characteristic of lymphogranuloma venereum. If suppuration develops, it may occur successively in multiple foci. The femoral and iliac glands may also be enlarged. A lymphangitis may rarely appear at the site of entry and extend along the shaft of the penis in which one or more bubonuli may develop. In women, inguinal lymphadenitis is rare; it occurs only when the primary lesion is on the vulva or in the anterior aspect of the vagina. The lymphatic drainage of the deeper lesions is toward the iliac and perirectal lymph nodes.

During the course of the lymphadenitis, mild constitutional signs and symptoms, consisting of irregular fever, chills, malaise, anorexia, myalgia, and arthralgia, may develop. A typhoidal state, meningism, and hepatosplenomegaly are rarely encountered. The *duration* of the adenopathy, which is self-limited, is 8 to 12 weeks. After suppuration and discharge the mass becomes shrunken and fibrotic.

ANORECTAL AND GENITAL SYNDROMES. The anorectal and genital syndromes are chronic manifestations of the disease. Anorectal lesions are more common in women; in men, they are often seen in homosexuals. In women, they develop either from direct implantation of the agent on the mucosa by rectal intercourse or by extension from the vagina, or from lymphatic anastomoses between the inguinal nodes and the perianal groups. The manifestations of rectal involvement are those of proctitis, a bloody or mucopurulent, rectal discharge with fever, pruritus, tenesmus, and alternating diarrhea and constipation. With the development of granulation tissue and, later on, fibrosis accompanied by permanent stricture formation, defecation becomes painful and the stools pencil thin. These changes are detectable by digital rectal examination. Proctoscopic examination shows an annular or tubular constriction from 4 to 10 cm. long; ulcerations may be seen. Papillomas of the anal mucosa and perianal region are common. Perirectal abscesses and rectovaginal and anal fistulae may occur. Polypoidal growths of the anus (lymphorrhoids) resemble hemorrhoidal tags.

Genital lesions are characterized by elephantiasic swelling of the penis or vulva, usually with superficial, painless, chronic ulcerations and fistulae; pedunculated and papillomatous growths often cover the affected area. In women, this picture is called esthiomene. Rectal stricture is often, but not always, associated with genital lesions. Malignant changes may develop in advanced and highly fibrotic lesions.

Systemic manifestations are less pronounced during the late stages than at onset and are often due to complications or secondary bacterial infection. Erythema nodosum, erythema multiforme, and exanthematous eruptions develop occasionally in the inguinal type and more frequently in women. Light sensitivity eruptions have been described.

Laboratory Diagnosis

The laboratory evidence of lymphogranuloma venereum by the Frei skin test, the complement-fixation test, or the culture of the causative organism is essential in order to confirm the clinical impression (Schachter et al., 1969). Alterations of the *peripheral blood* are not diagnostic but instead are indicative of an acute or chronic infectious process. The erythrocyte sedimentation rate is usually elevated in the late stages. In chronic cases, the hematocrit and hemoglobin values often indicate anemia. The albumin-globulin ratio is usually 1.1 or reversed. There is an elevation of the alpha-2 and gamma globulins in the acute cases. As the activity of the disease decreases, the serum proteins tend to return to normal levels.

The *Frei test,* a delayed intradermal reaction performed with a specific antigen, is the simplest and most effective diagnostic procedure. The antigen is readily available and consists of an inactivated suspension of the causative agent which has been cultured in yolk sacs of fertile chicken eggs. The test is performed by injecting 0.1 ml. of the antigen intradermally into the flexor aspect of the forearm. A few inches below the above test site, the same volume of a control material of chick embryo origin is injected; only by comparison of both reactions can the test be properly evaluated. A positive reaction is one presenting a papule or papule-vesicle of 7 mm. or larger in the antigen site at the end of 72 hours; the control test is usually non-reactive. Patients with allergies to eggs, chicken, or chicken feathers may give positive reactions to the control material. The ability to react to the Frei antigen develops two to three weeks after onset of the adenopathy. For this reason, a negative early test should be repeated if clinical appearance suggests the diagnosis of lymphogranuloma venereum. Intensive early therapy may prevent the Frei antigen from becoming positive and, exceptionally, may revert a positive test to negative.

Cross-reactions to the Frei antigen may be produced by agents of the same group which cause psittacosis, cat-scratch disease, trachoma, and viral pneumonias. Once the test becomes positive, the ability to react to the antigen may persist for many years. Therefore, clinical evidence of the disease is essential for the diagnosis, since a positive skin test indicates only that the patient has or has had an infection with a member of the lymphogranuloma venereum–psittacosis group. The test is of decided value when a negative reaction found at the onset of the disease is followed by a positive one when the test is repeated one or two weeks later. In exceptional cases, the *inverted Frei test* may be performed: pus aspirated from the unruptured suppurating adenopathy of the suspected case is prepared and is injected intradermally into the skin of a patient known to give a positive Frei test.

The *complement-fixation test* performed with antigen from a chick embryo is a useful procedure; other organisms of the lymphogranuloma venereum–psittacosis group can give a positive test. The test usually becomes positive within a month after the onset of the infection. Its interpretation is similar to that of the Frei test: a positive test indicates a present or previous infection; the degree of change in the titer of positivity of the complement-fixation test may be diagnostically helpful.

The search and culture of the causative agent is the most specific but the least practical diagnostic procedure. It requires laboratory personnel who are specialized in viral studies. Dunlop et al. (1969) have shown that the cell culture method for the detection and isolation of Chlamydia is more effective than yolk sac culture. Biologically false positive reactions of the serologic test for syphilis are occasionally found in patients with the inguinal type of infection; the titer is not high and tends to decrease within a few weeks. An increasing titer and/or a positive treponemal immobilization test (TPI) or FTA-ABS test will indicate a concomitant infection with syphilis.

Diagnosis and Differential Diagnosis

The primary lesion of lymphogranuloma venereum should be differentiated from that of syphilis, chancroid, herpes simplex, and traumatic infected erosions of the genitals. Its transient course and insignificant appearance make its diagnosis difficult. Intra-urethral lesions causing a discharge should be distinguished from gonorrhea and nonspecific urethritis of other causes.

In the early stages, the differential diagnosis of the inguinal lymphadenopathy is difficult, since it may resemble that of chancroid, severe herpes simplex, and syphilis; the lymphadenopathy of syphilis is rarely tender. Later on, the more characteristic matted-together nodes with multiple foci of suppuration are seen. The bubo of chancroid is usually a painful, single abscess–like swelling. The lymphadenopathy of syphilis consists of freely movable, shotty nodes. The overlying skin of these other conditions never presents the typical purplish-wrinkled appearance of lymphogranuloma venereum. The possibility of simultaneous venereal infections should always be kept in mind (Fig. 15–3

C). The lymphadenopathy of malignancies, especially the lymphomas, is usually chronic and painless.

Among the anorectal diseases to be considered in the differential diagnosis when there are anorectal manifestations present are the following: hemorrhoids, rectal polyposis, condyloma acuminata, gonococcal prostatitis, ulcerative colitis and Crohn's disease of the rectum, hidradenitis suppurativa of the anogenital type, and anal and rectal carcinoma. The possibility of carcinoma complicating lymphogranuloma venereum should always be considered when the bleeding granulomatous lesions do not heal with specific therapy (Levin et al., 1964). A biopsy is imperative. The clinical picture of elephantiasis with ulcerations of the genitals (esthiomene) may be identical to that of granuloma inguinale; the presence of rectal stricture favors the diagnosis of lymphogranuloma venereum. Elephantiasis due to filariasis should be considered in areas where this disease is endemic.

Treatment

Lymphogranuloma venereum responds to treatment with the sulphonamides and the broad-spectrum antibiotics; however, the response to therapy varies with the clinical types of the disease. The inguinal lymphadenopathy, which may resolve spontaneously, responds more satisfactorily to specific medication. Uncomplicated proctitis is curable but when the condition is more advanced, it becomes more refractory. The advanced fibrotic rectal strictures and elephantiasis of the genitals are not affected by medication; the treatment of these lesions is surgical.

Sulfonamide Group

These are still the drugs of choice because of their effectiveness, low cost, and the fact that they do not mask a concomitant syphilitic infection. Sulfadiazine, sulfathiazole, or sulfisoxazole (Gantrisin) may be used. The first dose is 4 gm. then 1 gm. four times daily for three to four weeks in the inguinal type. In the anorectal and genital syndromes, successive courses are advisable, often preceding and following surgical intervention.

BROAD-SPECTRUM ANTIBIOTICS. Broad-spectrum antibiotics are also effective. Tetracycline, chlortetracycline (Aureomycin), oxytetracycline (Terramycin), or chloramphenicol (Chloromycetin) may be given in doses of 2 gm. daily divided into four doses of 500 mg. each. Erythromycin and oleandomycin have been reported as being effective; penicillin and streptomycin are ineffective. In stubborn cases, sulfonamides and the above effective antibiotics may be administered in simultaneous or alternating courses. Collaboration with a surgeon is needed in advanced anorectal cases; colostomy or vulvectomy may be required.

LOCAL TREATMENT. In the inguinal type, the local therapeutic measures utilized are bed rest, icebag to the adenopathy, and aspiration (not incision) of fluctuating buboes. In the anorectal type, aspiration or drainage of abscesses and dilation of rectal strictures may be advisable.

REFERENCES

Abrams, A. J.: Lymphogranuloma venereum. J.A.M.A. *205*:199, 1968.

Anderson, K.: The cultivation from granuloma inguinale of a microorganism having the characteristic of Donovan bodies in the yolk sac of chick embryos. Science 97:560, 1943.

Asim, J.: Chancroid. Am. J. Syph. 36:483, 1952.

Barr, J., and Danielsson, D.: Gonococcal sepsis Lakarjisningen, Stockholm 68:4255, 1971.

Bedson, S. P.: The psittacosis-lymphogranuloma venereum group of infective agents. J. R. Inst. Public Health Hyg. 22:67, 99, 131, 1959.

Brown, W. M., Cowper, H. H., and Nodgman, J. E.: Gonococcal ophthalmia among newborn infants at L. A. General Hospital. Public Health Rep. *81*:926, 1966.

Davis, C. M.: Granuloma inguinale. J.A.M.A. *211*: 632, 1970.

Deacon, W. E.: Management of Chancroid, Granuloma Inguinale, Lymphogranuloma Venereum in General Practice. U.S. Department of Health, Education, and Welfare. Public Health Service Publication *225*:11, 1964.

Deacon, W. E., Beacock, W. L., Jr., Freeman, E. M., et al.: Fluorescent antibodies for detection of the gonococcus in women. Public Health Report 75: 125, 1960.

Dunlop, E. M. C., Hare, M. J., Darougar, S., et al.: Detection of Chlamydia (Bedsonia) in certain infections of man. II. Clinical study of genital tract, eye, rectum, and other sites of recovery of Chlamydia. J. Infect. Dis. 120:463, 1969.

Gougerot, H.: Bubons chancrelleux sans Chancre. Ann. des malad venerienne 8:459, 1925.

Greenblatt, R. B., and Sanderson, E. S.: The intradermal chancroid bacillary antigen as an aid in the differential diagnosis of venereal bubo. Am. J. Surg. *41*:384, 1938.

Handfield, H. H., Hodson, W. A., and Holmes, K. K.: Neonatal gonococcal infection (orogastric contamination with *Neisseria gonorrhoeae*). J.A.M.A. *225*: 697, 1973.

Holmes, K. K., Counts, G. W., and Beaty, H. N.: Disseminated gonococcal infection. Ann. Intern. Med. *74*:879, 979, 1971.

Holmes, K. K., Wiesner, P. J., and Pederson, A. H.: The gonococcal arthritis-dermatitis syndrome. Ann. Intern. Med. *75*:470, 1971.

Keiser, H., Ruben, F. L., Wolinsky, E., et al.: Clinical forms of gonococcal arthritis. N. Engl. J. Med. *279*:234, 1968.

Kerber, R. E., Rowe, C. E., and Gilbert, K. R.: Treatment of chancroid. Arch. Dermatol. *100*:604, 1969.

Kirkpatrick, D. J.: Donovanosis (granuloma inguinale): a rare cause of osteolytic bone lesions. Clin. Radiol. *21*:101, 1970.

Kvale, P. A., Keys, T. F., Johnson, D. W., et al.: Single oral dose ampicillin-probenicid treatment of gonorrhea in the male. J.A.M.A. *215*:1449, 1971.

Lal, S., and Nicholas, C.: Epidemiological and clinical features in 165 cases of granuloma inguinale. Br. J. Vener. Dis. *46*:461, 1970.

Levin, I., Romano, S., Steinberg, M., et al.: Lymphogranuloma venereum: rectal stricture and carcinoma. Dis. Colon Rectum *7*:129, 1964.

Lomholt, G.: Dermatology in Uganda. Int. J. Dermatol. *11*:156, 1972.

Marmar, J. L.: The management of resistant chancroid in Vietnam. J. Urol. *107*:807, 1972.

Metzger, A. L.: Gonococcal arthritis complicating gonorrheal pharyngitis. Ann. Intern. Med. *73*:267, 1970.

Miller, H.: Lymphogranuloma venereum and other inflammatory rectal strictures. Am. J. Proct. *16*:291, 1965.

Moulder, J. W.: Some basic properties of the psittacosis-lymphogranuloma venereum group of agents. Structure and chemical composition of isolated particles. Ann. N.Y. Acad. Sci. *98*:92, 1962.

Owen, R. L.: Rectal and pharyngeal gonorrhea in homosexual men. J.A.M.A. *220*:1315, 1972.

Pedersen, A. H. B., Wiesner, P., Holmes, K. K., et al.: Spectinomycin and penicillin G in the treatment of gonorrhea. J.A.M.A. *220*:205, 1972.

Rake, G., and Jones, H. P.: Studies on lymphogranuloma venereum. I. Development of the agent in the yolk sac of the chicken embryo. J. Exper. Med. *75*:323, 1942.

Rees, E.: Gonococcal bartholinitis. Br. J. Vener. Dis. *43*:150, 1967.

Riberiro, J.: Granuloma inguinale. Practitioner *209*: 628, 1972.

Rudolph, A. M.: Control of gonorrhea: guidelines of antibiotic treatment. J.A.M.A. *220*:1587, 1972.

Schachter, J., Smith, D. W., Dawson, C. R., et al.: Lymphogranuloma venereum. I. Comparison of the Frei test, complement fixation test, and isolation of the agent. J. Infect. Dis. *120*:372, 1969.

Schmidt, H., Hjorting-Hansen, E., and Philipsen, H. P.: Gonococcal arthritis complicating gonorrheal pharyngitis. Ann. Intern. Med. *73*:267, 1970.

Shapiro, L., Teisch, J. A., and Brownstein, M. H.: Dermatohistopathology of chronic gonococcal sepsis. Analysis of 12 new cases. Arch. Dermatol. *107*:403, 1973.

Sigel, M. M., (ed.): Lymphogranuloma Venereum. Epidemiological, Clinical, Surgical and Therapeutic Aspects Based on a Study in the Carribean. Coral Gables, Florida, University of Miami Press, 1962.

Storey, G.: Clinical manifestations of chancroid. Br. J. Urol. *42*:738, 1970.

Strakosch, E. A., Kendell, H. W., Craig, R. M., et al.: Clinical and laboratory investigation of 370 cases of chancroid. J. Invest. Dermatol. *6*:95, 1945.

Tahyer, J. D., and Martin, J. E.: Improved medium selective for cultivation of *N. gonorrhoeae* and *N. meningitidis*. Public Health Rep. *81*:559, 1966.

Thew, M. A., Swift, J. T., and Heaton, C. L.: Ampicillin in the treatment of granuloma inguinale. J.A.M.A. *210*:866, 1969.

Willcox, R. R.: A world look at the venereal diseases. Med. Clin. North Am. *56*:1057, 1972.

CHAPTER

16

BENIGN
RETICULOENDOTHELIAL DISEASES

Samuel L. Moschella

The reticuloendothelial system (Jandl, 1967; Marshall, 1956; Saba, 1970) consists of round or stellate cells that produce reticulum fibers and form the endothelial lining of blood spaces. In the broadest sense, the reticuloendothelial system is composed of mesenchymal cells which produce cells that form reticulum and then phagocytize and form immunologically active lymphocytes and plasma cells. The system is scattered throughout all tissue and is limited to the dermis of skin. The only exception is the monocyte, which appears to be derived, probably entirely, from the marrow (Van Furth, 1970). Although this system remains an enigma in regard to its response and functional capacities, progress has been made in understanding its functions of filtration, phagocytosis of toxic and infectious particles, and immunity. In the skin, it is distinguishable in the connective tissue near small blood vessels, may proliferate after suitable stimulation, and can differentiate into histiocytes, macrophages, and foam cells. Tissue macrophages have a hematogenous origin (peripheral blood monocytes) but also proliferate locally. Macrophages participate in the inductive phase of antibody synthesis. The heterophagic activity of the mononuclear phagocyte is fundamental for defense. Pinocytosis and phagocytosis are variants of endocytosis, with resultant intracellular digestion due to lysosomal enzyme activity. Plasma or serum factors called opsonins not only enhance phagocytosis but also provide a basis for the recognition of foreignness by the normal nonimmune host (Saba, 1970). The temporal changes of plasma opsonin levels as related to intravascular phagocytosis strongly suggest the presence and operation of a "negative feedback control system" which regulates the opsonin level and directly influences reticuloendothelial system activity.

The reticuloendothelial system can be altered by infection, presence of a foreign body, allergic or metabolic states, and neoplasia. Certain chronic inflammatory diseases have a distinctive pattern of inflammation that presents clinically as a tumor and histologically as a granuloma. The latter is characterized by focal, vascularized aggregations of histiocytes and hypertrophied fibroblasts that assume round to oval shapes with an abundant, ground-glass cytoplasm, resemble epithelial cells, and consequently are called epithelioid cells; the associated connective tissue changes consist of proliferation, new fiber formation, and degeneration such as necrobiosis or necrosis.

Benign reticuloendothelial diseases are classified in the following manner:

Benign Cutaneous Reticulosis (Inflammatory Hyperplasias)

    Histiocytoma (Localized, Generalized, Eruptive)

    Xanthogranuloma (Juvenile Nevoxantho-endothelioma)

    Xanthoma Disseminatum

    Multicentric Reticulohistiocytosis

    Pseudolymphoma (Spiegler-Fendt Sarcoid, Lymphadenosis Benigna Cutis, Lymphocytoma Cutis, Cutaneous Lymphoid Hyperplasia, Benign Lymphoid Hyperplasia)

    Pseudopyogenic Granuloma and Its Variants

    Persistent Insect Bite

    Histiocytosis X

        Letterer-Siwe Disease

        Hand-Schüller-Christian Disease

        Eosinophilic Granuloma

Granulomas

    Allergic or Hypersensitivity Granuloma

    Foreign Body Granuloma

    Sarcoidosis

    Palisading Granulomas

        Granuloma Annulare

        Necrobiosis Lipoidica

        Rheumatoid Nodules

    Infectious Granulomatous Diseases

        Chronic Granulomatous Disease

        Mycobacterial Infections

        Swimming Pool Granuloma

        Mycobacterial Phagedenic Ulceration

        Tuberculosis of the Skin

            Primary Inoculation Tuberculosis (Tuberculous Chancre)

            Miliary Tuberculosis of Skin (Hematogenous Primary Tuberculosis, Tuberculosis Miliaris Disseminatus)

            Lupus Vulgaris

            Tuberculosis Verrucosa Cutis

            Scrofuloderma

            Miscellaneous Tuberculous Lesions

            Anorectal

            BCG Vaccination

            Tuberculids

                Erythema Induratum

                Papulonecrotic Tuberculid

                Lichen Scrofulosorum

                Lupus Miliaris Disseminatus Faciei

Leishmaniasis

    Cutaneous Leishmaniasis

    American Leishmaniasis

    Disseminated Cutaneous Leishmaniasis

    Post-kala-Azar Dermal Leishmaniasis

Leprosy

Granulomatous Vasculitides

    Granuloma Faciale

    Erythema Elevatum Diutinum

    Granulomatous Arteritis

    Allergic Granulomatosis

    Wegener's Granulomatosis

    Midline Lethal Granuloma (Nonhealing Granuloma of the Nose)

    Giant Cell Arteritis (Temporal Arteritis, Cranial Arteritis, Polymyalgia Arteritica)

Takayasu Arteriopathy (Aortic Arch Syndrome)

Halogendermas

Orocutaneous Crohn's Disease

BENIGN CUTANEOUS RETICULOSIS (Inflammatory Hyperplasias)

HISTIOCYTOMA

Histiocytoma (subepidermal nodular fibrosis, dermatofibroma) is a common, acquired, circumscribed, and usually solitary proliferative tumor that often appears on the lower extremities (Fig. 16–1). Rarely, as many as 20 lesions may be present. These multiple, persistent histiocytomas differ from generalized eruptive histiocytoma in that they are not as widespread nor as symmetrical in distribution and they do not develop progressively and persist.

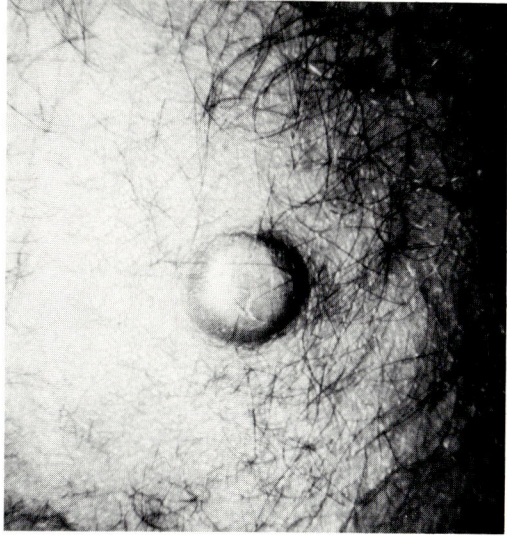

Figure 16–1 Histiocytomas (dermatofibroma). A classic asymptomatic slowly growing nodule of the lower extremity.

Generalized Eruptive Histiocytoma (Muller et al., 1967)

Generalized eruptive histiocytoma (GEH) is a rare, distinctive, syndrome seen in healthy adults. It is characterized clinically by multiple, symmetrical, papular lesions of the trunk and proximal part of the extremities (Figs. 16–2 and 16–3). The mucous membranes are rarely affected. The lesions may appear in hundreds to thousands, present as skin colored or bluish red, and appear nongrouped. No antecedent history of trauma is necessary. Histologically, the lesions appear as a mass of benign reticular histiocytic cells without fat, iron, or mucin, or changes in connective tissue or blood vessels. The clinical differential diagnosis is urticaria pigmentosa, syringoma, hemangioma, basal cell nevoid tumor, sarcoid, and lymphoma. The histologic differential diagnosis is histiocytoma, xanthogranuloma (nevoxantho-endothelioma), histiocytosis X, reticulohistiocytoma cutis, xanthoma disseminatum, granuloma annulare, and histiomonocytic reticulosis. The lesions undergo spontaneous resolution, leaving brown macules.

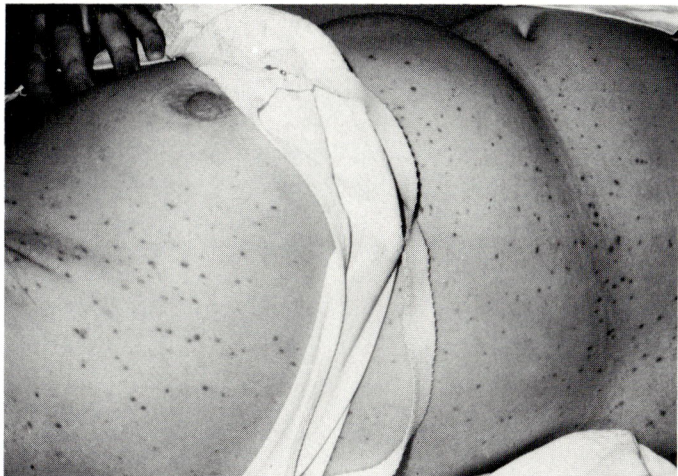

Figure 16–2 Generalized eruptive histiocytoma. Widespread, asymptomatic, papular eruption appearing in crops, which may clinically resemble xanthoma disseminatum or an eruptive xanthoma.

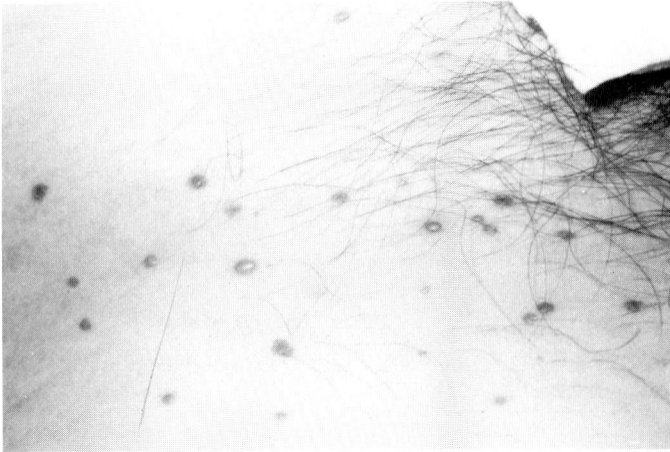

Figure 16–3   Close-up of lesions shown in Figure 16–2.

XANTHOGRANULOMA *(Juvenile Nevoxantho-Endothelioma)*

Xanthogranuloma (juvenile nevoxantho-endothelioma) is a benign, disseminated, xanthomatous-appearing eruption seen in healthy infants (Helwig and Hackney, 1954). It can present as a solitary lesion. The papules or nodules usually appear in early infancy but may develop in late childhood and early adulthood. It is probably a reactive granuloma, although some dermatologists believe that it may represent an incomplete or abortive expression of histiocytosis X.

Histology

The lesion is a poorly circumscribed, dermal nodule that initially consists of a large accumulation of histiocytes, without lipid infiltration, and a few lymphocytes and eosinophils. Later, xanthoma cells, fibrocytic cells, Touton giant cells, foreign body giant cells, some giant cells with the typical "wreath of nuclei," and lympho-histiocytic infiltrate that later is joined by plasma cells are seen. No histologic difference is present between the multiple, disseminate, and solitary lesions.

Clinical Manifestations

The skin lesions are multiple papules, red to yellow in color, and number from 1 to 100. During the first six months of life, the lesions tend to appear in crops. The scalp and face are more frequently involved (Fig. 16–4), but the lesions may also appear on the trunk and limbs. Iris and epibulbar involvement have been described as well. The lung, testes, pericardial area, and mouth are rarely involved. No dyslipidermia is present.

The clinical differential diagnosis of the disseminate small lesions is multiple hyperlipemic xanthomas, lymphocytomas, and urticaria pigmentosa; of the disseminate large lesions, myoblastoma, masto-

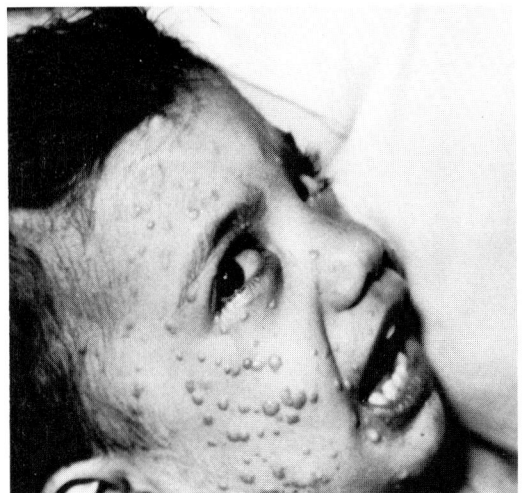

Figure 16–4   Juvenile xanthogranuloma. Asymptomatic papules of face which involuted spontaneously in one and one-half years.

cytosis, and malignant reticulosis; and of the isolated lesions, histiocytoma, spindle cell nevus, dermatofibroma protuberans, lymphosarcoma, and keratoacanthoma.

Treatment is not necessary because the lesions involute with no residua within a few months to several years.

XANTHOMA DISSEMINATUM

Xanthoma disseminatum (Altman and Winkelmann, 1962) is a rare, normolipemic, histiocytic, proliferative disorder in which lipid accumulation is secondary; it is characterized by disseminated xanthomatosis in predominantly young male adults.

Histology

Initially, a histiocytic proliferation is present, and later the appearance of the xanthoma cells, Touton giant cells, and inflammatory cells creates a picture similar to that of xanthoma tuberosum. At necropsy, other organs may be involved, especially the hypophysis and tuber cinereum.

Clinical Manifestations

The cutaneous eruption is characterized by yellow, reddish yellow, or brown papules or nodules that are symmetrically distributed in flexural areas, axillas, groins, neck, and cubital and popliteal fossae. Initially, these lesions are discrete but later coalesce to form verrucose plaques. One-third of the cases have mucous membrane involvement. The respiratory tract (mouth, pharynx, and upper respiratory tract), conjunctiva, and cornea may be involved. Diabetes insipidus is present in 40 per cent of the cases. Xanthosiderohistiocytosis (Halprin and Lorincz, 1960) was described as an unusual type of xanthoma disseminatum characterized by unique phagocytosis of iron by proliferative histiocytes, focal muscle wasting caused by the infiltrative process, and bone marrow involvement. The purplish brown nodules coalesce to form reticulate, greenish brown plaques on the face, chest, back, abdomen, and thighs.

Treatment

The prognosis is guarded. Although xanthoma disseminatum is a chronic, benign disease, it tends to persist indefinitely. After many years, it can involute spontaneously. Respiratory obstruction as a result of the disease is rare, and tracheostomy may be required.

MULTICENTRIC RETICULOHISTIOCYTOSIS

Multicentric reticulohistiocytosis (reticulohistiocytoma, reticulohistiocytic granuloma, lipoid dermato-arthritis, giant cell histiocytoma) is a rare, systemic disease characterized by polyarthritis of the hands and large joints and nodular infiltration of the skin, bone, and mucous and synovial membranes (Barrow and Holubar, 1969; Orkin et al., 1964). The cause of this disorder is unknown. The lesions consist of a granulomatous proliferation of lipid-laden histiocytes and multinucleated giant cell histiocytes to an unknown stimulus. The solitary reticulohistiocytoma of the skin appears as a single, asymptomatic, smooth erythematous nodule.

Pathology

The nodular infiltration of the skin, bone, and synovial membranes reveals the same histologic picture of many mononucleated or multinucleated giant cells, with voluminous, pale, eosinophilic granular cytoplasm having a ground-glass appearance. The nuclei are vesicular and contain prominent nucleoli. The early lesion contains a pronounced inflammatory response consisting of neutrophils, lymphocytes, and plasma cells. In the older lesions, fibrosis replaces the inflammatory response. On histochemical studies, the histiocytes and giant cells contain neutral fat, phospholipids, para-aminosalicylic reactive material, and sometimes iron.

Clinical Manifestations

The disease is worldwide and insidious in its onset. Two-thirds of cases present initially with polyarthritis which is followed by a nodular eruption in months or years. Three-quarters of the reported cases are women. The average age of the patient is 40 years. Constitutional signs of weight loss, weakness, and fever may be present. A pulmonary infiltrate of the lung may be seen on the roentgenogram. Laboratory studies may reveal a significantly elevated sedimentation rate, anemia, and hypercholesterolemia.

The yellowish to reddish papulonodules are located mostly on the face and hands but may also arise on ears, forearms, scalp, elbows, neck, trunk, shoulders, chest, abdomen, back, and legs. Small tumefactions resembling coral beads may appear around nail folds. The lesions can be 2 cm. or more in size and rarely necrose and ulcerate. The facial distribution may create a leonine facies. Plaque lesions of the neck and sacral areas have been described. Over 50 per cent of cases have mucosal involvement of the buccal mucosa, nasal septum, pharynx, larynx, sclera, tongue, gingiva, and especially the lips. Cystic swellings of tendon sheaths of the extensor or flexor aspect of the wrist may be seen. The nodules may disappear and recur later.

A symmetric, erythematous, tender, swollen, deforming polyarthritis that most commonly involves the interphalangeal joints and frequently results in shortened fingers and mutilation is seen. Other involved joints in the order of frequency include knees, shoulders, wrists, hips, ankles, feet, elbows, and spine, and occasionally the temporomandibular joint. Roentgenography of involved joints reveals resorption and destruction of articular surfaces and subarticular bone, with shortening of affected digits and secondary osteoarthritis.

The association of xanthelasma, hypertension, and carcinoma is greater than expected. The leonine facies and shortened fingers may suggest the diagnosis of leprosy except that in the latter disease the skin is tight over the fingers. Other conditions that may simulate this disease are gout, sarcoidosis, rheumatoid arthritis, tuberculosis, neurofibromatosis, xanthomatosis, eruptive histiocytoma, and myoblastoma.

The prognosis is good if the patient survives the early stage of the disease. Usually after seven or eight years the disease becomes quiescent, and the patient may be left with a crippling, mutilating arthropathy and disfigured skin.

Treatment

No treatment has proved to be effective. The systemic administration of corticosteroid is of questionable value; alkylating agents are worthy of further trial (Hanauer, 1972).

PSEUDOLYMPHOMA

Pseudolymphoma (Spiegler-Fendt sarcoid, lymphadenosis benigna cutis, lymphocytoma cutis, cutaneous lymphoid hyperplasia, benign lymphoid hyperplasia) is a reactive disease that responds to a known or unknown stimulus with the formation of localized or disseminate lesions that may have lymphoreticular, granulomatous, and follicular histopathologic patterns. Such lesions have been associated with irritation, trauma, infection, sunlight, insect bite, and such systemic diseases as lupus erythematosus and benign and malignant diseases of the lymphatic system. The pathogenetic mechanism is hyperplasia of preexisting, cutaneous lymphoid tissue. Lesions of lymphoid hyperplasia rarely undergo malignant transformation. These benign conditions may be confused clinically or histologically or both with lymphoma of skin. Among these reactive lymphoid hyperplasias that are clinically and histologically distinctive enough to be described as entities are lymphocytoma cutis, lymphocytic infiltration of the skin (Jessner and Kanof, 1953), and insect bite (arthropod) granuloma.

Lymphocytoma Cutis (Lymphadenosis Benigna Cutis, Spiegler-Fendt Sarcoid)

Lymphocytoma cutis is a condition of unknown origin whose clinical and histologic characteristics, course, and response to therapy suggest the diagnosis.

Histopathology

Below a subepidermal grenz zone, there is an infiltrate which consists of dense areas of lymphocytes with frequent follicular-like islands of pale cells and few eosinophils. The lymphocytes may rarely be located centrally and surrounded by histiocytes. A characteristic feature is the presence of large, pale reticulum cells, containing one or more round poly-chrome bodies which stain homogenously basophilic or eosinophilic; such poly-chrome bodies correspond to the Fleming bodies in mature lymph nodes (Mach and Wilgram, 1966). The benign lesions are differentiated from malignant ones by the higher incidence of epidermal, stromal, and vascular abnormalities and the presence of polymorphous well-differentiated cells; the malignant lesions have extensions of infiltrates into fat, abnormal reticulum cells, and frequent and abnormal mitoses (Caro and Helwig, 1969).

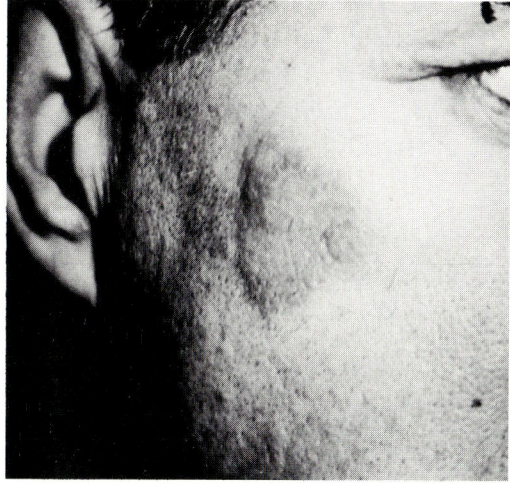

Figure 16–5 Lymphocytoma cutis. After failure of intralesional steroid therapy, the localized erythematous plaque responded quickly and completely to superficial radiation (total, 500 rads).

Clinical Manifestations

Two varieties of lesions have been described — a localized (miliary, papular, and tumid) type, and a disseminate type. The circumscribed or localized type is characterized by a purplish, yellow-brown, glistening papule or group of papules. A lesion can enlarge to a diameter of 5 cm. (tumid type). A localized miliary type which resembles lupus miliaris disseminatum may be seen. The localized type usually appears on the exposed areas, such as the face (Fig. 16–5), earlobes, and nose, as well as nipples and genitalia. The disseminate type is rarer and can occur in any site, especially the trunk and extremities. In the disseminate type, a number of patients have been reported to have lymphadenopathy, peripheral lymphocytosis, and a small increase in mature lymphocytes and reticulum cells in bone marrow. Both types are two to three times more frequent in women. The localized type appears in the late teens and early adulthood, and the disseminate tends to appear with greater frequency with advancing age.

The differential diagnosis of solitary, grouped, or tumid lesions is sarcoid, lupus erythematosus, granuloma faciale, lymphoma, or lupus vulgaris; of the localized miliary type, miliary sarcoid, miliary tuberculid, epithelioma adenoides cysti-cum, adenoma sebaceum, and syringoma; and of the disseminate type, generalized sarcoid, eruptive syringoma, leukemia and lymphoma cutis, and late syphilids.

Treatment

The prognosis of the localized type of lymphocytoma cutis is good, with occasional recurrence and spontaneous complete recovery after months or years or immediately after radiation treatment. The disseminate type tends to recur, spread, and persist throughout life, but pursues usually a benign course; rarely does it undergo malignant transformation, and it responds more slowly and less completely to radiation therapy.

Lymphocytic Infiltration of the Skin

Lymphocytic infiltration of the skin (Jessner and Kanof, 1953) is a benign, recurrent, raised-skin eruption of the face that histologically reveals a dermal infiltration of small lymphocytes beneath a normal epidermis. Although a relationship with polymorphous light eruption, discoid lupus erythematosus, and lymphocytoma cutis has been suggested, a significant number of patients have been found to have the described eruption without any evidence of these disorders or any others; consequently, this eruption appears distinctive enough at this time to be appreciated as an entity.

Histology

The epidermis is normal, and a periadnexal and perivascular accumulation of lymphocytes is present. Few histiocytes and plasma cells are present. No germinal centers are seen. Lymphocytic infiltration into the subcutaneous fat may be found. The histologic picture can resemble lupus erythematosus and polymorphous light eruption; the demonstration of fluorescent antibodies at the basement membrane or its thickening by the PAS (Periodic acid–Schiff) stain in lupus erythematosus helps to differentiate the two conditions.

Clinical Manifestations

The eruption is seen more commonly in men in the third and fourth decades and is characterized by discrete, flat or elevated, smooth, firm, pink to reddish brown asymptomatic papules that expand peripherally with central clearing. They may be solitary, aggregate, or numerous, and are located on the face, especially the malar areas, and on the forehead, neck, mastoid areas (Fig. 16–6), extremities, chest, and abdomen. The lesions tend to recur and persist for weeks to years. They heal spontaneously with no scarring and can reappear in the same area. Sunlight may aggravate the eruption.

Among the conditions to be considered in a differential diagnosis are lymphocytoma, plaque type of polymorphous light eruption, lupus erythematosus, sarcoidosis, granuloma faciale, lymphoma cutis, and drug eruption. Unlike lupus erythematosus, there is no follicular hyperkeratosis or atrophy on healing; it occurs on the back; no response to antimalarial treatment is observed; and no fluorescence or thickening of the basement membrane is seen. Lymphocytoma differs from lymphocytic infiltration in its histology, in its course, and in its response to therapy.

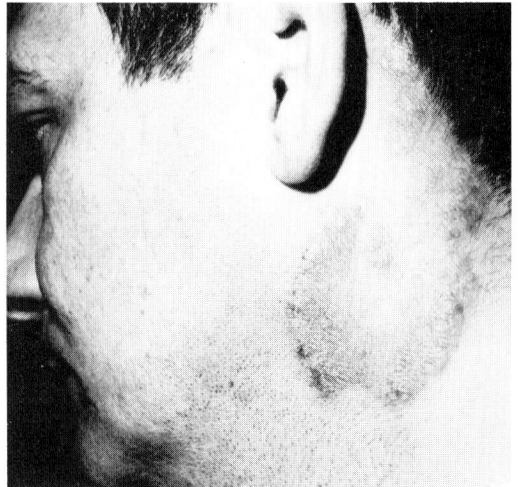

Figure 16–6 Lymphocytic infiltration of the skin. Erythematous plaque lesion in a favorite site with central clearing. The lesion was unrelated to light and was not affected by antimalarial therapy.

Treatment

No effective therapy is known. Despite its chronicity and tendency to recurrence, fortunately no scarring of skin or eventuation or association with a malignant lymphomatous process is present.

PSEUDOPYOGENIC GRANULOMA AND ITS VARIANTS

Pseudopyogenic granuloma (Jones and Bleehan, 1969) is probably a reactive condition, presently of unknown etiology, and is characterized by persistent angiomatous nodules and plaques about the head. The characteristic histopathologic changes are abnormal hypertrophic capillaries with swollen endothelial cells and a neighboring moderately dense lymphohistiocytic infiltrate, and a variable amount of eosinophils. The epidermis may be thickened or eroded. There is no damage to the skin appendages.

The eruption consists of persistent nodules and plaques about the ears and scalp. The lesions vary in size from 2 mm. to 1 cm. and are dull red or plum colored and usually sessile. They may be pruritic and bleed. The diseases to be considered in the differential diagnosis are malignant angioendothelioma, pyogenic granuloma, venous lakes, and glomus jugulare tumor.

Spontaneous resolution occurs. Complete excision has been therapeutically more effective than local x-ray therapy.

It has been suggested that subcutaneous angiolymphoid hyperplasia with eosinophilia (AHE) (Wells and Whimster, 1969), subcutaneous lymphoid hyperplasia with eosinophilia (LHE) (Wells, 1963), and eosinophilic lymphofolliculosis of the skin (Kimura's disease) (Kimura et al., 1948) are the same disease as pseudopyogenic granuloma (Kandil, 1970). These syndromes possess the same distinctive histologic features of angiolymphoid hyperplasia and a chronic inflammatory cellular infiltrate. The various differences of the syndromes are attributable clinically to the different tissue levels of involvement and histologically to the quantitative and qualitative cellular infiltrate which is proportional to the stage of evolution of the process. The lesions of AHE are single or multiple subcutaneous unencapsulated nodules of young adults, are confined to the head and neck, and may evolve and persist for 12 years or more. There may be an associated regional lymphadenopathy and a blood eosinophilia. The diseases to be differentiated from this syndrome are eosinophilic granuloma, lymphocytoma and follicular lymphoma, atypical granuloma pyogenicum, angiomatous lymphoid hamartoma, and persistent reactions to insect bites. Unlike pseudopyogenic granuloma, excision therapy has not been as effective as local radiotherapy.

PERSISTENT ARTHROPOD BITE
(Allen, 1948)

Many insects, especially ticks, produce a firm papule or nodule at the site of the bite that can ulcerate and persist for months or years. The lesions tend to be on the exposed area but can appear elsewhere. They tend to be solitary or few but can be multiple. The pathogenesis is unknown. In some way the stimulating agent or venom maintains the alterative response, even in the absence of recognizable remnants of the insect (especially arthropods). The major problem is the ability of this lesion to resemble clinically and histologically lymphoma cutis, especially

Hodgkin's disease and mycosis fungoides. If parts of the insects are found histologically in the dermis, surrounded by a wall of epidermis, the diagnosis is arrived at more easily. If the epidermis overlying the dermal infiltrate, which resembles lymphoma, is pseudocarcinomatous hyperplasia, the lesion is more likely to be an insect reaction. The histologic picture of persistent insect bite is a dense, dermal infiltrate that lies primarily about vessels, has no predilection for cutaneous appendages, and can extend into the subcutaneous fat. The infiltrate consists of eosinophils, plasma cells, lymphocytes, and histiocytes that may show some hyperchromatic nuclei, mitotic figures, and multinucleated giant cells that can resemble Sternberg-Reed cells. Karyorrhexis and phagocytosis of chromatin may occur. Large lymphoid follicles with germinal centers suggesting lymphocytoma cutis may be present. A histologic resemblance to facial granuloma or erythema elevatum diutinum may be present. The lesions can persist for years. They may respond, completely or temporarily, to intralesional corticosteroid therapy.

HISTIOCYTOSIS X

Histiocytosis X, proposed by Lichtenstein in 1953, describes an inflammatory, focal, or disseminate histiocytic proliferative disorder whose cause is unknown. Clinical manifestations vary with the number and degree of organ involvement. In general, four stages or degrees of clinical expression of this disease can be appreciated (Lichtenstein, 1964):

1. An acute, disseminate (multiple organ), rapidly progressive, proliferative reaction of histiocytes which is seen in the very young, is usually fatal, and is described as Letterer-Siwe disease.

2. A disseminate but more chronic histiocytic proliferative reaction is seen in the young and occasionally in adults, can be progressive and fatal in 50 per cent of cases, and is reported as Hand-Schüller-Christian disease.

3. A benign, chronic, usually solitary, histiocytic proliferative infiltrate, that can be multiple and disseminate, is seen in children and adults, usually involutes

spontaneously, and is described as eosinophilic granuloma.

4. A process that presents initially with one of the above patterns and subsequently develops features of another (transitional type) or presents initially with features of several of the above patterns (mixed type).

The conspicuous histopathologic changes appreciated are the initial proliferation of histiocytes and the subsequent granulomatous and xanthomatous reaction with varying amounts of eosinophils, neutrophils, lymphocytes, and plasma cells. Varying degrees of histiocytosis are present always. A histologic pattern predominates to a certain degree in the artificially established disease spectrum of histiocytosis X, but any pattern can be seen in any of these "diseases." The prognosis and type of treatment of this disease depend on the age of the patient at onset, the location, degree, and number of organs involved, the rate of progression, and the presence of anemia, thrombocytopenia, and infection.

Letterer-Siwe Disease

Clinical Manifestations

The disease appears usually in male children between three months and three years of age. The onset is acute and characterized by constitutional signs and extraosseous lesions. The fever may be 101° F. or higher. The cutaneous lesions (Ruch, 1957; Winkelmann, 1969) may precede the systemic signs of hepatosplenomegaly and lymphadenopathy by months. Roentgenologic evidence of pulmonary and osseous involvement may appear later. The most frequent cutaneous expression is a scaling, yellowish brown, usually purpuric, papular eruption that involves the scalp, neck, face, trunk, and buttocks (Fig. 16–7 A and B). Other visible expressions are necrotic lesions of the mouth, a vesiculopustular eruption, and nodules with or without ulceration. Only hemorrhagic lesions may be present. Purpura of the palms is reported as a bad prognostic sign. The differential diagnosis of the cutaneous lesions includes seborrheic dermatitis, Darier's disease, pyoderma, and purpuric disorders.

Histopathology

The histopathology is characterized initially by focal or disseminate aggregations of large, rounded, mononuclear cells with vesicular and lobulated nuclei and clearly demarcated nuclei; later a granulomatous or xanthomatous reaction with inflammatory cells, especially eosinophils, may be

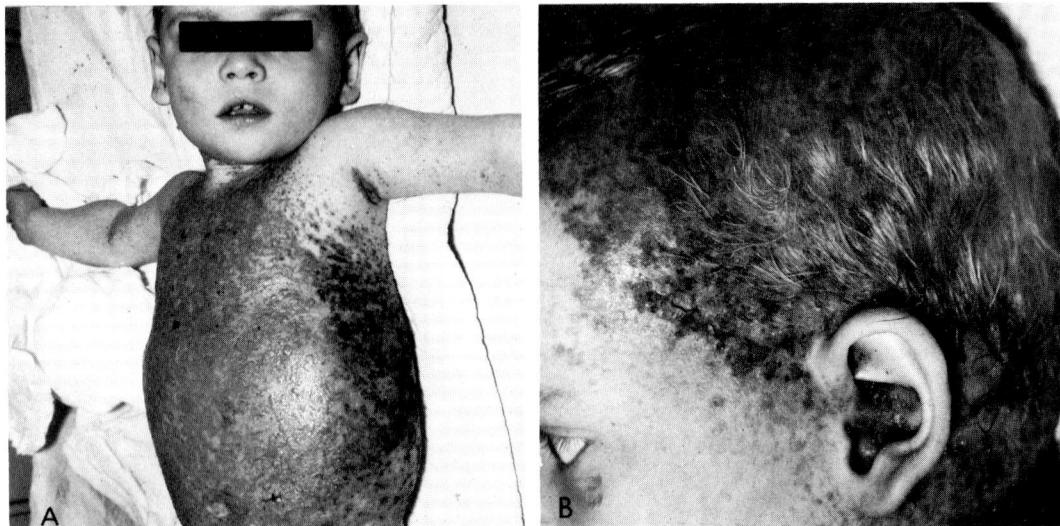

Figure 16–7 *A* and *B*, The Letterer-Siwe variant exhibiting the purpuric seborrhea–like dermatitis; hepatosplenomegaly was present. The patient in *A* died rapidly.

evident. Anemia, leukocytosis or leuko-penia, thrombocytopenia, and eosino-philia (in 10 per cent of cases) are seen. The disease is usually fatal within weeks to one year. Transition from this acute dis-ease to a more chronic disseminate dis-ease occurs. Secondary infections occur frequently.

Treatment (Winkelmann and Burgert, 1970)

No satisfactory form of treatment is available. When necessary, supportive therapy in the form of transfusions and antibiotics is essential. Although there are favorable reports in the literature, cortico-steroids are of questionable therapeutic value. Significant improvement of survival has been described through the use of 4-amino-N^{10}-methylpteroylglutamic acid (methotrexate) and particularly vinblastine sulfate (Velban), a mitotic spindle poison extracted from the periwinkle plant.

Hand-Schüller-Christian Disease

Clinical Manifestations

Although Hand-Schüller-Christian dis-ease may be seen in adults, it usually occurs in children between two and six years of age. The most frequent presenting clinical sign is a chronic otitis media with radiologic changes of the petrous and mastoid bones. The classically described triad of defects of cranial bone, exophthal-mos, and diabetes insipidus is rare. An eruption that resembles that seen in Letterer-Siwe disease but with less hemor-rhagic tendency is seen in one-third of pa-tients. Other skin eruptions, such as papulopustular and papulonodular lesions, have been described. Bronze pigmentation of the skin and xanthelasma are seen. Rare cases have been associated with rashes consistent with xanthoma dissemin-atum and nevoxantho-endothelioma. Plane, papular, and tuberous xanthomas and jaundice may occur secondary to biliary cirrhosis. The frequent skull in-volvement may be appreciated by palpa-tion of the soft tissue nodules overlying these bony defects. Ulceration of the mouth and gums is associated with ero-sions of the mandible and periodontal in-volvement, with resultant "floating teeth." Diabetes insipidus is found in 50 per cent of cases, pulmonary involvement in 30 per cent, and exophthalmos in 10 per cent. Anemia is infrequent, but when it is present it is reported to be a poor prognostic sign. On biopsy, any of the previously described histologic stages may be seen in the same or different le-sions. The course of the disease is chronic, with a mortality rate of 50 per cent, but spontaneous remissions and recoveries do occur.

Treatment

Supportive treatment should be initi-ated for anemia, secondary infection, and diabetes insipidus. Diabetes insipidus may best be treated by radiation therapy to the pituitary area, Pitressin therapy, or both forms of treatment. Other bone le-sions may best be treated by radiation therapy. Corticosteroids, folic acid antagonists, and vinblastine (Velban) have been effective agents.

Eosinophilic Granuloma

Eosinophilic granuloma is the least serious clinical expression of histiocytosis X. It usually presents as an isolated and, occasionally, multiple osteolytic lesion of one or more bones and may be associated with pulmonary or cutaneous involvement or both. The pulmonary and cutaneous le-sions can occur singly or together with-out bone changes (Fig. 16–8). Diabetes insipidus occurs secondary to involvement of the pituitary fossa. The greatest inci-dence is between the ages of two and five years, but it is seen in older children and adults. The osseous lesions are usually asymptomatic and involve the skull, pelvis, femur, and ribs. The lesions are usually found on routine examination or when the patient experiences a spontaneous frac-ture. The pulmonary involvement may cause clinical symptoms that resemble those of pulmonary tuberculosis. The re-sultant pulmonary fibrosis can cause re-spiratory insufficiency. Diffuse infiltra-tion of perihilar areas, nodules scattered

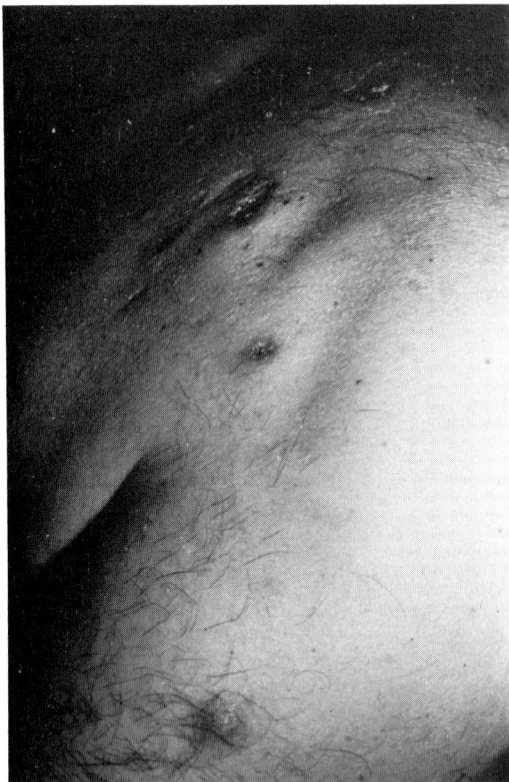

Figure 16–8 Nodulo-ulcerative lesions of the back which were histologically eosinophilic granuloma and were associated with multiple cystic pulmonary lesions.

throughout both lungs, or multiple cystic lesions giving a "honeycomb" appearance to the lungs may be seen on roentgenograms of the chest. Although all the cutaneous lesions of histiocytosis X have been reported, the most frequently observed lesion is the ulcerative mucocutaneous granuloma of the genitalia (Fig. 16–9) and oral cavity. Cutaneous sinuses extending from deep granulomatous lesions may develop. Histologically, a granulomatous reaction with eosinophils is conspicuous.

Treatment

Involution occurs in one to three years; deaths can occur. The preferred treatment for solitary lesions is usually radiation, but surgery may be performed. If there are multiple lesions present or organs involved, radiation treatment with or without systemic therapy (corticosteroids, methotrexate, and vinblastine) may be utilized.

GRANULOMAS

ALLERGIC AND NONALLERGIC GRANULOMAS

A granuloma (Forbus, 1955) is a focal, chronic, inflammatory reaction consisting of various cells, necrosis, and stromal proliferation. The cells are lymphocytes, plasma cells, eosinophils, and, especially, those of the reticuloendothelial system, mononuclear phagocytes, histiocytes, epithelioid cells, and giant cells.

It has been suggested that granuloma formation may be pathogenetically divided into two contrasting types, the allergic and nonallergic (Epstein, 1967). Only the allergic granulomas organize into nests of epithelioid cells. Among the so-called allergic or immune granulomas (Shelley and Hurley, 1971) are those produced by zirconium and beryllium and the etiologic agents of sarcoidosis and tuberculoid leprosy. The epithelioid and giant cells have the same characteristic ultrastructural features and are not phagocytic. These allergic granulomas develop slowly in response to trace amounts of material and have a prolonged course. The nonallergic granuloma (the so-called colloidal or phagocytic reactions) has a different cellular organization, can be produced in everyone (in contrast to the small number

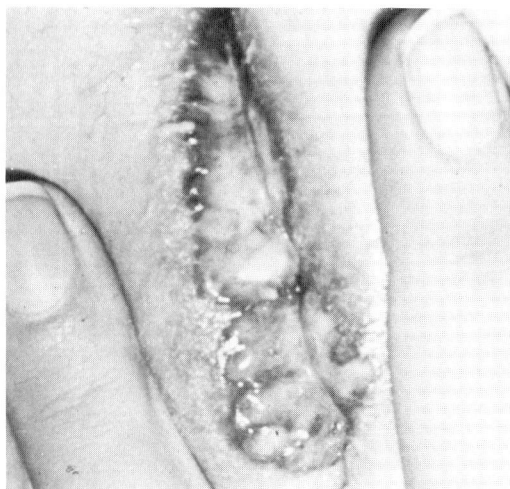

Figure 16–9 Ulcerated granulomatous plaque of the vulva which was clinically and histologically eosinophilic granuloma; no bone or lung lesions were noted.

in the allergic type), requires large quantities of insoluble but colloidizable material for induction, has epithelioid cells with characteristic microscopic and ultrastructural changes, and develops and resolves more quickly than the allergic type. Some examples of the nonallergic granuloma are the silica and sterate-palmitate granuloma. Some bacterial and fungal granulomas suggest additional or a combination of allergic and nonallergic mechanisms.

ALLERGIC OR HYPERSENSITIVITY GRANULOMA

Allergic or hypersensitivity granuloma is seen in beryllium and zirconium contamination of skin injuries, such as dermatitis and lacerations, and in some tattoos.

Four distinct types of cutaneous reactions to beryllium have been described: a contact allergic dermatitis occurring in workers handling the soluble salts, particularly fluoride and sulfate; cutaneous ulcers; granulomas (cuts by fluorescent lamps) resulting from trauma with soluble beryllium salts which are embedded in tissues; and "metastatic" granulomas associated with chronic pulmonary granulomatosis (berylliosis). The granulomas resulting from accidental contamination with beryllium phosphors heal and then discharge material for months or years. Biopsy reveals histologically a picture that can be confused with caseous tuberculosis or sarcoid. Beryllium can be demonstrated by analytic methods. Surgical excision results in cure; however, topical, intralesional, and systemic corticosteroids have been reported as being helpful.

Allergic granulomatous reactions to the cinnabar (mercuric sulfide) pigment of the red tattoos (Fig. 16–10), the chromium oxide (chrome green or Casalis green) pigment of green tattoos, and the cobalt blue pigment of light blue tattoos have been reported months to years after their acquisition. Other complications of tattoos include infections such as pyoderma, syphilis, hepatitis, leprosy, warts, vaccinia; allergic reactions resulting in dermatitis or the granulomas mentioned previously; photosensitivity dermatitis to yellow tattoos (cadmium sulfide); Koebner's phe-

nomenon for lichen planus, psoriasis, and lupus erythematosus; and foreign body reactions in the ocher tattoo caused by the high silica content.

Delayed granulomatous lesions develop weeks to months after frequent applications of extremely small amounts of the zirconium ion. Those that appeared in the axillae were secondary to the use of a stick-type of deodorant containing sodium zirconium lactate acid and were characterized by discrete papules 1 to 4 mm. in diameter. Similarly, repeated applications of hydrous zirconium oxide for poison ivy on the exposed areas may result in papular granulomas of the glabrous skin. After months or years, these lesions heal spontaneously. Topical, intralesional, and systemically administered corticosteroids are effective agents.

FOREIGN BODY GRANULOMA

When inoculated or implanted, exogenous materials which are foreign to the dermis or subcutaneous tissue persist and have the capacity to induce a foreign body granulomatous reaction. These materials include vegetable spines, metals, wooden splinters, silk or nylon sutures, paraffin, silicones, and silica. Endogenous materials, such as urates, oils and keratinous material from appendageal cysts, or tu-

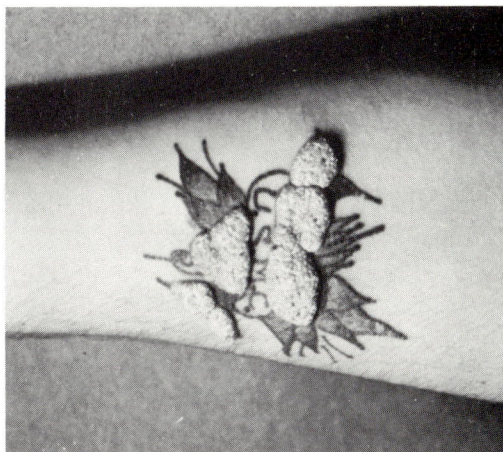

Figure 16–10 Allergic or hypersensitivity granulomas. Allergic reaction to the cinnabar (mercuric sulfide) pigment of a red tattoo.

mors, formed or deposited in the same areas, provoke a similar reaction. Clinically, the lesions may present as erythematous or noncolored visible nodules with or without an evident causative penetrant, or as an inflamed, indurated, or fluctuant plaque with or without drainage. Histologically, macrophages and foreign body giant cells surround and phagocytize the foreign material. Foreign body reactions to hair are seen in barbers, in whom interdigital sinuses of hands and toes may develop; in persons who milk cows, who may acquire sinuses of hands from fragments of cow hair; or in the anogenital area from an acquired pilonidal sinus. Metals which penetrate the skin may wander from the point of entrance.

Particles of gramineae inoculated into the skin by wheat stubble infrequently cause purplish red umbilicated nodules on the lower extremities (Pimentel, 1972). Intracellular plant material is identified within vacuoles of foreign body giant cells as rectangular, fasciculated "inclusion bodies" which are structurally similar to wheat stem. Excision of nodules is curative and the wearing of high boots is prophylactically effective.

The cactus granuloma, caused by the glochidium type of cactus spine, presents nonsuppurative, umbilicated papulonodular lesions with protruding, stubby, hairlike bristles. Upon penetration, the patient experiences an immediate burning sensation, redness, and swelling that subsides if the spine is removed in one to three days; local necrosis can result in spontaneous extrusion. Penetration of the skin by spines of cactus can also cause suppurative and verrucous lesions, ankylosis of interphalangeal joints, nerve paralysis with loss of sensation, and osteolytic lesions.

Silicon granulomas result from contamination of wounds by amorphous or crystalline silicon dioxide (quartz), magnesium silicate (talc), and complex polysilicates (asbestos). The silicon lesions usually appear in the exposed areas and tend to arrange themselves in parallel streaks. Talc granulomas complicate surgical wounds with the formation of a pseudotumor which is prone to suppurate. After a few weeks, months, or even years, a reddish violet or reddish yellow papulonodu-

lar lesion or plaque, resembling sarcoid, may develop within the scar or keloid. This lesion or plaque rarely recedes. It may remain firm or become fluctuant and can ulcerate and resemble a "rodent ulcer." The diagnosis is facilitated by the demonstration of colorless crystalline particles that measure up to 100 microns in length in some of the giant cells, appear as double refractory under polarized light, and are seen with spectrographic analysis of ashed tissue. Surgical excision is performed for symptomatic or cosmetic reasons.

The silicate in the bristly spines of sea urchins of the Mediterranean and tropical countries can cause cutaneous granulomas. The spines of many species are brittle and are retained in the wound. Foreign body granulomas develop months after injury (Fig. 16–11). Other resultant cutaneous lesions are hypersensitivity granulomas (sarcoidal) or an inclusion desmoid resulting from the implantation of fragments of epithelium into the depths of the wound. The foreign body granulomas usually persist but may spontaneously resolve. Intralesional steroid therapy may be helpful; if there is an unsatisfactory response, surgical excision may be performed.

The silica-headed darts of the cnidoblast cells of coral polyps may enter a traumatic laceration or unbroken skin. They release a toxic fluid that produces complete paralysis in small marine animals, is most likely irritating to human tissue, and produces an acute spreading cellulitis with lymphangitis and lymphadenopathy and, rarely, fever and malaise. A chronic deep ulceration (the so-called coral ulcer) occurs. Eventually, the wound becomes secondarily infected with staphylococci.

Silicone injections into the skin may result in siliconomas, foreign body granulomas caused by silicones. Silicones are long-chained polymers of dimethyl siloxane, and, as a clear injectable liquid, they are used to reconstruct congenital or surgically or traumatically acquired deformities, to remove facial wrinkles, or to augment breasts. The nodules and tumors that develop months later histologically have a "Swiss cheese pattern" and reveal luminous crystals in the giant cells and in the cellular infiltrate surrounding the nonstaining cavities.

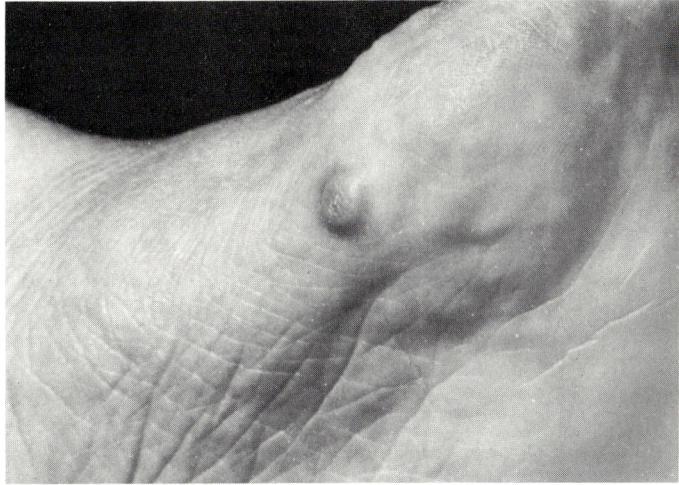

Figure 16–11 Foreign body granuloma (silicate). Three months after initial injury caused by stepping on a sea urchin, a granuloma resistant to intralesional steroid therapy developed and was subsequently excised.

The injection of oily substances such as paraffin, petrolatum, vegetable oil, mineral oil, lanolin, sesame oil, camphor oil, and beeswax, which were used in the past to repair cosmetic defects or as vehicles for repository therapy, or presently factitiously, subsequently produces a foreign body reaction. This foreign body reaction presents as nodules or plaques that may ulcerate or drain. Histologically, the tumor consists of many cavities filled with oily substances and multinucleated foreign body giant cells. Osmic acid stains animal and vegetable lipids but not mineral oils or paraffin, which stain orange with Sudan. If indicated, treatment is excision with plastic repair when it is necessary.

SARCOIDOSIS

Sarcoidosis (Besnier-Boeck and Schaumann's disease) is a systemic, inflammatory, granulomatous disease of unknown etiology. It has not been established as a single entity or syndrome resulting from multiple causes. Among the hypotheses (Siltzbach, 1969) entertained are that it is caused by a special form of tuberculosis, by an unidentified specific inciting agent such as atypical mycobacteria or pine pollen, or by a peculiar genetically determined host reactivity associated with unidentifiable hypersensitivity factors and immunologic abnormalities. In the past,

any noncaseating granulomatous process was diagnosed as sarcoidosis. As clinical and laboratory analysis improved, however, these processes were found to be caused by zirconium granules, talc and other crystals, tuberculosis, fungal infections, berylliosis, tuberculoid leprosy, syphilis, and some types of lymphoma. As these processes were removed from the so-called sarcoid spectrum, a uniform and characteristic process remained.

Pathology

The essential feature is the so-called hard tubercles, which are discrete aggregates of epithelioid cells and may coalesce. A narrow zone of lymphocytes may surround these masses. Central fibrinoid necrosis occurs, but caseation is absent unless tuberculosis develops later. The giant cells may include inclusion bodies, centrosomes, asteroid bodies, and Schaumann's bodies (conchoid bodies), which may represent a sequence. The constant histologic picture may be seen in almost any organ. Healing occurs with fibrosis. The constitutional manifestations, except initially, and the functional disabilities are the result of mechanical interference of organs by the granulomas or scars.

The histology of the skin lesions is not as consistent as in other organs; the granulomatous involvement may be less, the epithelioid cells more scattered, and the lymphocytes may be more and more diffuse. In lupus pernio, the capillaries in the upper dermis are dilated. The erythrodermic form of cutaneous sarcoid is characterized by small granulomas intermingled with histiocytes and lymphocytes.

Clinical Manifestations

Sarcoidosis is more common in the North Temperate Zone. It is frequent among the Scandinavians, the American Negro, and Caucasians of the southeastern section of the United States. In America, sarcoidosis is rare among the African Negro and does not occur in the American Indian. Its occurrence is unusual in children, and it is nine times more frequent in Negroes than in Caucasians and three times more frequent in women than in men.

The clinical picture (Longcope and Freiman, 1952; Scadding, 1967) is usually shaped by the activity, the degree, and the site of involvement. Among the organs involved are the lungs (Fig. 16–12), lymph nodes, eyes, skin, liver, spleen, kid-

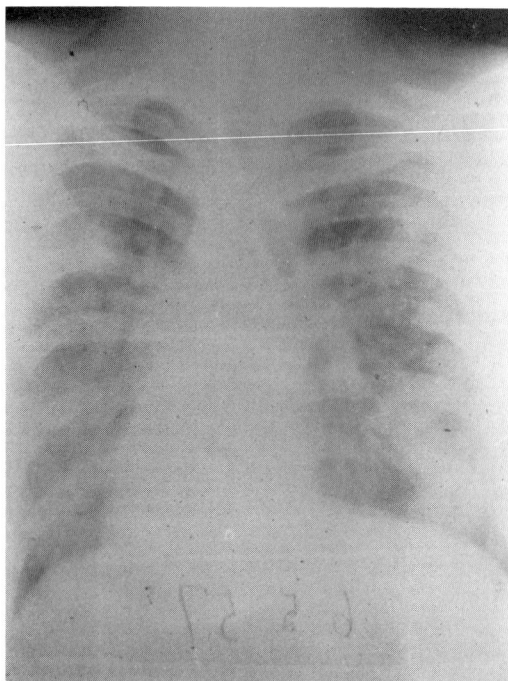

Figure 16–12 Extracutaneous sarcoidosis. Hilar and parenchymal involvement of the lungs.

neys, heart, salivary and lacrimal glands (Fig. 16–13), muscle, joints, bones (Fig. 16–14), and nervous system. The upper respiratory tract, thyroid, parathyroid, pancreas, and stomach are rarely involved. The disparity between the extensive involvement of organs and the mildness or even absence of symptoms is apparent. The seriousness of the disease depends upon the extent of impairment of function essential to life. Rarely does this disease pursue an unrelenting course with termination in death.

The early stage may be characterized by an asymptomatic bilateral hilar adenopathy with or without pulmonary involvement or symptomatic bilateral hilar adenopathy with fever, arthralgia or arthritis, and erythema nodosum. The intrathoracic involvement usually clears in about two years. If the disease persists, progressive pulmonary involvement, as well as that of other organs, may occur but subside after several years. The disease may continuously and progressively involve one organ.

Granulomatous involvement of the alveolar wall of the lung is the most common and can be the most important manifestation of the disease. If this parenchymal process becomes chronic and progressive, it can result in pulmonary emphysema and insufficiency, and cor pulmonale. Lymph nodes are enlarged in over 70 per cent of cases, are firm and rubbery, and do not break down. In about 25 per cent of cases, ocular lesions are present and are an acute granulomatous uveitis which may be the initial manifestation of the disease, lacrimal gland involvement, conjunctival infiltrations, keratoconjunctivitis sicca, and exophthalmos. Several syndromes of sarcoidosis are found that have an ocular component, namely, Löfgren's syndrome, consisting of erythema nodosum, bilateral hilar lymphadenopathy, and acute iritis; Heerfordt's syndrome, consisting of anterior uveitis, parotitis, and Bell's palsy, and Sjögren's syndrome without arthritis, consisting of keratoconjunctivitis sicca with enlargement of the parotid and lacrimal glands.

Although liver involvement is found in about two-thirds of cases by biopsy, hepatomegaly occurs in only about 20 per cent of cases; severe jaundice, cirrhosis, and

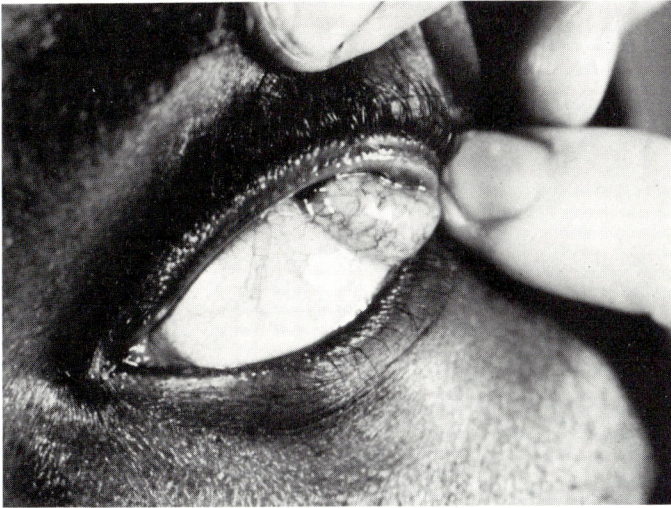

Figure 16–13   Extracutaneous sarcoidosis. Enlarged biopsy proved infiltration of the lacrimal glands.

hepatic failure are rare. Intense pruritus has been described as a presenting symptom. Splenomegaly is seen with about the same frequency and can result in "hypersplenism" with anemia, leukopenia and thrombocytopenia, Banti's syndrome, and spontaneous splenic rupture. Asymptomatic cystic bone changes of the distal phalanges of hands and feet are seen in about 10 per cent of patients. They appear as sausage swellings of the proximal interphalangeal joints. Joint involvement is

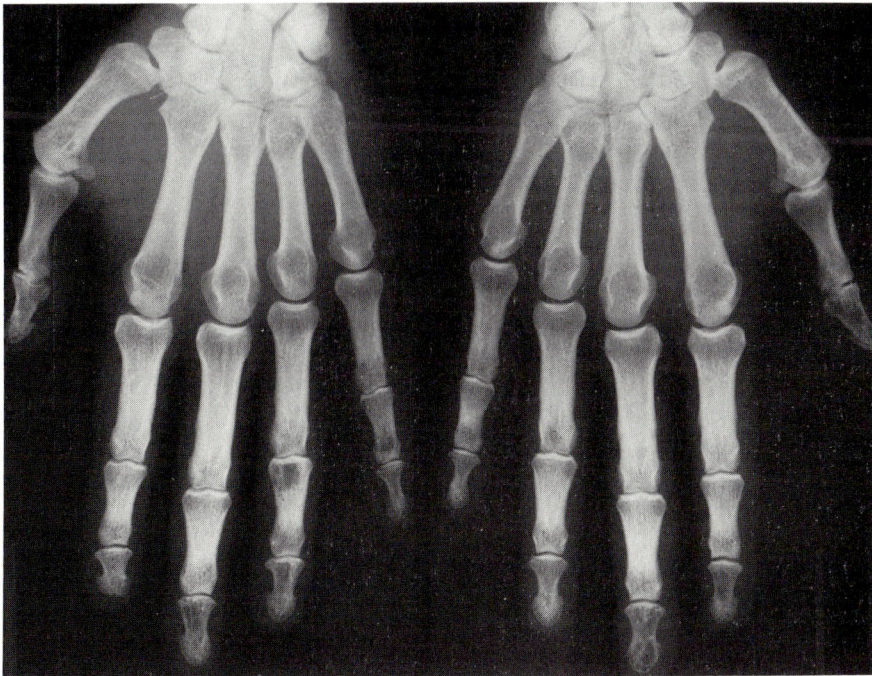

Figure 16–14   Extracutaneous sarcoidosis. Radiolucent defects of the phalanges, especially the terminal ones.

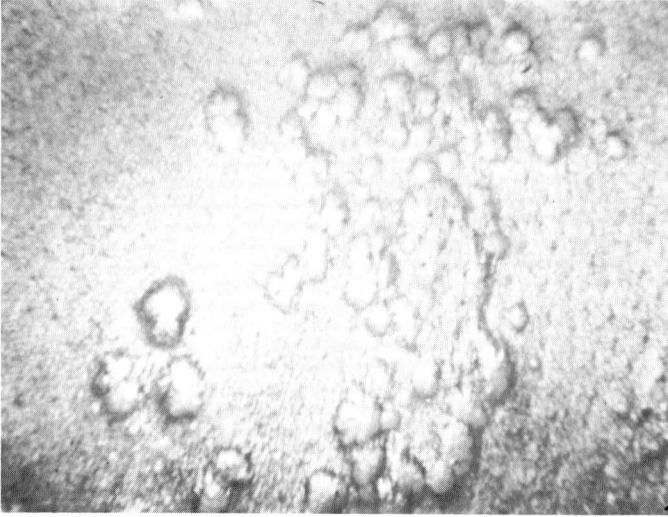

Figure 16–15 Cutaneous sarcoidosis. Grouped papules on the neck of a patient with pulmonary involvement.

appreciated as arthralgia or chronic migratory arthritis, with tubercles demonstrable histologically in the biopsied synovium. Despite the absence of muscle pain or weakness, sarcoid granulomas are seen in muscle biopsies. Nephrocalcinosis and renal calculi are secondary to hypercalcemia or hyperuricemia; granulomatous renal involvement is uncommon. Primary cardiac involvement may present clinically as conduction defects, paroxysmal arrhythmias, and myocardial failure. Pituitary lesions can produce diabetes insipidus.

Excluding erythema nodosum, sarcoidosis of the skin (James, 1959) occurs in approximately 30 per cent of patients with this disease. The commonest cutaneous expressions are a maculopapular eruption, plaques, cutaneous and subcutaneous nodules, and diffuse erythematous infiltration (Figs. 16–15 to 16–20); several differ-

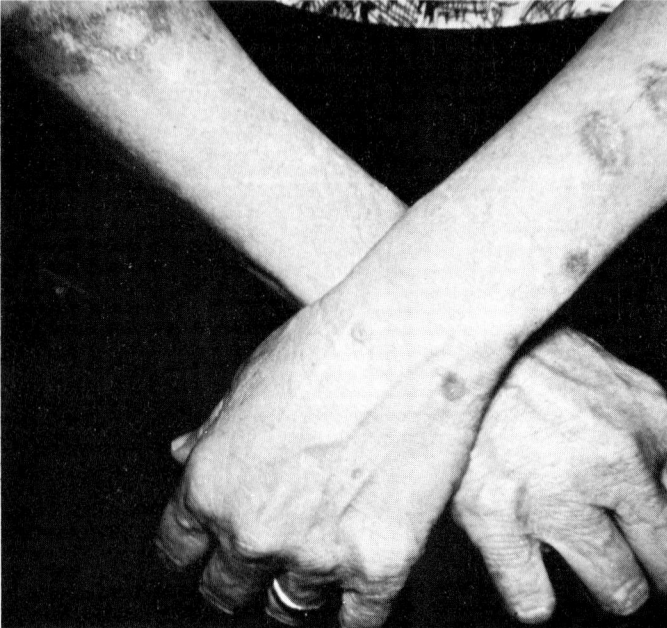

Figure 16–16 Cutaneous sarcoidosis. Erythematous plaques with central clearing on the arms and face.

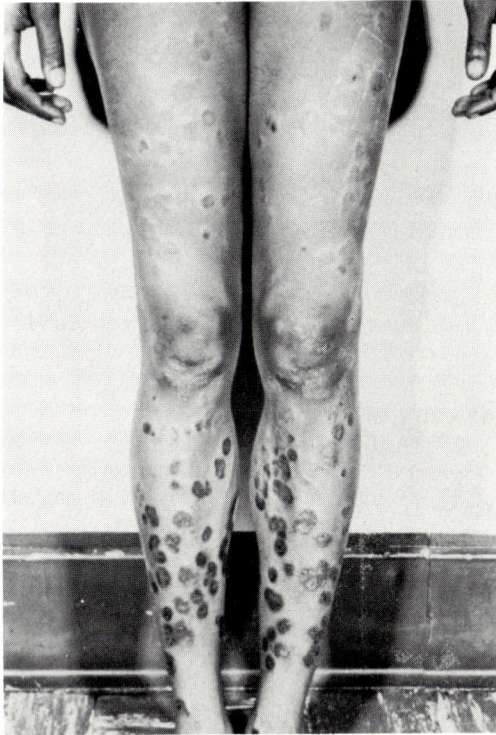

Figure 16–17 Cutaneous sarcoidosis. Hyperpigmented plaques with central clearing and hypopigmentation in the sites of involuting lesions.

plaque lesions may result from a coalescence of nodules or localized diffuse infiltration of the skin, forming placards of various shapes. These persistent purplish to brownish plaques tend to be bilateral, nearly symmetric, and commonly situated on limbs and buttocks. The lesion can be solitary and asymmetric on the face or have a characteristic annular pattern involving the forehead and scalp, with central atrophic scarring and alopecia. A rare, distinctive, nodular-plaque type of lesion, the so-called angiolupoid, is characterized by few persistent lesions with an associated livid hue, is localized to the malar area, bridge of the nose, or around the eyes, and predominates in women. A distinctive cutaneous nodular-plaque type of lesion, called lupus pernio, consists of soft, violaceous, acrally located lesions. They are symmetrically located on cheeks, ears, and dorsa of the hands and involve the nose, which may be bulbous with dilated venules. The involved digits of the hands and feet are usually fusiform and have bone cysts. The lesions occur in the chronic stage of sarcoidosis but may be the first manifestation of sarcoidosis. Lupus pernio may resolve with atrophy and may be the most disfiguring form of cutaneous sarcoidosis.

Subcutaneous, usually erythematous, nontender, indolent nodules are rarely seen. The lesions are roughly symmetric

ent types of lesions may be present at the same time. Among the miscellaneous and unusual lesions seen are "scar-sarcoidosis" (appearance of sarcoid in scars), the ulcerative and psoriasiform lesions, and the scarring alopecia of the scalp.

The papular lesions may range in size from that of a pinhead (lichenoid) to that of a pea. They may coalesce to form plaques that may clear centrally to become annular lesions. The lesions are initially erythematous or violaceous and assume a yellow to brown hue, are soft or firm, may appear in crops, and vary from a few to many lesions. They are seen predominantly on the face, especially about the eyelids and ala nasi, on the posterior aspect of neck and shoulder, and on the extensor surfaces of the extremities.

The nodular lesions are larger than the size of a pea, tend to be few in number and persistent, and are firm, soft, or rubbery in consistency. The distribution is similar to that of the papular lesions. They may heal with secondary anetoderma. The

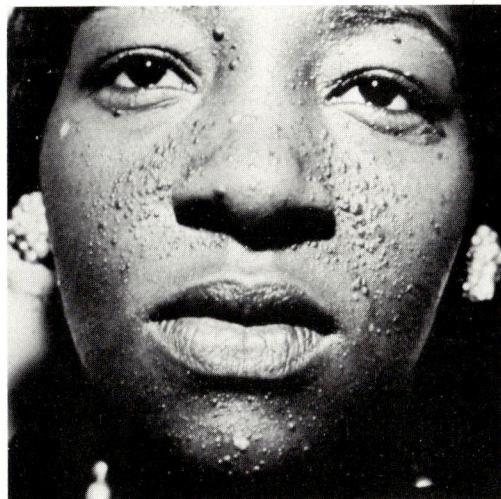

Figure 16–18 Generalized miliary sarcoidosis of the skin.

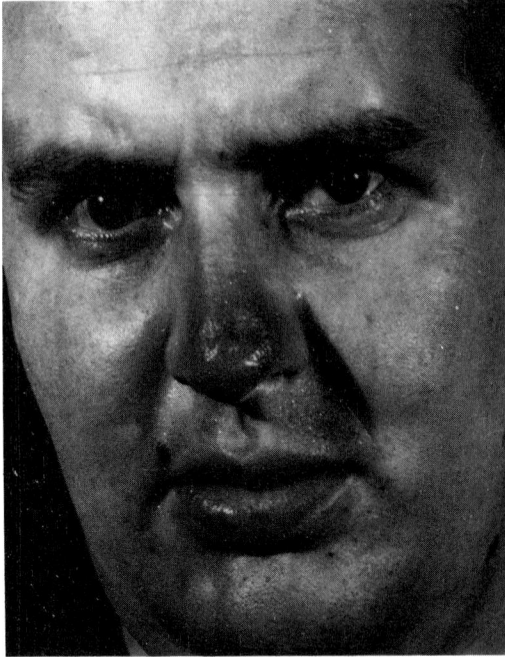

Figure 16–19 Diffuse bluish red infiltration of the nose, the so-called lupus pernio; the scars are biopsy sites.

in distribution on the extremities, can appear on the trunk, evolve slowly, and do not ulcerate. The overlying skin may appear normal.

A diffusely infiltrative, erythrodermic type of skin sarcoid is rarely seen and presents usually as an extensive erythematous scaling eruption of the extremities, particularly the lower extremities. Other signs of the disease, especially lymphadenopathy, are usually present. Sarcoidosis may appear in a scar, and it may be the only cutaneous manifestation. The scar becomes inflamed, infiltrated, and is initially purplish red and later brown in color.

Local and systemic sarcoidal reactions may be produced by certain infections and chemicals. Among the infections are those from mycobacteria (tuberculosis, leprosy, and atypical mycobacteria), syphilis, leishmaniasis, and deep mycotic infections (histoplasmosis, cryptococcosis, sporotrichosis); among the chemicals are beryllium, zirconium, and tattoo dyes. They resemble sarcoidosis clinically and histologically (Figs. 16–21 to 16–23).

The differential diagnoses of papular and nodular skin lesions of sarcoidosis include urticaria pigmentosa, histiocytoma, leiomyoma, syringoma, xanthoma, syphilids, leprosy (dimorphous or lepromatous), Kaposi's sarcoma, lymphoma cutis, lichen planus, polymorphous light eruption, lymphocytic infiltration of the skin, and disseminate granuloma annulare. The plaque lesions to be considered differentially are lupus vulgaris, leishmaniasis, lymphocytoma, lymphoma cutis, facial granuloma, polymorphous light eruption, erythematosus, necrobiosis lipoidica, erythema elevatum diutinum, and Kaposi's sarcoma. The annular lesions to be differentiated are tuberculoid leprosy, granuloma annulare, tertiary syphilid, lupus erythematosus, persistent gyrate erythemas, and lymphoma cutis.

The diagnosis depends on the confirmation of the clinical manifestations by histologic demonstration of epithelioid tubercles in the tissue biopsy or a positive Kveim reaction. The diagnosis is strongly suggested by the combination of bilateral hilar adenopathy, fever, and erythema nodosum with or without arthritis and anergy; unexplained uveitis with or without parotitis; sarcoid of skin and scars; and renal disease with hypercalcemia and normal serum phosphorus.

The essential histologic picture is most readily and easily obtained from tissue biopsy of the visible skin, conjunctival le-

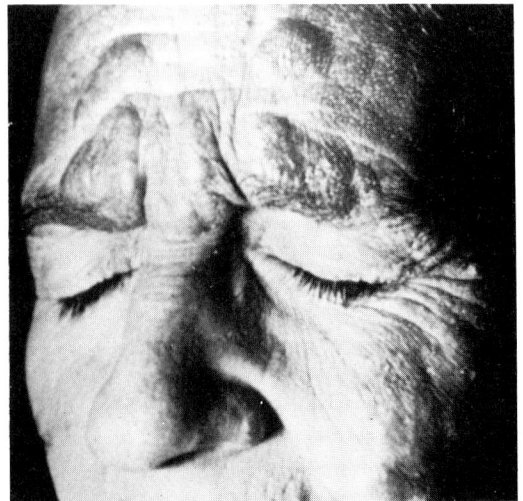

Figure 16–20 The "fleshy" plaque type of sarcoidosis of the skin.

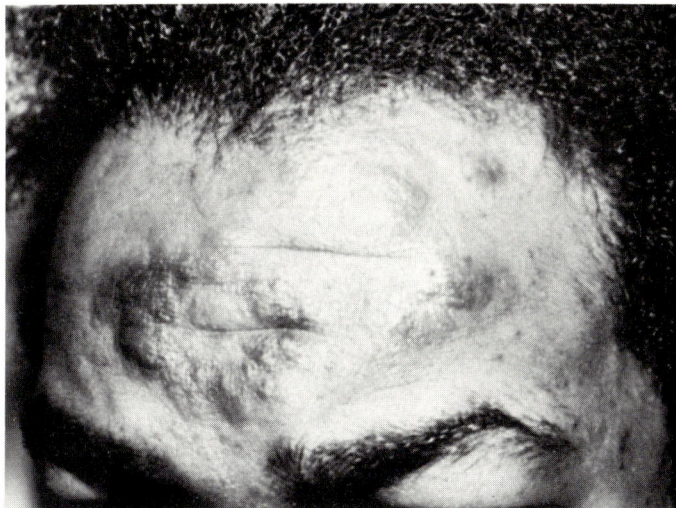

Figure 16-21 A patient with late secondary syphilid.

sions, and palpable lymph nodes. The highest positive diagnostic biopsy yield is found in the involved skin, palpable lymph nodes, and intrathoracic lesions (lung and lymph nodes). Biopsy specimens of liver and scalene fat pads reveal sarcoid granuloma in about 75 per cent of cases. In patients with erythema nodosum,

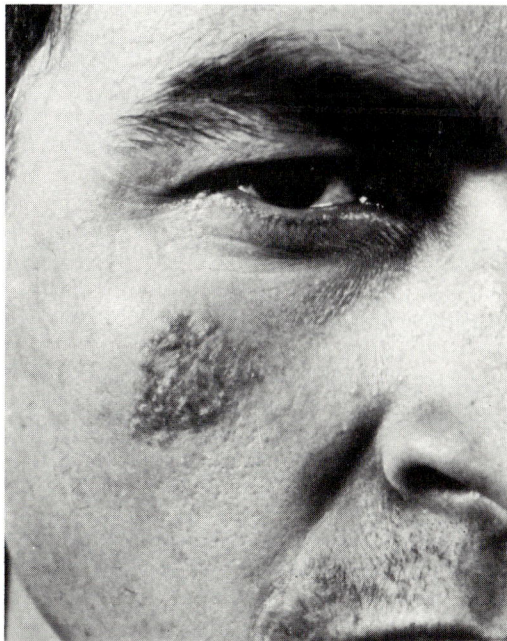

Figure 16-22 Leishmaniasis of the face of a Turkish sailor.

arthralgias, and arthritis, biopsy of the gastrocnemius muscle may show sarcoid granuloma histologically.

The Kveim test consists of an intracutaneous injection of 0.15 to 0.2 cc. of a standardized antigen, a 10 per cent heat-sterilized suspension of human sarcoid, spleen, or lymph node. It is believed to be a delayed reaction to some substance of the human sarcoidal tissue. In about 50 to 80 per cent of patients with sarcoid, a reddish brown papulonodular lesion arises at the injection site in 7 to 10 days and attains a diameter of 3 to 8 mm. in four to six weeks. On histologic examination, biopsy of the lesion must show epithelioid tubercles for the test to be considered positive. False positive reactions occur in 1 to 2 per cent, but false negative reactions are relatively frequent. The reaction is likely to be negative because of inadequate antigen, poor technique, steroid therapy, or inactivity of the disease.

Laboratory Findings

Leukopenia, hypochromic microcytic anemia, moderate eosinophilia, and hyperglobulinemia may be present. The blood sedimentation rate is elevated in 66 per cent of cases. In one-third of cases, the serum alkaline phosphatase level is elevated, even in the absence of clinically appreciable liver or bone disease. The serum uric acid level can be elevated with-

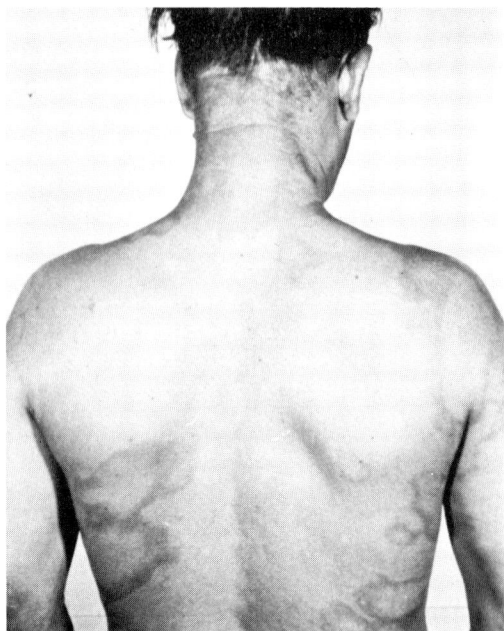

Figure 16–23 Borderline leprosy. Generalized annular lesions are centrally anesthetic.

out renal insufficiency. In about 90 per cent of cases, intrathoracic disease will be seen radiographically. In 25 per cent of cases, hypercalcinuria with or without hypercalcemia results from increased intestinal absorption caused by increased sensitivity to vitamin D. The cardinal immunologic features are significant elevations of the serum IgA, IgM, and IgG, impairment of delayed hypersensitivity reactions, preservation of circulatory antibody formation, and a delayed granulomatous response to intracutaneous injection of sarcoidosis tissue extracts. Tuberculin anergy is noted in 85 per cent of patients; anergy to other antigens, such as *Candida albicans* and mumps virus, also occurs.

Prognosis

In only a small percentage of patients does sarcoidosis become chronic. The decline of tuberculosis and the availability of corticosteroids have improved the outcome of the disease. The prognosis is stated to be better when the initial expression of the disease is cutaneous rather than pulmonary. Negroes tend to have the chronic progressive type of disease. Of the

untreated sarcoid patients, 10 per cent die within the first five years. The papular and nodular lesions clear in one-half to three or more years; plaque lesions are more persistent, and lupus pernio is the most chronic and resistant form. When skin lesions suddenly disappear, the onset of a complicating tuberculosis should be suspected (Cowdell, 1954).

Treatment

Patients with minimal symptoms require no treatment. Because of the variability of the course of this disease, the efficacy of drugs is difficult to evaluate; however, when therapy is indicated, the corticosteroids are the drugs of choice. Before one embarks on such a course of therapy, it is necessary to weigh the hazards of the required protracted steroid therapy, such as the endocrine side effects and the increased susceptibility to infections, against the presumed indications. The indications for corticosteroid therapy are (1) persistent constitutional signs, such as fever and weight loss; (2) acute and subacute ocular disease, especially iridocyclitis; (3) persistent hypercalcemia or hypercalciuria; (4) progressive pulmonary involvement; (5) symptomatic nervous system involvement; (6) myocardial involvement; (7) disfiguring cutaneous lesions of exposed areas; and (8) other vital organ involvement. Steroid therapy is required in only about one-third of patients with sarcoidosis. This drug reduces inflammation and gives symptomatic relief usually in two weeks; it must be administered systemically for at least six months and longer. It is administered locally in instances of anterior uveitis and skin lesions. Steroid therapy under occlusion may be tried for skin lesions, but intralesional steroid administration is more effective. Patients with a positive tuberculin skin test or evidence of active tuberculosis should receive antituberculous drugs. Chloroquine (Aralen), in view of its reported temporary results, lack of control studies, and ability to produce an irreversible retinopathy, has little if any justifiable therapeutic value. The status of immunosuppressive drugs requires further evaluation.

PALISADING GRANULOMAS

A group of cutaneous granulomatous diseases is discussed under the heading of palisading granulomas because, on histologic examination, they have characteristically a central zone of necrobiosis surrounded by inflammatory cells, especially epithelioid, in palisade fashion. Among these diseases are granuloma annulare, necrobiosis lipoidica, and rheumatoid nodules. Although at times basic clinical and histopathologic similarities are present, they are separate and distinct entities.

Granuloma Annulare

Granuloma annulare (Wells and Smith, 1963) is a benign, granulomatous process that usually involves the dermis, is clinically characterized by annularly grouped papules, and is of unknown etiology. Familial occurrence is rare. Its cause has been speculative, and it has been reported to be a constitutional alterative response to a variety of infections or toxic agents. The predilection of the eruption for the areas of trauma and exposure emphasizes the reported precipitating or localizing ability of physical trauma, insect bites, and sunlight. Since a relationship with diabetes mellitus has been appreciated in a significant number of cases, it is believed by some that all patients with granuloma annulare, especially the disseminate type, should be studied for the presence of diabetes. A similar pathogenesis for granuloma annulare, necrobiosis lipoidica, and rheumatoid nodule has been suggested because of the common histologic pattern based on the focal degeneration of collagen.

Pathology

The most common histopathologic presentation is many small foci of incomplete collagen degeneration; less commonly seen, but most easily recognized, are the one to several large, sharply demarcated areas of fibrinoid degeneration of collagen that are surrounded by a radially arranged infiltrate of histiocytes and chronic inflammatory cells. The homogeneous appearing material in the involved sites is diastase resistant, takes the PAS (periodic acid–Schiff) stain, and is probably fibrin. Perivascular lymphocytic cuffing may be seen in the vicinity of the necrobiosis.

Clinical Manifestations

Granuloma annulare appears to predominate in women. Of patients with granuloma annulare, 70 per cent are less than 30 years of age and more than 40 per cent are less than 15 years of age. Hand or arm involvement is found in 65 per cent of patients. Granuloma annulare can present with cutaneous lesions or subcutaneous lesions or both. The most readily appreciated lesion is the characteristic group of small, firm, flesh-colored nodules arranged in ring fashion on the hands or feet of children. The various clinical presentations of granuloma annulare may be classified into the papular, plaque, annular (Fig. 16–24), nodular, and disseminate types. The papular type is characterized by individual, flesh-colored, firm papules that measure a few millimeters in size, number one or more, are solitary, and have a predilection for the dorsal surface of the hands and feet, ankles, knees, and elbows.

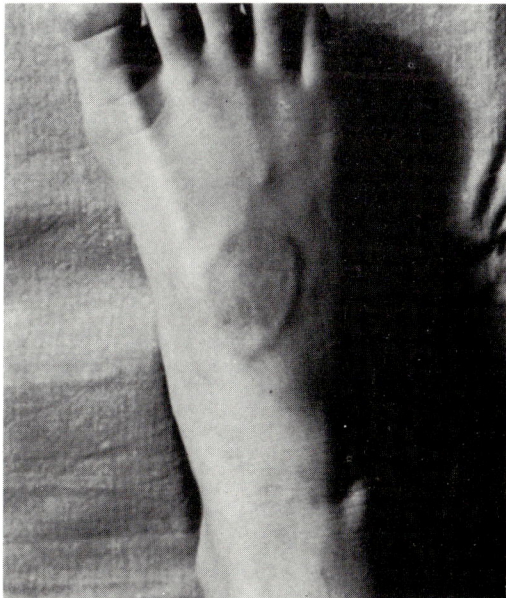

Figure 16–24 Granuloma annulare. A classic solitary annular lesion.

They may resemble verruca plana or lichen planus. In children, multiple pruritic "umbilicated" lesions have been described that reveal typical necrobiosis histopathologically, occur on the exposed skin, especially the extremities, and are associated with insect bites.

The plaque type is probably the most frequently found and is characterized by an elevated, flat, infiltrated area that, when put on the stretch, usually reveals coalescent flesh-colored or erythematous papules. One or more plaques may be present which may be accompanied by the other types of lesions. They usually appear on the extremities and the upper part of the trunk.

The annular type, as described, may be associated with the other types of lesions. A presumed atypical annular type, the so-called granuloma multiforme (Mkar disease; Leiker et al., 1964) has been described in Nigeria. Pruritus precedes the appearance of papulonodular circinate lesions; these lesions are multiple, may be gigantic in size (up to 15 cm. or more), are accompanied by plaques and nodules, and are located on the upper part of the trunk, face, and upper arms. Sensory changes are not evident in the lesions, sweating is not absent, and peripheral nerves not enlarged. The lesions heal spontaneously after months or years, with no residual scarring but often with some hypopigmentation. Among the diseases considered in the differential diagnosis are tuberculoid or borderline leprosy, sarcoidosis, and circinate syphilids.

The nodular type is characterized by the presence of superficial or deep nodules. These flesh-colored nodules, when superficially located, may be one or a few in number and are found especially on the hands and feet. When these nodules are deep, they may be confused with the juxta-articular rheumatic nodules in children and the rheumatoid nodules in adults. These so-called pseudorheumatoid nodules occur chiefly in children and rarely in adults. They tend to be single or multiple and to lie over the tibia, olecranon, skull, buttocks, and palms, and are often fixed to underlying bone. They may also have other types of granuloma annulare associated with them. They tend to regress after months to years. Among the other

diagnoses to be entertained in the differential diagnosis are juxta-articular nodules of the treponematoses (syphilis, yaws, pinta, bejel; Kalz and Newton, 1943), bacterial infection such as tuberculosis and leprosy, sarcoid of the Darier-Roussy type, parasitic disease such as onchocerciasis and filarial cysts, acrodermatitis chronica atrophicans, scleroderma, xanthomatosis, tophaceous gout, calcified hematomas, and benign tumors, such as dermatofibroma, fibrolipoma, and tendon sheath tumors.

A disseminate type of granuloma annulare (Stankler and Leslie, 1967) may be seen in women about 45 years of age and is characterized by a symmetric eruption involving especially the exposed areas (Fig. 16–25), wrists, forearms, thighs, and the upper trunk. The scalp and the palmoplantar surfaces are spared. The lesions are shiny papules that may remain solitary or coalesce to form plaques or annular and reticulate patterns (Fig. 16–26). The course tends to be chronic and lasts for years, with intermittent periods of remissions and exacerbations. The differential diagnosis includes lichen myxedematosus, lichen planus, sarcoidosis, papulonodular syphilids, tuberculids, and lymphoma cutis.

Treatment

The unpredictable behavior of the lesions of granuloma annulare and its 30 per cent recurrence rate make evaluation of any form of therapy difficult. The concept that any type of trauma, such as carbon dioxide, liquid nitrogen, intralesional saline, and also biopsy, would initiate resolution has not been substantiated by controlled studies. Corticosteroids administered by intralesional injection or by topical application followed by occlusion or by the use of adhesive tape containing corticosteroids are usually effective but not curative. The potential complication of dermal atrophy resulting from intralesional therapy must be weighed against the indications for therapy and its potential disfigurement or discomfort. In the disseminate cases, only a prolonged course of systemic corticosteroids can produce any significant results.

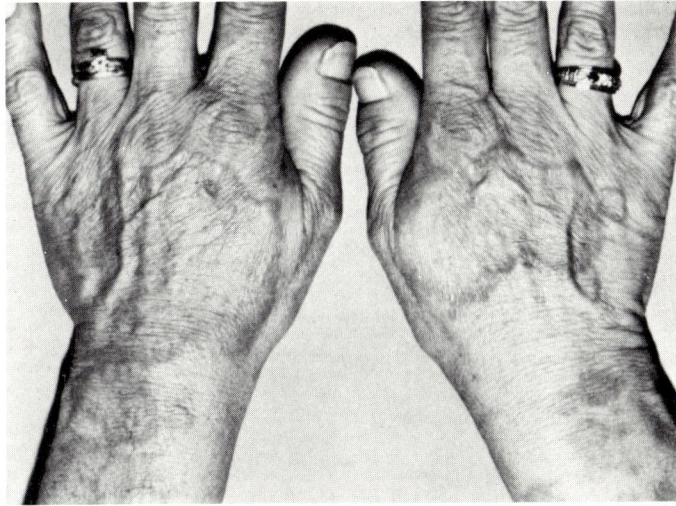

Figure 16–25 Granuloma annulare. Part of the disseminate presentation seen especially in the exposed areas of middle-aged women.

Necrobiosis Lipoidica

Necrobiosis lipoidica (Muller and Winkelmann, 1966) is a degenerative disease of dermal connective tissue characterized clinically by an inflammatory pretibial sclerodermiforme plaque and is often associated with diabetes mellitus.

The etiology is unknown. The development of necrobiosis lipoidica is not directly related to hyperglycemia and glycosuria. Many believe that the necrobiosis

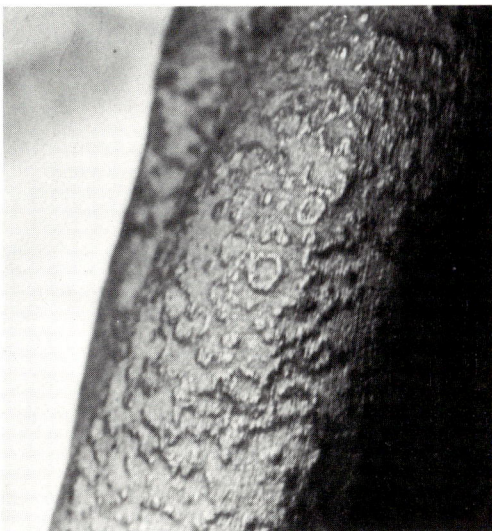

Figure 16–26 A diffuse, disseminated granuloma annulare consisting of small confluent annular lesions.

lipoidica of the diabetic and nondiabetic are the same disease in view of the similarity of the clinical appearance of the skin lesions, the genetic background for diabetes, and the histopathologic findings in patients with or without carbohydrate intolerance. Many of these initially nondiabetic patients are shown to have, on the basis of the results of standard and cortisone glucose tolerance tests and a family history of diabetes mellitus, current or prospective diabetes mellitus. Whether the necrobiosis of collagen is the result of occlusive vessel disease or whether the angiopathy is secondary to the inflammation resulting from the dermal degeneration is unsettled. The vessel changes seen in diabetes mellitus are part of the disease complex; the angiopathy can occur, however, before any clinically overt abnormality of carbohydrate metabolism is noted. It is believed that a glycoprotein is deposited in the blood vessel walls and between the collagen bundles, and that trauma often determines the site of necrobiosis. Over half of the reported cases with diabetes mellitus have evidences of the angiopathic stigmata of retinopathy, nephropathy, and neuropathy.

Pathology

Necrobiosis lipoidica is histologically characterized by epidermal atrophy, giant cells, tubercle formation, and inflammatory infiltrate, especially of the plasma cells. Necrobiosis lipoidica diabeticorum is characterized by prominent palisading of inflammatory cells about necrobiotic areas, mucinous material in areas of necrobiosis, and intimal proliferation and perivascular fibrosis of small vessels in the mid and deep corium. The walls of large vessels in the deep dermis may rarely be affected by a granulomatous giant cell reaction. Septal fibrosis and fibrotic replacement of fat lobules can occur. Lipid staining with scarlet red reveals numerous rust-brown lipid granules extracellularly in the areas of degenerative collagen. In necrobiotic lipoidica diabeticorum, more basophilic staining material is found, which is alcian blue positive at a pH of 2.5 and colloidal iron positive, and which has the histochemical properties of hyaluronic acid.

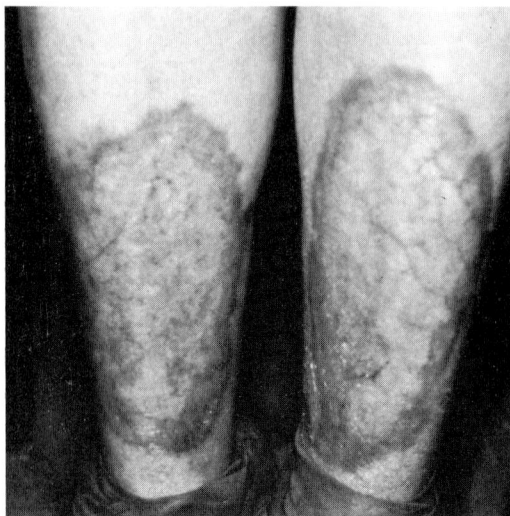

Figure 16–27 Necrobiosis lipoidica. Bilateral, symmetric, atrophic lesions in a diabetic woman.

Clinical Manifestations

The nondiabetic type of necrobiosis lipoidica has its greatest incidence in the 20-year-old to 40-year-old age group and is rarely seen in children. Necrobiotic lipoidica diabeticorum appears more frequently in children than in adults and has a peak incidence in persons between 50 and 60 years of age. Necrobiosis lipoidica and necrobiosis lipoidica diabeticorum cannot be differentiated clinically. The lesion begins as an erythematous papule in the pretibial area. As the lesion extends, it becomes a shiny, waxy, yellowish red sclerotic plaque with superficial telangiectatic vessels coursing over its surface and a violet-red margin. The central part of the lesion becomes slightly scaly, atrophic, and depressed. Ulceration and scarring of the lesion may occur. Although the pretibial area is the favorite site of involvement, any other part of the body may be involved, especially the thighs, popliteal areas, and dorsum of feet and arms. The lesions tend to be multiple, four or more, bilateral, and symmetric (Fig. 16–27).

The atypical forms of necrobiosis lipoidica are misdiagnosed because of their size, shape, location, or inflammatory or degenerative changes (Figs. 16–28 to 16–30). These lesions may be small and many, very inflamed, deeply nodular, diffusely and extensively sclerotic, severely ulcerated, and unusual appearing because of the presence of large amounts of lipid or hemosiderin. Among the striking atypical lesions are the deep and very inflamed indurated nodules of the extremities that clinically resemble nodular vasculitis and migratory panniculitis and the annular necrobiosis lipoidica of the face and scalp. The latter (Dowling and Jones, 1967) is seen mostly in women and, although this variant of necrobiosis clinically resembles cutaneous sarcoid, it differs from it in the absence of sarcoid elsewhere and the absence of the depression of the Mantoux sensitivity, in the presence of more typical lesions of necrobiosis elsewhere or their appearance sooner or later, and in a histopathology similar to diabetic necrobiosis with the unexplained and unusual number of asteroid bodies. In all the atypical lesions of necrobiosis, their association with more typical lesions and the presence of clinically appreciable lipid are helpful diagnostic features. The differential diagnosis of necrobiosis lipoidica includes morphea, sarcoid, granuloma annulare, rheumatoid nodule, stasis dermatitis, post-traumatic fibrosis with hemosiderosis, nodulo-ulcerative syphilids, tuberculids, ecthyma, nodular panniculitis, especially the migratory type, and xanthoma. The most common and po-

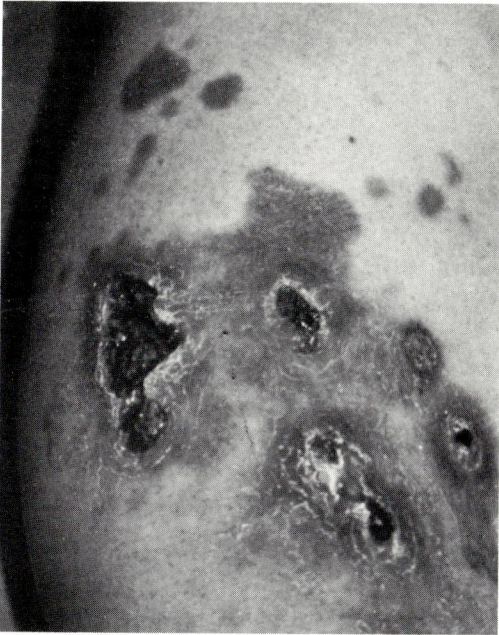

Figure 16-28 Necrobiosis lipoidica. Painful ulcerations of atrophic areas in a young diabetic woman.

tentially most severe complication of necrobiosis lipoidica of either the nondiabetic or diabetic type is ulceration. These ulcers are usually multiple, chronic, and recurrent over many years. Amputation of the lower extremity may be necessary because of severe unremitting ulceration or a complicating squamous cell carcinoma.

Granulomatosis disciformis chronica and progressiva, described by Miescher and Leder (1948), appears to be necrobiosis lipoidica because of its clinical similarity and the presence, histologically, of its more characteristic tuberculoid infiltrate.

Treatment

The lesions of necrobiosis lipoidica of the nondiabetic or diabetic type are chronic, but spontaneous resolution of the lesions after years has been reported. When diabetes mellitus is associated with necrobiosis, complete control of the diabetes does not affect the course of the disease. The only reason for treatment is to improve cosmetic appearance. Corticosteroids, under occlusion or intralesionally, are the only helpful measures. The ulcerations of the skin may require excision and graft, but recurrences occur.

Rheumatoid Nodules

Rheumatoid nodules are chronic inflammatory nodules that occur in 20 per

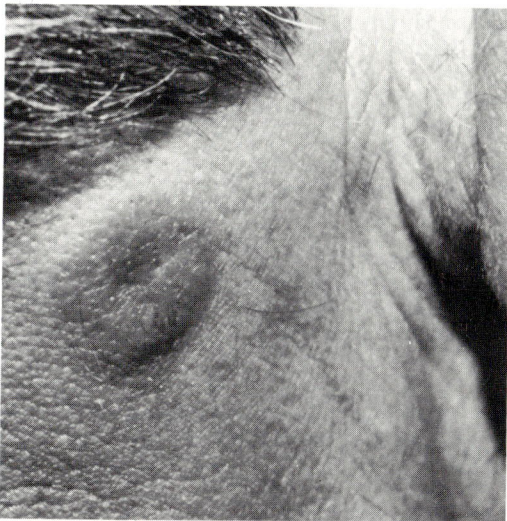

Figure 16-29 Necrobiosis lipoidica. An unusual location in a 45-year-old nondiabetic man; the lesion involuted spontaneously in four and one-half years.

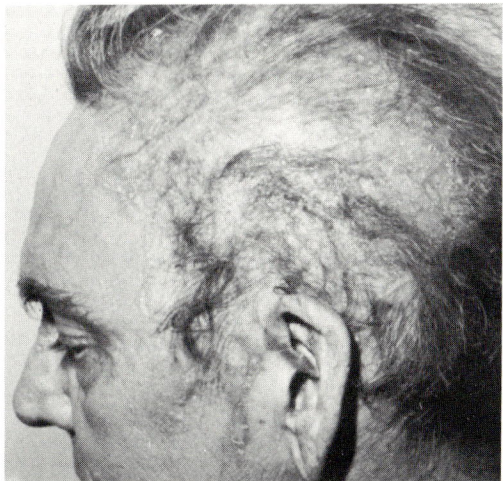

Figure 16-30 Necrobiosis lipoidica. Unlike similar lesions described about the face and scalp in women, this lesion was in a man, was extensive, and caused a diffuse scarring alopecia.

cent of patients with peripheral rheumatoid arthritis and are found characteristically in para-articular subcutaneous tissue but may be widely distributed in internal organs. They have been described in the pericardium, myocardium, endocardium, heart valves, visceral pleura, sclera, and dura mater.

The subcutaneous nodules are firm, large (several centimeters), nontender, lobulated and multicentric, multiple, freely movable, and cannot be sharply dissected from the underlying tissues, such as bursal walls, synovial membranes, tendon sheaths, and periosteum. Occasionally they can undergo central necrosis with softening, ulceration, and fistula formation. The sites of predilection appear to be areas subjected to mechanical pressure and repeated minor tumor. They are most commonly located about the elbows (Fig. 16–31), hands (Fig. 16–32), ankles, and feet. In addition to these more typical sites, the ear and the palms and soles may be involved. They rarely occur in the sclera but can produce scleromalacia or scleromalacia perforans, with resultant blindness. Nodules occur in adults who have relatively severe rheumatoid arthritis invariably associated with significant levels of rheumatoid and antinuclear factors. They occur infrequently in patients with systemic lupus erythematosus and, reportedly, in polymyalgia rheumatica, the so-called anarthritic rheumatoid syndrome. These nodules constitute a part of the widespread rheumatoid vasculitis syndrome characterized by skin lesions, multiple subcutaneous nodules, peripheral neuropathy, episcleritis, pericarditis, and a high mortality rate. Among the examples of necrosis and ulceration of subcutaneous or intracutaneous rheumatoid nodules caused by vasculitis are those tender erythematous nodules of the digital pads and points of pressure of the palms and soles that develop on their surfaces central hemorrhagic vesicles that heal in a few weeks, leaving small pigmented scars. The rheumatoid nodule is a proliferative and degenerative lesion that persists unpredictably for months and years but occasionally parallels the activity of the underlying disease.

When rheumatoid nodules appear in the two unusual sites, namely, the bridge of the nose and the ears, they have a tendency to ulcerate and resemble basal cell carcinoma. It appears that trauma caused by the wearing of glasses and the pressure of pillows during sleep condition their appearance. The differential diagnosis of the ear lesions are tophaceous gout and chondrodermatitis helicis chronica.

Patients with classic rheumatoid arthritis and many rheumatoid nodules may have striking subcutaneous linear bands that are histologically compatible with the rheumatoid granuloma (Dykman et al., 1965). They tend to be multiple, slightly erythematous and cordlike, measure 3 to 4 mm. in width, and extend from the axillae to the iliac crests.

The rheumatoid nodules over bony

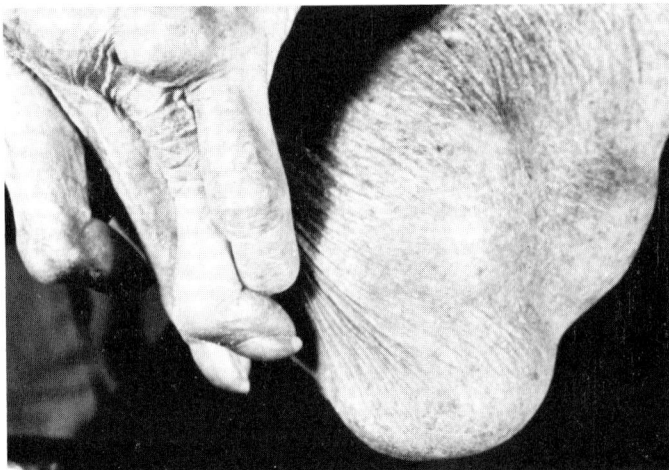

Figure 16–31 Patient with severe rheumatoid arthritis of many years' duration with marked joint deformities.

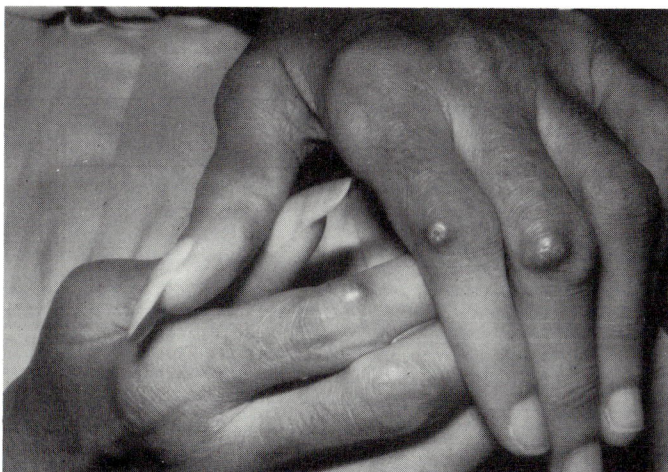

Figure 16–32 Multiple and generalized nodules especially of the fingers in a young woman with rheumatoid arthritis of three years' duration and thyroiditis of three months' duration.

prominences may cause cortical bone erosion of the subjacent bone as the result of repeated mechanical pressure. The benign lesions that can produce similar surface erosion of bone are juxta-articular chondromas, glomus tumors, nerve sheath tumors, inclusion cysts, pigmented villonodular synovitis, gouty tophi, and ganglia. The differential diagnosis of rheumatoid nodules includes the nodule of rheumatic fever and Still's disease, atypical granuloma annulare and necrobiosis lipoidica, and juxta-articular nodules. The rheumatic nodules are not as large nor as firm as the others, have the same distribution, occur more frequently in older children and young adults, appear more quickly and resolve more promptly, and differ histologically in that they are more exudative with less necrobiosis and cellular palisading. The nodules of Still's disease (juvenile rheumatoid arthritis) resemble those of rheumatic fever. The juxta-articular nodules are similar in appearance and distribution but differ as to cause, behavior, and histopathology; they usually appear several years after the responsible primary infection but may occur within the first year.

Histopathology

In the subcutaneous tissue and deep corium, a process appears that initially resembles granulation tissue and results in the formation of a fibrovascular nodule.

Necrobiosis or fibrinoid necrosis appears initially in the thickened vessels and spreads peripherally. Fibrocytes, histiocytes, and mononuclear cells arrange themselves in palisade fashion about the necrobiotic areas. Reticulum fibers and some residual collagen fibers can also be identified in the necrobiotic areas. Calcification of rheumatoid nodules rarely occurs.

INFECTIOUS GRANULOMATOUS DISEASES

Groups of biological agents have the capacity to produce specific morphologic reactive disease patterns. For example, certain infective bacteria evoke a focal suppurative necrotizing process; others, a spreading cellulitis; and still others, a relatively specific granuloma.

The reticuloendothelial system in virtually all organs and tissues of the body helps to repel many biological invasions by the phagocytic activity of its cells. This system was first appreciated when foreign particulate matter (India ink) was introduced into the circulation and was phagocytized in one hour by its cells. When an infective organism gains entry into the body, these cells may destroy it before it does any tissue damage. Unfortunately, certain parasites or bacteria resist phagocytosis, or, if they survive within the cell, they may multiply and spread through lymphatics to distant sites. It is virtually impossible to be certain of the precise etiology of a disease from the observed histologic response unless the responsible agent is appreciable with routine stain or is demonstrated by special stains. A diagnosis of the disease is determined from a consideration of the incidence, the clinical findings, and, finally, from the laboratory data, which include cultural, biochemical, serologic, and special histologic studies, and animal inoculation.

Chronic Granulomatous Disease

Chronic granulomatous disease is a familial entity inherited in an X-linked pattern. It is seen mainly in male infants, brothers, and some females and has been reported in adults (Balfour et al., 1971). The disease usually presents as a severe, recurrent, chronic granulomatous reaction to a number of bacteria of low virulence. Patients with chronic recurrent bacterial infections and focal granulomas should be suspected of having this disease. A defect of the disease resides in the peripheral polymorphonuclear leukocytes and monocytes which appear to be morphologically normal but have a functional deficit. These leukocytes are able to ingest but are incapable of killing certain bacteria, fungi, and, possibly, viruses. The defective bactericidal capacity may be due to the lack of hydrogen peroxide production by the leukocytes. Bacteria that produce hydrogen peroxide "correct" the intracellular deficit and are killed; those that do not, such as staphylococci, Klebsiella, Aerobacter, Salmonella, and Serratia, survive and infect. The leukocytic metabolic defect, that is, the inability to operate the hexose monophosphatase shunt during phagocytosis and to oxidize nicotinamide adenine dinucleotide (NADH) and nicotinamide adenine dinucleotide phosphate (NADPH), can be diagnostically utilized by the demonstration of the failure of the leukocytes to reduce nitroblue tetrazolium dye from the colorless to the deep blue state during phagocytosis (NBT test). The cellular and humoral immune responses are normal; all the serum immunoglobulins are markedly elevated. The organs predominantly involved are the skin, lymph nodes, liver, spleen, lung, and bone marrow, with granulomatous and infectious inflammatory processes. Among the cutaneous lesions seen are infectious eczematoid dermatitis, particularly about the orifices of the face; scrofulous lesions of the cervical and inguinal nodes; pyodermas (paronychia, impetigo, ecthyma, and a tendency for these conditions to be superimposed on other lesions); small indolent papules about the margins of the eyelids and lips; apple jelly–like nodules about the face; progressive ulcerative granulomatous lesions, as well as erythematous draining plaque (resembling erythema induratum) of the lower extremities; and a widespread eruption suggestive of sarcoidosis (Windhorst and Good, 1971).

Most of the infants do not survive to adolescence; however, this disease may first appear in adults and have a relatively mild course. The prognosis of this disease may be favorably affected by the prompt recognition of the offending organism and the immediate institution of appropriate antibiotic and vigorous supportive therapy.

Mycobacterial Infections (Table 16–1)

The mycobacteria are mainly a group of saprophytic or nonpathogenic organisms, such as *Mycobacterium smegmatis*, *M. phlei*, *M. butyricum*, and a few pathogenic myocobacteria, such as *Mycobacterium tuberculosis (avium, bovis, M. hominis*, cold-blooded strain), *M. paratuberculosis* (atypical), and *M. leprae*. These gram-positive, acid-fast rods are characterized by their slow uptake of bacterial dyes and their resistance to decolorization with acid alcohol that is the result of the mycolic acid in the bacillus and is responsible for the title "acid fast." The pathogenic organisms are more acid fast than the saprophytes. Although some have not successfully been cultured on artificial media, the majority can be cultured. The pathogenic members of this genus produce characteristically granulomatous lesions that can be disseminate in some. Those that are pathogenic for man are mainly *M. tuberculosis*, the human and bovine strains, and *M. leprae*. There is a growing number of the so-called atypical, anonymous, or unclassified mycobacteria

TABLE 16–1 CLINICAL AND LABORATORY CHARACTERISTICS OF
MYCOBACTERIAL INFECTIONS

Mycobacterium	*Significant Laboratory Observations*	*Animal Pathogenicity*	*Human Disease*
M. tuberculosis	Dry, rough, luxuriant, cream-colored colonies; visible growth at 37° C. in two to four weeks; niacin test positive; neutral red test positive	Guinea pig and mice	All organs and systems susceptible
M. bovis	As in *M. tuberculosis* except niacin test negative	Guinea pig and mice	
Group I (Photochromogens) M. kansasii	Usually dry, luxuriant colonies; light exposure produces yellow pigment; abundant catalase producer; neutral red test partially positive	Mice	Pulmonary disease; lymphadenitis; meningitis; bone and joint involvement; genitourinary disease; peritoneal disease; disseminated infection; verrucous granuloma of skin; sporotrichoid infection of skin; carpal tunnel syndrome
M. balnei	As in *M. kansasii;* grows at 30 to 33° C.	Only footpad of mouse	Swimming pool granuloma; sporotrichoid infection of skin
M. ulcerans	As in *M. kansasii;* optimum growth at 30 to 33° C.; neutral red test positive	Only footpad of mouse	Ulcerative granulomatous disease of skin
Group II (Scotochromogens)	Moist, smooth, luxuriant colonies; dark-adapted chromogenic (yellow to orange) colonies; unable to hydrolyze Tween 80	None	Cervical adenitis; pulmonary disease, especially complicating pneumoconiosis
Group III (Nonphotochromogens; Battey bacilli)	Predominantly smooth, sparse, white cream-colored, domed colonies; poor catalase producer; inability to hydrolyze Tween 80	Mice ±	Pulmonary disease; cervical adenitis; disseminated disease
Group IV (Rapid growers)	Usually moist, spreading, white to all colors colonies; primary isolation culture in three to five days; positive arylsulfatase test		Human pulmonary granulomatous disease; lymphadenopathy; systemic or inoculation cold abscess; sporotrichoid infection of skin; disseminated infection

being identified after isolation from infected tissue (Timpe and Runyon, 1954).

Because of the presently effective control of tuberculosis in cattle, the human strain of tuberculosis (Robbins, 1967) is responsible for most of the clinical mycobacterial infection in the United States. The *M. tuberculosis* organism is a slender, curved rod up to 10 microns in length and less than 1 micron in width; it is aerobic, multiplies at a significant rate of between 35 and 44° C., grows best in fairly high oxygen tension, is fairly resistant to drying, and can survive for days in ordinary room temperatures and humidity and for months in the dark. Fatty acids, local acidosis, and increasing anaerobiosis in foci of tuberculous infection may be responsible for the progressive disappearance of tubercle bacilli in central areas of necrosis. The organism consists of carbohydrates, proteins, and lipids. The carbohydrate fraction is capable of evoking a polymorphonuclear exudation; the tuberculoproteins evoke an immediate neutrophilic response followed by an accumulation of monocytes; and the lipids evoke the transformation of mononuclear phagocytes and macrophages into epithelioid cells. The more virulent strains are richer in lipids. The virulence or destructiveness of the tubercle bacillus is probably the result of an acquired sensitization or susceptibility of the host.

These microorganisms multiply in the tissue of the host, are phagocytized by macrophages, and continue to grow within these cells for 10 to 14 days until suddenly the organisms cause cell death and necrosis. This pathogenic process is accompanied by the clinical appearance of sensitization to the tuberculoprotein. Virulence of the organism appears to depend on many related factors, such as its capacity to proliferate in the host, to induce sensitization, to block the activity of defensive white cells, and to resist adverse local influences. The human susceptibility to tuberculosis depends on natural and acquired factors. Negroes, young adults, and children are more prone to infection. Not only genetic and hereditary factors but also malnutrition, fatigue, debilitation, intercurrent disease or infection (diabetes, lymphoma, and measles), intensity of exposure to bacilli, immunologic impairment by disease or drugs, and corticosteroids may influence the individual's susceptibility or handling of the infection.

Once a person becomes sensitized to the tubercle bacilli, he remains so even though all the organisms are destroyed. Anergy may be produced by an overwhelming tuberculosis or an intercurrent infection. This tuberculin sensitivity acquired from a previous inoculation or natural invasion may be demonstrated by a variety of techniques: intracutaneous inoculation, using measured amounts of tuberculoprotein, old tuberculin (second strength is Mantoux test) or purified protein derivative, or patch testing with a concentration of tuberculoprotein. The allergy is of the fixed cell, delayed hypersensitivity type. In the sensitized individual, there is a quicker inflammatory response, a greater amount of caseous necrosis, increased local tissue destruction, and a concomitant fibroproliferative response that hinders local and nodal extension. Although immunity and allergy can be separated, they both play supporting roles in the acquired resistance to infection; the allergy hastens cellular response, and immunity makes these cells effective. Consequently, in high-risk situations, clinicians inoculate tuberculonegative in-

dividuals with a vaccine of living but avirulent tubercle bacilli known as bacille Clamette Guérin (BCG).

There are two basic patterns of tuberculous infections. The first is known as primary or childhood tuberculosis, and the second is reinfection, secondary, or adult tuberculosis. The primary tuberculosis is the first seeding of the body by tubercle bacilli; the source of the organism is outside the body. Reinfection is the phase that results from reactivation of primary tuberculosis or reinfection. Its source is either endogenous or exogenous, and it occurs most commonly after adolescence — endogenously less than 40 years of age and exogenously more than 40 years of age. Miliary tuberculosis may result when the organism spreads through the lymphatics or blood to distant organs, particularly the lymph nodes, liver, spleen, kidneys, adrenals, and prostate, which become seeded with many characteristic, minute, yellowish white, barely visible foci. The most commonly isolated organs infected with tuberculosis are the skin, meninges, kidneys, bones, fallopian tubes, and epididymis. Although caseation necrosis is pathognomonic of tuberculosis, such a granulomatous process is seen in other mycobacterial infections, atypical sarcoidosis, leishmaniasis, and nonspecific granulomatous responses to foreign bodies, lipids, and certain fungi. Presumptive evidence is obtained by the demonstration of the tubercle bacilli by the acid-fast stain (Ziehl-Neelsen) of the histologic section or of bodily exudates or excreta. Fluorescent microscopic techniques have been shown to be an effective and rapid means of identification of mycobacteria in tissue sections, excreta, or secreta. A positive culture or successful guinea pig inoculation will provide absolute proof and exclude other mycobacterial infections.

With proper treatment (Table 16–2) the prognosis for recovery is excellent. In more than 95 per cent of patients, sputa will be negative in six months; however, poor treatment tends to result in resistant organisms. The drugs (Lester, 1970; Johnston and Hopewell, 1969) used initially in the treatment of tuberculosis are called "primary drugs"; they are isoniazid (INH), para-aminosalicylic acid (PAS), and streptomycin (SM). Ethambutol hydrochloride (Myambutol) and rifampin (Rimactane) may also be considered primary drugs. Because of the presence of naturally occurring drug-resistant tubercle bacilli, it is necessary for each treatment program to contain at least two effective drugs at all times. An initial, largely susceptible bacillary population can be converted into a totally resistant strain when isoniazid alone is given.

Since tuberculin converters have small numbers of bacilli, isoniazid alone is effective, but when a pulmonary lesion is roentgenographically appreciated, it is indicative of a large number of organisms and at least two drugs must be used. Isoniazid kills most. Mycobacteria and para-aminosalicylic acid inhibit the isoniazid-resistant organism. If para-aminosalicylic acid is intolerable, streptomycin or ethambutol hydrochloride may be substituted. With the recommended dosage and periodic visual acuity examination, the incidence of complicating retrobulbar neuritis from ethambutol hydrochloride may be reduced.

A 24-month course of chemotherapy has a relapse rate of only 2 per cent. In far-advanced cavitary tuberculosis, pyrazinamide is useful. The drugs that are relegated to a second line of defense because they are less tuberculostatic and have a greater toxicity are ethionamide (Trecator), cycloserine (Seromycin), kanamycin, and viomycin. When the patient's bacillary population increases after an initial decrease, a new drug must be instituted. Ethambutol hydrochloride, rifampin, and pyrazinamide may then be used as primary drugs. Rifampin should be used in patients in whom resistance to the organism has developed or who are intolerant of ethambutol hydrochloride. Chemoprophylaxis (Grzybowski, 1967) is strongly recommended for persons who not only have a positive tuberculin skin test but also are in the following categories: (1) they require long-term corticosteroid therapy for another disease; (2) they have a gastrectomy; (3) they have an unstable diabetes mellitus; (4) they have a reticuloendothelial disease, such as leukemia or Hodgkin's disease; (5) they are to have cancer chemotherapy or immunosuppressive therapy; (6) they have silicosis; (7) they are to have a rubeola vaccination or

do have a rubeola or pertussis infection; or (8) they are pregnant. The prophylactic therapy should be continued during the disease or the other special drug program for 6 to 12 weeks after clearing of infection and stoppage of the other drug.

When certain drugs were found to be therapeutically effective in human tuberculosis and more rapid, reliable, and inexpensive techniques for growth of bacilli were developed, varieties of mycobacteria other than *M. tuberculosis* and *M. bovis* which are capable of producing disease in man indistinguishable clinically, radiologically, and pathologically from tuberculosis were identified. They are not considered variations of the tubercle bacilli and are distinct and separate; yet, they are not accurately classifiable. These organisms exist in nature as saprophytes or animal pathogens and usually have a low virulence. Appropriate underlying conditions, such as carcinoma of the bronchus, tracheostomy, silicosis, and metabolic diseases in the host, may predispose to infection. Because of the lack of a standard animal test for mycobacterial pathogenicity, it is often difficult to differentiate the pathogenic from the saprophytic mycobacteria. The consistent association of these recovered organisms with the clinical, bacterial, and pathologic picture must be evaluated before declaring their responsibility for human diseases. The etiologic significance of these organisms depends on the number of colonies per culture, repeated cultural positivity, cultural recovery from involved tissue, and absence of other possible etiologic agents. The strains causing the diseases (mycobacteriosis) have been called atypical, anonymous, and unclassified (Chapman, 1967).

Timpe and Runyon (1954) proposed a provisional categorization of these organisms into four large groups based on pigmentation and morphology. Despite the superficiality of the groups, they have proved useful for identification and reference. There may not be homogeneity of species in each group. This general grouping has further been validated by biochemical and serologic studies as well as by mycobacteriophage susceptibility patterns. Four groups were described: group I—the photochromogens that become chromogenic with light exposure, group II—the scotochromogens that develop pigmenta-

TABLE 16-2 Summary of Antituberculosis Drugs

Drug	Site of Inhibitory Action	Dose
Isoniazid (INH)	Desoxyribonucleic acid synthesis; intermediary metabolism	Children—Oral, 10 to 20 mg./kg./day (not over 400 mg./day) Adults—3 to 5 mg./kg./day (usually 300 mg./day)
Sodium para-aminosalicylic acid (PAS)	Intermediate metabolism	Children—Oral, 200 to 300 mg./kg./day Adults—200 mg./kg./day (usually 9 to 12 gm./day)
Streptomycin	Protein synthesis	Children—Parenteral, 20 to 40 mg./kg./day Adults—15 mg./kg./day for two to three months then b.i.w. or t.i.w.
Ethambutol	Ribonucleic acid synthesis	Oral, 15 to 25 mg./kg./day
Pyrazinamide	Unknown	Children—Oral, 30 to 35 mg./kg./day Adults—40 mg./kg./day
Ethionamide	Protein synthesis	Adults—Oral, 15 mg./kg./day
Rifampin	Inhibits DNA-dependent bacterial RNA polymerase	Children—10 to 20 mg./kg./day (not to exceed 600 mg./day) Adults—600 mg./day
Cycloserine	Cell wall synthesis	Children—Oral, 5 to 10 mg./kg./day Adults—15 mg./kg./day

Summary of Other Antituberculosis Drugs
Kanamycin, viomycin and capreomycin are administered parenterally in about the same dosage, have toxic and allergic reactions similar to streptomycin but with greater frequency, and have an increased incidence of nephrotoxicity.

tion without light exposure, group III— the nonphotochromogens that are without pigmentation and are not light conditioned, and group IV—the rapid growers that are usually not very pigmented and grow rapidly in two to four days. These unclassified mycobacteria differ from the tubercle bacilli as follows:

1. Nontransferable from man to man.
2. Diminished virulence for man and experimental animals; fail to elicit progressive disease in guinea pigs but are pathogenic for mice.
3. Less regular morphologic variations.

4. Development of pigment in cultures.
5. Fail to produce nicotinic acid in culture and have the capacity for production of strong catalase activity.
6. Capacity to grow at room temperature.
7. Relative insusceptibility to isoniazid and para-aminosalicylic acid, less often to streptomycin.

These mycobacteria (Runyon, 1965) may produce pulmonary disease, cervical adenitis, osteomyelitis, fatal miliary tuberculosis, and skin infections that may present as cutaneous granulomas, ulcers, and abscesses (Figs. 16–33 to 16–37).

TABLE 16–2 SUMMARY OF ANTITUBERCULOSIS DRUGS *(Continued)*

Reactions (Toxic and Allergic)	Frequency	Precautions
Peripheral neuritis	0.3 per cent	Prevented by 50 mg.
Toxic encephalopathy	Rare	pyridoxine a day
Hypersensitivity (fever, hepatitis, skin rashes—within first three months of therapy)	0.1 per cent	
Gastrointestinal distress	10 per cent	Give with meals or with
Goitrogenic and hypothyroid effect	0.1 per cent	antacids
Depressed prothrombin and proconvertin activity	Rare	
Anemia (G6PD)	Rare	
Hypersensitivity (fever, skin rashes, hepatitis, blood dyscrasias within first three months of therapy)	8 per cent	Stop immediately
Vestibular toxicity	10 to 15 per cent	Routine BUN and audiometry
Tinnitus	10 to 15 per cent	
Pain at injection site	10 to 15 per cent	
Hypersensitivity (fever, skin rashes, hepatitis, lymphadenopathy within first three months)	5 per cent	
Retrobulbar neuritis with loss of visual acuity and color vision	Less than 5 per cent	Monthly visual acuity test
Hypersensitivity (skin rash)		
Hepatitis	5 per cent	Monthly SGOT
Hyperuricemia ± arthritis		
Hypersensitivity (fever, skin rashes, arthralgias, photosensitivity)	10 per cent	Serum uric acid determinations
Gastrointestinal distress	50 per cent	Administer with meals or
Hepatitis	5 per cent	antacids; monthly SGOT
Hypersensitivity (stomatitis, purpura, skin rashes)		
Gastrointestinal disturbances	?	Increases requirement of coumarin-type anticoagulant, excreta and secretions discolored orange-red
Central nervous system symptoms plus generalized numbness		
Hypersensitivity (fever, skin rashes, sore mouth)		
Hematologic problems (thrombocytopenia, leukopenia, anemia)		
Headaches, anxiety, and convulsions	5 to 10 per cent	Contraindicated in patients with history of psychiatric disturbances or epilepsy; monitor renal function; pyridoxine advised if used with INH
Hypersensitivity (fever, skin rashes)		

The unclassified mycobacteria, most commonly scotochromogens and less frequently Battey bacilli and *M. kansasii* (group II), may cause cervical lymphadenitis. The infection is characterized by a lack of other organ involvement and contact exposure to tuberculosis. It is seen usually in children from one and one-half to nine years of age. The oropharynx is thought to be the portal of entry. The nodes under the mandible are involved. The infection progresses more rapidly and suppurates earlier than tuberculous adenitis. There is no fever or leukocytosis, and group I beta-hemolytic streptococci are not demonstrable by throat culture. The results of tuberculin skin test (PPD-S) may be positive or negative, but the skin test reaction utilizing purified protein derivatives of the responsible infection group, that is, scotochromin (PPD-Scot), is usually greater. A multinodular cutaneous and subcutaneous lymphatic form of infection, resembling sporotrichosis, may be produced by unclassified mycobacteria of group I (*M. kansasii* and *M. balnei*) and group IV. Other organisms which can mimic this form of sporotrichoid infection

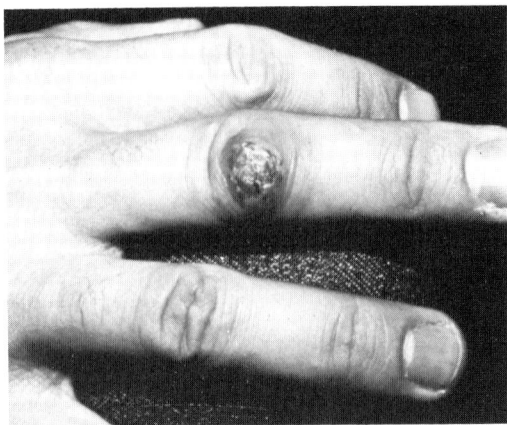

Figure 16–33 Inoculation of atypical mycobacterium (*M. marinum*) acquired from cleaning a fish tank.

are *M. tuberculosis, Pasteurella tularensis, Scopulariopsis blochi, Nocardia brazilensis,* syphilis, yaws, and cutaneous leishmaniasis. Most of group IV mycobacteria derived from clinical specimens appear to be saprophytes; however, *M. fortuitum* and *M. abscessus* were reported to have produced deep, painful bumps with indefinite margins or superficial pealike swellings that may suppurate, drain, and result in fairly large ulcers after injections of drugs and vaccine.

Patients with disseminated mycobacteriosis tend to have severe underlying disease, such as Hodgkin's disease or lymphosarcoma, that usually has been treated with immunosuppressive agents or radiation. It appears that a disturbance of the patient's immune system is responsible for the invasion by these opportunistic mycobacteria.

The histopathologic picture of human tissues infected with groups I, II, and III mycobacteria resembles that produced by *M. tuberculosis,* but group IV mycobacteria do not produce characteristic caseating granulomatous disease.

Skin antigens PPD-Y (*M. kansasii*), PPD-Gaus or PPD-Scot (group II), PPD-B (group III Battey organism), and PPD-F (*M. fortuitum*) are available, but their clinical usefulness is limited because of cross reactions between the different antigens and the high reactor rate. There appears to be some clinical specificity in that the skin test of the pathogen is usually larger than other positive tests. Although antibiotic and chemotherapeutic

resistance is generally characteristic of unclassified mycobacteria, treatment should be individualized and based on drug sensitivity to the primary as well as to the principal secondary antituberculous drugs. A combination of two or three drugs to which the organism is susceptible or partially susceptible should be part of the therapeutic regimen; therapeutic benefit has been noted despite in vitro evidence of drug resistance. Streptomycin and isoniazid have been useful, and cycloserine has been reported as helpful against organisms of groups I and II. A combination of ethambutol and rifampin was curative in a case of sporotrichoid infection of the arm with *M. balnei.* As a result of the limited effectiveness of antimicrobial therapy, local surgical resection of lesions, when feasible and practical, is recommended.

Swimming Pool Granuloma (Philpott et al., 1963)

Following abrasions in swimming pools, a chronic granulomatous infection at the traumatized sites may develop and resemble clinically and histologically that of tuberculosis. Similar lesions are acquired by abrasions from a fish tank. Inoculation with *M. balnei* (Sommer et al., 1962) and possibly other unclassified mycobacteria are responsible.

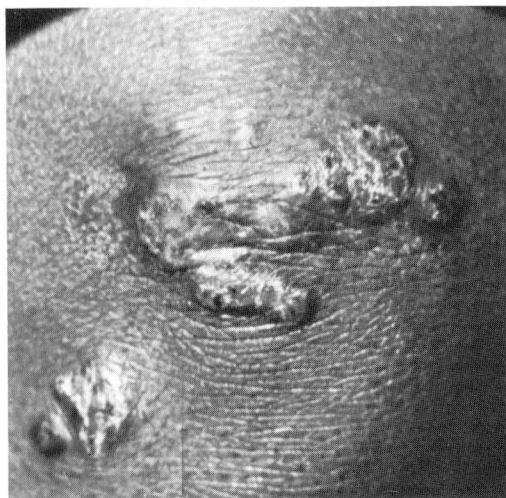

Figure 16–34 Inoculation of atypical mycobacterium (*M. marinum*) acquired from an abrasion in a swimming pool.

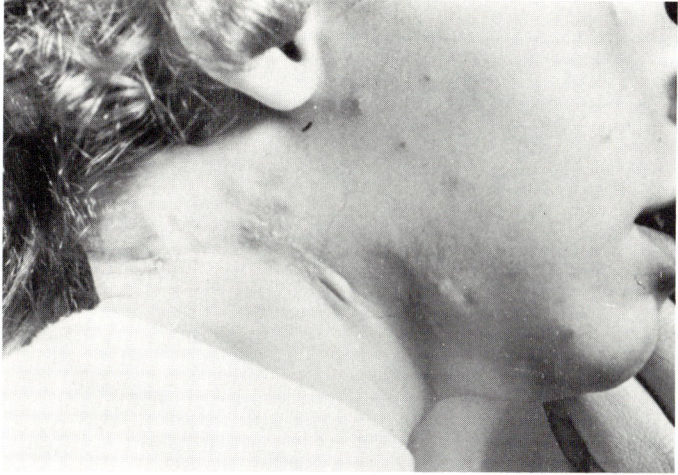

Figure 16–35 Scrofula-like syndrome from a scotochromogen (group II). The patient responded to drainage and excision and streptomycin and INH combination therapy in 18 months.

The bacilli of *M. balnei* are longer and wider than those of *M. tuberculosis* and sometimes have transverse bands. They are probably natural inhabitants of fresh water. Abundant cultural growth is obtained at 30 to 33° C. The growth which is best obtained by direct inoculation of biopsied material is visible between the eighth and fourteenth day. A positive culture is obtained in more than 70 per cent of cases. The fresher the lesions, the more numerous the yield of colonies on culture. No growth is obtained at 37° C.; this probably accounts for the failure of the bacilli to spread systemically. The color of the colonies changes characteristically from white to yellowish orange after exposure to light. *M. balnei* infection may cause Mantoux conversion in a small number of cases. Human infection with *M. balnei* does not create permanent immunity. BCG (tuberculin) immunization of mice can protect them against infection with *M. balnei*.

Histopathology

The older lesions show histologically a more typical tuberculoid structure with Langhans' giant cells. Fibrinoid masses, but no typical caseation necrosis, are seen. The granulomatous process may extend throughout the dermis and subcutaneous tissues. Organisms may be seen intracellularly within the histiocytes.

Clinical Manifestations

The classic clinical picture is characterized by the appearance of reddish papules or pustules that grow to the size of a pea in about three weeks following the abrasion of skin at the point of trauma—

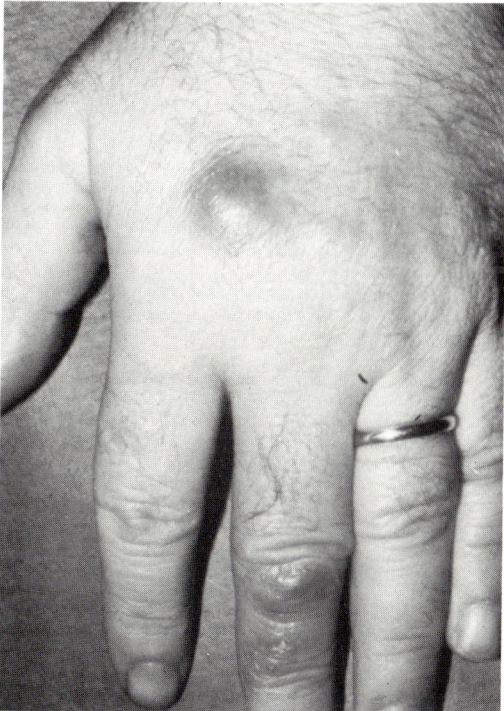

Figure 16–36 Sporotrichoid infection, in this case due to *M. marinum* acquired while cleaning a fish tank; similar lesions may be caused by *M. kansasii*. The lesions responded to a combination of rifampin (Rifadin) and ethambutol hydrochloride (Myambutol). The organisms were insensitive to old, first-line antituberculous drugs.

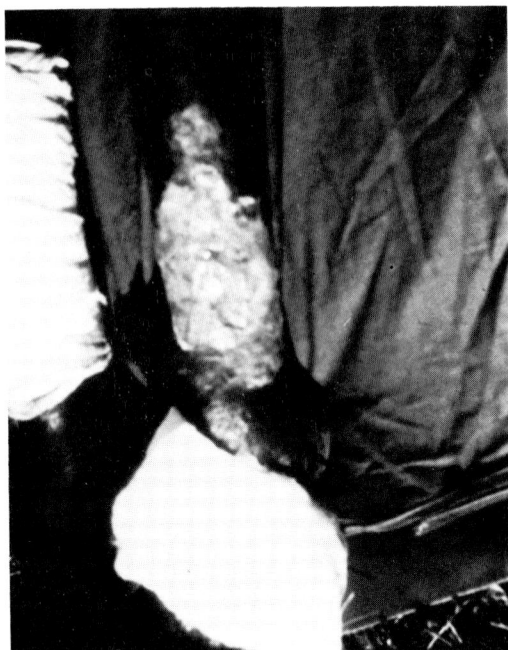

Figure 16–37   Chronic mutilating ulceration of the skin due to *M. ulcerans* in a patient from Uganda.

elbows (70 per cent), knees, dorsa of hands and feet, and nose. Some of the lesions may break down and become covered by brownish crusts. The lesions tend to be solitary; multiple lesions are infrequent. They may ascend proximally and resemble a sporotrichoid infection. Regional lymphangitis and lymphadenopathy have not been described. Local and systemic complaints are absent. *M. kansasii* inoculated traumatically into the skin can cause an indolent verrucous granuloma. The swimming pool granuloma tends to heal spontaneously within a few months to two years, although an exceptional instance was reported to have persisted for 17 years.

Treatment

There is no specific treatment. The organisms are partially susceptible to streptomycin but are resistant to isoniazid, para-aminosalicylic acid, and thiacetazone. Heat applied locally is sometimes helpful. Surgical excision may be satisfactory in a few cases, but recurrences are seen. Preventive measures consist of disinfection (chlorination) and exclusion of individuals with skin lesions from swimming pools (Sommer et al., 1962).

Mycobacterial Phagedenic Ulceration

Mycobacterial phagedenic ulceration is a chronic ulceration of the skin caused by unclassified mycobacteria and first described in Australia and later in Mexico, the Congo, and Uganda. The isolated organism in Australia was called *M. ulcerans* and that in the Congo, *M. buruli*. Despite the essential similarity of the organisms and the ulcers they produce, they are probably different and distinct species.

M. ulcerans grows best at 30 to 33° C. and not at all at 37° C. This probably accounts for the localized nature of this disease and its failure to disseminate. The infection is usually initiated through a scratch or an abrasion and presents as a papule that ulcerates and progresses to a large, deep, undermined ulcer with a necrotic base. The spreading ulcerative granulomatous process often destroys the subcutaneous tissue including fascia and muscle. The legs are most commonly affected. Satellite lymphadenopathy and systemic complaints or involvement do not occur. The ulcers are teeming with organisms. Histologically, there is marked necrosis of the skin and tuberculoid reaction. The ulceration may heal after many months. Although the organism is usually insensitive to the current antituberculous chemotherapeutic agents, sensitivity studies should be carried out in an attempt to obtain some adjunctive drug help. The only effective therapy presently available is wide surgical excision and skin grafting.

M. buruli was isolated from necrotizing skin ulcers seen in Central Africa (Connor and Lunn, 1966). Large numbers of acid-fast bacilli are found in the base of the ulcers. They grow best at 32 to 33° C., resemble closely *M. ulcerans*, but reportedly differ in certain growth requirements and biochemical tests. It has been suggested that the organisms cause widespread necrosis by elaborating a toxic substance. The mode of transmission of this infection is unknown. Constitutional signs or symptoms are absent. The ulcers are seen primarily on the extremities of children; involvement of the face and thorax has been described. The lesion begins as a small subcutaneous nodule on which a blister develops. The resultant ulceration enlarges through continuous necrosis and sloughing. The ulcer may progressively burrow through subcutaneous tissue, destroy muscle, and occasionally produce osteitis, with slow lysis of underlying bone. Lymphatic and systemic spread do not occur. Two unusual features, the early extensive and reversible calcification of diseased tissues and the distant appearance of small, subcutaneous granulomas that usually have extensive hairiness of the overlying skin, are seen. Histopathologically, necrosis is centered in the subcutaneous tissue, with colonies or individual bacilli in the necrotic tissue. When the ulcer begins to heal, a diffuse granulomatous reaction at the periphery of the necrotic fat and in the upper corium and tuberculoid granulomas, which are less conspicuous than those in *M. ulcerans*,

are seen. The ulcers may heal spontaneously after a number of months or years. The subsequent scarring can cause secondary lymphedema or contractures which can result in functional problems. B663 (Lamprene), a phenazine derivative, is the drug of choice and should be given for at least four weeks before performing the debridement and grafting that are necessary for complete healing.

Tuberculosis of the Skin (Table 16–3)

Cutaneous tuberculosis (Dowling and Wetherley-Mein, 1954; Pillsbury et al., 1956; Wilkinson, 1968), which has been rare in the United States, is declining the world over because of the availability of effective antitubercular drugs, elimination of infected milk herds, and an elevation of living standards. In the skin, tuberculosis presents itself in an astonishing variety of clinical expressions that have given rise to an unwieldy, overextended number of descriptive terms and bewildering classifi-

TABLE 16–3 CLASSIFICATION OF TUBERCULOSIS OF THE SKIN

Types	Mode of Infection or Spread	Bacilli Demonstrable	State of Immunity	Tuberculin Sensitivity	Histologic Caseation
True Cutaneous Tuberculosis					
Primary tuberculosis					
Tuberculous chancre	Inoculation	+++	+++	0 (initially)→ + (late)	+++
Miliary	Hematogenous	++	0	0 (terminal anergy)	+++
Secondary tuberculosis					
Lupus vulgaris	Inoculation	± (with difficulty)	+++	+++	+
Tuberculosis verrucosa cutis	Inoculation	+	+++	+++	++
Scrofuloderma	Local extension	++	+++	+++	+++
Tuberculous gumma	Hematogenous	++	+	+	+++
Tuberculosis cutis orificialis	Local extension	++	+	0 (terminal anergy or +++)	+++
Tuberculids					
Papular forms					
Lupus miliaris disseminatus facei	Hematogenous	0	+++	+++	++
Papulonecrotic tuberculid	Hematogenous	0	+++	+++	+++
Lichen scrofulosorum	Hematogenous	0	+++	+++	0
Nodular					
Erythema induratum	Hematogenous	± (sometimes)	+++	+++	+++

Code: 0 = Absent
   + = Slight
   ++ = Moderate
   +++ = Considerable

cations. Furthermore, the relationship of the so-called tuberculids to infection with *M. tuberculosis* is most uncertain.

The potentiality of the skin to react in many different ways to a single disease agent is nowhere better illustrated than in tuberculosis. Tuberculosis of the skin may present clinically as plaques, ulcers, verrucous lesions, nodules, papillomatous tumors, vegetative reactions, and cicatricial infiltrates.

The response of the host to infection with the tubercle bacillus is dependent on whether or not the host is encountering the organism for the first time. Koch observed that an indolent ulcer slowly developed in cutaneously inoculated guinea pigs, followed by rapid involvement of the regional lymph nodes, and finally death of the animal through dissemination of the lesions. In contrast, a quite different sequence of events is observed when animals previously infected with nonlethal strains are reinoculated skinwise. An inflammatory lesion rapidly develops at the inoculation site, soon ulcerates, and heals. There is little or no involvement of the regional lymph nodes, and when dissemination to other organs occurs, it is greatly delayed and reduced in degree.

That the immunity is only partial is shown by the tendency of reinfected animals eventually to die from disseminated tuberculosis. In man, too, there is good evidence that those who have recovered from a primary attack of tuberculosis acquire an increased resistance to re-infection. This is the basis for BCG vaccination in humans. It is necessary to emphasize that the immunity is only partial and may not control the disease completely.

Primary Inoculation Tuberculosis (Tuberculous Chancre)

Tuberculous chancre develops as a result of inoculation into the skin or, less frequently, into the mucosa of an individual who has not previously been infected or who has not acquired a natural or artificial immunity to the tubercle bacillus. Although this primary lesion occurs mainly in children since they are more likely to come in contact with the organism for the first time, adult cases are becoming relatively more common because of the number of adults who have a negative reaction to the Mantoux test. The inoculation occurs on the exposed areas, especially the extremities (Fig. 16–38), from cuts, scratches, insect bites, the result of a ritual circumcision, injections with inadequately sterilized syringes, or ear piercing. The adult infections are more frequently seen in physicians who accidentally inoculate their skin or mucous membrane with contaminated instruments or through mouth-to-mouth resuscitation. With the decline of tuberculosis following the advent of effective chemotherapeutic agents and the increased protection with BCG, the tuberculous chancre has become rare.

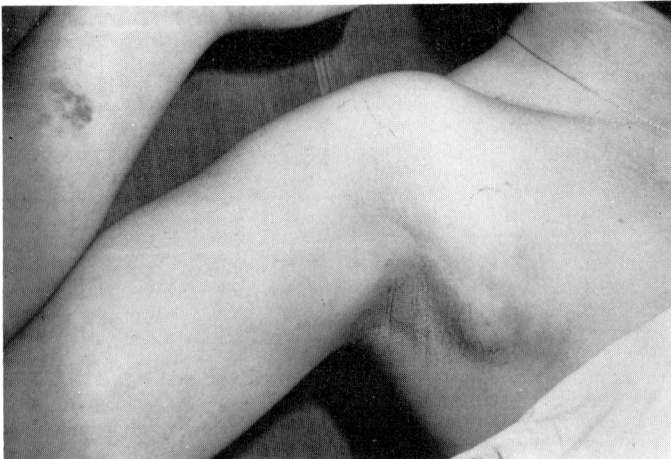

Figure 16–38 Tuberculous chancre. A laboratory technician accidently inoculated herself and presented with the primary chancre complex, ulcer of the skin, and an enlarged slightly tender proximal node.

infection with cervical adenitis as part of the primary tuberculous complex; less frequently, an existent pulmonary focus was the cause of infection. Scrofuloderma, presently less common in underdeveloped countries, no longer predominates in children and is associated with manifest tuberculosis elsewhere in the body, mostly of the lung in over 90 per cent of the cases.

HISTOPATHOLOGY. A chronic inflammatory response surrounds the characteristic necrotic tract of tissue extending throughout the dermis up to the overlying ulcerated skin. Collections of epithelioid cells usually surround some of the areas of caseation necrosis. Acid-fast bacilli are usually seen with the use of special stains.

CLINICAL MANIFESTATIONS. Painless swelling appears in the neck, resulting from an enlarged node or group of discrete or matted palpable nodes. There is bluish nodulation of the involved skin overlying the infected node, joint, or bone. The underlying mass, which is fixed to the skin, suppurates and burrows to the skin surface, with sinus and ulcer formation. Multiple sinuses that extend directly to the underlying focus usually form. The soft, undermined ulcers tend to be arranged in linear fashion. As a result of progression and scarring, irregular cicatricial bands and nodules form. Fungating tumors may result from the development of excessive granulation tissue.

The differential diagnosis consists of conditions that are characterized by suppurative lymphadenitis with cutaneous sinus formation, such as tularemia, cat-scratch fever, lymphopathia venereum, coccidioidomycosis, histoplasmosis, South American blastomycosis, actinomycosis, nocardiosis, dental sinus, and hidradenitis suppurativa.

TREATMENT. Incision and drainage of abscesses are not necessary. Selection of the antituberculous chemotherapy depends most often on the nature of the associated tuberculous infection. Usually, isoniazid alone is sufficient for tuberculosis lymphadenitis; however, if sinus formation is present, a two-drug regimen is preferred.

Miscellaneous Tuberculous Lesions

ANORECTAL TUBERCULOSIS. Anorectal tuberculosis is rare. Like other forms of intestinal tuberculosis, it is usually associated with active pulmonary tuberculosis. The mode of infection is the swallowing of infected sputum and occurs independently of tuberculous involvement higher in the gastrointestinal tract. It occurs more frequently in men than in women. The clinical expressions are tuberculous ischiorectal abscess and fistula-in-ano. Multiple fistulas are rare and are usually associated with extensive tuberculosis of the entire colon. The tuberculous abscess is treated by incision and drainage, and chemotherapy. The tuberculous fistulas are excised, and chemotherapy is given concurrently.

BCG VACCINATION. BCG vaccination (vaccination with attenuated bacille Calmette Guérin) has the ability to stimulate

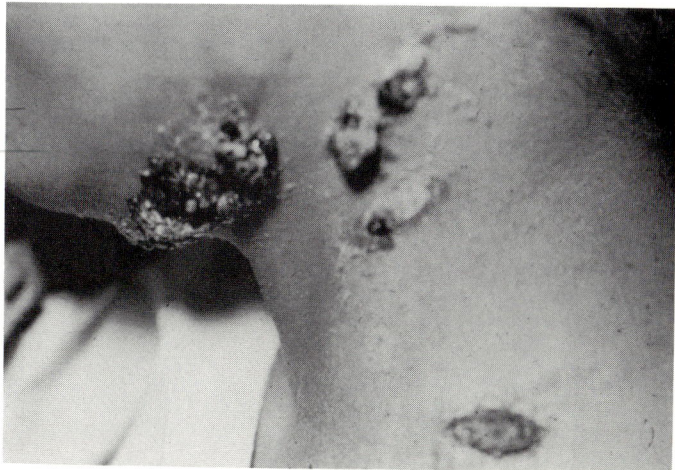

Figure 16–48 Scrofuloderma. Tuberculous cervical lymphadenitis with secondary impetiginization of the skin adjacent to sinuses.

tubercle formation and hypersensitivity to tuberculin, and to induce specific immunity in humans. The vaccine (USP) is prepared from the Glaxo substrain of a Danish strain of BCG bacillus. The organisms are harvested from culture by centrifugation and freeze-dried. The Glaxo freeze-dried BCG vaccine is as effective and satisfactory as the Danish liquid BCG vaccine. The listed indications for BCG vaccination are (1) children living in highly endemic areas and adults unavoidably and continually exposed to open cases of tuberculosis, (2) physicians and other medical personnel, and (3) institutionalized persons with frequent or consistent exposure to those with infectious disease.

The immunizing dose of BCG is 0.1 mg. intradermally. In the tuberculin-negative person, vaccination produces a small red papule in 7 to 10 days that enlarges to 8 to 11 mm. in about five weeks, ulcerates, and heals in three months. The tuberculin test should be performed two to three months after vaccination. If results are negative, vaccination should be repeated.

The contraindications to BCG vaccination are (1) tuberculin-positive individuals, (2) persons with fresh smallpox vaccination, (3) burn patients, and (4) patients taking corticosteroid therapy for chronic disease, those with hypogammaglobulinemia, or patients with diseases that adversely affect their natural immunologic capacity.

The incidence of undesirable reactions is related to the number of viable organisms in the immunizing dose, technique of administration, and the immuno-allergic state. The cutaneous complications (Dostrovsky and Sagher, 1963) may be described as nonspecific and specific lesions. Among the nonspecific are a group of hypersensitivity reactions, urticaria, erythema multiforme, Schoenlein-Henoch purpura-like syndrome, abscesses at the site of inoculation due to secondary infection, and keloid formation. The specific changes are excessive and protracted ulceration at the site of inoculation which is usually produced when vaccine is injected too deeply or administered to patients with a positive tuberculin skin test, autoinoculation ulcers, lupus vulgaris at the inoculation site which should be treated with isoniazid, lichen scrofulosorum, and

sarcoid reaction at the inoculation site. Regional lymphangitis and lymphadenitis with or without scrofuloderma rarely occur.

TUBERCULIDS (Van Der Lugt, 1965). The existence of tuberculids is presently uncertain and unconvincing. Most textbooks list four tuberculids—erythema induratum, papulonecrotic tuberculid, lichen scrofulosorum, and lupus miliaris disseminatus faciei. In the past, the prerequisites set for the diagnosis of tuberculids were (1) lesions are present that have the described clinical characteristics of the so-called tuberculids, (2) tuberculoid structure is seen on histologic examination, (3) the tuberculin skin test is usually strongly positive, and (4) an active tuberculous focus is demonstrable. Against the concept of tuberculids, the following facts are advanced: (1) some of the tuberculids, for example, papulonecrotic and lichen scrofulosorum–like lesions, have been seen in other diseases, (2) classic tuberculoid structure may be seen in patients with no history or clinical evidence of tuberculosis; for example, lupus miliaris disseminatus faciei, (3) the patients are often tuberculin negative, and (4) if there is an original tuberculous focus, it is often not clinically active at the time of the development of the eruption (tuberculid). Erythema induratum has not been accepted as a tuberculid by many physicians because (1) material from their cases which was inoculated into guinea pigs failed to produce an infection, (2) material injected into a special culture medium failed to produce a growth, (3) the frequency of the presence of tuberculosis was no greater than in the general population, and (4) the disease did not respond to antituberculous drugs but did to corticosteroid agents.

The clinical and histologic resemblance of some cases of pityriasis lichenoides et varioliformis and nodular dermal allergid to papulonecrotic tuberculid raises the question of the validity of the existence of the latter condition. The clinical and histologic pattern of lichen scrofulosorum strongly suggests the lichenoid type of sarcoidosis. The status of lupus miliaris disseminatus faciei as a tuberculid is confusing because the tuberculin tends to be weakly positive or negative, the histologic picture is one of a caseating or sarcoidal granuloma, and the Kveim test has been reported as negative in some of these cases.

The possibility that the tuberculids are the result of an embolic reaction to other mycobacteria has been advanced to explain the self-resolving course, the histologic features, the confusing results of tuberculin testing, and the lack of response to therapy.

If an eruption is presumed to be a tuberculid, a response to antituberculous therapy has been offered by some as reasonable proof of its existence.

Erythema Induratum. Erythema induratum (Bazin's disease, tuberculosis cutis indurativa) is a disorder characterized by painful, indolent, indurated plaques and nodules with a tendency to ulceration on the calves of young and middle-aged women. The failure to make a diagnosis is attributed to the declining incidence of tuberculosis and the occurrence of clinical conditions that resemble erythema induratum in nontuberculous patients.

Histopathology. The disease is located initially in subcutaneous tissue and later in the dermis. Vascular changes are characterized by endothelial proliferation of arteries and veins with obliteration, thrombus formation, and necrosis. The presence of tuberculoid infiltrate and caseation necrosis favors the diagnosis of erythema induratum. In late stages, the subcutaneous fat is replaced by fibrosis and atrophy (Wücher atrophy). *M. tuberculosis* is reportedly rarely found in the involved tissue.

Clinical Manifestations. The lesions of erythema induratum may be nodules with or without ulceration; plaques are dusky, indolent, and tender, and are located on the legs (Fig. 16–49) and feet. The ulcers are irregular and shallow, have a bluish edge, and rarely exceed 3 to 4 cm. in size. The lower extremities tend to be erythrocyanotic. The deeply infiltrated nodules and plaques gradually extend to the surface and necrose, although resorption of the lesions can occur without ulceration. Peripheral vascular stasis and cold weather may unfavorably influence the course of the disease. Initial regression may occur during warmer temperature. The disease is chronic and recurrent. In the majority of the patients, a personal or family history of tuberculosis is reported. None of these patients has clinical or radiologic evidence of active disease. They have a positive tuberculin skin test. The relationship of the nodular expression of the disease to nodular vasculitis is undeterminable. It has been stated that the uniform response to adequate antituberculous treatment justifies the diagnosis of erythema induratum.

The differential diagnoses are gumma, nodular panniculitides (erythema nodosum, Weber-Christian disease), and nodular vasculitides (so-called nodular vasculitis, thrombophlebitis), granulomatous diseases of the lower extremities with

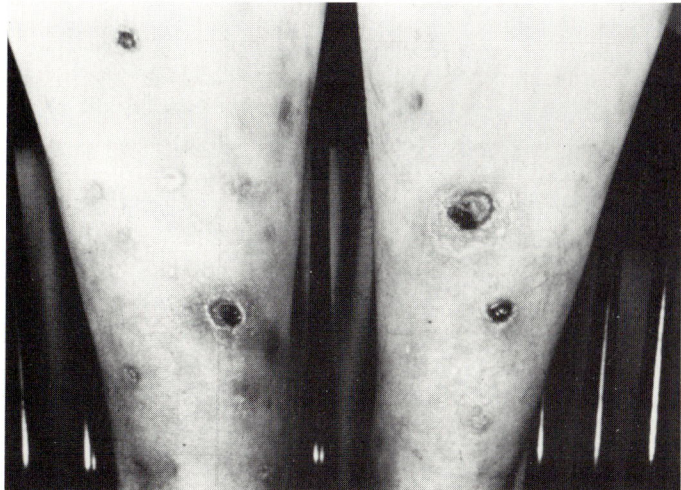

Figure 16–49 The controversial tuberculous panniculitis involving the posterior legs of a middle-aged woman; the biopsy showed tuberculoid infiltrate with caseation necrosis. No organisms were demonstrable; the inoculation of the guinea pig was unsuccessful. The patient responded to INH therapy.

ulceration, and stasis ulcers. Sometimes the clinical picture may simulate papulonecrotic tuberculid, especially when the lesions are papular or small nodules, and scrofuloderma.

Papulonecrotic Tuberculid. Papulonecrotic tuberculid is an eruption characterized by symptomless papules appearing in symmetric crops, necrotizing, and healing spontaneously with superficially depressed scars.

Histopathology. The early changes consist of vasculitis in the upper and middle corium; it is characterized histopathologically by endothelial swelling, thickening of vessel walls, and infiltration of walls with mononuclear cells. Obliteration of the vessels leads to necrosis of the upper dermis and epidermis. A dermal inflammatory cell infiltrate with epithelioid and giant cells and, occasionally, tubercle formation surrounds the area of necrosis. Tubercle bacilli are never seen with special stains.

Clinical Manifestations. The disorder occurs most commonly in young adults but is seen in children and infants. The papules, which may be initially colorless, are dusky red, 5 to 10 mm. in diameter, and may be capped early by a pustule. Central necrosis with ulceration and subsequent depressed small scars are seen (Fig. 16–50). The lesions, which may be few or numerous, appear in showers and symmetric crops on the dorsa of the hands and feet, elbows, knees, ears, and, sometimes, penis. The crops heal spontaneously in a few weeks, occasionally months, and, rarely, years. An active focus or a history of tuberculous infection and a strongly positive tuberculin skin test are usually present. It is usually necessary to correlate the clinical and other laboratory findings to differentiate papulonecrotic tuberculid from other types of allergic granulomatous vasculitis. The response of this disease to antituberculous therapy is offered to support its status as a tuberculid.

Lichen Scrofulosorum. Lichen scrofulosorum has been described as an eruption characterized by clusters of lichenoid papules on the trunk of children with tuberculous disease.

Histopathology. The cellular infiltrate which is localized about appendages in the superficial corium and in the dermal pap-

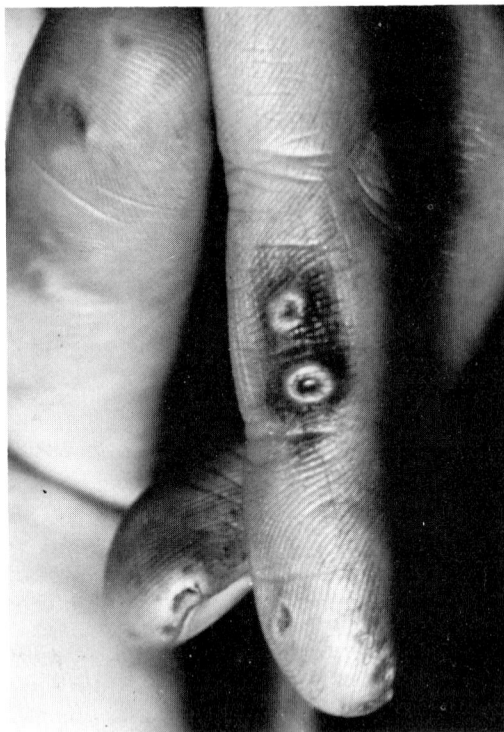

Figure 16–50 The nodulo-ulcerative lesions (papulonecrotic tuberculids) are presumably "diminutive" lesions of erythema induratum.

illae is predominantly epithelioid cells with some Langhans' giant cells and a thin mantle of lymphocytes. Caseation necrosis but no acid-fast bacilli is seen.

Clinical Manifestations. This so-called tuberculid had frequently been described in children who had caseous tuberculous lymph nodes or bone or joint tuberculosis. It was believed to be due to the hematogenous dissemination of the tubercle bacilli in strongly tuberculin-sensitive individuals. Skin testing was carried out cautiously in order to avoid severe local and systemic reactions. However, the status of lichen scrofulosorum has been confused because it has more recently been described in children with no evidence of tuberculosis and a negative tuberculin and Kveim skin test (Wilkinson, 1968).

The eruption consists of indolent, firm, flat-topped, lichenoid papules that are 1 to 2 mm., rarely exceeding 5 mm., in diameter and are of normal skin color or red; it tends to be follicular. An occasional minute pustule may be present. The lesions may be sparse or thickly set into scaling discoid plaques. It becomes more extensive over weeks and then slowly involutes within months without scarring. There may be recurrences. The eruption is indistinguishable from the lichenoid type of sarcoid. It may clinically resemble the lichenoid "id" and secondary eruptions of treponemal infections, lichen nitidus, and drug rashes. No therapeutic response to isoniazid or other antituberculous drugs has been reported.

Lupus Miliaris Disseminatus Faciei. Lupus miliaris disseminatus faciei is a papular eruption that involves the central part of the face of adults and heals spontaneously with scarring. Paradoxically, there are caseating tubercles histologically, but the patient often has a negative history for tuberculosis and a negative skin test to tuberculin. The Kveim reaction has been reported as negative. It has been classified as a variant of "lupoid" rosacea and even as a papular dermatosis of unknown origin.

Histopathology. A tubercle or a small nodule of tuberculosis infiltrate, which usually has caseation necrosis in moderate amounts and is situated about blood vessels, occupies the upper corium.

Clinical Manifestations. This condition predominates in young adults but may be seen in adolescents. The eruption consists of bright red, soft papules that later turn brown and appear as an apple jelly color on diascopy. The papules occur singly or in crops about the eyelids, cheeks, angles of the mouth and paranasal and mental areas, are pinhead to millet seed or larger in size, and spread occasionally to involve the neck and adjacent mucous membranes of the nose and lips. They disappear spontaneously in about a year, leaving small pitted scars. The diseases that may be entertained in the differential diagnosis are acne vulgaris, "lupoid" rosacea, perioral dermatitis, lupus vulgaris, papular syphilid, and sarcoidosis. The eruption does not respond to antituberculous drugs.

LEISHMANIASIS

The flagellate protozoa, which live in the blood and tissues of the human host, belong to the family Trypanosomatidae; the genera Leishmania and Trypanosoma are the only members of the family. Leishmaniasis (Faust and Russell, 1964) is a group of infections of man and certain animals caused by a flagellated parasite of the genus, all the species of which live alternately in the blood or other tissues of the vertebrate and the intestines of the insect. In the leishmanial stage of the life cycle, the parasite is a nonflagellated organism with a round or ovoid body measuring 1.5 to 5.0 mm., a spherical vesicular nucleus, and a smaller kinetoplast complex. It occurs only intracellularly in mammals. The organism in the leptomonad stage is slender and elongated, has a centrally placed vesicular nucleus, and has a single anterior flagellum arising from a well-developed kinetoplast. It is seen in insect hosts and cultures but never in man.

The biting flies of the genus Phlebotomus are responsible for the transmission of the parasites. These flies are small, hairy, and remain near breeding areas because they are weak fliers. Man, dog, and rodents are the main endemic reservoirs for the microorganisms of Leishmania; such other animals as cats, monkeys, guinea pigs, Chinese and European hamsters, the gerbil, and certain species of squirrels are also variably susceptible. The Phlebotomus fly acquires the protozoan by ingestion from the infected skin or blood of the reservoir host. In the insect's intestine, the microorganisms of Leishmania become leptomonads, and when the insect feeds on man, these leptomonads gain access to the body of man and localize in his reticuloendothelial system where they multiply as Leishmania.

The diagnosis of leishmaniasis is based on the demonstration of the parasite in the stained smears of material aspirated from cutaneous lesions, lymph nodes, bone marrow or spleen, and from spinal fluid, or in stained tissue or in culture. The Giemsa, Wright, or Feulgen stains are used to demonstrate the organisms in smears and tissues. With the use of these stains, the cytoplasm of these organisms appears blue, the nucleus pink, and the kinetoplast a deep red. The NNM (Nicolle-Novy-MacNeal) medium, consisting of bactoagar, sodium chloride, sodium hydroxide, distilled water, and rabbit or guinea pig defibrinated blood with added antibiotics, or chick embryo medium is used for culture.

As with the malarial parasites, there are possibly many different strains of Leishmania adapted to the local varieties of vectors, with varying virulence for human beings and animals. Although the organisms are morphologically similar, the differences are seen in the clinical manifestations of the infection, in the immunologic studies in animals and man, and in the geographic distribution of the infections. Innate in the metabolic and genetic constitution of these different strains of parasites are the enzymes or other unknown factors governing the migration of the parasite to the viscera or its localization to superficial dermal layers. The four main clinical expressions of leishmaniasis are shown in Table 16–4.

In oriental sore, only the exposed skin areas are affected; in the Central and South American (mucocutaneous) type, not only the exposed skin but also the mucous membrane of the nose, mouth, and pharynx may become involved; in dermal leishmaniasis, a disseminated nodular eruption appears predominantly on exposed areas; and in kala-azar, involvement of the liver, spleen, and marrow is seen. Cases have been reported, however, of the so-called American mucocutaneous type associated with visceral lesions (Shanbrom et al., 1956) as well as cases of kala-azar with ulcerations of skin and mucous membranes and dermal nodules (Kirk, 1942).

Animals which have recovered from *L. tropica* acquire an immunity against reinfection but not against *L. donovani;* however, *L. donovani* infections give an animal immunity against *L. donovani*

but not against *L. tropica*. It has been reported that surviving visceral leishmaniasis confers lifelong immunity against all types of leishmaniasis, and patients with the American form of cutaneous leishmaniasis have successfully been inoculated with *L. tropica* and vice versa. For ethical and practical reasons, no one has challenged patients with *L. donovani*, since its course is so variable and treatment often ineffective. Since immunity appears to be lifelong against infections of some strains of parasites of cutaneous and mucocutaneous leishmaniasis and in endemic areas, vaccination with some endemic strains may be effective prophylactically.

The delayed skin reaction (the Montenegro test, Leishman reaction) is positive in the majority of cases of cutaneous leishmaniasis. The skin positivity appears while the cutaneous eruption is still active and remains positive long after spontaneous cure. It is usually negative during the febrile phase of visceral leishmaniasis and often becomes positive after cure. A commercially prepared solution containing five to eight million phenol-killed leptomonads of *L. donovani* (Kenya strain) per cubic centimeter is a source of antigen for skin testing. There is no consistently effective therapeutic drug; the pentavalent organic antimonials are most frequently used, and less frequently pyrimethamine (Daraprim), chloroquine (Aralen), aromatic diamides, and amphotericin.

Cutaneous Leishmaniasis

Cutaneous leishmaniasis (old world type, oriental sore, Aleppo or Delphi boil, Bouton d'Orient) is endemic in countries bordering the Mediterranean and in Asia Minor and Central and South America. The incubation period, which varies with the strain of *L. tropica* and number of inoculated organisms, is from a few days to a year with an average of about two months. Children are affected more than adults. Contact infection is reported; the infection is inoculable and auto-inoculable. The skin, which on histopathology is initially infiltrated with large histiocytes filled with many Leishman-Donovan bodies, ulcerates.

TABLE 16–4 CLINICAL EXPRESSIONS OF LEISHMANIASIS

Type	Common Name	Etiologic Agent
Cutaneous	Oriental sore	*L. tropica*
Mucocutaneous	American	*L. braziliensis*
Dermal	Post-kala-azar dermal leishmaniasis	*L. donovani*
	Disseminated cutaneous leishmaniasis	*L. braziliensis*
Visceral	Kala-azar	*L. donovani*

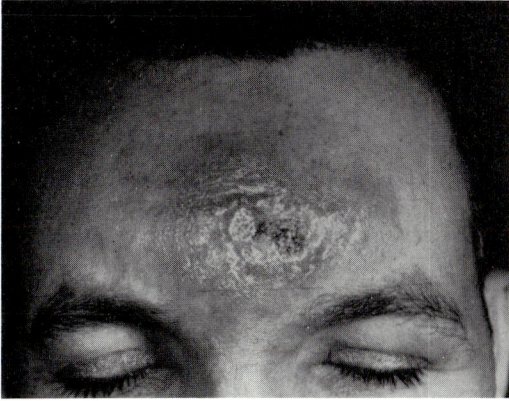

Figure 16–51 The inoculation site or sites of cutaneous leishmaniasis can appear as furuncles. The infection was acquired while the patient was visiting endemic areas in the Near East.

The four clinically distinctive forms of cutaneous leishmaniasis are (1) the wet (rural, major) type (Figs. 16–51 and 16–52), (2) the dry (urban, minor) type (Fig. 16–53), (3) leishmaniasis recidivans (tuberculoid type, chronic lupoid leishmaniasis), and (4) the lepromatoid type (Manson-Bahr, 1964). A comparison of the clinical aspects of the wet and dry types of cutaneous leishmaniasis is presented in Table 16–5. Although the lesions may extend locally to involve adjacent mucosa, they remain self-limited.

Leishmaniasis recidivans (chronic lupoid leishmaniasis) is a relapsing form of leishmaniasis which is a peculiar host reaction and not the result of strain differences of the parasites, which probably survive for years in the host. A similar lesion may be produced by natural or accidental reinfection in patients who have had leishmaniasis recidivans. In the incompletely healed oriental sore, in or near the resultant scar, or in distant normal skin, brownish red or yellow papules appear and coalesce to form a ring or plaque which appears most frequently on the face, can worsen in summer, and even ulcerate. These apple jelly nodules resemble those seen in lupus vulgaris. A tertiary syphilid, lupus erythematosus, and psoriasis may enter into the differential diagnosis of this lesion. The course of the disease is very chronic, and the lesion may enlarge considerably. On histopathology, tubercles composed of epithelioid cells and giant cells are seen; demonstrating organisms on microscopic examination or attemping to culture them is most difficult. The Leishman skin test is strongly positive.

The lepromatoid type of cutaneous leishmaniasis (pseudolepromatous cutaneous leishmaniasis) is characterized by symmetrically distributed papules, nodules, and plaques on the face and extremities and is so called because of its clinical and histologic resemblance to lepromatous leprosy (Balzer et al., 1960). Mucous membranes, viscera, or lymph

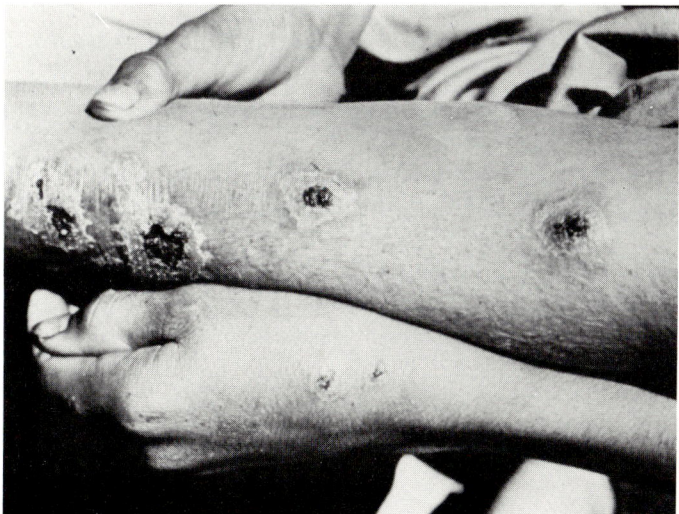

Figure 16–52 The furunculoid type ("multiple furuncles") of cutaneous leishmaniasis.

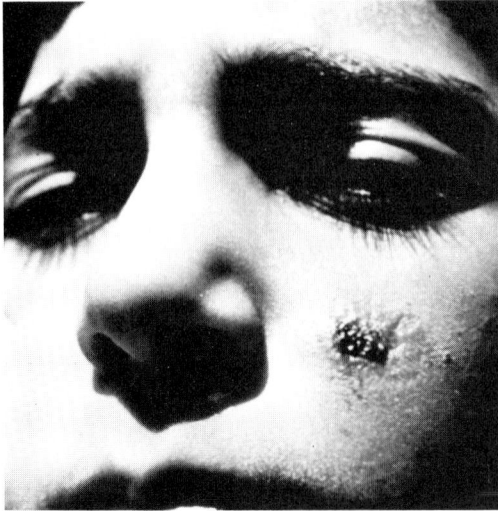

Figure 16–53 A Middle East child with a noduloulcerative lesion of cutaneous leishmaniasis of an exposed site. In older persons, it can be confused with basal cell cancer.

nodes are not involved. It has been described in Africa and is believed to correspond to the disseminated cutaneous leishmaniasis described in Bolivia and Venezuela. The eruption can resemble that of post-kala-azar dermal leishmaniasis seen in India and Africa.

American Leishmaniasis (Goldman, 1947)

American leishmaniasis (mucocutaneous, South American, new world, espundia,

uta, chiclero ulcer) is widely distributed throughout Central and South America with the exception of Chile. Although the commonest etiologic agent is *L. braziliensis*, other strains, such as *L. mexicana* causing chiclero ulcer and *L. braziliensis pifanoi* causing leishmaniasis tegumentaria diffusa, are seen. Various species of Phlebotomus have been reported as vectors. Dogs and wild rodents serve as reservoir hosts. The disease is endemic in damp, forested areas, and its incidence is greatest after the rainy season. About two to three months after a bite of the Phlebotomus in an exposed area, an erythematous nodule appears, ulcerates, resembling an oriental sore (Fig. 16–54), and heals spontaneously within one to two years. Because of a secondary infection, the lesion may appear impetiginoid, ecthymoid, and frambesiform. Lymphangitis and lymphadenitis may be primary or secondary to a complicating infection. In the so-called lymphangitis type, nodules may appear about the initial lesion, ulcerate, and clinically resemble sporotrichosis. Unlike the infection due to *L. tropica*, there is a great tendency to affect mucous membranes, either through local (uta, Figs. 16–55 and 16–56) or later after healing "metastatic" (espundia) spread.

Geographically, the disease may have a characteristic clinical presentation, such as an ulcerative destructive granulomatous lesion of the ears seen in the chicleros of Yucatan and Central America (Fig. 16–57), uta and espundia in Peru, a yaws-

TABLE 16–5 CLINICAL ASPECTS OF WET AND DRY TYPES OF CUTANEOUS LEISHMANIASIS

	Wet (Rural) Type (L. Tropica Var. Major)	*Dry (Urban) Type (L. Tropica Var. Minor)*
Incubation	One to four weeks, rarely greater than two months	Greater than two months, usually over one year
Nature of eruption	Localization — Extremities, head	Face
	Characteristics — Furunculoid nodules which ulcerate; can number more than 30 lesions; satellite lymphatic nodules as well as lymphadenitis	Few nodules which slowly become plaques and ulcerate; secondary satellite nodules not frequent
Seasonal variation	Incidence greatest June through October	Perennial
Pathology	Few organisms; tuberculoid pattern is exceptional	Many organisms, regularly tuberculoid
Host reservoir	Rodents	Man and dogs
Immunity	*L. tropica* var. major protects against reinfection and infection with *L. tropica* var. minor	*L. tropica* var. minor infection protects against reinfection

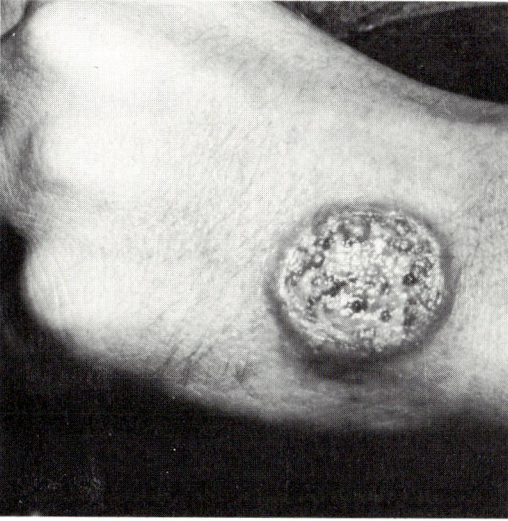

Figure 16-54 The most common expression of cutaneous leishmaniasis in Central and South America—a sharply defined infiltrated ulcer.

The differential diagnosis of American leishmaniasis consists of tropical ulcer, cancrum oris, syphilis, yaws, leprosy, tuberculosis, granuloma inguinale, pyoderma vegetans, myiasis, rhinoscleroma, and deep mycotic infections (South American blastomycosis, histoplasmosis, sporotrichosis). Although antimony is effective in the cutaneous type, relapse tends to occur even after adequate treatment in the mucosal type. The prognosis is good if treatment is started before the mucous membranes are involved. When the antimony preparations fail or the patient is debilitated, a trial of amphotericin B is recommended.

like lesion in Guiana, and less severe types in Panama and Costa Rica. The secondary mucosal lesions appear years later and affect the upper respiratory tract. Infiltration occurs initially, and then necrotic ulceration with marked deformity of nasal septum, nasopharynx, larynx, and mouth is seen.

Disseminated Cutaneous Leishmaniasis (Convit and Kerdel-Vegas, 1965)

Disseminated cutaneous leishmaniasis (Leishmania tegmenta diffusa, disseminated anergic leishmaniasis, leishmaniasis cutis diffusa, leishmaniasis cutanea pseudolepromatosa) is a form of generalized cutaneous leishmaniasis found in Central and South America (especially Venezuela and Brazil), India, Sudan, and Ethiopia (Fig. 16–58). It is caused by strains of *L. tropica* and *L. braziliensis*. The histopathologic picture is characterized by

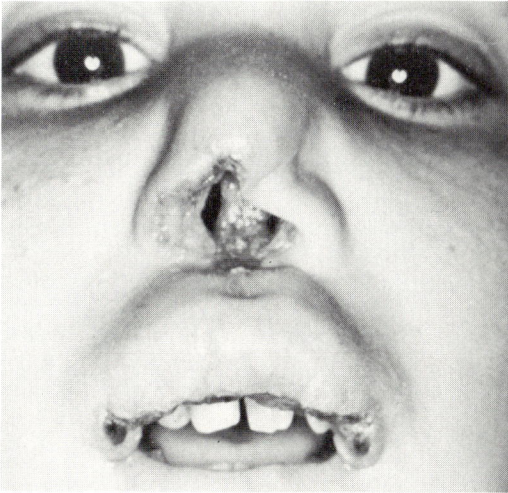

Figure 16-55 Mucocutaneous leishmaniasis. Marked involvement of the naso-oral mucosa in a Central American youth; the initial nasal infiltration extended to involve the other areas. The disease required intermittent courses of amphotericin B.

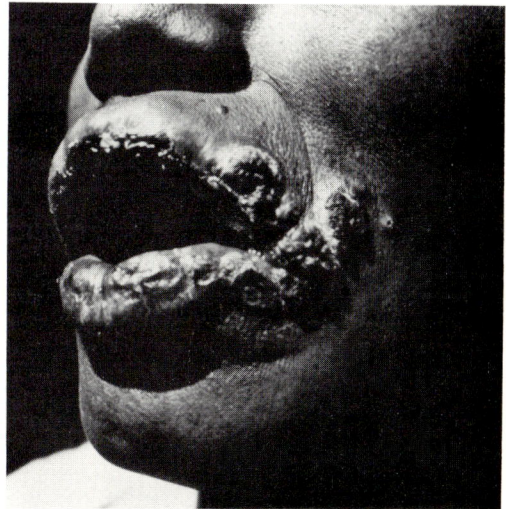

Figure 16-56 Mucocutaneous leishmaniasis. Vegetative disease of the skin and labial and oral mucosa in an African.

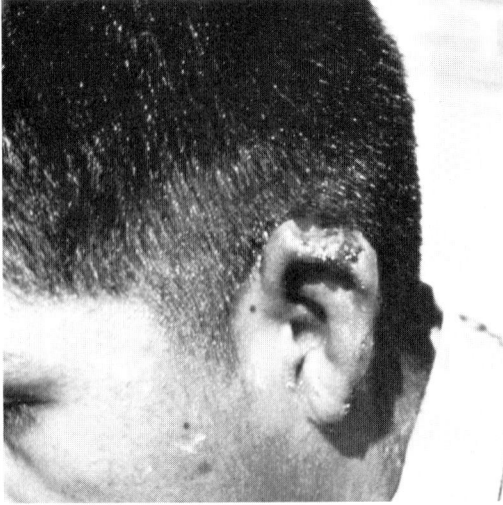

Figure 16–57   The common site of cutaneous leishmaniasis — the ear (the chiclero ulcer) — in the chicleros, the chicle workers of Central America.

granulomatous formation which has cells containing large protoplasmic vacuoles filled with numerous leishmania.

The disease begins as a single lesion which may be an ulcer, macule, nodule, or plaque. Satellite lesions are followed by other distant lesions. Discrete, nonulcerative lesions of the nasal mucosa may be present. The lesions predominate on the exposed surface and gradually increase so that all parts of the body are involved, except the scalp, armpits, and inguino-crural areas. The eruption becomes verrucoid over bony prominences and rarely ulcerates. The process is extremely slow, chronic, and progressive but can evolve more rapidly. There are no subjective symptoms. No systemic involvement is apparent. The Montenegro (Leishman) skin test is negative throughout the course of the disease. The differential diagnoses are lepromatous leprosy, xanthoma tuberosum, sarcoidosis, keloids, generalized nodular type of paracoccidioidal granuloma, Lobo's keloid blastomycosis, post-kala-azar dermal leishmaniasis, and lymphoma cutis. This disease is incurable in the advanced stage. Antimony preparations are effective only in the early stage. Patients with this disease present a public health hazard since the skin is heavily infested and is a reservoir for transmission by the Phlebotomus.

Visceral Leishmaniasis (Cahill, 1963)

Visceral leishmaniasis (kala-azar, Dumdum fever) is widely distributed with sharply limited endemicity in Asia, along the Mediterranean coast, and in Africa and South America. In India, the disease is transmitted from man to man while in some endemic areas of China, the Mediterranean countries, and Brazil, the dog is an animal reservoir. Since the lesion in the reservoir dog is predominantly cutaneous, the Phlebotomus vector has direct access to the infected macrophages. In the Mediterranean area and China, it is most commonly observed in children, and in India, in young adults. The incubation period is from one to four months but has been reported up to ten years (Cahill, 1963). Although the infection is typically insidious, it may have a sudden onset. The initial lesion, which is hardly noticed, is a cutaneous nodule which lasts one to two weeks. When the infection is fully established, irregular undulant fever, cachexia, dysentery, epistaxis, pigmentation, edema of

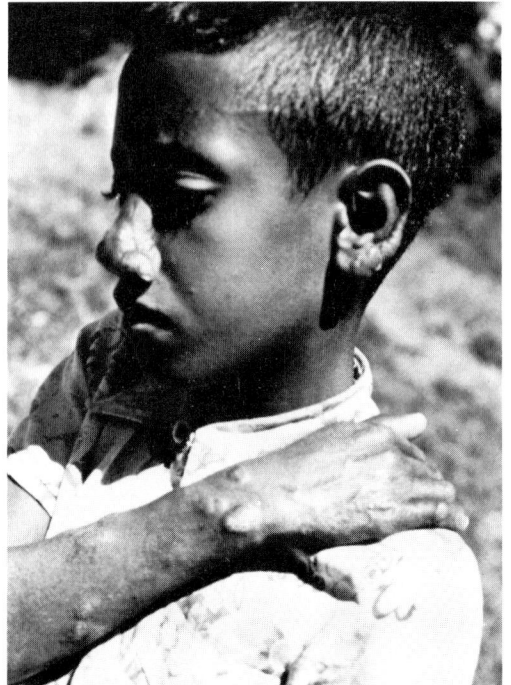

Figure 16–58   Generalized nodules and plaques of disseminated cutaneous leishmaniasis on the face and extremities. It resembles lepromatous leprosy and is resistant to all forms of therapy.

skin, hepatosplenomegaly, lymphadenopathy, anemia with leukopenia, hypoproteinemia with specific increase in "slow gamma" region, as well as presence of macroglobulins and cryoglobulins, are appreciated. A characteristic grayish discoloration of the skin is most noticeable on the hands, the nails, the forehead, and central line of the abdomen and has resulted in the condition being called the "black disease." Cutaneous ulceration and oronasal lesions have been reported. A definitive diagnosis depends upon the demonstration of *L. donovani* in stained smears of peripheral blood, splenic or liver pulp, lymph node juice, sternal bone marrow, or nasal secretions, or in culture of such material. Animal inoculation in the hamster, which is preferred, is not usually used because the time interval for diagnosis is several months. The complicating purpura, gingivitis, stomatitis, and trophic cutaneous changes are attributed to nutritional deficiencies. Cancrum oris, pneumonia, dysentery, hemorrhage, anemia, myocardial degeneration, and toxemia can be complicating terminal events. Post-kala-azar dermal leishmaniasis may develop after incomplete therapy. The differential diagnoses are malaria, typhoid and paratyphoid fevers, relapsing fever, undulant fever, dysentery, tuberculosis, infectious mononucleosis, and leukemia. Pentavalent antimonials are the drugs of choice. Recovery from this disease appears to be followed by a lasting immunity.

Post-Kala-Azar Dermal Leishmaniasis (Napier and Das Gupta, 1930)

Post-kala-azar leishmaniasis (dermal leishmanoid) is a sequela of treated, untreated, or symptomless kala-azar in endemic areas. This condition, a form of clinical relapse resulting from an incomplete cure, presents with a characteristic cutaneous eruption resulting from the infection of the skin by previous visceral infecting organisms. All ages, sexes, and races are susceptible. In India and Pakistan, the eruption occurs one to two years after the signs and symptoms of visceral infections have disappeared. In the Sudan, it occurs toward the completion of treatment or one to two weeks after discharge from treatment. The lesions seen are depigmented macules, malar erythema, nodules, and, less frequently, the verrucose, papillomatous, hypertrophic, and xanthomatous types.

The depigmented lesions are seen more commonly in the younger patient, usually appear below the shoulders, on the back, arms, and thighs, and contain a few organisms which are best demonstrable by culture. They may initially be pinpoint size and increase to 1 cm., are multiple, and may coalesce. In India and Pakistan, the initial depigmented macules later become slightly raised and are the prenodular lesions (Fig. 16–59).

In the Sudan, the pigmentary changes usually occur after the appearance of the nodular lesions. An erythematous eruption may appear early on the cheeks (as a butterfly rash), on the upper and lower lip areas, on the tip and sides of the nose, and on the chin. The nodules are soft, yellowish pink, the size of a split pea, may coalesce to form plaques, and do not break down. They can occur on all parts of the body, but the nose, chin, and cheeks are the usual sites, have demonstrable organisms, and are seen in older patients. The less frequently seen eruptions are the

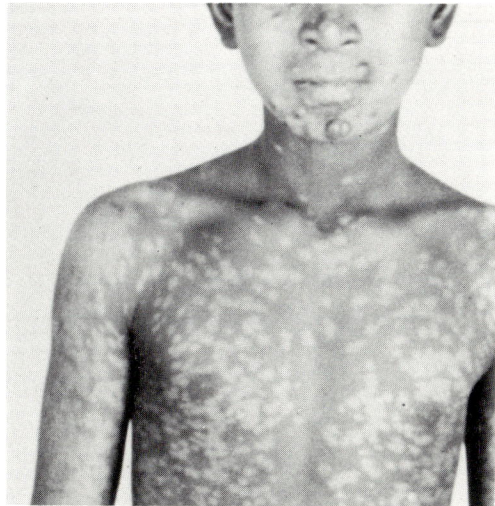

Figure 16–59 There were not only the initial disseminated and generalized depigmented lesions of post-kala-azar dermal leishmaniasis but also the nodulation of the face, especially the chin, in this Indian youth.

verrucoid at the root of the nails of the fingers and toes, the papillomatous on nose and chin, the hypertrophic (resembling lymphatic obstruction) of the eyelids and ala nasi, and the widely scattered xanthomatous. The differential diagnoses are lepromatous leprosy (Fig. 16–60) and xanthomatoses. The macular hypopigmented lesions may remain relatively refractory to therapy but the papular and nodular eruptions respond quickly to pentavalent antimony compounds.

LEPROSY

Leprosy is a chronic, infectious, and communicable disease that affects the cooler tissues of the body (the skin, mucous membranes of the upper respiratory tract, superficial nerves, eyes, superficial lymph nodes, and testes) and exhibits during its slow and insidious course episodes of acute and subacute change (the so-called reaction — Cochrane and Davey, 1964; Guinto and Binford, 1965; Trautman and Enna, 1971).

Distribution

The disease is widespread in tropical and subtropical countries and endemic in some temperate ones. The total number of cases in the world is estimated to be about 10 million; the greatest number is found in the African countries. There are about 2.5 million persons with leprosy in India, about 600,000 in Southeast Asia, about 200,000 in the Americas, and about 2500 registered cases in the United States. Among United States veterans with military service since 1940, there have been about 90 cases reported. In most statistics dealing with the prevalence of leprosy, the estimated number is usually given as at least twice that of the registered cases. In the United States, indigenous cases are found in southeast Texas, Louisiana, and Hawaii.

Epidemiology

As far as is known, the infection occurs only in man. The lepromatous type is considered to be the principal source. The risk of infection is four times higher for persons living in close contact with persons having lepromatous leprosy than with those who have the tuberculoid type. Some insects have been suspected of being vectors. The incubation period between infection and first sign of disease is about 3.5 years. No racial resistance exists. Lepromatous leprosy is much more frequent in men than in women. Leprosy in endemic areas is usually contracted in childhood, but a variable degree of exposure in adult life may result in infection. Prolonged residence in an endemic area is usually necessary for infection but not essential. It has been estimated that in endemic areas leprosy develops in 60 per cent of progeny of infected parents. Conjugal leprosy has a reported incidence of 5 per cent; this supports the view that adults are relatively insusceptible. A genetically determined inability to resist the invasion of *Mycobacterium leprae* successfully is suggested to be significantly responsible for infection and would reconcile many discrepancies in the epidemiology of leprosy.

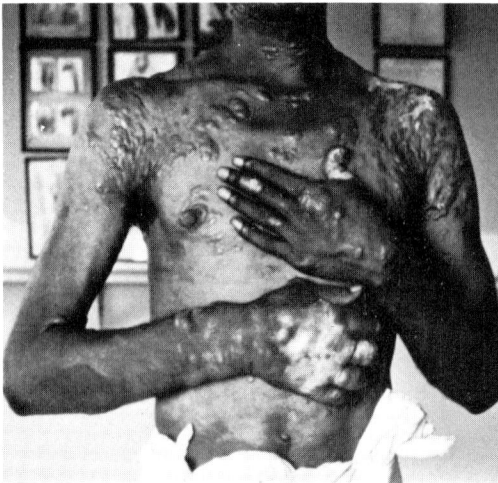

Figure 16–60   The acral distribution of nodules of post-kala-azar dermal leishmaniasis resembling lepromatous leprosy in an Indian.

Etiology

M. leprae is a gram-positive bacillus which resists decolorization when treated with weak acids and with alcohol after being stained with carbolfuchsin. Large, opaque polar bodies similar to those observed in *M. tuberculosis* have been demonstrated by electron microscopy. An estimate has been made that 1 gm. of leproma (lepromatous cutaneous nodule) may contain 5 million bacilli. *M. leprae* has multiplied in the foot pads of mice and in the ears of hamsters but has not produced progressive disease in these animals. Armadillos have been inoculated successfully and have developed the lepromatous form of this disease (Kirchheimer and Storrs, 1971). Attempts to transmit leprosy to human beings by inoculation with lepromatous material have been unsuccessful; there are scattered reports of leprosy resulting from accidental or artificial inoculation. Koch's postulates have not been fulfilled.

Pathogenesis

The bacilli that have a predilection for nerve tissue enter the nerve twigs close to the site of cutaneous inoculation or are carried from another portal of entry by way of the bloodstream to the Schwann cell of the peripheral nerve. The type of disease produced depends on the inherent resistance of the host and its effect on the bacilli-laden target cell, the Schwann cell, and organ. In lepromatous leprosy, in which the resistance is low, some of the Schwann cells become macrophages and transport the bacilli to other parts of the nerve, or to other nerves or organs; the intraneural bacilli can extend to the posterior ganglia. The bacilli-filled macrophages rupture and scatter their bacilli, which are rephagocytized by fresh histiocytes and further disseminated. In persons with high "tissue" resistance, the infected Schwann cells become fixed epithelioid cells, and giant cells form through their coalescence. This "anchored" infection, localized to an area of skin and underlying superficial nerves, is called tuberculoid leprosy.

A type of leprosy that is clinically and histologically between lepromatous and tuberculoid leprosy and called dimorphous or borderline is associated with an unstable immunologic state. Indeterminate (uncharacteristic) leprosy appears to be transitory; that is, it is initially characterized by minimal localized skin and nerve involvement and subsequently may eventuate into one of the other types, depending on the immunologic background of the host. The pattern of distribution of the skin lesions and areas of anesthesia corresponds to the cooler regions of the body where the *M. leprae* prefer to multiply; this is supported by thermographic studies (Hastings et al., 1968).

Pathologic Findings

Lepromatous leprosy is characterized histologically by a thinning of the epidermis, a subepidermal clear area, a diffuse dermal infiltrate consisting of sheets of foamy macrophages that contain large numbers of singly or clumped bacilli, and nerves that contain bacilli and no inflammatory infiltrate (Table 16–6). Fibrocytes are found at the periphery of healing lesions or throughout the lesion in relapse. The fibrocytes contain "viable" organisms and are the principal pathologic response of the so-called histoid variety of lepromatous leprosy.

In tuberculoid leprosy, there are foci of epithelioid cells that contain Langhans' giant cells, concentrate about neurovascular elements, invade papillae, contain no bacilli, and have a moderate perigranulomatous distribution of lymphocytes; additionally, there is diffuse granulomatous infiltration of cutaneous nerves with rare "cold abscess" formation.

The borderline (dimorphous) leprosy has histologic features of lepromatous (BL) or tuberculoid (BT) leprosy. In the BL variety, the histiocytes, some of which are foamy and contain bacilli, predominate; masses of lymphocytes surround the nerves and diffusely infiltrate the granuloma, and the cutaneous nerves contain bacilli and little if any cellular infiltrates. In the BT variety, the epithelioid cell granuloma tends to be more diffuse and less localized to the neurovascular elements, there is a free, narrow subepidermal zone, lymphocytes are predominantly perigranulomatous, Langhans' giant cells are scarce, and the cutaneous nerves are diffusely infiltrated with cells and may contain a few bacilli. The histopathologic picture of uncharacteristic (indeterminate)

TABLE 16–6   Histopathology of Nonreactive Leprosy

Histologic Changes	Indeterminate	Tuberculoid (TT)	Borderline Tuberculoid (BT)	Typical Borderline (BB)	Borderline Lepromatous (BL)	Lepromatous (LL)
Clear subepidermal zone	0	0	2+	2+	3+	4+
Bacterial index	0–1+	0	0–2+	1–3+	3–4+	5–6+
Composition of granuloma						
Epithelioid cells	0	4+ (focal)	3+ (focal)	3+ (diffuse)	1+ (difuse)	0
Langhans' giant cells	0	4+	2+	0	0	0
Foamy histiocyte	±	0	0	±	2+	4+
Globi	0	0	0	±	2+	4+
Histoid cell fibrocytes	±	0	0	0	2+	4+
Lymphocyte distribution						
Perigranuloma	0	2+	3+	2+	0	0
Diffusely infiltrative	0	0	0	1+	3+	2+
Periappendageal	2+	0	0	0	0	0
Nerve involvement						
Perineural cuffing	1+	0	0	2+	2+	1+
Schwann cell proliferation	1+	0	0	2+	2+	1+
Granuloma infiltration	0	4+	2+	0	0	0–1+ (late)
Nerve abscess	0	4+	1+	0	0	0–rare (reaction)

leprosy shows nonspecific infiltration of histiocytes and lymphocytes around cutaneous appendages and nerves which may appear normal in hematoxylin and eosin stain but may reveal a few bacilli with Fite-Faraco stain.

Clinical Manifestations

The cutaneous manifestations depend on the type of leprosy, the duration of the disease, the degree and extent of nerve damage, the presence or absence of reaction, and the effect of therapy (Table 16–7).

Neural involvement is an early and major expression of the disease (Moschella, 1966). The clinical signs of leprous neuropathy are palpable or visible neural enlargement or tenderness or both, anesthesia, anhidrosis, muscular atrophy, and trophic disturbances of skin and joints (Table 16–7; Chatterji, 1937). In a patient with suspected leprosy, the presence of one or several tender, enlarged nerves is strong presumptive evidence of the disease. The common palpable nerves are the great auricular (Fig. 16–61), the ulnar, and the common peroneal nerves. The cardinal symptom is anesthesia. The sensory losses are light touch, heat, pain, and pressure. The autonomic fibers are also involved early in the disease. The clinical manifestations are anhidrosis and

a change in the texture of the skin, which becomes dry and rough. More severe autonomic distribution results in vasomotor disturbances, which are characterized by cyanosis, edema, and elephantiasis of extremities. The skin of the lower extremities can become ichthyotic and sclerodermatous. The factors that affect nerve paralysis are tissue reactions, size of the nerve, and proximity of the nerve to the body surface.

Some of the more obvious clinical manifestations of muscular paralysis and atrophy are widening of the palpebral fissure, drooping of eyelids and commissure of the mouth, inability to raise eyebrows or to close eyes tightly, flattening of thenar and hypothenar eminences, "grooving" between metacarpal bones, slight flexion contracture of the fifth finger, external rotation of the thumb, clawhand (Fig. 16–62), drop foot, and "cock's gait." Severe trophic disturbances can cause bone changes with characteristic concentric absorption of phalanges and metacarpal and metatarsal bones, painless plantar ulceration, and neuropathic joint. The plantar ulcer (Fig. 16–63) is the most common major foot problem. The main sites of ulceration are the skin of the first, second, and fifth metatarsal heads, the heel, the interphalangeal joint of the big toe, and the tips of the toes. The neuropathic joint of Charcot results from severe and long-standing deep sensory loss.

If a diagnostic skin lesion is not available, a biopsy of a nerve that subserves no important function (for example, the sural) is a practical and valuable diagnostic procedure because bacilli in nerves are the first and last evidence of infection, and specific histologic changes are seen in tuberculoid leprosy.

The clinical changes appreciated in nonreactive leprosy are lesions of the anterior chamber of the eye; alopecia; macules that may be hypochromic or hyperchromic with or without inflammation; diffuse infiltration of the skin; annular, plaque, or nodular lesions; auricular involvement; and nasopharyngeal ulceration. The changes seen in reactive leprosy are exacerbations of old lesions, appearance of new lesions, vesicular and erythematous nodose lesions with or without suppuration and ulceration, fever, iritis, lymphadenitis, orchitis, and mastitis.

Eye involvement in leprosy is frequent and may be the result of the presence of bacilli in the eye; it may also occur secondary to involvement of the fifth and seventh nerve or as a hypersensitivity reaction of ocular tissues to the leprous infection. The fifth nerve involvement causes corneal and conjunctival anesthesia, and seventh nerve involvement

TABLE 16–7 CLINICAL CHARACTERISTICS OF LEPROSY

	Indeterminate (Uncharacteristic)	Tuberculoid (TT)	Borderline or Dimorphous (BB)	Lepromatous (LL)
Course	Unstable — Regresses or progresses into more definitive type	Stable — Severe cases can have high morbidity	Unstable — BT⇆BB⇆BL; change with treatment	Spectrally stable; progressive
Skin	Usually singly; hypopigmented or erythematous; ill-defined or well-defined borders; hypoesthetic	Asymmetric; single to few hypopigmented scaling macules with raised border; well-defined margins; plaques with pebbly surface; annular lesion	Multiple, widespread, asymmetric, thick, succulent; ill-defined plaques; dimpled nodules; lesions or areas may be hypoesthetic	Small, widespread, shiny, ill-defined, symmetric macules; diffuse infiltration; plaques, nodules
Nerve involvement	Slight and symmetric	Sudden, severe, asymmetric; occasionally intraneural "cold abscess"	Symmetric, more rapid than (LL)	Slow and symmetric
Complications	None	Tuberculoid reaction (tuberculoid reactivation); low resistant tuberculoid reaction — Akuter-Schub (reactional tuberculoid leprosy)	Nonpitting edema of hands and feet; reactive dimorphous leprosy; erythema nodosum (BL)	Eye, upper respiratory tract, bone involvement; plantar ulcers; Charcot joints; testicular atrophy; gynecomastia; reactions (acute exacerbation, hypersensitivity reactions, histoid variety); secondary amyloidosis
Bacterioscopy	Few, if any	No bacilli; few during reactions	Many bacilli	Abundant bacilli
Histopathology	Banal round cell infiltration about appendages and in nerves	Epithelioid cell granulomas with Langhans' giant cells; extends into papillary stroma; destroys nerves early	Features of both tuberculoid and lepromatous (dimorphous); depends on which predominates	Diffuse infiltrate of foamy macrophages; nerves infiltrate; no infiltrate; subepidermal clear zone
Lepromin reaction	Negative or weakly positive	Positive, usually strongly	Negative or weakly positive	Negative
Treatment	DDS, 200 mg. a week until signs of activity gone; 100 mg. a week for two years	DDS, 200 mg. a week until signs of activity gone; then 100 mg. a week for 12 years	DDS, 300 to 400 mg. a week until disease inactive, then 200 mg. a week for 10 years	Low dose initially with gradual build-up to 600 mg. a week; when disease inactive, 100 mg. twice a week for life
Prognosis	Good; may regress spontaneously	Good; can heal spontaneously but occasionally severe morbidity due to irreversible nerve damage	Guarded; reactions can significantly increase morbidity and course of disease	Guarded; complications of amyloidosis, tuberculosis, and severe reactive episode (Lucio's phenomenon) can be fatal

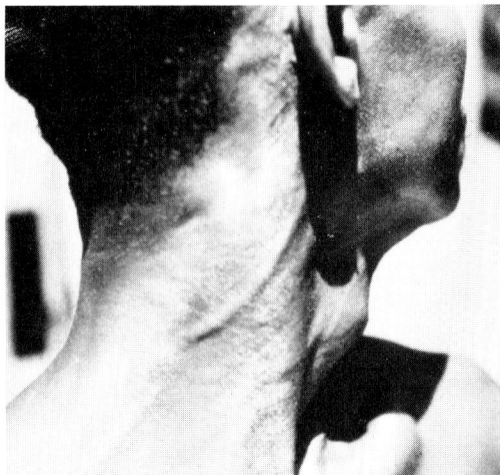

Figure 16–61 Visibly enlarged great auricular nerve in a patient with lepromatous leprosy.

causes lagophthalmos. With simultaneous involvement of the fifth and seventh nerve, exposure keratitis is most likely to occur. The gross changes due to direct infection of the eyeball with bacilli are pannus, miliary lepromata (iris "pearls"), and nodular lepromata. Acute, diffuse, plastic iridocyclitis ("red eye") is the result of a hypersensitivity of the uveal tract possibly to the breakdown products of *M. leprae* elsewhere in the body.

INDETERMINATE (UNCHARACTERISTIC) LEPROSY. Indeterminate leprosy consists usually of a single macule (Fig. 16–64), but there may be a few asymmetrically distributed, flat, smooth, usually hypopigmented and occasionally erythematous, well-defined or ill-defined macules located in the exposed areas. The lesion may be hypoesthetic or anesthetic. The histamine skin test, which can evaluate damage to sympathetic nerves in the skin, may be helpful for diagnosis in the absence of appreciable sensory changes. One drop of 1 to 1000 solution of histamine diphosphate is placed in the macule and another on an adjacent control area, and the skin is lightly pricked with a needle through each drop. A bright flare is seen in one to two minutes in the normal skin and is faint to absent in the diseased skin. There is usually no associated nerve enlargement. Bacilli are usually absent on

examination of skin smear of the macule, but, on histopathologic examination of involved skin, they may be seen in the nerves. The lepromin skin may show positive or negative reaction. The lesion may regress spontaneously or may progress and evolve into one of the more definitive types of leprosy.

TUBERCULOID LEPROSY. Tuberculoid leprosy involves nerves and skin. It may present only or initially as a purely neural disease with sensory and motor changes; later, the skin lesions, macules, or plaques develop. They tend to be solitary, hypopigmented or erythematous, dry, anesthetic (less so on the face), alopecic, and anhidrotic, and have a somewhat rough surface with clearly defined margins that tend to be raised, with a flat central area. The plaques may have a pebbly surface. The lesions can be extensive and larger than any other form of cutaneous leprosy,

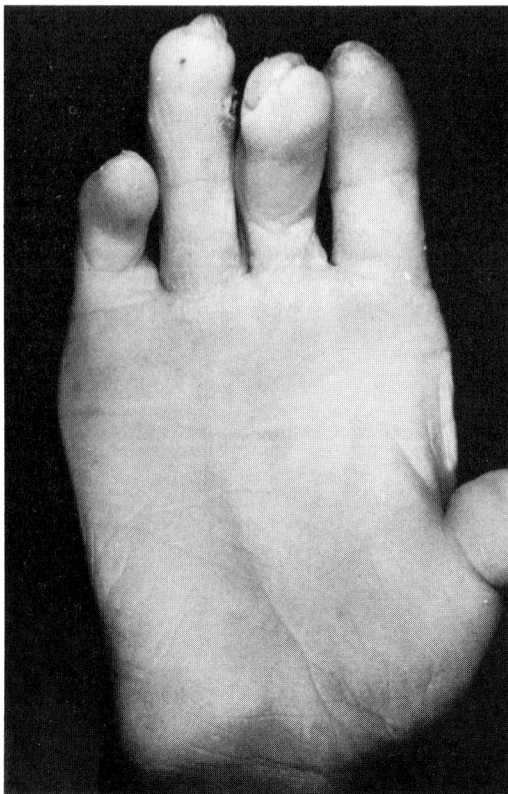

Figure 16–62 Leprosy. Advanced changes of the hands resulting from ulnar and median nerve involvement.

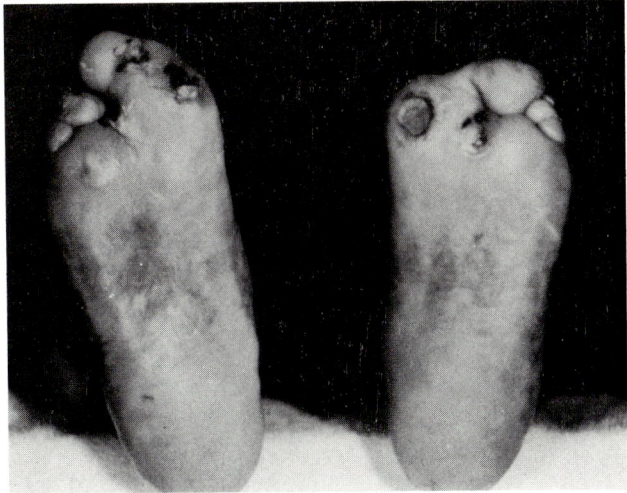

Figure 16–63 Leprosy. Painless plantar ulcerations and disfigurement of toes result from the respective involvements of the common peroneal (sensory) and the posterior tibial (motor) nerves.

up to 30 cm. in diameter. They are confined to the buttocks (Fig. 16–65), posterolateral aspect of the extremities, back, and face. Superficial nerves supplying the region may be palpable, visible, or both,

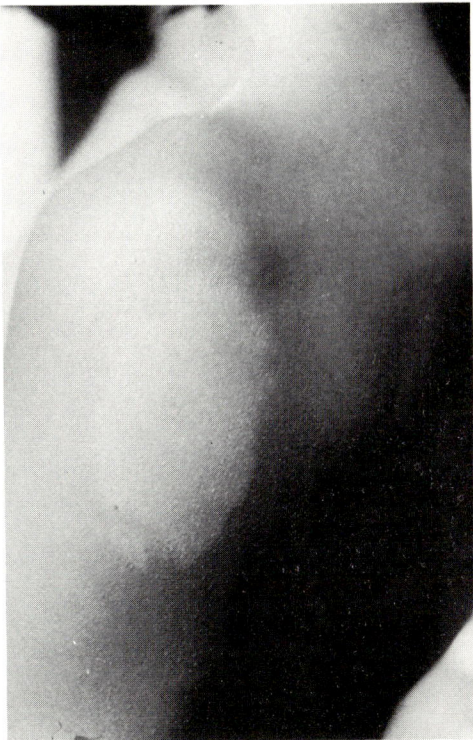

Figure 16–64 Solitary hypopigmented smooth anesthetic macule of leprosy; skin scrapings and biopsy did not reveal the presence of acid-fast bacilli.

especially in the vicinity of the lesion. The skin smears for bacilli are negative, and the lepromin skin test is always positive.

BORDERLINE (DIMORPHOUS) LEPROSY. Borderline leprosy, like tuberculoid leprosy, affects nerves and skin and exhibits clinical and histologic features of both lepromatous and tuberculoid leprosy. The clinical characteristics, such as the number of lesions, their size, margins, surface, and sensory changes, are intermediate or favor those of tuberculoid or lepromatous leprosy.

The skin lesions are usually plaques or annular lesions and less frequently macules or nodules; they are multiple and have a widespread asymmetric distribution. The plaque lesions are thick and succulent and are often without significant impairment of sensation, taper peripherally toward normal skin, and have ill-defined margins, a smooth surface, and a violaceous or brownish (sepia) hue. The macules are hypopigmented or erythematous. The nodules are less numerous in comparison to those of lepromatous leprosy and have dimpling at the summit. The so-called immune areas (warmer parts of the body, intergluteal and flexural areas, upper eyelids, midback, palms, and soles) may become involved. A characteristic and common eruption that has a "Swiss cheese" appearance is the erythematous, annular ("inverted saucer") lesions enclosing sharply hypopigmented areas and

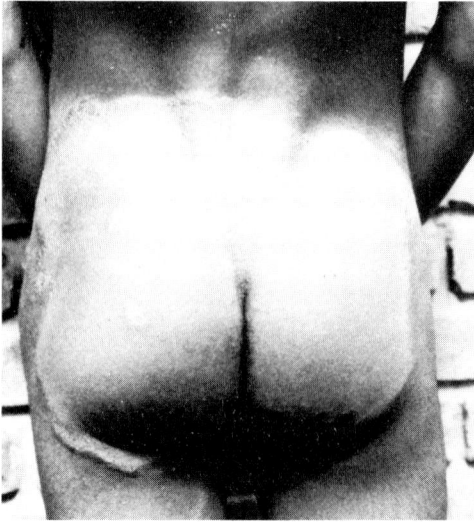

Figure 16–65 Sharply infiltrated scaling anesthetic plaques of leprosy that revealed, histologically, tuberculoid granulomas and nerve replacement by this process.

having a vague outer border (Fig. 16–66). The earlobes are usually involved unilaterally and not bilaterally as in lepromatous leprosy. Nonpitting edema of the hands and feet is more frequently seen than in any other type of leprosy. The borderline lepromatous (BL) variety is rarely complicated by erythema nodosum leprosum (ENL) reaction.

The skin lesions usually contain many bacilli, but scraping of nasal mucosa yields no bacilli. The lepromin skin test, the results of which are usually negative, can be weakly positive. Patients with borderline leprosy are infectious and respond to therapy more quickly than do those with lepromatous leprosy.

LEPROMATOUS LEPROSY. Lepromatous leprosy presents initially with cutaneous and mucous membrane lesions and subsequently with neural, ocular, reticuloendothelial, osseous, and testicular changes. The cutaneous lesions seen are macular, plaque, and nodular, as well as diffusely infiltrative. The clinical expression of this type of leprosy may be so subtle that the only presenting signs appreciated are those of the complicating lepra reaction, erythema nodosum leprosum, or Lucio's phenomenon. The macules, which are usually the earliest

expression, are small, multiple, ill-defined, hypopigmented or hyperpigmented or erythematous, shiny, symmetrically distributed, and without sensory changes. They are best appreciated on the face, extremities, and buttocks, but spare the warmer parts of the body (so-called immune areas).

As the disease progresses, plaques and nodules, which may coalesce, appear. The nodules are best seen about the rim of the ear and on the chin, elbows, buttocks, knees, and dorsa of hands and feet. The pure diffuse type occurs rarely and is characterized by diffuse infiltration of the skin. One suspects this type if he palpates the skin or appreciates the development of alopecia, nasal and laryngeal complaints, and clinical evidence of superficial neuropathy. The face has a puffy myxedematous appearance. The skin may be sclerodermatous with widespread small telangiectasis. A unique complication of this subtype of leprosy is the reactional state of erythema necroticans (so-called Lucio's phenomenon). Erosions of the diseased nasal mucosa may cause epistaxis, destruction of nasal supportive tissue, perforation and saddle nose deformity; laryngeal lesions may result in hoarseness and stridor; eye involvement creates pain, photophobia, loss of visual acuity, glaucoma, and blindness; secondary testicular atrophy results in sterility, impotence, and gynecomastia; lymph node and liver in-

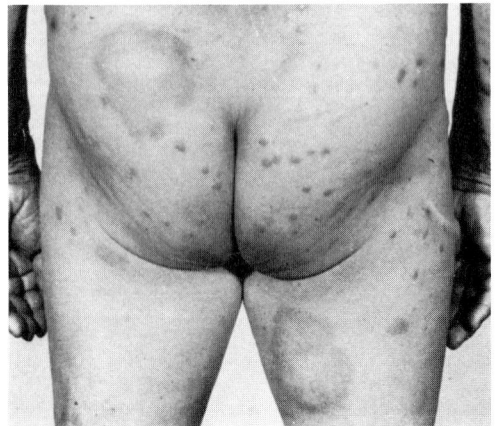

Figure 16–66 Erythematous anesthetic annular lesions of leprosy with a sharp inner and irregular outer border; biopsy of a lesion revealed a few acid-fast bacilli.

filtration cause lymphadenopathy and hepatomegaly; and leprous infiltration of hairy areas is responsible for alopecia, especially of the lateral third of the eyebows and of the eyelids, body hair, and, rarely, scalp, Ichthyosiform skin changes may appear on the lower extremities. Digital, carpal, and tarsal destruction and absorption are caused by bacillary invasion, neurovascular disease, and repeated painless trauma that results in aseptic necrosis and complicating osteomyelitis. In advanced lepromatous leprosy, brawny edema of lower extremities may be seen. Although anesthesia may be seen early in the disease, the symmetric, widespread, superficial neuropathy evolves slowly and insidiously, and its consequences are appreciated later. Stigmata of "burnt out" lepromatous leprosy are alopecia, anhidrosis, asteatosis, "cigarette-paper" skin, secondary cutis laxa, and destruction of nose, ears, digits, and joints of feet.

Large numbers of bacilli are found in all active, lepromatous skin and nasal lesions. The lepromin skin test always gives negative results.

Classification of Leprosy

The type of leprosy acquired is probably directly related to the degree of susceptibility, resistance, or immunity possessed by the individual. The current classification, based on the host's degree of resistance, describes a continuous spectrum between the two stable extremes, tuberculoid and lepromatous leprosy, which are regarded as the poles. Between the low-resistance lepromatous leprosy and the high-resistance tuberculoid leprosy lies an unstable, dynamic, intermediate group, which has features of both poles and is called dimorphous or borderline. A five-group system of classification (TT, BT, BB, BL, LL) has been advanced to supply the needed flexibility (Ridley and Jopling, 1966).

The stable polarized types (tuberculoid and lepromatous leprosy) and two unstable groups (uncharacteristic and borderline) have already been described and outlined (Table 16–7). The BT variety of borderline leprosy differs from tuberculoid leprosy (TT) in that the lesions of

BT are usually not so large and are more numerous, their surface is less dry, their borders are not so well-defined, and the thickened nerves are more numerous but not so irregularly thickened. Satellite lesions appear adjacent to larger lesions. The histologic distinction has already been described. A few organisms can be demonstrated in nerve bundles, and results of the lepromin skin test are positive but not strongly.

The BL variety of borderline leprosy differs from lepromatous leprosy in that the lesions of BL are not as many or as shiny for the duration of the infection, are succulent, and are not truly bilaterally symmetric; the plaques tend to be larger and to have a punched-out appearance (annular) and are partially anesthetic. Other clinical features distinguishing BL from LL leprosy are the "dimpled" center of the nodules, the earlier thickening of the superficial nerves, and the absence of the classic lepromatous features, such as madarosis, bilateral auricular involvement, keratitis, nasal ulceration or saddle deformity, and leonine facies (Fig. 16–67). Like leproma-

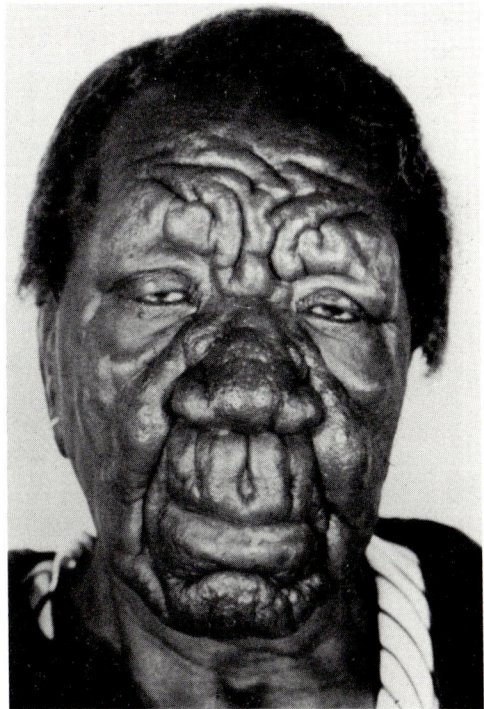

Figure 16–67 Advanced lepromatous leprosy of many years' duration resulting in leonine facies.

tous leprosy, the lepromin skin test usually gives negative results but may become weakly positive with effective treatment.

Diagnosis

An accurate diagnosis, as in other diseases, is made by a complete history, physical examination, and effective use of laboratory facilities. An advanced case of leprosy with obvious skin and nerve lesions is not a problem to the alert physician; the diagnostic problem is the patient with an early infection characterized by skin lesions which are not striking accompanied by an absent or minimal sensory deficit. The fact that the patient came from an endemic area or had a family exposure to leprosy should create an awareness for and reinforce the consideration of leprosy in the entertained differential diagnosis. The diagnosis of leprosy depends on the demonstration or appreciation of one or all of the following signs: *M. leprae* in skin smear or in the histopathologic examination of involved tissue, impairment of cutaneous sensitivity, and thickened and tender superficial nerves.

To demonstrate the presence of *M. leprae*, a skin smear, also known as "skin scraping," is taken. The suspected lesion or skin is picked up between two fingers, rendered avascular by squeezing, and incised with a size 15 Bard-Parker blade. The inflicted wound should be about 5 mm. long and 3 mm. deep and scraped several times in one direction by the blade, which is held at right angles. The gathered fluid and pulp are smeared on a glass slide, heat fixed, and stained by the Ziehl-Neelsen method; however, the preparation should not be decolorized too long because *M. leprae* is much less acid-fast than *M. tuberculosis*. Wade's modification of the Fite-Faraco stain is recommended for tissue staining for bacilli, because Ziehl-Neelsen's stain is not sensitive enough to be used on paraffin sections of tissue, particularly if bacilli are scarce (Wade, 1952). Scrapings of the nasal mucosa are usually avoided because nonpathogenic, acid-fast diphtheroid bacilli, indistinguishable from *M. leprae*, may be found. The sites that should be examined for bacilli are cutaneous or palpable lesions or, if none are present, areas of anesthesia; otherwise, the skin of earlobes, elbows, knees, and buttocks is the preferred location for investigation. At least six sites should be examined before the effort is considered fruitless.

Skin smears are necessary not only to make the diagnosis of leprosy but also to assess the type of leprosy, the severity of the infection, and the response to treatment. Healing, effectiveness of therapy, or both are reflected in the number of bacteria (bacterial index—BI) and the bacterial morphology (morphologic index—MI; Ridley, 1955). The bacterial index is expressed by word, by number code on a semilogarithmic scale, or by both:

Very numerous (6+)—more than 1000 bacilli per oil immersion field.
Numerous (5+)—100 to 1000 bacilli per oil immersion field.
Moderate (4+)—10 to 100 bacilli per oil immersion field.
Few (3+)—1 to 10 bacilli per oil immersion field.
Very few (2+)—10 to 100 bacilli per entire slide (100 field).
Rare (1+)—1 to 10 bacilli per entire slide.

The staining characteristics and morphology of *M. leprae* are probably an indication of the viability of the organism (Waters and Rees, 1962). Viable bacilli are "solid staining"; that is, there is uniform staining of the entire bacillus. Nonviable bacilli are nonsolid staining and may present as a uniform staining fragment, a failure to stain uniformly, or a beading or fragmentation of the bacilli. The MI is reported as the average percentage of the number of solid staining forms per 100 total bacilli examined; when there are less than 100 total bacilli, solid forms per total number of bacilli found are reported. A logarithmic index of bacilli (LIB) in biopsies, representing the number of bacilli per unit area of a section, has been recommended as the most practical and accurate laboratory tool for the assessment of alteration in bacterial density and size of granuloma.

The definitive diagnosis, classification, prognosis, and response to therapy can best be appreciated by biopsy of skin lesion. Occasionally, the clinical picture of an inactive case of leprosy may be confusing to an examining physician, but the histologic evidence of cutaneous nerve destruction or the presence of fragmented bacilli in nerves is helpful. Nerve biopsy of a thickened great auricular at the neck, the radial at the wrist, the superficial peroneal, and, preferably, the sural at the ankle may be necessary to confirm the diagnosis of tuberculoid or borderline neural leprosy. Enlarged lymph nodes may contain *M. leprae* and contribute to the diagnosis of leprosy on biopsy.

The lepromin (Mitsuda) skin test is a nonspecific test that has no diagnostic significance, is useful for classification, and is a measure of tissue "resistance." It consists of not only killed bacilli but also human tissue. An injection of 0.1 cc. of standardized lepromin is given intradermally. In 24 to 48 hours there may be a tuberculin-like reaction, the Fernandez reaction, which is of unknown significance. The test results are reported as positive if after three weeks an indurated area or papule, 3 mm. or greater in diameter, appears at the injection site; it is graded on the basis of size — 3 to 5 mm. is 1+; more than 5 mm., 2+; and any size papule that ulcerates is 3+.

The demonstration of the multiplication of *M. leprae* in the foot pad of the mouse (Shepard, 1960) has resulted in the application of this procedure to screen experimental drugs, to detect resistant bacilli, to evaluate drug resistance and efficacy of vaccines and the effect of physical forces on infectability of bacilli, and to explore the role of arthropods in the transmission of leprosy.

Differential Diagnosis

In areas in which the incidence of leprosy is low, the index of suspicion is low and the diagnosis is not made because of the wide spectrum of the cutaneous manifestations of leprosy. The differential diagnosis is as follows:

1. Macular lesions

   A. Achromic — Vitiligo, nevus anemicus, pityriasis simplex, tinea versicolor, morphea, postinflammatory leukoderma (for example, seborrheic dermatitis, atopic eczema).

   B. Hyperchromia — Café-au-lait, parapsoriasis en plaque, postinflammatory melanosis (lichen planus and fixed drug eruption).

2. Papular lesions

   Disseminated granuloma annulare, sarcoidosis, lichen planus, papular treponemal lesions, leishmanids, appendageal hamartomas (leiomyomas and syringomas).

3. Plaque lesions

   A. Annular — Tinea corporis, pityriasis rosea, lichen planus, figurative erythema, granuloma annulare, sarcoid, and lymphoma cutis.

   B. Solid — Benign and malignant lymphocytic infiltrations of skin, psoriasis, sarcoid, mastocytosis, facial granuloma, infectious granulomas (mycobacterial, treponemal, mycotic, and leishmanial), and lymphoma cutis.

4. Nodules

   Acne vulgaris, xanthomatosis, granulomas (sarcoid, histiocytosis, mycosis, treponematoses, leishmaniasis, and onchocerciasis), erythema elevatum diutinum, pretibial myxedema, lichen myxedematosis, neurofibromatosis, Kaposi's sarcoma, and lymphoma cutis.

Among the conditions to be considered in the differential diagnosis of leprous neuropathy are polyneuropathy caused by chronic intoxication, infections, metabolic disturbances, so-called auto-immune disease, nutritional deficiencies, syringomyelia, neurofibromatosis, entrapment syndromes, Dejerine-Sottas disease, and Raynaud's disease. The Charcot's joint of leprosy is to be differentiated from that of tabes dorsalis, diabetes mellitus, nutritional neuritis, syringomyelia, multiple sclerosis, and intra-articular injections of corticosteroid.

Reactional Leprosy (Ridley, 1969; Tolentino, 1965)

During the chronic course of leprosy, sudden episodes of exacerbation or changes of the chronic disease and the appearance of new lesions, either indicating a progression of the infectious process or representing a complicating hypersensitivity phenomenon, are called reactions (Tables 16–8 and 16–9). Two types of cutaneous expressions are appreciated. In one, the lesions of tuberculoid, borderline, or lepromatous leprosy become more erythematous and swollen and similar new

TABLE 16–8 LEPROSY IN REACTION

	Immunologic Nature of Infection (Infection vs. Host)	Hypersensitivity Phenomena
Mediation	Cell mediated	Humoral immune mechanism
Classification	Tuberculoid in reaction; reactional tuberculoid (Akuter-Schub); borderline reaction (downgrading and reversal reactions); acute lepromatous infiltration; histoid response	Erythema nodosum leprosum and its variants; erythema necroticans (Lucio's phenomenon)
Clinical characteristics	Abrupt onset; inflammatory edema of lesions; extension of old lesions, appearance of new lesions, ulcerations of lesions; tender thickening of nerves; fever	Acute onset; constitutional signs and symptoms; cutaneous lesions (nodose ± suppuration, vesiculobullous-pustular, ischemic ulcerations), neuritis, peripheral edema, iritis, mastitis, orchitis, arthritis, lymphadenitis
Histopathology	Edema; increased lymphocytic infiltration; reversal reaction; increased epithelioid response; bacilli diminished; downgrading reactions; loss of compact focalization; more foreign body giant cells; increased vacuolization of macrophages; increased number of bacilli	Occurs in inapparent lesions; edema; early polymorphonuclear leukocytes predominate; vasculitis (proliferative, allergic, necrotizing); thrombosis of blood vessels; dermal necrosis; panniculitis
Lepromin	Lessened reactivity in downgrading states and increased response in reversal states	No effect
Treatment	Initially reduce or discontinue DDS; systemic corticosteroid; in histoid response, another antileprotic drug (B-663)	Aspirin, antimalarials, antimonials, thalidomide, corticosteroids, B-663

lesions may appear. In the other type, the cutaneous lesions, resembling those of the erythema group (mainly erythema nodosum but also erythema multiforme and erythema necroticans), appear in lepromatous leprosy; rarely, in the borderline leprosy (BL type), erythema nodosum lesions may appear. They are associated with the presence of bacterial antigen and an alteration in the immunologic balance between host and bacillus. The former,

which usually occurs during the early stage of the disease and has bacilli that are predominantly solid, is presumed to be immunologically mediated by cells, and the latter, which occurs later in the disease and has bacilli that are mostly fragmented and granular, is presumably mediated by humoral mechanisms.

There is no general acceptable classification of these reactions. Eight categories that are distinct from simple activity or

TABLE 16–9 HISTOPATHOLOGY OF REACTIVE LEPROSY

Histologic Changes	Acute Exacerbation	Lepra Reaction
Epidermal changes	Blistering, ulceration	Blistering, pustulation, ulceration
Bacterial index	± (Indeterminate) − 4+ (LL)	No increase
Cellular response	Lymphocytes	Early — Polymorphonuclear leukocytes, eosinophils, mast cells; later — lymphocytes, plasma cells, fibroblasts
Dermal and hypodermal changes	Dermal edema (diffuse); neural edema and necrosis; fibrosis	Dermal edema (focal); neural edema and cellular infiltration; chronic granulomatous panniculitis; septal fibrosis
Blood vessel changes	Endothelial swelling	Endothelial swelling; cellular infiltration; hypersensitivity angiitis, proliferative angiitis; obliterative endophlebitis or endarteritis

regression of the infection can be appreciated and classified as follows:

1. Tuberculoid leprosy
   A. Tuberculoid reactivation.
   B. Reactional tuberculoid (Akuter-Schub).
2. Borderline leprosy
   A. Tuberculoid borderline (BT).
   B. Typical borderline (BB).
   C. Borderline lepromatous (BL).
3. Lepromatous leprosy
   A. Acute lepromatous infiltration with or without ulceration of the skin or acute exacerbation (AE).
   B. Erythema nodosum leprosum.
   C. Lucio's phenomenon (necrotizing vasculitis).

The histopathologic picture of the reactional states (Table 16–9) reflects the clinical picture. The acute exacerbation of the present lesions with the associated appearance of new but similar lesions is seen in all types of leprosy (for example, in tuberculoid leprosy, the Akuter-Schub); the histopathology of these lesions reveals dermal and neural edema, endothelial swelling of the blood vessels, a cellular response of lymphocytes, and an increase in the bacterial index. In lepromatous leprosy, vasculitis of the allergic, necrotizing, and proliferative types is seen and is associated early with a polymorphonuclear infiltrate, even with abscess formation, and eosinophilic and mast cells; later, it is associated with lymphocytic and fibroblastic infiltration (Mabalay et al., 1965), and occasionally, especially in Lucio's phenomenon, with a wedge-shaped necrosis of the dermis. The histoid response presents with spindle-shaped histiocytes arranged in an interweaving pattern with large numbers of solid-staining bacilli and is seen in lepromatous leprosy in relapse due to drug resistance (Mansfield, 1969; Wade, 1963).

The most severe reactions tend to occur in those patients who have borderline leprosy, while in those with the polar groups, especially the tuberculoid, the reactions tend to be less severe. In patients with arrested disease, reversal reactions and erythema nodosum leprosum tend to develop.

In indeterminate (uncharacteristic) leprosy, no reactions are described because, when they appear, the disease has been transformed into one of the three major forms of leprosy. In tuberculoid leprosy in reaction, the plaques become bright red, thickened, and raised, with well-marked margins, scaling, and occasional ulceration. The involved nerves become swollen, thickened, and very tender, with rare caseation that presents as a fluctuant swelling. A few smaller tuberculoid lesions may appear elsewhere. Some subsiding plaques initially clear centrally. The reactional tuberculoid leprosy, Akuter-Schub, consists of reactivation of initial, large, typical lesions, the appearance elsewhere of numerous, bright red, succulent, sharply defined papules and nodules, and aggravation of the involved nerves (Fig. 16–68). There may be an associated fever. During the reaction the lesions may harbor a few bacilli. The lepromin skin test becomes weaker. This can be a manifestation of the transition from indeterminate to tuberculoid leprosy.

Reactions that clinically, histologically, and immunologically move the patients toward the tuberculoid pole have been described as "reversal reactions" and those that move the patients toward the lepromatous pole have been described as "downgrading reactions." Reversal reactions occur in patients with BL and BB types of

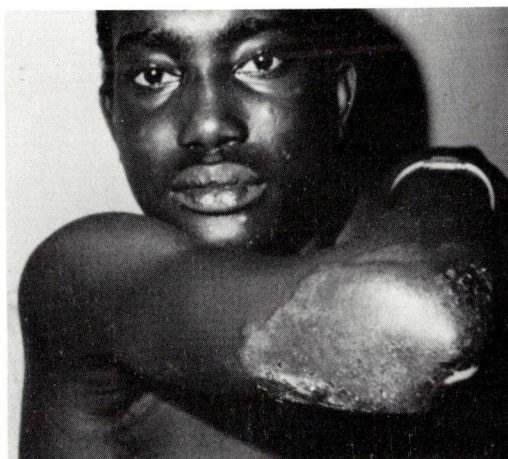

Figure 16–68 Tuberculoid leprosy in reaction characterized by acute edema and ulceration of the original anesthetic plaque with the appearance of distant new lesions of the face. There was also an acute swelling of the adjacent ulnar nerve with abscess formation.

disease when the number of bacilli is effectively reduced by therapy, and there is an associated increase of immunity. The downgrading reactions are seen in untreated patients in the BT and BB stages of leprosy who have an increase in the number of bacilli and a decline in immunity. The clinical features of borderline (Fig. 16–69) or near borderline reactions are characterized by erythema and edema of skin lesion that may become ulcerated. Severe involvement may be accompanied by fever, gross edema (face, hands, and feet), and nerve involvement. The extent and duration of skin and nerve involvement are greater than in tuberculoid leprosy because of the more widespread involvement.

Acute lepromatous infiltration occurs as a sudden exacerbation and a rapid extension of preexisting lepromatous lesions. There may be an acute, diffuse, erythematous thickening of skin and an aggravation of plaques and nodules, especially on the face, ears, and extremities. Multiple ulcerations in the center of the lepromatous plaques and nodules may occur with little systemic disturbance (Karat et al., 1967).

There is a variety of leprosy in which the so-called histoid lepromas are seen (Chaudhury, 1971; Rodriguez, 1969). When these lesions are many and of sudden onset (eruptive), the eruption can be described as a type of reaction and is a highly active process (Fig. 16–70). Although the histoid lepromas are seen

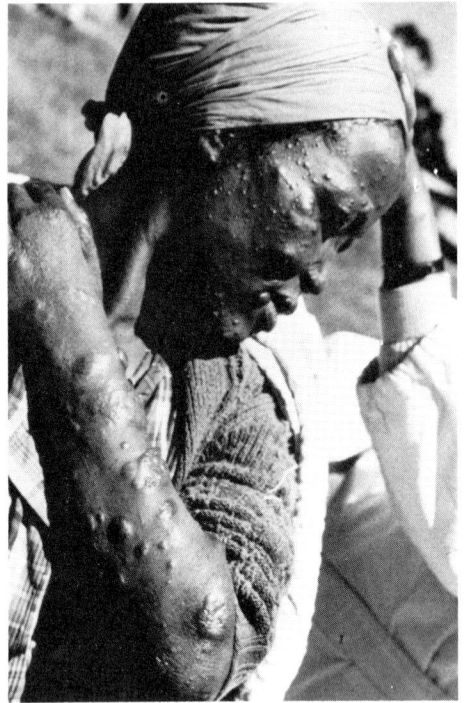

Figure 16–70 After 15 years of intermittent treatment with sulfones for lepromatous leprosy, the patient experienced the acute appearance of new nodules and plaques with significant increase of intact acid-fast organisms that were resistant to maximum doses of sulfones; an instance of resistant lepromatous leprosy.

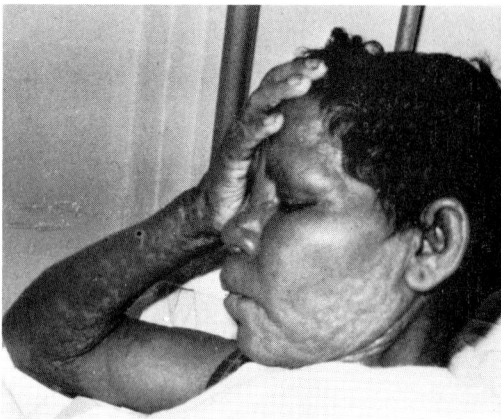

Figure 16–69 Borderline leprosy in reaction with acute inflammation and edema of the lesions of the face and extremities.

mainly in lepromatous leprosy which has become resistant to sulfone therapy, they may occur in relapsed and untreated cases of borderline and lepromatous leprosy. They are called histoid lepromas because they consist histologically of spindle-shaped histiocytes arranged in intervening patterns with the longer appearing acid-fast bacilli aligned both intracellularly and extracellularly along the long axis of these cells; the bacilli may appear in bundles but may rarely appear as globi. The clinical lesions of this type of leprosy are the classic histoid leproma, the soft histoid leproma (Rodriguez, 1969), and the subcutaneous nodules. The classic and most common lesion is the erythematous, shiny, smooth, hemispheric papule with slight constriction around its base. The soft nodules are flatter, less defined, and may coalesce. The subcutaneous nodules vary from 1 to 3 cm. in diameter and are usually firm and nontender; however, they may suppurate, ulcerate, and drain. The lesions tend to be located around the joints of the extremities, especially the elbows and wrists, and the trunk can be involved in the more extensive eruptions. The lesions respond to treatment but can persist in resistant and untreated cases. The epidemiologic significance of this type of leprosy is very important and is being examined.

Erythema nodosum leprosum (ENL) is seen most commonly in lepromatous leprosy (Fig. 16–71) and rarely in BL leprosy. This type of reaction occurs later in treatment when the ratio of the dead (fragmented and granular) bacilli to the viable (whole and intact) bacilli is greatly increased. It may be precipitated by physical or emotional stress, intercurrent infections, vaccination, and pregnancy, especially immediately postpartum (Pettit and Waters, 1967). It is characterized by the appearance of few or many erythematous, tender nodules or plaques, 1 to 5 cm. in diameter, that are widely distributed but predominate on the extremities and face. The eruption can at times present as a polymorphous erythema and rarely as a vesicular or bullous eruption with hemorrhage, ulcerations, or pustules, or as a panniculitis with or without suppuration.

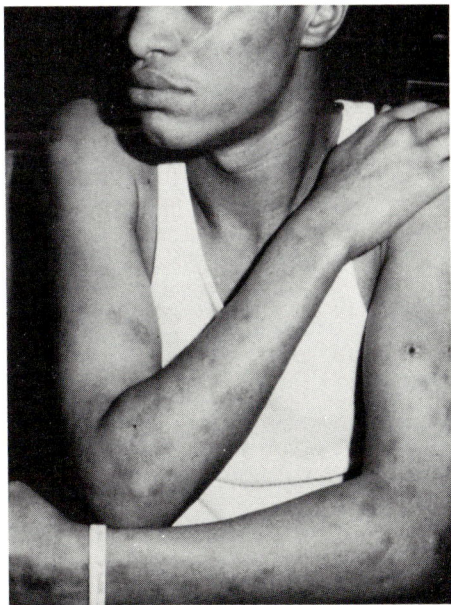

Figure 16–71 A patient with diffuse lepromatous leprosy experiencing erythema nodosum leprosum.

The individual lesions last a few days to a week, but crops of lesions may continue to appear for weeks, months, and, rarely, years. Patients with the more severe disease have fever up to 105° F., chills, generalized malaise, painful nerve swelling, peripheral edema, myalgia, arthralgia or arthritis, dactylitis (Fig. 16–72), bone pain, especially of the tibia, mental depression, and skin lesions that tend to become necrotic or ulcerative. Iridocyclitis, epistaxis, hoarseness or laryngeal stridor, mastitis, orchitis, lymphadenitis, and hepatosplenomegaly may be a part of the reaction. Leukocytosis is present, and cryoproteinemia (Matthews and Trautman, 1965) has been described. In the subacute but more often in the chronic reactive state, although the erythema nodosum–like lesions continue to be seen, small, violaceous or erythematous, subcutaneous lepromatous nodules (chronic nodular panniculitis) appear and coalesce to form infiltrative plaques, which become fixed to underlying tissue, feel leathery, and tend to ulcerate. These skin changes are associated with aggravation and accentuation of neural, mucosal, and osseous involvement. This phase of reaction, the so-called progressive lepra reaction, is very resistant to therapy and results in a worsening of the lepromatous process and a deterioration of the patient's condition; death may result from physical stress and debilitation, intercurrent infection, or secondary amyloidosis.

Lucio's phenomenon (erythema necroticans, Fig. 16–73) is a special type of reaction that is seen most frequently in Latin American countries (Moschella, 1966). The patients have diffuse infiltration of the skin which has a shiny, waxy appearance and is best appreciated only by touch. In the early stages, the face (la lepra bonita), hands, and feet may have a myxedematous appearance; later, the skin of the hands and feet usually becomes atrophic and ichthyotic. There is a slow, progressive loss of eyebrows, eyelashes, and, later, all the body hair. The scalp hair usually remains intact. Telangiectases may occur on the face and trunk. A severe, destructive rhinitis is usually present. There is anhidrosis of the involved skin. Numbness of the extremities is a frequent complaint.

When Lucio's phenomenon occurs, it does so about three to four years after the first manifestation of this subtype of lepromatous leprosy. Early in the reaction, the lesions tend to be few, but later they become more numerous. They are erythematous, slightly infiltrated, tender, irregularly shaped, often triangular, and measure from 1 to 5 cm. in diameter. They often appear on the body in a certain pattern, first the feet, then the legs, hands, thighs, buttocks, arms, trunk, and, rarely, the face. They have a central necrosis with or without antecedent blistering. The eschar may be shed, revealing a superficial or sometimes deep ulceration and healing with scar formation. The resultant scars are usually superficial (the "cigarette-paper" or "onion-skin" type), but occasionally they may be thick and radiating. Because the lesions appear in crops, all stages of clinical evolution are appreciated. Healing of a lesion usually occurs within two to four weeks. If patients with Lucio's phenomenon are given a lepromin skin test, they usually have an intensive local skin reaction (the Medina-Ramirez reaction), which occurs within four to six hours, persists for days, and is a reproduction of a diminutive lesion of Lucio's phenomenon.

The clinical differential diagnoses of reactive states include those conditions associated with edematous cutaneous lesions, angioedema, and cellulitis; those associated with various erythemas, serum sickness, erythema multiforme, and erythema nodosum; those associated with vesicular, bullous, and pustular lesions, erythema multiforme bullosum, dermatitis

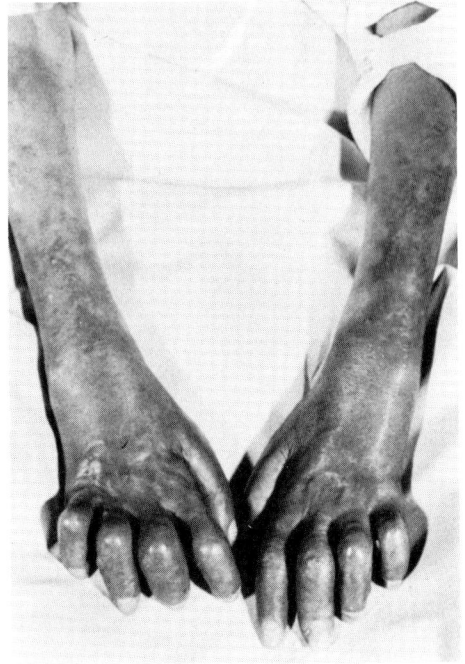

Figure 16-72 Acute dactylitis of erythema nodosum leprosum in a patient with lepromatous leprosy.

herpetiformis, varicella, rickettsialpox, pustular psoriasis, and subcorneal pustular dermatosis; those associated with "palpable" purpura and purpuric papules and nodules, Schoenlein-Henoch purpura, pityriasis lichenoides et varioliformis acuta, cutaneous allergic vasculitis (Ruiter), erythema elevatum diutinum, and diseases with dysproteinemia; those conditions resembling connective tissue syndromes, rheumatoid arthritis, systemic

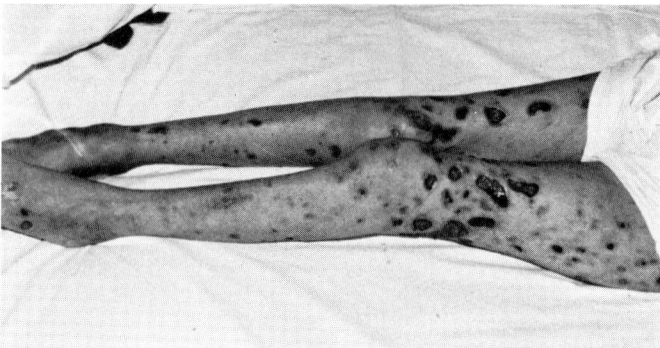

Figure 16-73 Lucio phenomenon (erythema necroticans) in a woman with diffuse lepromatous leprosy.

lupus erythematosus, scleroderma, and periarteritis nodosa; those associated with panniculitis, panniculitis secondary to other infections, malignancy, vasculitis, pancreatic disease, and Weber-Christian disease; and those associated with necrotic ulceration, ecthyma, pyoderma, ecthyma gangrenosum, ischemic ulcerations caused by underlying vasculitis, dysproteinemic syndromes, intravascular coagulopathy, deep mycoses, gummatous lesions, lymphoma cutis, and factitia.

Therapy

There is no satisfactory therapy; all the drugs used, except rifampin, are bacteriostatic. The search for a cure is limited because of the lack of an easy and practical method for cultivation and the present inability to infect easily available animals satisfactorily with the bacilli. The use of drugs effective against other pathogenic mycobacterial infections, for example, isoniazid (INH), has been disappointing. The current clinical factor used to appraise the effectiveness of a drug is the ability of the drug to affect the bacterial and morphologic indexes and to precipitate a lepra reaction (Shepard and Chang, 1964).

Originally, the more expensive parent sulfones, for example, glucosulfone (Promin), sulfoxone (Diasone), and Sulphetrone, were used because they were believed to produce less toxicity; however, when the parent substance DDS (4,4′-diaminodiphenylsulfone, DADDS [diacetyl DDS]) was found useful in a lower dosage, it became the drug of choice, since it can be given orally, parenterally, or depotwise, is inexpensive, and is easy to obtain (Levy, 1967). The basic philosophy in therapy is to start with a small dose and to maintain the smallest amount necessary. Presently, study trials of low doses are being investigated in an attempt to appraise their therapeutic efficacy and effect on the reaction rate, but the possibility of promoting the emergence of a resistant organism is not being ignored.

For patients who cannot be trusted to take medication or for logistic reasons, parenterally administered DDS in the form of an acetyl derivative (DADDS) is being used (Shepard et al., 1968). The amount and duration of treatment depend on the type and state (uncomplicated or reactive) of the leprosy. Treatment of indeterminate and tuberculoid leprosy consists initially of DDS, 25 mg. for four weeks, followed by 50 mg. a week for four weeks, then 100 mg. twice a week until the disease has become inactive, and finally 100 mg. a week for two years. Patients with dimorphous leprosy should initially be given 25 mg. twice a week for four weeks, followed by 50 mg. twice a week for four weeks, 100 mg. twice a week for four weeks, and then 100 mg. three to four times a week until the disease is inactive, at which time the dose can be reduced to 100 mg. twice a week for 10 years. In lepromatous leprosy, the initial treatment is similar to borderline leprosy except, if the dose of 100 mg. three to four times a week is well tolerated, the amount taken can gradually be increased over the next two months to 600 mg. a week; after the lepromatous type becomes inactive, the dose can be reduced to 100 mg. twice a week for life. The adverse reactions to the sulfones are gastrointestinal intolerance, hemolytic anemia, methemoglobinemia, agranulocytosis, hepatitis, neuritis, psychosis, and skin eruptions. The rashes described have been fixed drug eruption, erythema multiforme, including Stevens-Johnson syndrome, and toxic epidermal necrolysis.

In the event of an adverse drug reaction or resistance to DDS, the alternative drugs are B-663 (Lampren) and rifampin, and if intolerance or toxicity to either develops, thiambutosine (Ciba 1906, DPT), streptomycin with or without INH, ethambutol (Myambutol), and cycloserine may be tried.

The phenazine compound known as B-663 (Lampren) is a rimino compound that uniquely benefits not only the clinical and bacteriologic picture but also the reactive leprosy because of its anti-inflammatory property (Waters, 1969). It is believed to be therapeutically comparable to DDS, less likely to precipitate a lepra reaction, and is especially effective against ENL and acute leprous neuritis. In uncomplicated leprosy, B-663, 100 mg. three times a week, is recommended, and in sulfone-resistant leprosy, 100 mg. six times a week is given. In reactive leprosy, including ENL, B-663, 200 mg. three times a week, is prescribed for three weeks, and if there is no response, the dose is raised 100 mg. a day each week but should not exceed 600 mg. a day. In general, the maximum dose required is 400 mg. a day. When attempting to cut the dose, a reduction of 50 mg. a day at three-week intervals is advocated. In the chronic reaction that is being controlled by the combination of steroid and B-663, the steroid dosage should be cut gradually after a month of stability, and if a relapse should occur, it should be treated by raising only the dose of B-663. The side effects of B-663 therapy include upper gastrointestinal distress, cutaneous pigmentation, xeroderma and ichthyotic eruptions, and pruritus. After about three months of therapy, the skin becomes pink to red and later slate gray over the areas of maximal leprous involvement. The pigmentation is more appreciable in light-skinned patients. The red-brown color disappears in about six months and the darker patches a year after the cessation of therapy.

Rifampin, 600 mg. per day by mouth, is being evaluated as a first-line drug. Thiambutosine (4-butoxy-4'-dimethyl-amino-N, N-diphenylthiourea, known also as Ciba 1906 or DPT) is effective in all types of leprosy; a dose of 0.5 gm. is taken orally and is gradually increased to 3 gm. daily — the maximal dose. It is capable of producing reactions but less frequently than DDS. Two drawbacks to its use are the appearance of drug resistance after prolonged treatment (about two years) and its relatively high cost. When streptomycin with or without INH or ethambutol is used, it should be prescribed as for tuberculosis. Cycloserine is effective; the maximal daily dose is 1 gm., but its usefulness is limited because of its potential toxicity and high cost. Because of the development of resistance, the secondary drugs (thiambutosine, streptomycin, ethambutol, and cycloserine) are only temporarily effective. Cyclic drug therapy is advocated, with each course lasting less than two years.

In tuberculoid and borderline leprosy in reaction, fever and constitutional symptoms are unusual. The important complication to be treated is damage to motor nerves. If the problem is painful, edematous, or ulcerative skin lesions only, the dose of DDS should temporarily be reduced or discontinued. However, at the first sign of accompanying or aggravating motor nerve damage, DDS should be discontinued and systemic corticosteroid therapy initiated. If there is solitary nerve involvement, intraneural corticosteroid injections may be tried in lieu of systemic steroid. After the exacerbation has subsided completely, the dose of DDS should be raised slowly over a six-month period. As in all types of reactions, a precipitant cause, such as another infection, should be searched for.

Management of erythema nodosum leprosum depends on its severity. For mild cases, the patients may be treated with large doses of aspirin, indomethacin (Indocin), or antimalarials in the above sequence while continuing DDS. In moderately severe cases, if none of the forementioned measures is helpful, a course of trivalent organic antimony compounds, such as stibophen, is recommended. Stibophen, 2 to 3 cc., is given intramuscularly every other day for six to eight injections; a second course can be given if necessary after an interval of six weeks. Severe or chronic erythema nodosum should be treated preferably with thalidomide, or B-663, or systemic corticosteroids with reduced dose of DDS. Antimetabolites, such as azathioprine (Imuran) and methotrexate, are of questionable efficacy.

Thalidomide appears to be the most effective agent with the fewest side effects for ENL (Sheskin and Convit, 1969); B-663 is not as rapidly effective and has the unpleasant complication of cutaneous pigmentation; and systemic corticosteroid therapy is used hesitatingly because of the usually required prolonged therapy with its unfavorable side effects and the tendency toward relapse upon its discontinuance.

Thalidomide has not been useful in the reactions of tuberculoid and borderline leprosy. DDS can be continued during thalidomide therapy, which has no antileprosy effect. The clinical response and blood sedimentation rate are the criteria used to adjust dosage. Effective therapy results in defervescence, clearing of reactive skin lesions, and improvement of neuritis. The thalidomide dose is 400 mg. a day until the reactional syndrome is controlled; it is gradually reduced until

50 mg. a day, as a maintenance dose, is reached. The side effects during therapy are drowsiness, dizziness, and constipation; fortunately, the neuropathy reported in other treated conditions has not been appreciated in leprosy. Because of its teratogenic effect, a contraceptive should be prescribed.

Unfortunately, systemically administered corticosteroids are the only effective drugs available for the treatment of Lucio's phenomenon. Specific antileprosy medication probably should be discontinued during this type of reaction.

Leprosy is best controlled by treating the infected and following up closely the contacts. BCG vaccination, DDS, and their combination are being evaluated as to their prophylactic value (Bechelli et al., 1970; Long, 1969). The oral prophylactic dose of DDS is 10 mg. a week for each year of age, with a maximum of 150 mg. a week.

GRANULOMATOUS VASCULITIDES

Granuloma Faciale

Granuloma faciale (Johnson et al., 1959) is a chronic, indolent, therapeutically resistant dermatosis whose diagnosis is based on histologic findings. The etiology is unknown. There are no associated or underlying systemic lesions. Both sexes are affected. Although middle-aged and elderly persons are most often affected, it may be seen in children. Negroes do not seem to be afflicted. Sunlight and heat can aggravate the eruption. It is a slowly progressive eruption that remains periodically static.

Pathology

There is a subepidermal grenz zone. Eosinophils and polymorphonuclear cells predominate early in the granulomatous infiltrate; later, lymphocytes, plasma and mast cells, and fibroblasts are found. The adnexa are spared. Significant but not constant changes seen are fragmentation of polymorphonuclear cells and perivascular acidophilic material (not in the blood vessel walls as in erythema elevatum diutinum). The differential microscopic diagnoses include erythema elevatum diutinum, histiocytosis X, and syphilis.

Clinical Manifestations

The lesions of granuloma faciale tend to be single but may be multiple (Fig. 16–74). They begin as red, circumscribed macules that become raised and nodular, vary in size from a few millimeters to 8 cm., and can gradually cover large areas of the face. The lesions have an exaggeration of their follicular orifices and feel soft or moderately firm. The eruption usually appears on the nose, malar prominences, forehead, preauricular areas, and chin but has been described on the back of the trunk and

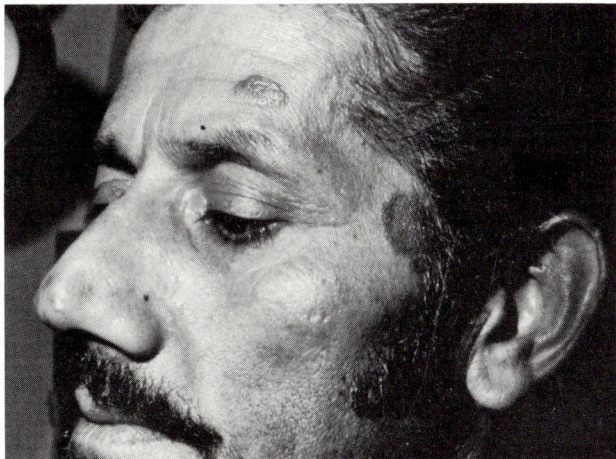

Figure 16–74 Cutaneous granulomatous vasculitis (granuloma faciale). Asymptomatic brown plaques of the face showed improvement with intralesional corticosteroid therapy.

hands. Patients are usually asymptomatic, but some may complain of itching, burning, stinging, and tenderness. The lesions rarely ulcerate or resolve spontaneously. The differential clinical diagnoses include sarcoidosis, lupus erythematosus, mycosis fungoides, benign lymphocytic infiltration of the skin, lymphoma, polymorphous light eruption, fixed drug eruption, and leprosy.

Treatment

The eruption is usually resistant to therapy. Roentgen therapy and antimalarials are ineffective. In some patients, the disease has been improved by cryotherapy and in others the disease has cleared completely when intralesional corticosteroid therapy was given. Surgical excision and graft have been advocated by some, but recurrences have been observed in the sites.

Erythema Elevatum Diutinum

Erythema elevatum diutinum (Haber, 1955; Mraz and Newcomer, 1967) is a rare, chronic, cutaneous disease that is listed among the chronic, small vessel, cutaneous vasculitides of unknown etiology.

Histopathology

The early histopathologic changes are a widespread endothelial swelling of small blood vessels, a deposition of eosinophilic fibrinoid (so-called toxic hyalin) material around and within blood vessels, and an infiltrate consisting mainly of neutrophils, variable amounts of lymphocytes and histiocytes, and a few eosinophils and plasma cells. There may be leukocytoclasis (fragmentation of neutrophilic nuclei, the so-called nuclear dust). A fibroproliferative response occurs later. Extracellular cholesterosis, regarded as a rare variant of erythema elevatum diutinum, differs histologically from the latter by the deposition of free and esterified cholesterol extracellularly between the collagen bundles. Foam or giant cells are absent.

Clinical Manifestations

This chronic disease affects persons between the ages of 30 and 60 years; the youngest reported patient is five years of age (Winston, 1964), and the oldest is 64 years. The sex incidence is equal. The disease tends to appear earlier in women. An associated recurrent polyarthritis has been recorded. The eruption is characterized by symmetric acral nodules and plaques which may occur singly or together. They are grouped in the neighborhood of the small and large joints and appear mainly on the hands, fingers, wrists, elbows, ankles, toes, Achilles tendons, and, less frequently, on the buttocks, nose, ears (Fig. 16–75), and penis; the trunk is usually spared. The lesions are generally oval but may be irregular, gyrate, or annular. Their color is red, but they may be yellow or ivory. Superficial scaling and purpura have been noted. The lesions may vary in size during the day. They may reappear in former sites after disappearing completely. Residual pigmentation with or without slight atrophy is seen. Verrucoid plaques and nodules may appear over the bony prominences of the extremities, ulcerate, and discharge material; this is the clinical picture of a described variant of erythema elevatum diutinum, the so-called extracellular cholesterosis (Fig. 16–76).

The differential diagnoses are lymph-

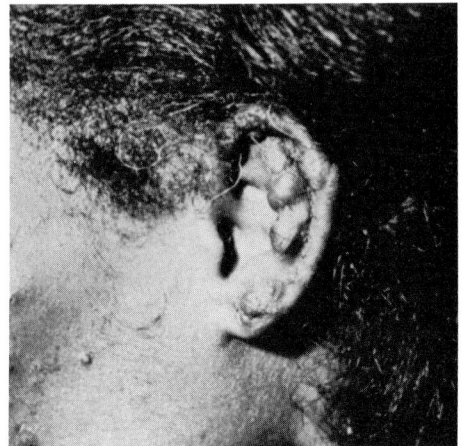

Figure 16–75 Cutaneous granulomatous vasculitis (erythema elevatum diutinum). Erythematous nodules of the ears, fingers, elbows, knees, and toes were present in this black woman.

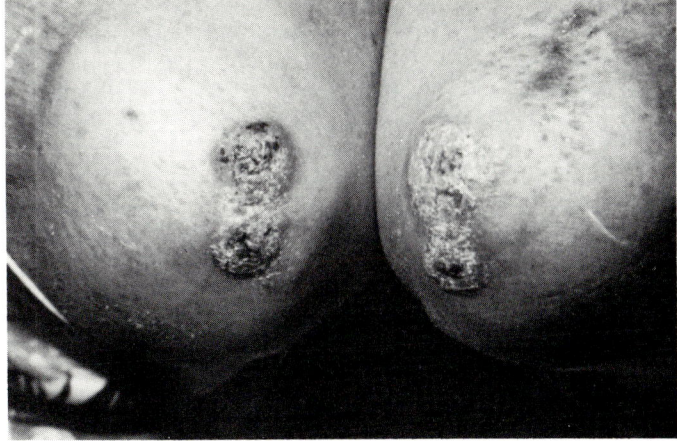

Figure 16–76 Cutaneous granulomatous vasculitis (erythema elevatum diutinum). Verrucoid nodules and plaques were present on the elbows, knees, and plantar aspect of the feet; the lesions, on histopathologic examination, revealed intracellular and extracellular cholesterosis.

oma cutis, mycosis fungoides, idiopathic hemorrhagic Kaposi's sarcoma, granuloma annulare, sarcoidosis, leprosy, tophaceous gout, and xanthoma tuberosum.

Treatment

The disease tends to be chronic and progressive over a period of 5 to 10 years and eventually tends to resolve spontaneously. No effective treatment has been reported. Systemically administered antimalarials and topically and intralesionally applied corticosteroids have been unsuccessful. For cosmetic or physical reasons, surgical excision of lesions may be attempted.

Granulomatous Arteritis

The term granulomatous arteritis (pathergic granulomatosis, noninfectious necrotizing granulomatosis) is used to describe a group of diseases that are characterized histologically by a necrotizing angiitis of medium-sized and small-sized arteries with vascular and extravascular granulomas. This group includes allergic granulomatosis (Churg and Strauss, 1951), Wegener's granulomatosis, cranial arteritis (giant cell arteritis), and Takayasu's arteriopathy. Because of the resemblance of these conditions to periarteritis nodosa, they have been described as variants or atypical expressions of periarteritis nodosa. At the present stage of our knowledge,

however, there is sufficient clinical and histologic evidence to respect them as separate entities. Among other unrelated conditions characterized by a vasculitis and granuloma formation are the various nodular vasculitides of the lower extremities, the necrotizing eosinophilic granulomatosis, and the rare association of granulomatous disease with hypogammaglobulinemia.

Necrotizing eosinophilic granulomatosis (Fossgreen, 1962) is a disease of the reticuloendothelial system with features characteristic of the allergic vasculitides and granulomatosis. The absence of Sternberg-Reed cells and other anaplastic features differentiates it respectively from Hodgkin's disease and malignant reticulosis. This disease reportedly evolves stepwise into a more obvious malignant lymphoma and an ultimate leukemic reticulosis (Lupovitch et al., 1965).

Vigorous corticosteroid therapy is generally advocated early for this group of granulomatous arteritides, and if no significant improvement occurs, a trial of alkylating agents or immunosuppressants is recommended.

Allergic Granulomatosis

Allergic granulomatosis (Churg and Strauss, 1951; Sokolov et al., 1962), which has protean systemic manifestations, occurs at any age and more commonly in women than in men. Two basic histopathologic lesions are appreciated: necrosis and granulomatous infiltration of the wall of medium-sized and small-sized vessels, and extravascular granuloma, consisting of fibrinoid degeneration of the infarcted collagen with eosinophils and epithelioid and giant cells. Patients may have hay fever and a history of drug sensitivity. They have fever, a significant eosinophilia, and a long history of asthma. Recurrent episodes of pneumonia with the clinical and roentgenographic characteristics of the Löffler's type occur. The cutaneous lesions are erythema multiforme, palpable purpura, and hemorrhagic and necrotic (Fig. 16–77), as well as subcutaneous, nodules. There may be gastrointestinal, central and peripheral nervous system, as well as renal, involvement. With the appearance of systemic manifestations, the patients survive three months to five years; the majority usually die in one to two years. Cardiac failure and cerebral hemorrhage are the most common causes of death. Systemic corticosteroid therapy has been lifesaving and has helped arrest the fulminating diffuse vasculitis.

Wegener's Granulomatosis

Wegener's granulomatosis (Mills, 1965; Tuhy et al., 1958) is a rare and fatal disease characterized by necrotizing granulomas of the upper or lower respiratory tract, generalized necrotizing angiitis of arteries and veins, and focal or diffuse necrotizing glomerulonephritis. It differs histopathologically from periarteritis nodosa by the presence of necrotizing vasculitis not only of medium-sized arteries but also of smaller blood vessels and by the presence of confluent areas of necrosis surrounded by granulation tissue (necrotizing granulomas). A history of atopy is usually not elicited. The onset of the disease is between 25 and 55 years of age, mainly in the fourth and fifth decades. Males predominate. The patients have fever and malaise. Wegener's granulomatosis presents usually and initially with upper respiratory tract involvement accompanied by rhinorrhea, epistaxis, nasal obstruction, and resistant sinusitis. The necrotic ulcerative process of the nasopharynx is consistent with one of the types of midline lethal granuloma (Fig. 16–78). Pulmonary involvement is characterized by cough, hemoptysis, and pleuritic pain. Roentgenologically, nodules, diffuse infiltration, or thick-walled cavities which are misinterpreted as being metastatic disease or infectious granulomas are seen. Any organ may be involved. Arthritis occurs. The cutaneous manifestations (Reed et al., 1963) are urticaria, polymorphous erythemas, vesicular and papulonecrotic eruptions, and pyoderma gangrenosum (Fig. 16–79). Buccal ulcerations are frequently seen. Renal failure, which is the most frequent cause of death, occurs usually within five months of the diagnosis of the disease. Scattered reports have appeared of survivals of 8 to 12 years without any therapy in the limited forms of Wegener's granulomatosis (Cassan et al., 1970).

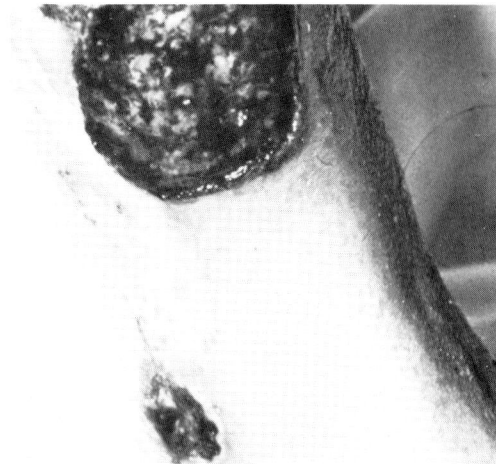

Figure 16–77 Systemic granulomatous vasculitis (allergic granulomatosis). Large, generalized, sharply defined ulcerated plaques in a child with asthma.

Treatment

There is no specific treatment. For the localized granulomatous lesions of the head and neck, radiation therapy has produced a temporary regression of the disease process in some cases. For the more limited forms of this disease, corticosteroids have been helpful and have ap-

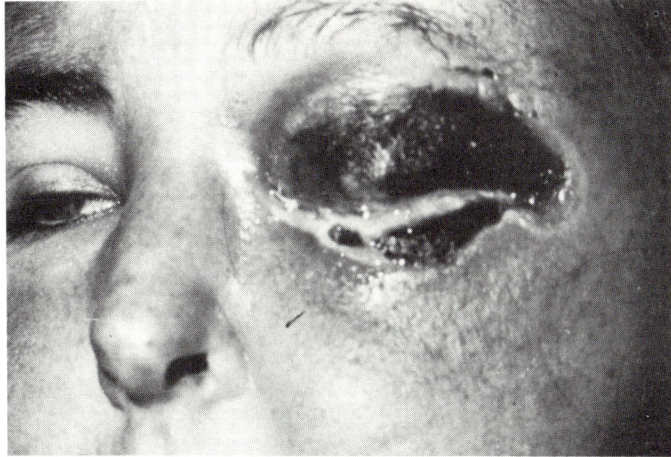

Figure 16–78 Systemic granulomatous vasculitis. Necrotizing destructive process of the nose and periorbital sinuses with extension to the orbit; this was reported as a midline lethal granuloma which may be a variant of Wegener's disease or eventuate into a lymphoma.

peared to prolong survival. Unfortunately, the glomerulitis is unaffected by steroids. Alkylating agents, chlorambucil (Leukeran), and nitrogen mustard have proved effective in some cases. Antimetabolites capable of immunosuppression and azathioprine (Imuran) with glutamine antagonist (Duazomycin A) have been reported as effective in advanced Wegener's granulomatosis with renal involvement (Aldo et al., 1970; Kaplan et al., 1968).

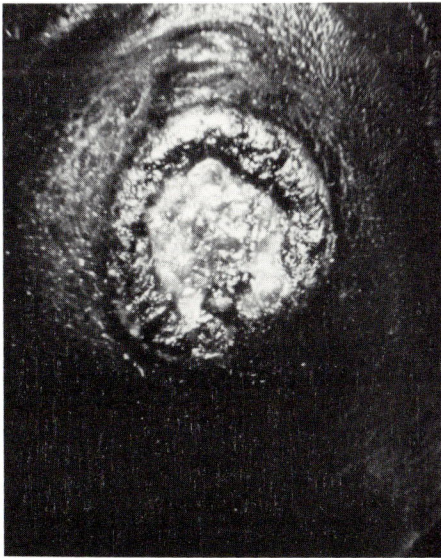

Figure 16–79 Systemic granulomatous vasculitis. Cutaneous expression of Wegener's disease; pulmonary nodulation with cavitation was present.

Midline Lethal Granuloma (Nonhealing Granuloma of the Nose)

Lethal midline granuloma is a clinical term used to describe a rapidly destructive process of the nose, paranasal sinuses, and facial tissues (Fig. 16–78). Among the midline diseases to be excluded are treponemal infections (syphilis, yaws, bejel), mycobacterial infections (tuberculosis, leprosy), sarcoidosis, mucocutaneous leishmaniasis, rhinosporidiosis, South American blastomycosis, phycomycosis, necrotizing fasciitis, noma, rhinoscleroma, myiasis, and basal cell carcinoma. After the described destructive granulomatous diseases and carcinoma are ruled out, three different clinicopathologic entities must be considered (Kassel et al., 1969). These include (1) midline malignant reticulosis (nonhealing granuloma of the nose, Stewart type); (2) Wegener's granulomatosis, which is usually a systemic disease and may present as a rhinogenic giant cell granuloma; and (3) a malignant lymphoma, usually reticulum cell sarcoma.

The nonhealing granuloma of the nose of the Stewart type begins initially as an indurated swelling of some part of the nose, becomes ulcerated, and progressively destroys soft tissue, cartilage, and bone. It may extend to involve the paranasal sinus, the orbit, oral cavity, pharynx, and even the brain. The overlying skin of the face or mucosa of the oral cavity or pharynx becomes necrotic, sloughs, and leaves a deep irregular ulcer. Histologically, there is a dense accumulation of pleomorphic cells, consisting predominantly of mature and immature lymphocytes with a sprinkling of bizarre reticulum cells. Necrosis is not limited to the ulcerated surface; a considerable part of the involved tissue reveals confluence of stellate areas of necrosis. Vascular thrombosis in the affected areas is responsible for the necrosis of soft tissue and bone. The disease tends to remain localized. Death usually results from secondary infection. If the patient lives long enough, this pleomorphic reticulosis eventuates into a malignant reticulosis or lymphoma (Eichel et al., 1966, 1968), or spread may occur. The five-year survival rate for patients with lethal midline granuloma treated with tumoricidal x-ray therapy has been significantly greater than for those with the lymphoma type. It has been suggested that steroids and alkylating or immunosuppressive agents may be relatively more effective in the Wegener's type (Raitt, 1971).

The nonhealing granuloma of the nose of the Wegener's type presents as a granulomatous disease of the upper respiratory tract with subsequent development of confluent, necrotic lesions of the lungs. The responsible necrotizing granulomatosis and angiitis further involve the systemic vasculature. The presence of multinucleated giant cells, although not pathognomonic, is helpful in the correct interpretation of the clinical picture. When the giant cells are close to vessels, the condition is distinguished from giant cell arteritis by the absence of breakdown of elastic tissue in the artery wall as seen in true giant cell arteritis. The destruction of tissue is not as extensive as in the Stewart type in which there is a greater tendency to involve cartilage and bone.

Giant Cell Arteritis (Temporal Arteritis, Cranial Arteritis, Polymyalgia Arteritica)

Giant cell arteritis (Meadows, 1966) is a widespread, granulomatous arteritis of large, medium, and small vessels, especially of the cranium; it is of unknown etiology and affects the elderly.

Histopathology

The disease is a necrotizing panarteritis with granuloma and giant cell formation. There is intimal thickening, fibrinoid necrosis and disruption of the elastic lamina by cellular infiltration of polymorphonucleocytes, histiocytes, and giant cells, as well as a patchy inflammatory exudate of lymphocytes and eosinophils and fibrosis of the adventitia.

Clinical Manifestations

The disease affects persons between the ages of 60 and 85 years, and the sex incidence is equal. Clinical signs and symptoms result from gradual arterial occlusion. Although the temporal (Fig. 16–80), occipital, and facial branches of the external carotid artery and ophthalmic branch of the internal carotid arteries are mainly affected, arteries of the brain, limbs, muscles, heart, and abdominal viscera may be involved.

Lassitude, weakness, vague muscle aches and pains, and depression are usually described. The acute clinical presentation is characterized by headache,

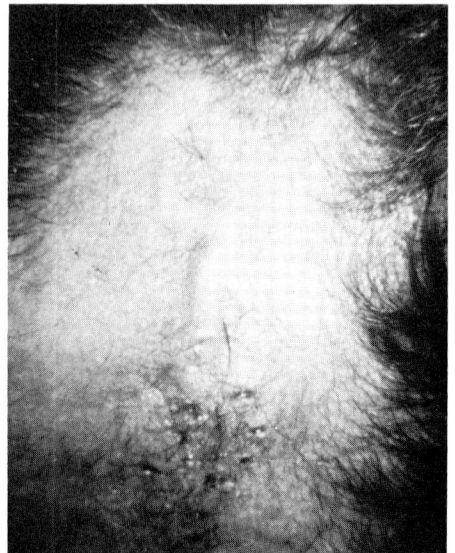

Figure 16–80 Systemic granulomatous vasculitis (temporal arteritis). Unilateral tenderness and prominence of the temporal artery; there were an associated polymyalgia rheumatica and a dramatic response to systemic corticosteroid therapy.

fever, glossitis, blindness (unilateral, bilateral, transient, partial), ophthalmoplegia, and deafness with or without pain and vertigo. The systemic lesions are polyarthritis, coronary occlusion, cerebral ischemia or stroke with mental changes, peripheral neuritis, and lymphadenopathy. There is frequently fever, elevated erythrocyte sedimentation rate, mild anemia, and polymorphonuclear leukocytosis. It has been reported that 40 per cent of patients with temporal arteritis will have polymyalgia rheumatica. The involved superficial temporal artery is swollen, nodular, and thick, has a diminution or loss of pulsation, and may rarely be associated with palpable purpura, hemorrhage, bullae, and necrotic ulcers of the scalp, which may be bilateral and massive, or of the anterior part of the tongue, or elsewhere (Kinmont and McCallum, 1964). The interval between the onset of headache and blindness is between one and three months and is unlikely to occur after six months. The disease is usually self-limiting and tends to burn itself out after months to a year or more. If death occurs, it may be the result of cerebral infarction, coronary occlusion, dissecting aneurysm, or a celiac or mesenteric thrombosis.

Treatment

As soon as the diagnosis is established, systemic steroids, initially in large doses (60 to 120 mg.), should be given, and when the disease process is controlled, as reflected by the clinical course and the erythrocyte sedimentation rate, the dose should be tapered gradually. A period of 6 to 12 months of therapy is usually required, with a maintenance dose of 10 to 20 mg. per day and adjunctive measures to reduce the side effects of prolonged steroid administration.

Takayasu's Arteriopathy (Aortic Arch Syndrome)

Takayasu's disease (Strachan, 1964), like temporal arteritis, is a rare granulomatous vasculitis and is one of the disorders of the so-called aortic arch syndromes, disorders resulting from the occlusion of the vessels arising from the arch of the aorta. It affects mostly women between 11 and 60 years of age. The clinical features are mainly the result of chronic hypoxia of the head and arms due to occlusion of the primary and secondary branches of the aortic arch. Two phases which have been described in this disease are the early systemic or prepulseless phase and the late occlusive or pulseless stage (Strachan, 1964). The signs and symptoms of the early systemic stage are fever, fatigue, cough, pleurisy with or without effusion, hemoptysis, pericarditis, polyarthralgia, arthritis, painful erythematous nodules of legs or ulcers, and Raynaud's phenomenon. The patients have a persistently elevated erythrocyte sedimentation rate, moderate anemia, and plasma protein abnormalities. During this prepulseless phase, the condition simulates systemic lupus erythematosus, rheumatoid arthritis, Still's disease, periarteritis nodosa, giant cell arteritis, and erythema nodosum.

The late phase is characterized by disorders resulting from vascular stenosis or occlusion of the aorta and its ocular, cerebral, abdominal, extremity, and myocardial branches. With limbal involvement, intermittent claudication, paresthesias, pallor, and gangrene are noted. In the middle aged and elderly, the condition resembles atherosclerosis. The patients die of heart disease. The life expectancy after onset is 1 to 15 years. Among the recommended treatments are systemic corticosteroids, long-term anticoagulation, and endarterectomy.

HALOGENODERMAS

Nodular, fungating, and papilliform cutaneous lesions have been induced by halogens (bromides, iodides, and, rarely, chlorides—Montgomery, 1967). They occur after prolonged ingestion and most frequently in adults, especially women. In infants, the lesions appear on the face as well as other areas and tend to be condylomiform. They may be carbuncle-like, the size of a nut, or flattened plaques with a cribriform surface with multiple, small but visible abscesses or pustules. The iododerma tends to be less verrucose and to ulcerate, and it may have an annular

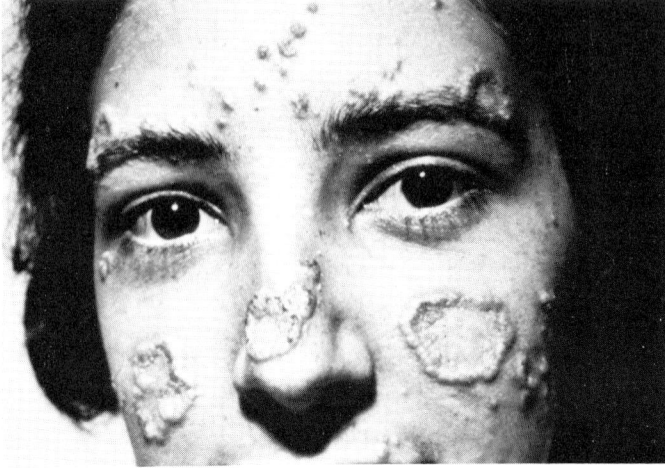

Figure 16–81 Halogenodermas. Patient had been taking iodides as adjunctive therapy for asthma. A pustular eruption of the face developed; some of these lesions were annular.

configuration (Fig. 16–81). The lesions may be few or numerous. In adults, the mucosa of the mouth and tongue may be involved and resemble the syphilitic gumma. They may be associated with other types of lesions; acneiform and vegetating lesions occur more frequently with bromism, and bullae more frequently with iodism. Löffler's syndrome has been associated with iododerma. The lesions may clinically resemble blastomycosis, pyoderma blastomycetica (Fig. 16–82), pemphigus vegetans, pyoderma gangrenosum, and mycosis fungoides.

The histopathologic picture is characterized by a papillomatosis or pseudoepitheliomatosis hyperplasia with intra-epidermal abscesses; iododerma shows less epithelial proliferation. The dermal infiltrate consists of neutrophils, lymphocytes, plasma cells, and histiocytes. In bromoderma, there may be numerous dermal neutrophils and abscesses. In iododermas, there may be many histiocytes, some of which may show mitotic figures and hyperchromic nuclei and resemble the histiocytes of mycosis fungoides. There is vascular proliferation with endothelial swelling. Features of allergic vasculitis, hemorrhage, hyaline changes in vessel walls, and disintegration of cells of infiltrate with varying degrees of nuclear dust may be seen.

If the lesions are few, they may be treated by topical or occlusive or intralesional corticosteroids or both; if nu-

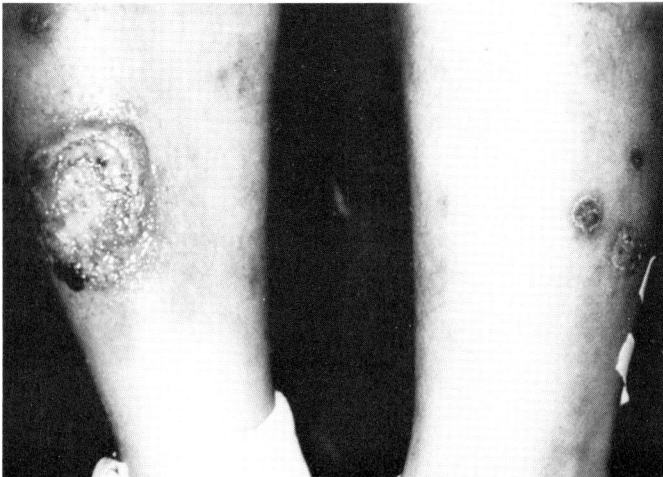

Figure 16–82 Halogenodermas. When bromides were used as a sedative, furunculoid lesions and a vegetative plaque of the lower extremities developed.

merous, systemic corticosteroids may be tried. The elimination of halogens is hastened by the daily administration of sodium or ammonium chloride.

OROCUTANEOUS CROHN'S DISEASE

Crohn's disease is a nonspecific, granulomatous, inflammatory condition mainly of the small bowel, especially the terminal ileum; any part of the gastrointestinal tract may become involved, however. Cutaneous (Mountain, 1970) or oral (Stankler et al., 1972) involvement by the disease process rarely occurs. The cutaneous lesions are perineal, parastomal, and metastatic and are characterized by florid granulation tissue surrounded by edematous, dusky red skin. The perineal lesion, which is the most common, may extend widely into the groin and even into the anterior abdominal wall. The parastomal ulceration is usually in continuity with the adjacent diseased bowel. The metastatic lesion is remote from the gastrointestinal tract, is separated from it by normal skin, and favors the intertriginous areas. The oral ulceration tends to be linear, with a cobblestone appearance. The diagnosis is based on the appearance and location of the lesions, the demonstration of the underlying bowel disease, and the presence of sarcoid granulomata in the histologic examination of the skin biopsy. Treatment consists locally of repeated curettage of the lesions, the necessary medical or surgical management or both of the adjacent bowel disease, and the use of systemic corticosteroids and immunosuppressants.

REFERENCES

Aldo, M. A., Benson, M. D., Comerford, F. R., et al.: Treatment of Wegener's granulomatosis with immunosuppressive agents. Description of renal ultrastructure. Arch. Intern. Med. *126*:298, 1970.

Allen, A. C.: Persistent "insect bites" (dermal eosinophilic granulomas) simulating lymphoblastomas, histiocytoses, and squamous cell carcinomas. Am. J. Pathol. *24*:367, 1948.

Altman, J., and Winkelmann, R. K.: Xanthoma disseminatum. Arch. Dermatol. *86*:582, 1962.

Balfour, H. H., Jr., Shehan, J. J., Speicher, C. E., et al.: Chronic granulomatous disease of childhood in a 23-year-old man. J.A.M.A. *217*:960, 1971.

Balzer, R. J., Destombes, P., Schaller, K. F., et al.: [Pseudolepromatous cutaneous leishmaniasis in Ethiopia.] Bull. Soc. Pathol. Exot. *53*:293, 1960.

Barrow, M. V., and Holubar, K.: Multicentric reticulohistiocytosis. A review of 33 patients. Medicine *48*:287, 1969.

Bechelli, L. M., Garbajosa, G., Uemura, K., et al.: BCG vaccination of children against leprosy. Bull. WHO *42*:235, 1970.

Cahill, K. M.: The human Trypanosomatidae. III. Leishmaniasis: Kala-azar. N. Y. State J. Med. *63*: 3405, 1963.

Caro, W. A., and Helwig, H. B.: Cutaneous lymphoid hyperplasia. Cancer *24*:487, 1969.

Cassan, S. M., Coles, D. T., and Harrison, E. G., Jr.: The concept of limited forms of Wegener's granulomatosis. Am. J. Med. *49*:366, 1970.

Chapman, J. S.: Atypical mycobacterial infections; pathogenesis, clinical manifestations, and treatment. Med. Clin. North Am. *51*:503, 1967.

Chatterji, S. N.: Neural affections in leprosy and their diagnosis, pathology, and treatment. Int. J. Lepr. *5*:329, 1937.

Chaudhury, D. S., Chaudhury, M., and Armah, K.: Histoid variety of lepromatous leprosy. Lepr. Rev. *42*:203, 1971.

Churg, J., and Strauss, L.: Allergic granulomatosis, allergic angiitis, and periarteritis nodosa. Am. J. Pathol. *27*:277, 1951.

Cochrane, R. G., and Davey, F. T., (eds).: Leprosy in Theory and Practice. 2nd ed. Baltimore, Williams & Wilkins Co., 1964, 660 pp.

Connor, D. H., and Lunn, H. F.: Buruli ulceration. A clinicopathologic study of 38 Ugandans with Mycobacterium ulcerans ulceration. Arch. Pathol. *81*: 183, 1966.

Convit, J., and Kerdel-Vegas, F.: Disseminated cutaneous leishmaniasis; inoculations to laboratory animals, electron microscopy and fluorescent antibodies studies. Arch. Dermatol. *91*:439, 1965.

Cowdell, R. H.: Sarcoidosis, with special reference to diagnosis and prognosis. Q. J. Med. *23*:29, 1954.

Dostrovsky, A., and Sagher, F.: Dermatological complications of B.C.G. vaccination. Br. J. Dermatol. *75*:181, 1963.

Dowling, G. B., and Jones, E.: Atypical (annular) necrobiosis lipoidica of the face and scalp. A report of the clinical and histological features of 7 cases. Dermatologica *135*:11, 1967.

Dowling, G. B., and Wetherley-Mein, G.: In MacKenna, R. M. B., (ed.): Modern Trends in Dermatology. 2nd ed. London, Butterworth, 1954, p. 111.

Dykman, C. J., Galens, G. J., and Good, A. E.: Linear subcutaneous bands in rheumatoid arthritis: an unusual form of rheumatoid granuloma. Ann. Intern. Med. *63*:134, 1965.

Eichel, B. S., and Mabery, T.: The enigma of the lethal midline granuloma. Laryngoscope *78*:1367, 1968.

Eichel, B. S., Harrison, E. G., Jr., Devine, K. D., et al.: Primary lymphoma of the nose including a relationship to lethal midline granuloma. Am. J. Surg. *112*:597, 1966.

Epstein, W. L.: Granulomatous hypersensitivity. Progr. Allergy *11*:36, 1967.

Faust, E. C., and Russell, P. F.: Craig and Faust's Clinical Parasitology. 7th ed. Philadelphia, Lea and Febiger, 1964, pp. 104–130.

Forbus, W. D.: Granulomatous inflammation—a clinical and pathologic challenge. Am. J. Clin. Pathol. *25*:427, 1955.

Fossgreen, J.: Eosinophilic granulomatosis. An unusual case with changes in the intestines, mesenteric lymph nodes, ovaries, bladder and heart. Acta Pathol. Microbiol. Scand. 56:143, 1962.

Friedmann, I.: The pathology of midline granuloma. Proc. R. Soc. Med. 57:289, 1964.

Goldman, L.: Types of American cutaneous leishmaniasis-dermatological aspects; review. Am. J. Trop. Med. Hyg. 27:561, 1947.

Grzybowski, S.: Chemoprophylaxis of tuberculosis. Clin. Notes Resp. Dis. 5:3, 1967.

Guinto, R. S., and Binford, C. H.: Leprosy. MB-10, Dept. of Medicine and Surgery, Veterans Administration, Washington, D.C., 1965.

Haber, H.: Erythema elevatum diutinum. Br. J. Dermatol. 67:121, 1955.

Halprin, K. M., and Lorincz, A. L.: Disseminated xanthosiderohistiocytosis (xanthoma disseminatum). Report of a case and discussion of possible relationships to other disorders showing histiocytic proliferation. Arch. Dermatol. 82:171, 1960.

Hanauer, L. B.: Reticulohistiocytosis remission after cyclophosphamide therapy. Arthritis Rheum. 15:636, 1972.

Hastings, R. C., Brand, P. W., Mansfield, R. E., et al.: Bacterial density in the skin in lepromatous leprosy as related to temperature. Lepr. Rev. 39:71, 1968.

Helwig, E. B., and Hackney, V. C.: Juvenile xanthogranuloma (nevoxantho-endothelioma). Am. J. Pathol. 30:625, 1954.

Hunder, G. G., Disney, T. F., and Ward, L. E.: Polymyalgia rheumatica. Mayo Clin. Proc. 44:849, 1969.

James, D. G.: Dermatological aspects of sarcoidosis. Q. J. Med. 28:108, 1959.

Jandl, J. H.: The spleen and reticuloendothelial system. *In* Sodeman, W. A., and Sodeman, W. A., Jr.: Pathologic Physiology: Mechanisms of Disease. 4th ed., Philadelphia, W. B. Saunders Co., 1967, pp. 897–932.

Jessner, M., and Kanof, N. B.: Lymphocytic infiltration of the skin. Arch. Dermatol. 68:447, 1953.

Johnson, W. C., Higdon, R. S., and Helwig, E. B.: Granuloma faciale. Arch. Dermatol. 79:42, 1959.

Johnston, R. F., and Hopewell, P. C.: Chemotherapy of pulmonary tuberculosis. Ann. Intern. Med. 70:359, 1969.

Jones, E. W., and Bleehen, S. S.: Inflammatory angiomatous nodules with abnormal blood vessels occurring about the ears and scalp (pseudo or atypical pyogenic granuloma). Br. J. Dermatol. 81:804, 1969.

Kalz, F., and Newton, B. L.: Syphilitic juxta-articular nodules. Arch. Dermatol. 48:626, 1943.

Kandil, E.: Dermal angiolymphoid hyperplasia with eosinophilia versus pseudopyogenic granuloma. Br. J. Dermatol. 83:405, 1970.

Kaplan, S. R., Hayslett, J. P., and Calabresi, P.: Treatment of advanced Wegener's granulomatosis with azathioprine and duazomycin A. N. Engl. J. Med. 278:239, 1968.

Karat, A. B., Job, C. K., and Karat, S.: Acute lepromatous ulceration of the skin. Lepr. Rev. 38:25, 1967.

Kassel, S. H., Echevarria, R. A., and Guzzo, F. P.: Midline malignant reticulosis (so-called lethal midline granuloma). Cancer 23:920, 1969.

Kimura, T., Yoshimura, S., and Ishikawa, E.: Unusual granulation combined with hyperplastic change of lymphatic tissue. Trans. Soc. Pathol. Jap. 37:179, 1948.

Kinmont, P. D., and McCallum, D. I.: Skin manifestations of giant-cell arteritis. Br. J. Dermatol. 76:299, 1964.

Kirchheimer, W., and Storrs, E. E.: Hansen's disease transmitted to an armadillo. Presented at Meeting of Joint Leprosy Research Conference, United States-Japan Cooperative Medical Science Program, Bethesda, Maryland, 1971. (Unpublished data).

Kirk, R.: Studies in leishmaniasis in the Anglo-Egyptian Sudan; cutaneous and mucocutaneous leishmaniasis. Trans. R. Soc. Trop. Med. Hyg. 35:257, 1942.

Leiker, D. L., Kok, S. H., and Spaas, J. A.: Granuloma multiforme, a new skin disease resembling leprosy. Int. J. Lepr. 32:368, 1964.

Lester, W.: Chemotherapy of tuberculosis. Clin. Notes Resp. Dis. 9:3, 1970.

Levy, L.: The efficacy of sulfone therapy in leprosy. Int. J. Lepr. 35:563, 1967.

Lichtenstein, L.: Histiocytosis X; integration of eosinophilic granuloma of bone, "Letterer-Siwe disease," and "Schüller-Christian disease" as related manifestations of single nosologic entity. Arch. Pathol. 56:84, 1953.

Lichtenstein, L.: Histiocytosis X (eosinophilic granuloma of bone, Letterer-Siwe disease, and Schüller-Christian disease). Further observations of pathological and clinical importance. J. Bone Joint Surg. (Am.) 46:76, 1964.

Long, E. R.: On simultaneous BCG vaccination and DDS chemoprophylaxis. Int. J. Lepr. 37:412, 1969.

Longcope, W. T., and Freiman, D. G.: A study of sarcoidosis based on combined investigation of 160 cases including 30 autopsies from Johns Hopkins Hospital and Massachusetts General Hospital. Medicine 31:1, 1952.

Lowney, E. D., and Simons, H. M.: "Rheumatoid" nodules of the skin: their significance as an isolated finding. Arch. Dermatol. 88:853, 1963.

Lupovitch, A., Katase, R. Y., Randall, H. P., et al.: Malignant lymphoma presenting as necrotizing eosinophilic granulomatosis. J.A.M.A. 192:285, 1965.

Mabalay, M. C., Helwig, E. B., Tolentino, J. G., et al.: The histopathology and histochemistry of erythema nodosum leprosum. Int. J. Lepr. 33:28, 1965.

Mach, K. W., and Wilgram, G. F.: Characteristic histopathology of cutaneous lymphoplasia (lymphocytoma). Arch. Dermatol. 94:26, 1966.

Mansfield, R. E.: Histoid leprosy. Arch. Pathol. 87:580, 1969.

Manson-Bahr, P. E.: Variations in the clinical manifestations of leishmaniasis caused by *L. tropica*. J. Trop. Med. Hyg. 67:85, 1964.

Marshall, A. H. E.: An Outline of the Cytology and Pathology of the Reticular Tissue. London and Edinburg, Oliver and Boyd, 1956, 274 pp.

Matthews, L. J., and Trautman, J. R.: Clinical and serological profiles in leprosy. Lancet 2:915, 1965.

Meadows, S. P.: Temporal or giant cell arteritis. Proc. R. Soc. Med. 59:329, 1966.

Miescher, G., and Leder, M.: Granulomatosis discriformis chronica et progressiva (Atypishe tuber-kulose). Dermatologica 97:25, 1948.

Mills, C. P.: Wegener's granulomatosis. Br. J. Dermatol. 77:203, 1965.

Montgomery, H.: Dermatopathology. New York, Hoeber Medical Division, Harper and Row, 1967, pp. 225–228.

Moschella, S. L.: Leprosy and the military physician. Milit. Med. 131:525, 1966.

Moschella, S. L.: The lepra reaction with necrotizing skin lesions. A report of six cases. Arch. Dermatol. 95:565, 1967.

Mountain, J. C.: Cutaneous ulceration in Crohn's disease. Gut 11:18, 1970.

Mraz, J. P., and Newcomer, V. D.: Erythema elevatum diutinum. Presentation of a case and evaluation of laboratory and immunological status. Arch. Dermatol. 96:235, 1967.

Muller, S. A., and Winkelmann, R. K.: Necrobiosis lipoidica diabeticorum. A clinical and pathological investigation of 171 cases. Arch. Dermatol. 93:272, 1966.

Muller, S. A., Wolff, K., and Winkelmann, R. K.: Generalized eruptive histiocytoma. Enzyme histochemistry and electron microscopy. Arch. Dermatol. 96:11, 1967.

Napier, L. E., and Das Gupta, C. R.: A clinical study of post-kala-azar dermal leishmaniasis. Indian Med. Gaz. 65:249, 1930.

Orkin, M., Goltz, R. W., Good, R. A., et al.: A study of multicentric reticulohistiocytosis. Arch. Dermatol. 89:640, 1964.

Ormsby, O. S., and Montgomery, H.: Diseases of the Skin. 7th ed. Philadelphia, Lea and Febiger, 1948, pp. 224–225, 227–229.

Pettit, J. H., and Waters, M. F.: The etiology of erythema nodosum leprosum. Int. J. Lepr. 35:1, 1967.

Philpott, J. A., Jr., Woodburne, A. R., Philpott, O. S., et al.: Swimming pool granuloma. A study of 290 cases. Arch. Dermatol. 88:158, 1963.

Pillsburg, D. M., Shelley, W. B., and Kligman, A. M.: Dermatology. Philadelphia, W. B. Saunders Co., 1956, pp. 516–540.

Pimentel, J. C.: The "wheat-stubble sarcoid granuloma": a new epithelioid granuloma of the skin. Br. J. Dermatol. 87:444, 1972.

Raitt, J. W.: Wegener's granulomatosis: treatment with cytotoxic agents and adrenocorticoids. Ann. Intern. Med. 74:344, 1971.

Reed, W. B., Jensen, A. K., Konwaler, B. E., et al.: The cutaneous manifestations in Wegener's granulomatosis. Acta Derm. Venereol. (Stockh.) 43:250, 1963.

Ridley, D. S.: Bacteriological interpretation of skin smears and biopsies in leprosy. Trans. R. Soc. Trop. Med. Hyg. 49:449, 1955.

Ridley, D. S.: Reactions in leprosy. Lepr. Rev. 40:77, 1969.

Ridley, D. S., and Jopling, W. H.: Classification of leprosy according to immunity. A five-group system. Int. J. Lepr. 34:255, 1966.

Robbins, S. L.: Pathology. 3rd ed. Philadelphia, W. B. Saunders Co., 1967, pp. 334–346.

Rodriguez, J. N.: The histoid leproma. Its characteristics and significance. Int. J. Lepr. 37:1, 1969.

Rook, A., Wilkinson, D. S., and Ebling, F. J. G., (eds.): Textbook of Dermatology. Vol. 1. Oxford, Blackwell Scientific Publications Ltd., 1968, pp. 665–681.

Ruch, D. M.: Cutaneous manifestations of Letterer-Siwe's disease. Arch. Dermatol. 75:88, 1957.

Runyon, E. H.: Pathogenic mycobacteria. Adv. Tuberc. Res. 14:235, 1965.

Saba, T. M.: Physiology and pathophysiology of the reticuloendothelial system. Arch. Intern. Med. 126:1031, 1970.

Sabin, T. D.: Temperature-linked sensory loss. A unique pattern in leprosy. Arch. Neurol. 20:257, 1969.

Scadding, J. G.: Sarcoidosis. London, Eyre and Spottiswoode, 1967, pp. 174–194.

Shanbrom, E., Minton, R., Lester, C., et al.: Visceral manifestations of American mucocutaneous leishmaniasis. Am. J. Med. 20:145, 1956.

Shelley, W. B., and Hurley, H. J.: The immune granuloma: Late delayed hypersensitivity to zirconium and beryllium. In Sampter, M., Talmage, D. W., Rose, B., et al., (eds.): Immunological Diseases. 2nd ed. Boston, Little, Brown and Co., 1971, pp. 722–734.

Shepard, C. C.: The experimental disease that follows the injection of human leprosy bacilli into foot-pads of mice. J. Exp. Med. 112:445, 1960.

Shepard, C. C., and Chang, Y. T.: Activity of antituberculosis drugs against Mycobacterium leprae. Int. J. Lepr. 32:260, 1964.

Shepard, C. C., Tolentino, J. G., and McRae, D. H.: The therapeutic effect of 4,4'-diacetyldiamino-diphenylsulfone (DADDS) in leprosy. Am. J. Trop. Med. Hyg. 17:192, 1968.

Sheskin, J., and Convit, J.: Results of a double blind study of the influence of thalidomide on the lepra reaction. Int. J. Lepr. 37:135, 1969.

Siltzbach, L. E.: Etiology of sarcoidosis. Practitioner 202:613, 1969.

Sokolov, R. A., Rachmaninoff, N., and Kaine, H. D.: Allergic granulomatosis. Am. J. Med. 32:131, 1962.

Sommer, A. F., Williams, R. M., and Mandel, A. D.: Mycobacterium balnei infection. Report of two cases. Arch. Dermatol. 86:316, 1962.

Stankler, L., and Leslie, G.: Generalized granuloma annulare. A report of a case and review of the literature. Arch. Dermatol. 95:509, 1967.

Stankler, L., Ewen, S. W. B., and Kerr, N. W.: Crohn's disease of the mouth. Br. J. Dermatol. 87:501, 1972.

Strachan, R. W.: The natural history of Takayasu's arteriopathy. Q. J. Med. 33:57, 1964.

Timpe, A., and Runyon, E. H.: Relationship of "atypical" acid-fast bacteria to human disease; preliminary report. J. Lab. Clin. Med. 44:202, 1954.

Tolentino, J. G.: Acute manifestations of leprosy. Int. J. Lepr. 33:Suppl.:570, 1965.

Trautman, J. R., and Enna, C. E.: Leprosy. In Tice's Practice of Medicine. Vol. 3, Chap. 33, New York, Harper & Row, 1971, pp. 1–38.

Tuhy, J. D., Maurice, G. L., and Niles, N. R.: Wegener's granulomatosis. Am. J. Med. 25:638, 1958.

Van Der Lugt, L.: Some remarks about tuberculosis of the skin and tuberculids. Dermatologica 131: 266, 1965.

Van Furth, R.: Origin and kinetics of monocytes and macrophages. Semin. Hematol. 7:125, 1970.

Wade, H. W.: Demonstration of acid-fast bacilli in tissue sections. Am. J. Pathol. 28:157, 1952.

Waters, M. F.: G 30 320 or B 663 — lampren (Geigy). Lepr. Rev. *40*:21, 1969.

Waters, M. F., and Rees, R. J.: Changes in the morphology of *Mycobacterium leprae* in patients under treatment. Int. J. Lepr. *30*:266, 1962.

Wells, G. C.: Subcutaneous lymphoid hyperplasia with eosinophilia. Proc. R. Soc. Med. *56*:728, 1963.

Wells, G. C., and Whimster, I. W.: Subcutaneous angiolymphoid hyperplasia with eosinophilia. Br. J. Dermatol. *81*:1, 1969.

Wells, R. S., and Smith, M. A.: The natural history of granuloma annulare. Br. J. Dermatol. *75*:199, 1963.

Wilkinson, D. S.: Tuberculosis of the skin. *In* Rook, A., Wilkinson, D. S., and Ebling, F. J. G., (eds.): Textbook of Dermatology. Vol. 1. Oxford, Blackwell Scientific Publications Ltd., 1968, p. 675.

Windhorst, D. B., and Good, R. A.: Dermatologic manifestations of fatal granulomatous disease of childhood. Arch. Dermatol. *103*:351, 1971.

Winkelmann, R. K.: The skin in histiocytosis X. Mayo Clin. Proc. *44*:535, 1969.

Winkelmann, R. K., and Burgert, E. O.: Therapy of histiocytosis X. Br. J. Dermatol. *82*:169, 1970.

Winston, M. I.: Erythema elevatum diutinum. Arch. Dermatol. *89*:888, 1964.

CHAPTER

17

DISEASES OF THE PERIPHERAL VESSELS AND THEIR CONTENTS

Samuel L. Moschella

Peripheral vascular disease is the term used to describe blood flow disturbed by the structural or functional abnormalities of the peripheral vessels (Allen et al., 1962). Most of the patients affected by this condition suffer from the effects of ischemia or hyperemia resulting from abnormal dilatation, the so-called erythromelalgia. The symptoms and signs of peripheral vascular disease include the following: (1) coldness of the extremities, their temperature being related to the amount of blood flow through them; (2) intermittent claudication, which is the painful cramping of muscles during activity, indicates an imbalance existing between the blood supply and metabolic requirements and is the result of organic obstruction rather than sympathetic activity; (3) pain, which is present at rest, is agonizing and is associated with sudden arterial occlusion from thrombosis or embolism, indolent ulceration or gangrene, or ischemic neuritis; (4) skin color changes, that is, cyanosis and

rubor which is a persistent dull red or reddish blue discoloration of a cold extremity; (5) trophic changes, which include atrophic, shiny, hairless, tightly drawn skin prone to indolent ulceration and dystrophic nails; (6) venous filling which is quicker from below when the blood flow is greater and vice versa; (7) diminished pulsation of arteries; and (8) local gangrene and ulceration which indicate an underlying ischemia resulting from obliterated or thrombosed vessels.

The peripheral vascular diseases reviewed in this chapter are those resulting from abnormal vasoconstriction, post-traumatic reflex, sympathetic dystrophy, acrocyanosis, ergotism, and methysergide maleate toxicity; those resulting from vasodilation (erythromelalgia); and those resulting from organic arterial obstruction, arteriosclerosis obliterans, thromboangiitis obliterans, arterial embolism, peripheral arteritis, and gangrene in systemic infections such as typhoid fever, typhus, pneumonia, influenza, cholera, bacterial endocarditis, septicemia, trichinosis, scarlet fever, and rickettsial and viral diseases.

Acrocyanosis is a symmetric persistent coldness and cyanosis of the distal areas of extremities. It is a vasospastic disturbance of the smaller arterioles of the skin with secondary dilatation of the capillary beds and subpapillary venous plexuses. Association with asthenia, endocrine disorders, and anxiety states has been described. The condition is seen more frequently in female adolescents but may occur at any age. The involved hands and feet are mottled blue and red, sweat profusely, may swell (especially in cold weather), and may be slightly hyperesthetic. It is intensified by cold and emotion and relieved by warmth. Raynaud's disease differs because of its intermittent nature and greater pallor and discomfort. Trophic changes, ulceration, and gangrene do not occur in acrocyanosis. Patients with this condition are prone to acquire chilblains. It may be associated with livedo reticularis. For treatment, only reassurance and protection are necessary.

The post-traumatic reflex sympathetic dystrophy syndrome (De Takats, 1965) is neurovascular, occurring after injury or operation of the extremities and may be associated with rheumatoid arthritis and the shoulder-hand syndrome. When severe excruciating burning pain is the chief symptom, it has been called causalgia. The clinical characteristics are initially those of vasodilatation, elevated local temperature, hyperhidrosis, and edema, and later those of vasospasm, coldness of the extremities, cyanosis, atrophy of the skin, and Raynaud's phenomenon. There are local trigger points of exacerbation. The syndrome may be associated with acute bone atrophy (Sudeck's osteoporosis). The symptoms may be aggravated by emotional tension, weight bearing, dependency of the extremity, and cold. Satisfactory clinical response has been achieved by sympathectomy.

ERGOTISM AND METHYSERGIDE MALEATE TOXICITY

Peripheral vasoconstriction may follow the use of ergot and its derivates and methysergide maleate. Ergotism is an acute or chronic intoxication caused by the ingestion of grain or its products infected with the ergot fungus (*Claviceps purpurea*). Epidemics of ergotism resulting from ingestion of infected food were seen in Europe. Presently, intoxication is seen sporadically following the repeated administration of ergot in abortion and ergotamine in pruritus or migraine. Prolonged spasm of blood vessels may produce intimal damage and subsequent distal thrombosis. Toxicity is characterized by gastrointestinal necrosis and peripheral vascular signs and symptoms. The patients may experience vomiting, colic, diarrhea, headache, vertigo, paresthesias, convulsive seizures, psychic disturbances, coldness and cyanosis of extremities, Raynaud's phenomenon, intermittent claudication, absences of peripheral pulsations, and gangrene of digits, nose and ears (Fig. 17–1).

Symptoms related to vasoconstriction of small and large arteries are seen in approximately 7 per cent of patients who are receiving methysergide maleate (1-methyl-lysergic acid butanolamide) in large doses, but they have also been seen in patients taking an amount as small as 1 mg. (Graham, 1964).

Treatment consists of protection from cold and the use of vasodilator drugs and anticoagulants.

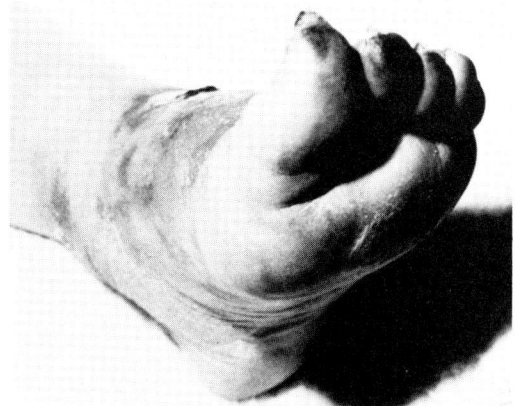

Figure 17–1 Female adult consumed large doses of ergotamine tartrate regularly for years for migraine headaches; personality and behavioral change and gangrene of the digits of the feet developed.

COMPLICATIONS OF ACCIDENTAL INTRA-ARTERIAL INJECTIONS OF MEDICATIONS

Accidental intra-arterial injections of medications can cause ischemia and gangrene of an extremity (Hager and Wilson, 1967). Small arteries, arterioles, and capillaries are involved initially. An inflammatory response in the vessels to the drug leads to arteriospasm followed by intravascular thrombosis. Among the incriminated compounds are thiopental sodium, contrast media, promazine hydrochloride, chlorpromazine hydrochloride, ether, mephenesin, amobarbital sodium, and propoxyphene. There is immediate severe burning in the hand and forearm, an initial flushing followed by blanching and cyanosis, and a patchy bluish or blue-green mottling distal to the injection site. Edema of the forearm, which can be extensive, is rarely present. Ischemic changes and a variable amount of gangrene of the hand or forearm supervene. Therapy is directed toward elimination of arterial spasm, prevention of thrombosis, and restoration of blood flow to the limb. The therapeutic measures used are extensive fasciotomy, arteriotomy, intra-arterially administered procaine and papaverine hydrochloride, vasodilators, injection of adventitia with lidocaine, administration of dextran 40 by intravenous drip, anticoagulation, sympathetic block, and sympathectomy.

ERYTHROMELALGIA

Erythromelalgia is a condition characterized by paroxysmal vasodilation with redness, burning pain, and increased warmth of the involved extremities.

The etiology is divided into the primary or idiopathic erythromelalgia and secondary erythromelalgia. The primary type occurs in otherwise healthy persons without any evidence of vascular or neurologic disease. Secondary erythromelalgia has been associated with occlusive vascular disease, polycythemia vera or thrombocythemia, gout, organic neurologic disease, and heavy metal poisoning (mercury, arsenic, thallium). The increased temperature of the skin is diagnostically the most important of all the disturbances of this syndrome. The reason for the sensitivity to warmth is not understood. The temperature at which the distress is produced lies within the range of 32° C. to 36° C. (89.6° F. to 96.8° F.); it varies in different persons and in different areas of the same patient.

Clinical Manifestations

The disease rarely affects children. Men and women are both afflicted, usually at middle age or later. The involved feet and hand are red or cyanotic, warm or hot to the touch, and "burning." The arterial pulsation is increased locally and the affected area frequently sweats profusely. Trophic changes, ulceration, and gangrene are not common in the primary type but may occur in the secondary type. The onset is gradual; the disease remains mild for years but may become so severe and continuous as to result in total disability. The attacks last for minutes to several hours. They are induced by stimuli which produce vasodilation or engorgement, such as local heat, warm environment, exercise, standing, or dependency of extremities.

The disease must be differentiated from painful paresthesias of cold limb syndromes and acrocyanosis and from the red, painful, but cold extremities of thromboangiitis obliterans and arteriosclerosis obliterans. Although glomus tumor and arteriovenous fistula produce an increase in temperature, venous engorgement and local pulsation are present, and the nature of the pain is different.

Treatment

Treatment is not uniformly helpful. Attacks may be aborted by rest, elevation, and cold application. Aspirin has relieved pain. Vasoconstrictors (ephedrine) and even vasodilators (isoproterenol and nitroglycerin) have been reported as being helpful (Babb et al., 1964). In severe cases, liberal amounts of aspirin and sedation may be required. Nerve blocks or section as well as sympathectomy sometimes help.

ARTERIOSCLEROSIS OBLITERANS

Arteriosclerosis obliterans describes an occlusive arterial disease of large and medium-sized arteries of the extremities which is caused by either atherosclerosis (focal plaque-like lesions of intima) or medial arteriosclerosis (medial coat vessel changes of medium-sized arteries) or both. This disease is responsible for three-fourths of all the cases of occlusive disease of extremities. Arteriosclerosis of small digital arteries of the hands and feet is rare, but thrombotic occlusion of these vessels may occur when extensive obstruction of the larger proximal arteries is present.

Arteriosclerosis predominates in men between 50 and 70 years of age and is being recognized more frequently in patients in the fourth decade of life. Diabetics have a higher incidence and severity. The relationship of hypertension to arteriosclerosis obliterans has not been established. In patients who continue to smoke, the incidence of amputation is greater. The symptoms, which result from the ischemia of tissues, are intermittent claudication, rest pain, pain of ulceration and gangrene, pain of ischemic neuropathy, pain of disuse atrophy, sensitivity to cold, and stiffness of joints from prolonged disuse or muscular weakness. The signs of occlusive arterial disease include impaired arterial pulsation, especially of the posterior tibial, popliteal, and femoral arteries; systolic bruits; postural and other color changes; thermal and trophic changes; atrophy of muscles, soft tissues, and skin; and xanthomata. Redness, bluish discoloration, pallor, or mottled duskiness of the skin occurs. Abnormal pallor is seen on elevation and rubor on dependency, and the filling of the superficial veins is delayed.

The changes in temperature in arteriosclerosis obliterans are best appreciated by comparing the differences between the two feet. The trophic changes include scarring and shrinkage of digits, deformed nails, and ulceration and gangrene which appear first in terminal toes. Hypoesthesia and hyporeflexia of the ischemic neuropathy must be differentiated at times from those of diabetes mellitus. Edema of the foot and leg occurs in advanced cases and is attributable to capillary atony, venous thrombosis, or lymphangitis secondary to infection. The association of venous thrombosis with arteriosclerosis oblit-

erans results from ischemic damage to the endothelium, hypercoagulability of blood, and the slowdown of blood flow due to arterial occlusion.

The laboratory studies which may be helpful are roentgenograms of extremities to detect arterial calcification, examinations for diabetes mellitus, determination of plasma lipids, and special studies to investigate for polycythemia. Because of the frequent association of coronary arteriosclerosis and myocardial infarction, electrocardiography is performed. Arteriography gives information about the site and extent of an occlusive arterial lesion and is indicated especially when reconstructive surgery is contemplated.

Treatment

Arrest of the progress of the disease is accomplished by control of abnormal lipid and carbohydrate metabolism. Environmental control measures, such as avoidance of cold exposure, trauma, local and external heat, and smoking, as well as excessive sedentary activity, are recommended. At rest, the extremity should be held horizontal or slightly below. The infected lesions should be kept open and moist and treated vigorously with appropriate antibiotics. The use of anticoagulant therapy to protect against thrombosis is controversial. Surgery may be recommended to restore circulation by thromboendarterectomy, excision and graft replacement, or by-pass. The preganglionic sympathectomy usually increases blood flow to the skin and allows superficial ulcers to heal more quickly. Extensive involvement of vessels may cause gangrene which often necessitates amputation.

THROMBOANGIITIS OBLITERANS (Buerger's Disease)

Thromboangiitis obliterans (McKusick et al., 1962) is a segmental thrombosing of medium and small arteries and, less commonly, veins and rarely affects the large vessels of both with acute and chronic inflammation. The extremities are chiefly involved, the viscera rarely. There is no accumulation of lipids or deposits of calcium in the vessels. Although the disease predominantly affects the lower extremities, it may begin in the small arteries of the hands. Thrombosis of the mesenteric, coronary, cerebral, and renal arteries is unusual. The etiology is unknown. Smoking has a deleterious effect and may be one of the most important responsible factors. The disease has practically never been seen in nonsmokers. It occurs predominantly in young male adults between 25 and 40 years of age but may have its onset as early as age 17 and as late as age 75. It is seen most frequently among Jews.

Clinical Manifestations

The clinical manifestations are coldness and postural color changes of the involved extremities, pain, trophic changes, recurrent superficial migratory phlebitis (Fig. 17–2), arteriolar spastic phenonemon, and

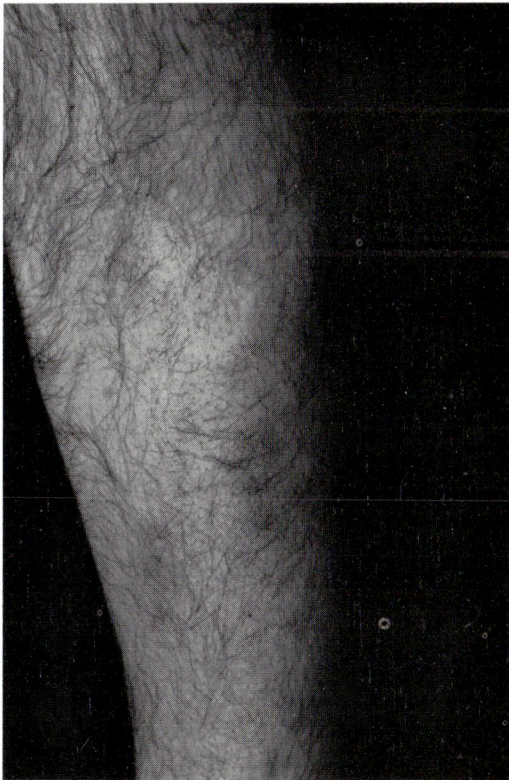

Figure 17–3 *A* and *B*, Thromboangiitis obliterans (Buerger's disease). Changes of digits resulting from thrombosis of medium and small arteries.

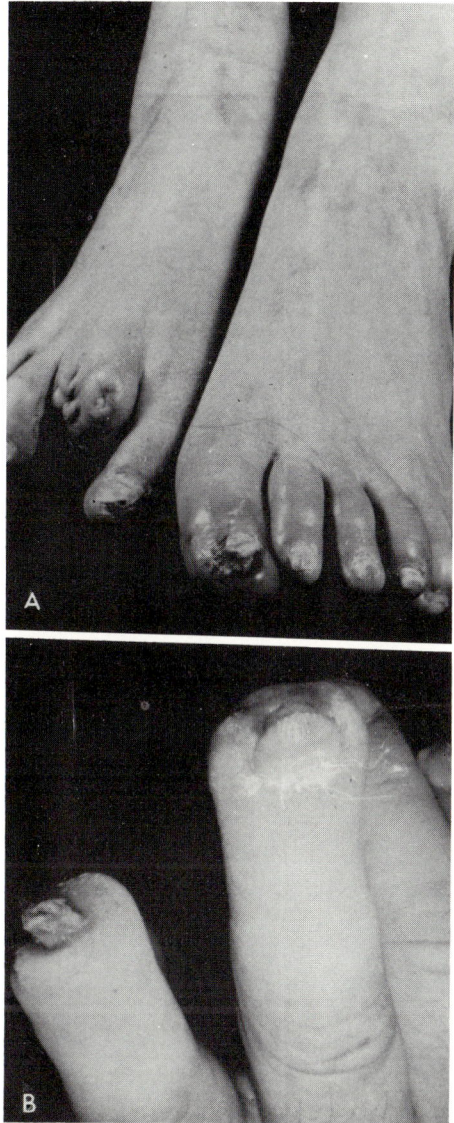

Figure 17–2 Recurrent episodes of superficial phlebitis developed in a young male patient who was a heavy smoker; these were followed by gangrenous changes of digits, initially of toes and later fingers.

gangrene (Fig. 17–3). The duration and degree of resultant peripheral ischemia determine the degree of rubor, the trophic skin and nail changes, and the wasting of muscles. Pain, which is the result of thrombosis and ulceration, is present at rest, is worse at night, and is constant. The crampy pain and muscle fatigue experienced during exercise result from intermittent claudication. The paroxysmal lancinating pain and associated paresthesias, the blanching cyanosis, the mottling of extremities, and the excessive sweating are the results of ischemic neuropathy. The superficial migratory phlebitis may precede or accompany arterial involvement, presents as tender red elevated linear areas about 1 cm. in diameter, involves the small superficial veins of feet or lower legs, disappears gradually over two-week to three-week periods, and recurs at irregular intervals with new lesions. Arteriolar spasm contributes to the severity of ischemia and may produce cold sensitivity and Raynaud's phenomenon. Mechanical, chemical, and thermal trauma initiates ulceration frequently in the region of the nails, the tips of the digits, the foot, and rarely the leg.

Treatment

Treatment consists of abstinence from tobacco, analgesics for pain, prophylactic and local measures for ulceration and gangrene, sympathectomy, and amputation. Sympathectomy has been helpful when vasospasm is prominent. Amputation is deferred until conservative therapy fails. Gangrene and intractable pain are indications for amputation. Unlike arteriosclerotic gangrene, the resistance to infection is rather high and collateral circulation is usually good, so that minor amputations may be more successful.

ARTERIAL OCCLUSION (Arterial Embolism and Thrombosis)

Embolism and thrombosis are the chief causes of arterial occlusion of the extremities. The occurrence of sudden arterial insufficiency without physical findings of an underlying severe peripheral vascular disease suggests an embolus. The origins of emboli include the mural or valvular thrombi of the left side of the heart, detachment of atheromatous material, paradoxical emboli from the right side of the heart through a patent foramen ovale, and myxoma of the left atrium. Among the miscellaneous and unusual causes for sudden occlusion are amniotic

fluid, air, tumor, fat, bile, and accidental intra-arterial injections of bismuth and metallic mercury. Predisposing factors are atrial fibrillation, bacterial endocarditis, and coronary occlusion with mural thrombosis. The embolus obstructs the blood flow through the involved vessel and causes, within a few hours, secondary thrombosis below and sometimes above the obstructed site. Secondary vasospasm is presumed to be an important contributory factor to the ischemia of the affected limb.

Clinical Manifestations

The intensity of the clinical manifestations of arterial occlusion due to embolism and thrombosis is proportional to the size and extent of the artery obstructed, the adequacy of collateral circulation, the presence of previous distal occlusive disease, and arteriospasm. Prolonged and severe ischemia can produce intimal changes not only of arteries but also of veins, with resultant venous thrombosis. Among the appreciable clinical changes are lowered surface temperature, pallor, collapsed superficial veins, decrease or loss of sensation, reflexes, and muscular strength, and absence of pulsation. At first, no pain is present at the site of embolization, but tenderness usually develops in a few hours. The initial pallor is followed by a blotchy cyanosis, and later, if treatment is delayed or ineffective, massive gangrene with mummification and blister formation occurs.

Several syndromes resulting from occlusion of specific peripheral arteries by embolism or thrombosis can be appreciated clinically. The anterior tibial compartment syndrome (Cobbet and Wallace, 1965) is the result of the occlusion of the anterior tibial artery. These patients initially experience paresthesias, pain, tenderness, and swelling of the anterior surface of the leg. Later, fever, drop foot and inability to flex toes, absence of pulsation of the anterior tibial artery, and finally gangrenous changes of the erythematous, edematous skin occur.

Atheroembolism, embolization (Carvajal et al., 1967; Retan and Miller, 1966; Young et al., 1963) of the atheromatous material from aortic and arterial atheromatous plaques with impaction within small arteries and arterioles of various organs and tissues, is being appreciated clinically with increased frequency (Fig. 17–4). The manifestations are paroxysmal painful ischemia of the feet and legs, livedo reticularis and gangrene despite the presence of adequate arterial pulses, hypertension and impaired renal function, abdominal pain, gastrointestinal hemorrhage, pancreatitis, and, occasionally, neurologic symptoms and retinal emboli. This condition has been misdiagnosed as polyarteritis nodosa, various types of peripheral vasculitis, and a complication of subacute bacterial endocarditis. In elderly patients with suspected multiple system embolization, biopsy of the muscle from the involved regions shows the intra-arteriolar acicular clefts typical of cholesterol crystals.

Anatomic thrombosis of arteries with resultant occlusion occurs in the inflammatory diseases (thromboangiitis obliterans, periarteritis nodosa, nonspecific arteritis), in the degenerative conditions (arteriosclerosis, cystic medial necrosis, dissecting hematoma), in situations precipitated by trauma (the thoracic outlet, compression syndromes, external trauma, intra-arterial insertions of needles and catheters), and in hematologic states or diseases (polycythemia vera and other myeloproliferative disorders, thrombophilia, cryoglobulinemia, thrombotic thrombocytopenic purpura, intravascular coagulopathy states).

Treatment

The most essential factor in caring for patients with vascular occlusion is the institution of treatment as soon as possible. The involved extremity should not be elevated or subjected to heat exceeding 32.2° C. (90° F.). Vasomotor dilators, such as alcohol and intra-arterially administered papaverine and tolazoline, anticoagulant therapy, treatment of underlying medical conditions, and embolectomy are the recommended immediate measures. Sympathectomy, cardiac valvuloplasty, correction of existing arterial aneurysms, and long-term anticoagulant therapy are indicated or recommended prophylactic measures. The position of thrombolytic therapy (for example, streptokinase) in the management of thromboembolic occlusive vascular disease and dipyridamole in thromboembolic prophylaxis is being evaluated.

VASCULITIS

CLASSIFICATION OF PRIMARY INFLAMMATORY VASCULITIS

Obliterative type
  Local
      Atrophie blanche
      Hypertensive ischemic ulcer
      Livedo reticularis

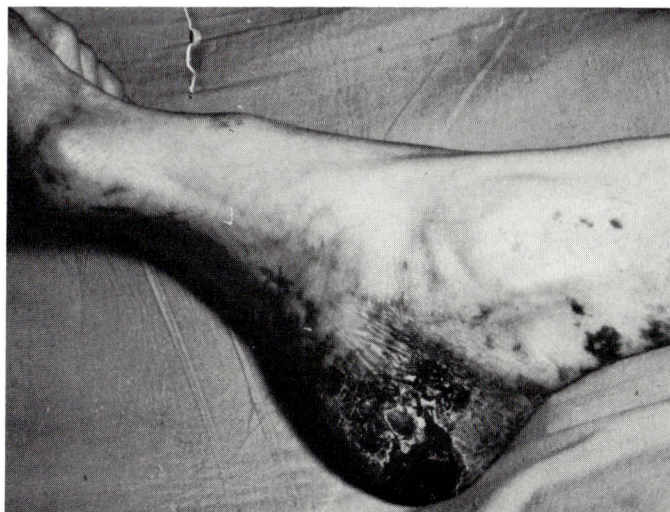

Figure 17–4 Atheroembolism. Gangrenous changes of skin secondary to atheroemboli; biopsy of proximal muscle revealed intra-arteriolar acicular clefts typical of cholesterol crystals.

Systemic
  Thromboangiitis obliterans
  Malignant atrophic papulosis
Necrotizing type with or without granu-
loma
  Leukocytoclastic angiitis
    Skin: Pityriasis lichenoides
    Systemic: Schoenlein-Henoch,
      cutaneous systemic angiitis,
      collagen diseases, dyspro-
      teinemias, infectious diseases
Large and smaller vessels: Polyarteritis
nodosa, malignant granulomatosis (Churg
and Strauss, Wegener's)
  Giant cell arteritis

Atrophie Blanche

Atrophie blanche (Gray et al., 1966; Nelson, 1955) is a distinctive entity that consists of periodic ulcerations of the lower leg with characteristic scarring.

Women in the third decade of life are most frequently affected. Because it may become worse during the summer, atrophie blanche may have to be differentiated from livedo reticularis with summer ulcerations; however, the disease does not have livedo reticularis clinically. In some cases, it has been associated with varicose veins and has been described as a localized expression of hypersensitivity.

On histopathologic examination, superficial capillary endothelial proliferation, extravasated red cells, perivascular inflammation, fibrosis, accumulation of fibroid material in and about the lumina of superficial blood vessels, and segmental infarction of epidermis and superficial corium are present.

The lesions appear on the lower legs, ankles, and dorsa of the feet and present as small erythematous telangiectatic areas that develop central, tender, hemorrhagic crusts or painful, burning ulcerations measuring usually 1 to 5 mm. (Fig. 17–5). They heal with irregular atrophic white scars with hyperpigmented telangiectatic borders; the central areas may have pigmented spots or small crusts. Larger superficial ulcers may develop in preexisting patches. The lesions take months to heal and may continue to appear for years.

There is no specific treatment. Symptomatic relief may be obtained by local,

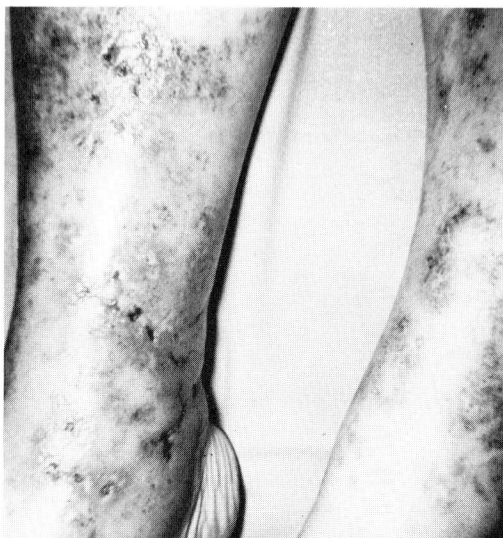

Figure 17–5 Atrophie blanche in a 32-year-old woman with no varicose veins. Tender erythematous telangiectatic, purpuric lesions are seen. Painful ulcerations developed.

with or without occlusion, and intralesional corticosteroids. Rest and supportive bandages or stockings have been ineffective. Systemic corticosteroid therapy is helpful while being administered.

Hypertensive Ischemic Ulcer

Hypertensive ischemic ulcer (Schnier et al., 1966) results from infarction of skin from arteriolar occlusion as part of a long-standing hypertensive vascular disease (Fig. 17–6). The disease predominates in women between the ages of 50 and 70 years. These women have had essential hypertension for a long time and usually have hypertensive (group 2) fundal changes. There is no evidence of disturbance of major arterial, venous, or lymphatic circulation. Peripheral pulses are palpable. Ulceration results either from minor trauma to the skin with impaired vasculature or from spontaneous cutaneous infarction from the occlusion of arterioles or small arteries as a result of the intimal proliferation of the vessels. An increase in the thickness of the arteriolar wall, hyaline degeneration of media, intimal proliferation, and mild periarteritis are noted histologically.

The ulcer appears most often on the lateral surface of the ankle and leg and less commonly on the posterior, medial, and anterior aspect of the ankle or leg. A painful erythematous plaque appears initially. In 7 to 10 days, the center of the lesion becomes blue and purpuric or develops a hemorrhagic bulla and eventually a necrotic eschar which sloughs, leaving a superficial or deeply punched-out ulcer; occasionally, the lesion remains surrounded by poor granulation tissue. The ulcers can measure from 1 to 10 cm. in diameter. They are sensitive and painful. Brown pigmentation caused by hemosiderin and melanin surrounds the longstanding ulcers. A characteristic clinical feature is the development of satellite lesions resulting from episodic and irregular extension of the skin infarction. The ulcers heal usually within three months and remain healed, but recurrences may appear in the same or opposite leg. Like other ischemic ulcers, they do not seem to support infection.

These ulcers must be differentiated from stasis ulcers resulting from chronic venous insufficiency; ischemic ulceration due to pernio, frostbite, livedo reticularis, drug intoxication, and chronic occlusive arterial disease; from those of infectious or drug-induced granulomatous processes; epitheliomas; lymphoma cutis; and factitial ulcers.

Treatment is aimed at clearing up any infection, relieving pain, stimulating healing, and increased blood supply. Among the measures utilized are analgesics, vasodilators, sympathectomy, prophylaxis against precipitating factors of gangrene, and antihypertensive therapy.

Livedo reticularis

Livedo reticularis (Champion, 1965) is a reddish blue mottling or reticular network pattern of the skin of the extremities. It is presumed that the pattern of discoloration is the result of the interference of the assumed cone arrangement of the cutaneous blood supply. Insufficiency of arterial supply leads to dilation of the small vessels, especially in the peripheral parts of the cones. The obstruction in the artery or arteriole is the result of either spastic or organic factors. Livedo reticularis, which can be a physical sign of physiologic and pathologic states, can be classified according to cause as follows:

1. Physiologic: Cutis marmorata.

2. Idiopathic or primary: Localized disease of skin.

3. Symptomatic or secondary: Result of a systemic vascular disease.

4. Congenital livedo reticularis.

When the livedo is widespread and symmetric, it is rarely associated with

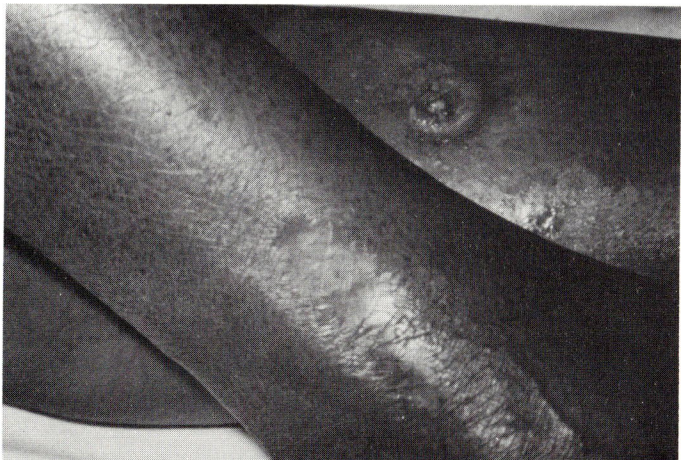

Figure 17–6 Hypertensive ischemic ulcer. Middle-aged black woman with hypertension of 15 years' duration has recurrent painful necrotic ulcerations of lower legs.

systemic disease; however, when it is patchy, asymmetric, or associated with erythematous nodules or digital gangrene, an underlying systemic disease must be searched for.

Cutis marmorata is a transitory mottling of the skin which occurs on exposure to cold, is seen frequently in children, and is only temporarily cosmetically significant.

Idiopathic (primary) livedo reticularis is characterized by symmetric erythematous bluish mottling of the lower and, less frequently, the upper extremities, and occasionally the lower trunk. It persists despite temperature changes (Fig. 17–7). It affects young persons and middle-aged women. The degree of involvement is accentuated by cold. Patients with this condition may complain of coldness, numbness, dull pain, and paresthesias of the extremities, especially on exposure to cold. An associated edema of the skin of the ankles, feet, and legs may be present. Recurrent ulcers of the skin of the legs and, less frequently, of the digits may appear in the winter and occasionally in the summer. An associated mild hypertension may be present. The larger limbal, dorsal pedis, posterior tibial, and popliteal arteries are not involved. The disease may remain stationary or progressive. A marked arteriolitis and venulitis with thrombosis is seen histologically. Steroid therapy has been ineffective. Prolonged anticoagulant therapy or sympathectomy may relieve the symptoms and promote healing of the ulcerations. Several cases have been reported to result in amputation because of intractable pain, extensive painful ulceration, and gangrene.

Symptomatic livedo reticularis may be caused locally by pernio and systemically by arteriosclerosis, arteritis, and intravascular occlusion. It is characterized by persistent bluish red mottling which may be asymmetric and may be accompanied by erythematous plaques or nodules which can ulcerate and reflect the patchy involvement of the cutaneous and subcutaneous vascular system. Recurrent ulceration and gangrene of digits may be complications. Among the diseases which are responsible for these clinical changes secondary to arteritis are periarteritis nodosa, the so-called collagen disease (LE, rheumatoid arthritis, dermatomyositis, and rheumatic fever), the infections of syphilis and tuberculosis, intravascular occlusion by arterial emboli of atheromatous material, gas, or chemicals, thrombocytosis, cryoglobulinemia as seen in multiple myeloma, and intravascular coagulopathy associated with infections, hemolysis, and tumors.

Congenital livedo reticularis is a rare vascular developmental defect which is characterized by localized or extensive cutaneous bluish mottling, is present at birth, may be associated with atrophy of the skin, and is not associated with any other disorder (Fig. 17–8). The eruption tends to persist indefinitely, but some fading may occur. Although its appearance may be alarming, systemic involvement has not been reported. Calcinosis cutis may complicate the condition. No effective treatment is known.

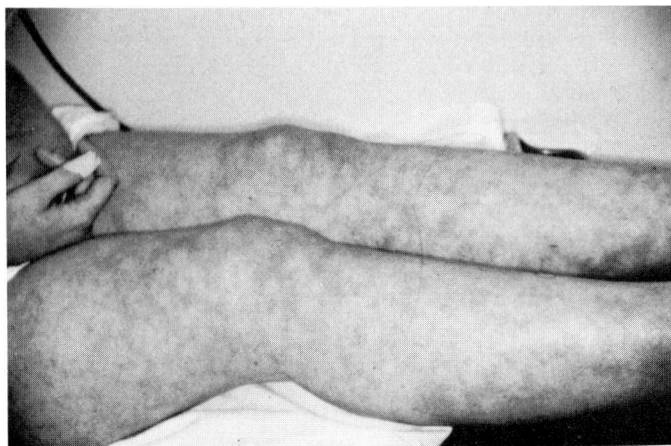

Figure 17–7 Livedo reticularis. Young woman with idiopathic (primary) livedo reticularis; biopsy revealed vasculitis of arterioles and venules.

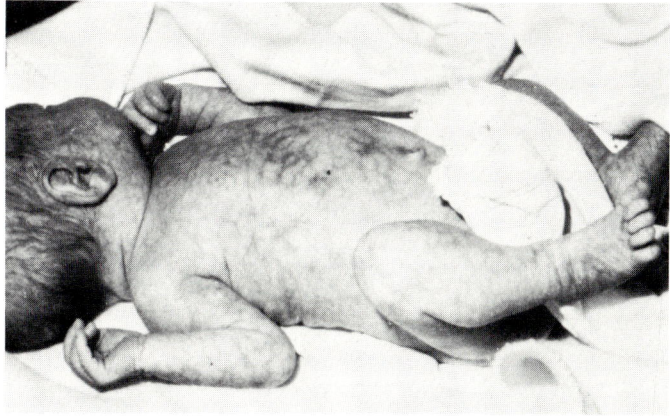

Figure 17–8 Rare case of congenital livedo reticularis; no underlying or associated conditions were appreciable.

Malignant Atrophic Papulosis (Degos' Syndrome)

Malignant atrophic papulosis (Strole et al., 1967) is a fatal disease characterized by an endovasculitis of skin, gastrointestinal tract, and, less frequently, other viscera. The cause is unknown. The basic pathogenic mechanism is vascular obliteration from endovasculitis and thrombosis with resultant ischemic infarction of involved tissues. Histologically, there is small arterial endothelial swelling and proliferation, which may be associated with fibrinoid necrosis of the intima and thrombosis. Fibrosis occurs between the intima and internal elastic lamina. Inflammation or necrosis in the media or adventitia of the vessels is significantly absent. Wedge-shaped infarcts result, consisting of acellular homogenous collagen with the broad base located at the epidermis. The mucin deposition in the dermis is secondary to the necrobiosis. Analogous infarction of other organs, especially the intestines, exhibits histologically a more pronounced perivascular infiltrate. Later, veins are involved to a lesser degree. It remains to be proved whether malignant papulosis can be considered a form of vasculitis (Strole et al., 1967).

The eruption consists of asymptomatic crops of erythematous papules which evolve slowly over a period of weeks and months, become umbilicated with characteristic porcelain-white centers; a few disappear, leaving small white scars (Fig. 17–9). The papules measure 2 to 5 mm. in size and may coalesce. There is an average of 30 lesions, and there may be as many as 100. The eruption involves the entire skin except the face, palms, and soles, is more proximal than distal, and involves the back more than the front.

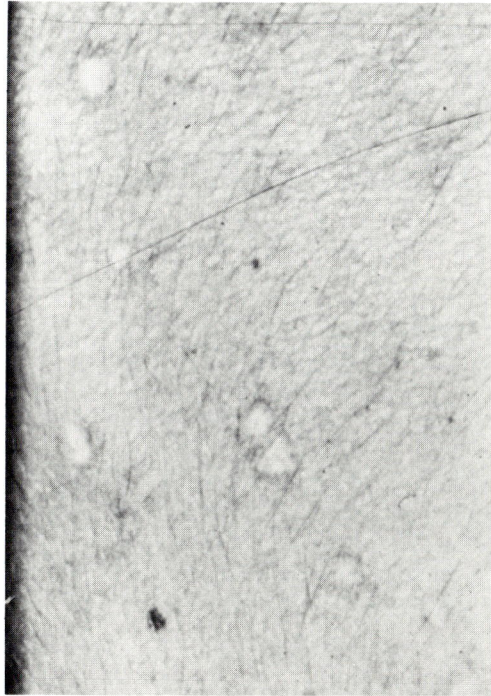

Figure 17–9 Malignant atrophic papulosis (Degos' syndrome). The erythematous papules that developed the characteristic porcelain-white centers are demonstrated; the patient had bulbar conjunctival lesions and showed no evidence of systemic disease at that time.

Lesions of the oral mucosa and lips may occur. Urticaria-like, ulceropustular, and gummatous nodular lesions have been described. The lesions may appear in crops for years.

A few months after the appearance of skin lesions, the patient may experience abdominal complaints. The gastrointestinal symptoms include nausea, vomiting, abdominal pain and colic, diarrhea, ileus, melena, and malabsorption. These symptoms may occasionally precede the skin lesions. The onset of these complaints signals the impending fatal ending within a few months from hemorrhage, perforation, and peritonitis. The neurologic symptoms are headache, numbness of the extremities, ataxia, and diplopia. Retinal and scleral plaques and microaneurysms of the bulbar conjunctival vessels have been described. Other viscera which may be involved are the heart, kidneys, pericardium, and bladder. A few patients have survived for six years or more. No effective therapy is known.

Pityriasis Lichenoides

Parapsoriasis is divided into two groups. One consists of parapsoriasis en plaque and lichenoides, which may be complicated later by lymphoma cutis, and the other is the guttate type with an acute or chronic course. Parapsoriasis guttata may consist of papulosquamous (guttate type), and hemorrhagic, varioliform, necrotic, and pustular (pityriasis lichenoides type) lesions. Because of the presence of a lymphocytic vasculitis in pityriasis lichenoides et varioliformis acuta (PLEVA) and pityriasis lichenoides chronica, it has been recommended that these two conditions be separated from the parapsoriasis group. PLEVA is more severe clinically and histologically than pityriasis lichenoides chronica; transitions between the two related conditions do occur, however.

PLEVA. PLEVA is an acute polymorphous eruption which heals with superficial scarring and pigmentation. The cause is unknown, and it has not been associated with any underlying diseases. Histologically, there is a vasculitis characterized by invasion of the capillary walls by lymphocytes, extravasation of erythrocytes, obliteration of the dermo-epidermal junction, and severe intercellular and intracellular edema in the epidermis with vesicle formation and necrosis. The vasculitis usually differs from the so-called allergic type by the absence of neutrophils, "nuclear dust," and fibrinoid deposits within and around the blood vessels; however, these features have been seen in some cases. The eruption is generalized, and its lesions appear in successive crops so that they are in all stages of development. Although the individual lesions persist about two weeks, the disease, because of the continuous appearance of new lesions, may last several months to years. Patients with this condition may experience some itching or burning of the rash; they are usually asymptomatic, however. In more severe cases, patients may experience fever, malaise, and other constitutional symptoms which may precede or accompany the eruption; painful joint swellings have also been reported.

PLEVA is more common in children and young adults. An erythematous and edematous papule measuring 2 to 4 mm. in size is the primary lesion. It becomes hemorrhagic, may vesiculate, rarely forms frank bullae (Fig. 17–10) develops a central necrotic crust (Fig. 17–11), and heals with a varioliform scar. The eruption tends to be widespread, affecting the trunk, thighs, upper arms, and flexors. The palms, soles, and mucous membranes of the oral cavity and genitalia are occasionally involved; the face and scalp are generally spared. When PLEVA presents as a varicelliform eruption, it is to be differentiated from chickenpox and rickettsialpox. When necrotic papules predominate, conditions associated with necrotizing angiitis of small vessels are to be considered.

There are several reports of a condition which clinically resembles PLEVA and has not only the associated lymphocytic vasculitis but also a distinguishing and striking infiltrate of large, highly atypical histiomonocytic cells. The eruption is benign, continuous, and self-healing and has been described as Mucha-Habermann's disease, simulating lymphoma cutis (Verallo and Haserick, 1966) and lymphomatoid papulosis (Macaulay, 1968). PLEVA is self-limited and may last

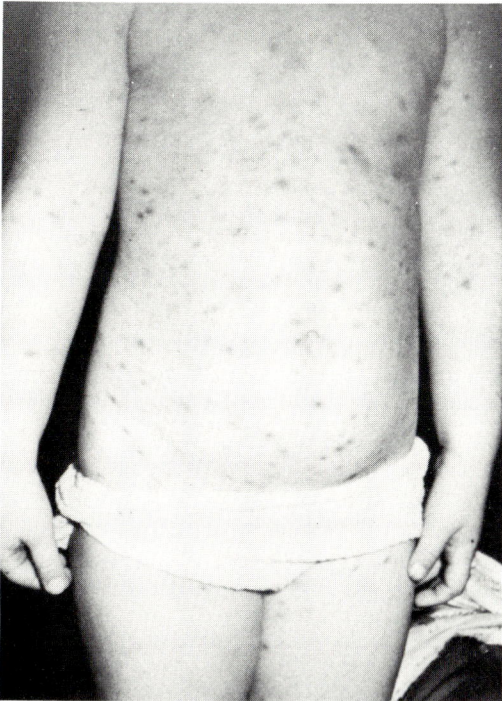

Figure 17–10 Pityriasis lichenoides. Widespread mildly pruritic erythematous papules with or without hemorrhage with a distribution following the lines of cleavage; the eruption cleared spontaneously in four months.

weeks to years; the more severe cases may be improved temporarily during systemic corticosteroid therapy, which does not modify its course. Topical crude coal tar followed by ultraviolet therapy may be of some benefit.

PITYRIASIS LICHENOIDES CHRONICA. Pityriasis lichenoides chronica of Juliusberg is a milder monomorphous eruption and is probably a less intense expression of the same disease process as that of PLEVA. Histologically, the degree of lymphocytic vasculitis and the extravasation of red blood cells are less. It affects mainly adolescent males, rarely infants, but has been reported at birth. The eruption appears in crops and is less acute and extensive than that of PLEVA. The lesion is a scaly, reddish brown papule which is 3 to 10 mm. in diameter, evolves slowly over three to four weeks, flattens out, and leaves some residual pigmentation. The eruption predominates on the trunk and clears within six months but may recur in crops for years. The lesions of pityriasis

lichenoides chronica are different from those of guttate parapsoriasis which are fawn colored and almost macular, have a tenacious micaceous scale, and are relatively fixed and persistent. A very severe ulcerative pityriasis lichenoides associated with persistent fever has been described (Degos et al., 1966). The diseases to be considered in the differential diagnosis of pityriasis lichenoides chronica are guttate psoriasis, papular pityriasis rosea, lichen planus, secondary syphilis, and insect bites.

Topical therapy, with or without occlusion, or intralesional steroid and tar therapy with ultraviolet light may be tried. These therapeutic measures may be temporarily effective and do not appear to modify the course of the disease.

Cutaneous Systemic Vasculitis

Eruptions due to vasculitis are among the most striking and challenging. The term *vasculitis* is used to describe a group of diseases characterized by an idiopathic primary inflammation of blood vessels and having many common clinical features. Their onset may be acute or insidious. Persons between the ages of 3 months and 80 years may be affected, but the incidence is greatest in middle-aged men. The cutaneous lesions tend to be petechial or hemor-

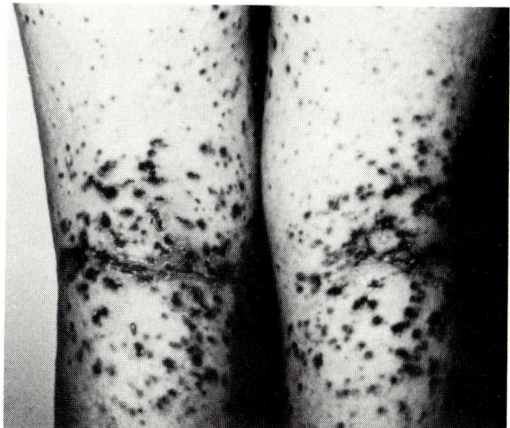

Figure 17–11 Widespread hemorrhagic vesiculopapular eruption favoring the flexural areas; because of its polymorphous and acute nature, it was described as pityriasis lichenoides et varioliformis acuta (PLEVA).

rhagic and palpable and may include livedo reticularis. There may be fever, arthralgias, myalgia, neuropathy, renal disease, asthma and pulmonary infiltrates, myocardial infarction and chronic heart failure, abdominal pain and mesenteric infarction, and variable central nervous system complaints. Laboratory studies may reveal leukocytosis, eosinophilia, telescoped urine, (urinary sediment with red blood cell casts), and histologic evidence of vasculitis in the biopsies of skin, muscle, kidney, liver, rectum, and testes. Systemic corticosteroids may be helpful. Antimetabolites have been reported as useful, especially in the granulomatous types.

The dermatologist may be consulted when the presenting condition affects the small-sized and medium-sized blood vessels of the dermis and subcutaneous tissue (Table 17–1). The cutaneous manifestations are usually signs of a complex pathologic process which not only affects the skin but also accompanies or heralds a systemic disorder. As a result of the lack of knowledge, many of the associated clinical manifestations and syndromes are presently not acceptable as diseases. Attempts have been made to classify these conditions for prognostic, therapeutic, and investigational purposes. Simplification of these endeavors is prevented by the current state of knowledge and the clinical overlap of the conditions. Present classifications are based on the clinical presentation, histopathology, and cellular response.

The cutaneous expressions are dependent on the type and severity of the reaction, the nature and frequency of the responsible insult, the size and depth of the involved vessels, and the extent of impairment of the vasculature. The cutaneous blood vessels have a limited number of ways to react. When the small superficial vessels are involved, purpura, erythematous macules and papules, hemorrhagic vesicles or bullae, and superficial ischemic infarctive ulcerations are seen clinically. When the deeper and larger vessels of the dermis and subcutaneous tissues are involved, one sees clinically Raynaud's phenomenon, pernio, livedo reticularis, tender erythematous nodules with or without ulceration, digital thrombosis, gangrene, and suppurative and nonsuppurative panniculitis. Unfortunately,

TABLE 17–1 Dermatologic Spectrum of Vasculitis

Dermatopathy
  Capillaritis (lymphocytic type)
      Purpura pigmentosa chronica (so-called Shamberg's disease and its variants)
      Pityriasis lichenoides et varioliformis acuta
  Capillaritis (leukocytoclastic type)
      Granuloma faciale
      Erythema elevatum diutinum
      Benign leukocytoclastic vasculitis of small vessels—the so-called Gougerot-Ruiter type
Systemic disease
  Leukocytoclastic angiitis of small vessels
      Allergic vasculitis (Schoenlein-Henoch purpura)
      Cutaneous—systemic vasculitis (hypersensitivity angiitis of Zeek, systemic vasculitis of McCombs)
      Angiitis of connective tissue disease (rheumatoid arthritis, systemic lupus erythematosus)
      Angiitis of malignant lymphoproliferative diseases and adenocarcinoma
  Necrotizing angiitis of medium-sized vessels and its variants
      Periarteritis nodosa
      Allergic granulomatosis
      Wegener's granulomatosis
      Giant cell arteritis
  Dysproteinemia with vasculitis
      Hypergammaglobulinemic purpura of Waldenström
      Cryoglobulinemia, cryofibrinogenemia
      Livedo vasculitis
  Intravascular coagulopathy (vascular damage, slowing of blood, hypercoagulable state) including thrombotic thrombocytopenic purpura
  Septic vasculitis
      Bacterial (meningococcemia, gonococcemia, staphylococcemia, pseudomonas septicemia)
      Viral (ECHO 9, Coxsackie A9, arbor viruses)
      Rickettsial (Rocky Mountain spotted fever)
      Fungus (phycomycosis, aspergillosis, cephalosporiosis)

any classification based on the cutaneous manifestation fails to project the generally systemic and overlap nature of these conditions.

The term *vasculitis* or *angiitis* is used to describe the inflammatory changes in and around blood vessels which are primary and not secondary to embolization or inflammation in the neighboring tissues. Two types of small-vessel vasculitis are mainly appreciated: (1) a proliferative and obliterative vasculitis accompanied by lymphocytes, and (2) a necrotizing vasculitis associated with polymorphonuclear cells and immunoglobulins, complement, and fibrin in and about the walls of skin blood vessels. In any variety of angiitis neither capillary, venule, nor artery is the sole primary site. Small veins and capillaries are usually affected in necrotizing vasculitis of the skin (Copeman and Ryan, 1970). Fibrinoid change is seen not only in necrotizing but also in other types of angiitis. The nuclear fragmentation (leukocytoclasia), characteristically seen in necrotizing vasculitis, results from the destruction of young polymorphonuclear leukocytes.

When the endothelium is damaged, as in vasculitis, fibrin or platelets or both are deposited on or within the walls of the involved blood vessels. There are conditions which cause excessive fibrin and platelet deposition that are not associated with angiitis. A classification of vasculitis based on the mechanisms responsible for the initiation, enhancement, and modification of fibrin and platelet deposition has been advanced to augment therapeutic and investigative approaches (Copeman and Ryan, 1970). Among the factors which initiate fibrin and platelet deposition are the injuries to the vessel wall by immune complexes, bacterial endotoxins, and ischemic, pharmacologic, and biochemical insults. Among those factors which enhance fibrin and platelet deposition are fibrinolysis and its impairment, coagulopathies, blood viscosity, and blood flow; those which modify the pathology are red and white blood cell extravasation, alteration of macrophage activity, release of vasoactive substances from platelets, and the secondary epidermal and fat changes. Macrophages remove agents which tend to cause or enhance inflammation. Phagocytosis is essential for the clearance of fibrin or platelet factors. Blocking of the reticuloendothelial system is one of the best ways of encouraging angiitis.

Prognosis depends on the extent and degree of extracutaneous lesions, especially of vital organs. Clinical clues which signal a serious disease and a guarded prognosis include a widespread bullous and infarctive eruption, deep ulcerative or granulomatous lesions of the nose or mouth, hemorrhagic infarctive lesions of the tips of the fingers and toes, and digital gangrene. Systemically, severe degrees of renal involvement, pulmonary infiltra-tive disease, gastrointestinal hemorrhage, and coronary ischemia or occlusion indicate a grave condition, and, laboratory-wise, hematuria, elevated blood urea nitrogen, highly elevated sedimentation rate, and presence of rheumatoid factor and LE cells signal a serious disease.

Leukocytoclastic Angiitis

Leukocytoclastic angiitis (Alarcón-Segovia and Brown, 1964; Braverman, 1970; McGrae and Winkelmann, 1963), which is the commonest form of vasculitis, involves the small vessels of the skin and internal organs and has a specific histopathologic picture which resembles that of the Arthus reaction and experimental serum sickness.

On histopathologic study, two striking features are noted—the small vessel changes and the neutrophil infiltration. The small vessels (capillaries, venules, and arterioles) have endothelial swelling and the deposition of fibrinoid material in and around their walls. The infiltrate consists mainly of neutrophils, which are perivascular but frequently invade the vessel walls, varying amounts of eosinophils, and some lymphocytes. Many scattered nuclear fragments, so-called nuclear dust, which result from nuclear disintegration (karyorrhexis or leukocytoclasia) are characteristically seen.

Necrotizing angiitis is probably pathogenetically initiated by an Arthus type of reaction, and the inflammatory response is perpetuated by either repeated small Arthus reactions or a local Shwartzman reaction at the same site. It is presumed that antigen-antibody complexes in the vessel wall fix complement components C1-4-2-3, which activate and release the complement complex of C5-6-7, which is the chemotactic factor attracting neutrophils. Polymorphonuclear leukocytes phagocytize and catabolize the immune complexes and release proteolytic enzymes which damage the vessel walls.

Leukocytoclastic angiitis (Winkelmann and Ditto, 1964) is an acute, subacute, or chronic syndrome which exhibits a spectrum of cutaneous, visceral, and transitional forms. It may be idiopathic or associated with drug therapy and various diseases. The reported responsible drugs are sulfonamides, penicillin, quinine, quinidine (Fig. 17–12), phenylbutazone, phenothiazine, thiazides (Fig. 17–13), mycins, and iodides (Fig. 17–14). The described associated diseases are periarteritis nodosa and its variants, LE (Fig. 17–15), rheumatoid arthritis (Figs. 17–16 and 17–17), scleroderma, dermatomyositis, Sjögren's disease, chronic ulcerative colitis, hemolytic anemia, dysproteinemia (cryoglobulinemia and purpuric hyperglobulinemia of Waldenström), leprosy (Fig. 17–18), tuberculosis, syphilis (Fig. 17–19), carcinoma, lymphoma (Fig. 17–20), and leukemia.

The names for leukocytoclastic angiitis, used synonymously, depend on the specialty of the reporting physician. Dermatologists have coined the terms arteriolitis allergica (Ruiter), nodular dermal allergid (Gougerot and Duperrat, 1954), monopentasymptom complex (Gougerot and Blum, 1950), and dermatitis nodularis necrotica (Werther). Internists

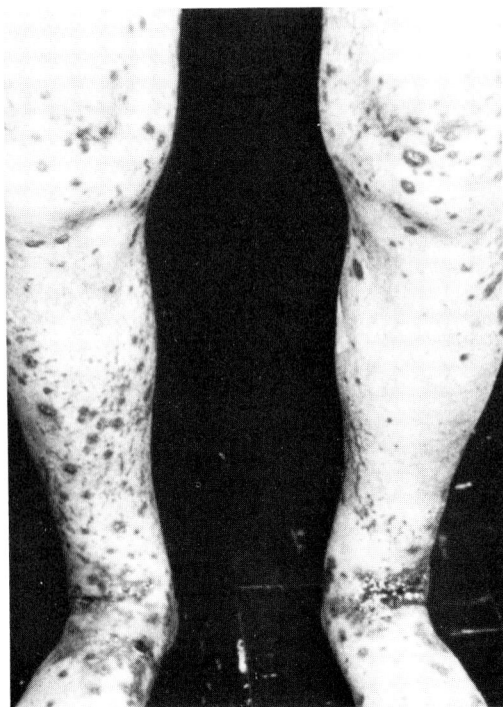

Figure 17–13 Acute heart failure developed in a hypertensive patient and he was given Hydrodiuril; after five days a hemorrhagic vesiculobullous eruption on the edematous lower extremities developed.

and pathologists have used allergic angiitis, systemic allergic vasculitis (McCombs, 1965), hypersensitivity angiitis (Zeek, 1953), anaphylactoid purpura (Schoenlein-Henoch purpura), and "microscopic" periarteritis nodosa.

Among the previously mentioned syndromes with an identical histopathologic picture, two major types appear: one consistent with the clinical picture of Schoenlein-Henoch purpura, and the other consistent with the remaining syndromes listed previously. Acute febrile neutrophilic dermatosis, a rare and unknown entity, is best classified among the leukocytoclastic angiitides.

SCHOENLEIN-HENOCH PURPURA (ANAPHYLACTOID PURPURA, ALLERGIC PURPURA). Schoenlein-Henoch purpura (Ackroyd, 1953; Allen et al., 1960; Cream et al., 1970; Gairdner, 1948) is a necrotizing angiitis involving the small vessels, especially the capillaries, in the upper dermis. It affects primarily children, boys (Fig. 17–21) more often than girls, and young adults. The disease usually has an acute onset and may recur or become chronic. No antecedent illness may be present, but it may follow within a week to three weeks an acute streptococcal or upper respiratory infection. Food allergy is rarely responsible. The peak incidence of disease occurs during the months of March, April, and May.

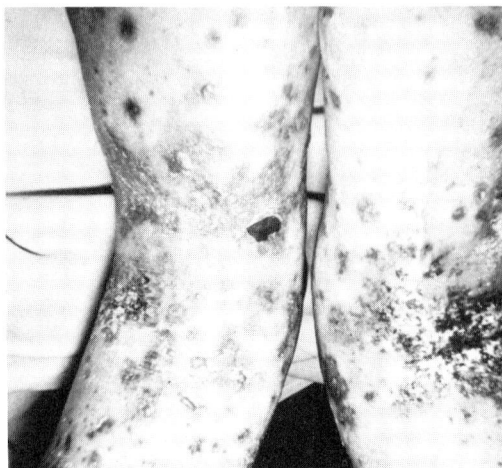

Figure 17–12 Cardiac arrhythmia developed in this patient and he was given quinidine. After seven days, a widespread hemorrhagic papulovesicular eruption, hematuria, and occult melena developed.

The eruption consists of erythematous macular, papular, and urticarial lesions with purpura, and infrequently hemorrhagic vesicles, bullae, and ulcers. In children less than three years of age, edema of the scalp, periorbital areas, hands, feet, and scrotum unassociated with cardiac or renal disease is seen. The lesions appear in crops over days to weeks and have a predilection for the extensor surfaces of the limbs and back and, uncommonly, the face and mucous membranes. They tend to be profuse about the ankles, knees, and elbows. A prodrome of headache, anorexia, and fever occurs. Gastrointestinal lesions occur more frequently in older children. The abdominal problems are of variable severity and consist of colic, vomiting, diarrhea, hematemesis, melena, and, rarely, intussusception. Renal involvement is characterized most commonly by microscopic hematuria with proteinuria; gross hematuria occurs. It is often self-limiting, and, if hematuria continues, it portends a poor prognosis

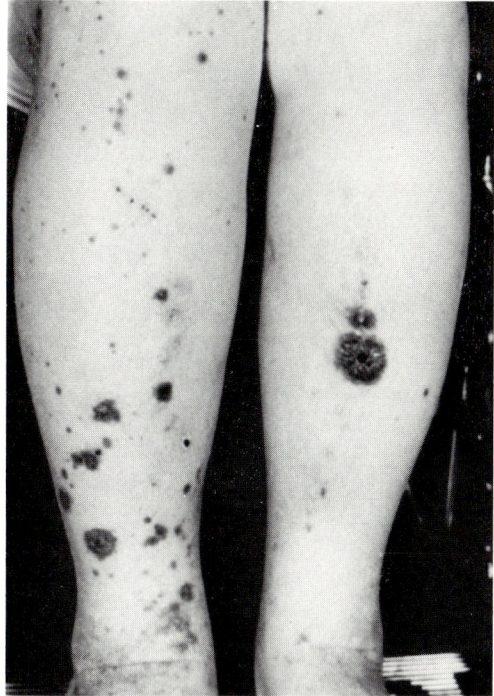

Figure 17–15 Hemorrhagic bullous eruption of the legs and a glomerulitis with hematuria developed in a middle-aged woman with systemic lupus erythematosus.

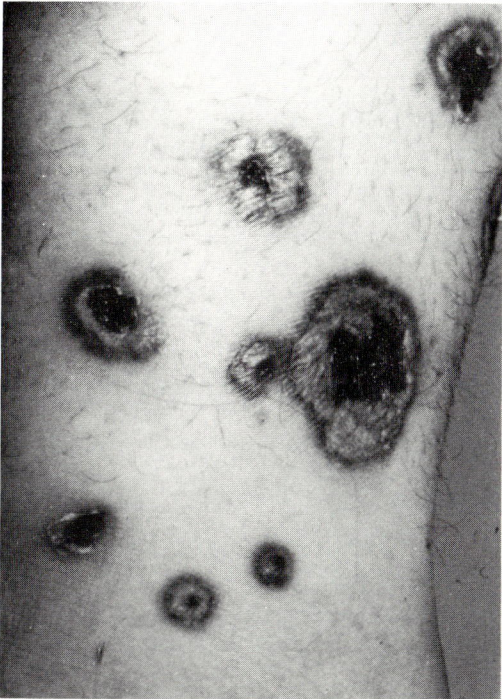

Figure 17–14 Patient was being prepared for thyroid surgery with saturated solution of potassium iodide; during the second week, hemorrhagic necrotic bullae of the extremities developed.

because of advanced glomerular disease. Tender articular swelling of the knees, elbows, ankles, and joints of the hands occurs, persists for a few days, and may recur.

The differential diagnosis of this entity is leukemia, glandular fever, Waldenström's purpura, systemic lupus erythematosus (SLE), thrombotic thrombocytopenic purpura (TTP), subacute bacterial endocarditis, meningococcemia, rickettsial diseases, and bacterial and viral infection with disseminate intravascular coagulation.

The disease is usually self-limited and lasts a few weeks but may recur for weeks and months. The prognosis depends on the severity of the renal involvement. The acute manifestations can be suppressed by systemic corticosteroid therapy, which appears to have no effect on the prognosis or natural course of the disease.

CUTANEOUS SYSTEMIC ANGIITIS. Cutaneous systemic angiitis (Braverman, 1970) affects the small vessels throughout the dermis and occasionally the subcutis.

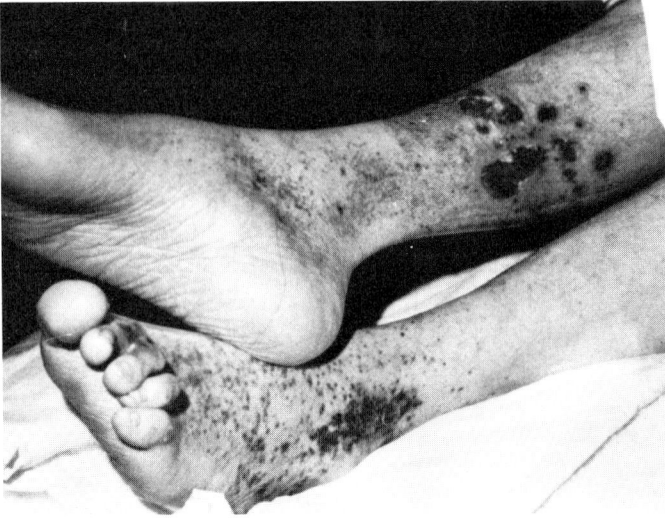

Figure 17-16 Patient had deforming rheumatoid arthritis especially of the hand and less of the feet, rheumatoid nodules of the elbows, and a high titer of rheumatoid factor and palpable purpura and ulcerations of the legs.

Figure 17-17 A 15-year-old boy developed rheumatoid-like arthritis, hemorrhagic plaques of the legs, and a peripheral neuropathy following a beta-hemolytic streptococcal infection of the throat. Histopathologically, biopsy of nerve and muscle revealed periarteritis nodosa and skin leukocytoclastic angiitis.

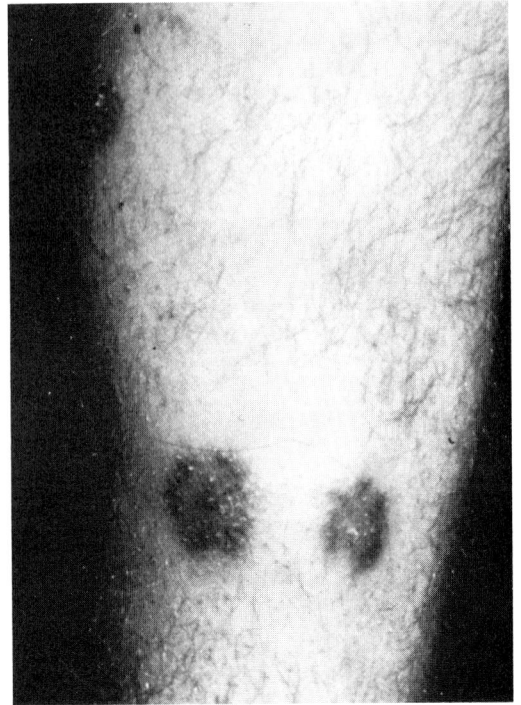

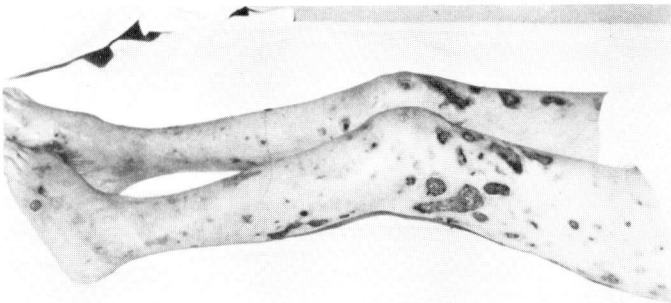

Figure 17-18 Patient had diffuse lepromatous leprosy and Lucio's phenomenon (erythema necroticans) which was misdiagnosed as pyoderma and factitial dermatitis.

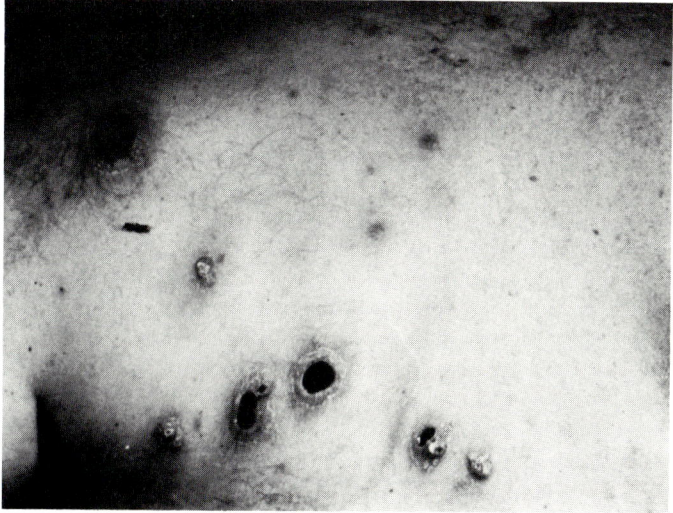

Figure 17–19 Late necrotic nodular syphiloderm.

Drugs and infections have been most frequently implicated. In most instances, the eruption continues despite the discontinuance of the drugs. In a majority of the

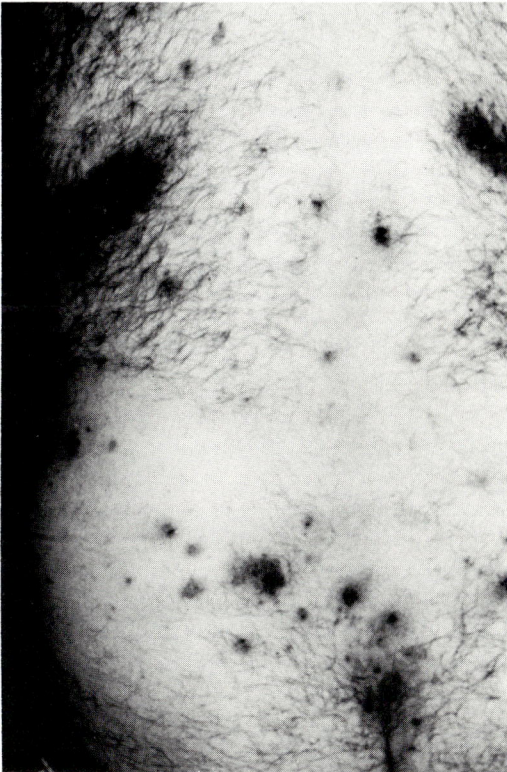

Figure 17–20 Patient presented with purpuric plaques which initially exhibited a necrotizing angiitis on histopathologic study; however, rebiopsy five months later revealed not only the vasculitis but also the presence of lymphosarcoma.

cases, no causal associations can be made. Various names have been coined for this condition, depending on the nature of the onset, the extent and degree of cutaneous and systemic involvement, and the course. There is a predilection for adults between the ages of 30 and 60 years; however, both the young and old may be affected. Both sexes are equally susceptible. The disease may be acute, subacute, chronic, or recurrent, and the eruptions limited or extensive. The more acute the process, the more likely it is to be associated with constitutional symptoms of fever, malaise, arthralgia, and myalgia and with a more severe and extensive cutaneous eruption.

The diagnostic clinical lesion is palpable purpura. The other lesions seen are erythematous macules, papules, urticaria, and nodules, which are usually purpuric, hemorrhagic vesicles and bullae, and necrotic ulcerations. In the more chronic eruptions, the papules may coalesce to form plaques. The lesions appear in crops and subside in two to three weeks. When the eruption is chronic and systemic involvement is minimal or absent, the clinical picture is that described by Gougerot and Blum (1950) as monopentasymptom complex or by Ruiter (1954) as arteriolitis allergica. When the eruption consists of many tender nodules which result from small-vessel involvement at the dermal subcutaneous border and may ulcerate, it resembles the condition reported as nodular dermal allergid by Gougerot and Duperrat (1954) and that reported as derma-

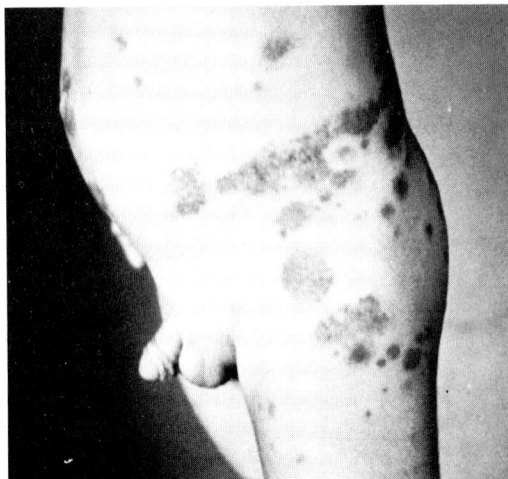

Figure 17–21 After a streptococcal infection of his throat, a 14-year-old boy developed Schoenlein-Henoch purpura (anaphylactoid purpura) and associated urticarial erythematous lesions with purpura, painful articular swelling, and microscopic hematuria.

titis nodularis necrotica by Werther (Duemling, 1930).

The most commonly involved systems are the joints, kidneys, peripheral nerves, lungs, gastrointestinal tract, and heart. Just as the skin eruptions, the systemic manifestations may be acute or chronic and mild or severe. The arthritis resembles that seen in collagen diseases and can persist between attacks. Renal involvement occurs frequently, presents histologically as a focal necrotizing glomerulitis or a diffuse glomerulonephritis, may continue for months to years, and may result in death from chronic renal insufficiency. Although peripheral neuropathy is the main manifestation of nervous system involvement, patients may exhibit central nervous system signs and symptoms, such as headaches, mental confusion, delirium, and diplopia. Gastrointestinal involvement results in abdominal pains, diarrhea, hematemesis, and melena. As a result of coronary vessel involvement, the patient with this condition may experience congestive heart failure, arrhythmias, pericarditis, angina, and myocardial infarction. When the severity of the systemic involvement overshadows that of the skin and the course of the disease is fulminant with death from uremia, the clinical picture resembles the hypersensitivity angiitis de-

scribed by Zeek (1953). The cases described as systemic allergic vasculitis by McCombs (1965) were less severe, more chronic, and resulted in fewer fatalities than those of Zeek (1953).

The most frequently observed abnormal laboratory tests are an elevated sedimentation rate, hypergammaglobulinemia, and eosinophilia, which occurs in about 10 to 20 per cent of patients. Patients with mixed cryoglobulinemia of IgG and IgM immunoglobulins may experience arthralgias, palpable purpura of the lower extremities, visceral angiitis resulting from necrotizing angiitis, Sjögren's syndrome, thyroiditis, glomerulonephritis with renal death, anemia, hypergammaglobulinemia, presence of antinuclear factors, and depressed serum complement levels.

The treatment in the form of occlusive topical and systemic corticosteroids is suppressive and appears to have no effect on the duration or prognosis of the disease. Elastic support stockings are a helpful measure for the cutaneous lesions of the lower extremities.

Acute Febrile
Neutrophilic Dermatosis

Acute febrile neutrophilic dermatosis (Goldman and Moschella, 1971; Sweet, 1968) is a rare, unusual, self-limiting illness which is characterized by a high, persistent fever with no appreciable internal organ involvement and by painful nodules and plaques with a consistent histopathologic picture and a tendency to recur.

On histopathologic examination of skin lesions, there are vasodilation, endothelial swelling, and focal or massive infiltration of polymorphonuclear leukocytes in the upper and mid-dermis. There may be numerous pyknotic polymorphonuclear leukocytes near the center of the infiltrate, resembling the formation of an incipient abscess. The condition is probably a hypersensitivity reaction to agents as yet undiscovered.

Usually an antecedent upper respiratory infection occurs about two weeks before the onset of the skin lesion. The disease predominantes in middle-aged women, who constitute 90 per cent of the reported cases. They have a persistent fever of 100 to 102° F., no chills, and malaise. On physical examination, no systemic signs are appreciated. The cutaneous lesions are dull red, tender, and painful edematous nodules which coalesce to form plaques (Fig. 17–22). Vesicles or small sterile pustules may appear on the surface of the lesions. The plaques appear asymmetrically and centrifugally on the extremities, face, and neck and vary in size from 0.5 to 4.0 cm. in diameter. The active disease, fever, and skin lesions subside spontaneously, usually in four to eight weeks, although it has been reported to persist for up to six months. No scarring is present. The only significant laboratory abnormalities are leukocytosis and an elevated sedimentation rate. The differential diagnosis includes atypical erythema multiforme, erythema nodosum, erythema elevatum diutinum, granuloma faciale, and bromoderma.

The disease tends to recur in at least one-third of the cases, and each time there is usually an antecedent upper respiratory tract infection. It responds to systemic corticosteroids, which may have to be administered for weeks to minimize relapse. Intralesional steroid therapy is

effective local treatment for the cutaneous lesions.

Periarteritis Nodosa

Periarteritis nodosa (Frohnert and Sheps, 1967; Rose and Spencer, 1957; Zeek, 1953) is a widespread segmental necrotizing panarteritis of the medium and, less frequently, the small arteries with signs and symptoms from infarction and scarring of involved organs and systems. The cause of this disease is unknown but it is believed to be the result of a hypersensitivity reaction. The onset may be preceded by a chronic upper respiratory tract infection, such as bronchiectasis, an acute hemolytic streptococcal infection, or an attack of rheumatic fever. Among the many drugs which have been incriminated etiologically are sulfonamides, penicillin, streptomycin, chlorpromazine, hydantoin derivatives, hydralazine, phenylbutazone, uracil compounds, guanethidine, corticosteroids, and others, but no consistent relationship has been established. Lesions indistinguishable from those of periarteritis nodosa have been seen in patients with rheumatoid arthritis, rheumatic fever, SLE, scleroderma, and TTP.

Pathology

On histopathologic examination, the involved medium and small muscular arteries demonstrate initially swelling and edema of the media and subendothelial deposition of hyaline material which disrupts the internal elastic lamina. The subsequent necrotizing inflammatory process involves the entire vessel wall. The associated cellular infiltrate consists largely of neutrophils and a few eosinophils and, later, lymphocytes, monocytes, and plasma cells. The lesions heal with fibrosis, recanalization, and aneurysmal dilatation. Intimal proliferation is followed by thrombosis and infarction. There is segmental involvement of the vessels at the site of branching. The more commonly involved organs are the musculoskeletal system, peripheral nerves, kidneys, gastrointestinal system, lungs, heart, testes, and brain. It can be distinguished from the hypersensitivity angiitis of Zeek, which is char-

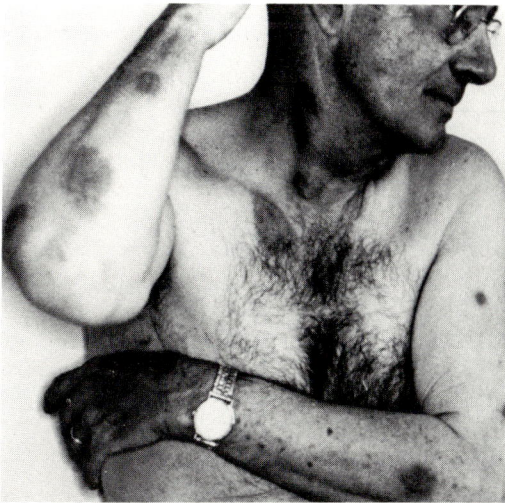

Figure 17–22 Acute febrile neutrophilic dermatosis (Sweet's disease). Middle-aged man who, after a viral upper respiratory tract infection, noticed fever, plaques, and nodules which resembled erythema nodosum; histopathologic examination revealed acute febrile neutrophilic dermatosis.

acterized by small artery and vein involvement with an intense cellular reaction, especially eosinophils, and histopathologic changes of the same age.

Clinical Manifestations

Periarteritis nodosa is usually a fatal protean multisystem disease. It is ordinarily acute but can be insidious or chronic; there may be temporary and, infrequently, complete remissions. The disease process may be confined to one organ or system for a variable period of time. It may be fatal within a few weeks, but patients with this condition have survived for 10 years or more. The constitutional signs and symptoms are fever, malaise, weight loss, excessive sweating, tachycardia, and aching extremities. Periarteritis nodosa may present clinically as a nonspecific acute or chronic febrile illness, atypical abdominal illness, primary renal disease, peripheral polyneuritis or polymyositis or both, bronchial asthma with focal pulmonary infiltrates, and myocardial infarction. The disease is three times more frequent in men than in women, and it has been reported in patients from 3 months to 78 years of age, with a peak incidence between 20 and 50 years of age. All races may be affected.

The muscle changes may be due to a myopathy secondary to vessel changes or a nonspecific wasting which results from the severe illness. The joint involvement may be acute, resembling that of rheumatic fever, or subacute or chronic, resembling that of rheumatoid arthritis.

The kidneys are involved in about 50 per cent of the cases. This involvement is the commonest cause of death, recovery is rare, and hypertension is a complication. Two distinct lesions are appreciated: a characteristic glomerulitis and a polyarteritis of the renal arteries which causes cortical infarction.

The peripheral neuropathy is usually bilateral, asymmetric or symmetric, and of the mixed type (motor and sensory). The lower extremities are especially afflicted. The central nervous system may be affected and can cause convulsions, vertigo, subarachnoid hemorrhage, hemiplegia, cerebellar signs, and visual disturbances.

Abdominal pain, which is seen in about one-half of the patients, is often sharp, periumbilical, or in the right upper quadrant. The patients experience anorexia, nausea, vomiting, and blood diarrhea. The disease may affect the gastrointestinal tract, liver, pancreas, and spleen. Hemorrhage and perforation of the bowel occur. Other lesions seen are thrombosis and infarction of the liver and spleen, perihepatitis, perisplenitis, and pancreatitis with subsequent fibrosis. Steatorrhea has been reported (Carron and Douglas, 1965).

Lesions occur in the coronary vessels and cause myocardial infarction and, rarely, angina. Congestive heart failure may complicate the infarction or the hypertension. Periarteritis nodosa in infants frequently involves the coronary arteries and results in sudden, unexpected death.

The pulmonary arteries are spared, but the bronchial arteries can be affected. When pulmonary lesions occur, they usually precede involvement of other organs and are associated with asthma, a fleeting pulmonary infiltration of Löffler's type, and eosinophilia. The disease may affect the ovaries, testes, and epididymis.

Cutaneous involvement (Beliasario, 1960; Fisher and Orkin, 1964) occurs in about 25 per cent of cases. The type of lesion seen depends on the stage and severity of the disease and the depth of the involved vessel. The commonest eruption is characterized by tender, erythematous, cutaneous, and subcutaneous nodules which are of varying size, occur in crops and groups which are seen more commonly on the lower extremities about the knees and feet, and may break down and ulcerate (Fig. 17–23). Similar nodules may be palpable along the brachial and intercostal arteries. In the more chronic cases, a reticulate livedo may accompany the nodules; this type of eruption may be associated with an underlying specific myopathy and may be the only clinical manifestation of periarteritis nodosa. Other cutaneous lesions seen are those of diffuse erythema, urticaria, scarlatiniform and morbilliform exanthemata, palpable purpura, Schoenlein-Henoch–like purpura, ecchymosis, and gangrene, which are associated with underlying systemic visceral lesions. The erythematous macules may develop hemorrhagic bullae which result

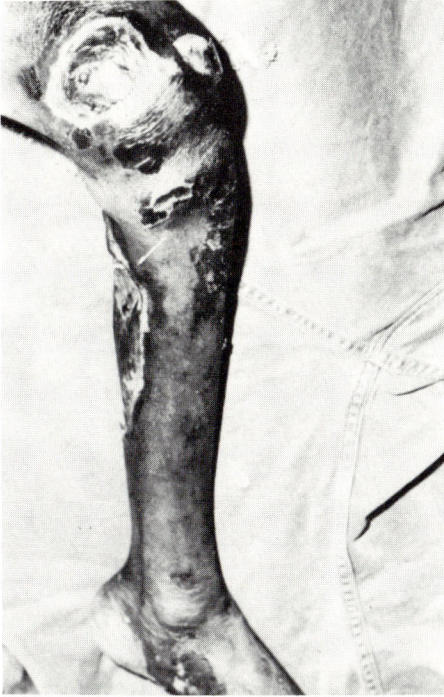

Figure 17–23 Periarteritis nodosa. Diffusely infiltrated hemorrhagic plaques which became large ischemic ulcerations developed in a 37-year-old asthmatic patient; subsequently, perforation of the small bowel developed from the disease process.

in crusted necrotic ulcerations. An erythema nodosum–like eruption has been described. Other extremity changes seen are Raynaud's phenomenon, persistent coldness and blueness, absorption of terminal phalanges, and acral necrosis and gangrene.

The differential diagnoses of the systemic disease are trichinosis, typhoid fever, dysentery, tuberculosis, meningitis, cholecystitis, appendicitis, and acute nephritis. The differential diagnoses of the diseases associated with similar cutaneous lesions include dermatomyositis, SLE, cryoglobulinemia, Schoenlein-Henoch purpura, and the necrotizing angiitides.

Laboratory studies reveal leukocytosis with a predominance of polymorphonuclear leukocytes, eosinophils, anemia resulting from blood loss or renal insufficiency, an elevated blood sedimentation rate, and an increase of serum globulin. Biopsy of the clinically involved muscles, liver, testes, and rectum is performed to establish the diagnosis.

Those persons afflicted do not survive more than 6 to 12 months and rarely more than 10 years; spontaneous remissions can occur. Death results from renal involvement in about 65 per cent of cases, from myocardial infarction in about 15 per cent, and from gastrointestinal and central nervous system lesions in the remaining.

Treatment

Systemic corticosteroid therapy in adequate large doses suppresses and controls many symptoms but must be continued over long periods to prevent exacerbations. Steroid therapy should be initiated early and vigorously. That corticosteroids increase survival has been controversial, and it has been suggested that their use results in the postponement of death. It has been reported recently that corticosteroid therapy gives a five-year survival in approximately 50 per cent of the patients in contrast to only about 15 per cent survival in the untreated cases.

PURPURA

Purpura (Harrington, 1957, 1967) is the discoloration of skin and mucous membranes resulting from intracutaneous and subcutaneous bleeding. It appears as petechiae or ecchymoses. Petechiae are small pinpoint hemorrhages and result from vascular or platelet abnormalities, while ecchymoses are larger extravasations of red blood cells, appear as bruises, and are the usual form of bleeding into the skin of patients with clotting disorders. Purpura (Bowie and Owen, 1968) may occur spontaneously or after innocuous trauma and results from vessel wall damage, defective number or function of blood platelets, faulty coagulation, defective quality of perivascular support, or a combination of these faulty hemostatic factors (Table 17–2). The hemorrhagic disorders may be acute or chronic, primary or secondary, and congenital or familial. Although purpura is usually asymptomatic, the lesions may be tender and palpable as in the vasculitides, or paresthetic as in acute erythrocyte sensitization. Bruising without evidence of a hemorrhagic dis-

TABLE 17–2 CLASSIFICATION OF PURPURA

Primary vascular purpura (extravascular)
    Purpura simplex, senilis cachectica, Cushing's syndrome, myxedema, rheumatoid arthritis, and glucocortical therapy
    Hereditary disorders of connective tissue, Ehlers-Danlos and Marfan's syndromes, osteogenesis imperfecta
Secondary vascular purpura
    Mechanical (orthostasis, local obstruction, embolism, factitia)
    Infectious — Embolism, toxin, purpura fulminans
    Metabolic — Scurvy, diabetes mellitus, uremia
    Immunologic — Schoenlein-Henoch purpura, serum and drug sensitivity, auto-erythrocyte and DNA hypersensitivity
    Associated with various forms of vasculitides
    Carcinomatous — Tumor or fibrin embolism
    Toxic — Venoms
Platelet abnormalities
    Thrombocytopenia
        Decreased production — Idiopathic marrow infiltration (malignancy), marrow depression (drugs, radiation), megaloblastic anemias, splenomegaly, and decrease of "thrombopoietin"
        Increased destruction — Excessive sequestration, primary and secondary auto-immune mechanisms, accelerated intravascular coagulation, transfusion reactions, thrombotic thrombocytopenic purpura, auto-antibodies for platelets
    Thrombocythemia — Myeloproliferative disorders, carcinoma
    Thrombopathy — Phospholipid defect, Glanzmann's thromboasthenia
        Primary (congenital) — Hereditary thrombasthenia and thrombocytopathia
        Secondary (acquired) — Dysproteinemia (cryoglobulinemia, macroglobulinemia, hyperglobulinemia), metabolic states (uremia, liver disease)
Coagulopathies
    Defects of factors VIII (hemophilia), IX (plasma thromboplastin component, Christmas disease), XI (plasma thromboplastin antecedent)
    Hypoprothrombinemias
        Congenital — Congenital deficiencies V, VII, X
        Acquired — newborn, vitamin K deficiency, anticoagulant drugs
    Fibrinogen disorders — Congenital and acquired (defibrination syndrome) hypofibrinogenemia, factor XIII deficiency
Circulating anticoagulants
Dermatologic purpura — Purpura pigmentosa chronica

order may occur in normal persons, depending on the character of their skin and their age, weight, and other variables.

The events responsible for preventing the escape of cells from the vessels or sealing of vascular perforations are reflex vasoconstriction of vessel walls and chemical forces attracting platelets to each other and to the denuded subendothelial collagen. Adenosine diphosphate and triphosphate (ADP and ATP), which are contained in platelets, are strong platelet aggregators. Upon contact with collagen, the platelets swell and release vasoconstrictive amines, notably serotonin (5-hydroxytryptamine), "platelet factor 3" (a phospholipoprotein necessary for generating the clotting mechanism), and thrombosthenin (a contractile protein leading to retraction of the clot). The repair process proceeds with inhibition of excessive coagulation by anticoagulants and finally with dissolution of the clot by fibrinolytic enzymes.

Among the laboratory tests used to investigate and establish the cause of purpura are the following: examination of peripheral blood smear, bone marrow examination, platelet count, bleeding and coagulation time (the latter in glass and nonwettable tubes), capillary fragility, clot retraction, one-stage prothrombin time, partial thromboplastin time, thromboplastic generation tests, and assays for fibrinogen and fibrinolysis.

The commonest clinical manifestations of primary vascular purpura are easy bruising, spontaneous ecchymoses, and, less frequently, petechiae and hematomas. The mucous membranes can be involved. They may occur without any discernible blood or capillary abnormalities. Among these conditions are purpura simplex and those associated with states or disease characterized by connective tissue alterations. Purpura simplex is seen in healthy women about menstrual time and appears as easy bruising (the so-called devil's pinches). In old (Fig. 17–24) and cachectic persons, atrophy of the skin and loss of subcutaneous fat and skin elasticity permit the skin to be susceptible to minor trauma with the formation of petechiae and ecchymoses along the veins of the hands, forearms, legs, and feet. Similar lesions are seen in patients who have Cushing's syndrome, myxedema, rheumatoid arthritis, or have been receiving prolonged topical fluorinated corticosteroid or systemic glucocorticoid therapy which affects adversely extravascular tissues through its hormonal antianabolic effects.

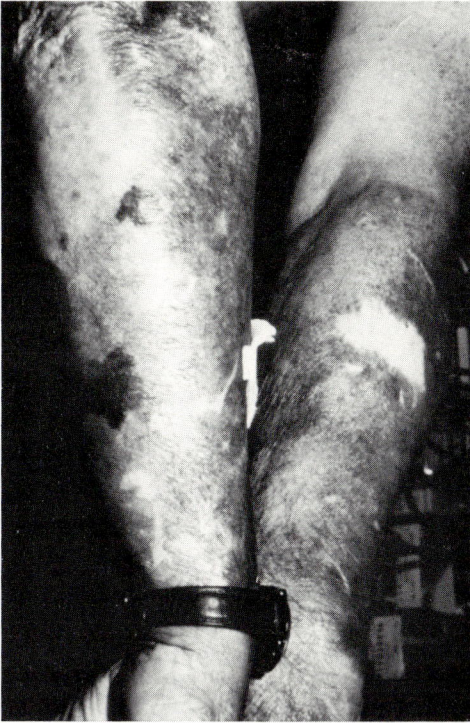

Figure 17–24 Purpura in an elderly woman. The so-called senile purpura characterized by ecchymotic areas, triangular scars, and hyperpigmentation; prolonged systemic or topical corticosteroid therapy in sufficient amounts can produce a similar change.

The heritable dysplastic mesenchymal disorders of Ehlers-Danlos syndrome, pseudoxanthoma elasticum, osteogenesis imperfecta, and Marfan's disease can be associated with extravascular hemostatic defects. Ehlers-Danlos syndrome is associated with increased fragility of subcutaneous vessels, and easy bruisability, subcutaneous hematomas, petechial and gingival bleeding, and various abnormalities in the clotting mechanisms and in platelets have been described. In osteogenesis imperfecta, subconjunctival hemorrhages and hematomas may be seen.

Secondary vascular purpura may be caused by (1) mechanical factors which may be orthostatic, locally obstructive, embolic, or factitial; (2) infectious complications of septic embolization (Fig. 17–25), toxicity, and purpura fulminans; (3) metabolic purpura seen in scurvy (Fig. 17–26), diabetes mellitus, and uremia; (4) immunologic states such as Schoenlein-Henoch purpura, serum and drug sensitivity, and auto-erythrocyte and DNA hypersensitivity; (5) the various vasculitides; (6) carcinoma; and (7) toxic venoms.

Purpura secondary to trauma of violent muscular contractions, whoop, Valsalva's maneuver, convulsions, or the constrictive forces of tourniquets and the like (Fig. 17–27) is the result of the rupture of capillaries in the afflicted sites (usually the head, neck, and upper extremities). Crops of petechiae due to prolonged coughing or vomiting (Fig. 17–28) may be seen in the face and neck and are a result of loose tissue in the areas. Purpura may develop in some persons without any appreciable bleeding or coagulable defects on the lower extremities after prolonged standing. An example of factitial purpura is the "battered child" syndrome, which is characterized by the sudden appearance of crops of ecchymoses in a child who was physically beaten by an emotionally disturbed parent. Neoplastic disease may cause purpura through embolization of tumor or fibrin from the aseptic vegetations on the heart valves which may be seen in

Figure 17–25 Purpura of the nails, the splinter hemorrhages of septic embolization resulting from subacute bacterial endocarditis.

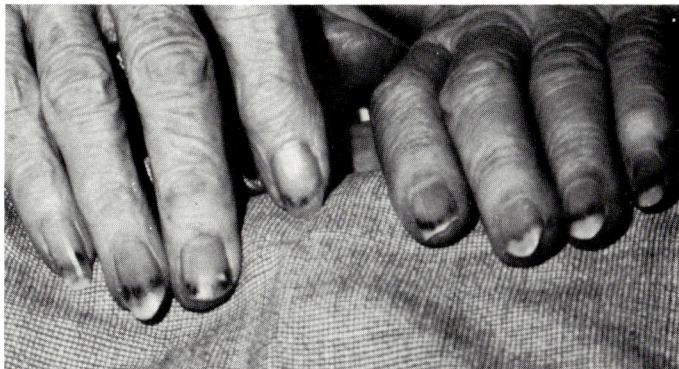

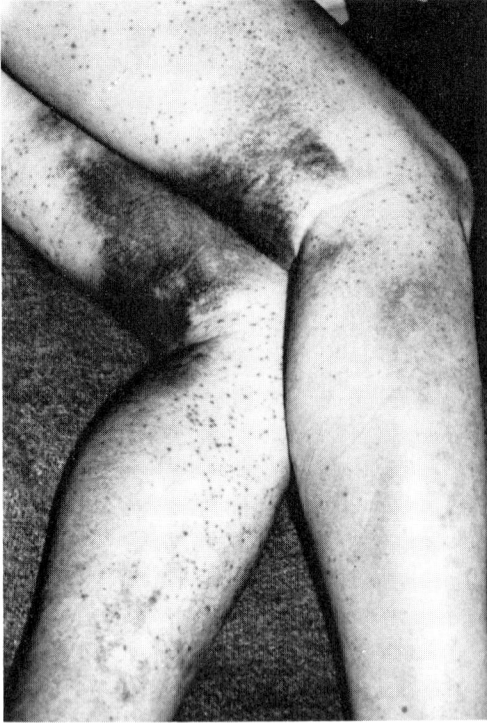

Figure 17–26 Purpura in a patient who had chronic ulcer disease and whose diet was free of vitamin C for years; the purpura of the skin in scurvy appears in the keratotic follicles and as ecchymoses.

any wasting disease. Microemboli from atheromatous plaque fragments, lipids from fatty acids liberated by hydrolysis of lipids after injury to bone, or gas emboli (the "bends") can cause petechiae.

Infectious diseases may induce purpura through high fever, minute infarctive thrombi, toxins, septic emboli, thrombocytopenia, damage to blood vessel endothelium, and intravascular coagulation. High fever can cause increased capillary fragility with resultant purpura. Rickettsial and malarial organisms invade the endothelium of blood vessels and can cause infarctive thrombosis with hemorrhage. Some infectious agents, such as those of epidemic hemorrhagic fever and Weil's disease, have an extraordinary capacity to damage endothelium. In the absence of thrombocytopenia, the purpura associated with acute infectious diseases is usually attributed to the effect of toxins on the vascular endothelium. The erythrotoxin of scarlet fever is capable of inducing widespread capillary damage. There is

often purpura about the ankles and areas distal to physical constrictive sites; in severe cases, the purpura may be extensive and associated with mucosal bleeding.

A purpuric eruption may be seen in typhoid fever, meningococcemia, pneumococcemia, the sepsis of pseudomonas and clostridium, and in the exanthemata of varicella, vaccinia, variola, rubella, and rubeola, as well as in the arborvirus infections, such as hemorrhagic fever. The bleeding, especially when it is severe, may be the result of a disseminated intravascular coagulation. The cutaneous manifestations of the consumptive coagulopathy caused by infection are purpura, ecchymosis, necrosis of skin, and gangrene of digits and extremities. The classic cutaneous expression of this phenomenon is purpura fulminans, sometimes called purpura hemorrhagica, purpura necrotica, or purpura gangrenosa. This syndrome is seen most often in children during the convalescent stage of various infectious diseases. It is characterized by the abrupt appearance of localized areas of massive, tender, intracutaneous and subcutaneous hemorrhage, which symmetrically involves the extremities, especially the site of pressure, and tends to progress and coalesce, and by intense systemic symptoms of fever, chills, and prostration. Central nervous system symptoms, hemorrhagic shock, coma, and finally death usually occur within the first 48 to 72 hours. In the ecchymotic (blueblack) regions surrounded by a halo of warm erythema, a hemorrhagic bulla or necrosis or both may develop.

In advanced cases of purpura fulminans, the indurated lesions may surround an extremity completely and result in ischemic gangrene that frequently necessitates amputation. Lesions of the kidney, intestine, and lung have been described. Therapy consists primarily of anticoagulation with heparin, elimination of the underlying disease, and judicious supportive care. The local destructive process of skin and subcutaneous tissue may cause residual scars with contractive and functional impairment.

Among the metabolic conditions that can be associated with purpura are scurvy, diabetes mellitus, Cushing's syndrome, exogenous hypercorticoidism, and uremia. Vitamin C deficiency, which has been

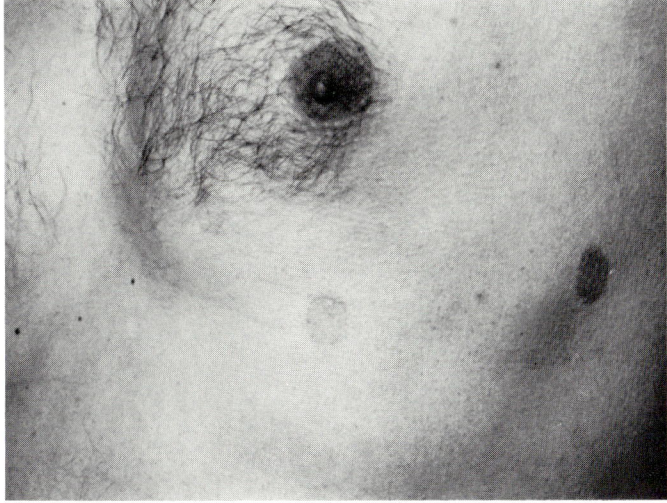

Figure 17–27 Purpura from trauma induced by suction cups used to fix chest leads utilized for electrocardiography.

thought to result in faulty cement substance between endothelial cells, loss of vascular support from impaired collagen synthesis, a thrombopathy (poor aggregation of platelets upon addition of ADP), and a mild thrombocytopenia, can cause petechiae. The cause of purpura in diabetes mellitus is unknown. The friability of the skin has been advanced as being responsible for the purpura seen in Cushing's syndrome or exogenous hypercorti-

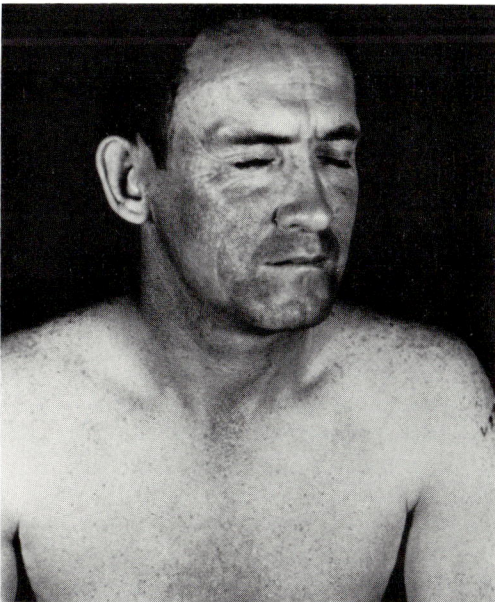

Figure 17–28 Purpura of the face secondary to the physical force of prolonged vomiting.

coidism. In uremia, not only purpura of the skin and mucous membranes but also large subcutaneous extravasations are seen; the abnormal bleeding commonly present is attributed to platelet quantitative or qualitative phospholipid abnormalities or their inadequate release.

Immunologic mechanisms have been implicated for the cause of purpura in allergic vasculitis (Schoenlein-Henoch purpura), serum and drug reactions, and auto-erythrocyte and DNA hypersensitivity. Schoenlein-Henoch purpura (anaphylactoid or allergic purpura) is believed to be the result of an immunologic insult (Arthus-like reaction) to the host's vascular endothelium. Among the causes are bacteria (streptococci, tubercle bacilli, bacterial vaccines), drugs (antibiotics, analgesics, sedatives, anticonvulsants, heavy metals, diuretics), foods (berries, pork, nuts), insect bites, and serum sickness.

Purpura resulting from such drugs as iodides, belladonna, phenacetin, acetylsalicylic acid, and chloral hydrate is mainly idiosyncratic or may be due to a resultant thrombocytopenia which may be dose related or may depend on host sensitivity. Among the drugs which frequently cause thrombocytopenia are those used in leukemia, Hodgkin's disease, cancer, and immunosuppression (for example, nitrogen mustard and antimetabolites). When thrombocytopenic purpura due to drugs is dose related, an accompanying anemia or leukopenia may be present. Some drugs like Sedormid (allylisopropylacetylcarbamide) cause only hypersensitive thrombocytopenic purpura; others may cause not only the hypersensitive thrombocytopenia but also leukopenia or aplastic anemia. At least two mechanisms are suggested to explain the thrombocytopenia. One damages megakaryocytes, and the other destroys platelets. Allylisopropylacetylcarbamide and quinidine result in immunologic agglutination and lysis of platelets. The responsible drug combines haptenically with platelets which agglutinate and are lysed by antibodies in the presence of complement. Certain drugs, such as carbromal (Fig. 17–29) and phenacetin, may cause a distinctive clinical picture which is characterized by an erythematous eruption with purpura due to a capillaritis, resembling Schamberg's disease or itching purpura.

Two conditions characterized by autosensitivity, one to erythrocyte stroma (Gardner and Diamond, 1955) and the other to DNA on intradermal testing, are

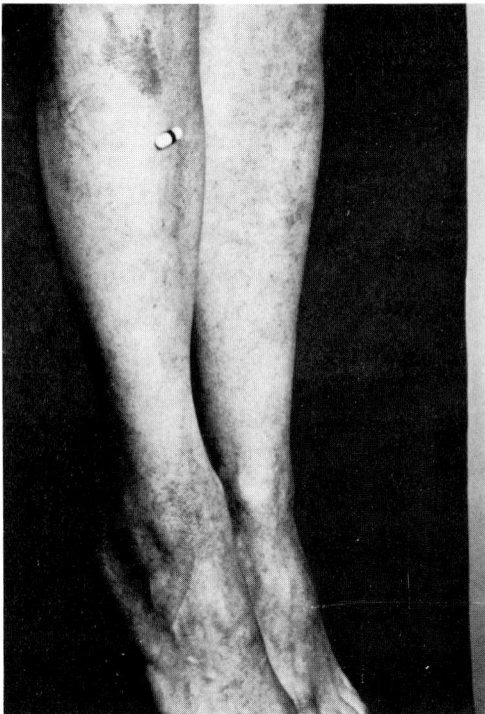

Figure 17–29   Drug-induced purpura. Carbromal, a sedative, can produce an erythematous purpuric eruption that may resemble Schamberg's disease.

associated with tender ecchymoses. The former may be a psychosomatic disorder (Ratnoff and Agle, 1968). It is seen in women between the ages of 19 and 54 years. It is related to trauma and usually appears initially on the lower extremities and later the face and trunk. The painful bruises tend to be multiple and may appear in a linear fashion, creating a ladder effect. Generalized abdominal complaints associated with nausea and vomiting, as well as syncopal attacks, occur. Gastrointestinal and intracranial bleeding have been reported. There are periods of remissions and attacks, and their intensity is related to the degree of emotional stress.

Patients with autosensitivity to erythrocyte stroma have a high incidence of conversion reactions, psychosomatic symptoms, dissociative episodes, and difficulties in emotional adjustment. Biopsy reveals extravasation of red blood cells. Patients react, on intradermal skin testing, not only to red blood cell stroma but also reportedly to its lipid constituents and even hemoglobin (Groch et al., 1966). The patients and the disease are resistant to psychotherapy. No significant response is seen to corticosteroids.

DNA autosensitivity appears to be a localized hypersensitivity to the patient's leukocytes or a solution of autologous or heterologous desoxyribonucleic acid (Levin and Pinkus, 1961). The spontaneous, painful, erythematous swelling and extensive ecchymosis usually involve the extremities but may involve the trunk and face. The condition may resemble or be related to SLE (Chandler and Nalbandian, 1966) because of the sensitivity to sunlight, renal involvement, and the nonspecific symptoms of fever, malaise, fatigue, muscle pain, headache, and arthralgia; however, the antinuclear factor titer (ANFT) and LE tests reveal negative findings. The condition responds dramatically to antimalarials. DNA autosensitivity appears to be distinctly different from auto-erythrocyte sensitization.

Palpable purpura may result from an inflammatory vasculitis of small vessels of the necrotizing, lymphocytic, and granulomatous types, or from a dysproteinemic state. These conditions must be differentiated from intentionally produced purpura, the so-called factitial purpura.

Neoplastic disease (carcinoma, leukemia, lymphoma, myelomatosis, and giant hemangioma) may cause purpura not only by tumor and fibrin embolism but also by dysproteinemia, disseminated intravascular coagulation, and fibrinolysis. The viperine, croataline, and arachnid (spiders and scorpion) venom can injure endothelium of capillaries and veins, have an anticoagulant effect, and cause disseminated intravascular coagulation (DIC) and consequently purpura.

Purpura may result from platelet abnormalities due to a decrease (thrombocytopenia) or an increase (thrombocythemia) in circulating platelets or to a disturbance in their physiologic function (thrombopathy and thrombasthenia). Although petechiae and ecchymoses are most typical, visceral bleeding, such as menorrhagia and melena, and intracranial hemorrhage, are seen. In thrombocytopenia, there is a decrease in platelet count, the tourniquet test is positive, the bleeding time is prolonged, the prothrombin conversion is impaired, and there is an absence or diminution of clot retraction; however, the clotting time is usually normal. The thrombocytopenia may result from decreased platelet production or an increased destruction of platelets. Platelet production can be reduced when the marrow is infiltrated with leukemic cells, metastatic carcinoma, sarcoid, lymphoma, granulomatous disease, or fat-laden histiocytes (in the lipidoses), or when it is sclerosed through irradiation. A reduction in platelet production also occurs when the marrow becomes aplastic from the exposure to chemicals and the use of oncolytic drugs as well as others such as chloramphenicol (Fig. 17–30), in certain deficiency states causing megaloblastic anemias and scurvy, and in certain conditions such as idiopathic thrombocytopenia, splenomegaly, uremia, acute infection, congenital aplasia, lack of circulating thrombopoietin, and Hegglin's anomaly (faulty maturation of platelets and granulocytes). Thymic tumor may have an anemia and, less frequently, thrombocytopenia.

The normal life span of platelets is 8 to 10 days. Increased destruction of platelets may result from sequestration, as in splenomegaly and extensive hemangiomas, immunologic mechanisms, massive blood

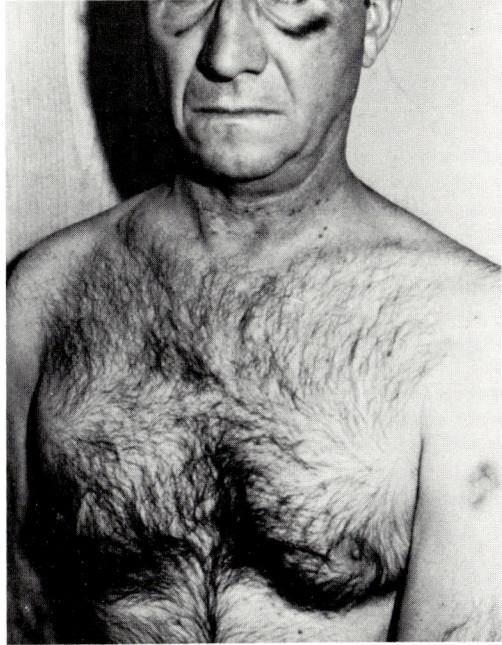

Figure 17–30 Chloramphenicol produced aplastic marrow with resultant purpura seen in this patient as scattered ecchymotic areas.

transfusions, intravascular coagulation, and TTP. The thrombocytopenia in uremia is probably partly the result of accelerated thrombolysis. In Aldrich's syndrome, the eczematous boy who has an increased susceptibility to infection may have thrombocytopenia. Among the immunologic conditions is the rare neonatal thrombocytopenia which is the result of an iso-immune phenomenon akin to erythroblastosis fetalis. The primary idiopathic auto-immune thrombocytopenic purpura is probably the result of an antiplatelet factor which appears to be a 7S type of immunoglobulin which causes clumping of platelets. The thrombocytopenia associated with Coombs' positive hemolytic anemia is described as the Evans-Fisher syndrome. A secondary immunologic mechanism appears to be responsible for the thrombocytopenia seen in lymphoproliferative disorders, multiple myeloma, macroglobulinemia, and SLE. Repeated transfusions, probably as a result of antibody formation, may cause a rapid disappearance of platelets. DIC, which is associated with an increased physiologic utilization of platelets, occurs in TTP. In

DIC, the excessive blood coagulation with fibrinous occlusion of blood vessels causes paradoxically severe hemorrhage resulting from depletion of clotting factors.

Idiopathic thrombocytopenic purpura is usually an auto-immune disorder characterized by petechiae and ecchymoses in the skin and mucous membranes and hemorrhage in and from internal organs. It most commonly affects children and premenopausal women. The onset in infants and children may follow an upper respiratory tract infection. The onset may be mild or severe and without prodromata. The more chronic forms are more likely to occur especially in women after puberty. There may be a history of easy bruising, epistaxis, and menorrhagia. Melena and hematemesis are less frequent manifestations. The signs and symptoms reflect blood loss or focal complications. The patient appears to be well. The commonest skin lesions are petechiae (Fig. 17–31), but ecchymoses, suffusions, and hematuria occur. Splenomegaly is rare. The diagnosis is based on a low platelet count without any discernible cause, an abundance of megakaryocytes in the marrow, no evidence of a blood dyscrasia, and a negative LE test. Although spontaneous remissions and exacerbations occur, the remissions tend to be incomplete. Treatment consists of corticosteroid therapy, splenectomy which results in a prompt response in

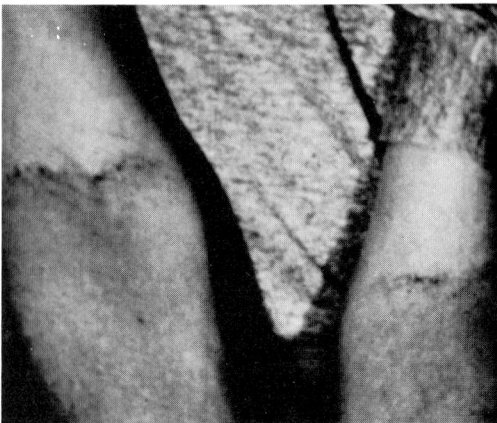

Figure 17–31 Idiopathic thrombocytopenic purpura. The patient had a history of easy bruising and menorrhagia. The tourniquet test (Rumpel-Leede test) was performed. The area below the tourniquet developed many nonpalpable petechiae.

three-fourths of the patients, and immunosuppressants, such as cyclophosphamide and azathioprine.

DIC (Deykin, 1970; Siegel and Brodsky, 1970), a clinical condition that has variously been described as the generalized Shwartzman reaction, the defibrination syndrome, and consumption coagulopathy (Rodriguez-Erdmann, 1965), is caused by the entry of a critical amount of clot-promoting material which initiates rapid coagulation (Rodriguez-Erdmann, 1965). As fibrin, the end product of coagulation, continues to accumulate, certain coagulation factors are consumed faster than they are replaced and the blood becomes incoagulable. The reticuloendothelial system is capable of removing fibrin macromolecules, activated clotting factor, and endotoxin, and its "blockade" seems to be necessary for the generalized Shwartzman reaction to occur. Fibrinolysis (Pechet, 1965) is a secondary physiologic response to intravascular coagulation. Intravascular coagulation produces a sequence of changes resulting from a complex series of enzymatic reactions which convert prothrombin to the proteolytic enzyme thrombin which affects fibrinogen with the ultimate formation of fibrin clots. In this process, the coagulation factors consumed are platelets, factors V and VII, prothrombin, and fibrinogen.

Among the disease processes which trigger this intermediary, pathogenic mechanism are intravascular hemolysis, tissue thromboplastin, bacterial endotoxin, proteolytic enzymes, particulate or colloidal matter, anoxia and anoxemia, endothelial damage, and ingestion of certain lipid substances. Intravascular consumption has been observed in the following conditions: gram-negative and gram-positive septicemia, viral, rickettsial, and fungal infections, malaria, miliary tuberculosis, cardiac surgery, abruptio placentae, amniotic fluid embolism, missed abortion, carcinomatosis, promyelocytic leukemia, hemolysis, transfusion reaction, hemolytic uremia syndrome, purpura fulminans, fat embolism, and the Kasabach-Merritt syndrome (giant cavernous hemangioma filled with fibrin thrombi, Fig. 17–32).

The clinical manifestations range from transient abnormal laboratory tests to fatal

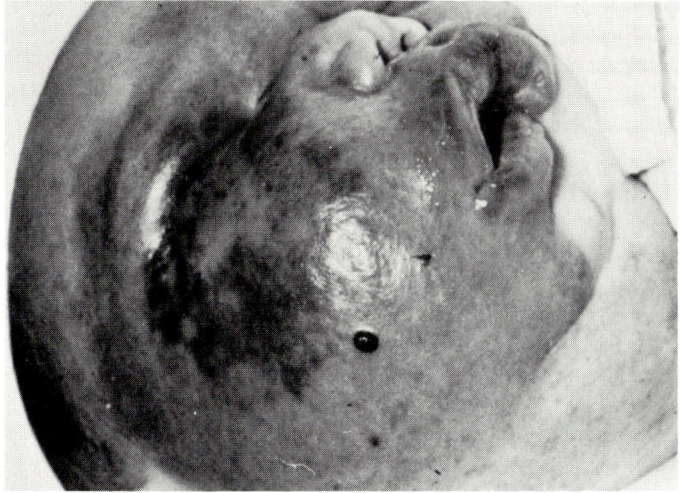

Figure 17–32 Sudden extensive swelling of the existing cavernous hemangioma with thrombosis and subsequently fatal hemorrhage in a six-month-old male infant.

hemorrhage or thrombosis. The patient may suffer shock, bleeding tendency, oliguria or anuria, back pain, convulsions, coma, nausea, vomiting, diarrhea, abdominal pain, cyanosis, and dyspnea. The cutaneous manifestations are petechiae, ecchymoses, ischemic necrosis of skin, hemorrhagic or necrotic infectious exanthemata, purpura fulminans (Fig. 17–33), and symmetric peripheral purpura. The

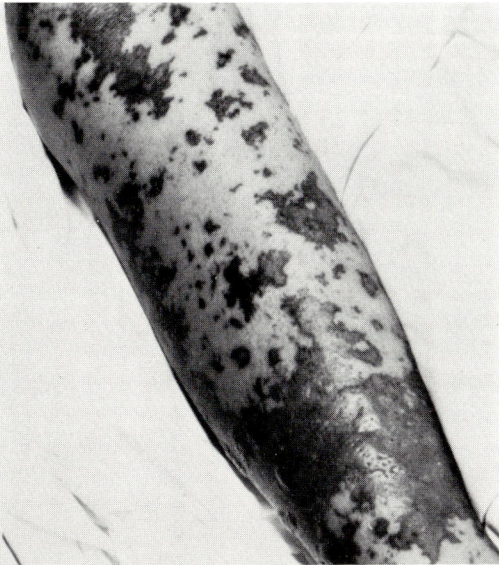

Figure 17–33 Patient had acute meningococcemia which was complicated by disseminated intravascular coagulopathy which presented clinically as purpura fulminans.

clinical tests for evidence of DIC are those to evaluate the depletion of clotting factors, such as phase-contrast microscopy platelet count (platelets), prothrombin time (prothrombin and factor V), partial thromboplastin (factor VII), and the thrombin time (fibrinogen), and those to evaluate the secondary fibrinolysis, such as protamine precipitation of plasma (circulating split products of fibrin) and euglobulin clot lysis time (absence of primary fibrinolysis; Table 17–6, p. 902). On examination of the blood smear, erythrocyte fragmentation with the formation of helmet and blister cells is observed.

Therapy consists of treatment for the underlying disease, administration of heparin for the intravascular coagulation, and other necessary supportive measures.

TTP is a febrile entity with thrombocytopenic purpura, "microangiopathic" hemolytic anemia, and neurologic and renal manifestations (Amorosi and Ultmann, 1966). The pathologic findings demonstrate widespread hyaline (fibrin on immunofluorescent technique), occlusion of terminal arterioles and capillaries, and an accompanying endothelial proliferation. In the kidney, microaneurysms and pretubular glomeruloid structures have been reported as being specific (Orbison, 1952). Biopsy of bone marrow or lymph node or splenectomy may be diagnostic. At autopsy, the heart, kidneys, adrenals, pancreas, and brain are found to be involved most frequently. Although the etiology and pathogenesis are unknown, the histologic changes are compatible with intravascular coagulation being a pathogenic factor.

TTP has been associated with SLE, glomerulonephritis, Coombs-positive hemolytic anemia, some diseases affecting blood vessels (for example, aspergillosis), diseases with microangiopathic hemolytic anemia, and epidemic virus infection with hemolytic uremia syndrome. The disease affects predominantly females between 10 and 40 years of age. The signs and symptoms include fever, fatigue, pallor, weakness, purpura, headache, mental changes, syncope, visual changes, seizures, coma, cranial nerve palsies, paresthesias, vertigo, nausea, vomiting, abdominal pain, jaundice, arthralgias, and myalgias. Petechiae, ischemic hemorrhagic blistering with necrosis of skin, and extensive gangrene of subcutaneous tissue also occur. The laboratory studies reveal anemia (probably the result of hemolysis), elevated reticulocyte count, alteration of red blood cells (schistocytes, burr cells, helmet cells, microspherocytes, and triangular erythrocytes), indirect reacting bilirubin, leukocytosis, thrombocytopenia, proteinuria, hematuria, pyuria and casts, and azotemia.

The differential diagnosis of TTP includes idiopathic thrombocytopenic purpura (ITP), idiopathic auto-immune hemolytic anemia, symptomatic hemolytic anemia, SLE, periarteritis nodosa, drug eruption, septicemia, and leukemia.

TTP is usually rapidly and progressively fatal within three months. The prognosis is better when there is an appreciable and treatable underlying or associated disease. Large doses of adrenocorticosteroids with or without splenectomy have been used therapeutically. In view of the intravascular thrombosis, heparinization is being recommended and evaluated.

Thrombocytosis may be accompanied paradoxically by a hemorrhagic tendency. When the direct platelet count is 1,000,000 per cubic millimeter, a hemorrhagic tendency occurs; it is especially likely to occur when the levels are twice this or more. These very high platelet counts are seen in the myeloproliferative disorders (primary thrombocythemia, polycythemia vera, chronic myelocytic leukemia, and myelofibrosis with myeloid meta-

plasia), after splenectomy, and, rarely, in chronic granulomatous or malignant diseases.

The primary thrombocythemia is seen in either sex over the age of 30 and is characterized by spontaneous bleeding of variable severity, splenomegaly, and thrombocytosis. Spontaneous bruising with extremely large hematomas occurs frequently, purpura of skin and mucous membrane is infrequent, and digital gangrene (Fig. 17–34) has been described. Gastrointestinal bleeding, which can be massive, is most frequent, but hematuria, hemoptysis, menorrhagia, and bleeding after minor trauma and surgery have been seen. The platelets in thrombocythemia are thrombopathic, and, in the test tube, excessive platelets inhibit thromboplastin generation test. The associated thrombosis results from the increased amounts of platelets.

The commonest thrombosis appears in the splenic vein, that of the hepatic and penile veins may also be present, and involvement of the superficial and deep veins of the legs is seen less frequently. The occurrence of thrombocytosis of more than 400,000 in some patients with various malignancies (of lung, breast, ovary, stomach, and pancreas) may be responsible for the associated migratory thrombophlebitis. Radioactive phosphorous is often thera-

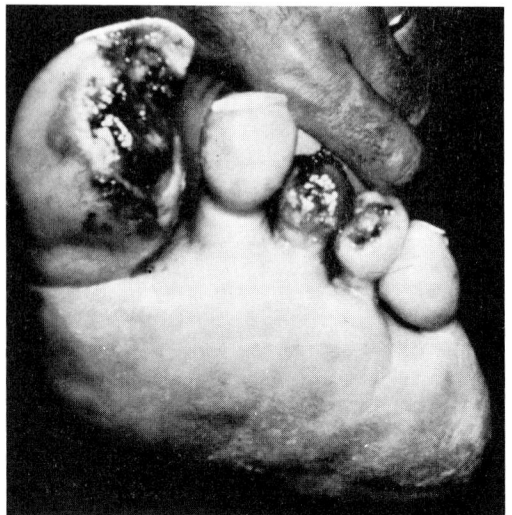

Figure 17–34 Primary thrombocythemia in a 42-year-old man with a history of spontaneous bruising, gastrointestinal bleeding, and gangrene of toes.

peutically effective; the alkylating agent, busulfan, is less helpful.

Although the term *thrombopathy* has been applied to disorders characterized by deficient platelet functional activity, it is used here to describe the qualitative platelet disorders (thrombocytopathia), the functional platelet disorders with or without deficiency of the plasmatic coagulation factors, especially VII and IX (the so-called compound platelet diseases), and those disorders with thrombasthenia characterized by non-adhesive platelets (the so-called thrombopathic thrombasthenia). These disorders may be congenital (primary) or acquired (secondary). They may present clinically with petechiae and ecchymoses, spontaneous bleeding from the mucous membrane and internal surfaces of the body, and post-traumatic and postoperative bleeding. Glanzmann's thrombasthenia denotes various hemorrhagic states characterized by normal bleeding time, platelet count, and coagulation time but with poor clot retraction and abnormal structure of platelets. Among the varieties is the Glanzmann-Naegeli type in which small round platelets are present or increased and their adhesiveness and agglutinability are impaired. In another group, enzymatic deficiencies and reduced levels of ATP are present. In other cases, defective utilization of ATP occurs.

The acquired deficit thrombopathy may be seen in liver disease, azotemia, and scurvy. An acquired functional thrombopathy is frequently associated with dysproteinemia which not only inhibits platelet function by coating the platelets with abnormal globulin (for example, macroglobulinemia) but also induces other hemostatic defects. Capillary anoxia may develop when macroglobulins complex with plasmatic coagulation factors, with a resultant hyperviscosity. Purpura on exposed areas may appear when cryoglobulins precipitate upon exposure to cold.

Hypergammaglobulinemic purpura of Waldenström (Alper et al., 1966; Capra et al., 1971; Kyle et al., 1971) is a chronic benign disease characterized by recurrent purpura predominating in young women with diffuse hypergammaglobulinemia (polyclonalgammopathy). The etiology and pathogenesis are unknown; Sjögren's syndrome, in its complete or incomplete

forms, collagen disease, chronic lymphatic leukemia, reticulum cell sarcoma, and multiple myeloma develop subsequently in some of these patients. On histopathologic examination, there may be a mild endothelial proliferation and thickening of the vessel wall with perivascular and vascular infiltration by lymphocytes and monocytes, red cell extravasation, and hemosiderin deposition about dermal vessels, or there may be a necrotizing vasculitis with fibrinoid material within and around the involved vessel walls.

The main clinical expression of the disease is purpura, which develops rapidly, may recur for as long as 20 years, causes a burning sensation or pruritus of the involved sites, and heals with residual pigmentation. It involves especially the lower extremity with a stasis gradient picture but also may affect the trunk and arms. The liver and skeletal system are not involved; splenomegaly and lymphadenopathy may occur. There is a heterogeneous or polyclonal hypergammaglobulinemia with a broad-based peak similar to that of LE, cirrhosis, and infections. Data suggest that antigammaglobulins of the IgG (γG) type account for most of the gamma globulin elevation characteristic of this disorder. Significant titers of rheumatoid factors are usually found. A mild anemia and a leukopenia may be present. The blood sedimentation rate is markedly accelerated. The platelets are quantitatively, qualitatively, and functionally normal. The marrow studies are unremarkable, no significant amounts of cryoglobulins are present, and no coagulation or bleeding defects are appreciable. There is capillary fragility and a positive tourniquet test.

The prognosis for the disease is good but it lasts for years. Treatment consists of the use of elastic stockings and elevation of the legs. Secondary hyperglobulinemic purpura, which usually appears after the age of 40, may be associated with sarcoidosis, collagen diseases, chronic infections, hepatic diseases, leukemia, lymphoma, and multiple myeloma.

Primary macroglobulinemia or Waldenström's macroglobulinemia (McCallister et al., 1967; Rosen, 1962) is a chronic progressive disorder characterized by the neoplastic proliferation of lymphocytoid cells and large amounts of IgM globulins and classified as a plasma cell dyscrasia. On sternal marrow examination, there is an increase of small atypical "plasmacytoid" lymphocytes and plasma cells; the small lymphocyte, which has a dense pyknotic nucleus and is probably a degenerating cell, is most typical for macroglobulinemia. Histologic studies of lymph nodes reveal a proliferation of lymphocytic plasmacytic cells which tend to assume a follicular hyperplastic pattern, reveal on immunofluorescence the synthesis of IgM globulin, and may contain intranuclear and intracytoplasmic diastase-resistant, PAS-positive staining material. Whether this disease is a reactive or an autonomous neoplasia is presently indeterminable. Some of the cases are initially benign and transform into other more malignant neoplastic forms of plasma cell dyscrasia.

The disease affects both sexes, is slightly more prominent in men, and generally appears between the ages of 40 and 70 years. It usually begins insidiously and ultimately progresses rapidly; complete remissions or recoveries are unknown. The patients may experience fatigue, malaise, weight loss, lassitude, visual disturbances, and increased susceptibility to infections. Purpura is uncommon and cutaneous hematomas are rare. Recurrent epistaxis, gingival and mucosal bleeding, and massive gastrointestinal bleeding occur. When the macroglobulin has the property of cryoglobulin, Raynaud's phenomenon, urticaria, necrosis and ulceration of the skin, and leg edema may be seen. On funduscopic examination, the retinal veins are engorged and have the appearance of "link sausage," and there may be exudates, papillitis or papilledema, venous thrombosis, retinal detachment, and macular degeneration. Lymphadenopathy and splenomegaly, which resemble those conditions seen in lymphoma and lymphatic leukemia, are present but differentiate primary macroglobulinemia from multiple myeloma. The serum hyperviscosity is responsible not only for the ocular and neurologic manifestations but also for the cardiac failure with dyspnea and pulmonary hypertension.

The neurologic manifestations of primary macroglobulinemia result from strokes, acute focal and multifocal brain syndromes, progressive coma (coma paraproteinemia), neuropathies, subarachnoid hemorrhages, or combinations of them. Among the mental changes observed are disorientation, progressive alterations of personality, and organic psychoses. Roentgenographic examination reveals generalized osteoporosis, and the punched-out bone lesions of multiple myeloma are rarely seen. Mickulicz's and Sjögren's syndromes have been described (Kappeler et al., 1958).

Anemia, which is the commonest clinical manifestation, is the result of accelerated red blood cell destruction, blood loss, and decreased erythropoiesis. The excessive IgM macroglobulin coats red blood cells and causes the elevated blood sedimentation rate, rouleaux formation, autoagglutination, positive Coombs' test, positive STS, positive rheumatoid factors, and difficulties in cross matching of blood. The complexing of macroglobulins with serum proteins can interfere with hemostatic factors (fibrinogen, prothrombin, and factors V, VIII, and others). The coating of platelets by the abnormal globulins may induce thrombocytopenia. Leukocytosis with lymphocytosis occurs, and occasionally pancytopenia may be seen.

Bence Jones proteinemia is present in about 10 per cent of patients with this condition and, unlike multiple myeloma, renal complications are unusual. Amyloidosis has been seen in only a few cases. When the macroglobulinemia is elevated in excess of 15 per cent of serum gamma globulins (macroglobulins usually contitute up to 5 per cent of serum gamma globulins), it is highly suggestive of primary macroglobulinemia in contrast to the secondary type associated with neoplastic diseases (multiple myeloma, reticulosis, carcinoma of the bronchus, uterus, larynx, biliary tract, and prostate), collagen diseases (SLE, polyarteritis nodosa, rheumatoid arthritis, and Sjögren's and Felty's syndromes), infections (kala-azar, chronic hepatitis, toxoplasmosis, congenital syphilis), and miscellaneous conditions, such as cirrhosis and the nephrotic syndrome. The Sia water test, which is the appearance of a rapidly settling precipitation upon the addition of a drop of serum in water, is the simplest but least specific and reliable test for abnormal proteins; it can be negative in macroglobulinemia.

Death occurs from sepsis, pneumonia, thrombosis or hemorrhage, cachexia, congestive heart failure, or coma.

Treatment is directed to the associated anemia and bleeding manifestations and the problems and syndromes created by increased plasma viscosity. When the central nervous system and ocular involvement is severe, plasmapheresis is initiated until chlorambucil, the main therapeutic measure for macroglobulinemia, has been administered adequately. Prednisone may be helpful in controlling the capillary bleeding.

The term *cryopathy* is used to describe all the conditions or disorders associated with cold sensitivity. A modification of a reported classification (Ritzmann and Levin, 1961) is:

Cryoglobulinemias
Cryofibrinogenemia
Paroxysmal cold hemoglobinuria
Collagen disorders (associated with Raynaud's phenomenon or dysproteinemia or both)
Idiopathic or essential Raynaud's disease and phenomenon
Other cryopathies: Familial cold allergy, cold allergy (physical allergy)

Patients with cold intolerance, which may be seasonal, may have the following signs and symptoms: cyanosis, numbness, and Raynaud's phenomenon of the extremities; urticaria; purpura of the skin and mucous membranes; vascular occlusions producing visual and auditory disturbances, ulceration, necrosis, and gangrene of skin; fever and chills; and the symptoms of pulmonary infarction, hemolytic anemia, and hemoglobinuria.

Cryoglobulinemia (Barnett et al., 1970) is an essential (idiopathic) or secondary disorder characterized by the presence of serum immunoglobulins which precipitate or gel on cooling and redissolve on warming. These cryoprecipitates may contain a single immunoglobulin (IgG, IgA, or IgM) or a mixture of immunoglobulins (IgG-IgM or IgG-IgA). In the mixed type, the presence of both immunoglobulins is required for the occurrence of cryoprecipitation. Cryoglobulins must be distinguished from cold agglutinins and cryofibrinogen but may be associated with them and may even be the cold agglutinin.

Since the macroglobulin may also be a cryoglobulin, it is difficult to separate the properties of the two. In contrast to the typical homogeneous cryoglobulins which are demonstrated by precipitation at 4° C. and return to solution when warmed to 37° C., the mixed complexes may not dissolve upon heating to 37° C. Large amounts of cryoglobulins are seen in patients with multiple myeloma or Waldenström's macroglobulinemia and lesser amounts (less than 25 mg. per 100 ml.) in the other associated disorders. The combinations of IgG-IgM or IgG-IgA cryoglobulins account for one-third of all cases of cryoglobulinemia and are significantly associated with the connective tissue diseases.

A classification of cryoglobulinemia (Phelps and Geokas, 1963) is:

Essential cryoglobulinemia
    Asymptomatic
    Associated with peripheral vascular manifestations, visceral thrombosis, cold hemagglutination or hemolysis or both
Secondary cryoglobulinemia
    Neoplastic diseases: Multiple myeloma, chronic lymphatic leukemia, polycythemia vera, Hodgkin's disease, lymphosarcoma, and widespread malignancies
    Collagen diseases: Rheumatoid arthritis, LE, periarteritis nodosa, Sjögren's syndrome, rheumatic fever
    Infectious diseases: Kala-azar, subacute bacterial endocarditis, malaria, leprosy, syphilis, cytomegalovirus, infectious mononucleosis
    Other diseases: Cirrhosis of the liver, coronary artery disease

The signs and symptoms are probably produced by in vivo precipitation or gelling of the cryoglobulins, resulting in sluggishness of the circulation and, in some instances, thrombosis by circulating immune complexes (the mixed types of cryoglobulins consisting of antigens, antibodies, and complement components) which can clinically produce vasculitis, glomerulonephritis, synovitis, serositis, purpura, hyperviscosity syndromes, Raynaud's phenomenon, deficient exocrine function (Sjögren's disease), anemia, leukopenia, and thrombocytopenia. The cutaneous manifestations (Ellis, 1964) include

Raynaud's phenomenon, acrocyanosis, livedo reticularis, petechiae, purpura, ecchymosis, urticaria, ulceration of the skin, and gangrene of the digits with subsequent amputation (Fig. 17–35). Cryoglobulinemia may resemble clinically factitial ulcerations (Baughman and Sommer, 1966). The systemic symptoms are chills and fever, oronasal bleeding, decreased visual acuity, deafness, dyspnea, melena, and those of stomatitis, vascular occlusion, pulmonary infection, and hemoglobinuria. Laboratory examinations reveal rouleaux formation, pseudoagglutination of red blood cells, and an elevated sedimentation rate.

The syndrome described as "arthralgia-purpura-weakness" cryoglobulinemia (Meltzer and Franklin, 1967) has not only the symptom complex of cold intolerance but also arthralgia, purpura of the lower extremities, weakness, mixed cryoglobulin with rheumatoid factor activity, and low serum complement levels. Other clinical findings have been hepatomegaly, splenomegaly, lymphadenopathy, Sjögren's syndrome, rheumatoid arthritis, thyroiditis, glomerulonephritis with hematuria, leg ulcers, inflammatory vasculitis, peripheral neuritis, hemolytic anemia, presence of serum antinuclear antibodies, immunoglobulin deposits in glomeruli, and renal tubular acidosis. Immunoglobulins in cutaneous vessels, seen by immunofluorescent techniques; microangiopathic erythrocyte changes; and a relationship of skin lesions to trauma have been demonstrated (Mathison et al., 1971). There may be an associated chronic infection, such as blastomycosis, syphilis, and toxoplasmosis. In view of the findings of immunoglobulins in the glomeruli, of low serum complement titers, and of the soluble IgM, anti-IgG complexes suggest disorder of immune complexes of the Arthus reaction type.

The disease may exist for years with minimal clinical manifestations or can be fatal within months as a result of renal failure. As a part of therapy, cold is to be avoided. Corticosteroids have been used but without any significant clinical or laboratory improvement. Penicillamine and chlorambucil with or without corticosteroids have not been effective therapeutically. A trial of alkylating agents, especially cyclophosphamide, and possibly splenectomy, have been recommended. Plasmapheresis has been used as a temporary measure. The leg ulcers have been treated by elevation of the legs, wearing of elastic stockings, topical application of 0.25 per cent silver nitrate solution, and anticoagulant therapy (bishydroxycoumarin). Sympathectomy has not been of benefit.

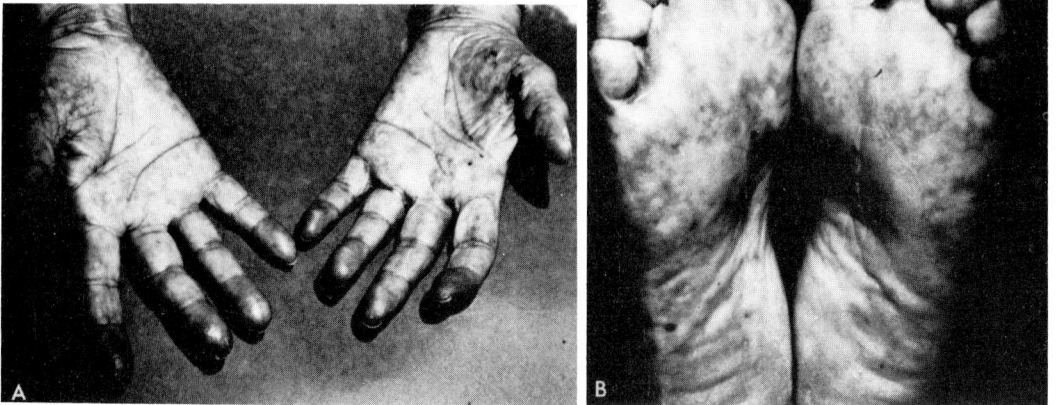

Figure 17–35 *A* and *B*, Secondary cryoglobulinemia. A 47-year-old man with multiple myeloma who had cryoglobulinemia which was associated with Raynaud's phenomenon of the hands, acrocyanosis of the toes, livedo reticularis of the arms and legs, and purpura and ecchymoses of the extremities.

Crystalglobulinemia (Grossman et al., 1972) is a cryopathic syndrome characterized by repeated episodes of widespread cutaneous purpura and necrotic ulcerations of the skin and the presence in the serum of a homogeneous (IgG3K) cryoglobulin that spontaneously forms crystals. The patient with this condition may have a pruritic erythematous rash on the face, ears, and buttocks; ulcerations are usually seen on the lower extremities but may also appear on the ears and breasts. The kidneys and other organs are not involved. The serum is turbid because the cryoproteins form aggregates or microcrystals at temperatures as high as 33° C. The deposition of the cryoprotein in blood vessel walls initiates a vasculitis. The tests for antinuclear antibody, LE cells, Bence Jones protein, and cold agglutinins are negative. The bone marrow aspirate is normal. The normal serum complement and absent rheumatoid factor differentiate crystalglobulinemia from the mixed type (IgG-IgM or IgG-IgA) of essential cryoglobulinemia in which vasculitis and glomerulitis occur. Treatment with moderately high doses of prednisone and plasmapheresis has been effective in controlling the disease; cyclophosphamide therapy has been unsuccessful.

Cryofibrinogenemia

In cryofibrinogenemia, a gelatinous flocculent material precipitates when the heparinized plasma is chilled to 4° C. and dissolves upon warming to 37° C. In healthy persons, the amount of reversible cold-precipitable fibrinogen rarely exceeds 400 mg. per 100 ml. Cryofibrinogenemia may occur without an associated underlying disease or may be secondary to pulmonary, gastric, ovarian, and metastatic carcinoma of the prostate (Fig. 17–36), chronic lymphatic leukemia, fibrosarcoma, and acute rheumatic fever. Both primary and secondary cryofibrinogenemia may be associated with cold sensitivity and the chronic paradox of intravascular clotting appearing simultaneously with a hemorrhagic diathesis. It has been emphasized (Kalbfleisch and Bird, 1960) that screening procedures for cold precipitable protein must use plasma and serum instead of

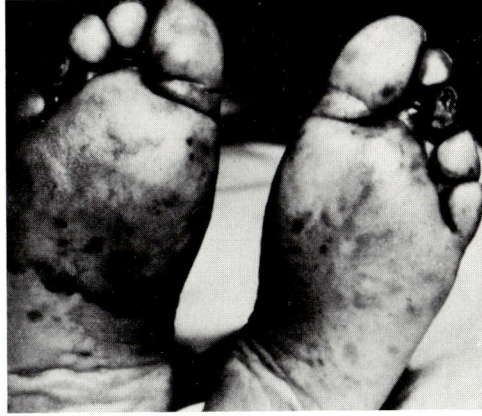

Figure 17–36 Cryofibrinogenemia secondary to prostatic carcinoma. Elderly man with widespread metastases of prostatic carcinoma with cold sensitivity (Raynaud's phenomenon) and gangrene of digits experienced a terminal gastrointestinal hemorrhage.

serum alone. The cold precipitable plasma protein migrates electrophoretically similar to fibrinogen, has the clotting properties of fibrinogen, and possibly some prothrombin and accelerator factor activity (Kalbfleisch and Bird, 1960).

Cold Agglutinin Syndrome

The cold agglutinin syndrome consists of cold agglutinin disease with a chronic increase of cold agglutinins, viral infections with an acute increase of cold agglutinins, and lymphoma with a subacute increase of cold agglutinins. These may be associated with the signs and symptoms of cold sensitivity plus necrosis and gangrene of acral areas (fingers, toes, ears, and nose). Hemolysis and hemoglobinuria may occur as a result of the simultaneous increase of titers of hemolysins. The higher the titer of cold agglutinins, the higher the thermal range at which cold agglutinins are active. Agglutination and hemolysis may occur at temperatures up to 20° C. and rarely as high as 30° C. Death has occurred even at summer temperatures.

Hemorrhage Resulting From Coagulopathies

The disorders of coagulation (Ratnoff, 1968; Roberts and Brinkhouse, 1968; Rossi et al., 1972; Tocantins and Kazal, 1964) may be heritable or acquired (Table 17–7). The defective hemostasis may be the result of coagulable defects caused by inadequate production of one or more procoagulant substances, the depletion of clotting components from increased utilization, the presence in the blood of inhibitors of coagulation, or the activation of the proteolytic mechanism of the plasma. The heritable conditions are mostly the result of impaired synthesis of organic clotting factors and usually present as deficiencies of a single clotting factor in contrast to the acquired disorders which generally have multiple defective components of the clotting system. The pattern of inheritance helps assess the nature of the clotting disorder. Deficiency of Christmas factor (factor IX) and deficiency of the antihemophiliac factor are inherited as X chromosome–linked recessive traits, and are autosomal recessive. These autosomal recessive traits are rare and are found often in the offspring of consanguineous unions. The hemorrhagic syndromes produced by isolated deficiency of various clotting factors are similar, and thus differentiation on a clinical basis is not possible. The usual clinical expression is hemorrhage into the skin (ecchymosis) in contrast to the petechiae of the platelet or vascular disease.

The final insoluble fibrin clot in the process of coagulation is generated extrinsically in the adjacent tissue or intrinsically within the damaged vessel through a sequential cascade of enzymatic activations of various plasma proteins which constitute the coagulation factors. The defective coagulation is the result of deficiencies of one or more of the components of the three useful and arbitrary conceptual reactions—the formation of prothrombinase, thrombin, or fibrin. Prothrombinase (thromboplastin generation) is the activity responsible for the conversion of prothrombin to thrombin and is appreciated by delayed clotting of whole blood, retarded thromboplastin generation, deficient prothrombin utilization, and prolonged partial thromboplastin time. In the second stage, prothrombin is converted to thrombin and is associated with prolonged prothrombin time. In the third stage, conversion of fibrinogen to fibrin occurs and is manifested by the deposition

of little or no fibrin, the retardation of clotting after adding thrombin to plasma, and the formation of abnormal clots. The specific deficiencies are identified by determining if connection occurs when the patient's plasma is mixed with that of a known coagulation defect.

The basic tenet of treatment for these deficiencies is replacement of missing factor in amounts to maintain "hemostatic" level by using fresh or stored plasma or blood or specific concentrates, depending on the deficiency. The problems in the use of plasma component treatment of bleeding disorders include the short survival of coagulant activity, the variable recovery of clotting activity, protein contaminants (presence of other clotting factors), drug idiosyncrasies (pyrogens), and viral hepatitis.

Hereditable Disorders of Coagulation

Von Willebrand's disease (pseudohemophilia, vascular hemophilia) is a disorder characterized by a prolonged bleeding time (not seen in other hemophilioid diseases) with a normal platelet count and a factor VII deficiency. It is transmitted as an autosomal dominant trait with variable expressivity and occurs with equal frequency in women and men. The disease begins in early life and is manifested by cutaneous and mucous membrane bleeding, easy bruisability, hematomas, occasionally petechiae, rarely hemarthrosis, and urogenital and gastrointestinal hemorrhage. Fresh and stored blood and plasma transfusions and plasma components are used in treatment.

Hemophilia is a variable, severe, familial disorder of coagulation characterized by a deficiency of factor VIII (antihemophilic factor or AHF deficiency). It occurs in 1 out of 25,000 men and is transmitted by women. Infants tend to have hematomas into soft tissues; the scalp may be distorted by subcutaneous hemorrhage. In later life, hemarthrosis is characteristic, and the hemorrhages tend to dissect through subcutaneous tissues along fascial planes and into muscles with pseudotumefactions, muscular contractures and deformities, and clawhand. The enormous hematomas reabsorb but may calcify, leaving firm masses. Severe anemia can occur without external evidence of blood loss. Difficulty in eating and swallowing may result from hemorrhage into the lax tissue of the oropharynx. The character of the bleeding and the family history suggest the diagnosis which is confirmed by the use of tests that detect abnormalities of the first stage of coagulation or measure factor VII of plasma. Treatment consists of fresh plasma, exchange transfusion, and concentrates of antihemophilic factor.

Acquired Disorders of Coagulation

Acquired disorders of coagulation can result from vitamin K deficiency, liver disease, hypofibrinogenemia or dysfibrogenemia, defibrinating syndrome, circulating anticoagulants, and fibrinolytic disorders.

CIRCULATING ANTICOAGULANTS. A severe bleeding tendency may result from the presence in blood of heparin or abnormal complex proteins which interfere with the clotting process. The circulating anticoagulants exert their inhibitory effects in several ways: (1) inactivation of the hemophilic factor by an agent which has characteristics of an antibody is seen in classic hemophilia, SLE, penicillin reactions, and post partum, and occurs idiopathically; (2) interference with formation of the prothrombin-converting principle which is seen in plasma of patients with SLE who also usually have a positive STS and cryoglobulinemia suggestive of a generalized derangement of protein synthesis; (3) hyperheparinemia which results from parenteral administration of heparin and interferes with thromboplastin generation as well as the conversion of fibrinogen to fibrin.

INTERFERENCE WITH SYNTHESIS. Bishydroxycoumarin and related compounds do not directly affect coagulation but interfere with the synthesis of the clotting factors. A rare, presently unexplainable complication of coumarin congeners in anticoagulant therapy is the sudden, localized, hemorrhagic, gangrenous necrosis of skin, usually of the lower half of the body. The lesion or lesions appear on the third to sixth day of administration and heal in about five weeks despite the continuation of therapy. On histo-

pathologic study of these lesions, occlusive thrombi are seen in capillaries, venules, and occasionally veins.

Purpura Pigmentosa Chronica (Idiopathic Pigmented Purpuric Dermatoses)

Purpura pigmentosa chronica is a group of benign, usually asymptomatic dermatoses of unknown etiology (Randall et al., 1951). They are unassociated with an underlying systemic disease or medication and have close clinical and histopathologic similarities. The cutaneous clinical manifestations result from an increased capillary fragility or permeability or both as well as from dilatation and proliferation of the capillaries in the upper dermis. The basic histologic process is a lymphocytic vasculitis. Important localizing factors are gravity and increased venous pressure. There are no underlying hematologic, coagulatory, bleeding disorders or deficiency of coagulation factors, and the platelets are normal in number, morphology, and function. The tourniquet test usually gives positive results.

The primary clinical lesion is a patch of purpuric puncta with pigmentation from hemosiderin; telangiectasis occurs as a result of capillary dilatation. The purpuric, fawn-colored macular lesions may assume annular and serpiginous patterns, become confluent, and have central clearing with slight atrophy and lichenoid papules. When the eruption is pruritic, scaling macules, papules, and lichenification may be seen. The conditions to be differentiated are drug reactions, purpuric contact allergic dermatitis (clothing), and hyperglobulinemic states.

The drug reactions, which can cause similar eruptions, result from the carbromal components of acetylcarbromal, meprobamate, and mephesin (Rosenthal and Burnham, 1964), and present clinically as a pruritic pigmented purpuric lichenoid eruption. Clothing purpura (Greenwood, 1960) is an acute or chronic dermatosis appearing mostly in middle-aged men whose skin is irritated by underlying woolen garments, especially in the lower extremities. A sensitivity to wool oil is demonstrable. The eruption is characterized by papules, purpura, and pityriasis rosea–like lesions. Hypergammaglobulinemic purpura is characterized by petechiae which are more diffusely scattered over the legs and are not accompanied by brown-yellow patches. Stasis purpura (angiodermatitis, dermite ocre of Favre) is an asymptomatic eruption appearing mainly in men with varicose veins (Mali et al., 1965). The purpuric macules involve the lower legs as well as the feet and toes and may extend along the superficial varicosities. There may be an associated stasis dermatitis, edema, sclerosis, and ulceration. Treatment is directed to the underlying venous and cutaneous problems.

Treatment of these so-called idiopathic pigmented purpuric dermatoses which may persist for months to years is symptomatic. Systemic corticosteroid and topical steroid therapy, including occlusion, temporarily clears the eruption which relapses on discontinuance of therapy. Gradient pressure stockings, topical antiinflammatory or antipruritic preparations, and oral antipruritics, when necessary, are recommended supportive measures.

The current philosophy and concept of these purpuric dermatoses consider them to be variants of the same pathologic process; however, the typical or classic examples of these eponymous entities are sufficiently clinically distinctive to warrant a brief description of their salient clinical features.

Schamberg's progressive pigmented purpuric dermatosis is usually an uncommon asymptomatic disease of adolescent and young adult men and is characterized by orange-colored to fawn-colored macules with cayenne pepper spots within or on their borders (Fig. 17–37). The eruption is localized to shins, ankles, and dorsa of feet and toes. Its course is chronic, and the disease may persist for years and then clear spontaneously.

Pigmented purpuric lichenoid dermatosis of Gougerot and Blum resembles Schamberg's disease except that it favors older men (between 40 and 60 years of age), is associated with lichenoid papules in the petechiae-containing macules, has a more exaggerated histologic process, tends to be more extensive, involving thighs, trunk, and upper extremities, and tends to be less chronic.

Purpura annularis telangiectodes (Majocchi's disease) is an asymptomatic eruption seen in adolescent and young men and is characterized by brownish yellow macules which contain red punctiform and follicular spots (cayenne pepper spots) and telangiectases and develop central clearing with slight atrophy. The eruption persists for months to years and may spread centrifugally.

Itching purpura (Lowenthal, 1954) – eczematid-like purpura (Doucas and Kapetanakis, 1953); disseminated pruritic angio-

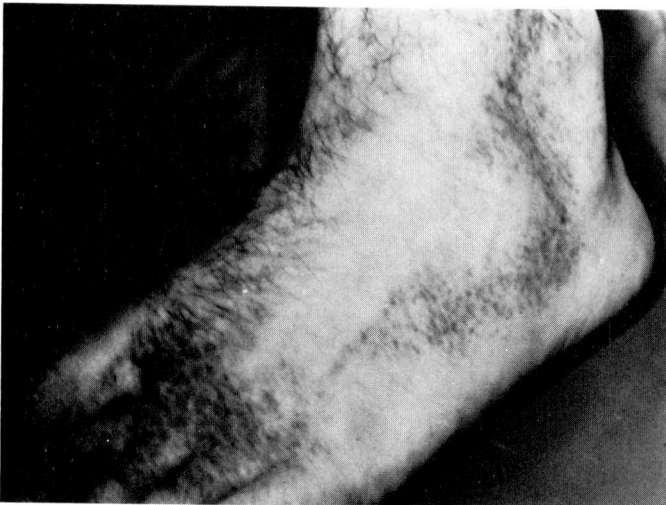

Figure 17–37 Purpura pigmentosa chronica (Schamberg's disease). A 24-year-old white man with asymptomatic purpura and pigmentation that began on his toes and has extended to below his knees.

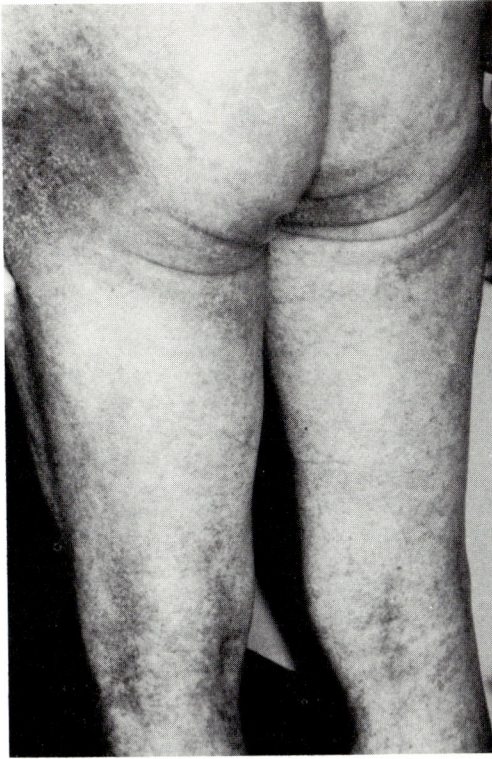

Figure 17–38 A 34-year-old white man with disseminated pruritic purpura has no discernible underlying disease or history of drug ingestion. The eruption responded to systemic and local (under occlusion) interrupted courses of corticosteroid therapy and cleared after eight months of such therapy.

dermatitis—is an extremely pruritic eruptive hemorrhagic dermatosis which tends to affect male adults (Fig. 17–38). On histopathologic examination, one sees not only capillaritis but also epidermitis. The eruption consists of erythematous, fawn-colored macules which contain punctate purpura. Lichenoid papules may be scaly and become lichenified from scratching. It is usually localized to the legs, with dissemination to the thighs, trunk, upper extremities, and, in the more severe cases, the large flexural areas, and is more pronounced at the sites of friction. It persists for months with marked fluctuations and episodic recurrences, especially during the spring and summer, and clears spontaneously. Local corticosteroid therapy with or without occlusion causes improvement of the eruption, which flares upon its discontinuance.

TELANGIECTASIA

Telangiectasia is a permanent dilatation of the cutaneous venules. They may appear as fine wires, heavy cords, or as spiders which are characterized by an accentuated pulsating punctum with radiating limbs. Telangiectasia (McGrae and Winkelmann, 1963; Shelley, 1971) may be divided etiologically into two groups—a primary group of unknown etiology and a secondary group resulting from or associated with known disease.

CLASSIFICATION OF TELANGIECTASIA

Primary
  Nevoid states
        Nevus flammeus, spider telangiectasis
        Idiopathic spider angioma
        Angioma serpiginosum
        Hereditary hemorrhagic telangiectasia
        Ataxia telangiectasia
        Syndromes with telangiectatic erythemas: Bloom's, Rothmund-Thomson, hereditary sclerosing poikiloderma, Cockayne's, dyskeratosis congenita, xeroderma pigmentosum
  Generalized or unilateral essential telangiectasia
  Poikiloderma atrophicans vasculare
Secondary
  Physical exposure: Sunlight or tar or both, radiodermatitis, Hartnup disease
  Rosacea and rosacea-like syndromes: Polycythemia vera, prolonged local or systemic corticosteroid therapy, carcinoid syndrome, mastocytosis, drug therapy
  Secondary poikilodermic states: Physical exposure, collagen diseases (LE, dermatomyositis, scleroderma, Sjögren's syndrome, parapsoriasis en plaque, lymphoma)
  Mastocytosis
  Varicose veins
  Associated with malignancy (basal cell carcinoma, carcinoma telangiectaticum)
Spider angioma is a type of telangiectasia which persists as an elevated pulsating

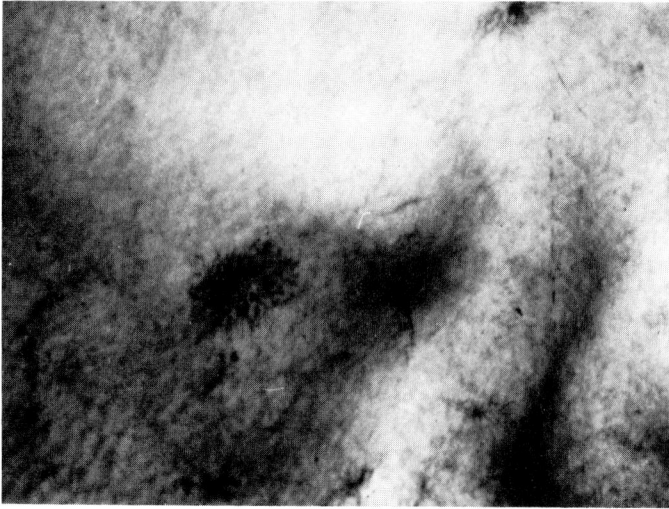

Figure 17–39 Spider angiomata were seen on the face and trunk, mainly the chest, in a patient with advanced cirrhosis of the liver.

punctum with symmetrically radiating thin branches (Fig. 17–39). The central arteriole can proliferate to a degree to produce the elevated mass which looks like a strawberry nevus and can measure up to 2 cm. in diameter. It appears most commonly on the exposed areas—the face, arms, and hands—and, rarely, below the umbilicus. The mucous membranes of the lips and nose may be involved. The lesions tend to be solitary, but, when numerous, they are most commonly associated with liver disease. In children and adolescents, they are usually idiopathic or nevoid, and in adults, they are associated with pregnancy, cirrhosis, and metastatic carcinoma of the liver. In pregnancy, they usually appear during the first few months and usually disappear within six weeks after delivery. The lesions may resemble the nonpulsatile telangiectases of hereditary hemorrhagic telangiectasia.

Angioma serpiginosum is a nevoid disorder which is a dilatation of capillaries and appears clinically as deep, erythematous, nonpalpable, grouped, asymptomatic puncta arranged in a macular, linear, mottled, or netlike pattern. It usually begins in childhood or early adult life, and females are predominantly affected. The lower legs and buttocks are most frequently involved, extension and presentation on the trunk and arm occur, and mucous membranes are not affected. The eruption often begins unilaterally. Although the lesions

are not purpuric, they do not usually blanch. The condition starts as one or several small lesions which extend peripherally so that serpiginous borders are created over the period of months to years. The puncta may spontaneously clear, traces may persist indefinitely, and slight atrophy may occur.

Hereditary hemorrhagic telangiectasia is a dominantly inherited disorder affecting blood vessels throughout the body. Twenty per cent of patients with this condition are unaware of a family history. The homozygous state is probably lethal. In women, it often becomes more prominent during pregnancy. It is characterized histopathologically by large, irregular, thin-walled blood vessels. The widely disseminated telangiectases are almost invariably seen in the mucous membranes of the nasal septum, mouth, and oropharynx; other viscera, such as the gastrointestinal tract, adrenal glands, brain, lungs, spleen, liver, and retina, may be involved. The disease usually presents in childhood or puberty as recurrent epistaxis (Fig. 17–40); however, hemorrhage can occur from any noncutaneous involved site. Telangiectases which involve the skin of the upper half of the body—face, lips, conjunctivae, ears, fingers, nail beds, forearms, and upper trunk (Fig. 17–41)— are usually not seen before puberty and appear especially during the third and fourth decades.

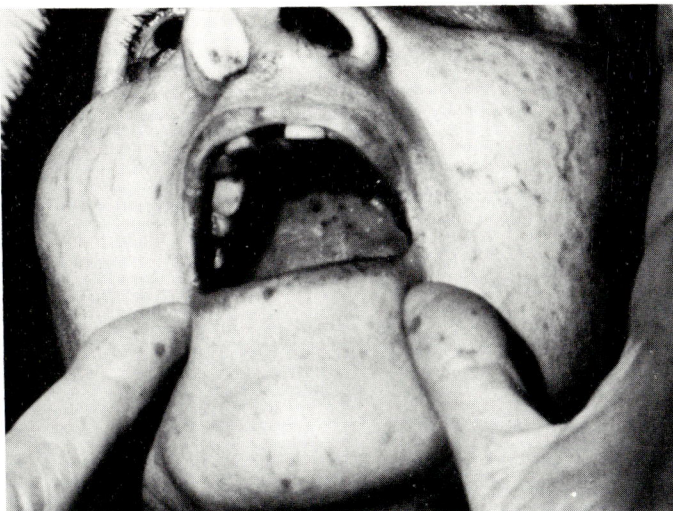

Figure 17–40 Hereditary hemorrhagic telangiectasia. A 45-year-old woman who has had recurrent epistaxis for 20 years and had first noted telangiectases of her skin and mucous membranes in her early twenties; her father had a similar problem.

The earliest cutaneous lesions are bright red nonpulsatile puncta or linear macules which measure 2 to 3 mm. in diameter. They rarely appear spiderlike or nodular and do not pulsate. When the patient is anemic, the cutaneous telangiectases may become invisible. Arteriovenous fistulas may appear in the lungs and brain. The pulmonary lesion presents radiologically as a coin lesion (Figs. 17–42 and 17–43), and extensive clubbing, cyanosis, and polycythemia are seen. Asymptomatic gastrointestinal tract bleeding occurs in about 15 per cent of patients with hereditary hemorrhagic telangiectasia. Hepatic telangiectases and arteriovenous anastomoses have been seen in the liver with an associated hepatomegaly and cirrhosis. Aneurysms of the aortic arch or of the splenic or hepatic artery, which often have thin walls, are liable to spontaneous rupture and can be visualized with angiography. The disease does not affect longevity, and the mortality rate is less than 10 per cent.

Treatment is directed to cauterization of lesions to arrest bleeding or for cosmetic appearance. Secondary anemia is treated by transfusions when necessary.

Ataxia Telangiectasia

Ataxia telangiectasia (cephalo-oculocutaneous telangiectasia, Louis-Bar syndrome) is a rare familial syndrome characterized by progressive cerebellar ataxia, oculocutaneous telangiectasia, recurrent sinopulmonary infections, immunologic defects, and an unusual form of diabetes mellitus. It appears to be an autosomal recessive trait. The earliest sign is ataxia, which is usually seen at 12 to 18 months of age but can occur later. The cerebellar component expresses itself by clumsiness, swaying head and trunk, abnormal gait, ataxic intentional movements, nystagmus,

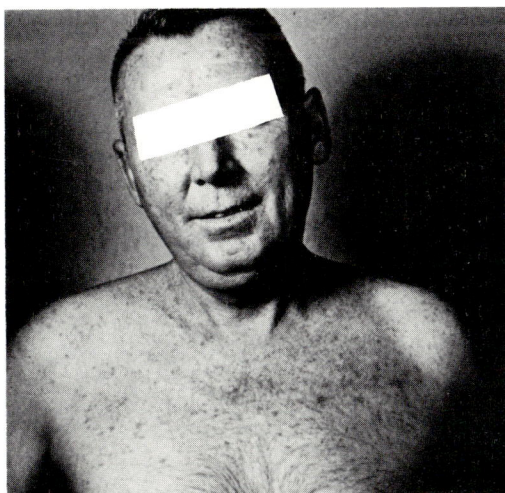

Figure 17–41 A 50-year-old man with increasing dyspnea on exertion and slight clubbing of fingers had telangiectases of the face, chest, fingers, lips, and tongue.

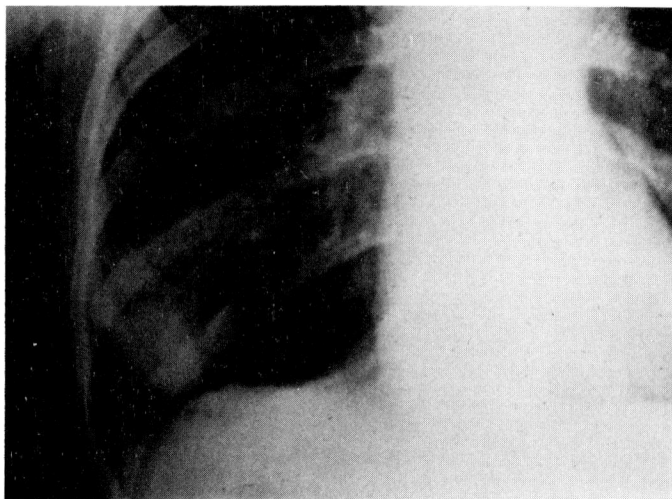

Figure 17–42 A coin lesion in the right chest which was shown by pulmonary angiography to be an arteriovenous shunt.

and slurring speech. Mental deterioration can occur. The telangiectases are fine wiry elongated vessels involving the bulbar conjunctivae and pinnae, and shorty stubby vessels appear symmetrically on the eyelids, butterfly area of the face, post-auricular area, neck, V of chest, the dorsa of hands and feet, and the popliteal and cubital fossae (Fig. 17–44). They appear at four to five years of age and as late as eight years and may occasionally be noted before or simultaneously with ataxia. Mucous membranes may be involved, but epistaxis, hemoptysis, hematemesis, and melena are rare. Sinopulmonary infection, including bronchiectasis, occurs in 75 per cent of cases, and the terminal event in this disease is pneumonia.

Among the immunologic defects seen are deficiency of immunoglobulin A (IgA), structural anomalies of the thymus and lymph nodes, prolonged survival of skin homografts, impaired lymphocyte transformation, and lymphopenia. Of those patients who survive to the late teens, malignant lymphoma develops in many. The associated diabetes mellitus is characterized by hyperglycemia with only rare glycosuria, absence of ketosis, marked hypersecretion of insulin, and peripheral resistance to the action of insulin. Other dermatologic findings, such as diffuse poliosis, café-au-lait spots, excessive dryness of skin and hair, disturbances of pigmentation, and eczema are seen in 40 to 60 per cent of patients. The only therapy is that directed to a complicating infection.

Among the hereditary telangiectatic syndromes with telangiectatic erythema and growth retardation are Bloom's syndrome, Rothmund-Thomson syndrome, hereditary sclerosing poikiloderma, Cockayne's syndrome, and dyskeratosis congenita. (See Chap. 20.)

Generalized or Unilateral Essential Telangiectasia

Generalized or unilateral essential telangiectasia is characterized by extensive

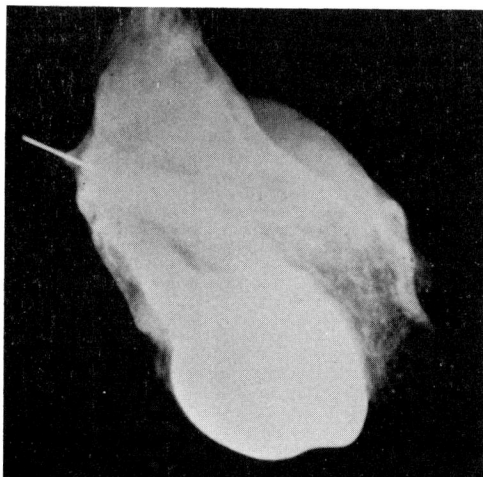

Figure 17–43 Arteriovenous shunt.

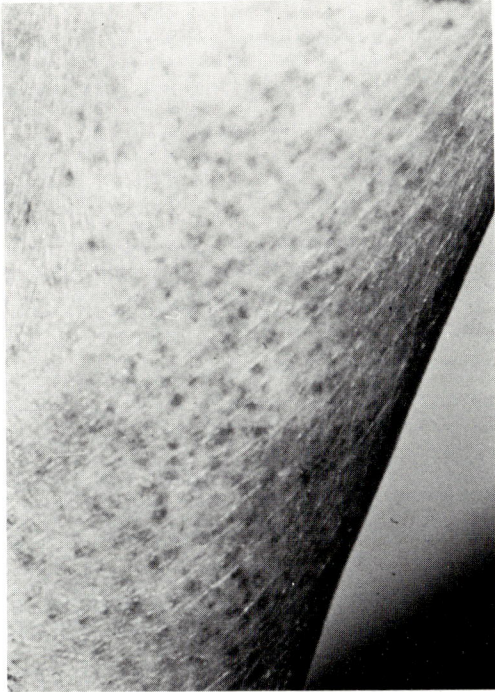

Figure 17–44 A six-year-old girl with ataxia telangiectasia characterized by ataxia, swaying of the head and trunk, nystagmus, and telangiectases of the conjunctivae and face, especially the butterfly area, and flexures of the arms.

sheets of telangiectases covering almost the entire surface of the lower extremities; it may spread insidiously over the trunk and upper arms (Fig. 17–45) and is associated with other changes in the skin. No familial incidence is noted. It occurs most frequently in women in late childhood to 60 years of age. Sensations of numbness, tingling, or burning of the lower extremities may occur. The eruption may be unilateral. The lesions are linear and may contain angiomas. The eruption progresses slowly and persists for from 3 to 40 years. The distribution and lack of hemorrhages differentiate it from hereditary hemorrhagic telangiectasia. Varicose veins are not associated with it. A case of essential progressive telangiectasia was successfully treated with tetracycline (Shelley, 1971).

Poikiloderma Atrophicans Vasculare

Poikiloderma atrophicans vasculare is a chronic, slightly scaling, patchy dermatitis

with hyperpigmentation and hypopigmentation, atrophy, fine telangiectases, and occasionally small bright red papules; it may be generalized or localized. The affected areas appear erythematous, have a cigarette paper–like wrinkling, and simulate radiodermatitis. It appears at any age but is seen most frequently in middle-aged persons. The eruption is symmetrically distributed on breasts (Fig. 17–46), buttocks, and in flexural areas and rarely involves mucous membranes. The condition tends to be permanent, the original patches remain for years, and others may appear later. It may be an idiopathic disease or may be associated with collagen diseases (LE, dermatomyositis), lymphomas (Hodgkin's disease, and particularly mycosis fungoides), and genodermatosis (Rothmund-Thomson syndrome, and hereditary sclerosing poikiloderma [Weary et al., 1969].)

In the idiopathic cases, the histopathologic picture consists of atrophy of epider-

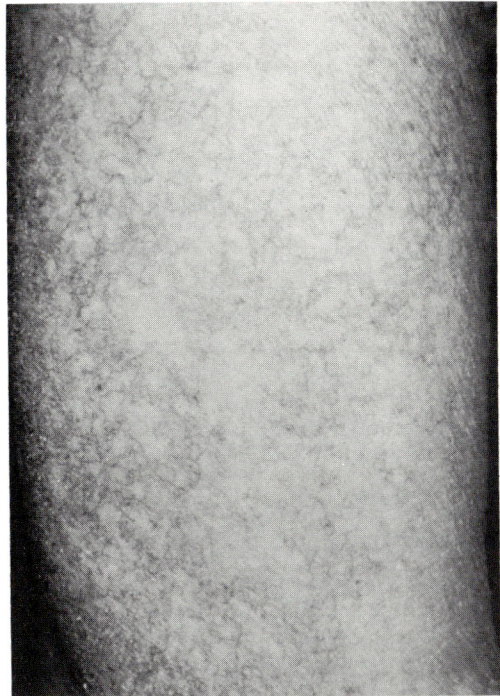

Figure 17–45 A 32-year-old woman with telangiectases on the lower extremities which spread to involve the trunk and upper extremities; she also complained of burning and tingling of her lower extremities; no underlying or associated disease was appreciated.

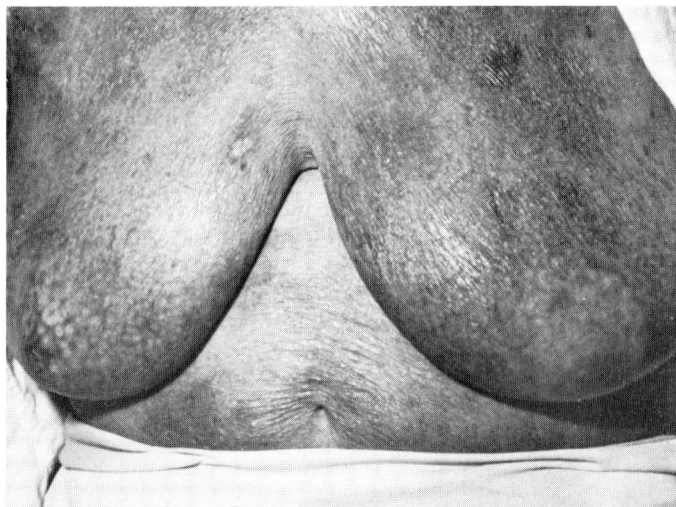

Figure 17–46 A 57-year-old woman had patchy disseminate poikiloderma of the skin; two years later mycosis fungoides developed in the areas.

mis with hydropic degeneration of basal cells and a dense bandlike infiltrate which lies in the upper dermis, invades some areas of the epidermis, and consists mainly of lymphocytes, some histiocytes, and plasma cells and melanophages. Idiopathic poikiloderma atrophicans vasculare may antedate the complicating cutaneous or systemic lymphoma for years. The poikilodermatous changes which complicate lesions of parapsoriasis en plaque–like lesions usually signal the presence of an underlying lymphoma. The poikilodermatous lesions associated with lymphoma are very pruritic, occur on covered areas, and have lymphomatous histopathologic changes; these characteristics are in contrast to those lesions associated with dermatomyositis or LE, which appear late in the course of the underlying disease, are relatively asymptomatic, and complicate an existing dermatosis on the exposed areas but can appear spontaneously on the trunk and have the same histopathologic picture as the idiopathic type.

Secondary Telangiectasia

Secondary telangiectasia may result from aging of the skin, physical insults, and chronic vasodilatation or may be associated with certain diseases. Owing to radiation (Fig. 17–47), telangiectases, as a part of the poikilodermic picture, are seen in poikiloderma of Civatte, radiodermatitis, erythema ab igne, and Hartnup's syndrome. They are also seen in rosacea and rosacea-like states of polycythemia vera and in long-term local or systemic corticosteroid therapy and may result from the prolonged vasodilatation appreciated in the carcinoid syndrome, mastocytosis (Fig. 17–48), and drug therapy.

The collagen diseases, LE, dermatomyositis, scleroderma, and Sjögren's syndrome may be associated with telangiectases with or without erythema. A variant of mastocytosis seen in adults, telangiectasis macularis eruptiva perstans, has characteristically telangiectatic lesions. Patients with varicose veins may have localized areas with superficial arborization of venules and capillaries about the lower extremities.

Erythema ab igne is an erythematous reticular pigmented dermatosis with telangiectases usually seen on the legs of young women who have repeated and prolonged exposure to infrared radiation which is below the threshold capacity to burn. It is also seen in other areas similarly exposed to the frequent and prolonged application of the hot water bottle for pain.

In persons who handle coal tar products, such as asphalt, pitch, creosote, or mineral oils, cutaneous changes consisting of atrophy, telangiectases, lichenoid papules, and follicular keratoses can develop slowly

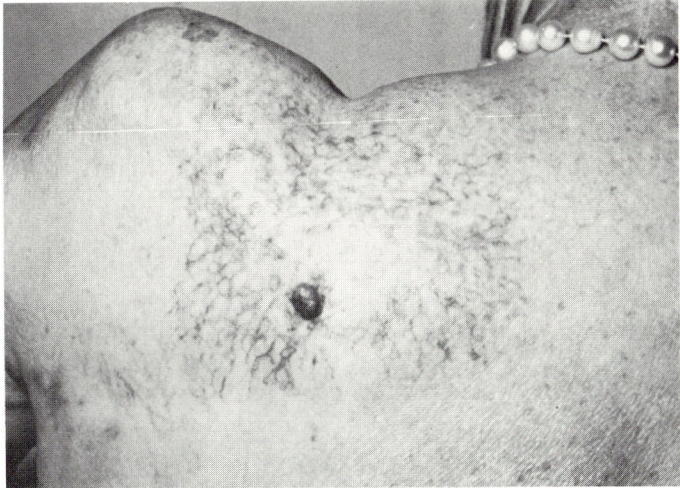

Figure 17–47 Secondary telangiectasia. A 58-year-old woman had radical mastectomy of the right breast followed by radiation for carcinoma of the breast; 15 years later, telangiectasia, atrophy, and basal cell epithelioma in one of the originally irradiated areas (right shoulder) developed.

on continuous exposure in the uncovered areas.

In middle-aged women, a condition called poikiloderma of Civatte (erythromelanosis colli) is seen. The eruption is reddish brown, with reticulated pigmentation and telangiectases, and has a symmetric sun-exposed pattern involving the face and neck with striking absence in the area shaded by the chin.

DISEASES OF PERIPHERAL VEINS

Although veins resemble arteries, they have thinner walls, a weaker middle muscular coat, and semilunar valves which are seen particularly in the smaller veins and their junction with larger branches. These valves prevent reflux of blood, especially in the legs where they and the calf muscle pump, the so-called venous heart, must counter the gravitational pressure. There are three systems of veins—a deep system, a superficial system which dilates under prolonged back pressure, and the communicating veins, which connect the two systems and are involved in the postthrombophlebitic syndrome. The venous diseases to be described are those of dilatation or thrombosis or both.

CLASSIFICATION OF DISEASES OF PERIPHERAL VEINS

Varicose veins
Thrombophlebitis and associated entities
    Superficial thrombophlebitis, for example, Mondor's disease

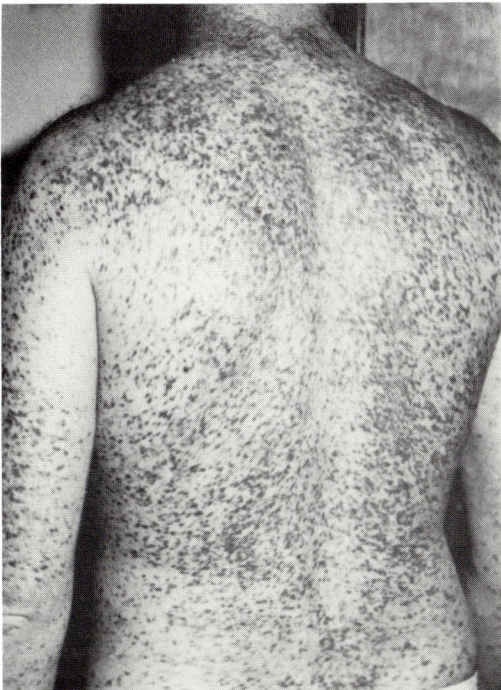

Figure 17–48 This 38-year-old man has an extensive pigmented telangiectatic eruption (telangiectasia macularis eruptiva perstans) and experienced pruritus and significant whealing of skin upon stroking and pressure.

Post-thrombophlebitic syndrome
Phlegmasia cerulea dolens
Vena caval syndrome
Venous lakes
Arborizing venules
Arteriovenous shunts

The venous flow in the extremities may be affected either by intrinsic disorders resulting from disease of the walls, an abnormality of blood, or extrinsic disorders resulting from venous invasion or external pressure. Venous blockage as a result of thrombosis or external pressure, and the dilatation secondary to hydrostatic forces, as seen in varicose veins, produce various disabling conditions whose severity depends on the degree of stasis.

Varicose Veins

Varicose veins are dilated and tortuous superficial veins, especially of the lower extremities. They result either from the combination of constitutionally defective valves with postural strains, especially occupational, or from obstructive deep venous states which produce compensatory enlargement of the superficial circulation.

The increased blood flow from the hydrostatic pressure occurs in the rare congenital arteriovenous fistula or in acquired conditions, such as the postphlebitic syndrome or pregnancy and the extrinsic obstruction of the inferior vena cava as a result of thrombophlebitis, abdominal malignancies, ascites, and abdominal aneurysm. The tendency is inheritable, and the disorder occurs four times more frequently in women, appears rarely before adolescence, and frequently complicates deep vein thromboses. The extremities are warm, and the arterial pulses are good. The great saphenous vein and its tributaries are most commonly involved. Patients may experience fatigue of muscles, muscle cramps at night, and edema at the end of the day. Extensive varicose veins may not be symptomatic. When the communicating vein or the arteriovenous connection becomes varicose, ulceration of the skin may occur.

Treatment of varicose veins may be conservative or surgical. The conservative measures are rest periods with elevation of the legs, exercises, and elastic stockings. Ligation and stripping can prevent or arrest the breakdown of the tributaries of the varicose veins. Incompetent great or small saphenous veins are usually detrimental because of the retrograde flow which, if marked, will overload the deep veins with an increase of venous insufficiency. Since the varicose veins resulting from deep venous obstruction are compensatory, ligation and stripping do not help the extremities.

Thrombophlebitis

Venous obstruction may be caused by phlebothrombosis, a condition in which clotting appears on the wall of a relatively noninflamed vein, and by thrombophlebitis, a condition in which thrombus forms on an inflamed intima. The former condition has little or no clinically appreciable local reaction and has a greater tendency to embolization than thrombophlebitis, which has classic local and systemic signs and symptoms of inflammation. Among the predisposing factors of thrombophlebitis are idiopathic venous stasis associated with prolonged bed rest or external pressure, local injury to endothelium by trauma, administration of various solutions and medications, or bacteria, thrombophilia, blood changes which favor coagulation, thromboangiitis obliterans, Behçet's disease, and infective fevers. Conditions in which a thrombophilic or hypercoagulable state exists include pregnancy (last two trimesters), estrogenic and progestational medications), postoperative period, cancer, especially carcinoma of the pancreas, and ulcerative colitis and pancreatitis.

The signs and symptoms develop acutely and persist for one to three weeks and depend on the size of the involved vessel. Constitutional reactions are usually minimal, but chills, high fever, and severe malaise are seen in suppurative thrombophlebitis. When the superficial veins are involved, it may be felt as a tender cord and usually leaves no clinical residua. When the deeper branches of the popliteal area are involved, local tenderness of the calf and pain on dorsiflexion of the foot are present, and residual manifestations of chronic venous insufficiency result from luminal constriction and valvular incompetency caused by fibrosis. A sudden extensive venous thrombosis and arterial vasospasm may cause the limb to become cold, pale, and pulseless. Treatment is directed toward removing the underlying cause, preventing pulmonary embolism by anticoagulant therapy and surgery, and relieving edema. Other measures of therapy are bed rest, local heat, and, rarely, sympathetic block to abolish reflex arterial vasospasm.

Thrombophlebitis migrans refers to multiple episodes of involvement of large and small veins throughout the body over a period of months to years. It may be idiopathic or associated with infections, malignant disease, Behçet's disease, or thromboangiitis obliterans. Migratory recurrent superficial thrombophlebitis involves the superficial veins of the extremities, abdominal wall, and flanks and presents as successive crops of tender, linear, or nodular lesions which may resemble clinically erythema nodosum, nodular vasculitis, and various panniculitides. The superficial thrombophlebitis may antedate any signs or symptoms of carcinoma, especially of the pancreas, stomach, or the lung. Carcinoma is considered one of the commonest causes of thrombophlebitis. In contrast to idiopathic thrombophlebitis, carcinogenic thrombophlebitis may show less inflammatory reaction, does not respond to anticoagulants, and may be the result of a hypercoagulable state. Heparin, Butazolidin, and fibrolysin may be helpful.

Mondor's disease, superficial thrombophlebitis of the thoracoepigastric veins (Johnson et al., 1962), is a special, rare, benign type of thrombophlebitis, the so-called string phlebitis, which may be related to direct mechanical or surgical trauma or to physical muscle strain from work or sports. It presents clinically as a tender, painful, subcutaneous cord 3 to 5 mm. in diameter, which usually is aligned between the anterior axillary line or breast and the lower costal or margin umbilicus; it may extend to the axilla and be bilateral, and it persists for one to six weeks and may remain palpable for months. Multiple recurrences are rare. It should not be confused with carcinoma of the breast or lymphangial spread of carcinoma.

Post-thrombotic (postphlebitic) syndrome occurs after a deep vein thrombosis, is caused by greatly increased venous pressure in the deep and communicating veins, and results in chronic venous insufficiency. Other conditions which may be associated with chronic venous insufficiency are varicose veins with incompetency of valves, extensive hemangiomas, and congenital or acquired arteriovenous fistulas.

The clinical manifestations of this syndrome are edema, pigmentation, dermatitis, and indurated cellulitis. Edema is the essential expression and the other signs do not appear until orthostatic edema has been present for a long period. Purpura and pigmentation follow and appear usually above the ankle (Fig. 17–49). A chronic eczematous dermatitis and ulceration with scar formation occur in areas of marked congestion. Pruritus may antedate or accompany the dermatitis, which may become lichenified. The longer the lymphedema persists, the more likely is the development of complicating subcutaneous fibrosis and hypertrophied and pachyder-

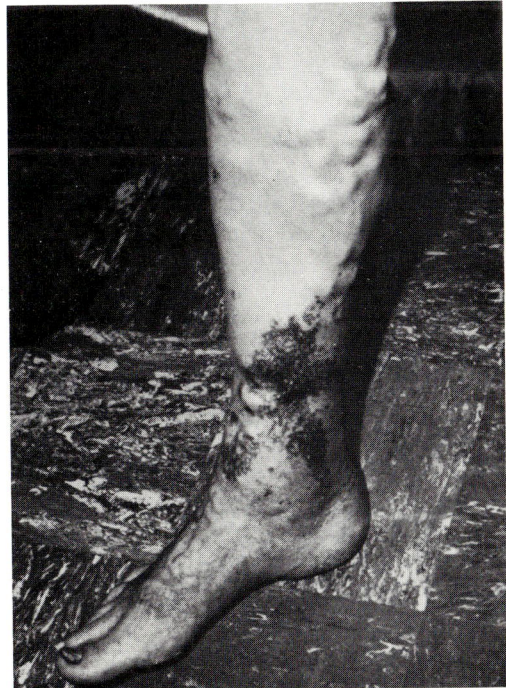

Figure 17–49 Stasis eczema with pigmented purpura.

matous skin. A low-grade inflammatory state may produce a hard, brawny induration of the skin and subcutaneous tissue, the so-called indurated cellulitis; it is seen most frequently proximal to the internal malleolus but can affect other areas and even the entire circumference of the leg and create the "champagne bottle" or "piano leg" appearance. It can be painful and disabling. At the sites of trauma, ulceration commonly develops, may be chronic and disabling, can become secondarily infected, and heals with an atrophic scar. The ulcers appear about the malleoli, especially the internal one (Fig. 17–50), and vary greatly in size; their healing may be impaired by the scar tissue of secondary infection. The ulcers are never as painful as the ischemic ones.

Among the unusual complications are pseudoepitheliomatous hyperplasia which may resemble epithelioma, subcutaneous calcification which can be widespread and interfere with the healing of an ulcer, bone changes resulting from periostitis seen beneath the chronic ulcer, and the development of an epithelioma which is characterized clinically by a vegetative lesion failing to respond to ulcer therapy (Fig. 17–51). Atrophie blanche may be associated with the stasis syndrome (Fig. 17–52).

Therapy is directed to the treatment of

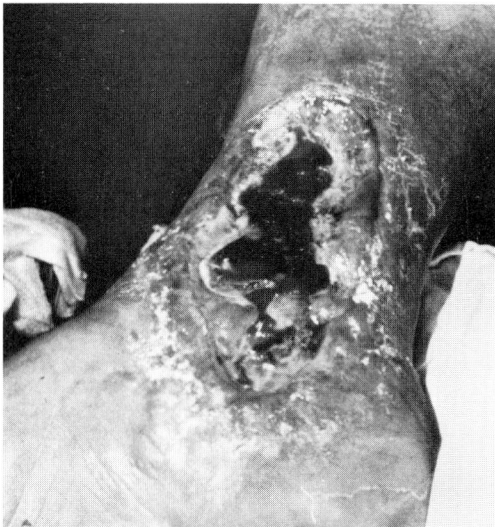

Figure 17–51 Patient had stasis ulcer of three years' duration; the border of the lesion was biopsied and the pathological report was pseudoglandular squamous cell carcinoma.

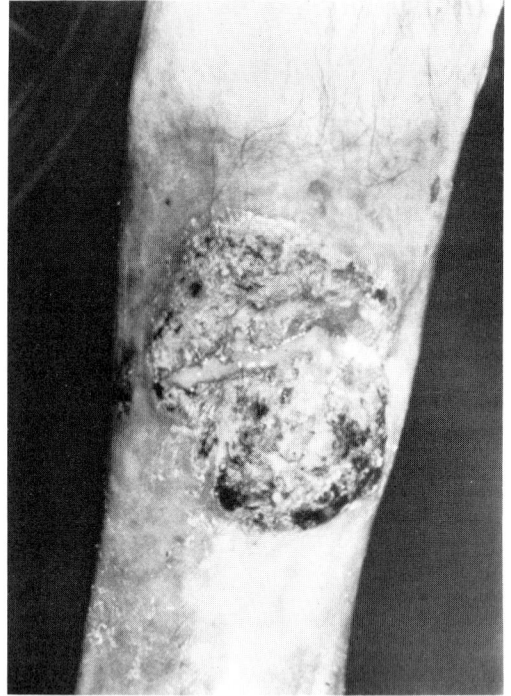

Figure 17–50 Classic stasis ulcer with superimposed gram-negative infection.

edema and ulcer by bed rest, elevation, supporting bandages and stockings, and diuretics; to the treatment of secondary infection by soaks and topically applied and systemic antibiotics; to the treatment of symptomatic calcification by surgical removal; and to the treatment of resistant ulcer or epitheliomatous complication by excision and grafting. The affected areas are susceptible to sensitization reactions to applied medicaments (Fig. 17–53).

Phlegmasia Cerulea Dolens

Phlegmasia cerulea dolens, the so-called gangrene of venous origin (Stallworth et al., 1965), is a rare, severe, extensive thrombotic disease of deep veins with discoloration of the involved limb. The femoral, iliac, intercommunicating, and multiple superficial veins may be involved. Vasospasm of arteries and veins occurs. The disease most frequently appears in patients between the ages of 40 and 50 years, and the sexes are equally affected. In most of the cases, an antecedent thrombophlebitis, a disease (for example, acquired hemolytic anemia, malignancies, ulcerative colitis, pneumonia, heart failure, diabetes, and tuberculosis), or an operation immediately precedes its acute onset.

Phlegmasia cerulea dolens presents initially with acute pain in the extremity which becomes tremendously edematous and demonstrates a bluish violet discoloration. As the condition progresses, bullae and ischemic necrosis of the skin, paresthesias, and motor paralysis may develop. The ischemia and gangrene are probably the result of obstruction of blood flow at the arteriole-capillary-venule level possibly due to spasm or stasis and thrombosis. The left lower leg is involved three times more frequently than the right one. The pulses are bounding except when the edema is such that the pulses are difficult to appreciate. Gangrene of toes and foot may occur and is similar to that of peripheral

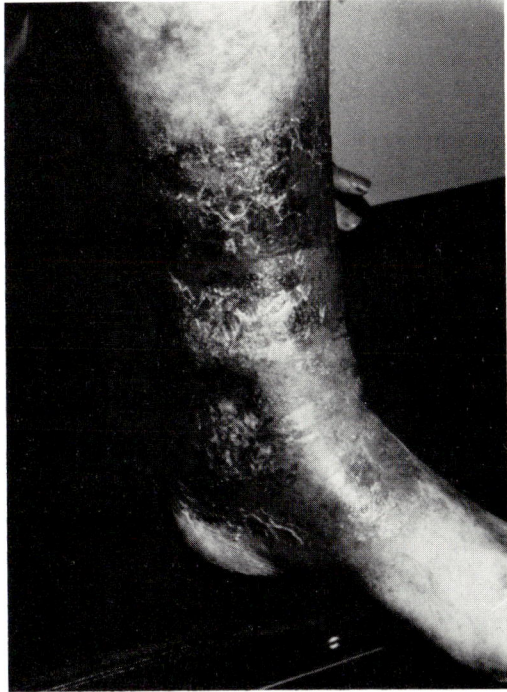

Figure 17-53 Contact dermatitis superimposed upon the stasis dermatitis and caused by neomycin.

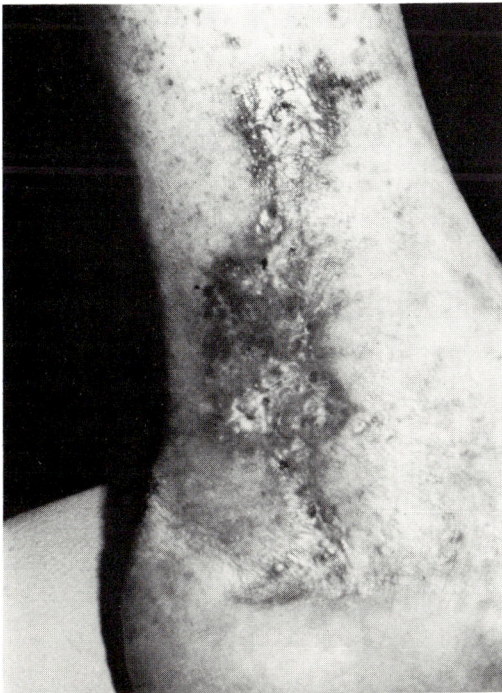

Figure 17-52 Atrophie blanche characterized by superficial painful ulcers caused by local small vessel occlusion in the lower foot of an extremity of a patient with varicose vein disease.

arterial disease. This gravid disease state is frequently complicated by shock, gangrene, and pulmonary embolism which is often fatal. The post-thrombotic syndrome develops in about half of those persons who survive.

Among the medical and therapeutic measures are elevation of the involved extremity, heparinization, and infusion of dextran 75. Among the surgical procedures utilized have been sympathetic blockade or sympathectomy for the vasospasm, thrombectomy, fasciotomy, and amputation. The underlying or associated condition should be treated if or when possible.

Vena Caval Syndrome (Superior and Inferior)

When the superior vena cava is completely obstructed, a classic and easily appreciable syndrome is seen; however, if the obstruction is incomplete or the disease is insidiously progressive, the diagnosis is less obvious (Effler and Groves,

1962). The clinical picture is determined by the suddenness of the occlusion and the functioning collateral circulation. The causes of the obstruction are primary (carcinoma of the lung, lymphoma) and secondary (metastatic) malignancy, inflammatory conditions (chronic fibrous mediastinitis, such as tuberculosis and histoplasmosis), constrictive pericarditis, thrombophlebitis, and benign tumors (aortic aneurysm).

Malignant tumors, especially bronchogenic carcinoma (Fig. 17–54), cause more than 75 per cent of all instances of vena caval obstruction. Since the occurrence of bronchogenic carcinoma is five times greater in men than in women, malignant vena caval obstruction is predominately a masculine disease. When the obstruction is relatively complete, edema and a dusky cyanosis of the face, neck, thorax, and upper extremities are noted which are aggravated by the horizontal position. Edema of the eyelids, suffusion of conjunctival vessels, and dilated cutaneous venules (venous stasis) of the chest wall may occur. The distended skin may be painful. Dyspnea may be present. The increased venous pressure in the cerebral veins may cause headache, drowsiness, stupor, loss of consciousness, and convulsions. With gradual obstruction, cyanosis and dyspnea are much less evident but are made more prominent by recumbency or exercise. The point of obstruction determines the pattern of the collateral veins. Thoracotomy, venous pressure determination, and vena cavography are useful diagnostic measures. When the condition is present for longer than six months, the primary lesion is usually benign and is compatible with long life. However, if carcinoma of the lung is present, superior vena caval syndrome is an ominous sign, and the patients rarely survive longer than 10 weeks. Therapy (surgery, radiotherapy, chemotherapy, and a combination) depends on the nature of the lesion.

The obstruction of the inferior vena cava is most frequently caused by thrombosis or thrombophlebitis (Fig. 17–55). The thrombosis most commonly results from extension of the older thrombi in one or both iliac veins. Among other causes are extrinsic pressure from enlarged organs (liver and pancreas), benign tumors (aneurysm), ascites, malignancy (gastrointestinal carcinoma, lymphoma, renal carcinoma), and inflammatory fibrosis (adhesive bands, retroperitoneal fibrosis, and old inflammatory processes). Renal cell carcinoma tends to invade the renal vein and extends into the inferior vena cava. The thrombosis may be associated with a hypercoagulable state.

Multifocal fibrosclerosis (Carton and Wong, 1969) is used to describe a group of fibrosing conditions consisting of chronic mediastinal fibrosis, retroperitoneal fibrosis, pseudotumor of the orbit, sclerosing

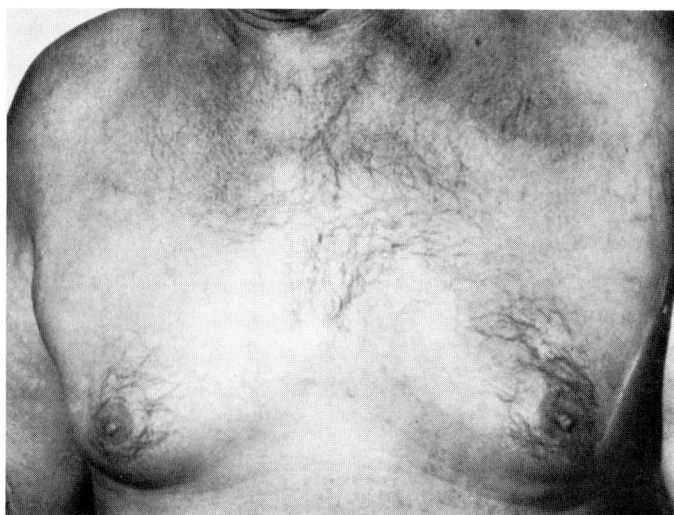

Figure 17–54 Superior venal caval syndrome with dusky cyanosis and edema of the upper chest, neck, and face and showing prominent venous pattern caused by bronchogenic carcinoma.

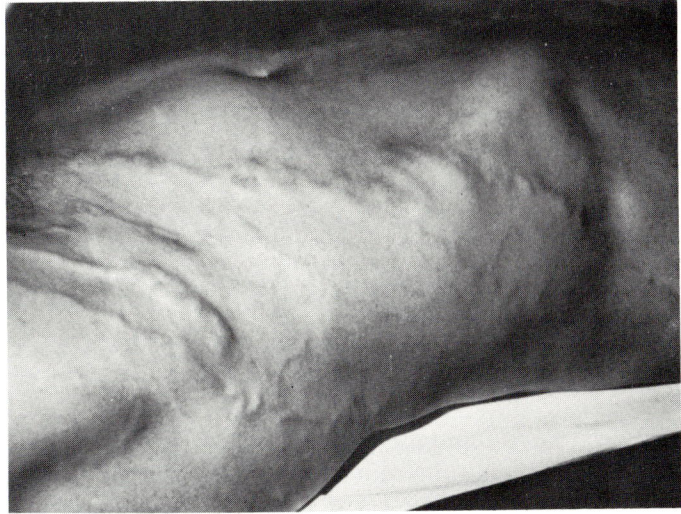

Figure 17–55 Inferior venal caval syndrome with varicose veins of the extremities and dilated veins of the lower trunk secondary to thrombosis of the inferior vena cava.

cholangitis, Riedel's struma of the thyroid, and generalized vasculitis.

When thrombosis is the cause of this syndrome, the signs and symptoms appear more suddenly than those produced by the extrinsic pressure of tumors. The clinical picture in the absence of pulmonary embolism is characterized by bilateral swelling of the lower extremities, marked prominence of the superficial veins of the legs, dilated and tortuous superficial veins extending up to the thorax, and edema of the lumbosacral area. Venography is one of the most helpful measures in identifying the obstruction and differentiating extrinsic from intrinsic causes. When the occlusion is the result of thrombosis or thrombophlebitis, the patient may live for years. The recanalization and collateral circulation may reduce the orthostatic pressure in the legs, but the dilated veins persist. The therapeutic approach is similar to that of the superior vena caval syndromes. Adequate elastic bandages or hose may prevent the severe complications of chronic venous insufficiency of the legs.

Venous Lakes

Venous lakes are greatly dilated thin-walled venules without vascular proliferation and are a type of senile angioma seen on the face and ears of elderly people.

Arborizing Venules

Among the arborizing venules are the progressive, symmetric venous telangiectases seen in families and occurring usually in the same areas and the usually symmetric, branching, linear venous telangiectases seen on the medial aspect of the thighs, especially of women.

Arteriovenous Fistula

Arteriovenous fistula (Gomes and Bernatz, 1970) has been described as a pulsating angioma, cirsoid aneurysm, and arteriovenous shunt between arteries and veins without the arterial blood traversing a capillary network. It may be congenital or acquired and single or multiple. The congenital type is present from birth and is usually multiple and associated with birthmarks, such as telangiectases, port wine stain, cavernous hemangioma, or diffuse hemangiomas. In the affected regions, an increased growth of hair and sweating may be noted. Bruits and thrills are not produced because the communications are multiple and narrow.

The acquired type of arteriovenous fistula is almost invariably caused by a penetrating wound made by a bullet or stabbing and is usually single and saccular. The size and location of the fistula affect the hemodynamics and the resultant disease. The skin near the fistula may be red or cyanotic, tender, warm, and edematous. The traumatic fistula is accompanied by a continuous murmur and usually a thrill. The venous pressure in the involved area is great and is the result of the complicating chronic venous insufficiency. Varices, edema, stasis pigmentation, and indurative cellulitis with or without ulceration may be seen. The ulcer is more distal and warm (the "hot" ulcer) than that of the post-thrombophlebitis or varicose ulcer. The decreased capillary flow may cause not only shallow indolent ulcers but also rarefaction of bone and unilateral arthritic changes. This shunting of arterial blood from the capillary can produce gangrene of the digits and distal part of the extremity. Depending on the size, duration, and location of the fistula, cardiac enlargement and failure may occur. The exact location, number, and size of the communications can be appreciated by arteriography. A single fistula is amenable to surgery if the collateral circulation is adequate; multiple fistulas are less amenable.

LYMPHEDEMA (Allen et al., 1962; Kinmonth et al., 1962)

The lymphatic system is a vast, intercellular vascular network which collects tissue, fluid, and lymph from the extravascular spaces and conducts them by valved channels of increasing size to regional lymph nodes and then through lymphatic trunks to the subclavian veins. The lymph flow depends on muscular contractions, respiratory movements, and gravity. Most organs have lymphatic capillaries; in the skin, they are numerous in the dermis and subcutaneous tissues. The lymphatic capillaries remove plasma proteins and particulate matter from the extravascular spaces either across or between the endothelial cells. The superficial dermal plexus can be visualized by intradermal injection of blue-violet or saccharated iron oxide, and a radiopaque substance is injected into a lymphatic trunk on the dorsum of the foot to visualize the lymphatic trunks and nodes. The lymphatic function has been evaluated by studying the rate of

clearance of I^{131} albumin from the extravascular tissues.

Lymphedema is soft-tissue swelling caused by increased accumulation of lymph as a result of inadequate lymphatic drainage. It may be divided into primary and secondary forms. Primary or idiopathic edema can be subdivided into the congenital type which is present at birth, lymphedema praecox appearing after birth to age 35, and lymphedema tarda (Fig. 17–56) appreciated after the age of 35. The congenital lymphatic abnormalities based on lymphangiographic studies have been described as aplastic, hypoplastic, hyperplastic, and dermal backflow. When several members within a family are affected, it has been called Nonne-Milroy-Meige's disease. The age at onset and severity tend to be similar in a family.

The clinical presentation of the familial type is not unlike the nonfamilial expression. Three-quarters of the patients are women. The most frequent sites of involvement are the legs, but the arms, genitalia, and face may be involved. The swelling appears about the ankle and gradually extends upward. Both lower extremities may eventually be involved. Trauma has frequently been described as the precipitant. The swelling is at first soft, disappears during rest, and becomes firm with the passage of time owing to the complicating reactive fibrosis. Hot weather, menses, and gestation may accentuate the edema. The chronically, firmly enlarged hyperkeratotic, warty ("mossy") skin (Fig. 17–57) has been referred to as elephantiasis. Alterations of the skin by lymphedema, trauma, fissuring, and epidermophytosis permit the entry of bacteria, especially hemolytic streptococci, and less frequently staphylococci, into the involved part to cause lymphangitis and recurrent cellulitis.

Secondary lymphedema may be noninflammatory, resulting from some extralymphatic process, or secondary to an inflammatory process. Lymph vessels may be compressed by direct invasion of lymphatics or lymph nodes by neoplasms, surgical extirpation of nodes, fibrosis resulting from radiation therapy, and scars. Unexplained unilateral lymphedema in a person over the age of 40 may be the first expression of a neoplasm. Prostatic car-

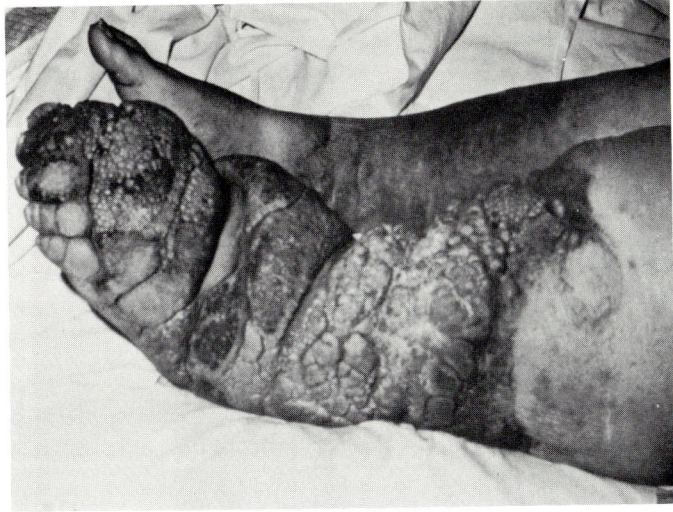

Figure 17–56 Lymphedema tarda in a 38-year-old man; there is involvement of both legs.

cinoma (Fig. 17–58) is the most responsible malignancy in men and lymphoma is the most responsible in women.

Secondary lymphedema of the inflammatory type may result from recurrent lymphangitis or cellulitis (the commonest cause), lymphogranuloma venereum, filariasis, and chronic venous insufficiency. The sexes are equally affected, and it rarely appears before the age of 40. Both legs are rarely affected except when the disease is caused by infection. Irregular recurrences are the result of reinfection from outside or intermittent activity of foci in the extremity. The edema fluid, which is rich in proteins, is an excellent culture medium and also stimulates fibrosis. The thick, coarse skin tends to develop ulceration and erysipeloid infections, and the resultant changes produce the picture of elephantiasis.

Middle-aged persons and even children may experience the yellow nail syndrome which is characterized by lymphedema, usually of the legs, and nail changes. The lymphedema usually affects the hand and face and may be universal; recurrent pleural effusions occur infrequently. The involved nails are smooth, thickened, excessively curved on the long axis, and pale yellow or yellowish green, and may become loose and be shed; these changes may reverse spontaneously.

Another rare complication of chronic

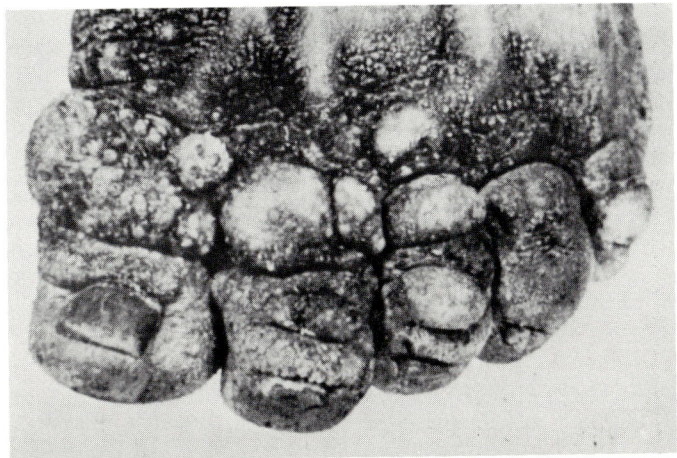

Figure 17–57 Mossy foot seen in chronic lymphedema of the lower extremity.

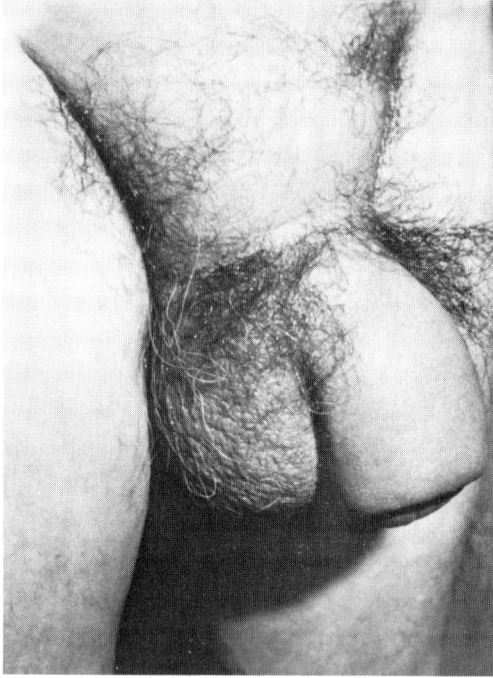

Figure 17–58   Secondary lymphedema of the genitalia and pubic area resulting from metastatic prostatic carcinoma.

lymphedema is lymphangiosarcoma which usually occurs after a radical postmastectomy and is characterized clinically by blue-red or purple well-defined macules or papules (Danese et al., 1967). These lesions appear on the arm, forearm, or hand in crops and may coalesce, spreading to the chest wall and shoulder girdle, or metastasize. Lymphangiosarcoma does not complicate the lymphedema of filariasis or venous stasis but rarely does complicate congenital lymphedema. Although the lymphangiosarcoma unassociated with malignancy tends to run a slower course, 50 per cent of all known cases have died two years after its onset regardless of therapy.

The treatment of lymphedema is aimed at keeping the tissues free of edema in order to prevent fibrosis and recurrent bacterial infections. Frequent elevation of the involved extremity, use of elastic bandages or stockings, diuretics, and a diet low in salt are routine therapeutic measures. Epidermophytosis should be treated vigorously and controlled. Long-term intermittent antibiotic prophylaxis is advis-

able for recurrent lymphangitis. Factors which aggravate the edema include excessive use of the limb, local heat, generalized heating, puncture wounds, and constriction of the limb. The basic surgical procedures are to improve lymphatic drainage by omental transposition or by the transfer of a buried dermal flap or to remove the severely edematous and fibrotic subcutaneous tissue in order to improve the size and appearance of the grossly distorted limb and to reduce recurrent cellulitis and lymphangitis. The therapeutic management of lymphangiosarcoma is uniformly poor.

NODULAR VASCULITIDES

A variety of chronic syndromes characterized by a group of inflammatory, visible, or palpable nodules have been referred to as nodular vasculitides. The nodules are red and tender, predominate on the lower extremities (Wilkinson, 1954) but may also appear on the arms and trunk, may suppurate or ulcerate or both, and demonstrate histopathologically a variable degree of vasculitis in the small or medium-sized blood vessels with inflammation and fibrosis of the subcutaneous tissue. The classification of the nodular vasculitides is arbitrary and describes either a primary vasculitis or one secondary to an adjacent inflammatory process. The associated panniculitis in the syndromes has a histologic resemblance; therefore, it is of little assistance in differentiating the various clinical expressions. Since the cause and nature of the vascular injury are obscure in many of the cases, a classification has to be empirical (Table 17–1). This group of conditions must be differentiated further from other inflammatory nodules of the extremities (Table 17–3).

A variant of classic erythema nodosum has been described as chronic erythema nodosum, subacute nodular migratory panniculitis, erythema nodosum migrans (Bäfverstedt), and erythema nodosum perstans (Vilanova and Piñol Aguadé, 1959). The descriptive names attempt to point out salient clinical features of the disease. It differs from acute erythema nodosum mainly by its protracted course, lasting continuously or intermittently for months to several years, and its migratory pattern. The lesions tend to coalesce with one another or to extend gradually centrifugally, forming lumpy, deep-seated plaques. The lesions are moderately tender in contrast to the usually exquisitely painful classic erythema nodosum and lack the latter's bruising changes. The cause of this variety is unknown, and the

TABLE 17–3 CLASSIFICATION OF
INFLAMMATORY NODULES OF EXTREMITIES

So-called "nodular vasculitis"
    Variants of erythema nodosum
    Erythema induratum
    Recurrent superficial migratory phlebitis
    Nodular vasculitis
    Erythrocyanosis with nodules

Small vessel vasculitis
    Erythema nodosum and its variants (subacute nodular migratory panniculitis of Vilanova, erythema nodosum migrans of Bäfverstedt)
    Nodular dermal allergide
    Nodular erythrocyanosis
    Livedo reticularis

Superficial phlebitis (small and medium-sized vessels)
    Idiopathic recurrent migratory thrombophlebitis
    Those associated with malignancies, reticuloses, thromboangiitis obliterans, ulcerative colitis, Behçet's disease, thrombocythemia

Arteritis with or without granuloma
    Polyarteritis nodosa
    Allergic granulomatosis
    Wegener's granulomatosis

Panniculitides (primary or secondary)
    Infectious: Erythema induratum (Bazin), erythema nodosum leprosum, typhus, disseminated sporotrichosis
    Connective tissue diseases: Lupus erythematosus, scleroderma, periarteritis nodosa
    Carcinogenic: Metastatic emboli, subcutaneous nodular fat necrosis (carcinoma of pancreas)
    Physical agents: Trauma, cold, factitial
    Poststeroid panniculitis
    Idiopathic panniculitides: Local or disseminated, suppurative or nonsuppurative, subcutaneous lipogranulomatosis of Rothman-Makai, systemic nodular panniculitis (Weber-Christian disease)

Miscellaneous
    Trichophyton granuloma
    Sarcoidosis (Darier-Roussy)
    Deep fungal (nocardiosis) and bacterial abscesses (staphylococcal, *Pseudomonas aeruginosa*)

histologic picture is not significantly different from erythema nodosum except for a greater frequency of foci of granulomatous inflammation with giant cells.

The disease usually develops in young Caucasian women 1 to 20 days after an upper respiratory tract infection. Except for the cutaneous nodules, no other signs and symptoms are noted. Unlike erythema nodosum, the lesions appear commonly on the calves and buttocks. Like acute erythema nodosum, it responds to low doses of corticosteroids but tends to relapse upon their withdrawal. The title "subacute nodular migratory" (Vilanova and Piñol Aguadé, 1959) has been used to describe slowly expanding, unilateral, and sometimes solitary tender red nodules. There is an elevated sedimentation rate; the patient may respond to systemically administered iodides; and it may resemble cellulitis or superficial phlebitis.

Erythema induratum has been used to describe syndromes (erythema induratum of Bazin, erythema induratum of Whitfield, and nodular vasculitis) which are characterized by chronic, recurrent, tender, bluish nodules or infiltrated plaques which appear on the lower leg, especially the calf, in crops, have a variable tendency to ulceration, and are associated with cold, venous stasis, or tuberculous adenitis or pulmonary tuberculosis or history of same. Using immunofluorescent techniques, 7S gamma globulins and beta 1C globulin component of the complement system have been demonstrated in the vascular and perivascular tissue of the lesions (Stringa et al., 1966).

In erythema induratum of Bazin, the nodules are more prone to ulcerate than the other members of this group, and these indolent ulcers heal slowly, leaving depressed, hyperpigmented scars. Crops of new nodules may be precipitated by exposure to cold. The involved, usually fat legs show an associated violaceous or perniotic appearance, edema, and a coolness to touch.

The relationship of erythema induratum of Bazin with tuberculosis has been controversial. Among the factors suggesting this possibility are the presence of a tuberculoid infiltrate, epithelioid and giant cells in or about vessels in the subcutaneous tissue, evidence in some patients of a distant active foci of tuberculosis, the frequently positive tuberculin skin tests, and the response of some patients to a course of antituberculous therapy. However, the infrequent isolation of the tubercle bacilli or successful inoculation of guinea pigs or both casts doubts. It has been suggested that an allergic reaction to tuberculous protein, a tuberculid, or other hematogenous antigens may be responsible. The lesions may initially improve during the warmer months. An adequate course of antituberculous therapy is indicated. In this group have been included patients with quiescent or active tuberculosis in whom multiple small indolent nodules on the lower extremities develop which resemble the papulonecrotic tuberculid.

The nodules of erythema induratum of Whitfield are more acute, tender, and diffuse than those of Bazin, do not ulcerate, and have histologically less tuberculoid granuloma. No erythrocyanosis, precipitation by cold, or association with tuberculosis is noted. Venous stasis has been stressed as an important pathogenic factor. The course of this disorder is chronic, with a gradual decline and eventual disappearance within several years. In severe cases, bed rest and elevation of legs followed by ambulatory use of elastic bandages or stockings provide some symptomatic relief and improvement.

The relationship of nodular vasculitis to erythema induratum of Whitfield is uncertain—are they the same disease? The lesions clinically and histologically resemble each other. The histopathology reveals a significant amount of dermal and subcutaneous vasculitis with perivascular lymphocytic cuffing and less granulomatous infiltrate and not infrequently a patchy fibrinoid necrosis of the vessels. In nodular vasculitis, there is no association with cold, venous stasis, tuberculosis, or other systemic diseases except hypertension. The disorder eventually clears after several years. Corticosteroids given systemically, intralesionally, and topically under occlusion may be temporarily ameliorative. Bed rest and elastic bandages and stockings are effective supportive measures.

Nodular vasculitis has been described in patients who have had poliomyelitis or are paraplegics and who have severe erythrocyanosis about the lower legs. These patients are usually fat, middle-aged women. On histopathologic examination, dermal and vascular edema and vasodilatation are noted; occasionally, thrombosis with infarction, extravascular red blood cells, and necrotizing vasculitis are seen in severe cases. In young women, the nodules may appear in paralyzed, thin, cold legs, even in the absence of erythrocyanosis. During cold exposure, the nodules may appear not only in and beyond the areas of erythrocyanosis but also on the buttocks and knees. Ulceration of nodules seldom occurs, and, when it does, it is superficial and heals easily with rare scar formation. Adequate protection against cold is the effective therapeutic measure.

NECROSIS OF THE SKIN

Necrosis is the death of a cell or group of cells that form part of the living body. The morphologic changes associated with this dynamic process can occur suddenly. Six types of necrosis include coagulative, caseous and gummatous, liquefactive (or colliquative), fibrinoid, enzymatic, and gangrenous. Coagulative necrosis is seen most frequently and is usually the result of arterial obstruction or inherent vascular diseases that cause anemic or ischemic infarction. Caseous necrosis, in which tissue has a cheesy appearance, is characteristically seen in tuberculosis but may also be seen in tularemia, plague, sporotrichosis and other deep fungal infections, lymphopathia venereum, and cat-scratch fever. Despite its histologic caseous appearance, syphilitic necrosis is called gummatous because of its rubbery consistency.

Although liquefactive necrosis is best appreciated in the brain, it can be seen in dead skin softened and liquefied by neutrophils that are rich in lysozymes and have responded to a secondary pyogenic infection. Fibrinoid necrosis is a misnomer and does not apply to true necrosis. In the so-called hypersensitivity diseases, the inflammatory lesions that have a fibrinoid appearance in the connective tissue and blood vessels are probably the result of a focal precipitate of fibrin. Local and distant foci of enzymatic necrosis (fat necrosis, lipolytic necrosis) result from the release of lipases and other enzymes locally or into the vascular system after pancreatic destruction. Focal necrosis of adipose tissue seen in so-called traumatic fat necrosis and subcutaneous fat necrosis of the newborn are clinically and histologically different from enzymatic lipolytic necrosis. Gangrenous necrosis results from massive necrosis of the skin with a superimposed saprophytic infection. Dry gangrene (mummification) describes necrosis of the tissue of the extremities resulting from vascular occlusion. Wet or moist gangrene occurs when bacteria invade dead tissue, producing putrefactive change. When the gas-forming group of saprophytes, for example, *Bacillus welchii*, invade ischemic tissue, gas gangrene occurs.

Necrosis of the skin (Moschella, 1969) may involve part or all of the epidermis, the dermis, and the underlying panniculus. In 1956, toxic epidermal necrolysis was reported. It clinically resembles scalding of the skin and is characterized histologically by necrosis of the epidermis with only minimal changes in the dermis. It is believed to be a toxic or hypersensitivity eruption resulting mainly from the use of drugs or from staphylococcal infections.

The four basic activities of cells are (1) production of energy needed for vital metabolic processes, (2) synthesis of enzymatic and structural proteins, (3) maintenance of the chemical and osmotic homeostasis of the cell, and (4) reproduction. Injury or death of cells occurs as a result of derangements of these vital functions at a molecular level. Factors that adversely influence cellular functions include ischemia, physical agents, chemical agents, microbiologic agents, derangements in the immune mechanism, and genetic defects.

The conditions which can produce local anemia and ischemia, namely vasospastic disorders, embolization, primary vascular diseases, vasculitides of the so-called acquired connective tissue diseases, dysproteinemias, and disseminated intravascular coagulation, can also cause necrosis of the skin, and they have been discussed elsewhere. A classification of necrosis of the skin is presented in Table 17–4.

Physical Agents

Physical agents capable of causing necrosis of the skin include extremes of heat and cold, trauma, pressure (Figs. 17–59 and 17–60), radiant energy, and electrical energy. These agents may act directly upon the cells themselves or may act indirectly by increasing the metabolic activity of cells so that their blood supply is inadequate or by altering the environment so that it becomes unsuitable for the survival of cells.

Chemical Agents

Cells and tissues can be destroyed by inorganic and organic chemicals of endogenous or exogenous origin. If sufficiently concentrated, almost any substance can affect cells adversely. When chemical escharotics (for example, monochloracetic, dichloracetic, and trichloroacetic acids and carbolic acid) and vesicants (for example, nitrogen mustard and 5-fluorouracil) are applied locally, they can necrotize skin. If sulfobromophthalein (Fig. 17–61) and Levophed escape into the tissue about the site of an intravenous injection, necrosis of the skin appears. In patients in shock, necrosis has developed about the site of an intravenous infusion of norepinephrine. A rare complication of coumarin congeners in anticoagulant therapy is sudden, localized, hemorrhagic, gangrenous necrosis.

Venoms of certain snakes (water moccasin), spiders (*Loxosceles reclusa*), and jellyfish (Portuguese man-of-war) have a local necrogenic and proteolytic activity. The bite of the brown spider (*Loxosceles laeta*) can cause a gangrenous eschar that will reveal a deep ulcer when shed (Fig. 17–62). Satellite lymphadenopathy does not occur. The patient may experience nervousness, insomnia, and possibly an elevation of temperature. In the rare viscerocutaneous loxoscelism, he may experience high fever, hematuria, anuria, cyanosis, and icterus, followed by death within 24 hours after the bite. The systemic component lasts five to seven days. The ulcer

TABLE 17–4   Causes of Necrosis of Skin

Anemic or ischemic infarction
  Vasospastic disorders
    Raynaud's syndrome
    Hypertensive ischemic ulcer
    Ergotism
    Accidental intra-arterial injection
 	
  Embolization
    Atheromatous
    Thromboembolic (infected or noninfected)
    Fat and gases
 	
  Primary vascular diseases
    Arteriosclerosis obliterans
    Thromboangiitis obliterans
    Malignant atrophic papulosis (Degos)
    Phlegmasia cerulea dolens
 	
  Vasculitides of so-called acquired connective tissue
    diseases
    Polyarteritis nodosa
    Systemic lupus erythematosus
    Rheumatoid arthritis
    Temporal arteritis
    Wegener's granulomatosis
 	
  Dysproteinemias
    Cryoglobulinemia
    Cryofibrinogenemia
 	
  Disseminated intravascular coagulation (consumption coagulopathies)
    Human equivalents of Sanarelli-Shwartzman
      reaction (GSR)
    Infusion of exogenous or endogenous thromboplastin
    Fat embolism
    Kasabach-Merritt syndrome
 	
  Physical Agents
    Extremes of heat and cold
    Trauma
    Pressure
    Radiant energy
    Electrical energy
	Chemical Agents
	    Topical escharotics and vesicants
	    Oral coumarin congeners
	    Intravenous norepinephrine or misdirected
	      BSP and Levophed
	    Venoms of snakes, spiders, and marine life
	    Abnormal circulating enzymes
	
	Microbiologic agents
	  Bacterial infections
	    Anthrax
	    Diphtheria
	    Group A beta-hemolytic and microaerophilic
	      anhemolytic streptococcus
	    Necrobacillosis (fusospirochetal gangrene)
	    Pseudomonas aeruginosa
	    *Mycobacterium tuberculosis, M. leprae, M.
	      ulcerans*
	
	  Viral infections
	    Herpes zoster
	    Vaccinia
	
	  Treponemal infections
	    Syphilis
	    Yaws
	    Bejel
	    Endemic syphilis
	
	  Rickettsial infections
	    Rocky Mountain spotted fever
	    Typhus
	
	  Protozoan infections
	    Amebiasis cutis
	    Bilharziasis cutis
	
	  Fungal infections
	    Nocardiosis
	    Actinomycosis
	    Sporotrichosis
	    Histoplasmosis (especially African type)
	    Cryptococcosis
	    North American blastomycosis
	    South American blastomycosis
	    Mucormycosis

of the skin heals spontaneously in six to eight weeks, occasionally with keloid formation. Skin grafting may be necessary.

The association of pancreatic disease with subcutaneous fat necrosis is rare. Multiple nodose lesions that may suppurate, drain, and result in punched-out ulcers may develop in patients with pancreatitis or carcinoma of the pancreas.

Microbiologic Agents

Bacteria, treponemas, viruses, rickettsiae, protozoa, and fungi can cause necrosis of the skin. When the organism produces an exotoxin (for example, *Bacillus anthracis, Corynebacterium diphtheriae*) or endotoxin, the mechanism, direct interference with essential cellular enzymatic activity, is easily understood. In some parasites for which no toxins have been identified, the mechanism is poorly understood. Toxins usually act not only locally but also on distant parts through both their primary toxic action and their secondary interference with circulation. Some of the bacterial and viral organisms produce a local or systemic vasculitis through invasion of vessels or the initiation of the

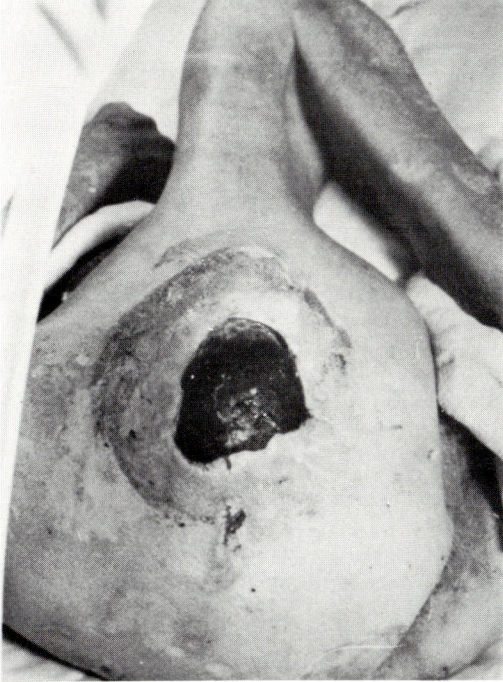

Figure 17–59 Decubitus ulcer in a debilitated elderly man who had progressive renal failure.

theria. Both diseases are accompanied by systemic symptoms. The cutaneous lesion is painless and that of diphtheria may be anesthetic. Patients with cutaneous anthrax tend to have a greater amount of local edema and satellite lymphadenitis.

Infectious gangrene may be acute, as seen in amebic and fusospirochetal gangrene. Necrotizing fasciitis (Beathard and Guckian, 1967), also called hospital gangrene, necrotizing erysipelas, and streptococcal gangrene, is a fulminating group A beta-hemolytic streptococcal infection of the superficial and deep fascia that results in thrombosis of subcutaneous vessels and gangrene (Fig. 17–63). Within 40 to 96 hours, the site of trauma changes from an erythematous, edematous, painful lesion to a bluish black patch that has irregular, ill-defined borders and usually hemorrhagic bullae. The involved region becomes numb and anesthetic because of damage to the local cutaneous nerves by the disease process. A probe or hemostat can easily be passed along the fascial planes above the deep fascia. Patients with

Sanarelli-Shwartzman reaction with necrosis of the skin. The caseous necrosis seen in tuberculosis, late syphilis, and some deep mycotic infections possibly represents a hypersensitivity phenomenon. Cytopathic viruses (for example, herpes zoster and vaccinia) probably destroy cells by adversely affecting vital intracellular metabolism through the incorporation of the viral RNA and DNA into the RNA messenger system or DNA of the host. Some nontoxic constituents or products of bacteria that are determinants of pathogenicity are coagulase, streptococcal fibrinolysin (streptokinase), deoxyribonuclease (streptodornase), and hyaluronidase.

Among the bacterial infections that can produce necrosis of the skin are those caused by *B. anthracis*, *C. diphtheriae*, *Streptococcus pyogenes* (group A beta-hemolytic streptococcus), hemolytic microaerophilic streptococcus, *Fusobacterium fusiforme* (Vincent's bacillus), *Pseudomonas aeruginosa*, and *Mycobacterium tuberculosis*, *M. leprae*, and *M. ulcerans*. A leathery eschar surrounded by vesicles in an exposed region is the classic clinical expression of cutaneous anthrax or diph-

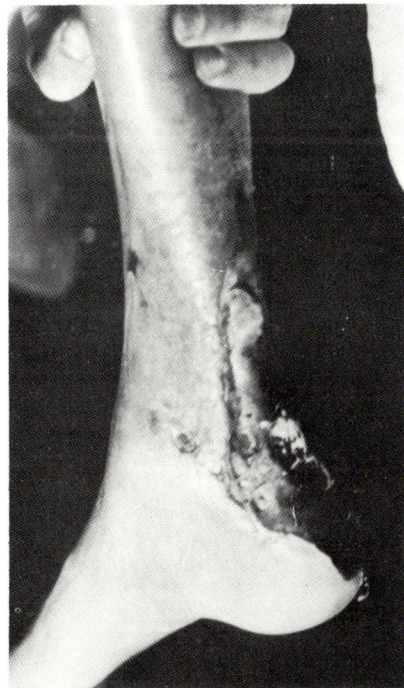

Figure 17–60 Pressure ulceration resulting from too tightly applied plaster cast for fracture of the ankle.

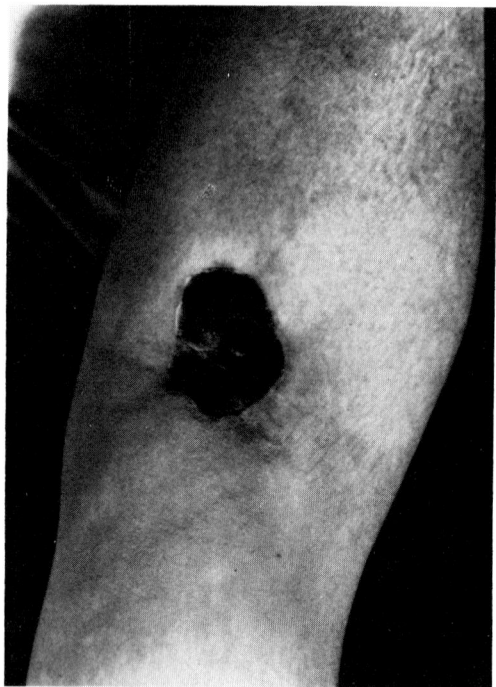

Figure 17–61 Escape of sulfobromophthalein into tissue about the site of intravenous injection resulted in necrotic eschar.

necrotizing fasciitis have a moderate fever but a tremendous amount of prostration. The high mortality and morbidity rates may be the result of failure to make an early diagnosis.

Fournier reported an acute gangrene (Fournier's gangrene) localized to the scrotum (Thomas, 1956); association with gangrene of the penis and abdominal wall was described subsequently. It was originally called spontaneous because of failure to demonstrate a cause. It has been associated with local trauma (mechanical, chemical, thermal), underlying urinary tract disease (paraphimosis, penile erosion, inguinal adenitis, prostatovesiculitis, epididymitis, periurethral extravasation of urine), distant acute inflammatory processes (perforative retrocecal appendicitis, acute hemorrhagic pancreatitis); it also is seen following operative procedures (circumcision, herniorrhaphy, hemorrhoidectomy, incision of perirectal abscess, injection of a hydrocele, abdominoperineal resection). The clinical appearance, course, and treatment are those of necrotizing fasciitis.

Bacterial synergistic gangrene is caused by anaerobic cocci mixed with *Straphylococcus aureus*, hemolytic streptococci, and *Proteus vulgaris*. A deep, painful ulcer with gangrenous margins may arise around retention sutures after abdominal operations and become very extensive; this condition is called postoperative synergistic gangrene. Amebic gangrene of the skin appears rarely about the anus as a complication of gastrointestinal amebiasis or on the abdominal wall secondary to drainage of an amebic abscess of the liver or an operation on the intestine. Fusospirochetal gangrene may follow a human bite; it appears rarely as a severely destructive stomatitis (noma, fusospirochetal gangrenous stomatitis) in a child with a debilitating disease. When gangrenous tissue is crepitant, it is because of the presence of gas-producing organisms.

Pseudomonas aeruginosa is usually an avirulent secondary contaminant of superficial wounds and burns, but serious and even fatal infections may occur in infants and adults whose resistance is impaired by other disease. Factors predisposing to septicemia and toxemia include malignant disease; low white blood cell count; previous treatment with systemic corticosteroids, broad-spectrum, antibiotics, or antimetabolites; and extensive burns. The organism tends to multiply in the walls of

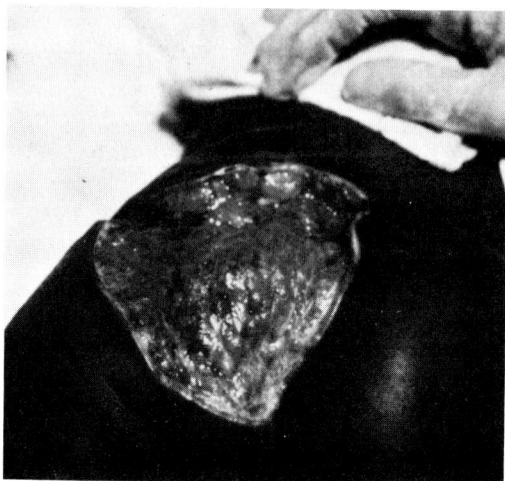

Figure 17–62 Granulation of ulcer after removal of hemorrhagic necrotic eschar; the lesion was produced by the bite of the brown recluse spider (*Loxosceles laeta*).

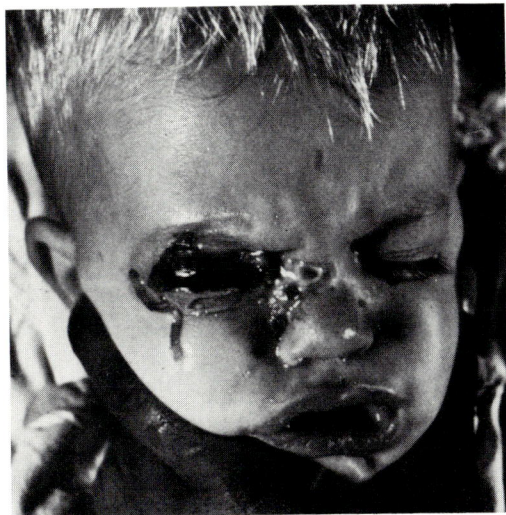

Figure 17–63 A three-year-old boy sustained a black eye by a fall; 48 hours after trauma, hemorrhagic bullae, high fever, and chills developed. A necrotizing fasciitis due to group A beta-hemolytic streptococci (necrotizing erysipelas) was diagnosed and successfully treated by surgical debridement and high doses of penicillin.

small blood vessels, producing vasculitis of the arterial and venous walls with secondary thrombosis and infarct necrosis. The septicemia may result in petechiae, subcutaneous indurated cellulitis, and ecthyma gangrenosum (Fig. 17–64). The subcutaneous indurated cellulitis is not pathognomonic, is more necrotic than suppurative, and may involve the epidermis. Ecthyma gangrenosum is specific and almost pathognomonic. These lesions may be single or multiple and tend to be located on the buttocks and extremities. They begin as tense, occasionally grouped vesicles on an erythematous base. After the vesicles become purulent or hemorrhagic, a punched-out, indurated ulcer with a necrotic base results. Patients with septicemia caused by pseudomonas may experience intravascular coagulation with a resultant generalized Shwartzman reaction that can be appreciated clinically as purpura fulminans and purpura necrotica.

Mycobacterial infections caused by *Mycobacterium tuberculosis, M. leprae,* and *M. ulcerans* can cause necrotic ulceration. Patients with lepromatous leprosy may experience the unusual type of lepra reaction characterized by necrotizing skin lesions. Infection with *M. ulcerans* causes a chronic, necrotizing ulceration of the extremities, especially in children. It begins as a painless, subcutaneous nodule that ulcerates. The necrosis is believed to be caused by a toxic substance elaborated by the bacillus. The ulcer requires months to heal, and complicating contractures and lymphedema may occur.

In the late stages of the treponemal infections — syphilis (Fig. 17–65), yaws, bejel, and endemic syphilis — fluctuant subcutaneous nodules, which usually commence in the skin but can extend from gummas of underlying bone, necrose to form chronic, indolent ulcers. Because of their cytopathic ability, infection with the herpes zoster and vaccinia viruses can produce necrotic skin lesions. In addition to the spreading necrosis at the site of vaccination (vaccinia gangrenosa), meta-

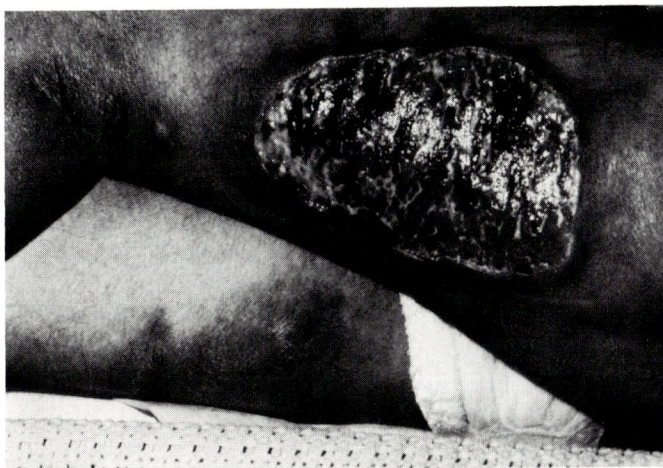

Figure 17–64 A 25-year-old woman with advanced Hodgkin's disease had been receiving triple chemotherapy; pseudomonas septicemia and subcutaneous abscesses occurred; ecthyma gangrenosum developed in the sites of the drained abscesses.

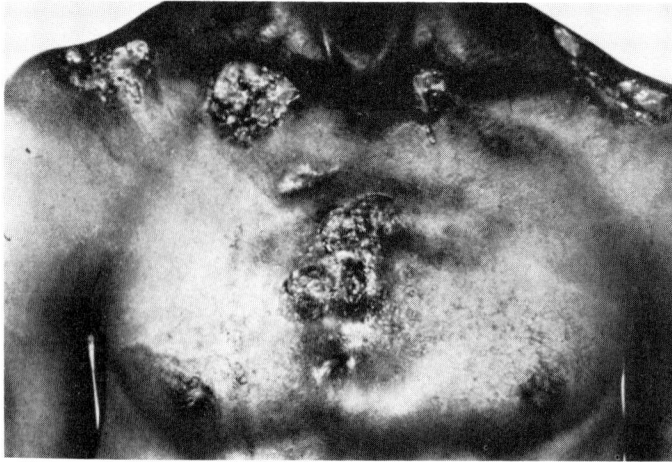

Figure 17–65 A 52-year-old black man with disseminated gummata of tertiary syphilis.

static necrotic lesions may appear elsewhere on the body. In Rocky Mountain spotted fever and typhus, necrotic ulceration of the scrotum has been seen.

Deep mycotic infections can cause necrosis of the skin. The systemic mycotic infections capable of producing such lesions include nocardiosis, actinomycosis, sporotrichosis, histoplasmosis, cryptococcosis, and North American and South American blastomycosis. Phycomycosis is caused by several members of the class of Phycomycetes (true fungus) that are commonly saprophytic but can be opportunistic—that is, able to cause superficial and visceral infection when tissue resistance is lowered by local or systemic factors. Predisposing factors for visceral involvement include debilitation resulting from diabetes mellitus, lymphoma, leukemia, and extensive burns, and therapy with antibiotics, steroids, antimetabolites, chemotherapy, and radiation. Landau and Newcomer (1962) classified phycomycosis into four types: craniofacial (orbital, nasal and paranasal sinus, palatal, pharyngeal, laryngeal, and brain involvement; Fig. 17–66); thoracic (pulmonary involvement); abdominopelvic (gastrointestinal involvement); and dermal (subcutaneous nodule). The commonest clinical expression of visceral involvement is the craniofacial type which is usually characterized by infection of an orbital and nasal cavity in a patient with uncontrolled diabetes who later dies from meningoencephalitis. The hyphae of the invading organism have a predilection to grow in and along blood

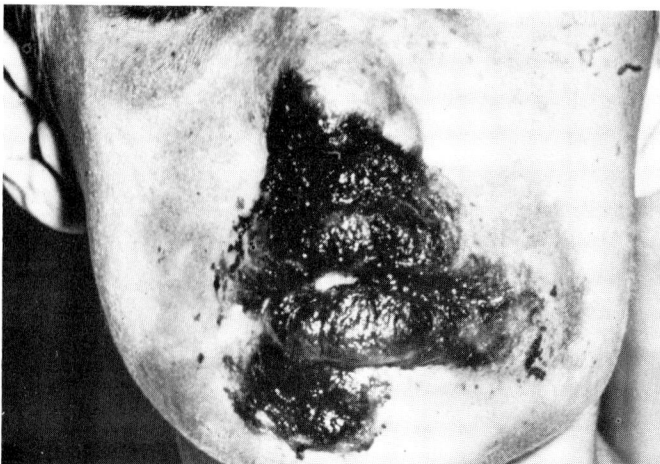

Figure 17–66 A 14-year-old boy with monocytic leukemia had necrotizing granulomatous disease of the midline of the face; hyphae were seen in thrombosed vessels, and the fungus Mucor was grown on culture (mucormycosis).

vessels; this permits hematogenous dissemination and frequently results in vascular occlusion and ischemic necrosis.

LEG ULCERS

Although the stasis ulcer is the commonest chronic ulceration of the leg, the other chronic leg ulcers can be difficult to diagnose unless one can appreciate the nature of the lesion or its underlying cause. History, physical examination, laboratory studies, cultures, and skin biopsy are diagnostically helpful. The causes of leg ulcers

(Table 17–5) are traumatic, vascular, infectious, hematologic, metabolic neurologic, drug induced, and neoplastic and include a miscellaneous group of conditions.

Certain diagnostic clues may be obtained from the history, appearance, and location of the ulcer. History can reveal the racial (sickle cell disease) or familial (spherocytosis) background; a description of the initial appearance of the ulcer helps to appreciate the distortion by infection or medication; knowledge of the precipitating event (for example, trauma, bites, cold exposure) aids in making the diagnosis; and the ulcer with the slower onset

TABLE 17–5 CAUSES OF LEG ULCERS

Traumatic: Mechanical, physical, chemical, irradiative

Vascular
Small vessels
Vasculitis: Allergic and necrotizing angiitis, those associated with connective tissue diseases, malignant atrophic papulosis
Embolism: Infections (subacute bacterial endocarditis), tumor
Livedo reticularis
Chronic pernio
Hypertensive ischemic leg ulcer
Atrophie blanche
Raynaud's disease
Large vessels
Thromboangiitis obliterans
Arteriosclerosis obliterans
Chronic venous insufficiency (stasis ulcer)
Periarteritis nodosa with or without granuloma
Arteriovenous fistula

Infections
Bacteria: Ecthyma, *Pseudomonas aeruginosa*, diphtheria, anthrax, tularemia, tuberculosis, atypical mycobacteria, leprosy, tropical ulcer
Treponemal infections (syphilis, yaws)
Mycoses: Chromoblastomycosis, blastomycosis, coccidioidomycosis, histoplasmosis, sporotrichosis, nocardiosis, actinomycosis, Madura foot
Protozoa: Leishmaniasis (cutaneous, mucocutaneous, kala-azar)
Animal and marine life: Bites or venoms

Hematologic diseases or states
Hemoglobinopathies: Sickle cell anemia (30 to 50 per cent), hereditary spherocytosis, thalassemia (major and minor)
Dysglobulinemias (hypogammaglobulinemia, cryoglobulinemia, and macroglobulinemia)
Thrombocythemia, polycythemia vera
Felty's syndrome
Coagulation disorders
Microthrombotic angiopathy

Metabolic states
Diabetes mellitus: Necrobiosis lipoidica diabeticorum, diabetic dermopathy, peripheral neuropathy
Porphyria cutanea tarda
Carcinosis cutis
Tophaceous gout
Gaucher's disease

Neurologic diseases
Tabes dorsalis
Syringomyelia
Spina bifida
Hereditary sensory radicular neuropathy
Primary amyloidosis (especially familial)
Congenital indifference to pain

Drug induced
Ergotism
Halogenoderma
Barbiturate intoxication
Methotrexate

Neoplasms
Epithelioma: Melanoma, squamous cell carcinoma, basal cell cancer, and complications of Marjolin's ulcer
Cutaneous lymphoma (mycosis fungoides, lymphosarcoma)
Kaposi's sarcoma
Metastatic carcinoma
Lymphangioendothelioma and lymphangiosarcoma

Miscellaneous
Lichen planus
Pyoderma gangrenosum
Panniculitides (primary and secondary)
Epidermolysis bullosa
Werner's syndrome
Acrodermatitis chronica atrophicans

and greater pain, relieved somewhat by dependency, points to an ischemic cause. On physical examination, the location and the appearance of the ulcer and the condition of the surrounding skin may give further diagnostic clues. The stasis ulcer has a predilection for the skin about the internal malleolus because this is the area drained by the saphenous systems and the communicating veins in the lower leg. When the ulcer appears pale with purpura or has a hemorrhagic eschar, the arterial blood supply is impaired; if the ulceration contains red or pink granulation tissue, such as seen in stasis ulcers, the arterial blood supply is good. In stasis ulcer disease, the surrounding skin is pigmented and edematous; in scleroderma and Werner's disease, it is sclerotic; and in acrodermatitis chronica atrophicans, it is atrophic.

Laboratory studies, such as hemoglobin determination and analyses, demonstration of sickling, osmotic fragility of red blood cells, white blood cell count, coagulograms, serum protein electrophoresis, cryoglobulins, blood sugar, serologic tests for syphilis, ANFT, LE tests, bacteriologic and mycologic studies, and skin biopsies which may show the presence of vasculitis, infectious agents, metabolic conditions (necrobiosis lipoidica, calcinosis cutis, tophaceous gout), panniculitis, and lichen planus are diagnostically helpful or conclusive.

CUTANEOUS MANIFESTATIONS OF HEMATOLOGIC DISORDERS

Associated with Anemias (Burns et al., 1970; Tables 17–6 and 17–7)

The cutaneous manifestations of hematologic disorders are those associated with anemias of the microcytic hypochromic type resulting from chronic blood loss or iron deficiency, of the macrocytic type resulting from low production of red blood cells, and of the normocytic type resulting from acute blood loss or increased destruction.

IRON DEFICIENCY SYNDROME. Among the cutaneous manifestations is pallor of the skin, mucous membranes, nail beds,

TABLE 17–6 COMPARISON OF CHANGES IN COAGULATION FACTORS*

Activity	Consumption Coagulopathy	Fibrinolytic State
Platelets	Decreased	Normal
Fibrinogen	Decreased	Decreased
Prothrombin	Decreased	Normal
Factor V	Decreased	Decreased
Factor VIII	Decreased	Decreased
Fibrinolysis	Variable	Increased
Antithrombin	Decreased initially	? Normal
Cryofibrin	Present	Absent

*Modified from Rodriguez-Erdmann, F.: N. Engl. J. Med. *273*:1376, 1965.

and conjunctivae. The skin may have a green or brown tint; vitiligo occurs. The tongue may be sore with mild papillary atrophy. The nails can be dull, brittle, flattened or concave, and longitudinally ridged; onycholysis occurs.

The Plummer-Vinson syndrome, which predominates in women, is characterized by hypochromic anemia, dysphagia, esophageal stricture or web in the postcricoid region, spoon nails, and inflammation of the tongue, mouth, and lips with atrophy. Cancer of the upper gastrointestinal tract may develop.

PERNICIOUS ANEMIA. The classic clinical presentation is the triad of anemia, sore tongue, and numbness and tingling of the extremities; the disease is usually seen more often in men over 40 years of age. There may be a lemon tint to the skin and sclerae. Isolated or diffuse areas of pigmentation, as well as vitiligo (10 per cent of cases), and Sutton's (halo) nevus are seen (Grunnet et al., 1970). The classic description of blue eyes, blond hair, premature graying, and facies (wide set eyes in a short broad face) is infrequently seen. The tongue may be episodically beefy red with shallow ulcerations, the mucous membranes are pallid, and the lips may be inflamed. Hyperthyroidism and diabetes mellitus are relatively frequent accompaniments. The laboratory findings include macrocytic anemia, histamine-fast achlorhydria, megaloblastic marrow, decreased levels of serum vitamin B_{12}, and reduced excretion of orally administered radioactive vitamin B_{12} (Schilling test).

HEREDITARY APLASTIC ANEMIA (FRANCONI'S ANEMIA). This anemia is an autosomal recessively inherited syndrome characterized by retarded growth, patchy brown pigmented skin, congenital malformations (microcephaly, microphthalmia, splenic atrophy, renal anomalies, and hypogenitalism), pancytopenia, and chromosomal breaks in fibroblast and lymphocyte cultures. Individuals with Franconi's syndrome often die from acute leukemia, or squamous cell carcinoma may develop. Patients with the rare syndrome of dyskeratosis congenita may have a similar aplastic anemia.

Increased Numbers of Red Blood Cells (Polycythemia)

Polycythemia vera is seen usually in middle-aged men who experience headache, dizziness, vertigo, visual disturbances, weakness, lassitude, dyspnea, and epigastric distress and have the classic ruddy cyanosis. The associated cutaneous changes are attributed to (1) increased blood viscosity and vascular distention with resultant rubor of skin and mucous membranes, rosacea, spider nevi, hemangiomas, hemorrhages, ecchymosis, acne urticata, erythroderma, erythromelalgia, and pruritus, (2) changes of blood vessels with the development of varicosities, thrombophlebitis, ulcerative nodules, Raynaud's syndrome, and scleroderma-like lesions, and (3) impaired temperature control resulting from capillary dilatation and causing intolerance to cold and itching and burning sensations (the post-bathing pruritus syndrome).

Acne urticata polycythemia (Baxter and Lockwood, 1958) is a chronic severely pruritic eruption characterized by pale red wheal-like papules which are sometimes surmounted by vesicles, appear in crops, and favor the face and extensor aspects of the extremities. Scars and hyperpigmentation result from excoriations. Heat, especially from hot baths, aggravates the condition. The increased histamine levels seen in the blood, mainly the white blood cells, and urine have correlated with the pruritus, urticaria, and upper gastrointestinal distress which may be controlled by cyproheptadine.

Secondary polycythemia (erythrocytosis), which develops from lowered oxygen tension, impaired pulmonary ventilation, defective cardiovascular structure, hemoglobinopathy, and humoral substances (renal, hepatic, or cerebral in origin, producing erythropoiesis) gives rise to signs and symptoms of the primary type as well as clubbing of the terminal digits.

Genetic Red Cell Diseases (Hemoglobinopathies)

Signs result from vascular occlusion by aggregates of defective red cells.

SICKLE CELL ANEMIA. The sickling phenomenon occurs more easily in the presence of a higher percentage of hemoglobin S (Hb S) and is influenced by reduced pH and stasis which exaggerate deoxygenation of hemoglobin. The sickled red blood cells become trapped in small vessels, leading to further stasis, deoxygenation, decreased pH, increased sickling, thrombosis, and infarction. The Negro patients tend to have an asthenic habitus (long extremities and short trunk) and may have bony deformities (dorsal kyphosis, lumbar lordosis, scoliosis, saber shins, and tower-shaped skull). The mucous membranes, nail beds, and palms are pale; the conjunctivae are icteric; and the lower legs are hyperpigmented. Three-quarters of the patients with sickle cell disease develop chronic leg ulcers (Fig. 17–67) and only about 3 per cent with the trait develop leg ulcers. These punched-out ulcers tend to be unilateral, are generally proximal to the malleoli, and heal with thin atrophic scars. Attacks of joint, bone, and abdominal pain occur.

HEREDITARY SPHEROCYTOSIS. Hereditary spherocytosis, which results from an abnormal cell membrane and not a hemoglobin defect, is primarily a disease of northern Europeans, is inherited as an autosomal dominant disorder, and appears at any age. The disease is characterized by anemia, jaundice, splenomegaly, and spherocytes. The skeletal abnormalities noted are tower-shaped skull, brachydactyly, and polydactyly. Epicanthal folds, dental abnormalities, and palatal deformities are seen. Leg ulcers, which may be preceded by a dusky blueness and are similar to those of sickle cell anemia, are uncommon.

THALASSEMIA. Thalassemia is a complex hereditary hemolytic anemia with the

TABLE 17–7 DIFFERENTIATION OF SOME HEMORRHAGIC DISORDERS

Disorder	Deficient Factor	Clotting Time	Partial Thromboplastin Time	Thrombin Time
Hemophilia A (classic)	Antihemophilic (AHF), VIII	Normal to prolonged	Prolonged	Normal
Hemophilia B (Christmas disease)	Plasma Thromboplastin component IX, Christmas factor	Normal to prolonged	Prolonged	Normal
Hemophilia C (PIA deficiency)	Plasma thromboplastin antecedent (PTA), XI	Slightly prolonged	Slightly prolonged	Normal
Vascular hemophilia (von Willebrand's disease)	Antihemophilic globulin (AHG)	Variable	Usually moderately prolonged	Normal
Congenital hypothrombinemia	Prothrombin, II	Normal to prolonged	Prolonged	Normal
Factor V deficiency	Accelerator globulin (AcG), proaccelerin	Normal to prolonged	Prolonged	Normal
Factor VII deficiency	Serum prothrombin conversion accelerator (SPCA)	Normal	Normal	Normal
Stuart disease	Stuart or Power factor	Normal to prolonged	Prolonged	Normal
Factor XIII deficiency	Fibrinase, fibrin stabilizing factor	Normal (clot soluble in SM urea)	Normal	Normal
Congenital afibrinogenemia and hypofibrinogenemia	Fibrinogen deficiency	Prolonged or incoagulable	Prolonged or incoagulable	Prolonged or incoagulable
Glanzmann's disease	Abnormal structure of platelets impaired clot retraction	Normal	Normal	Normal
Thrombocytopenia	Platelets	Normal	Normal	Normal

(Table 17–7 continued on the opposite page)

basic genetic defect involving the rates of synthesis of the individual polypeptide chains with a secondary basic impairment of alpha or beta chain and protoporphyrin synthesis and an increase of Hb F and Hb A_2.

The homozygous form of beta-thalassemia (thalassemia major, Cooley's anemia) appears in infancy or childhood and presents with physical underdevelopment, prominent frontal bossae and cheek bones, epicanthal folds with "mongoloid facies," icterus, and hepatosplenomegaly, Cardiomegaly, cardiac decompensation, edema, serous effusions, and ecchymoses may be present.

Thalassemia trait (minor) is an expression of a heterozygous state affecting adolescents who may be asymptomatic completely or have a mild disorder of easy fatigability, splenomegaly, anemia, and icterus.

Thalassemia may occur with other hemoglobinopathies. Thalassemia Hb S disease (microdrepanocytosis) combines usually to a lesser degree the features of thalassemia and sickle cell anemia. Chronic leg ulcers and splenomegaly, as well as periodic painful crisis (bone, joint, back, and abdominal pain), are seen. The sickling phenomenon, hypochromic microcytosis, target cells, and stippling are present.

Immunologic Diseases of Erythrocytes

PAROXYSMAL (COLD) HEMOGLOBINURIA. Paroxysmal (cold) hemoglobinuria is the result of an autohemolysin and a 7S gamma globulin, which combines with erythrocytes at lower temperatures, fixes complement, and produces hemolysis upon warming. It may occur idiopathically, in syphilis, especially the congenital type,

TABLE 17-7 DIFFERENTIATION OF SOME HEMORRHAGIC DISORDERS—*Continued*

Prothrombin Time	Serum Prothrombic Activity	Bleeding Time	Treatment
Normal	Normal to prolonged	Normal	Fresh or fresh frozen plasma or AHF concentrate
Normal	Normal to prolonged	Normal	Whole blood; plasma up to seven days, fresh frozen plasma
Variable	Normal to prolonged	Variable	Fresh or frozen plasma
Prolonged	Normal to prolonged	Prolonged	Fresh or frozen or ANF concentrates
Prolonged	Normal	Normal	Whole blood; fresh plasma up to three weeks old
Prolonged	Normal	Normal	Whole blood; plasma up to seven weeks old
Prolonged	Normal	Normal	Whole blood; fresh plasma or frozen plasma
Prolonged	Prolonged	Normal	Whole blood or plasma up to seven days old; fresh frozen plasma
Normal	Normal	Normal	Whole blood or plasma (also facilitates healing of wounds)
Prolonged or incoagulable	Normal	Normal or may be prolonged	Fibrinogen concentrates
Normal	Normal	Prolonged	Unsatisfactory
Normal	Elevated	Long	Corticosteroids, splenectomy immunosuppressants, platelet transfusions

and in other infections, especially post-viral states. During the paroxysmal episodes of hemolysis, fever, chills, headache, vomiting, muscular aching and cramping, passage of dark urine, urticaria, asthma, unusual sensitivity to frostbite, and Raynaud's phenomenon are seen. On physical examination, icterus and hepatosplenomegaly are often present. The direct Coombs' test is positive during the acute phase only. Circulating hemolysins are demonstrable in the blood. The peripheral blood picture is that of hemolytic anemia. In the urine, red blood cells, oxyhemoglobin and methemoglobin, red blood cell "ghosts," and albumin are found. Immersion of hands or feet in cold water for 10 to 20 minutes may produce an attack (Rosenbach test).

COLD HEMAGGLUTININS SYNDROME. Cold hemagglutinins syndrome is caused by hemagglutinins which are 19S or alpha M globulins and agglutinate erythrocytes of all groups at temperatures of 0° to 5° C. A rare chronic primary type is seen in elderly persons and a secondary type is associated with infections (primary atypical pneumonia, infectious mononucleosis, trypanosomiasis), collagen diseases, malignant tumors (carcinoma, lymphoma, and myeloma), and cirrhosis of the liver. When a high enough titer of hemagglutinins is present, agglutination occurs in the cooler parts of the body. The resultant clinical manifestations depend on the intensity of the process and include acrocyanosis, Raynaud's syndrome, acral ulcerations and, rarely, gangrene.

PAROXYSMAL NOCTURNAL HEMOGLOBINURIA (PNH). Paroxysmal nocturnal hemoglobinuria is a rare nonfamilial disease which is characterized by chronic

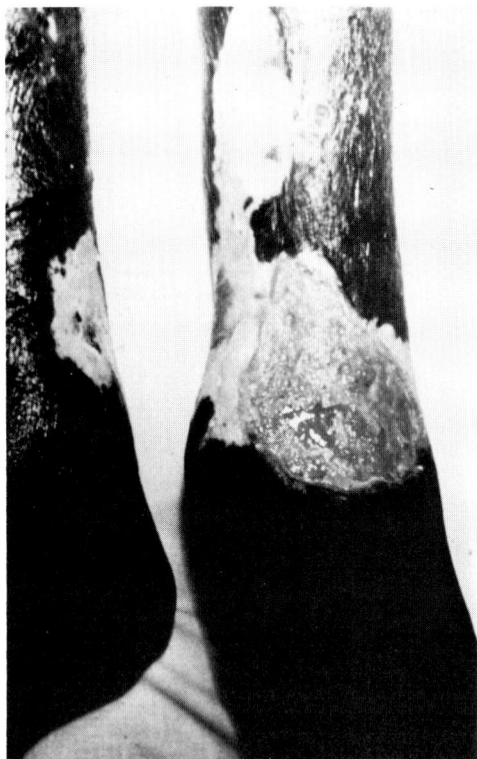

Figure 17–67   Patient with sickle cell anemia had chronic leg ulcers for five years.

hemolysis with hemoglobinemia, methemalbuminemia, and hemoglobinuria, and usually occurs at night. Both sexes are affected equally, and it appears most commonly during the third and fourth decades of life. The hemolysis, which is increased during sleep, is presumably the result of lowered blood pH and an intracorpuscular defect. The urine passed upon arising is usually brown. Exacerbations of the disease are associated with infections, injections of vaccines, operations, and transfusions. The skin can be pale, jaundiced, or may have a peculiar bronze coloration. Functional heart murmurs and hepatosplenomegaly may be present. Neutropenia and thrombocytopenia are commonly seen. The urinary urobilinogen is elevated, and free hemoglobin is demonstrated in urine on spectroscopic examination.

Among the diagnostic laboratory aids are the acid hemolysin test of Ham, the thrombin test of Crosby, and the heat resistant test of Hegglin.

AUTO-ERYTHROCYTE SENSITIZATION (Ratnoff and Agle, 1968). This syndrome, which is believed to be the result of sensitization to extravasated red blood cells, is characterized by painful recurring ecchymoses following minimal trauma in hysterical, masochistic women.

UNTOWARD REACTIONS TO TRANSFUSIONS. Febrile reactions are caused by hemolytic transfusion resulting from an incompatibility in the ABO system, sensitivity to leukocytes and platelets, and bacterial pyrogens. Allergic reactions characterized by generalized pruritus, urticaria, bronchospasm, and anaphylaxis are due to the transfer of reagins and, rarely, anti-IgA in IgA-deficient recipient. Air embolism is a rare complication, and fat embolism may complicate bone marrow transfusion under positive pressure. Large numbers of transfusions can cause hemosiderosis which resembles hemochromatosis. Among the diseases transmitted are syphilis, malaria, serum hepatitis, and brucellosis.

Chemical (Enzymatic) Disturbances of Erythrocytes

ERYTHROPOIETIC PORPHYRIA. Erythropoietic porphyria is a rare, inborn error of metabolism which is transmitted as an autosomal recessive trait and is characterized by photosensitivity. The clinical manifestations include erythrodontia, hypertrichosis, pruritus, and erythema with development of subepidermal vesicles and bullae which heal with residual pigmented mutilatory scarring. The urine has a classic pink to burgundy color.

ERYTHROPOIETIC PROTOPORPHYRIA. Erythropoietic protoporphyria is a dominantly inherited disorder especially of men, and clinically, upon exposure to sunlight, causes itching, burning, or tingling of exposed areas followed by erythema, urticarial edema, and often an eczematous eruption. Hyperpigmentation, purpura, lichenification, and scarring may be secondary sequelae.

ERYTHROPOIETIC COPROPORPHYRIA. Erythropoietic coproporphyria is a third type of congenital erythropoietic porphyria and occurs clinically as itching, burning, and swelling after exposure to sunlight.

LEAD POISONING. An increased

amount of lead in tissue can cause toxicity. Inorganic lead may be absorbed from the respiratory and gastrointestinal tract, and organic lead may be absorbed percutaneously. The poisoning may be acute or chronic from prolonged exposure. The clinical manifestations may be divided for descriptive purposes into three forms — alimentary, neuromuscular, and encephalopathic.

In the chronic disease, the skin is often damp and cool and has pallor in the absence of anemia. The nail bed may be cyanotic, and the gingival margins may reveal a stippled bluish black pigmentation ("lead line"). Stippling of the retina adjacent to the optic disc has been described as an early sign.

Laboratory studies reveal normochromic microcytic anemia, decreased red blood cell life span, and osmotic and increased mechanical fragility. Basophilic stippling of red blood cells is nonspecific but may be the initial clue. Increased erythrocytic protoporphyrin occurs without photosensitivity. Epithelial changes of the proximal and convoluted renal tubules produce amino-aciduria and renal glycosuria. The diagnosis is made by determination of the content of lead in the blood and urine. The prognosis is serious in the encephalopathic type, with a mortality rate of 25 per cent and a significant amount of residual morbidity. Symptomatic treatment and chelation with the calcium salt of ethylene diaminotetraacetic acid, by calcium disodium edetate USP (CaEDTA) or by penicillamine are the current therapeutic approaches.

CARBOXYHEMOGLOBINEMIA (Long, 1969). Carbon monoxide has 300 times more affinity for hemoglobin than oxygen. In carbon monoxide poisoning, the severity of the signs and symptoms is proportional to the concentration of carbon monoxide and is increased by the presence of anemia and exercise. Sixty per cent saturation of the blood produces unconsciousness and, in higher concentrations, death. The symptoms include headache, nausea, excessive sweating, blindness, deafness, convulsions, incontinence, collapse, and unconsciousness. Cherry red skin color with suffusion of mucous membranes is the commonest skin sign. Other cutaneous manifestations include small hemorrhages, edema, vesicles and bullae, alopecia, and leukonychia. Necrosis of sweat glands, a striking histopathologic feature, results from pressure. Temperature above 102° F., neurologic abnormalities, cardiac irregularities, skin lesions, and leukocytosis with lymphopenia signal a poor prognosis.

METHEMOGLOBINEMIA (Jaffé and Heller, 1964). Symptoms of poisoning appear when the level of methemoglobinemia reaches 20 to 50 per cent. In mild cases, cyanosis is the main sign. In severe cases, the syndrome of acute hypoxemia occurs and is characterized by weakness, fatigue, exertional dyspnea, headache, dizziness, blurring of mentality, tachycardia, and, in extreme cases, coma and death. If the venous blood retains its brownish hue after shaking with air for 15 minutes, suspicion is confirmed.

SULFHEMOGLOBINEMIA. When cyanosis occurs without evidence of cardiac or pulmonary dysfunction, methemoglobinemia or sulfhemoglobinemia should be suspected. Many of the compounds that produce methemoglobinemia cause sulfhemoglobinemia, the diseases frequently coexist, and the signs and symptoms are similar. Hand spectroscopy reveals the absorption band at 630 mm. for methemoglobin and that of sulfhemoglobin at 618 mm. There are no measures to convert sulfhemoglobin to hemoglobin.

Extracorpuscular Hemolyzing Infectious Agents

Malaria produces anemia by destruction of erythrocytes, and the degree of anemia correlates with the intensity of infection. Jaundice may develop.

BABESIASIS. Babesiasis is a rare protozoan infection which resembles malaria, is transmitted by ticks, and can cause jaundice.

BARTONELLOSIS. Bartonellosis (Van der Walle, 1957) is a noncontagious bacterial disease limited to western South America and is characterized by two distinctive clinical phases. The initial stage is a severe febrile state (Oroya fever) with a very high mortality rate in contrast to the secondary and benign stage with its characteristic generalized verruga peruana. The organism parasitizes the red blood cells, causing increased mechanical fragility and sequestration in the spleen, liver, and the reticuloendothelial system. (See also Chap. 11, section III.)

Conditions Associated with Leukocytosis or Leukopenia

LEUKOCYTOSIS (Acute Febrile Neutrophilic Dermatosis; Sweet's Syndrome – Goldman and Moschella, 1971). This syndrome is characterized by tender erythematous nodules and plaques with or without vesiculation which have a marked neutrophilic dermal infiltrate by polymorphonuclear leukocytosis and a dramatic response to intralesional or systemic corticosteroid therapy.

Eosinophilia is seen in pruritic states, urticaria, angioedema, erythema multiforme, exfoliative dermatitis, dermatitis herpetiformis, pemphigus, Löffler's syndrome, scarlet fever, scabies, trichinosis, cysticercosis, pernicious anemia, Hodgkin's disease, periarteritis nodosa, and sarcoidosis.

NEUTROPENIA. Periodic or cyclic neutropenia (Levy and Schetman, 1961) is a cyclic autosomal dominant disorder which usually begins at infancy but may occur at any age, persists for decades, and is characterized by regular symptomatic episodes of neutropenia. The cycle is 21 days, with extremes of 14 to 45 days, and lasts 5 to 10 days. The clinical manifestations include fever, malaise, severe aphthosis, gingivitis, and infections of the pharynx, rectum, and skin, especially of the intertriginous areas. Arthralgia, abdominal pain, lymphadenopathy, and splenomegaly have been described. The leukopenia is 2000 to 4000 leukocytes per cubic millimeter with often severe neutropenia. There may be a compensatory monocytosis and an eosinophilia in the recovery phase. Bone marrow studies have revealed a cyclic arrest of the entire neutrophilic series. As the child with this disorder grows older, the associated conditions become less severe; this suggests that adaptive immune mechanisms provide the protection normally assumed by the granulocytes. Splenectomy has little therapeutic value except occasionally in patients with splenomegaly. Corticosteroid therapy gives only symptomatic relief.

Felty's syndrome (Ruderman et al., 1968) is a clinical variant at the most severe end of the spectrum of rheumatoid arthritis and exhibits an unusual reticuloendothelial stimulation manifested by hypersplenism with neutropenia. Brownish pigmentation of the skin of the extremities, leg ulcers, pyoderma, gingivitis, stomatitis, oral ulcerations, Sjögren's syndrome, and rheumatoid nodules are seen.

SLE is a so-called acquired connective tissue disease with multisystem clinical manifestations and frequently with a mild to moderate leukopenia. The cutaneous manifestations seen in 70 to 80 per cent of cases are lesions specific for lupus erythematosus: for example, the erythematous malar and nasal (butterfly or batwing) flush or the characteristic discoid lesions; those seen in other connective disorders: for example, facial and periorbital edema, erythema of the face, palms, digits, and periungual area with linear telangiectasia, telangiectases of exposed areas and hands, and rheumatoid nodules; and those of the associated vasculitis, such as palpable purpura, hemorrhagic bullae, livedo reticularis, ulcerations of the legs, palms, and digits, digital gangrene, and Raynaud's phenomenon. Other cutaneous lesions include a maculopapular eruption simulating a drug eruption, variants of the discoid lesion of the hypertrophic or profound type or both, acute violaceous reactive papules or plaques, urticaria, generalized hyperpigmentation, photosensitivity, and Sjögren's syndrome. Mucosal ulcerations and scarring and patchy or diffuse alopecia with or without scarring are seen.

Deficiency of Neutrophil (Windhorst, 1970)

An intrinsic deficiency of neutrophil may be reflected by defective neutrophil mobilization, phagocytosis, bacterial activity, and chemotaxis and is seen in such diseases as fatal granulomatous disease of childhood, "lazy-leukocyte" syndrome, and Chediak-Higashi syndrome.

FATAL (CHRONIC) GRANULOMATOUS DISEASE OF CHILDHOOD – FGD (Windhorst and Good, 1971). Fatal (chronic) granulomatous disease of childhood is a sex-linked disease affecting young boys. It is characterized by a defect in the intracellular killing processes of phagocytic cells with severe, recurrent, and chronic granulomatous reactions to some common bacteria of low virulence. In the study of patients with increased susceptibility to invading microorganisms, one must consider not only abnormalities of phagocytosis by leukocytes, serum immunoglobulins, and lymphocyte function but also disorders of leukocyte function, such as disorders of degranulation, specific deficiencies of granule hydrolases, peroxidases, and bactericidal proteins.

Leukocytes from patients with FGD have a genetic defect of oxidase activity, fail to produce hydrogen peroxide, and do not kill certain bacteria. The biochemical defect appears to be somewhere in the electron transport system in which the TPN-TPNH of the shunt participates. Since the tetrazolium dyes are substances that are known to act as hydrogen ion acceptors for both DPNH and TPNH, the characteristic defect is demonstrable by the failure of leukocytes to reduce during phagocytosis nitro-blue tetrazolium dye (NBT test) from its colorless to its deep blue state. This leukocyte function test can detect the heterozygous female carriers of the trait. A number of clinically similar cases without any demonstrable in vitro defect of leukocyte function or metabolism as measured by tetrazolium dyes has been described in women, suggesting that the phenotype of chronic granulomatous disease may result from more than one genetic defect.

A chronic LE-like illness characterized by arthralgia, cutaneous lesions, and photosensitivity has been described in mothers of boys with chronic granulomatous disease (Schaller, 1972). The organs involved are skin (pyodermas, purulent granulomas), lymph nodes (scrofula-like), liver (diffuse granuloma, liver abscess), spleen (diffuse granuloma), lung (acute and chronic interstitial infiltrative granulomatous process with occasional abscesses), and bone marrow (granulomatous osteomyelitis); rarely, gastrointestinal and pericardial involvement occurs. The cutaneous lesions are the early manifestations of this syndrome. Among the skin lesions are an infectious eczematoid dermatitis, particularly about the orifices of the head, seborrheic folliculitis, miliaria pustulosa, paronychia, impetigonization, ecthyma, scrofulous lesions of cervical and inguinal lymph nodes, and, more infre-

quently, cutaneous granulomas suggesting the apple jelly nodules of lupus vulgaris, sarcoidosis, and progressive purulent granuloma and erythema induratum–like lesions on the legs. The sites of injections in the buttocks remain nodular for months and may drain for weeks; similarly, the fluctuant draining lymph nodes may take months to heal.

The histopathologic picture for this syndrome consists of varying degrees of histiocytic infiltration, foreign body giant cells, and extensive accumulation of neutrophils with necrosis. The common streptococcal and pneumococcal pathogens are effectively handled. The more commonly associated infections are those from staphylococcus, Klebsiella, Aerobacter, Salmonella, and Serratia species. The skin lesions may heal completely. Hyperglobulinemia is present. Most deaths are the result of an acute pulmonary insult superimposed upon a chronic process. Prompt recognition of the infectious organism and immediate initiation of appropriate and vigorous antibiotic therapy will improve the prognosis.

"LAZY-LEUKOCYTE" SYNDROME (Miller et al., 1971). "Lazy-leukocyte" syndrome is seen in children who have a primary or presently undefinable defect of neutrophilic function involving random mobility and chemotaxis and severe peripheral neutropenia. There is normal humoral and cellular immunity. The clinical picture is characterized by low-grade fever, gingivitis, recurrent stomatitis, and otitis. The infections and fever seem to result from the host's inability to release and mobilize neutrophils which have normal phagocytic and bactericidal activities; thus, the "lazy leukocytes" appear to have a primary cellular defect of chemotaxis.

CHEDIAK-HIGASHI SYNDROME (Windhorst et al., 1968). Chediak-Higashi syndrome is a rare autosomal recessive disorder which is characterized by oculocutaneous albinism with a lethal defect of leukocytes. The homozygous state is lethal. The syndrome is recognized by the appearance of giant granules in the cytoplasm of white cells from bone marrow and peripheral blood. These granules have been described in melanocytes, causing a color dilution, and in other cells. Ultrastructural cytochemical techniques have demonstrated the lysosomal nature of these granules (White, 1966). The hair, which may be sparse, is blond or gray. The presenting symptom may be ocular or cutaneous intolerance to sunlight. The multiple defects in host defenses with this syndrome which have a marked susceptibility to pyogenic infections are neutropenia, defective leukocyte migration, cellular defect in chemotaxis, failure in post-phagocytic degranulation, and diminished intracellular bactericidal degranulation which may be related to the ineffective delivery of lysosomal contents to the phagocytic vacuole (Wolff et al., 1972). This syndrome is also frequently associated with malignant lymphoma.

Cutaneous Conditions Associated with Lymphocytosis

Among the cutaneous conditions associated with lymphocytosis of the peripheral blood are acute infectious lymphocytosis associated with a morbilliform and maculopapular eruption, infectious mononucleosis associated with nonspecific eruptions in approximately 3 per cent of cases, German measles, secondary syphilis, and brucellosis with nonspecific eruptions in 8 per cent of cases.

Infectious mononucleosis (McCarthy and Hoagland, 1964) is probably caused by a virus of a herpes type (Epstein-Barr) or one related to it and may have edema of the eyelids, palatal enanthema (5 to 20 pinhead-sized red spots at the junction of the soft and hard palates), rubelliform or scarletiniform exanthem, urticaria, petechiae, purpura, ecchymoses, jaundice, and a biologic false positive test for syphilis.

Cases of Australian antigen (HAA)–positive hepatitis can have a lymphocytosis and may present prodromally urticaria, arthritis, skin nodules, and occasionally maculopapular eruptions. Immune complexes involving HAA have been described as responsible for the extrahepatic manifestations (Alpert et al., 1971).

Diseases with Cutaneous Lesions and Monocytosis

Monocytosis is present in subacute bacterial endocarditis, brucellosis, typhoid fever, Rocky Mountain spotted fever, typhus, kala-azar, Gaucher's disease, and monocytic leukemia.

REFERENCES

Ackyrod, J. F.: Allergic purpura, including purpura due to foods, drugs, and infections. Am. J. Med. *14*:605, 1953.

Alarcón-Segovia, D., and Brown, A. L., Jr.: Classification and etiologic aspects of necrotizing angiitides: An analytic approach to a confused subject with a critical review of the evidence for hypersensitivity in polyarteritis nodosa. Mayo Clin. Proc. *39*:205, 1964.

Allen, D. M., Diamond, L. K., and Howell, D. A.: Anaphylactoid purpura in children (Schoenlein-Henoch syndrome): Review with a follow-up of the renal complications. Am. J. Dis. Child. *99*:833, 1960.

Allen, E. V., Barker, N. W., and Hines, E. A., Jr., et al.: Peripheral Vascular Diseases. Philadelphia, W. B. Saunders Company, 1962, pp. 125–171.

Alper, C. A., Rosen, F. S., and Janeway, C. A.: The gamma globulins. II. Hypergammaglobulinemia. N. Engl. J. Med. *275*:591, 652, 1966.

Alpert, E., Isselbacher, K. J., and Schur, P. H.: The pathogenesis of arthritis associated with viral hepatitis. N. Engl. J. Med. *285*:185, 1970.

Amorosi, E. L., and Ultmann, J. E.: Thrombotic thrombocytopenic purpura: Report of 16 cases and review of the literature. Medicine *45*:139, 1966.

Babb, R. R., Alarcón-Segovia, D., and Fairbairn, J. F., 2nd: Erythermalgia. Review of 51 cases. Circulation *29*:136, 1964.

Barnett, E. V., Bluestone, R., Cracchiolo, A., 3rd, et al.: Cryoglobulinemia and disease. Ann. Intern. Med. *73*:95, 1970.

Baughman, R. D., and Sommer, R. G.: Cryoglobulinemia presenting as "factitial ulceration." Arch. Dermatol. *94*:725, 1966.

Baxter, D. L., and Lockwood, J. H.: Acne urticata polycythemica; report of a case. Arch. Dermatol. *78*:325, 1958.

Beathard, G. A., and Guckian, J. C.: Necrotizing fasciitis due to group A beta-hemolytic streptococci. Arch. Intern. Med. *120*:63, 1967.

Beeson, P. B., and McDermott, W. (eds.): Cecil-Loeb Textbook of Medicine. Philadelphia, W. B. Saunders Company, 1967.

Belisario, J. C.: Cutaneous manifestations in polyarteritis nodosa. Report of a case with livedo reticularis. Arch. Dermatol. *82*:526, 1960.

Bowie, E. J., and Owen, C. A., Jr.: Purpura: Diagnostic possibilities. Postgrad. Med. *43*:104, 1968.

Braverman, I. M.: Skin Signs of Systemic Disease. Philadelphia, W. B. Saunders Company, 1970, pp. 199–238.

Burns, R. E., Abraham, J. P., and Chapel, T. A.: Visible evidence of red cell disease. An exhibit from the Departments of Dermatology and Hematology, Henry Ford Hospital, Detroit, Michigan, 1970.

Capra, J. D., Winchester, R. J., and Kunkel, H. G.: Hypergammaglobulinemic purpura. Medicine *50*:125, 1971.

Carron, D. B., and Douglas, A. P.: Steatorrhoea in vascular insufficiency of the small intestine. Five cases of polyarteritis nodosa and allied disorders. Quart. J. Med. *34*:331, 1965.

Carton, R. W., and Wong, R.: Multifocal fibrosclerosis manifested by vena caval obstructions and associated with vasculitis. Ann. Intern. Med. *70*:81, 1969.

Carvajal, J. A., Anderson, W. R., Weiss, L., et al.:

Atheroembolism. An etiologic factor in renal insufficiency, gastrointestinal hemorrhages, and peripheral vascular diseases. Arch. Intern. Med. *119*:593, 1967.

Champion, R. H.: Livedo reticularis. A review. Br. J. Dermatol. 77:167, 1965.

Chandler, D., and Nalbandian, R. M.: DNA autosensitivity. Am. J. Med. Sci. *251*:145, 1966.

Cobbet, J. R., and Wallace, A. F.: Skin loss in the anterior tibial syndrome. Br. J. Plast. Surg. *18*:359, 1965.

Copeman, P. W. M., and Ryan, T. J.: The problems of classification of cutaneous angiitis with reference to histopathology and pathogenesis. Br. J. Dermatol. *82* (Suppl. No. 5):2, 1970.

Cream, J. J., Gumpel, J. M., and Peachey, R. D.: Schönlein-Henoch purpura in the adult. A study of 77 adults with anaphylactoid or Schönlein-Henoch purpura. Quart. J. Med. *39*:461, 1970.

Danese, C. A., Grishman, E., and Dreiling, D. A.: Malignant vascular tumors of the lymphedematous extremity. Ann. Surg. *166*:245, 1967.

Degos, R., Duperrat, B., and Daniel, F.: Le parapsoriasis ulcér-nécrotique hyperthermique. Forme suraiguë due parapsoriasis en gouttes. Ann. Derm. Syph. *93*:481, 1966.

De Takats, D. G.: Sympathetic reflex dystrophy. Med. Clin. North Am. *49*:117, 1965.

Deykin, D.: The clinical challenge of disseminated intravascular coagulation. N. Engl. J. Med. *283*: 636, 1970.

Doucas, C., and Kapetanakis, J.: Eczematid-like purpura. Dermatologica *106*:86, 1953.

Duemling, W. W.: Dermatitis nodularis necrotica: Report of a case and review of the literature. Arch. Dermatol. *21*:229, 1930.

Effler, D. B., and Groves, L. K.: Superior vena caval obstruction. J. Thorac. Cardiovasc. Surg. *43*:574, 1962.

Ellis, F. A.: The cutaneous manifestation of cryoglobulinemia. Arch. Dermatol. *89*:690, 1964.

Fisher, I., and Orkin, M.: Cutaneous form of periarteritis nodosa—an entity? Arch. Dermatol. *89*: 180, 1964.

Frohnert, P. P., and Sheps, S. G.: Long-term follow-up study of periarteritis nodosa. Am. J. Med. *43*:8, 1967.

Gairdner, D.: The Schönlein-Henoch syndrome (anaphylactoid purpura). Quart. J. Med. *17*:95, 1948.

Gardner, F. H., and Diamond, L K.: Autoerythrocyte sensitization; form of purpura producing painful bruising following autosensitization to red blood cells in certain women. Blood *10*:675, 1955.

Goldman, G. C., and Moschella, S. L.: Acute febrile neutrophilic dermatosis (Sweet's syndrome). Arch. Dermatol. *103*:654, 1971.

Gomes, M. M., and Bernatz, P. E.: Arteriovenous fistulas: A review and ten-year experience at the Mayo Clinic. Mayo Clin. Proc. *45*:81, 1970.

Gougerot, H., and Blum, P.: Un noveau cas de trisymptôme ou plutôt pentasymptôme. Bull. Soc. Franc. Derm. Syph. *57*:336, 1950.

Gougerot, H., and Duperrat, B.: Nodular dermal allergides of Gougerot. Br. J. Dermatol. *66*:283, 1954.

Graham, J. R.: Methysergide for prevention of headache; experience in five hundred patients over three years. N. Engl. J. Med. *270*:67, 1964.

Gray, H. R., Graham, J. H., Johnson, W., et al.: Atrophie blanche: periodic painful ulcers of lower extremities. A clinical and histopathological entity. Arch. Dermatol. *93*:187, 1966.

Greenwood, K.: Dermatitis with capillary fragility. Arch. Dermatol. *81*:947, 1960.

Groch, G. S., Finch, S. C., Rogoway, W., et al.: Studies in the pathogenesis of autoerythrocyte sensitization syndrome. Blood *28*:19, 1966.

Grossman, J., Abraham, G. N., Leddy, J. P., et al.: Crystalglobulinemia. Ann. Intern. Med. *77*:395, 1972.

Grunnet, I., Howitz, J., Reymann, F., et al.: Vitiligo and pernicious anemia. Arch. Dermatol. *101*:82, 1970.

Hager, D. L., and Wilson, J. N.: Gangrene of hand following intra-arterial injection. Arch. Surg. *94*:86, 1967.

Harrington, W. J.: The purpuras. DM 1, July, 1957.

Harrington, W. J.: Hemorrhagic disorders. *In* Beeson, B. P., and McDermott, W., (eds.): Cecil-Loeb Textbook of Medicine. Philadelphia, W. B. Saunders Company, 1967, pp. 1121–1138.

Jaffé, E. R., and Heller, P.: Methemoglobinemia in man. *In* Moore, C. V., and Brown, E. B., (eds.): Progress in Hematology. Vol. 4. New York, Grune and Stratton, Inc., 1964, pp. 48–71.

Johnson, W. C., Wallrich, R., and Helwig, E. B.: Superficial thrombophlebitis of the chest wall. J.A.M.A. *180*:103, 1962.

Kalbfleisch, J. M., and Bird, R. M.: Cryofibrinogenemia. N. Engl. J. Med. *263*:881, 1960.

Kappeler, R., Krebs, A., and Riva, G.: Klinik der Makro-globulinämie Waldström; Beschreibung von 21 Fällen und Übersicht der Literatur. Heln. Med. Acta *25*:54, 101, 1958.

Kinmouth, J. B., Rob, C. G., and Simeone, F. A.: Vascular Surgery. London, Edward Arnold (Publishers) Ltd., 1962.

Kyle, R. A., Gleich, G. J., Bayrd, E. D., et al.: Benign hypergammaglobulinemic purpura of Waldenström. Medicine *50*:113, 1971.

Landau, J. W., and Newcomer, V. D.: Acute cerebral phycomycosis (mucormycosis). Report of a pediatric patient successfully treated with amphotericin B and cycloheximide and review of the pertinent literature. J. Pediatr. *61*:363, 1962.

Levin, M. B., and Pinkus, H.: Autosensitivity to desoxyribonucleic acid (DNA). Report of a case with inflammatory skin lesions controlled by chloroquine. N. Engl. J. Med. *264*:533, 1961.

Levy, E. J., and Schetman, D.: Cyclic neutropenia. Arch. Dermatol. *84*:429, 1961.

Long, P. I.: Carbon monoxide poisoning. Arch. Dermatol. *100*:385, 1969.

Lowenthal, L. J. A.: Itching purpura. Br. J. Dermatol. *66*:95, 1954.

Macaulay, W. L.: Lymphomatoid papulosis. A continuing self-healing eruption, clinically benign—histologically malignant. Arch. Dermatol. *97*:23, 1968.

Mali, J. W., Kuiper, J. P., and Hamers, A. A.: Acroangiodermatitis of the foot. Arch. Dermatol. *92*:515, 1965.

Mathison, D. A., Condemi, J. J., Leddy, J. P., et al.: Purpura, arthralgia, and IgM-IgM cryoglobulinemia with rheumatoid factor activity. Response to cyclophosphamide and splenectomy. Ann. Intern. Med. *74*:383, 1971.

McCallister, B. D., Bayrd, E. D., Harrison, E. G., Jr., et al.: Primary macroglobulinemia. Am. J. Med. *43*:394, 1967.

McCarthy, J. T., and Hoagland, R. J.: Cutaneous manifestations of infectious mononucleosis. J.A.M.A. *187*:153, 1964.

McCombs, R. P.: Systemic "allergic" vasculitis. Clinical and pathological relationships. J.A.M.A. *194*:1059, 1965.

McGrae, J. D., Jr., and Winkelmann, R. K.: Generalized essential telangiectasia: Report of a clinical and histochemical study of 13 patients with acquired cutaneous lesions. J.A.M.A. *185*:909, 1963.

McKusick, V. A., Harris, W. S., Ottesen, O. E., et al.: Buerger's disease: A distinct clinical and pathologic entity. J.A.M.A. *181*:5, 1962.

Meltzer, M., and Franklin, E. C.: Cryoglobulins, rheumatoid factors and connective tissue disorders. Arthritis Rheum. *10*:489, 1967.

Miller, M. E., Oski, F. A., and Harris, M. B.: Lazy-leukocyte syndrome. A new disorder of neutrophil function. Lancet *1*:665, 1971.

Moschella, S. L.: The clinical significance of necrosis of the skin. Med. Clin. North. Am. 53:259, 1969.

Nelson, L. M.: Atrophie blanche en plaque. Arch. Dermatol. 72:242, 1955.

Orbison, J. L.: Morphology of thrombotic thrombocytopenic purpura with demonstration of aneurysms. Am. J. Pathol. 28:129, 1952.

Pechet, L.: Fibrinolysis. N. Engl. J. Med. *273*:966, 1024, 1965.

Phelps, M. D., Jr., and Geokas, M. C.: Circulatory problems in dysproteinemia. Med. Clin. North Am. *47*:353, 1963.

Randall, S. J., Kierland, R. R., and Montgomery, H.: Pigmented purpuric eruptions. Arch. Derm. Syph. 64:177, 1951.

Ratnoff, O. D.: An approach to the diagnosis of disorders of hemostasis. Mod. Treat. 5:11, 1968.

Ratnoff, O. D., and Angle, D. P.: Psychogenic purpura: A re-evaluation of the syndrome of autoerythrocyte sensitization. Medicine *47*:475, 1968.

Reed, W. B., Landing, B., Sugarman, G., et al.: Xeroderma pigmentosum. Clinical and laboratory investigation of its basic defect. J.A.M.A. *207*:2073, 1969.

Retan, J. W., and Miller, R. E.: Microembolic complications of atherosclerosis. Literature review and report of a patient. Arch. Intern. Med. *118*:534, 1966.

Ritzmann, S. E., and Levin, W. C.: Cryopathies: A review. Classification; diagnostic and therapeutic considerations. Arch. Intern. Med. *107*:754, 1961.

Roberts, H. R., and Brinkhous, K. M.: Blood coagulation and hemophilioid disorders. Postgrad. Med. *43*:114, 1968.

Rodriguez-Erdmann, F.: Bleeding due to intravascular blood coagulation. Hemorrhagic syndromes caused by consumption of blood-clotting factors (consumption-coagulopathies). N. Engl. J. Med. *273*:1370, 1965.

Rose, G. A., and Spencer, H.: Polyarteritis nodosa. Quart. J. Med. 26:43, 1957.

Rosen, F. S.: The macroglobulins. N. Engl. J. Med. 267:491, 1962.

Rosenthal, D., and Burnham, T. K.: Nonthrombocytopenic purpura due to carbromal ingestion. Arch. Dermatol. 89:200, 1964.

Rossi, E. C. (ed.): Hemorrhagic disorders. Med. Clin. North Am. 56:9, 25, 1972.

Ruderman, M., Miller, L. M., and Pinals, R. S.: Clinical and serologic observations on 27 patients with Felty's syndrome. Arthritis Rheum. *11*:377, 1968.

Ruiter, M.: Some further observations on allergic cutaneous arteriolitis. Br. J. Dermatol. 66:174, 1954.

Schaller, J.: Illness resembling lupus erythematosus in mothers of boys with chronic granulomatous disease. Ann. Intern. Med. 76:747, 1972.

Schnier, B. R., Sheps, S. G., and Juergens, J. L.: Hypertensive ischemic ulcer. A review of 40 cases. Am. J. Cardiol. 17:560, 1966.

Shelley, W. B.: Essential progressive telangiectasia. Successful treatment with tetracycline. J.A.M.A. *216*:1343, 1971.

Siegel, N. H., and Brodsky, I.: The diagnosis and treatment of disseminated intravascular coagulation. Med. Clin. North Am. *54*:555, 1970.

Stallworth, J. M., Bradhaum, G. B., Kletke, R. R., et al.: Phlegmasia cerulea dolens. A 10-year review. Ann. Surg. *161*:802, 1965.

Stringa, S. G., Bianchi, C., and Zingale, S. B.: Nodular vasculitis: Immunofluorescent study; 7S gamma-globulin and complement (beta-1c-globulin) in lesions of nodular vasculitis. J. Invest. Dermatol. *46*:1, 1966.

Strole, W. E., Jr., Clark, W. H., Jr., and Isselbacher, K. J.: Progressive arterial occlusive disease (Köhlmeier-Degos). A frequently fatal cutaneosystemic disorder. N. Engl. J. Med. 276:195, 1967.

Sweet, R. D.: Further observations on acute febrile neutrophilic dermatosis. Br. J. Dermatol. 80:800, 1968.

Thomas, J. F.: Fournier's gangrene of penis and scrotum. J. Urol. 75:719, 1956.

Tocantins, L. M., and Kazal, L. A., (eds.): Blood Coagulation, Hemorrhage and Thrombosis, Methods of Study. New York, Grune and Stratton, Inc., 1964.

Van der Walle, N.: Verruga peruana. Doc. Med. Geographica Tropica 9:149, 1957.

Verallo, V. M., and Haserick, J. R.: Mucha-Habermann's disease simulating lymphoma cutis: Report of two cases. Arch. Dermatol. 94:295, 1966.

Vilanova, X., and Piñol Aguadé, J.: Subacute nodular migratory panniculitis. Br. J. Dermatol. 71:45, 1959.

White, J. G.: The Chediak-Higashi syndrome: A possible lysosomal disease. Blood 28:143, 1966.

Wilkinson, D. S.: Vascular basis of some nodular eruptions of legs. Br. J. Dermatol. 66:201, 1954.

Windhorst, D. B.: Functional defects of neutrophils. *In* Stollerman, E., (ed.): Advances in Internal Medicine. Chicago, Year Book Medical Publishers, Inc., 1970, pp. 329–349.

Windhorst, D. B., and Good, R. A.: Dermatologic manifestations of fatal granulomatous disease of childhood. Arch. Dermatol. *103*:351, 1971.

Windhorst, D. B., Zelickson, A. S., and Good, R. A.: A human pigmentary dilution based on a heritable subcellular structural defect—the Chediak-Higashi syndrome. J. Invest. Dermatol. *50*:9, 1968.

Winkelmann, R. K., and Ditto, W. B.: Cutaneous and visceral syndromes of necrotizing or "allergic" angiitis: A study of 38 cases. Medicine *43*:59, 1964.

Wintrobe, M. M.: Clinical Hematology. 6th ed. Philadelphia, Lea and Febiger, 1967.

Wolff, S., Dale, D. C., Clark, R. A., et al.: The Chediak-Higashi syndrome: studies of host defenses. Ann. Intern. Med. 76:293, 1972.

Young, J. R., Humphries, A. W., DeWolfe, V. G., et al.: Peripheral arterial embolism. J.A.M.A. *185*:621, 1963.

Zeek, P. M.: Medical progress: Periarteritis nodosa and other forms of necrotizing angiitis. N. Engl. J. Med. 248:764, 1953.

INDEX

Note: In this index, page numbers in *italics* indicate illustrations; those followed by (t) indicate tables. The abbreviation vs. denotes differential diagnosis.

Dermatitis (*Continued*)
 poison oak, treatment of, 257
 primary irritant, crusting in, *184*
  in infant, 120, 313(t)
 procaine, *247*
 quinacrine hydrochloride, 375
 radiation, acute, 1450
  chronic, 1451, *1452, 1453*
 schistosomal, 1508, *1510*
 seborrheic. See *Seborrheic dermatitis.*
 sensitization, in lichen simplex chronicus, 294
 shoe, 252, *252*
 signs of, 279
 stasis. See *Stasis dermatitis.*
 stomal, 244
 suboccipital, 288, 293, *294*
 sweat retention in, 281
 treatment of, by radiation, 1683
 uncinarial, 1495
 water bath, 671
Dermatitis artefacta, 1556, *1559*
Dermatitis bullosa striata praetensis, 1108
Dermatitis cruris pustulosa et atrophicans, 1722
Dermatitis exfoliativa neonatorum, 397
Dermatitis gangrenosum, 526
Dermatitis herpetiformis, 474–476, *475, 476*
 distribution pattern in, 198, *198*
 histologic features of, 93
 juvenile, 476
 of hands and feet, 316
 urticaria in, 232
 vs. erythema multiforme, 389
 vs. herpes gestationis, 473
Dermatitis medicamentosa. See *Drug eruption(s).*
Dermatitis nodularis necrotica, 852, 855
Dermatitis papillaris capillitii, 1212, *1213*
 in blacks, 1720, *1720*
Dermatitis repens, 280, *523*
 of hands and feet, 315, 316(t)
 vs. pustular psoriasis, 418
Dermatitis vegetans, 518
 in anogenital region, 161
Dermato-arthritis, lipoid, 755
Dermatobia hominis, 1530
Dermatofibroma, *753,* 1368, *1369, 1370*
 histologic features of, 101, *102*
 pseudosarcomatous, 1374
Dermatofibrosarcoma protuberans, 1374, *1374*
Dermatofibrosis lenticularis disseminata, 1368
Dermatoglyphic pattern(s), 8, *8*
Dermatologic surgery, 1690–1703
 closure of wounds in, 1692
 excisions in, 1691–1695, *1693*
 punch biopsy in, 1691
Dermatologic therapy, 1608–1640
 intralesional, 1622–1623
 radionuclides in, 1688–1689
 systemic, 1623–1636
 topical, 1609–1622
Dermatologist, industrial, role of, *1457,* 1458
Dermatology, clinical vs. industrial, 1456
Dermatomyositis, 942–949
 classification of, 942
 clinical manifestations of, 944, *945–948*
 differential diagnosis of, 947

Dermatomyositis (*Continued*)
 edema in, 1294
 electromyography in, 948
 esophagus in, 941
 etiology of, 943
 Gottron papules in, 945, *946*
 histologic features of, 97
 in children, 123, 943
 incidence of, 945
 laboratory studies in, 947
 muscular involvement in, 945
 neoplasm in, 944
 pathology of, 944
 photosensitivity in, 341
 prognosis in, 948
 treatment of, 948
 vs. contact dermatitis, 241
 with internal malignancy, 1318
Dermatopathia pigmentosa reticularis, 1111
Dermatophytid(s), *142,* 660, *661*
 of hands, 649, *651,* 660
 types of, 661
Dermatophytosis. See *Tinea pedis.*
Dermatosis(es)
 acneiform, 1129–1145
  drug-induced, 1137
 acute febrile neutrophilic, 852, 856, *857,* 908
 ashy, of Ramirez, 387
 benign, radiation dosage for, 1677
 Bowen's precancerous. See *Bowen's disease.*
 bullae in, 91
 chronic, and squamous cell carcinoma, 1342
 chronic discoid and lichenoid, in aged, 131
 exudative, treatment of, 1611
 ichthyosiform. See *Ichthyosis(es).*
 idiopathic pigmented purpuric, 875
 in blacks, 1705
 industrial. See *Industrial dermatosis(es).*
 melanin and, in blacks, 1710
 subcorneal pustular, 477–479, *478, 479*
 transient acantholytic, 1075
 tropical, panoramic view of, 1540–1551, *1541–1550*
 vitamin A deficiency and, 1244
Dermatosis cinecienta, 387
 hyperpigmentation in, 1109
Dermatosis papulosa nigra, 128, *148,* 1326, *1327,*
 1718, 1719
Dermatostomatitis, 387
Dermis, 10–18
 adventitial, 10, *12*
 as origin of skin tumors, 1324
 cellular responses in, 75
 collagen synthesis in, 11
 connective tissue fiber proteins in, 11
 elastic fibers in, 13, *14, 15*
 embryonal, 2
 fibroblast in, 10
 ground substance in, 14
 papillary, 10, *11, 12*
 periadnexal, 10, *11, 12*
 reticular, 10
 reticular fibers in, 13
 thickness of, 10, *12*
Dermo-epidermal junction, formation of, 3
Dermographism, 230, *231*

Fibromatosis(es) (*Continued*)
  idiopathic gingival, of oral cavity, 1593
  infantile digital, 990, *990*
  juvenile, 1374
  palmar and plantar, 993
  penile, 993
Fibromatosis colli, 990
Fibrosarcoma, paradoxical, 1374
Fibrosclerosis, multifocal, 888
Fibrosis
  cystic, 1166
    altered eccrine secretion in, 1183
  in insulin fat atrophy, 998, 999
  mediastinal, chronic, 888
  nodular subepidermal, 1368
    histologic features of, 101
  periglandular, in lymphogranuloma venereum, 745
  retroperitoneal, 888
Fibrous dysplasia, polyostotic, café-au-lait spots in, 1101
Fibroxanthoma, atypical, 1374
Field effect, of ionizing radiation, 1449
Filariasis, 1499
Filiform wart(s), 574
Filtration, in x-ray therapy, 1666
Finger(s), fissures at proximal joint of, *182*
Fingernail(s), fungal infection of, *142*
  growth of, 1222. See also *Nail(s)*.
  ringworm of, 662, *664*
Fingerprint(s), individuality of, 8
Fire ant, bite of, 1537
Fish, venomous, disorders due to, 1539
Fish skin appearance, of ichthyosis, *181*
Fissure(s), at proximal joint of fingers, *182*
Fistula(s), arteriovenous, 889
    in hereditary hemorrhagic telangiectasia, 879, *880*
  congenital, of lower lip, 1049
Fistula dermatitis, 244
Fistula-in-ano, 797
502 A therapy, for furunculosis, 503
Flag sign, in kwashiorkor, 1240
Flagyl, in trichomoniasis, 1489
Flap(s), skin, 1696, *1697*
Flash burn(s), and leukoderma, 1123
Flat wart(s), 577, *577*
  treatment of, 579
Flatworm(s), cestodal, diseases due to, 1506
  trematodal, diseases due to, 1508
Flea(s), burrowing, 1534
  disorders due to, 1532
  human, 1532
  sand, 1534
  water, and dracunculiasis, 1504
Floating teeth, in Hand-Schüller-Christian disease, 761
Flora, of skin. See *Skin, flora of.*
Fluocinolone acetonide, in mycosis fungoides, 1433
  in psoriasis, 424
Fluorescent lighting, in clinical examination, 138
Fluorescent treponemal antibody-absorption test, 720, 721
Fluorescent treponemal antibody test, 720
5-Fluorocytosine, in dermatologic therapy, 1629
5-Fluorouracil
  cutaneous reactions due to, 378

5-Fluorouracil (*Continued*)
  in actinic keratoses, 1336
  in dermatologic therapy, 1699
  in keratoses, 331
  in skin cancer, 1619
  in solar keratoses, 331
Flushing, in carcinoid syndrome, 1310, *1311*
Fly(ies), disorders due to, 1528, 1530
Foam cell(s), 1272
Foam cell fat necrosis, 996
Focal dermal hypoplasia, 984, *984*, 985
  characteristics of, 877(t)
Fogo selvagem, 460, 465
Folic acid, deficiency of, oral manifestations of, 1601
Folinic acid, in toxoplasmosis, 1492
Follicle. See *Hair follicle.*
Follicular lymphoma, 1413–1415
Follicular occlusion triad, 517
Folliculitis, 499
  bacterial, *500*
  classification of, 492
  deep, 501
    histologic features of, 108
  gram-negative, 499
  granulomatous, 655
  in anogenital region, 161
  in contact dermatitis, 245
  in monomorphous lymphomas, 1409
  keloidal, 1212–1213, *1213*
  of scalp, 153, *157*, 500, *1195*
  oil, 1477
  perforating, 975
    of nose, 502
    vs. elastosis perforans serpiginosa, 101
  secondary, 517
  staphylococcal, 499
  superficial, 499
    histologic features of, 108, *108*
  vs. multiple sweat gland abscesses, 1188
Folliculitis decalvans, 506, *1194*
Folliculitis ulerythematosa reticulata, 1139
Folliculitis varioliformis, 505
Folliculopapular id, *661*
Fonsecaea compacta, 698
Fonsecaea dermatitidis, 698
Fonsecaea pedrosoi, 698
Fontana-Masson stain, as histochemical technique, 80(t)
Foot(feet)
  dermatitis of, 280, 314–318
    preventive methods in, 317
  dermatophytosis of, scaling of, *181*
  dermatoses of, *170, 171*
  effects of moisture on, 168
  eruptions of, diagnosis of, 168
  fox-hole, 1445, *1446*
  fungal infections of. See *Tinea pedis.*
  keratoderma of, in Reiter's syndrome, *400*
  Madura, 699
  mossy, 698
  nummular dermatitis of, *292*
  psoriasis of, *171*
  pustular eruptions of, 281
  ringworm of, 639
  superficial inflammatory conditions of, 168

Gonorrhea (*Continued*)
  incidence of, 730
  incubation period in, 731(t)
  laboratory diagnosis of, 734
  pathology of, 731
  sequelae of, 732
  Thompson two-glass urine test in, 732
  treatment of, 538, 735, 735(t)
Gomori's stain, as histochemical technique, 80(t)
Goose flesh, 20
Gopalan's syndrome, hyperhydrosis in, 1171
Gorham's disease, 1313
Gottron papule(s), in dermatomyositis, 945, *946*
Gougerot and Blum, pigmented purpuric lichenoid
    dermatosis of, 876
Gougerot-Carteaud syndrome, 1745
  vs. acanthosis nigricans, 1104
Gout, 1253, *1254–1256*
  and psoriasis, 412
  anhidrosis in, 1177
  edema in, 1294
  tophi of, on ear, 149
Gowers, panatrophy of, 999
Gnathostoma spinigerum, and gnathostomiasis, 1499
Gnathostomiasis, 1499
Graft(s), skin, 1695–1696, *1696*
Graft vs. host reaction, 1738–1739
Grafting, technique for, in common male baldness,
    1198
Grain(s), in Darier-White disease, 1075, *1077*
Grain itch, 1516
Granular cell myoblastoma, 1376
  of oral cavity, 1593
Granular cell schwannoma, 1376
Granular layer, in atopy, 1064
  analysis of, 1065(t)
Granule(s), Fordyce's 1593
Granuloma(s), 762–833
  allergic, 762, *763*
  cactus, 764
  definition of, 762
  eosinophilic, 760, 761, *762*
  foreign body, 763
    histologic features of, 105, *107*
  giant cell reparative, 1594
  histologic features of, 103
  Hodgkin's, 1417
  hypersensitivity, 763, *763*
  in mycobacterial ulceration, 789
  infectious, histologic features of, 103, *105*
  insect bite, 756
  lethal midline, 829
  Majocchi's, *653, 655, 657*
  Mycobacterium kansasii and, 788
  of nose, nonhealing, 829
  oily substances and, 765, 1005
  palisading, 773
    histologic features of, 105, *107*
  panniculitis with, 1006
  paracoccidioidal, oral manifestations of, 1574
  pseudopyogenic, 758
  pyogenic, *176, 507,* 1382, *1382*
    of nail, *1234*
  reticulohistiocytic, 755
  rheumatoid, 952

Granuloma(s) (*Continued*)
  scarring, depigmentation in, 1122
  sclerosing, 741
  silicon, 764, 1005
  swimming pool, 786, *786, 787*
    treatment of, 788
  talc 764
Granuloma annulare, *189,* 773, *773, 775*
  atypical, vs. rheumatoid nodules, 779
  dermal collagen in, 75
  differential diagnosis of, 774
  histologic features of, 105
  on hands, 141
  photosensitivity in, 343
  treatment of, 774
Granuloma Donovani, 741
Granuloma faciale, 825, *825*
  histologic features of, *96*
Granuloma fissuratum, 1594
Granuloma fungoides. See *Mycosis fungoides.*
Granuloma inguinale, 741–744, *742*
  clinical manifestations of, *742, 743*
  clinical variants of, 743
  definition of, 741
  differential diagnosis of, 744
  epidemiology of, 741
  etiology of, 741
  incidence of, 741
    in blacks, 1726
  incubation period in, 731(t), 743
  historical review of, 741
  laboratory diagnosis of, 743
  of anogenital region, *164*
  pathology of, 741
  treatment of, 735(t), 744
  vs. lymphogranuloma venereum, 749
Granuloma multiforme, 774
Granuloma pudendi chronicum, 741
Granuloma pyogenicum, 1594
Granuloma telangiectaticum, 1382
Granuloma venereum, 741
Granulomatosis
  allergic, 827, *828*
  lymphomatoid, 1740–1741
  necrotizing eosinophilic, 827
  noninfectious necrotizing, 827
  oral lesions of, 1588
  pathergic, 827
  Wegener's, 828, *829*
Granulomatosis disciformis, 777
Granulomatous disease
  chronic, 780
    of children, 215
      fatal, 908
  infectious, 779
Granulosis rubra nasi, 73, 1186
Graves' disease, 1282
  vitiligo with, 1118
Graying, of hair, 1121, 1214
Gray patch ringworm, 627
Greasiness, of skin, in seborrheic dermatitis, 283
Green bottle fly(ies), 1532
Green nail syndrome, 538
Grenz ray machine(s), 1673, 1674
Grenz ray therapy, 1673

Herxheimer effect, in onchocerciasis, 1502
Herxheimer reaction, 354
Hetrazan, in filariasis, 1500
  in trichinosis, 1506
Hexachlorophene, in sterilization of skin, 490
Hexapoda, disorders due to, 1522
Hexosamine, 1279
Hexuronic acid, 1279
Hidracanthoma simplex, 1350
Hidradenitis axillaris, 1160
Hidradenitis suppurativa, 1160–1164, *1548*
  abscesses of, *1161*
  and squamous cell carcinoma, 1342
  anogenital, 161, 1162
  apocrine system in, 73
  clinical manifestations of, 1161
  definition of, 1160
  diagnosis of, 1162
  differential diagnosis of, 1162
  epidemiology of, 1161
  etiology of, 1161
  historical aspects of, 1160
  in axilla, *144, 145*
  in follicular occlusion triad, 517
  in tropics, 135
  late, *1162*
  pathology of, 1162
  pathogenesis of, 1161
  prognosis in, 1164
  scarring of, *187*
  skin grafting in, *1696*
  treatment of, 1163
    by radiation, 1685
Hidradenoma(s), clear cell, 1350
  nodular, 1350
  solid-cystic, 1350
Hidradenoma papilliferum, 1349
Hidrocystoma, 1348
Hidromeiosis, 1185
Hidrotic ectodermal dysplasia, 1038, 1233(t)
Hilar adenopathy, in erythema nodosum, *394, 395*
Hilus cell tumor(s), 1218, 1220
Hippocratic nail(s), definition of, 1235
Hirsutism, 1215–1220
  definition of, 1216
  idiopathic, 1216
    diagnosis of, 1217
    treatment of, 1217
    vs. secondary, 1218
  menstrual abnormalities in, 1218
  oral contraceptives and, 378
  secondary, 1218, *1219*
    treatment of, 1220
Hirudinea, disorders due to, 1538
Histamine
  effect of cyclic-AMP on, 222
  in atopic dermatitis, 270
  in mast cell, 15
  role of, in anaphylactic syndrome, 224
    in antigen-antibody reactions, 212
    in inflammation, 214
  urticaria due to, 230
Histamine release test, for penicillin sensitivity, 368
Histamine skin test, in leprosy, 812
Histidinemia, hypopigmentation in, 1115

Histiocyte(s), fusion of, 75
  origin of, 15, *16*
Histiocytoma(s), 753, *753, 754*
  giant cell, 755
  histologic features of, 101
Histiocytoma cutis, 1368
Histiocytosis, oral lesions of, 1588
Histiocytosis X, 759
  eosinophilic granuloma, 761
  Hand-Schüller-Christian disease, 761
  Letterer-Siwe disease, 760
  vs. atopic dermatitis, 264
Histochemistry, techniques in, 80–81, 80(t)
Histopathology, of skin, 78–113
Histoplasma capsulatum, 684
Histoplasma duboisii, 687
Histoplasmosis, 684
  African, 687
  diagnosis of, 686
  erythema nodosum in, 394
  in children, 122
  incidence of, 684
  lesions in, 685
  oral manifestations of, 1575
  progressive, 685
  serologic reactions in, 686
  treatment of, 687
History, family, in dermatologic patients, 115
  medical, in dermatologic patients, 114–137
    objectives of, 115
Hive(s), definition of, 177
HL-A antigen(s), and psoriasis, 411
Hodgkin's disease, 1416–1419
  and exfoliative dermatitis, 451
  and herpes zoster, 571
  clinical manifestations of, 1417, *1417–1419*
  definition of, 1416
  etiology of, 1417
  histology of, 1417
  hypogammaglobulinemia in, 205
  incidence of, 1416
  pruritus in, 1555
  staging in, 1420(t)
  treatment of, 1419
  tuberculous tenosynovitis in, *793*
  vs. necrotizing eosinophilic granulomatosis, 827
Hodgkin's granuloma, 1417
Hoffmann-Zurhelle, nevus lipomatosus superficialis of, 1368
Homocystinuria, 1249
  characteristics of, 1250(t)
  hypopigmentation in, 1115
  treatment of, 1243
Honeycombed atrophy, 1139
Hongkong foot, 136
Hoof and mouth disease, vs. hand-foot-mouth syndrome, 599
Hookworm disease, 1494, 1495
Hordeolum, 502
Hormone(s). See also specific names.
  and acneiform eruptions, 1137
  and adipogenesis, 1001
  and hair growth, 37
  definition of, 1237
  disorders of, photosensitivity in, 339

Industrial dermatosis(es) (*Continued*)
  prevention of, protective ointments in, 1482
  rehabilitation in, 1483
  specific causes of, 1462–1478
    adhesives, 1469
    agricultural chemicals, 1473
    chemical agents, 1465
    dyes, 1468
    explosives, 1475
    infestations, 1465
    lacquers, 1475
    mechanical agents, 1463
    metals, 1465
    paints, 1475
    petroleum products, 1475
    physical agents, 1463
    plants, 1468
    plastics, 1469
    resins, 1469
    rubber, 1469
    solvents, 1478
    varnishes, 1475
  treatment of, 1484–1485
Infant(s). See also *Child(ren)*.
  anhidrosis in, 1178
  atopic dermatitis in, 120, 307, *310, 311*
  care of skin in, 313
  circumscribed neurodermatitis in, 121
  contact dermatitis in, 307
  cyanosis in, 1264
  dermatitis in, types of, 313(t)
  diagnosis of skin disease in, 118
  diaper rash in, 121
  eczema in. See *Eczema, infantile*.
  Gaucher's disease in, 1267
  generalized cutaneous candidiasis of, 671, *672*
  herpes simplex in, 561
  Kaposi's varicelliform eruption in, 562
  measles in, 594
  primary irritant dermatitis in, 120
  rubella syndrome in, 596
  scarring in, 121
  seborrheic dermatitis in, 120
  syphilis in, 716
  toxic erythema of, 396
  varicella in, 569
  yellowish discoloration of skin of, 127
Infection(s). See also specific names.
  bacterial. See *Bacterial infection(s)*.
  fungal. See *Fungal infection(s)*.
  immunity against, 216
  immunodeficiency and, 205(t)
  immunologic processes in, 216–218
  mycotic, 621–707
  predisposing conditions favoring, 217(t)
  ringworm, 625–666
  viral. See *Viral infection(s)*.
Infectious gangrene, 522
Infectious mononucleosis, 601–602
Infestation(s), insect, as industrial dermatosis, 1465
Infiltration, lymphocytic, of skin, 757, *758*
Inflammation
  as response to injury, 214–216
  degree of, defense status of host and, 217

Inflammation (*Continued*)
  disorders of, 199–238
  histologic changes in, 82
Inflammatory disorder(s), 385–408
Inflammatory reaction, factors modifying, 216
Infundibulofolliculitis, disseminate recurrent, 1213
    in blacks, 1717, *1718*
Infundibulum, of hair follicle, *37, 40*
Ingram technique in psoriasis, 424
Ingrown hair(s), 1212, *1212*
    in pseudofolliculitis barbae, 527, *528*
Inguinal adenitis syndrome, 746, *746, 747*
Inheritance, Mendelian patterns of, 1013
Injection(s), intra-arterial, accidental complications from, 839
Insect(s), disorders due to, 1522
    in tropical dermatology, 137
Insect bite(s)
    and papular urticaria, 1533, *1533*
    edema in, 1294
    general biology of, 1523
    in children, 128
    persistent, 759
    reactions to, on leg, *169*
    simulating lymphoma, 1415
    vesicular reaction to, *178*
Insecticide(s), dermatitis due to, 1473
Insulin
    and adipogenesis, 1001
    cutaneous reactions due to, 383
    injection of, and deep atrophy, 999
    level of, in lipoatrophy, 997
Insulin fat atrophy, 998
Interferon, in viral infections, 605
Intertrigo, 161, 519, *520, 521*
    candidal, 670
        treatment of, 675
    of toes, *170*
    treatment of, 520, 1614
Intralesional therapy, 1622–1623
Ioderma(s), treatment of, 370
Iodide(s), cutaneous reactions due to, 379, *380*
        lesions in, 831, *832*
    in sporotrichosis, 695
Iodochloroxyquinoline, in acrodermatitis entero-
        pathica, 1241
5-Iodo-2'-deoxyuridine, in viral infections, 604
Iodoform, in acrodermatitis enteropathica, 1241
Ionization, and percutaneous absorption, 66
Ionizing radiation. See *Radiation, ionizing*.
Iontophoresis, definition of, 1641
"Iris" lesion(s), of erythema multiforme, *389*
Iris "pearl(s)," 812
Iron colloidal technique, 80(t), 81(t)
Iron deficiency, and Plummer-Vinson syndrome, 1585
Iron deficiency syndrome, 902
Isomorphic phenomenon, in psoriasis, 416
Isoniazid, cutaneous reactions due to, 373, 376
    in tuberculosis, 784(t)
Isovaleric acidemia, odor in, 1148
Isthmus, of hair follicle, *37, 40, 43*
Itching. See also *Pruritus*.
    vs. pain, 19. See also *Pruritus*.
Itching eruption of axillae and pubes, chronic, 1156
Ito, nevus of, 1105, 1366

Necrobiosis lipoidica (*Continued*)
  differential diagnosis of, 776
  histologic features of, 75, 105
  of face, 776
  treatment of, 777
  ulcerations in, 777, *777*
Necrolysis, toxic epidermal, 359, 450, 895
Necrosis
  fat. See *Fat necrosis.*
  fibrinoid, in connective tissue disease, 913
  gummatous, 894
  of skin, 894–901
    bacterial infections and, 897
    causes of, 896(t)
    chemical agents and, 895, *898*
    microbiologic agents and, 896
    mycobacterial infections and, 899
    mycotic infections and, 900
    physical agents and, 895, *897*
    Pseudomonas aeruginosa and, *898*
    treponemal infections and, 899
    types of, 894
  with metastatic calcification, 1293
Necrotizing fasciitis, 510, 992, 1373
  clinical manifestations of, 897, *899*
Negro(es). See *Black race(s).*
Neisseria gonorrhoeae, 538, 729, 731
Neisseria meningitidis, and meningococcemia, 535, 536
Nelson's syndrome, melanosis in, 1106
Nemathelminthes, 1492
Nematocyst(s), 1537
Neomycin, and contact dermatitis, *887*
  in bacterial infections, 494
Neonate(s). See *Infant(s).*
Neoplasm(s). See *Cancer, Carcinoma(s), Sarcoma(s), Tumor(s).*
Neosporin, in hidradenitis suppurativa, 1163
Neotestudina rosatii, 701
Nephrosis, depigmentation in, 1122
Nephrotic syndrome, in systemic lupus erythematosus, 929
Nerve(s), autonomic, disturbances of, 1563
  cutaneous, formation of, 2, 18–20, *20*
Nervous system, in Behçet's disease, 403
Netherton's disease, 263, 1078
Neumann's pemphigus vegetans, 464
Neural crest, 2
  melanocytes from, 30, *30*
Neuralgia
  herpes zoster and, 571
  post-herpetic, 1563
  post-zoster, 573
  trigeminal, from stilbamidine, 683
Neurilemmoma, 1375
  of oral cavity, 1593
Neuritis, alcoholic, anhidrosis in, 1177
  hypertrophic interstitial, 1564(t)
Neurocutaneous syndrome(s), 1015–1026
Neurodermatitis. See also *Atopic dermatitis.*
  circumscribed, 293, *295*
    in infant, 121
  histologic changes in, *85*
  localized, 318

Neurodermatitis (*Continued*)
  localized, facial, 147
    in aged, 131
    of ear, 149
    of legs, 165
    of scalp, 151
    racial tendency in, 137
    with seborrheic dermatitis, 288
  polymorphic, 295
  psoriasiform, 418, *418*
Neuroectoderm, 2
Neurofibroma(s), 1021, 1375
  histologic features of, 102
  molluscoid, 1020
Neurofibromatosis, 1020
  bone involvement in, 1023
  café-au-lait spots in, 1022, *1023*, 1101
  clinical manifestations of, 1307
  endocrine abnormalities in, 1024
  giant pigmented nevus with, 1359
  in children, 128
  melanosomes in, 1088
  mode of inheritance in, 1020
  multiple, 1375
  neurologic manifestations of, 1024
  nodules of, *175*
  oral lesions of, 1593, *1593*
  pigmentary abnormalities in, 1022, *1023*
  tumors in, 1020, *1021*, *1022*
  vs. Albright's syndrome, 1313
  with internal malignancy, 1318
Neurofibrosarcoma, in neurofibromatosis, 1022, *1022*
Neurogenic skin disease(s), 1561–1564
Neuroma(s), plexiform, 1020
Neuropathy(ies), sensory, characteristics of, 1564(t)
  ulceration in, 1561
Neurosis, and atopic dermatitis, 273
Neurosyphilis, asymptomatic, 710
  congenital, 718
  in blacks, 1727
Neutropenia, 908
  cyclic, oral lesions of, 1585
Neutrophil, deficiency of, 908
Nevoid basal cell epithelioma syndrome, 1354
Nevoid lentigo(ines), 1097
Nevoid syndrome(s), with internal malignancy, 1318
Nevoxanthoendothelioma, 127
  juvenile, 754
Nevus(i)
  achromic, 1120, *1120*
  as epidermal appendageal tumor, 1345
  bathing-trunk, 1359
    with internal malignancy, 1318
  Becker's, 1101
  blue, 1365, *1366*
    malignant, 1366
  blue rubber bleb, 1386
  changes in, 1361
  connective tissue, 1312, 1367, *1368*
  definition of, 1327
  epidermal, 1327, *1328*, *1329*
  epithelioid cell, 1358
  flat pigmented, *173*
  giant congenital pigmented, 1359, *1360*

Psoralen(s), and phototoxicity, 333, *335*
Psoriasis, 410–427
  and fungal infection of nails, 665
  anhidrosis in, 1178
  annular patterns in, *189*
  anogenital, 161, 319
  arthritis in, 419
  bacteriology of, 416
  characteristics of, 1057(t)
  clinical manifestations of, 412
  colonization of *Staphylococcus aureus* in, 489
  congenital, 1068, *1071*
  diagnosis of, 422
  distribution pattern in, 192, *193*
  epidemiology of, 410
  etiology of, 411
  exfoliative, 419, 449
    treatment of, 453
  flexural, 415, 417
  guttate, 417
  hair in, 1191
  heredity in, 410, 411
  histologic changes in, 83, *84*
  histopathology of, 421
  historical features of, 410
  in atopic dermatitis, 261
  in blacks, 1732
  in children, 122
  inverse, 417
  Koebner phenomenon in, 416, *416*
  laboratory findings in, 422
  lesions of, 413, *413, 414*
    oral, 1584
  nail changes in, 415, *415*, 1229–1230, *1230*
  nummular, *414*, 417
  of axilla, *144, 145*
  of ear, *152*
  of elbow, *143*
  of hands and feet, 315
  of legs, 165, *166*
  of nails, *141*
  of palm, *141*, 418
  of scalp, 151
    vs. seborrheic dermatitis, 282
  of sole, *171*
  of trunk, 156, *160*
  papules of, *174*
  pathogenesis of, 411
  percutaneous absorption in, 67
  photosensitivity in, 343
  plaque, 417, *417*
  prognosis in, 426
  pustular. See *Pustular psoriasis.*
  race factor in, 116
  Reiter's syndrome and, 399
  scaling in, *181*
  seasonal factor in, 117
  seborrheic, 283, 417
  sites of predilection in, 414, *414*
  systemic associations in, 421
  treatment of, 422, 1614
    azaribine in, 1632
    by radiation, 1684
    by teleroentgen therapy, 1688

Psoriasis (*Continued*)
  treatment of, chemotherapeutic, 1747, 1748
    hydroxyurea in, 1631
    methotrexate in, 1630
    photosensitizers in, 1620
    systemic antibiotics in, 1627
    ultraviolet light in, 1659
    wet dressings in, 1611
  with discoid lupus erythematosus, 923
  vs. discoid lupus erythematosus, 917, *919, 920*
  vs. granuloma inguinale, 744
  vs. intertrigo, 520
  vitiligo with, 1119
Psychogenic skin disease(s), 1553–1560
Psychotherapy, in atopic dermatitis, 275
Pterygium unguis, definition of, 1236
  in lichen planus, 1232, *1232*
Puberty, cutaneous manifestations of, 1295
Pulex irritans, disorders due to, 1532
Punch biopsy, 1691
Purpura, 859–877
  anaphylactoid, 852, *856*
  classification of, 860(t)
  clinical manifestations of, 860
  clothing, 875
  definition of, 859
  drugs causing, 365(t), 863, *864, 865*
  eczematid-like, 876
  from infectious diseases, 862
  hypergammaglobulinemic, of Waldenström, 869
  in children, 124
  in chronic ulcer disease, *862*
  in metabolic diseases, 863
  in neoplastic disease, 861, 865
  in post-thrombotic syndrome, *885*
  in scurvy, 862
  laboratory tests for, 860
  nonthrombocytopenic, in systemic amyloidosis, 1287
  of legs, 165
  of nails, *861*
  of palms, in Letterer-Siwe disease, 760
  palpable, 864
  platelet abnormalities and, 865
  pruritic, 876, *877*
  psychogenic, 864
  Schoenlein-Henoch, 852, *856*, 863
  scurvy and, 75
  secondary vascular, 861
  senile, 860, *861*
  stasis, 876
  with malignancy, 1317
Purpura annularis telangiectodes, 876
Purpura fulminans, 534, 862
  in disseminated intravascular coagulopathy, 867, *867*
Purpura gangrenosa, 862
Purpura hemorrhagica, 862
Purpura necrotica, 862
Purpura pigmentosa chronica, 875, *876*
Purpura simplex, 860
Puss caterpillar, dermatitis due to, 1536
Pustular bacterid, treatment of, systemic antibiotics in, 1627